Immunology

'You can't quarantine congressmen, they've got immunity, or something . . .'

Colonel Wainwright Purdy III in the movie
The Teahouse of the August Moon

Immunology

SECOND EDITION

Jan Klein

Max-Planck-Institut für Biologic,
Abteilung Immungenetik,
Tübingen, Germany

Václav Hořejší

Institute of Molecular Genetics,
Academy of Sciences of the Czech Republic,
Prague

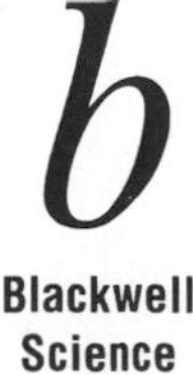

Blackwell
Science

Editorial Offices:
Osney Mead, Oxford OX2 0EL
25 John Street, London WC1N 2BL
23 Ainslie Place, Edinburgh EH3 6AJ
350 Main Street, Malden
MA 02148 5018, USA
54 University Street, Carlton
Victoria 3053, Australia

Other Editorial Offices:
Blackwell Wissenschafts-Verlag GmbH
Kurfürstendamm 57
10707 Berlin, Germany

Blackwell Science KK
MG Kodenmacho Building
7–10 Kodenmacho Nihombashi
Chuo-ku, Tokyo 104, Japan

First published 1990
Reprinted 1991
Paperback reissue 1991
Second edition 1997
Reprinted 1999

Set by Excel Typesetters Co., Hong Kong
Printed and bound in Italy by
Vincenzo Bona srl, Turin

DISTRIBUTORS

Marston Book Services Ltd
PO Box 269
Abingdon
Oxon OX14 4YN
(*Orders*: Tel: 01235 465500
Fax: 01235 465555)

USA
Blackwell Science, Inc.
Commerce Place
350 Main Street
Malden, MA 02148 5018
(*Orders*: Tel: 800 759 6102
617 388 8250
Fax: 617 388 8255)

Canada
Copp Clark Professional
200 Adelaide St West, 3rd Floor
Toronto, Ontario M5H 1W7
(*Orders*: Tel: 416 597-1616
800 815-9417
Fax: 416 597-1617)

Australia
Blackwell Science Pty Ltd
54 University Street
Carlton, Victoria 3053
(*Orders*: Tel: 3 9347 0300
Fax: 3 9347 5001)

A catalogue record for this title
is available from the British Library

ISBN 0-632-04228-1

Library of Congress
Cataloging-in-publication Data

Klein, Jan, 1936–
Immunology / Jan Klein, Václav Hořejší.
—2nd ed.
p. cm.
Includes bibliographical references
and index.
ISBN 0-632-04228-1
1. Immunology. I. Hořejší, Václav.
II. Title.
[DNLM: 1. Immune System
—physiology. 2. Immunity.
QW 504 K64ia 1997]
QR181.K52 1997
616.07′9—dc20
DNLM/DLC
for Library of Congress 96-17956
CIP

Contents

Preface

This second edition retains the organization of the first; it was chosen to reflect the logic of the discipline. The book is divided into two parts, the first being more static, the second more dynamic: the former represents the 'hardware' and the latter the 'software' of the discipline. The progression of the first, descriptive part, is from organs and tissues to cells and then to molecules. The description of molecules is in the order in which they become involved in the adaptive immune response (major histocompatibility complex molecules, T-cell receptors, immunoglobulins and others). Whenever possible, the description follows the path from a gene to a protein. The dynamic part, too, approximates the order of involvement of different cell types in the immune response, from macrophages, through T lymphocytes and then on to B lymphocytes, followed by the description of specific forms of immune response. This organization has necessitated a certain degree of overlap between some of the chapters, which we hope will be viewed by the reader as an advantage. A chapter of interest may be selected without the reader having to study the rest of the text.

Descriptions of methods and experiments have been largely delegated to figures and figure legends, as have explanations of basic terms and concepts with which some readers may be familiar, while others may need a review. We have chosen this arrangement to simplify the narrative. A glossary is not included in this book because new terms are defined when first introduced and the reader can locate definitions by consulting the index. Some explanatory comments are repeated to make each chapter as self-contained as possible.

The emphasis throughout this text is on facts; descriptions of hypotheses and speculations on controversial topics, no matter how currently fashionable, have been restricted to a minimum. Discoveries are not credited to individuals for the simple reason that in a text of this genre it is all but impossible to be fair in this regard. Most discoveries in immunology have been made by teams, often by several teams simultaneously, and to acknowledge each investigator would render the text unreadable; to give credit to a select few would be grossly unjust. For similar reasons, we have avoided citing original articles in Further reading sections; instead, we provide lists of reviews in which the reader will find specific references.

The descriptions focus on the human immune system, the subject of interest for clinically-oriented readers. We do, however, point out evolutionary interconnections wherever they are known. We have also included, as a preamble, a chapter on invertebrate immunity, an area still greatly undervalued but one with tremendous growth potential.

Lest our female readers be offended by the usage of 'he' in places, we hasten to explain that we have been guided by a simple rule: Male authors use 'he,' female authors use 'she.'

Anyone who has penned a text of similar magnitude knows that the period of writing constitutes a gap in one's personal life. In order not to strain social bonds to the breaking point, a great deal of tolerance and understanding on the part of one's immediate contacts is required. We have been extremely fortunate to have been accorded both by our families, friends and colleagues. We are embarrassed that we can offer them only a few sentences of appreciation in return and it is with profound gratitude that we acknowledge their support. We would like to single out particularly our secretaries, Ms Lynne Yakes and Ms Eva Tvrzníková. It is no exaggeration to state that without their patience, endurance and dedication we would have been unable to complete this work. Further, we thank our associates and colleagues who in various ways helped us in the writing. From J.K.'s side they are: Ms Donna Devine, Ms Moira Burghoffer, Dr Werner Mayer, Dr Colm O'hUigin and Dr Akie Sato; and from V.H.'s side, Dr Ivan Hilgert, Dr Pavla Angelisová, Mr Jan Josek, Dr Helena Tlaskalová and Dr Pavol Ivanyi.

Parts of the manuscript have been reviewed by Dr Bernhard Arden (Department of Immunology, Paul Ehrlich

Institute, Langen, Germany), Dr Bonnie B. Blomberg (Department of Microbiology and Immunology, University of Miami School of Medicine, Miami, FL, USA), Professor Hans G. Boman and Professor Dan Hultmark (Department of Microbiology, Stockholm University, Stockholm, Sweden), Dr Austin L. Hughes, Department of Biology, The Pennsylvania State University, University Park, PA, USA), Dr Masanori Kasahara (Department of Biochemistry, Hokkaido University School of Medicine, Sapporo, Japan), Dr Pawel Kieselow (Basel Institute of Immunology, Basel, Switzerland), Professor Peter Lachmann (MRC Group on Mechanisms in Tumour Immunity, Laboratory of Molecular Biology, Cambridge, England), Professor Fritz Melchers (Basel Institute of Immunology, Basel, Switzerland), Dr Kazuya Mizuno (Department of Microbiology and Immunology, Tokyo Metropolitan Institute for Neuroscience, Tokyo, Japan), Dr Keiko Ozato (National Institutes of Child Health and Development, NIH, Bethesda, MD, USA), Dr Jenny Pan-Yun Ting (UNC Lineberger Comprehensive Cancer Center School of Medicine, University of North Carolina, Chapel Hill, NC, USA), Dr Roy Riblet (Medical Biology Institute, La Jolla, CA, USA), Dr Ton Rolink (Basel Institute of Immunology, Basel, Switzerland), and Professor Rolf M. Zinkernagel (Institute of Pathology, University of Zürich, Zürich, Switzerland). Their helpful comments have saved us from making embarrassing mistakes. We are greatly obliged to them for their assistance.

To all those who suffered with us we offer a promise: *Parce, pater, virgis, iam numquam carmina dicam*; they may, however, not believe us.

Jan Klein
Tübingen

Václav Hořejší
Prague

chapter 1 Basic terms and concepts

Parasites, immunity, immunology

Organisms are *hosts* to a variety of other organisms, both small (*microorganisms*: viruses, bacteria and fungi) and large. Organisms that live in or on individuals of another species without providing any benefits to their hosts are *parasites*; those that harm the host (cause disease) are *pathogenic organisms* or *pathogens*. The entry (*invasion*) of a parasite into a host and its establishment resulting in disease is an *infection* (*infestation*) and the parasite is an *infectious agent*.

All organisms have their means of resisting infection. Bacteria have sets of restriction enzymes that digest foreign DNA of invading viruses (the enzymes 'restrict' the infectivity of the virus). They also produce proteinaceous compounds, *bacteriocins*, that inhibit or kill bacteria of other species. Plants have special sets of *resistance genes*, each turned on by a particular infectious agent and triggering a *hypersensitivity response* on activation. The gene instructs cells in the vicinity of the infected cell to die rapidly and other cells to produce chemicals that thicken their walls. The death of the cells (*necrosis*) deprives the invader of nutrients and the cells with thickened walls erect a cork-like barrier to prevent spreading of the infection. Plants also have numerous other means of protecting themselves against infection. Animals are particularly vulnerable to being overwhelmed by parasites because the conditions inside their bodies resemble those of tissue cultures, an optimal setting for an infection.

The body's power to resist infection and its ability to protect itself against reinfection is referred to as *immunity*. An alternative term is *defence reaction* (*response*), but the latter has a broader meaning because it includes protective measures against predators. For example, a bee sting is a defence reaction but not an immune reaction and mellitin, the main component of bee venom, is a defence substance but not an immune substance. On the other hand, not all forms of immunity constitute defence reactions, for some forms are detrimental to the body that has unleashed them. The word 'immunity' derives from Latin *immunis*, which means 'free of a burden', where the burden could be a tax imposed by the government or a disease. Individuals who are protected against reinfection by the same parasite are therefore said to be *immune*. The branch of biology that deals with the study of processes and substances associated with resistance to infection is called *immunology*. Some researchers prefer to restrict usage of the term 'immunity' to processes occurring in one group of animals only — that which includes humans — and view immunology primarily as a medical discipline. However, as the ability to resist infection is ubiquitous in the entire living world, such a restriction is not justified. All animals, plants and microorganisms are capable of developing some form of immunity.

Principle of non-adaptive immune responses

An animal body has set aside groups of substances and cells (and in some animals also tissues and organs) whose primary function is defence against parasites—the *immune system*. There are two basic strategies a body can use to protect itself against infection. The strategies have a series of characteristics, each of which has been used to name the two contrasting types of immune response.

The characteristics (and their names) of the first strategy are:

- the strategy does not change (adapt) in response to an infection (*non-adaptive immune response*);

• its power to discriminate between various parasites is low (*non-specific immune response*);
• the response does not need to be induced and is available instantaneously (*innate immune response*);
• the response is of a generalized type, i.e. it does not anticipate individual parasites (*non-anticipatory immune response*).

The contrasting characteristics of the second strategy are:
• the responses to infection and reinfection are qualitatively and quantitatively different, i.e. an adaptation has taken place (*adaptive immune response*);
• the response's power of discrimination is very high (*specific immune response*);
• the response requires time to develop during an infection, but on reinfection takes place instantaneously (*acquired immune response*);
• the response anticipates all possible parasite-derived stimuli (*anticipatory immune response*).

The various names for the two strategies are virtual synonyms; in this book we shall use the designations 'adaptive' and 'non-adaptive' responses. It appears that invertebrates are capable only of non-adaptive responses, whereas vertebrates possess both types of response.

To explain how the non-adaptive strategy may have evolved, let us consider a hypothetical, highly simplified situation (Fig. 1.1). Let us assume that at some point, a particular species became plagued by a parasite. The host was caught unprepared for this intruder and the parasite therefore spread virtually unopposed through the population, decimating it. However, individuals vary in the constituents of their bodies, and so it happened that a few individuals in the population possessed a variant of a protein in their tissue fluids that other individuals lacked and which, by chance, showed an attraction for one of the constituents of the parasite. There is nothing unusual about such occurrences. All molecules either attract or repel each other, depending on the distribution of electrical charges they carry and on other forces, but most of the time the strength of this interaction (*affinity*) is so low that the molecules virtually ignore each other. Occasionally, however, the attraction between two unrelated molecules becomes so strong that an unstable bond is formed between them. If one of the molecules happens to be larger than the other it is called a *receptor*; the molecule that binds to the receptor is then referred to as a *ligand* (Latin *ligare*, to bind). Sometimes, however, the ligand can be larger than the receptor and the terms are assigned by convention alone. If the receptor binds (*recognizes*) only one type of ligand and no other, it is said to be *monospecific*; if it binds several types, it is *polyspecific*; and if it discriminates between ligands poorly, it is said to be *non-specific*. In immunology, *specificity* therefore indicates the ability of a receptor to discriminate among ligands.

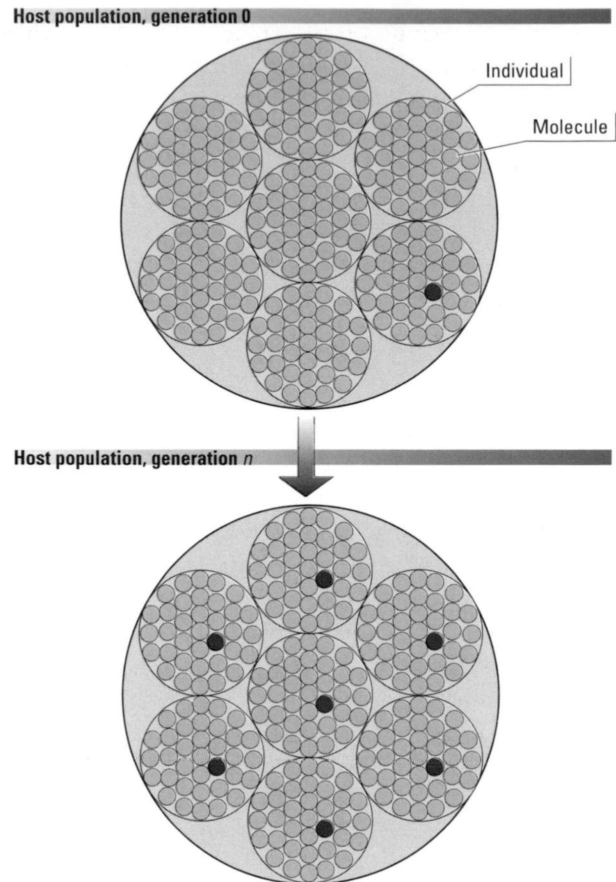

Figure 1.1 Evolution of the non-adaptive immune system. The large, medium, and small circles represent population, individual and molecule, respectively. The small dark red circle in the host represents a molecular variant (receptor) capable of binding a component (ligand) of a parasite that has infected individuals in the population. This binding ultimately leads to the elimination of the parasite from the host's body. Individuals possessing this receptor molecule become resistant to the parasite and survive the infection; others die. In the *n*th generation, the population consists of resistant individuals only. This cycle repeats itself when a new parasite or a new variant of the old parasite appears on the scene.

At any rate, let us assume that such a receptor–ligand relationship developed between a protein of our hypothetical host and a component of its parasite. If we call the parasite's component substance S1, we can say that the host's receptor displays anti-S1 activity, where the prefix *anti* signifies 'exerting energy in the opposite direction', here displaying the binding affinity for the particular ligand. In reality, of course, the interaction between the two molecules is mutual so we could also say that the ligand binds the receptor. The few individuals in the population who happen to have the interacting protein could not care less which binds which as long as binding occurs, because for them it may be a life-saving event — the receptor protein will coat the parasite, interfere with its activities and thus protect the host.

The individuals carrying the gene for the receptor protein may be the only ones to survive an infestation by that particular parasite. These individuals thrive, but only until another parasite or a variant of the original parasite finds its way into the new population; then the process starts all over again. Many individuals die because the parasite does not express the S1 component and the anti-S1 protein is ineffective against the new invader. Eventually, however, a few individuals will emerge that do have a protein with an affinity for the S2 constituent of the parasite. The anti-S2 protein may again interfere, in some other way, with the activities of the parasite and hence protect the host.

These cycles of decimation and rebirth in host populations are repeated again and again. Each time a new parasite appears on the scene, there is a catastrophe in the host population from which the host species may or may not recover, depending largely on luck — whether or not it will come up with a suitable anti-S protein or some other deterrent in time. It is a risky and costly system of defence, but one that apparently serves most, if not all, invertebrates (and also plants) well. The anti-S proteins that emerge from time to time to combat new parasites are probably not related to one another. The host will haphazardly use any protein that happens to have anti-S activity, so that sometimes the protein will be derived from one, and at other times from a different, protein family.

Evolution of adaptive immune responses

For reasons we do not quite understand, perhaps because their bodies are more complex or because they have fewer progeny, vertebrates, the small minority of animals with backbones, found the non-adaptive strategy of defence not fully satisfactory. In addition to the non-adaptive system, they therefore developed a new system, the main feature of which is that it anticipates all the S substances a parasite can carry. To be more precise, the system does not anticipate the entire S molecule (we can now call it *antigen*, an entity capable of eliciting an adaptive immune response) but rather a small part thereof. When a receptor binds a ligand, the interaction does not involve the entire molecule; instead, it involves a small region on the receptor's surface (the *combining site*) and a small region of the ligand's surface (the *epitope*, *antigenic determinant* or simply *determinant*, because it determines the binding capacity). These surfaces must be *complementary*, which means that one is moulded in a certain way and the other in the opposite way. Only complementary surfaces can come together close enough for the weak bonds between them to spring into action. The ease with which complementary surfaces come together is illustrated by the wizard of complementarity, the Dutch artist Maurits C. Escher, who even managed to unite angels with devils (Fig. 1.2)!

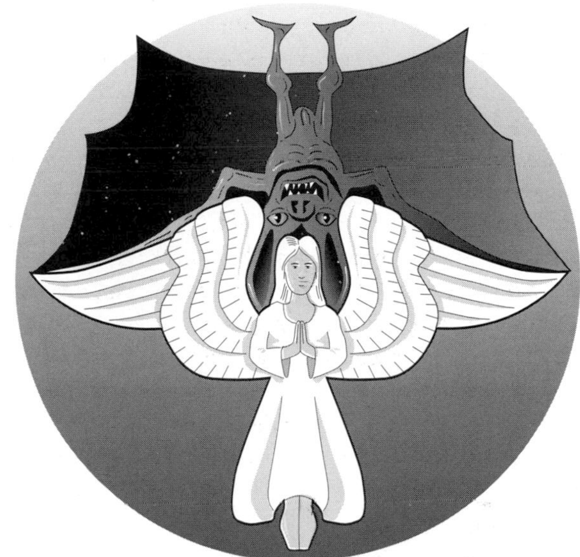

Figure 1.2 Complementarity of angels and devils in the eyes of Maurits C. Escher. Combining sites and epitopes must fit together.

Since there may be a finite number of epitopes, the vertebrates decided to make receptors for all, or almost all, of them[1] (Fig. 1.3). The immunologist, Niels Jerne, compared the vertebrate immune system to a glove factory. Of course, you can go ahead and custom-make gloves, but it is terribly inefficient and very expensive. So what did the entrepreneurs do? They built a factory in which gloves are mass produced in different sizes and forms. Each customer is then sure to find a pair that more or less fits his or her hands. This was also what the ancestors of contemporary vertebrates decided on; they set up a factory to make a *repertoire* of receptors that would fit any epitope. The factory thus anticipates all the possible needs for defence against parasites.

The adaptive system cannot manufacture receptors using one protein once and quite a different protein the next time. All the receptors have to be made from the same family of proteins so that their production can be coordinated and

[1] We use such phrases ('vertebrates decided') in a metaphorical sense only. In reality, of course, vertebrates did not 'decide' anything; it all happened by blind forces of evolution.

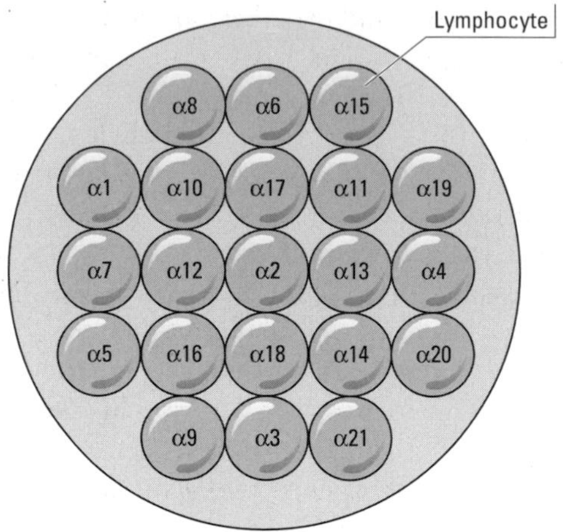

Figure 1.3 Abstract representation of the adaptive immune system. The large circle represents a collection of cells, the small circles represent lymphocytes, and α stands for 'anti' and indicates the ability of a receptor on the lymphocyte to bind a particular epitope (indicated by a number). Because the entire spectrum of epitopes is covered by the repertoire of receptors (combining sites), the host can be said to anticipate any foreign substance that a parasite might come up with.

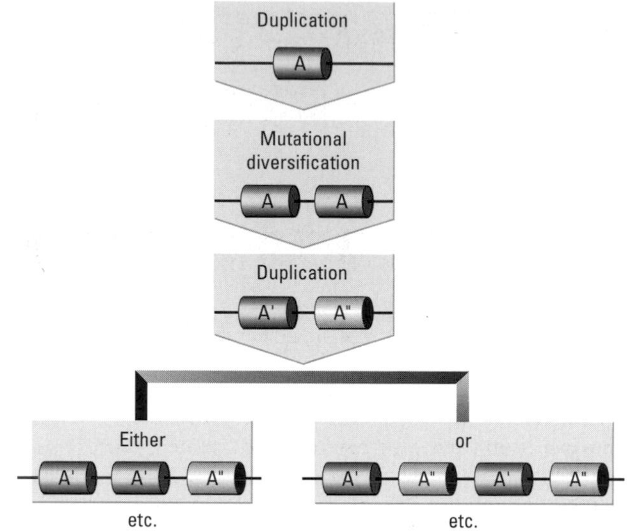

Figure 1.4 Gene duplication which generates a gene family. Each cylinder represents a single gene.

controlled. The origin of the protein family that the vertebrates decided to use for this purpose is not known. The proteins probably already existed in ancient invertebrates, but carried out some function possibly unrelated to defence. Perhaps they were receptors for transporting molecules across the plasma membrane, a function that all cells must be able to carry out. At any rate, in vertebrate ancestors these proteins were expropriated by the vertebrate's equivalent of the Pentagon, the adaptive immune system, for the purpose of defence.

Generation of diversity

Because a single family was to be used, a way had to be found of diversifying the proteins to generate the large number of different receptors required for the large number of epitopes. A system of *generation of diversity* (GOD) had to be invented. The generation of diversity takes place at the level of the genes coding for the receptors and not at the level of the receptors themselves. It relies on two principal mechanisms, one operating in the germ line and the other in the soma[2].

The first mechanism is the *multiplication of genes* and their mutational diversification. If the process starts from a single gene, an identical copy is first made of this gene (*gene duplication*), copies are then made of one or both of the duplicated genes, copies are made of the copies, and so on, until a *multigene family* is generated (Fig. 1.4). The individual members of the family may stay together in a single chromosomal region to form a *gene complex* or they may disperse throughout the genome. The multiplication process occurs over long periods, always one step at a time. The family remains unstable and continues to gain genes by further duplication (*expand*) or to lose them by deletion (*contract*). Gene duplication and deletion occur as a result of *unequal crossing-over (recombination)* between asymmetrically aligned chromosomes (chromatids; Fig. 1.5). During the evolution of the multigene family, the individual genes gradually accumulate mutations (different genes accumulate different mutations) and thus drift apart in terms of their nucleotide sequence and often also of their organization. Since mutations accumulate at more or less constant rates, genes separated from a common ancestor for a long time are less similar to one another than genes separated more recently. Gene duplications and gene families are, of course, not limited to the immune system; they are a common feature of genome evolution.

The second mechanism is *somatic diversification* of the receptor genes. Because the diversification occurs in the soma, it affects only some cell lineages but not others and it is not transmitted to progeny. Each individual has to go through this process on its own and must always start from scratch, so to speak. Since somatic diversification is never the same on repetition, no two individuals possess receptors

[2] Germ line (Latin *gignere*, to beget) is the lineage of cells leading from the fertilized egg or zygote to the functional germ cells (eggs and sperm); *soma* (Greek for body) is the collection of all the cells, except the germ cells, in an organism.

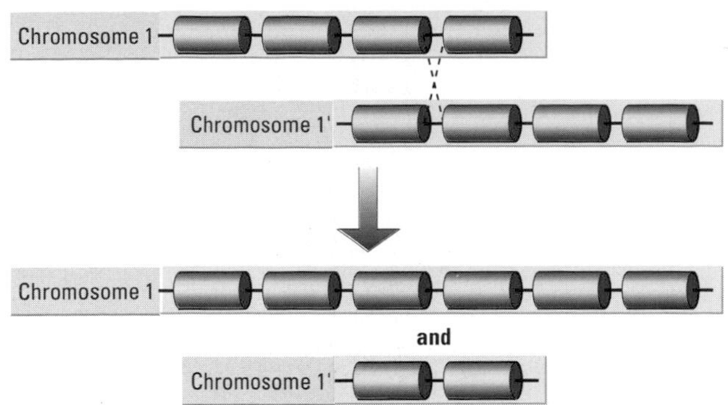

Figure 1.5 Expansion and contraction of gene families. Two homologous chromosomes, each carrying the same number of genes in a given family, align asymmetrically during meiosis. Such misalignment is possible because the individual genes closely resemble one another. Recombination between the misaligned chromosomes (dashed lines) produces two chromosomes of unequal length, one in which the number of genes has expanded from four to six, and the other in which the number has contracted to two.

that diversified in exactly the same way. The three known mechanisms of somatic diversification are shown in Fig. 1.6. In the first mechanism, the germ-line genes are arranged in pairs, one gene being shared by all the pairs (*constant* or C gene) and the other varying from pair to pair (*variable* or *V* gene). The basis of diversification is that different gene pairs are expressed in different cells (Fig. 1.6a). In the second mechanism, there is one master constant–variable gene pair that is expressed in all the specialized cells, and a set of extra *V* genes. In each cell, a short segment of one of the extra *V* genes (a different *V* gene in different cells) is copied into the master *V* gene (*gene conversion*; Fig. 1.6b). In the third mechanism, the *V* genes are split into pieces, a *V* gene is assembled from the pieces (different pieces come together in different cells) and the assembled *V* gene is expressed together with the single *C* gene (Fig. 1.6c). *V* genes diversified by one of these three mechanisms can also diversify further by accumulating *somatic mutations* during cell division.

The diversification of receptor genes occurs in specialized cells that have been set aside for just this purpose, the *lymphocytes*. As these cells differentiate and each of them expresses a particular receptor gene, they are subsequently excluded from expressing all other receptor genes. The progeny of a given cell will therefore express the same gene and the same receptor. It will thus form a *clone*, a group of cells that are all derived from the same ancestral cell. Since different cells express different receptors, the lymphocyte population of a vertebrate is a mosaic of clones covering all

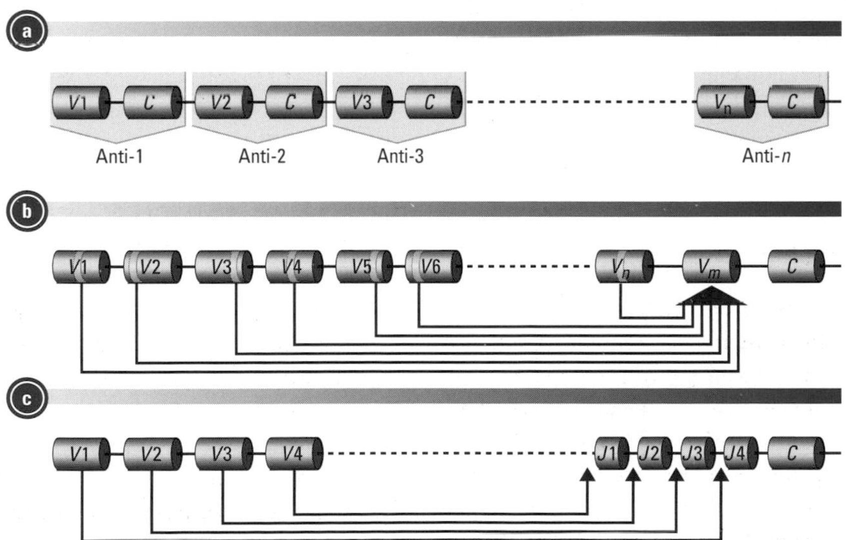

Figure 1.6 Three mechanisms of receptor gene diversification in lymphocytes. Each gene is represented by a cylinder. *C*, *J* and *V* are the constant, joining and variable genes, cylinder. Different numbers indicate that the genes differ from one another in their nucleotide sequence. 'Anti' indicates the specificity of the receptor. (a) Only one of the several *V–C* doublets is expressed in each lymphocyte; different doublets are expressed in different cells. (b) A segment from one of the V_n genes is copied into the master V_m gene (indicated by arrows), which is then expressed together with the *C* gene. (c) One of the *V* genes is transposed to the vicinity of one of the *J* segments and the *V–J* segment is expressed together with the *C* gene. Black dashed lines indicate unspecified lengths of DNA. In all three situations, the genes are selected for expression at random. Mechanisms (a), (b) and (c) are known to be used in the generation of immunoglobulin diversity in fish, birds and mammals, respectively.

the possible epitopes (see Fig. 1.3). It is like a store selling gloves of all possible sizes. The customer entering the store (the antigen or epitope binding to the receptor) selects a particular pair of gloves (a particular lymphocyte) and purchases it (stimulates the lymphocyte). The selected lymphocyte then divides and the progeny forms a clone of identical specificity (*clonal selection*; Fig. 1.7).

In addition to developing as a generator of diversity, lymphocytes have adapted to their function by acquiring a combination of properties not possessed by other cells. New lymphocytes are supplied continuously from undifferentiated stem cells. Lymphocytes themselves have the ability to either differentiate terminally or remain in a partially differentiated state for months or even years. They can also oscillate between a state of rest, in which they carry out housekeeping functions only, and a hyperactive state, in which they divide and secrete proteins (Fig. 1.8). Lymphocytes have the capacity to divide rapidly and repeatedly (*proliferate*), and thus to generate clones of considerable size. Finally, lymphocytes can exist in a state in which they move around a lot or in a state in which they settle down and remain in one place.

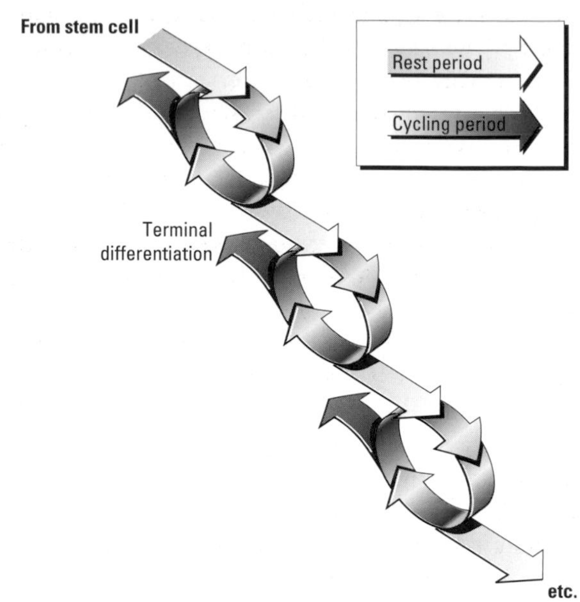

Figure 1.8 Oscillation of a lymphocyte between cycling and resting states. In the cycling period, the lymphocyte divides several times over. Some of the progeny from these divisions differentiate into effector cells, whereas other progeny turn into resting memory cells that can enter the cycling phase upon appropriate stimulation.

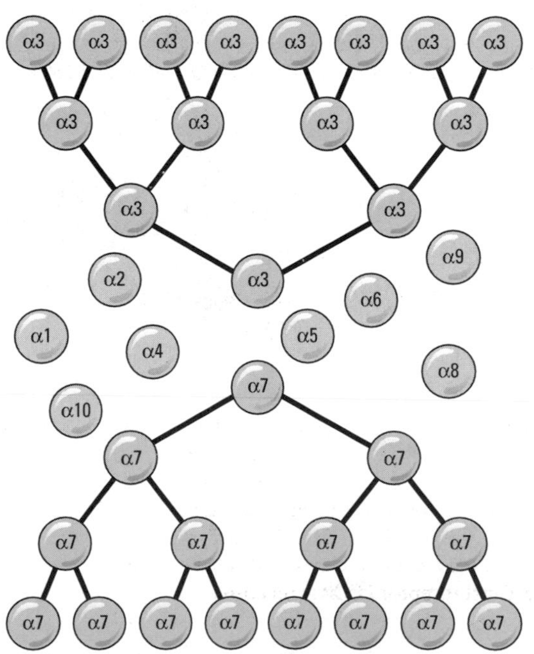

Figure 1.7 Principle of clonal selection. Circles represent individual lymphocytes with receptors for different epitopes (α, anti; 1, 2, 3, . . . , epitopes). Lymphocytes anti-3 and anti-7 have encountered their corresponding epitopes and have thus been selected to multiply. Each has produced a progeny of cells (a clone) with receptors identical to those of the original cell.

Displaying their trap-like receptors, the lymphocytes roam the body in endless migratory cycles, propelled by the blood and the lymph. Most of them never snap their traps and thus never realize their potential, but those few that encounter a complementary ligand become activated and initiate a defence reaction. However, because the initial encounter with the antigen involves only a few cells, it takes several days to multiply them into large clones required for the full-blown response. During this amplification period, the vertebrate relies on the non-adaptive response, which develops almost instantaneously and thus becomes the first line of defence. The situation changes, however, when an organism is attacked by the same parasite for the second or third time. Now the period required for the full development of the response is shortened considerably because the immune system retains an *immunological memory* of the initial experience that allows it to react swiftly to the renewed challenge. The organism is then said to have *acquired immunity* to the particular parasite. Because the organism has modified its behaviour (ability to deal with a particular parasite) so as to conform to the altered circumstances (the presence of the parasite in the environment), it can also be said to have *adapted* or to have developed *adaptive immunity*. Clonal selection (and hence specificity) and memory are the two hallmarks of the adaptive immune response.

There is, however, one hitch in the anticipatory response. Since the receptors cover the entire repertoire of epitopes, some of them are also bound to interact with the ligands of the body that manufactures them, i.e. to *self* structures. In other words, while most of the receptors will have affinities for foreign (*non-self*) substances, some of them will react with self substances, thus unleashing an attack on the body itself, i.e. they will cause *autoimmunity*. Such an attack must be prevented at all costs by making the potentially autoreactive cells tolerant of self components. Therefore, cells expressing receptors for self components must be either eliminated or prevented from responding. In the vertebrate immune system apparently both mechanisms operate to achieve *tolerance* of self.

However, the system does not recognize all potential epitopes of an antigenic molecule, self or non-self. Instead, it focuses on selected parts of the molecule, at least if the molecule is a protein. The focusing is accomplished by a complex process that involves at least three cell types and an intricate molecular machinery (Fig. 1.9). Antigenic proteins are first degraded (*processed*) into peptides and some of the peptides are then taken up by specialized *major histocompatibility complex* (MHC) molecules of *antigen-presenting cells* (APCs) to be presented to the *thymus-derived (T) lymphocytes*. The T cells recognize the peptide–MHC molecule assemblage via their *T-cell receptors* (TCR) and *co-receptors* and are thereby stimulated to differentiate into *effector cells*. Some of the effector T cells participate directly in the removal of the parasite, e.g. by killing the infected cells (*cytotoxic T lymphocytes*, CTL), while others help other lymphocytes, in particular the *bone marrow-derived (B) lymphocytes*, to complete their maturation into effector cells (*helper T* or *T_H cells*). B cells recognize unprocessed antigen via their *B-cell receptors* (BCR), also called *immunoglobulins,* and when differentiated into *plasma cells* secrete a soluble form of the receptor, *antibodies*, into the body fluids. The secreted antibodies, which like the membrane-bound BCR recognize free antigen without an *MHC context*, then become one of the effectors of the adaptive immune response.

The body of a multicellular animal consists of cells and body fluids or *humours*. Both elements are recruited into immune reactions so that, traditionally, immunologists distinguish between *cellular immune responses*, in which cells play a dominant part, and *humoral immune responses*, which are based primarily on molecules present in the body fluids. Both types of response, however, involve cellular and humoral factors, the difference being only in the degree to which the two components participate.

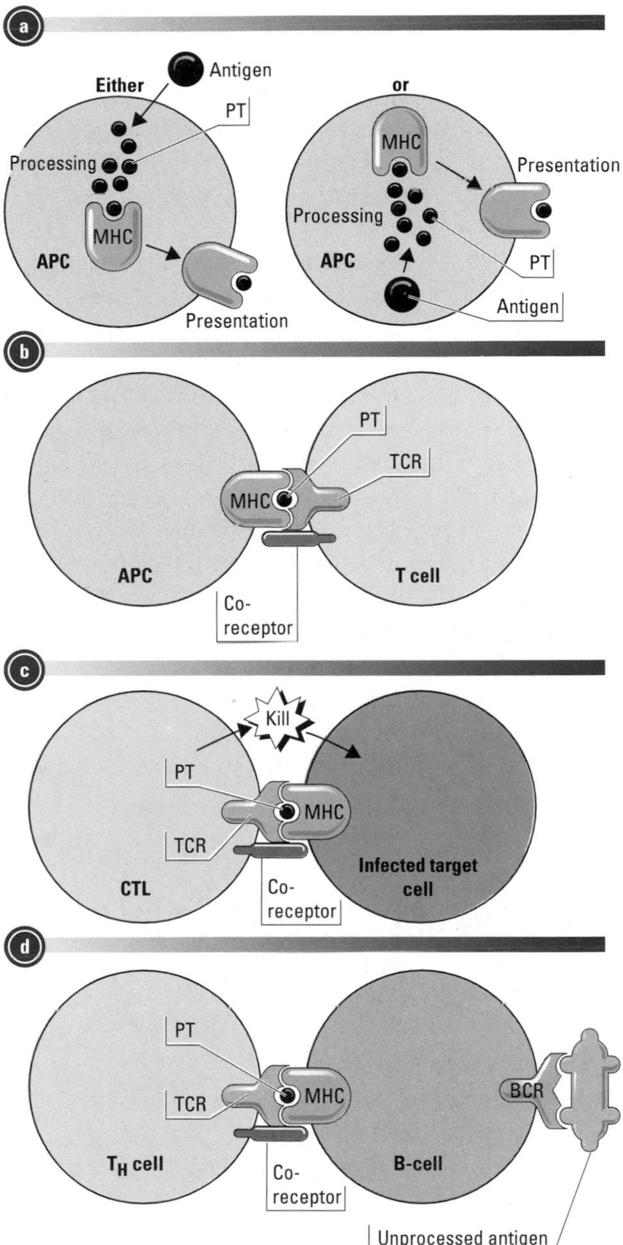

Figure 1.9 Initiation of adaptive immune response in vertebrates. (a) Antigen taken up by an antigen-presenting cell (APC) or derived from proteins inside the cell is processed into peptides (PT), picked up by major histocompatibility complex (MHC) molecules synthesized by the cell and displayed on the cell's surface. (b) The peptide–MHC molecule assemblage is recognized by the T-cell receptor (TCR) and co-receptor of the T lymphocytes. (c) The activated T lymphocyte differentiates into effector cells. One type of effector, the cytotoxic T lymphocytes or CTL, kills infected cells which are recognized when the TCR of the CTL reacts with the same peptide–MHC molecule assemblage that stimulated the original (naive) T lymphocyte. (d) Other types of effector T lymphocytes (helper T or T_H cells) help B lymphocytes that have bound free antigen via their B-cell receptors or BCR (immunoglobulins) to differentiate into antibody-producing plasma cells.

Further reading

Klein, J. (1989) Are invertebrates capable of anticipatory immune response? *Scandinavian Journal of Immunology*, **29**, 499–505.

Langman, R.E. (1989) *The Immune System. Evolutionary Principles Guide Our Understanding of this Complex Biological Defense System*. Academic Press, San Diego, CA.

chapter 2

Immune responses of invertebrates

Invertebrates played an important part in the early development of immunological research. Elie Metchnikoff's demonstration in 1883 that foreign objects introduced into starfish larvae are attacked by mobile amoeboid cells, *macrophages*, is generally considered as marking the beginning of cellular immunology, the branch of immunological sciences dealing with cellular reactions to infections. Later, however, the interest shifted almost exclusively to vertebrates or, more precisely, to mice and humans and studies of immune responses in invertebrates fell into neglect. A revival of invertebrate immunology began only some 20 years ago, but even then the studies remained mere imitations of mouse and human immunology. True progress in invertebrate immunology became possible only when the notion that invertebrates possess an immune system similar to that of vertebrates was abandoned and when sophisticated methods of molecular biology were used in the search for invertebrates' own systems. Although the studies are still in their infancy, the results from a handful of laboratories have revealed already a tremendous variety of means by which invertebrates protect their bodies against parasites. A brief description of some of the protective substances and mechanisms follows, most of which is taken from insect studies. All those discovered thus far are part of the non-adaptive strategy; no evidence of vertebrate-like adaptive responses has been found. Some of the invertebrate responses resemble vertebrate non-adaptive responses, while others do not; the latter may be restricted to particular invertebrate groups.

Cellular immune responses

It is not easy for a microorganism to reach the soft tissue of an insect, for the entire body surface of the potential host is covered by an impenetrable cuticle, which also lines the tubes of the breathing apparatus, various gland ducts and sense organs, as well as the beginning and end parts of the digestive tract. Only when the integrity of the entire cuticle is breached by an abrasion or a wound do microorganisms get their chance. Once inside the body, they are taken up by the fluid that irrigates the tissues and is collected in the vessels of the insect's circulatory system, the *haemolymph*[1]. In addition to the fluid phase, the haemolymph also contains cells, *haemocytes*, of which at least six types can be distinguished by their morphology and function: prohaemocytes, plasmatocytes, granulocytes (granular cells), coagulocytes (cystocytes), sphaerulocytes (sphaerule cells) and oenocytoids. Of these, the plasmatocytes and granular cells are most important in cellular immunity. In the absence of infection, the cells in the haemolymph carry out their everyday chores that are all part of the routine activities in a healthy body. Alerted by an infection, the cells assume extra duties. What exactly alerts the cells is not clear but, in principle, the signal may come from two sources: the injured

[1] In insects, the circulatory and respiratory systems are separated and the 'blood' (fluid in vessels) is combined with 'lymph' (tissue fluid) into haemolymph. The system of vessels is open, allowing the haemolymph to bathe the internal organs and fill the body cavity or haemocoel.

tissue may release substances normally absent in the haemolymph; and the invaders themselves may reveal their presence by releasing substances as part of their normal activities, or fragments of their disintegrating dead cells. These substances circulate through the body via the haemolymph and attract haemocytes to the site of injury and infection. What follows has only been roughly outlined in the case of invertebrate cells, but an analogous process has been studied in greater detail in vertebrates and will be described in Chapter 15. It is likely that the released substances induce the plasmatocytes in the haemolymph to express receptors with affinities for compounds either normally present on bacterial surfaces or taken up by the bacteria from the haemolymph. The interaction triggers a chain reaction in the plasmatocyte that leads to the reorganization of the cytoskeleton and the formation of extensions ('false feet' or *pseudopodia*), by which the cell surrounds and ultimately engulfs the bacterium (Fig. 2.1). In the cell, the bacterium remains in a bag (*vacuole*) lined by a fragment of the plasma membrane derived from the plasmatocyte's surface. The process of internalization of bacteria (or any other particulate matter) by cells is referred to as *phagocytosis* (from Greek *phagein*, to eat; *kytos*, cell). Cells capable of phagocytosis are *phagocytes* and the bag containing the ingested particle is a *phagosome*. The fate of microorganisms in insect phagosomes is not known. Vertebrate phagocytes are able to kill engulfed bacteria by releasing toxic substances (see Chapter 15) and it is possible that similar destructive mechanisms have evolved also in some invertebrates. However, sequestration alone is a protective mechanism. Phagocytosis is probably the most widespread form of immune response shared by all animal groups.

Phagocytosis disposes of individual cells. However, microorganisms can occur in the haemolymph in groups, either because they aggregate spontaneously or because they are clumped together by products of the host cells. The aggregates are too large to be engulfed by a single plasmatocyte and must therefore be disposed of in some other way. Before we describe the disposal of large particles, however, a word should be said about the aggregation process itself. A common instigator of cell aggregation in insects and other animals is the *coagulation* (*clotting*) process. The biochemistry of haemolymph clotting is poorly understood in insects, but has been elucidated reasonably well in the horseshoe crab *Limulus*, which, like insects, is an arthropod, but a member of another class (Fig. 2.2). The horseshoe crab clotting reaction is initiated, for example, by lipopolysaccharide (LPS, also called endotoxin; see Chapters 13 & 21), a major structural component of the outer wall in Gram-negative bacteria. (Recall that the stain invented by the Danish bacteriologist Hans C.J. Gram divides bacteria into two types: those that do and those that do not retain a dark purple colour after treatment with this concoction—the Gram-positive and the Gram-negative bacteria, respectively.) Some of the haemocytes circulating in horseshoe crab haemolymph contain bags (*granules*) loaded with at least 20 different proteins. They also express receptors on their surfaces that bind readily to the LPS component of the Gram-negative bacteria. The binding activates a biochemical pathway that leads to the fusion of the individual granules with the plasma membrane of the haemocyte, localized distribution of the membrane at the fusion site, and emptying of the granules' contents into the haemolymph (*exocytosis*; see Fig. 2.2). Among the released proteins are at least four that participate in the clotting process: factors B and C, proclotting enzyme and coagulogen. *Factors B* and *C* are enzymes whose active site

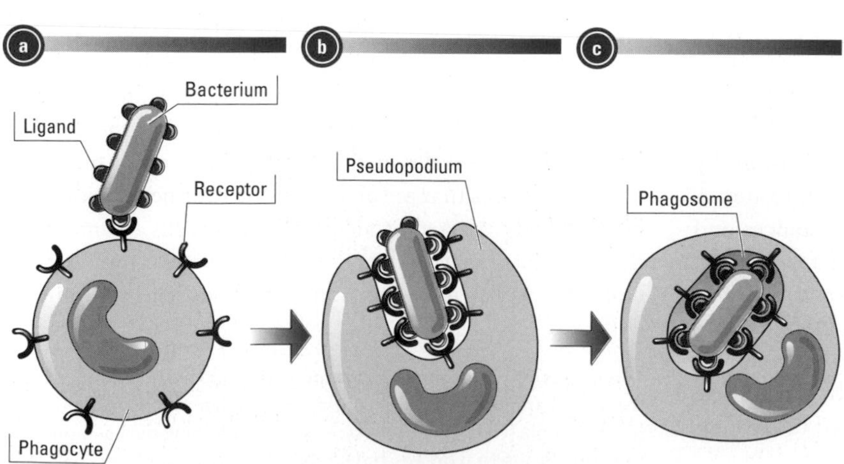

Figure 2.1 Diagrammatic representation of phagocytosis. (a) Receptors on the surface of a phagocyte bind a ligand on a bacterium. (b) The binding triggers rearrangement of the cytoskeleton network in the phagocyte and the formation of pseudopodia, which surround the bacterium. (c) The engulfed bacterium is sequestered into a membrane-bounded vesicle, the phagosome.

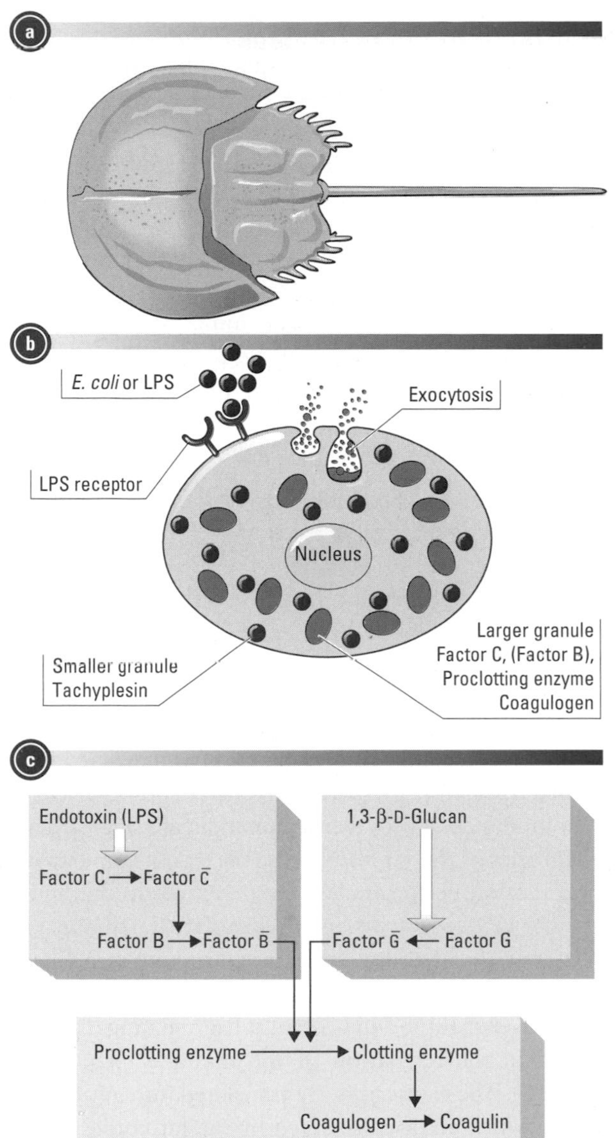

Figure 2.2 The clotting system of the horseshoe crab. (a) Horseshoe crab. (b) Activation of a haemocyte (granular cell) and subsequent degranulation by exocytosis. (c) The coagulation cascade 1,3-β-D-glucan is a component of the cell wall of certain fungi; LPS, lipopolysaccharide. Bar above a letter indicates active state. (b and c, based on Iwanaga, S. (1993) *Current Opinion in Immunology*, 5, 74.)

is characterized by the presence of the amino acid serine and which, when activated, cleave proteins (they are members of the family of *serine proteases*). However, factor C also contains segments (domains) that show sequence similarity not only with the C1 component of the vertebrate complement system (see Chapter 12), but also with some of the vertebrate blood-clotting factors (see Chapter 12) and carbohydrate-binding proteins called lectins (see Chapter 13). The factor is present in the granules in an inactive form (*zymogen*), but when released into the haemolymph activates itself with the help of LPS and then activates factor B. There is also another factor, G, whose localization has not yet been determined. Both active factors B and G activate the *proclotting enzyme*, turning it into a clotting enzyme, which subsequently turns the *coagulogen* into coagulin. Interactions of the coagulin molecules produce an insoluble gel, the clot, which traps cells and cellular fragments.

Nodular reaction

The clotting reaction is very swift: Within seconds of exposure to LPS, granular haemocytes can be seen emptying their granules into the haemolymph and clots become visible as they form around them. It is assumed that similar reactions also take place in the insect haemolymph and entrap invading microorganisms. The clot becomes a focus of further haemocyte activities that result in the formation of a *nodule*. Each nodule consists of entrapped aggregates of microorganisms that are too large to be engulfed and of plasmatocytes with engulfed single bacteria. All this is enclosed in a fibrous material presumably secreted by haemocytes arranged in several concentric layers around the entrapped material. The isolation inside the nodule prevents the bacteria from multiplying and limits their access to nutrients. It also makes them a clearly delineated target for an attack by noxious substances released by the haemocytes. This process ultimately results in the death of the bacteria, their degradation and subsequent resolution of the nodule, thus ending the nodular reaction.

Encapsulation reaction

When a large number of microorganisms or a multicellular parasite invade the body cavities of an insect, the nodule develops into a tight, multicellular sheath called a *capsule* (Fig. 2.3) and, concurrently, this *encapsulation reaction* is accompanied by melanization of the capsule's inner content. *Melanin* is a polymer of compounds ultimately derived from the amino acid tyrosine. Different variants of the polymer are pigments widely distributed in both the plant and animal kingdoms. In humans, for example, melanin is chiefly responsible for the colour of skin, hair and eyes; in insects, melanin tans the cuticle. A key enzyme in the biosynthetic pathway leading from tyrosine to melanin is *phenoloxidase* (*tyrosinase*) which, in some arthropods at least, is present in the granules of granular haemocytes in an inactive form called the *prophenoloxidase*. The granules also contain proteases, again

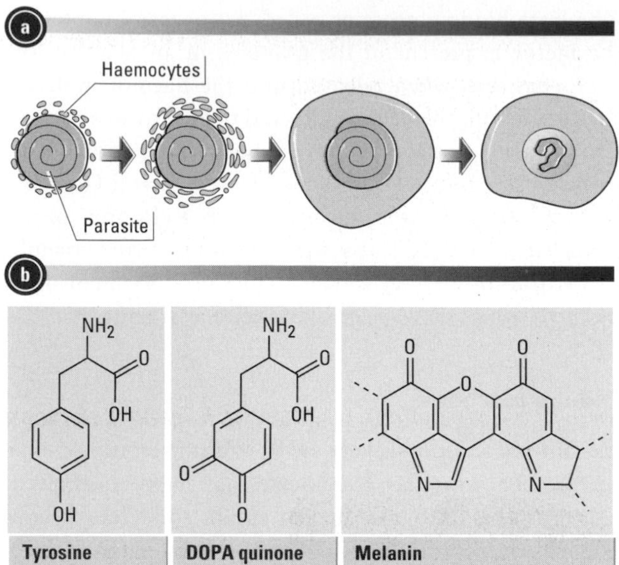

Figure 2.3 Encapsulation and melanization. (a) Stages in the formation of a capsule around a parasite (worm). From left to right: host's haemocytes surround the worm; the haemocytes arrange themselves in multiple layers and flatten; the capsular cells release toxic substances onto the parasite (among others, intermediates of melanin synthesis) and then die; the parasite dies and shrinks. (b) Starting compound, one of the intermediary substances and the end-product in the biosynthetic pathway of melanin synthesis. DOPA, 3,4-dihydroxyphenylalanine.

in inactive pro-enzyme forms, which convert the prophenoloxidase into active phenoloxidase. When the haemocytes degranulate on contact with bacterial substances and the contents of the granules are released onto the parasite, one of the proteases is activated by microbial cell wall components. The activated protease in turn activates another protease, which activates another, until the ultimate serine protease activates the phenoloxidase. This last enzyme then begins to oxidize phenols to quinones, which then polymerize non-enzymatically to melanin. The prophenoloxidase is a 'sticky' protein that attaches nonspecifically to microbes or multicellular parasites in the growing nodule or capsule. Melanin synthesis then proceeds on these surfaces, resulting in the melanization of the nodule or capsule. Although capsules have been demonstrated to form in the absence of melanization, melanin may help to form a mechanical barrier that restrains the activities of the entrapped parasite and the toxic intermediates of melanin synthesis may contribute to killing the parasite. The end result of the encapsulation reaction, the capsule, thus consists of an inner sheath of dark, melanized material and dead cells surrounded by a thick layer of haemocytes tightly adhering to one another and isolating the interior from the outside fluids.

Humoral immune responses

Although phagocytosis, nodule formation and encapsulation are accompanied by the release of a plethora of substances into the haemolymph, the actual effectors in these responses, and the agents that carry them out, are primarily cells, the *effector cells*. An infection, however, also triggers a response in which the effectors primarily take the form of substances released into the haemolymph, that is to say, by *humoral immune response*. The initial stimulus for the humoral immune response may be provided by the same substances that trigger the cellular response, i.e. LPS and peptidoglycans from the bacterial cell walls and 1,3-β-D-glucans from fungal cell walls. These structures normally do not occur in animal bodies and they are therefore easily identified as foreign during an infection. The identity of the receptors that bind the foreign substances and the site at which the binding takes place have not been established, nor is it known what happens after the initial recognition. Presumably, the ligand–receptor interaction generates a signal that is transmitted, via a chain of intermediates, to the *fat bodies*, which are present in various places in the body cavity (haemocoel) and function somewhat like the liver of vertebrates, by storing glycogen and other energy-rich compounds and by being metabolically highly active. In the nuclei of the fat body cells, the signal stimulates the appearance of specific *nuclear factors*, proteins that bind to particular DNA segments and thus initiate the transcription of the genes located downstream from them (see Chapter 6). The sequence of these DNA segments is similar to that of the NF-κB element found upstream from mammalian genes involved in the regulation of the immune response (see Chapter 8). The transcripts are translated into antibacterial proteins which are then secreted by the fat bodies into the haemolymph. The proteins are produced in an inactive form, presumably to avoid self-damage. When an appropriate stimulus is generated in the body, the preproproteins are processed proteolytically into their active forms.

The first antibacterial proteins appear in the haemolymph within a few hours after infection; their production peaks 3–6 days later and declines in the following 3–6 days. Eventually, the proteins disappear from the haemolymph altogether to reappear only after a fresh encounter with bacteria. When that happens, the dynamics of the response mirrors that following the first encounter — the organism retains no *memory* of the previous experience. However, since similar responses can be activated by a variety of stimuli, the immune system of an insect remains in an activated state for much of the host's lifespan. There is therefore no need for immunological memory in these organisms.

More than 50 antibacterial proteins and peptides have

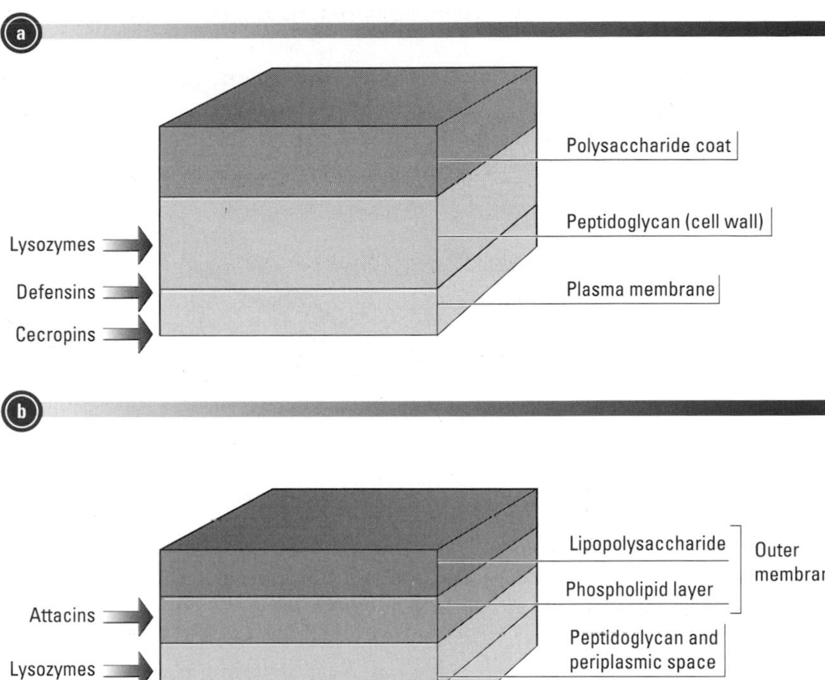

Figure 2.4 Structure of the envelope in (a) Gram-positive and (b) Gram-negative bacteria. The target layers of the main classes of inducible antibacterial proteins and peptides are indicated by arrows. (See also Fig. 21.34.)

been isolated from the insect haemolymph; they can be classified into four major groups according to their structure and function (Fig. 2.4): lysozymes, cecropins, defensins and attacins.

Lysozymes

Lysozymes are enzymes closely related to the so-called chicken (c)-type lysozymes in vertebrates. They act by breaking the bond between acetylmuramic acid and *N*-acetylglucosamine in the peptidoglycan layer of the bacterial cell wall (Fig. 2.5). (Their name derives from the observation that they rapidly dissolve bacteria growing in culture; Greek *lyein* means to dissolve and *zymé* is a 'ferment' and the root of the word 'enzyme'.) In a few bacteria the peptidoglycan layer is immediately accessible to the enzymes and these species are killed directly by lysozymes. In other bacteria, the peptidoglycan layer becomes accessible only after the cell wall has been damaged by other antibacterial proteins, for example cecropins and attacins. In some insects, lysozymes are induced by an encounter with bacteria; in others they are expressed constitutively and, paradoxically, their synthesis may even be shut off during an infection. In *Drosophila*, for example, lysozymes are encoded in at least seven genes expressed in different parts of the digestive tract, presumably as an adaptation to a microorganism-rich diet. One of the signs of a bacterial infection in *Drosophila* is cessation of lysozyme production in the insect's gut.

Cecropins

Cecropins are a family of peptides named after the cecropia moth, *Hyalophora cecropia*, from which they were first isolated (Fig. 2.6). The peptides, which are 35–39 amino acid residues long, are organized into two amphipathic α-helices interrupted by a flexible hinge region. (An *amphipathic* molecule has two parts with characteristically different properties: one part is water-soluble or *hydrophilic* and the other water-insoluble or *hydrophobic*; see Chapter 6, especially Fig. 6.33.) Their amphipathicity enables the molecule to penetrate bacterial membranes and create holes in them, thus killing the cells. The target of the cecropin molecules is the plasma membrane of Gram-positive bacteria and the inner membrane of Gram-negative bacteria (see Fig. 2.4). Several cecropins (designated A, B, C, D, etc.) have been isolated from the cecropia moth and their encoding genes are presumed to have arisen by duplication from a common ancestor. Cecropins have also been isolated from other insects and given different names such as lepidopterans, bacteriocidins, sarcotoxins and others. However, they are all members of the same family.

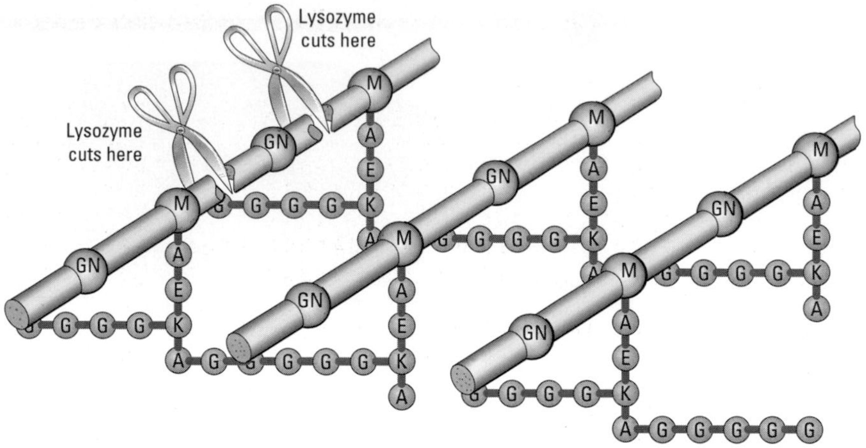

Figure 2.5 The site of lysozyme action in the peptidoglycan layer of the bacterial cell wall. Glycan strands (red bars) are composed of alternating *N*-acetylglucosamine (GN) and *N*-acetylmuramic acid (M) residues. The vertical lines emanating from M represent amino acid residues of the tetrapeptide subunit: A, alanine; E, glutamic acid; K, lysine. The horizontal lines represent the peptide cross-linking bridges consisting of five repeated glycine (G) residues. (See also Fig. 21.34.)

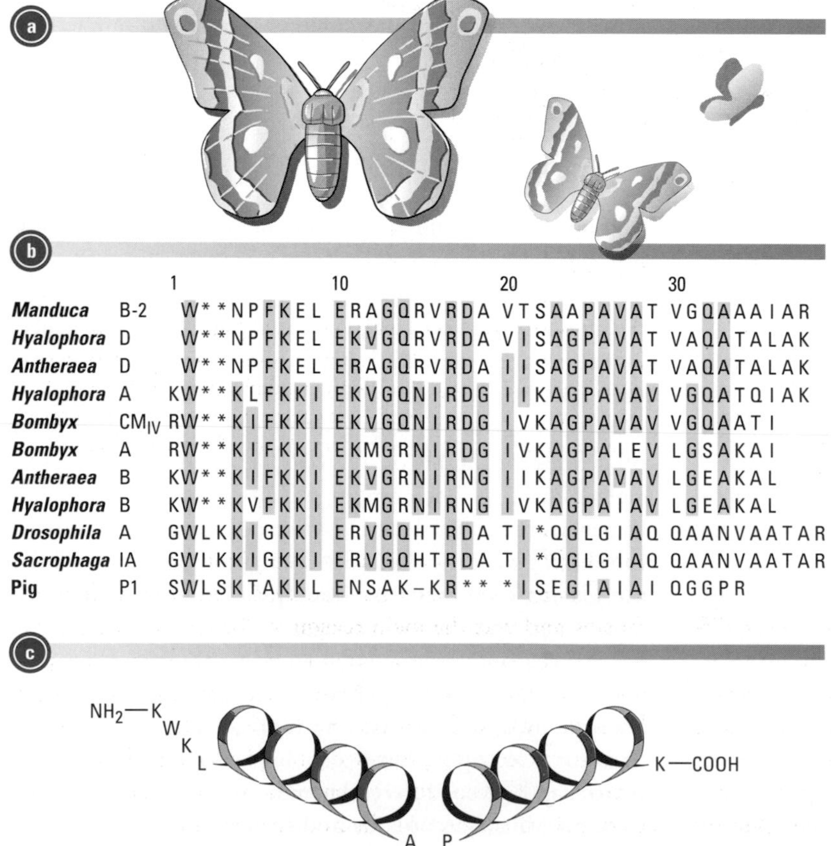

Figure 2.6 Cecropins. (a) The cecropia moth, *Hyalophora cecropia*. (b) Comparison of 11 cecropin amino acid sequences from six insects and one mammal. Residues shared by most of the sequences are highlighted. Asterisks indicate gaps introduced to achieve optimal alignment of the sequences. The positions are numbered from the N-terminus towards the C-terminus (see Chapter 6). The amino acid residues are given in the international one-letter code (see Appendix 1). (c) Model of three-dimensional structure of an insect cecropin peptide molecule. The first four amino acid residues of the N-terminus (NH_2) are non-helical; they are followed by an amphipathic α-helix (see Chapter 6) encompassing residues 5–21, a hinge region with alanine, glycine and proline, and then a second amphipathic α-helix (residues 25–37). Groups of hydrophilic and hydrophobic residues are indicated by red and grey lines, respectively. COOH, carboxyl terminus (see Chapter 6); A, G, K, L, P, W are abbreviations of amino acid residues (see Appendix 1). (b and c, from Bowman, H.G. *et al.* (1991) *European Journal of Biochemistry*, **201**, 223.)

Species	Name of peptide	Peptide sequence: Loop	α-helix	β-sheet
Phormia terranovae	Defensin A	ATCDLL*** *SGTGINHSA	CAAHCLIR*G	NR*GGYCNG* **KGVCVCRN
	Defensin B	ATCDLL*** *SGTGINHSA	CAAHCLLR*G	NR*GGYCNR* **KGVCVCRN
Eristalis tenax	Defensin	ATCDLL*** *SFLNVNHAA	CAAHCLSK*G	YR*GGYCDG* **KKVCNCR
Sarcophaga peregrina	Sapecin A	ATCDLL*** *SGTGINHSA	CAAHCLLR*G	NR*GGYCNG* **KAVCVCRN
	Sapecin C	ATCDLL*** *SGIGVQHSA	CALHCVFR*G	NR*GGYCTG* **KGICVCRN
Zophobas atratus	Defensin A	FTCDVLGFE IAGTKLNSAA	CGAHCLAL*G	RR*GGYCNS* **KSVCVCR
	Defensin B	FTCDVLGFE IAGTKLNSAA	CGAHCLAL*G	RT*GGYCNS* **KSVCVCR
Sarcophaga peregrina	Sapecin B	LTCEID*** *****–RS–L	CLLHCRLK*G	YLRA–YC*SQ Q*K–VCRCVQ
Aeschna cyanea	Defensin	GFGCPL**** *****–DQMQ	CHRHCQTITG	RS*GGYC*SG PLKLTCTCYR
Leiurus quinquestriatus	Defensin	GFGCPL**** *****–NQGA	CHRHCRSIRR	R**GGYCAGF F*KQTCTCYRN

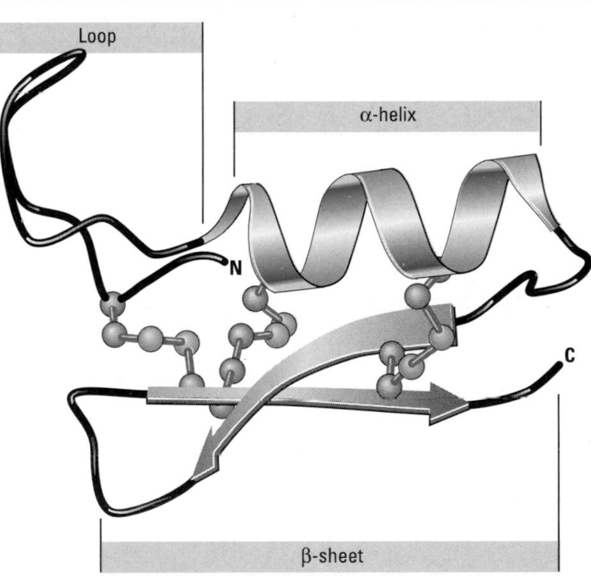

Figure 2.7 Defensins. (a) Comparison of 10 defensin amino acid sequences from six insect species. Residues shared by most of the sequences (among them the six cysteines) are highlighted. Asterisks indicate gaps introduced to achieve optimal alignment. The amino acid residues are given in the international one-letter code (see Appendix 1). The extent of each of the three domains (loop, α-helix, β-sheet) is delineated. (b) Model of the three-dimensional structure of an insect defensin molecule. The three intradomain disulphide bonds are highlighted. N- and C- are the amino and carboxyl termini of the protein (see Chapter 6). (Based on Sociancich, S. *et al.* (1994) *Parasitology Today*, **10**, 132.)

Defensins

Defensins (sapecins) are another family of at least seven different peptides ranging in length from 38 to 45 amino acid residues. There is also a group of mammalian defensins (see Chapter 15) originally believed to be related to insect defensins; in fact, they are not. Insect defensins consist of three distinct domains: a flexible N-terminal loop, a central amphipathic α-helix and a C-terminal antiparallel β-sheet (Fig. 2.7). Each peptide contains six cysteine residues forming three intramolecular disulphide bonds (a similar arrangement of cysteines also exists in mammalian defensins and was the main reason for believing that the two groups of peptides were homologous). Defensins are produced not only by fat body cells but also by certain haemolymph cells (thrombocytoids). They kill Gram-positive bacteria by puncturing the plasma membrane as do cecropins. Gram-negative bacteria seem to be protected from defensin attack by their outer membranes.

Attacins

Attacins are a rather heterogeneous group of proteins varying in size (M_r 9000–35 000), but rich in glycine residues (10–22%). They include *attacins* found in moths, *sarcotoxin II* and *diptericin* in flies, *coleoptericin* in beetles and others. The various proteins are united by a weak (13–35%) sequence similarity in the glycine-rich region (the G domain); some of them also share short stretches with high proline content (the P domain). Attacins act by blocking the synthesis of the major outer membrane proteins in dividing Gram-negative bacteria, thus disturbing the integrity of the cell wall and causing the bacteria to grow in long chains.

There is very little discrimination (specificity) in the insect antibacterial responses. Different bacteria induce the production of most of the proteins and the same protein once induced by one particular type of bacteria can act on unrelated bacteria. At most, the responses may differentiate between Gram-positive and Gram-negative bacteria. The advantage of the relative non-specificity of the response lies in the potential of the responses against different types of bacteria to enhance one another during an infection by more than one type of bacterium. Absence of memory and relative non-specificity are two characteristics of antibacterial responses and indeed of all non-adaptive responses.

Further reading

Boman, H.G., March, J. & Goode, J. (eds) (1994) *Antimicrobial Peptides*. Ciba Symposium no. 186. John Wiley & Sons, Chichester.

Boman, H.G., Faye, I., Gudmundsson, G.H., Lee, J.-Y. & Lidholm, D.-A. (1991) Cell free immunity in *Cecropia*. *European Journal of Biochemistry*, **201**, 23–31.

Ganz, T. & Lehrer, R.I. (1994) Defensins. *Current Opinion in Immunology*, **6**, 584–589.

Hoffmann, J.A. (1995) Innate immunity of insects. *Current Opinion in Immunology*, **7**, 4–10.

Hoffmann, J.A. & Hetru, C. (1992) Insect defensins: inducible antibacterial peptides. *Immunology Today*, **13**, 411–415.

Hoffmann, J.A., Natori, S. & Janeway, C. (eds) (1994) *Phylogenetic Perspectives in Immunity: the Insect-Host Defense*. R.G. Landes Biomedical Publisher, Austin, TX.

Hultmark, D. (1993) Immune reactions in *Drosophila* and other insects: a model for innate immunity. *Trends in Genetics*, **9**, 178–183.

Iwanaga, S. (1993) The *Limulus* clotting reaction. *Current Opinion in Immunology*, **5**, 74–82.

Johansson, M.W. & Söderhäll, K. (1989) Cellular immunity in crustaceans and the proPO system. *Parasitology Today*, **5**, 171–176.

Ratcliffe, N.A. (1985) Invertebrate immunity—a primer for the non-specialist. *Immunology Letters*, **10**, 253–270.

Sociancich, S., Bulet, P., Hetru, C. & Hoffmann, J.A. (1994) The inducible antibacterial peptides of insects. *Parasitology Today*, **10**, 132–139.

Wright, T.R.F. (1987) The genetics of biogenic amine metabolism, sclerotization, and melanization in *Drosophila melanogaster*. *Advances in Genetics*, **24**, 127–222.

chapter 3 Tissues and organs of the immune system

Circulatory systems

An efficient immune response is contingent upon the delivery of immune cells and molecules to the site at which a parasite has lodged itself; the fastest means of transport available to an organism are the extracellular fluids that bathe the tissues. To be able to transport material, the body fluids must be in motion. In the simplest animals, fluids move by diffusion, but in larger and more complex animals this mode of transport is too inefficient to serve all the needs of the organism. These animals have developed special circulatory systems, a set of plumbing conduits for transporting fluids over longer distances, while retaining the diffusion-based transport for shorter distances in the tissues themselves. The circulatory systems consist of vessels, chambers, sinuses[1] and usually also pumping organs (hearts). A consequence of the appearance of circulatory systems was the separation of the extracellular body fluids into two compartments: blood, the fluid (and everything suspended in it) largely confined to the vessels; and lymph[2], the fluid percolating for the most part around the tissues outside the vessels. Where there is no clear distinction between these two compartments, as in the case of insects for example, the fluid is referred to as haemolymph. The cells suspended in blood are the blood cells; those dominating the vertebrate lymph are lymphocytes[3]. The main vertebrate blood cells are erythrocytes, B lymphocytes (which can enlarge into blasts and differentiate in tissues into plasma cells), T lymphocytes, monocytes (which differentiate in tissues into macrophages), neutrophils, basophils and eosinophils. These will be described in Chapters 4 and 5.

There are two principal types of the circulatory system: open and closed (Fig. 3.1). In the *open circulatory system*, the pumping organ forces the fluid (blood) through a series of vessels, the arteries, to the tissues in the various parts of the body. There the vessels terminate, the fluid diffuses into the tissues and then oozes back into the heart through tissue spaces. There are no return vessels. In the *closed circulatory system*, most of the fluid never leaves the vessels, but passes instead through a system of hair-like, thin-walled vessels, the capillaries, followed by equally fine venules, and then returns to the heart through a second series of closed ducts, the veins. Some invertebrates (e.g. insects) have open circulatory systems, while others (e.g. annelids, represented by the earthworm) have closed systems; all vertebrates have closed systems.

1 The Latin word *sinus* refers to a hollow or a cavity. In anatomy and histology it describes dilatation of a vessel.

2 The Latin word *lymph* is derived from Greek *lyma*, which indicates the dirt removed by washing or dirty water, and the Greek *lonein* meaning to wash the body, to bathe.

3 Lymphocyte-like cells have also been described in invertebrates but there is no evidence that they are homologous to vertebrate lymphocytes.

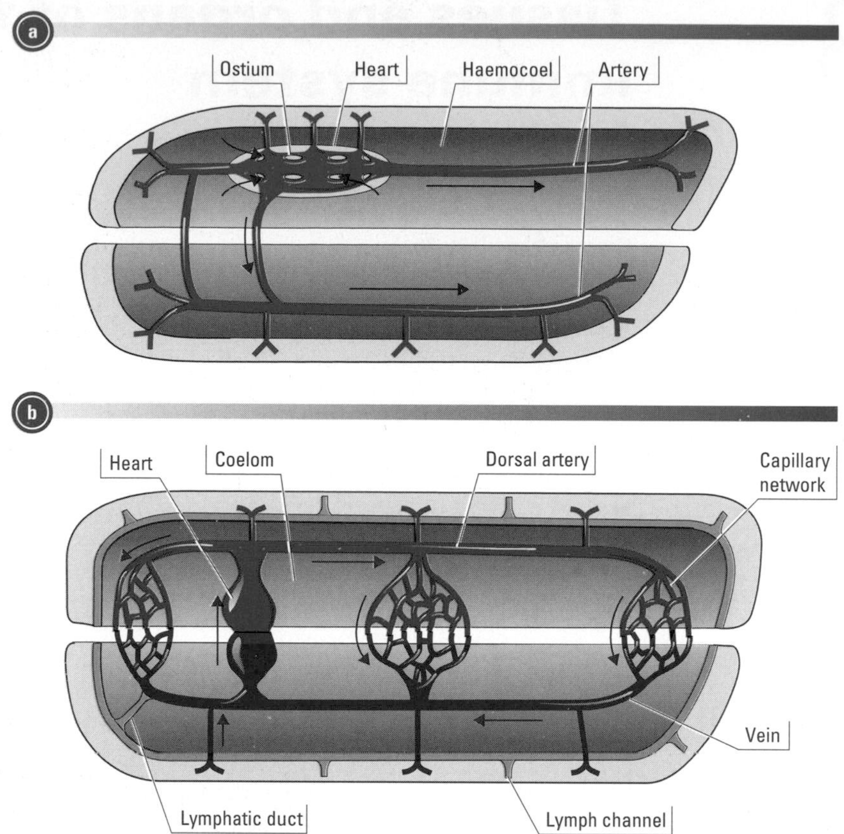

Figure 3.1 Diagrammatic representation of an open (a) and closed (b) circulatory system. Ostia are small orifices through which blood (haemolymph) returns to the heart. Arrows indicate direction of fluid movements. Coelom and haemocoel are body cavities. (Based on Prosser, C.L. (1973) *Comparative Animal Physiology*, 3rd edn. W.B. Saunders, Philadelphia.)

Lymphatic system

In more advanced vertebrates blood is pumped under pressure, so that with every heart beat more blood arrives in the capillaries than can possibly pass through. The extra volume of fluid seeps through the thin capillary walls into the surrounding tissue. Most of the fluid returns back into the venules immediately, between two heart beats, while the rest is drained by a system of lymphatic vessels. In the human body, the system begins with a turf of blind *lymphatic capillaries* (Fig. 3.2), which change into a mesh of delicate vessels, then into coarser vessels and finally into *lymphatics* of ever increasing bore. All the lymphatics eventually connect to one of two large lymphatic trunks, either the right lymphatic duct or the thoracic duct (Fig. 3.3). The *right lymphatic duct* drains the upper right part of the body, including the right side of the head, the neck, the heart, the lungs and part of the diaphragm; it empties into the right subclavian vein. The *thoracic duct*, which starts in its lower part as a dilated cisterna chyli, drains the rest of the body and empties into the left subclavian vein.

In the evolution of vertebrates, lymphatic vessels first appear in animals with well-developed blood capillaries—some cartilaginous fish and all bony fish; jawless fish lack lymphatic vessels altogether. The lymphatic system of the bony fish is relatively simple; it was only after vertebrates ventured on land and greatly expanded their blood capillaries that the lymphatics began to grow in complexity. In mammals, lymphatic vessels form a dense three-dimensional meshwork pervading the entire body and the lymphatics are frequently interrupted by filtering stations, the *lymph nodes*.

The fluid flowing in the lymphatic vessels is the *lymph*. When collected initially in the lymphatic capillaries, the lymph is largely cell-free, clear and colourless or yellowish. However, as it percolates through the lymph nodes, it collects cells, mainly lymphocytes brought into the node with blood, as well as large quantities of proteins, and thus becomes increasingly turbid. The lymph flowing through the lymphatic vessels of the intestine has a milky appearance because of a high content of fine droplets of fat. The composition of the lymph varies depending on the species, the tissue and the circumstances. The highest number of cells, primarily lymphocytes, is present in the lymph of the ducts.

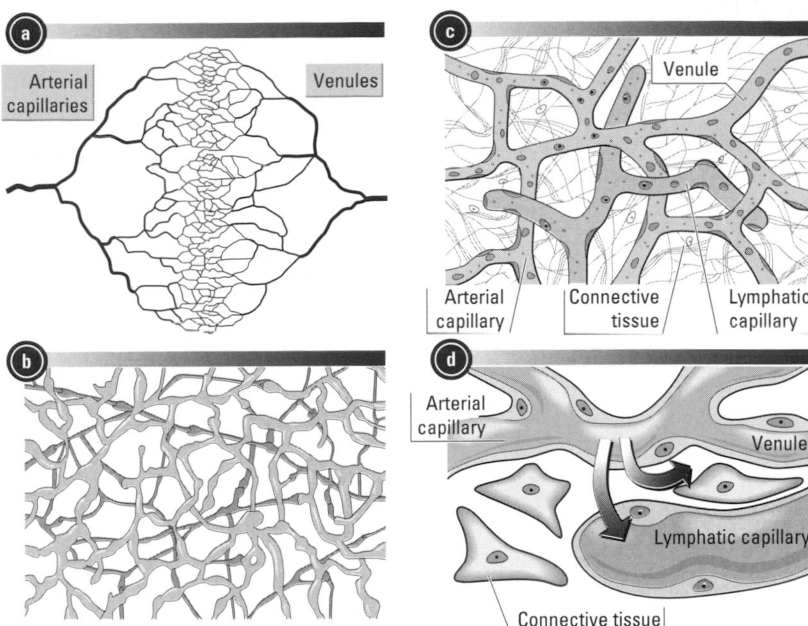

Figure 3.2 Interrelationship of blood and lymphatic capillaries in tissues. (a) Blood capillary bed. (b) Lymphatic capillary bed. (c) Intertwining of blood and lymphatic capillaries in connective tissue. (d) Distribution of fluid forced out of arterial capillaries (arrows). Most fluid returns into the blood circulation via the venules but some does seep into the lymphatic capillaries.

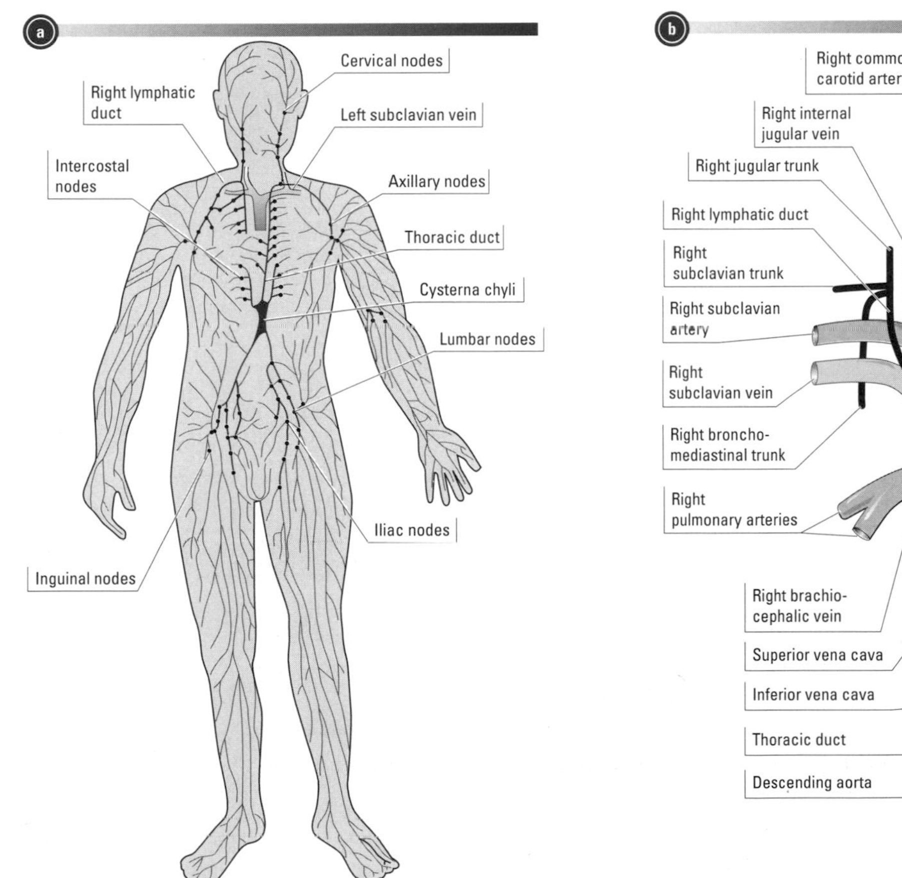

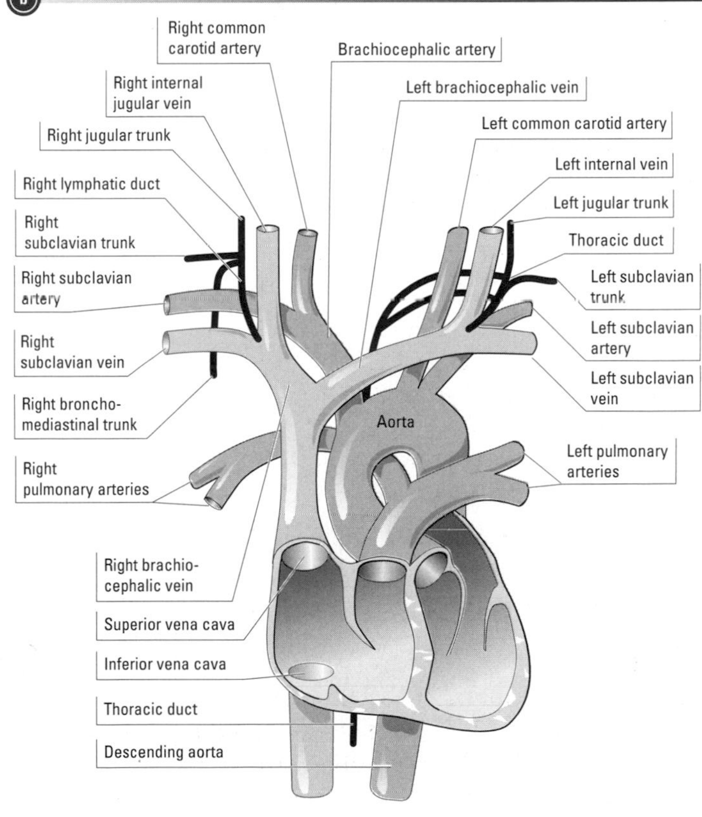

Figure 3.3 Human lymphatic system (a) and its connection to the bloodstream (b). The human body is divided into two parts by the lymphatic system, the larger part drained by the thoracic duct and the smaller part drained by the right lymphatic duct (a). The thoracic duct empties into the left subclavian vein; the right lymphatic duct, which drains the heart, the lungs, part of the diaphragm, the right upper part of the body and the right side of the head and neck, empties into the right subclavian vein (b).

Organs of immunity

The immune system of invertebrates consists of individual cells scattered throughout the body and molecules produced by some of these cells. Both the cells and molecules are delivered to the site of infection by the circulatory system. Although collections of immune cells can occur in different parts of an invertebrate body (in the fat bodies of insects, for example), the primary function of these parts is not defence against parasites. In the evolution of vertebrates, on the other hand, there is a trend towards a gradual organization of the immune system into body parts composed of several tissues and specializing mainly in defence, the organs of immunity (Fig. 3.4). Because their main components are lymphocytes, they are referred to as *lymphoid organs*. In the earliest vertebrates, the immune system probably consisted of unorganized assemblies of lymphocytes around the intestine and other tubes through which foreign matter can enter the body. Some of the lymphocytes may have circulated with blood and lymph, while others may have been more sessile forming *diffuse lymphoid tissues*. Later, some of the lymphocytes began to group into small spherical or oval clusters, the *lymphoid follicles*. The advantage in congregating together is that the lymphocytes can interact with one another more easily than when they are scattered around the body. Later still, the follicles themselves grouped into little nests or *patches*. Finally, the follicles began to surround themselves with membranes, grew in complexity and thus formed primitive *lymphoid organs*: the lymph nodes, the spleen, the thymus and in the birds the bursa of Fabricius. These different forms of lymphocyte organization still exist in the various classes of extant vertebrates and they are all still present in even the most advanced vertebrates.

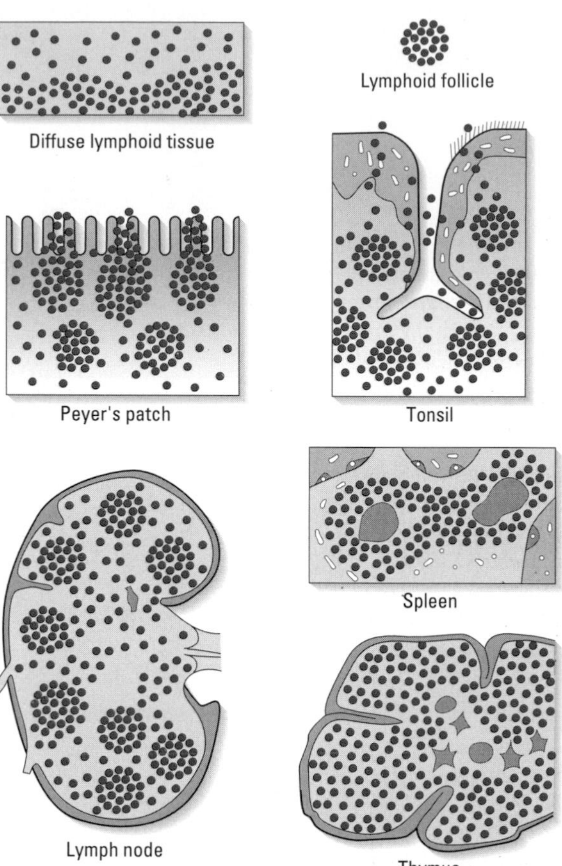

Figure 3.4 Schematic representation of the various types of lymphoid tissue occurring in the human body. Red dots indicate lymphocytes. (Modified from Elias, H., Pauly, J.E. & Burns, E.R. (1978) *Histology*, 4th edn. John Wiley & Sons, New York.)

Diffuse lymphoid tissue

Most body surfaces, outer or inner, are covered by *epithelium*, a sheet of polyhedral, tightly associated cells. Beneath this sheet is a layer of loose connective tissue[4], *lamina propria*, which is basically a three-dimensional meshwork of fibroblasts[5] and fibres. The meshes of the network are filled with ground substance and a variety of free cells, in particular lymphocytes (Fig. 3.5). The free lymphocytes are so dense in some places, particularly during an infection, that they are said to form a *diffuse lymphoid tissue*. The digestive tract contains a second dense accumulation of lymphocytes in the *tela submucosa*, a loose connective tissue rich in large blood and lymphatic vessels, nerves and fat cells. Diffuse lymphoid tissue can be found in virtually all vertebrates.

Solitary lymphoid follicles

Lymphocytes that have aggregated into a dense sphere or oval, usually surrounded by a network of draining lymphatic capillaries, are referred to as the *lymphoid follicle* (*lymphatic nodule*; Fig. 3.6). The follicles do not occupy fixed positions: they come and go, depending on the conditions in a given organ at a given time. They are found in the same places as the diffuse lymphoid tissue, being particularly abundant in the lamina propria of the digestive, res-

[4] Connective tissue is one of the four fundamental tissue types; it is characterized by loose connections among cells and large intercellular spaces filled with fibres and ground substance.

[5] Fibroblasts are plump, usually spindle-shaped cells with oval, pale-staining nucleus and varying numbers of cytoplasmic projections or processes by which they interconnect with one another. Their function is to produce extracellular fibres and amorphous ground substance.

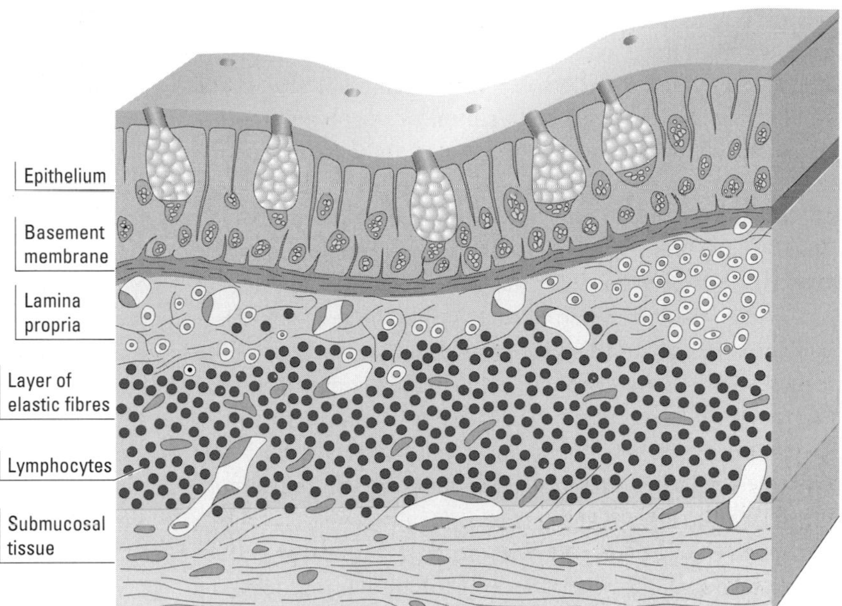

Figure 3.5 Diffuse lymphoid tissue in the mucous membrane covering the inner surface of adult human trachea (Based on Kampmeier, O.F. (1969) *Evolution and Comparative Morphology of the Lymphatic System*. Thomas, Springfield, IL.)

piratory and genital tracts, and in the tela submucosa of the intestine. Histologists have estimated that the bowels of a healthy child contain approximately 15 000 follicles.

Some of the follicles are uniformly dense over the entire space they occupy and these are called *primary follicles*. Others differentiate into a peripheral, more dense *mantle* and less dense *germinal centre* (see Fig. 3.6). The mantle often becomes polarized and crescent-shaped, being wider in the area in which the follicle faces the epithelium—it forms a cap. Sometimes the mantle is covered on the outside by a thin layer of elongated, densely apposed cells, the *capsule*. The germinal centre itself may differentiate into a more loosely arranged *light region* and a somewhat more closely packed *dark region*. The germinal centre is the site of B-cell proliferation; it contains B lymphocytes but few T lymphocytes. The light region is occupied primarily by differentiating and proliferating B lymphocytes, blast cells and some plasma cells, while the dark region contains large- and medium-sized lymphocytes, blast cells in the course of transformation into plasma cells and macrophages. Secondary follicles with germinal centres do not appear until after birth, when the animal is exposed to foreign matter from the environment; they do not develop in animals raised under sterile conditions.

Aggregated lymphoid follicles

The solitary follicles are like truffles scattered throughout the woods. Certain clusters of lymphoid follicles have

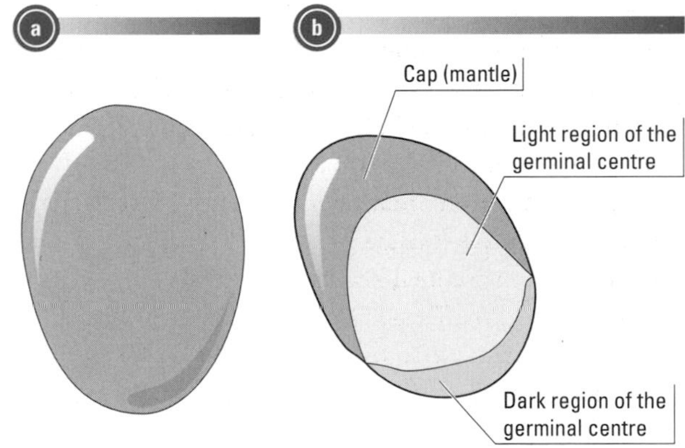

Figure 3.6 Primary (a) and secondary (b) solitary lymphoid follicle.

special names: tonsils, Peyer's patches and the follicles of the appendix.

Tonsils

The Latin word *tonsa* means a stake set up on the shore, and that is what the tonsils look like: six small stakes set up around the entrance to the upper part of the digestive tract. Some histologists refer to the ring as a 'chain of fortresses', which is also an apt designation. The ring consists of two palatine, one patch of lingual, one pharyngeal and two tubal tonsils (Fig. 3.7). The *palatine tonsils* are two almond-shaped bodies that can be seen on either side of the entrance to the throat in a wide-open mouth. They are also the 'tonsils' to which a layperson refers when he or she speaks of having them removed. Like almonds, they have a corrugated surface with cracks and pits (*crypts*) extending deep into them. The crypts often become filled with sloughed off epithelial cells, living and dead lymphocytes, and exuded fluid, which form an excellent culture medium for the growth of certain bacteria and fungi, a frequent cause of complications with palatine tonsils. The *lingual tonsil* is a collection of 35–100 discrete units found at the base of the tongue (Latin *lingua*, tongue). Each unit contains several lymphoid follicles and is demarcated by a single crypt. Since glands open into the crypts and their excretions flush out any accumulating material, inflammation of the lingual tonsil is rare. The *pharyngeal tonsil*, called *adenoids* when enlarged (Greek *adén*, gland), is situated on the rear wall of the pharynx. It consists of several folds radiating forward from the region in which the roof of the nasal pharynx joins the hind pharyngeal wall. The spaces between the folds resemble crypts of other tonsils. When enlarged, the pharyngeal tonsil may block the nasal passage and force mouth breathing. The *tubal tonsils* are located near the two openings of the auditory (Eustachian) tubes into the nasal cavity. The diffuse lymphoid tissue and the lymphoid follicles in the larynx wall are sometimes referred to as *laryngeal tonsils*.

The surface of a tonsil is covered by epithelium that also extends into the crypts. Underlying each tonsil and separating it from the muscular layer beneath it is a fibrous capsule that sends extensions (*septa*) into the tonsil's interior (Fig. 3.8). The space between the epithelium and the capsule is occupied by a loose connective tissue packed with lymphocytes. The band of diffuse lymphoid tissue condenses at places into lymphoid follicles (see Fig. 3.7). Each tonsil is surrounded by a network of draining lymphatic capillaries that collect fluid and cells from it and carry them to the nearest lymph node. The circle of lymph nodes, lymphatic capillaries and tonsils is called *Waldeyer's ring* (see Fig. 3.7e).

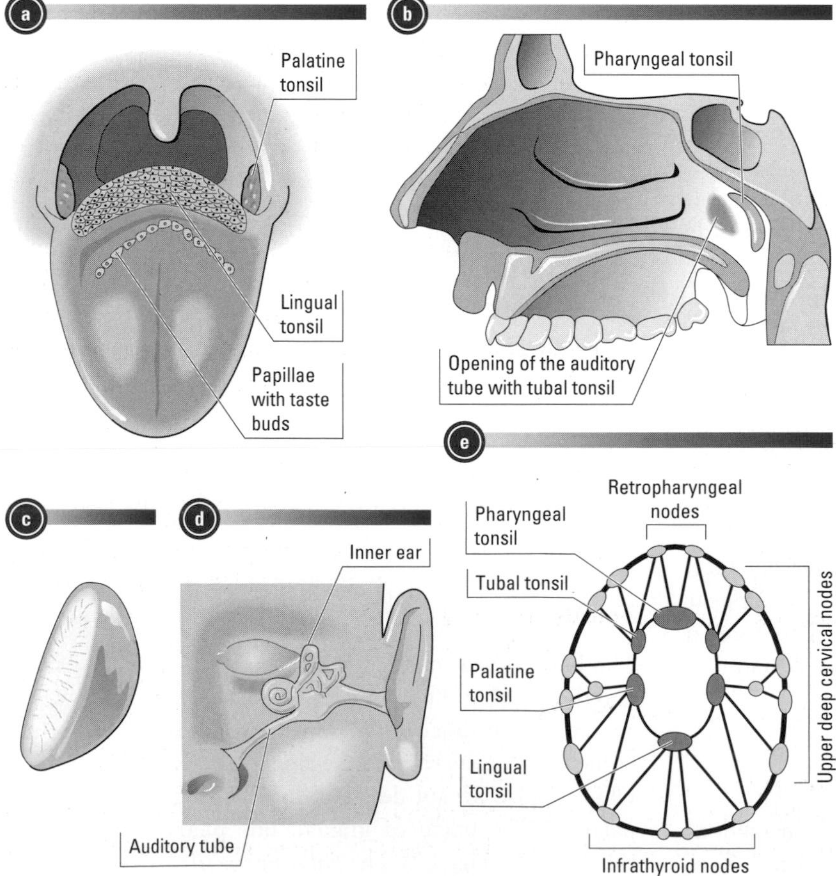

Figure 3.7 Human tonsils. (a) Palatine and lingual tonsils visible in an open mouth and on the tongue. (b) Section through the nose showing the location of pharyngeal and tubal tonsils. (c) Dissected out palatine tonsil ('the tonsil'). (d) Connection of the nasal cavity with the inner ear via the auditory tube. (e) Waldeyer's ring: the system of lymphatics and lymph nodes draining the tonsils.

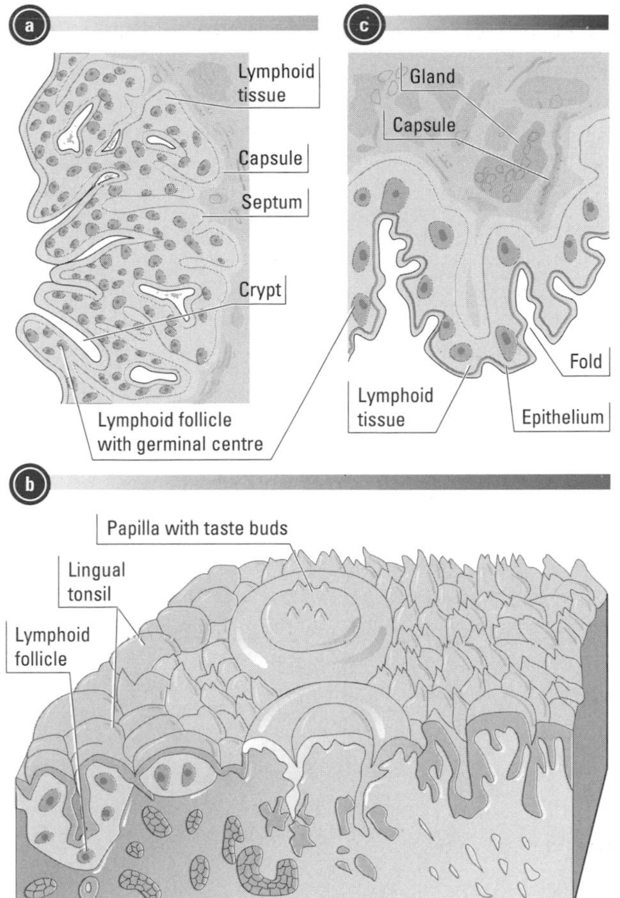

Figure 3.8 Structure of human tonsils. (a) Cross-section through a portion of the palatine tonsil. (b) Block of tissue from the tongue with lingual tonsil. (c) Cross-section through a portion of the pharyngeal tonsil. (Based in part on Kahle, W., Leonhardt, H. & Platzer, W. (1986) *Taschenatlas der Anatomie*, 5th edn. Georg Thieme Verlag, Stuttgart.)

Peyer's patches

The inner surface of the intestine is wrinkled into numerous folds and the folds are covered by finger-like projections, *villi* (Fig. 3.9a–c), which sway to and fro like the tentacles of a sea anemone, dipping into the foodstuff as it passes by. At the base of the individual villi are deep trenches, the crypts (Fig. 3.9d). The number and height of the folds and villi decrease from the duodenum towards the colon so that the large intestine has hardly any villi at all. The wall of the intestine consists of seven layers termed, from inner to outer surface, epithelium, lamina propria, lamina muscularis mucosae (together these three layers constitute the mucosal membrane), submucosa (connective tissue layer), circular muscle, longitudinal muscle, and serosa (outer epithelial layer). Of these seven layers, only the first three (the mucosal membrane) participate in the formation of the villi.

Each villus is supplied by a separate branch of blood capillaries and each is drained by a single lymphatic capillary projecting into it (see Fig. 3.9e). The capillary is called the *lacteal* because it is white, like milk (Latin *lac*, milk), from the content of absorbed fat globules. The lacteals drain into a network of thin lymphatic vessels spread out over the thick layer of smooth muscles in the mucosal membrane between the crypts (see Fig. 3.9f). Branches of this mucosal network penetrate the muscular layer and form another network of larger lymphatic vessels 'one floor below', in the submucosa. Branches from this second network then penetrate the muscular layers (circular and longitudinal), receiving additional lymphatic capillaries from the space between them, and drain into lymphatic vessels of the mesentery (the membrane attaching the intestine to the abdominal wall).

The submucosa contains rich diffuse lymphoid tissue with a dense sprinkling of solitary lymphoid follicles, particularly in the ileum. This part of the small intestine contains, in the wall opposite the mesentery, nests of lymphoid follicles called *Peyer's patches* after the Swiss anatomist Johann K. Peyer (1653–1712). Each patch is visible on the inner surface as a collection of bare, dome-shaped structures in the dense lawn of microvilli—like puffballs in the grass (Fig. 3.10). There are 20–30 such patches in the human intestine, each patch consisting of some 20 puffballs and each puffball containing one lymphoid follicle. The epithelium of the dome overlying each follicle is composed of specialized cells with many microfolds, the *M cells*. In contrast to the epithelium of the villi, the epithelium of the bare areas does not contain any mucus-secreting *goblet cells* and is not columnar. The M cells are thought to be involved in absorbing foreign matter and passing it on to the cells in the follicle (see Chapters 18 & 21). Each follicle is surrounded by a network of lymphatic capillaries that drain into the lymphatic vessels in the submucosa.

Vermiform appendix

The worm-like projection of the human large intestine, the appendix, is 10–15 cm long and up to 8 mm in diameter. Like the rest of the large intestine it lacks villi, but its wall consists of the same seven layers found elsewhere in the intestine. The lamina propria contains dense, diffuse lymphoid tissue packed with some 200 lymphoid follicles (Fig. 3.11). Because the crypts on the inner surface of the appendix resemble those of the tonsils, they are referred to as *abdominal tonsils*.

The diffuse lymphoid tissue of the lamina propria, the solitary lymphoid follicles, Peyer's patches and the appen-

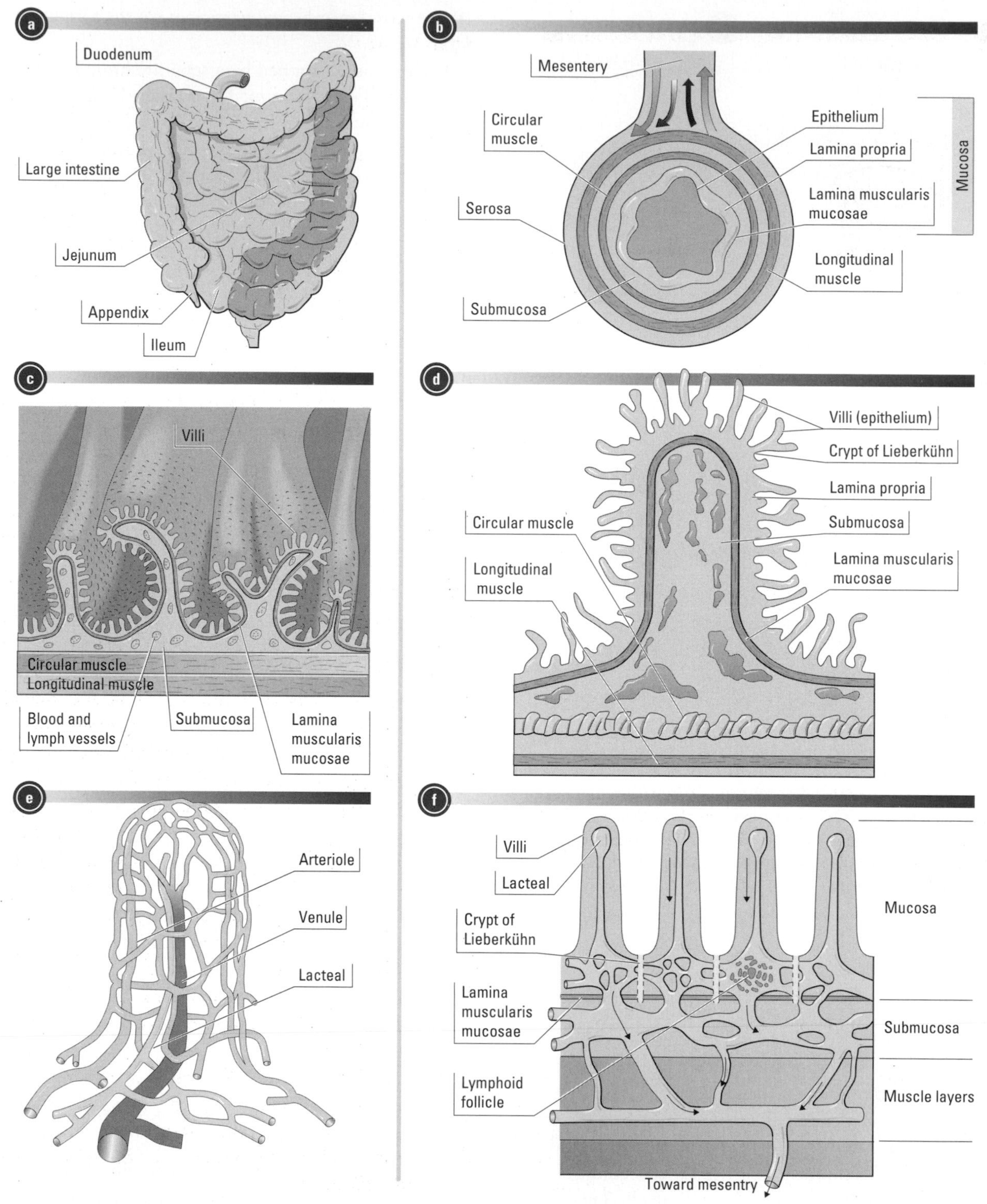

Figure 3.9 Organization of human gut. (a) Location of the intestine in the abdomen. (b) Cross-section through the intestine (jejunum) wall. Arrows indicate blood supply and innervation. (c) Inner surface of the small intestine (duodenum) with folds and villi. (d) Cross-section of a villus. (e) Blood supply and the lymphatic drainage of a villus. (f) Lymphatics of the intestine wall. (Modified from Kahle, W. *et al.* (1986) *Taschenatlas der Anatomie*, 5th edn. Georg Thieme Verlag, Stuttgart; Krstić, R.V. (1984) *Illustrated Encyclopedia of Human Histology*. Springer-Verlag, Berlin.)

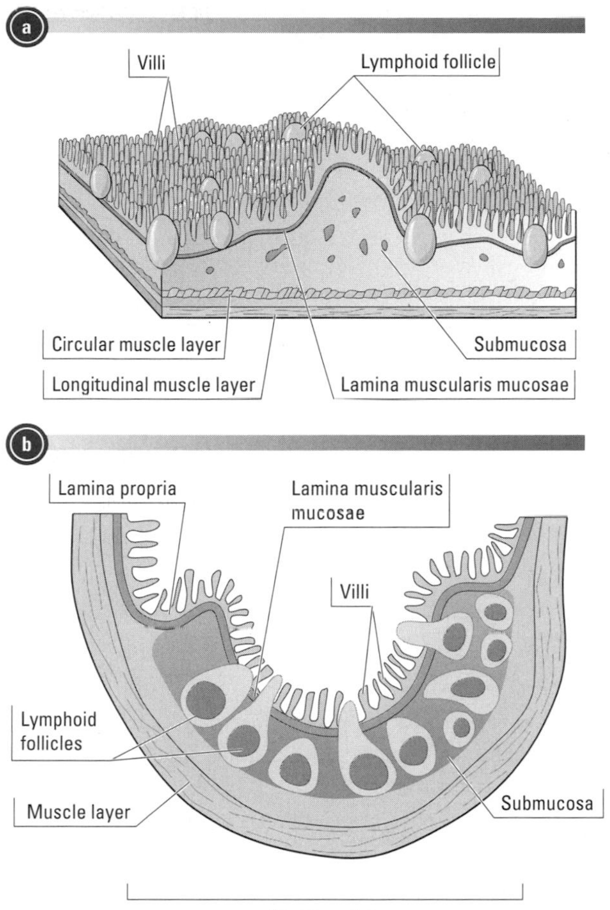

Figure 3.10 Peyer's patches. (a) Single Peyer's patch in the ileum of the small intestine. (b) Cross-section through the ileum opposite the mesentery with lymphoid follicles forming a Peyer's patch. (b, Modified from Krstić, R.V. (1984) *Illustrated Encyclopedia of Human Histology*. Springer-Verlag, Berlin.)

dix are all believed to belong to a single functionally interconnected system, the *gut-associated lymphoid tissue* (GALT). Some immunologists also include the tonsils and lymph nodes of the mesentery in this system. GALT is important in processing foreign matter entering the body from the gastrointestinal tract. A similar system, the *bronchial-associated lymphoid tissue* (BALT), may exist in association with the respiratory tract (Fig. 3.12) and may be primarily involved in handling inhaled foreign matter. Sometimes all these and certain other tissues are grouped together into a single system, the *mucosa-associated lymphoid tissue* (MALT). (Mucosa is the layer lining all body cavities, i.e. the gastrointestinal tract, the respiratory system and the genito-urinary system; it consists of an epithelium, lamina propria and sometimes a muscular layer. For further discussion of MALT, see Chapter 18.)

Lymph node

Lymph nodes are knots in the lymphatic net, the filtering stations through which lymph percolates on its way to the bloodstream. There are thousands of them, some as small as a pinhead, others as large as a walnut. They are so numerous that most of them do not even have a name, a rather unusual situation in anatomy. They are found everywhere in the body where lymphatics are also present (Fig. 3.13), but particularly large and numerous lymph nodes are present in the armpits (*axillary lymph nodes*), groin (*inguinal lymph nodes*), near the abdominal aorta (*coeliac lymph nodes*), in the neck (*cervical lymph nodes*), and in the mesentery (*mesenteric lymph nodes*; see Fig. 3.3). Lymph nodes filtering lymph from a particular region or organ are often simply referred to as *regional lymph nodes*.

Each lymph node is enveloped by a thin capsule that sends many projections or *trabeculae* into the node's interior (Fig. 3.14). The capsule and the trabeculae are made of dense connective tissue containing some fibroblasts and an occasional smooth muscle cell, but mainly many fine, elastic fibres. Adhering to the outer surface of the capsule is fat and loose connective tissue, so that the nodes are rarely free but rather embedded in the surrounding tissues. The inner surface of the capsule and trabeculae are lined by a sheet of flattened *littoral cells*, continuous with the endothelial cells lining the inner surface of the connecting lymphatic vessels. The origin of littoral cells (endothelial vs. reticular) is uncertain. In the capsule, the littoral cells rest on the *basement membrane*, a fine feltwork of microfilaments embedded in an acellular matrix; in the trabecular system, they rest directly on the individual projections. The number of *afferent lymphatic vessels* (Latin *af-*, to; *ferre*, carry) bringing lymph into each node and piercing the capsule varies depending on the node's size and location.

The 'meat' of the lymph node consists of a scaffolding (*stroma*) and free cells (the *parenchyma*). The stroma (*reticular tissue*) is a form of fibrous connective tissue consisting of a three-dimensional meshwork of reticular cells and reticular fibres. *Reticular cells* are star-shaped elements with a central nucleus and many long, thin cytoplasmic processes by which the individual cells interconnect. Running along the processes and in the space between the cells are bundles of *reticular fibres*.

The parenchyma consists of lymphoid cells; these are predominantly lymphocytes, but some macrophages and dendritic cells are also present. Depending on the relative density of the lymphoid tissue, the parenchyma can be divided into the peripheral cortex and the central medulla. The *cortex* (Latin, bark) can be subdivided further into the *outer cortex*, which contains lymphoid follicles and *inter-*

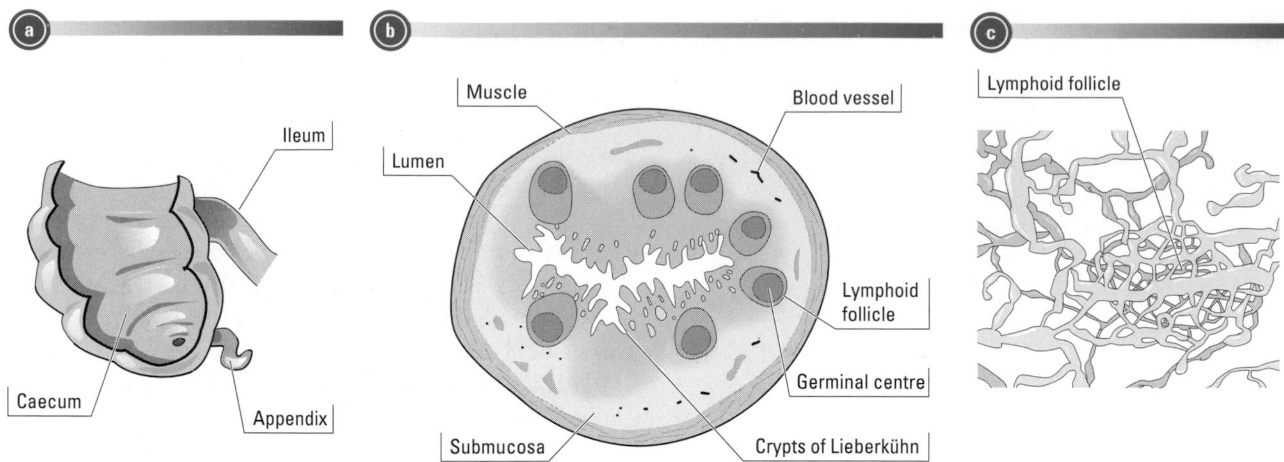

Figure 3.11 Human appendix. (a) Caecum (cut open) and vermiform appendix. (b) Cross-section through the appendix showing the accumulation of lymphoid follicles underneath the inner surface. (c) Lymphatic network surrounding lymphoid follicles in the appendix.

follicular (internodular) diffuse lymphoid tissue, and the *inner cortex* (*paracortical region, paracortex*), which is the diffuse lymphoid tissue beneath the band of follicles. Generally, the outer cortex is more dense than the inner cortex and the whole cortex is more dense than the medulla. The lymphoid follicles can be either *primary*, which are of a uniform density, or *secondary*, which are differentiated into a mantle and a germinal centre with light and dark zones. Occasionally, more dense aggregations of lymphocytes are also seen in the inner cortex of the *tertiary follicles*; these are always devoid of germinal centres. The entire follicle, but the germinal centre in particular, is penetrated by a meshwork of *follicular dendritic cells* that specialize in trapping foreign matter and delivering it to other cells, primarily B lymphocytes (see Chapter 17). In the *medulla* (Latin *medius*, middle), the parenchyma is frayed into a series of strands, the *medullary cords*. The different regions of the parenchyma differ not only in cell density but also in the type of cells they contain. The primary and secondary follicles contain mainly B lymphocytes; the interfollicular diffuse tissue of the outer cortex and the inner cortex contain for the most part T lymphocytes; and the medulla consists predominantly of blasts and plasma cells.

The reticular tissue and the parenchyma are less dense beneath the capsule and around the trabeculae. The relatively empty spaces form the *sinuses*, through which the lymph passes relatively unhindered. The space directly below the capsule is the *subcapsular (marginal) sinus*; that around the trabeculae the *intermediate sinuses*; and that between the medullary cords the *medullary sinuses*. All sinuses are lined with littoral cells and their spaces are crisscrossed by reticular cells and fibres. All the spaces are interconnected, allowing the lymph to pass from the afferent lymphatic vessel into the subcapsular sinus, from there into the intermediate sinuses, and finally into the medullary sinuses. It is collected at the *hilus* (Greek *kélis*, spot) and led away by one or more *efferent lymphatic vessels* (Latin *effere*, to bring out). The lymph, of course, also penetrates the lymphoid tissue but flows through it more slowly than through the sinuses, from the cortex to the medulla, and to the hilus.

Each lymph node is supplied with blood by a single artery that enters the node through the hilus, runs within the trabeculae, branches, and leaves the trabeculae in the medullary cords. On reaching the cortex, it branches further into capillary networks around the germinal centres of the lymphoid follicles. The arterial capillaries continue into postcapillary venules and veins, which then turn back, pass through the inner cortex and unite in the medullary cords into a larger vein that leaves the node at the hilus. The postcapillary venules of the inner cortex are lined with a special *high endothelium* (Fig. 3.15) which, as we shall learn later, plays an important part in lymphocyte circulation.

Besides providing a place of residence for lymphocytes and macrophages, lymph nodes perform three other functions: they trap infectious agents and other particulate matter brought in with the lymph; process the foreign material phagocytically; and provide the cellular scaffolding necessary for the interactions of immune cells.

During embryogenesis, lymph nodes arise from the mesenchyme in circumscribed areas between blood and lymphatic vessels (Fig. 3.16). In each of these areas, the mes-

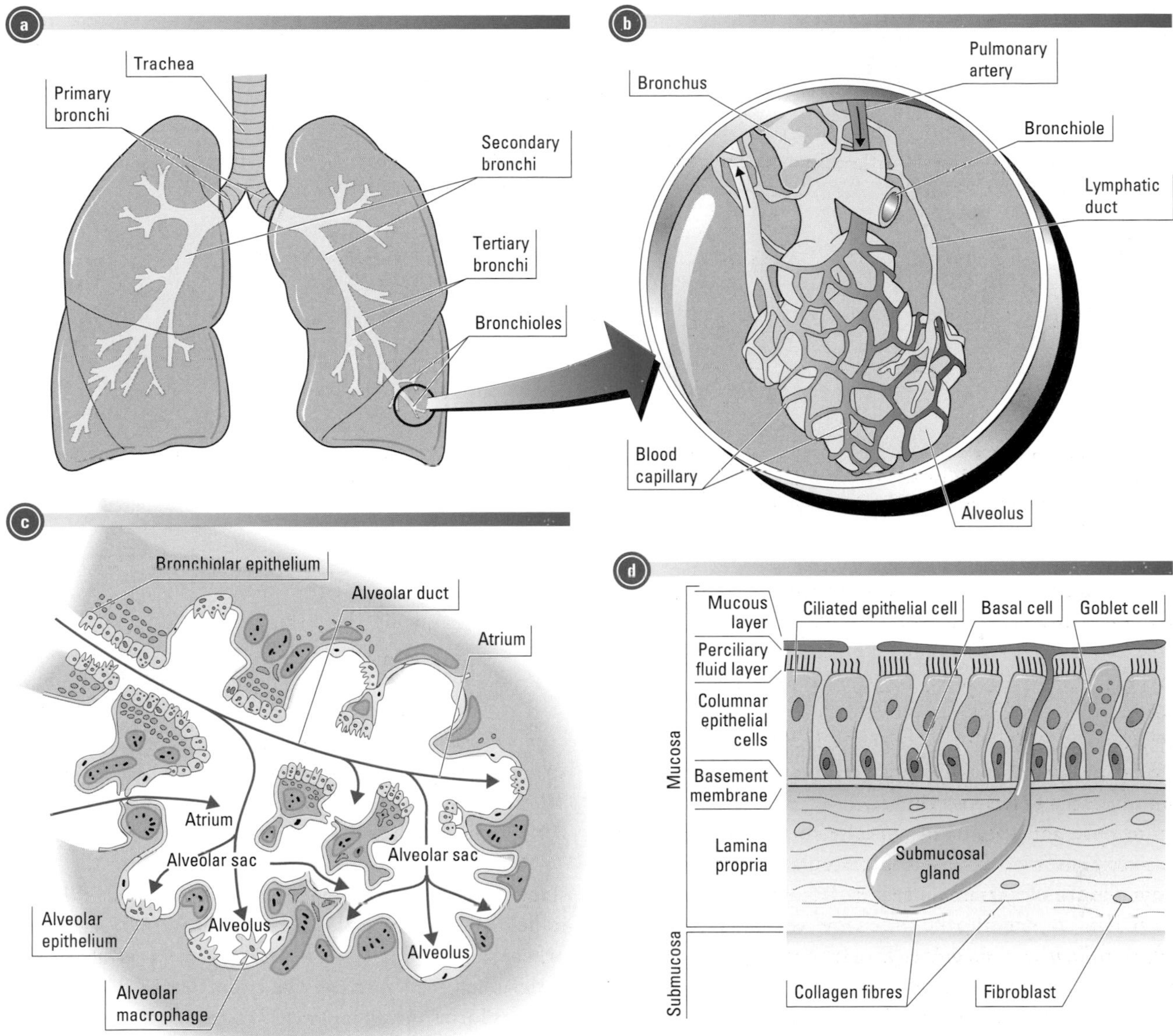

Figure 3.12 Organization of the human lower respiratory system, the site of the bronchial-associated lymphoid tissue (BALT). (a) Air-conducting tubes of the lungs. (b) Blood and lymphatic supply at the termination of bronchioles into alveoli. (c) Cross-section through a terminal bronchiole. (d) Bronchial mucosa. (Combined from different sources.)

enchyme condenses into a bulb-shaped primordium, which is infiltrated by blood-borne lymphocytes. The lymphatic vessel widens into a flat sac, indented by the outgrowth of the primordium. Cords of mesenchymal cells then invade the sac and divide it into a maze of channels and spaces—the future sinuses of the adult node. Some of the mesenchymal cells transform into connective tissue, which gives rise to the capsule on the primordium's surface and condenses into trabeculae inside, between the channels. Almost simultaneously, an ingrowth of blood vessels occurs along the developing trabeculae and into the primordium's interior.

Lymph nodes are a mammalian invention. Although accumulations of lymphoid tissues occur in some amphibians, crocodiles and some water birds, lymph nodes with their characteristic structure occur only in mammals.

Spleen

The spleen is an oblong, purplish body the size of a fist and thus the largest of all the lymphoid organs. It has a smooth

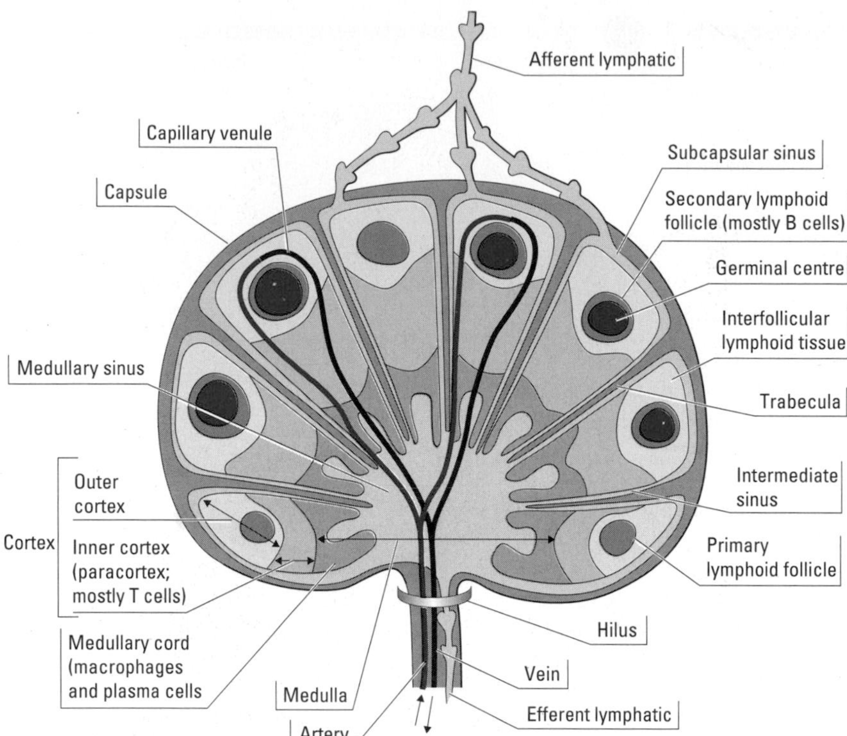

Figure 3.13 Lymph node organization.

surface except for an indented region, the hilus, where blood vessels enter and leave; there are no lymphatics leading into the spleen. In contrast to the lymph nodes, which are inserted in the lymph circulation, the spleen is inserted in the blood circulation.

Like the lymph node, the spleen is enveloped in a capsule and pervaded by trabeculae (Fig. 3.17). The latter form a dense bush that grows out of the hilus and connects with the capsule by its terminal twigs. The interior of the spleen not occupied by the trabeculae contains a delicate, three-dimensional lace of reticular tissue composed of reticular cells and reticular fibres. The meshes of the lace are filled with parenchyma, the free cells of the spleen.

The *splenic artery* splits into four to six branches (*trabecular arteries*) before it enters the hilus and these then enter the hollow spaces of the trabeculae. As the trabecular arteries leave the trabeculae, they are surrounded by a mass of lymphoid tissue, the *periarteriolar lymphoid sheath* (PALS). Since the arteries run through the centre of the PALS cylinder, they are, at this point, referred to as *central arteries*. The PALS has an inner and outer region that differ in their cellular composition. The inner PALS contains almost exclusively T lymphocytes, whereas the outer PALS contains a majority of T lymphocytes and a minority of B cells. Scattered throughout the PALS are spherical structures, the *lymphoid* (*Malpighian*) *follicles*, which resemble similar structures in the lymph nodes and elsewhere in the body. They are visible with the naked eye on the surface of freshly cut spleen as small (0.3–0.5 mm in diameter) white spots. The number of follicles varies, depending on the circumstances. A 20-year-old healthy person has 10 000–20 000 follicles in his or her spleen. The follicles can be classified as primary or secondary, the latter containing germinal centres surrounded by a mantle. The collection of PALS with the follicles forms the *white pulp*.

At one point, the central artery divides into four to ten *central arterioles*, also called *penicillar arteries* because they resemble a small brush (Latin, *peniculus*). These, too, are surrounded by a lymphoid sheath that is thinner than that of the central artery and conical rather than cylindrical. *Arterial capillaries* depart at right angles from the central arterioles and as they reach the surface of the lymphoid sheath they branch out into a network emptying into the *marginal sinus*, a system of irregular channels with walls penetrated by small ‘windows’. Surrounding the marginal sinus (and the PALS) is a sheath of macrophages with some scattered B lymphocytes, the *marginal zone*, which is thickest over the lymphoid follicles. The marginal sinus separates the marginal zone from the PALS on most of the white pulp surface. The central arterioles terminate in one of two ways: they either connect with long, irregularly shaped, intercommunicating channels, the *venous sinuses* (splenic sinusoids;

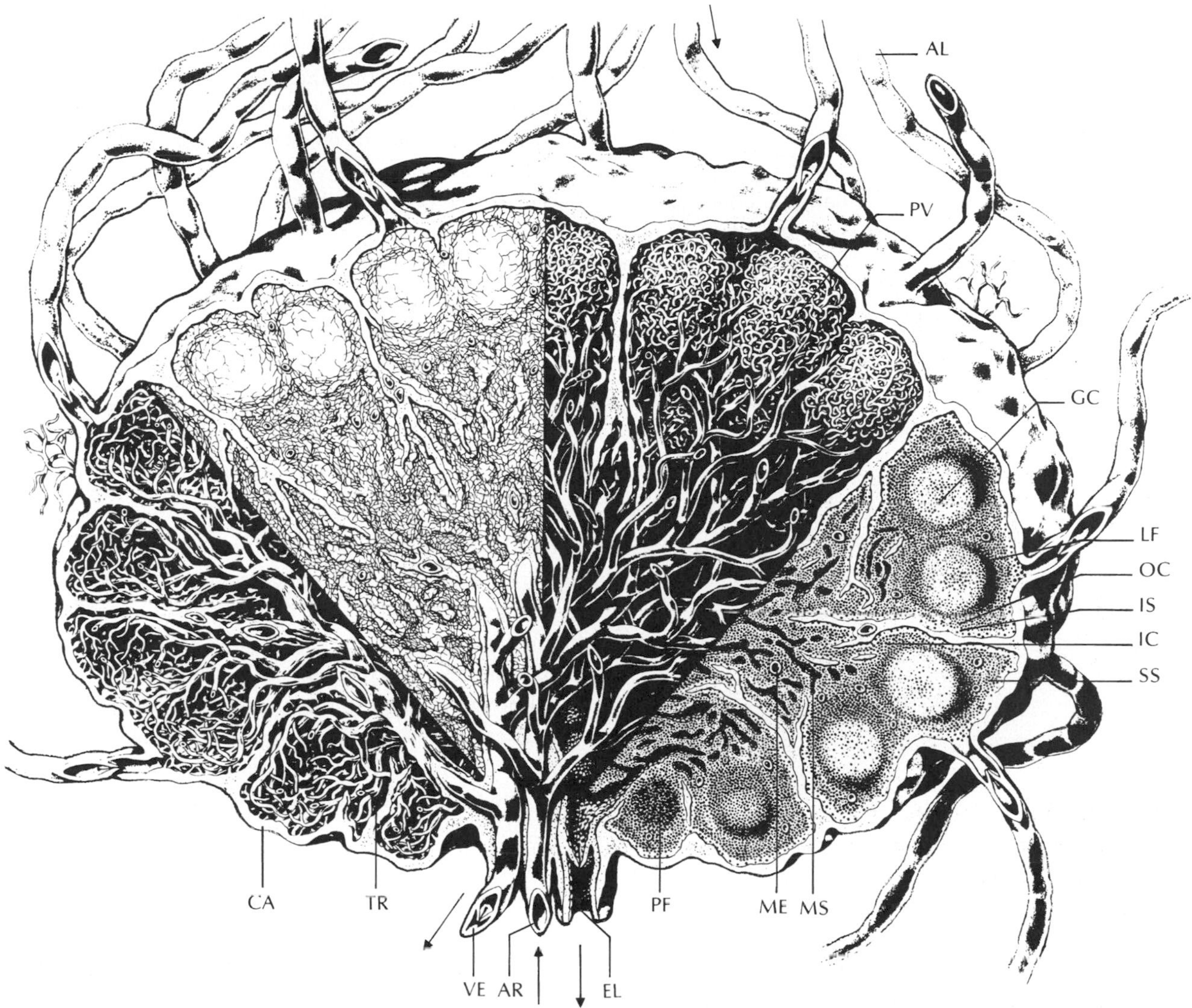

Figure 3.14 Human lymph node structure. The four sections show the main structural elements of the node, which are, from left to right: the trabecular system; the reticular tissue scaffolding; the blood vessels; and the parenchyma. AL, afferent lymphatic; AR, artery of the node; CA, capsule; EL, efferent lymphatic; GC, germinal centre; IC, inner cortex; IS, intermediate sinus; LF, lymphoid follicle (secondary); ME, medulla; MS, medullary sinus; OC, outer cortex; PV, postcapillary venule; PF, primary lymphoid follicle; SS, subcapsular sinus; TR, trabecula; VE, vein of the node.

note that here 'sinus' has a different meaning than in the lymph node); or they continue into arterial capillaries (terminal arterioles), which presumably terminate with open ends in the tissue between the venous sinuses—the *splenic (Billroth's) cords*. The blood released into these spaces is then collected by the venous sinuses. The sinuses are lined with endothelial cells supported on the outer surface by star-shaped reticular (adventitial) cells and a system of circularly arranged reticular 'ring' fibres, giving each sinus the appearance of a barrel with staves and hoops (Fig. 3.18). The endothelial cells rest on a membrane composed of fine fibres, the basement membrane, with many windows through which cells can pass. The splenic cords consist of macrophages, monocytes, lymphocytes, erythrocytes and other mature blood cells. The regions of the spleen containing the venous sinuses and the splenic cords are referred to as the *red pulp* because of the predominance of erythrocytes. The marginal sinus also drains into the venous sinuses. In the mouse, the white pulp connects with the red pulp via narrow *marginal zone bridging channels*. Near the trabeculae, groups of sinuses converge to form *pulp veins*, which immediately enter the trabecular system to become *trabecular veins*. The individual trabecular veins drain into one of the four to six branches of the *splenic vein*, which then leave the spleen at the hilus, ultimately becoming a single vein. The preceding description of the splenic circulation combines the *closed circulation hypothesis*, which holds that all the capillaries connect directly to the sinuses so that very little of the circulating blood is spilled into the tissues outside the sinuses, with the *open circulation hypothesis*, according to which all the capillaries open freely into the reticular tissue and that from there blood is collected by the sinuses. This combination, the *mixed circulation hypothesis*, reflects best the current status of knowledge, although the dispute among the proponents of the three hypotheses — a dispute that has lasted for over a century—cannot be considered resolved. The issue is complicated by the fact that the splenic circulation is organized somewhat differently in various species and that the blood flow through the spleen may change depending on the circumstances.

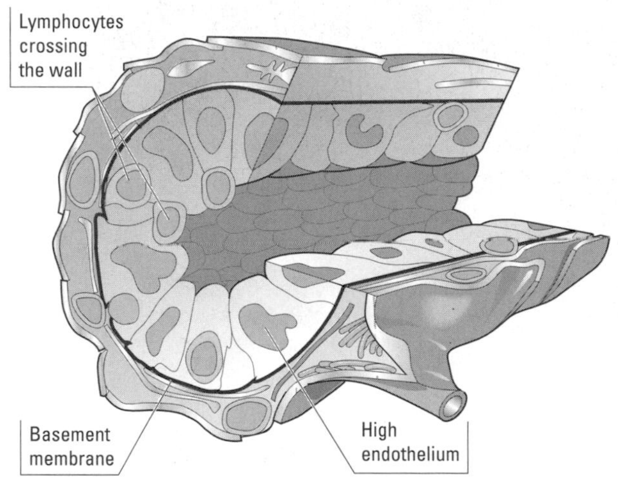

Figure 3.15 Postcapillary venule with high endothelium. Lymphocytes are shown crossing the wall on the way from the blood to the surrounding tissue. (Based on Weiss, L. & Greep, R.W. (1977) *Histology*, 4th edn. McGraw-Hill, New York.)

The spleen contains *efferent lymphatics* only. They start as blind sacs around the germinal centres in the PALS, in a manner not yet fully clarified, reach the trabeculae, and unite within the trabeculae into major vessels drained by the left *gastroepiploic lymph node* in the splenic hilus.

The ratio of white pulp to red pulp varies, depending on the immune status of an individual. Normally, the white pulp constitutes about 20% of the spleen, but in highly immunized animals it may comprise more than half the splenic volume. The histology of the white pulp changes with immunological stimulation. The hallmarks of this alteration are the emergence of blast cells in the PALS, cellular proliferation and the appearance of young plasma cells in the germinal centres, the appearance of intermediate and mature plasma cells in the marginal zone, and the passage of plasma cells into the red pulp.

Although the spleen is not essential for survival (an individual can lead a normal life without it), it nevertheless has an important function as a discriminatory filter for blood cells and fluids and as an organ of immunity. In its role as a filter, the spleen sorts the blood cells, sends them to different compartments, examines them for imperfections, stores some of them and concentrates others. The sorting process begins after the arterioles have discharged their content into the marginal sinuses and these into the spongework of the marginal zone. As the blood filters through the mesh, erythrocytes continue their movement towards the red pulp, push through the masses of macrophages filling the splenic

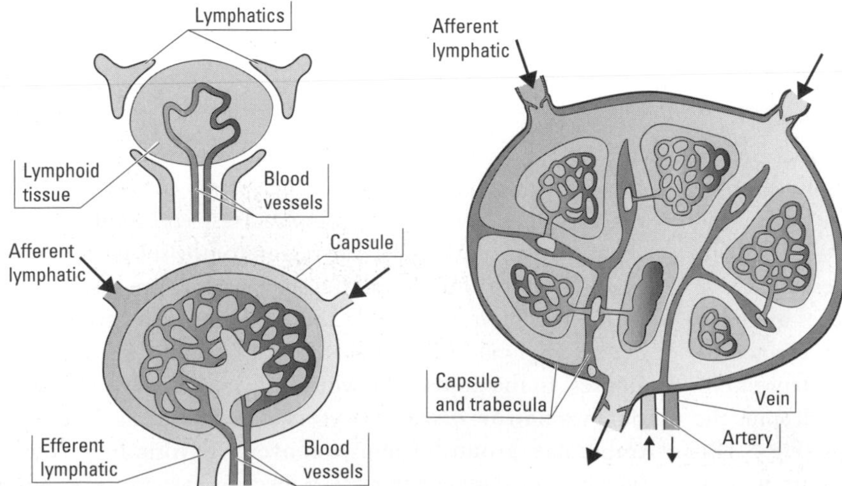

Figure 3.16 Embryonic origin of the lymph node. (From Arey, L.B. (1965) *Developmental Anatomy*, 7th edn. W.B. Saunders, Philadelphia, PA.)

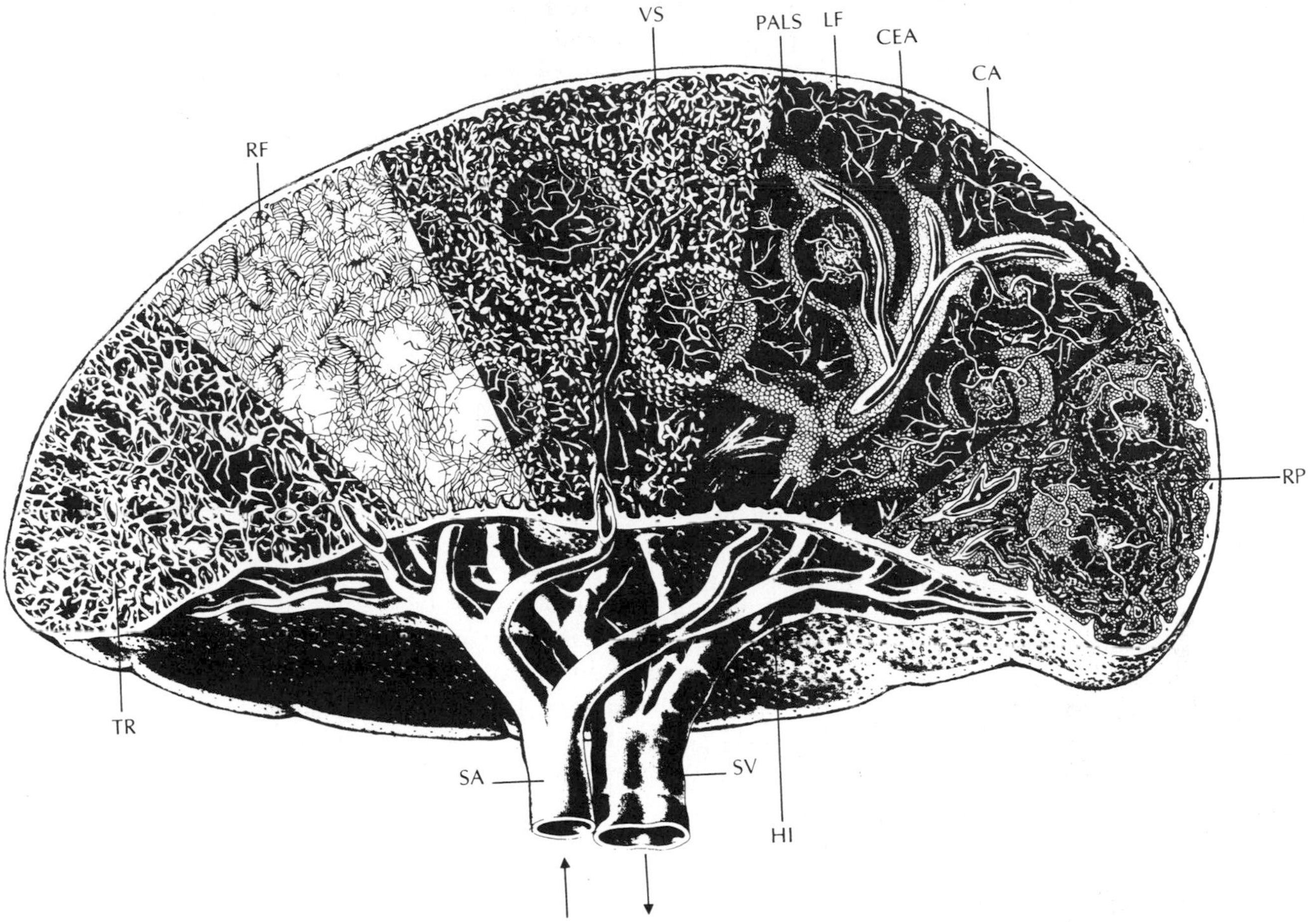

Figure 3.17 Overall organization of the human spleen. The five sections show the main structural features of the spleen, which are, from left to right: trabecular system; reticular tissue scaffolding; blood vessels; white pulp; and parenchyma. CA, capsule; CEA, central artery; HI, hilus; LF, lymphoid follicle, secondary, with germinal centre; PALS, periarteriolar lymphoid sheath; RF, reticular fibres; RP, red pulp; SA, splenic artery; SV, splenic vein; TR, trabeculae; VS, venous sinuses.

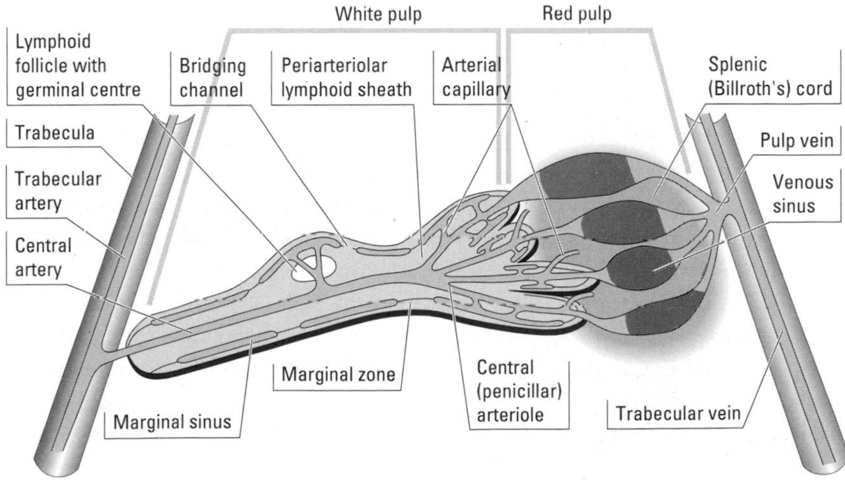

Figure 3.18 Details of spleen structure showing the blood circulation and organization of the white pulp.

cords and enter the sinuses. As the red cells squeeze through, the macrophages examine every one, like the blind Polyphemus feeling his sheep while searching for Odysseus. Cells showing any defect are checked and devoured on the spot. Lymphocytes are brought into the spleen by the arteries and arterioles; they enter the marginal sinus and then migrate to their respective domains, B cells to the follicles and T cells to the PALS (see also Chapter 17). They probably leave the white pulp by migrating via the marginal zone bridging channels to the red pulp, and then enter either the veins or the efferent lymphatics. Monocytes are removed from the circulation and set on a course that transforms them into macrophages. Blood plasma is taken up by the sinuses, only to be expelled again when they constrict and forced to move towards the lymphatic vessels, where it becomes part of the lymph. Any particulate foreign matter present in the blood is taken up by macrophages and destroyed. The immune function of the spleen is to trap and process particles and substances capable of eliciting immune responses and to provide a 'home' for lymphocytes and macrophages, a place where they can interact and go about the business of defence.

Phylogenetically, as well as ontogenetically, the spleen is derived from the gut. Its source is the mesodermal tissue that envelops the gastrointestinal tract of the oldest living vertebrates, such as the hagfish, lamprey and Dipnoi. In the hagfish, this tissue contains masses of differentiating blood cells that are organized into islets and cords around venous channels. In the lamprey, a step further towards complexity has been taken because the primordial spleen tissue is not so dispersed as in the hagfish, but concentrated largely in the *spiral valve*, an epithelial, corkscrew-shaped organ in the gut (Fig. 3.19). In the Dipnoi, the primitive splenic tissue is still embedded in the wall of the stomach but is clearly demarcated as a single body. The first clear separation of the spleen from the gut occurs in the oldest living bony fish, such as the sturgeon, in which the blood-forming tissue is assembled into a compact, discrete organ outside the gut, near the stomach–intestinal junction. From these fish onwards, all vertebrates possess a spleen as a distinct organ. In the majority of fish, urodele amphibians and reptiles, the spleen is elongated in shape and runs along a considerable length of the gut; in all other vertebrates, the organ has become much more compact. In fish and in some amphibians, the spleen pulp is predominantly red; noticeable white pulp begins to appear only in amphibians and reptiles.

In addition to spleen and bone marrow, some vertebrates have also used other sites and organs for blood formation, such as the portal system in the kidney of lampreys, many bony fish and amphibians; subcapsular and stromal areas of the gonads in cartilaginous fish; and the subcapsular region of the liver in bony fish, amphibians and turtles. A common feature of these sites is that they lie near venous sinuses in which the stagnant blood current seems to provide the necessary stimulus for blood formation.

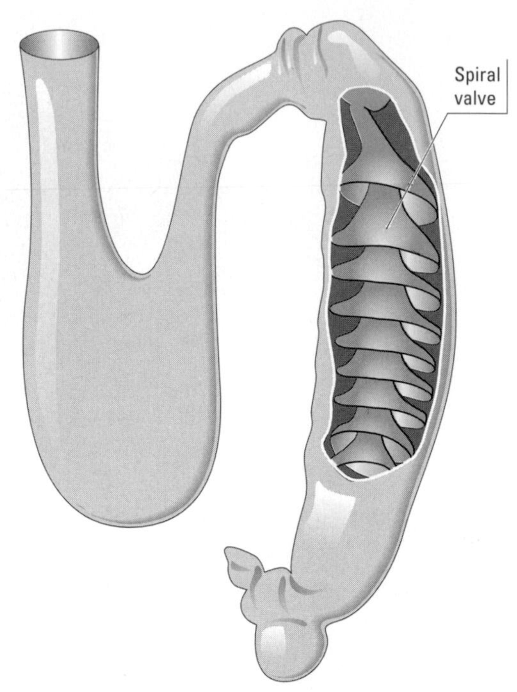

Figure 3.19 Spiral valve in the intestine of a shark. (From Klein, J. (1982) *Immunology: The Science of Self–Nonself Discrimination.* John Wiley & Sons, New York.)

Thymus

The thymus of a human newborn consists of two *lobes* resembling apposed pyramids. Its base rests on the heart-enveloping membrane, the pericardium, and its tips extend to the upper end of the breastbone (Fig. 3.20). Each lobe is enclosed in a connective tissue *capsule* that sends numerous *septa* into the organ's interior, thin partitions that divide the inner space into a multitude of tiny, interconnected chambers, the *lobules* (Figs 3.21 & 3.22). Most of the chambers are not completely enclosed by the septa. They either lack or have incomplete partitions on the side oriented towards the organ's centre. Most of the other partitions have small openings through which the chambers communicate. The lobules are filled with a meshwork of *epithelial cells* (not reticular cells, as in other lymphoid organs). It is, however, most uncharacteristic epithelium that pervades the thymus. Instead of consisting of closely apposed, flat or columnar cells with little space between them, as every decent epithelium does, the thymic epithelial cells are star-shaped and

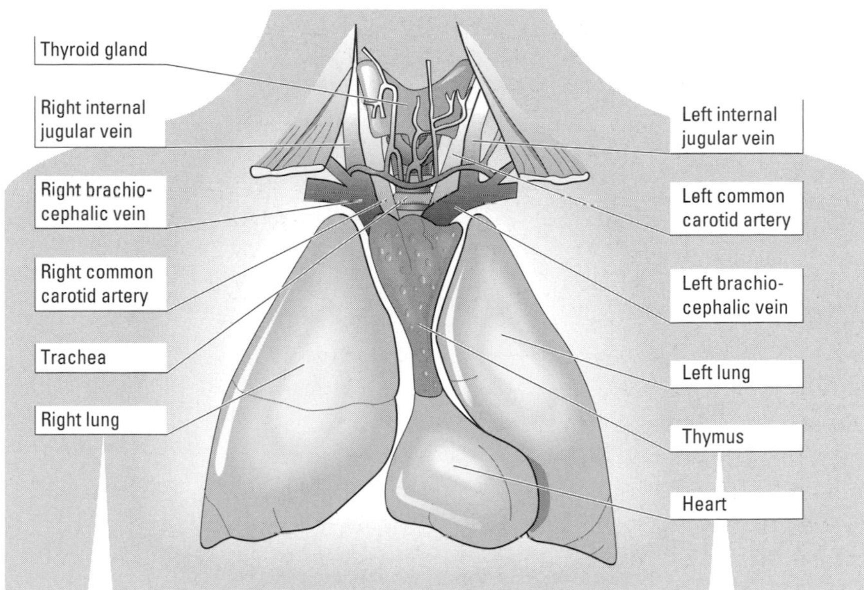

Figure 3.20 Location of the human adult thymus. (Modified from Lippert, H. (1983) *Anatomie*, 4th edn. Urban & Schwarzenberg, München.)

apposed only at the ends of their processes. The epithelial nature of these cells, however, is given away by *desmosomes*, the plaques that bridge the space between the adjacent membranes of the touching projections. The unnatural, spongy appearance of the thymic epithelium is caused by the lymphocytes, here called *thymocytes*, that fill the mesh of the three-dimensional lacework: thymocytes squeeze between the epithelial cells and push them apart.

In each chamber, more thymocytes are crowded in the periphery, the *cortex*, than in the centre, the *medulla*. The epithelial cell spongework is correspondingly more dense in the medulla than in the cortex. On histological preparations, the cortex can be recognized as the darkly staining region and the medulla as the pale region of each lobule. The medullas of the individual lobules are interconnected with each other by thin strands passing through the openings in the septa, the 'windows' of the chambers, and with the central medullary mass of each lobe by broad strands.

On sections, the pale medulla contains scattered dark spots, whose number increases with age. On closer examination, the spots (*Hassall's corpuscles*; named after the English chemist and physician, Arthur H. Hassall, 1817–1894) appear as little cabbage heads, each consisting of several layers of flattened, concentrically organized, epithelial cells. The innermost cells of the head often die and lyse, leaving a hollow space; the cells on the corpuscle's periphery sometimes fuse. The function of Hassall's corpuscles, if they have one, is unknown. They are sparse in some species (in healthy mice, for example) and abundant in others, especially after stress.

Each lobe is supplied by several blood vessels, small branches of the arteries that pass by the organ (see Fig. 3.22). The arteries pierce the capsule and enter the septa, in which they run all the way to the area occupied by the central medullary mass. There they leave the septa, turn back and run along the corticomedullary junction, separately in each chamber. On the way they branch out into numerous capillaries that cross the cortex, reaching the septal walls. There a few of the arteries connect to interlobal veins, while others turn back, cross the cortex again and turn into postcapillary venules that drain into veins running parallel to the arteries along the corticomedullary junction. The veins then enter the septa and there run parallel with the arteries. They leave the thymus at several points and connect to larger veins passing by the organ. The cortex is thus richly supplied with blood, while the medulla contains only a few arteries branching off from those that run along the corticomedullary junction. No lymphatics enter the thymus but a number of lymphatic capillaries begin in the medulla and the connective tissue of the septa. The lymphatics drain into lymph nodes of the mediastinum, the partition separating the two lungs.

The thymus, as a site where rites of T-cell maturation take place, is a very private abode, and to bring blood vessels into it amounts to taking a four-lane motorway through a Freemason's meeting place. To keep the would-be trespassers out of the thymus, the inner content of the thymic capillaries is separated from the surrounding parenchyma by at least four layers of tissue. The innermost of these is a layer of endothelial cells, which of course is present in all blood vessels, but is particularly cohesive in the thymic capillaries. Surrounding the endothelium is a basement

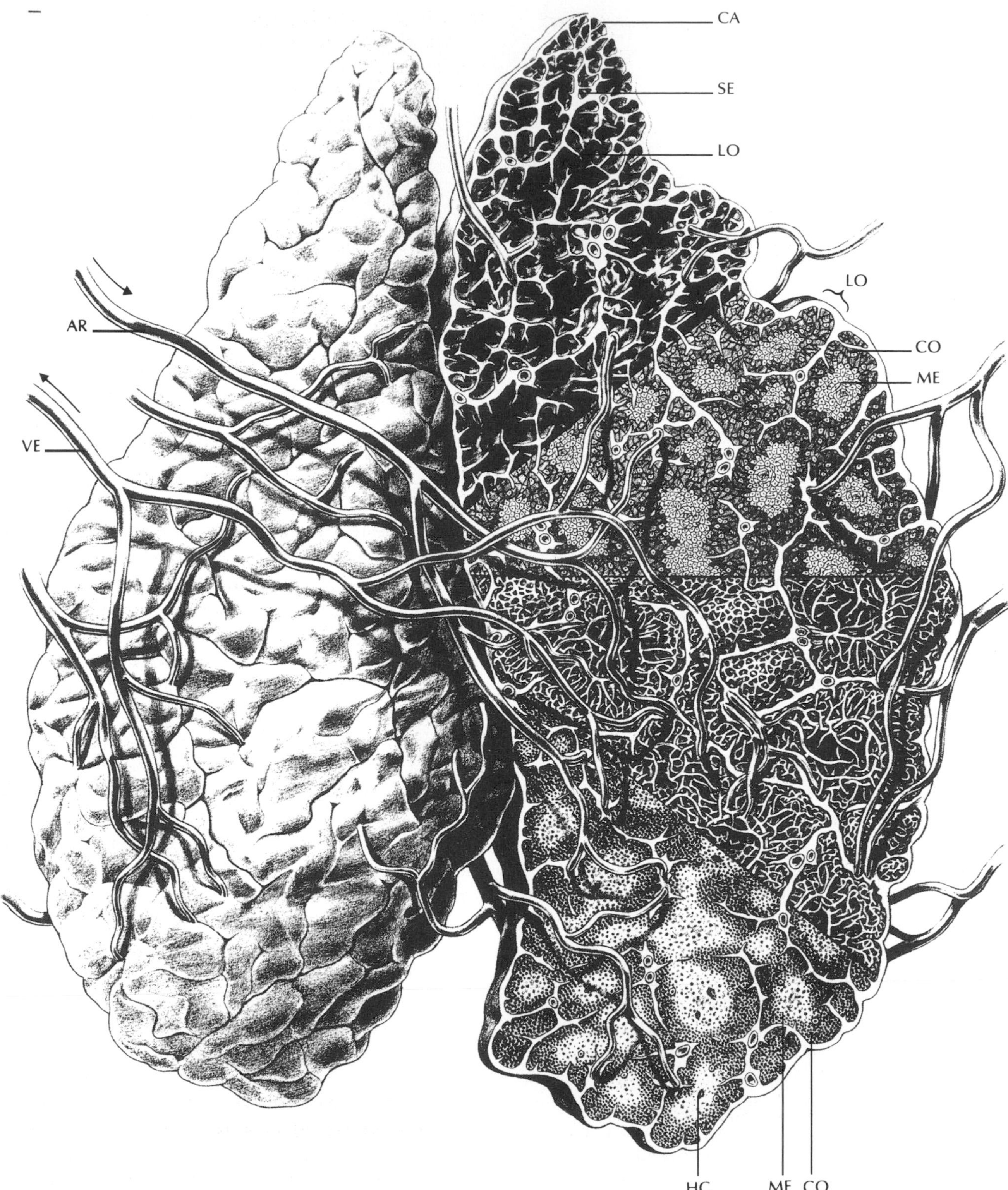

Figure 3.21 Overall organization of the human thymus. The figure shows the surface of one lobe and a sectional view through the second lobe. The four individual sections depict the main structural features of the thymus, which are, from top to bottom: capsule with septa; lymphoid cells; blood circulation; and parenchyma. AR, artery; CA, capsule; CO, cortex; HC, Hassall's corpuscle; LO, lobule; ME, medulla; SE, septa; VE, vein.

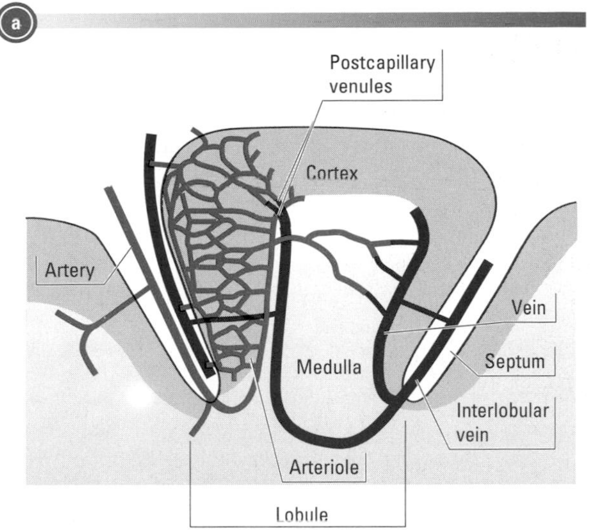

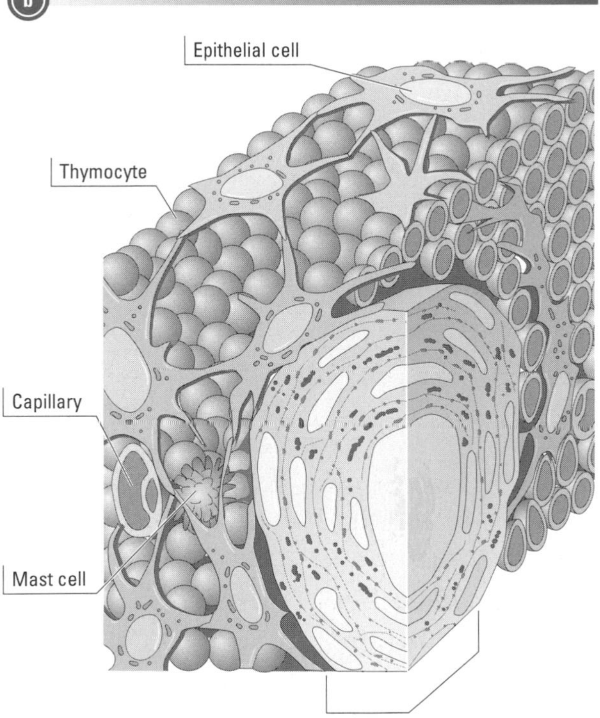

Figure 3.22 Two details of thymus structure. (a) Blood circulation through thymic lobule. (b) Epithelial cell network in the medulla filled with thymocytes. (a, modified from Krstić, R.V. (1984) *Illustrated Encyclopedia of Human Histology*. Springer-Verlag, Berlin; b, modified from Krstić, R.V. (1978) *Die Gewebe des Menschen und der Säugetiere*. Springer-Verlag, Berlin.)

membrane, followed by a perivascular space filled with connective tissue of the sort found in the septa and possibly continuous with extrathymic tissue. The final layer is another basement membrane generated by a single sheet of epithelial cells surrounding the capillary. In the cortex, the sheet is uninterrupted, whereas around the medullary vessels it has gaps, cracks and rifts. Blood cells normally cannot pass these fortified walls of the cortical capillaries or of the postcapillary venules — the walls constitute the *blood–thymus barrier*. Yet the barrier is not impenetrable, for experiments have shown that while the cortical blood vessels are permeable only to soluble, low-molecular-mass substances, the medullary vessels allow high-molecular-mass substances and even small particles and cells to pass through. The blood–thymus barrier is thus weaker in the medulla than in the cortex. Also, in the fetal and neonatal period, the thymic blood vessels appear to be more permeable to the passage of molecules and cells compared with later life; indeed, most lymphocyte precursors arrive in the thymus when it is not yet vascularized. At all stages of life, both the admittance of cells into, and the departure of cells out of, the thymus are highly selective processes. How this selective admission and departure are accomplished is not known, but some kind of Maxwell's demon must surely be at work here.

The overwhelming majority of the 'free' cells in the thymus are thymocytes; a small minority consists of macrophages and interdigitating cells. In the cortex, the *thymocytes* are so crowded that instead of being spherical, as one would expect from normal lymphocytes, they are polyhedral. They are literally packed into the cortex like sardines in a can. Most of these *cortical thymocytes* are small cells but the outer cortex also contains large *subcapsular lymphoblasts* that divide rapidly. Most cortical thymocytes are functionally immature cells that express receptors for the peanut agglutinin (PNA) and soybean lectins and synthesize the nuclear enzyme terminal deoxynucleotidyl transferase. In some species (e.g. mouse, rat, rabbit and Syrian hamster), the cells express receptors for hydrocortisone (a hormone produced by the cortex of the adrenal gland) and are lysed when the hormone is injected into the animals, i.e. they are cortisone-sensitive. Cortical thymocytes of humans, monkeys, guinea-pigs and horses do not express these receptors and are therefore cortisone-resistant. In the medulla, where the conditions are less crowded, the *medullary thymocytes* are round, small, do not express PNA and soybean lectin receptors, do not synthesize deoxynucleotidyl transferase, are cortisone-resistant in all the species and at least some of them are functionally mature.

The majority of the *macrophages* are present in the

medulla, but a few are also scattered throughout the cortex. *Interdigitating cells* are present only in the medulla. They are so designated because they possess many rod- or knob-like projections with which they contact one another. They may represent a subset of dendritic cells.

The human embryonic thymus develops from the gut wall during the fourth to fifth week of gestation. At this time, the primitive gut is a simple tube running the length of the embryo and opened in the middle into the yolk sac (see Chapter 4). The tube is lined with embryonic endoderm and is separated from the embryonic ectoderm covering the surface of the embryo by embryonic mesoderm (mes-

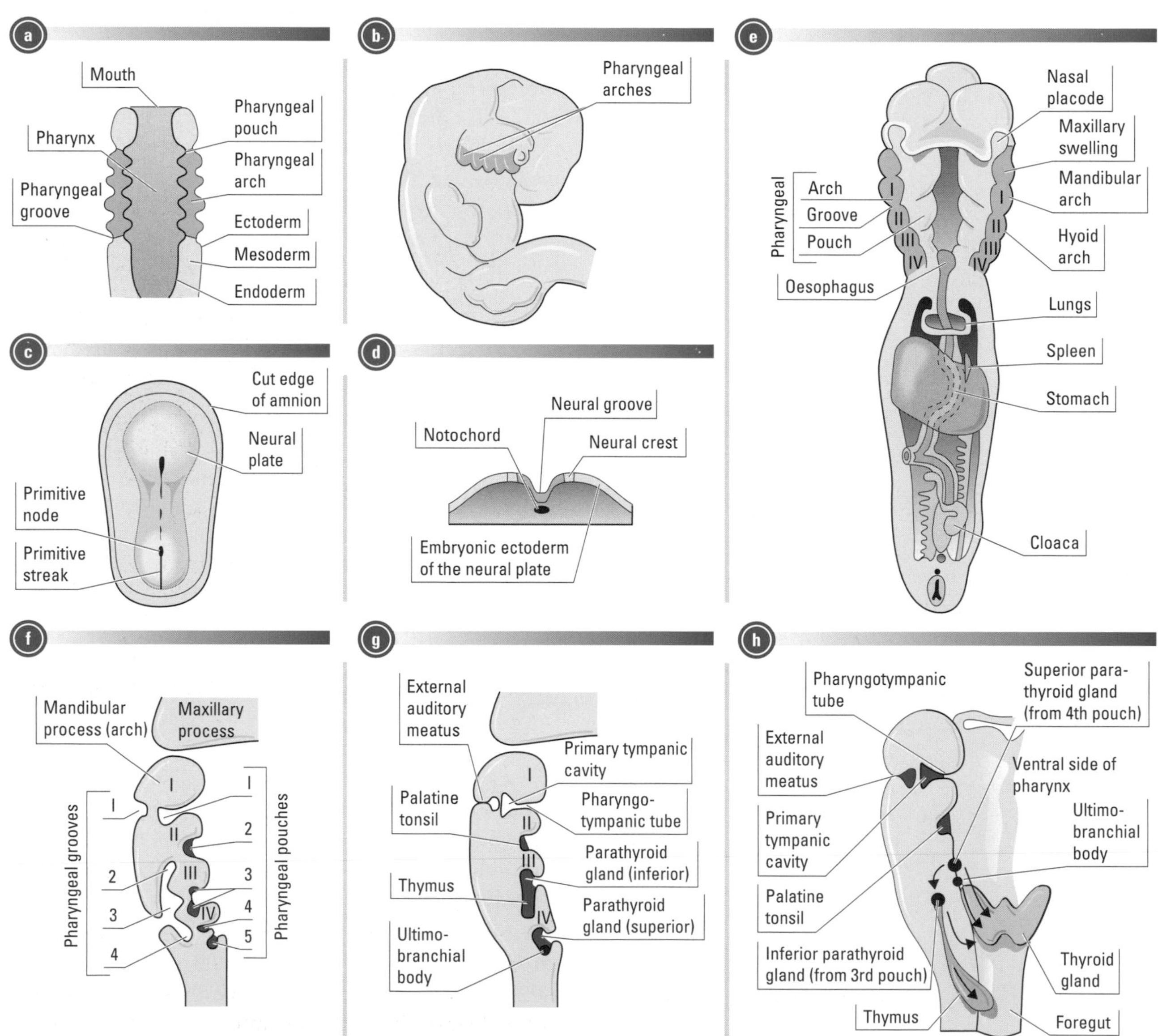

Figure 3.23 Development of the thymus in the human embryo. (a) Section through the head region of an early embryo. (b) External appearance of a 5-week-old embryo. (c) Back view of a 19-day-old embryo showing the region (neural plate) from which ectodermal cells migrate into the area of the pharyngeal pouches. (d) Cross-section of the embryo in (c) showing the origin of the neural crest. (e) Partially dissected early embryo exposing the primitive gut. (f)–(h) Consecutive stages in the development of pharyngeal grooves and pouches and in the development of the thymus from the third pharyngeal pouch. (The second arch grows over the third and fourth arches and buries the second, third and fourth pharyngeal grooves.) In (h), the thymus begins to migrate in the direction of the arrows. (Combined from different sources.)

enchyme). The development begins with four pairs of depressions[6] in the sides of the gut in the area of the future throat (pharynx). Similar depressions appear also on the outer surface of the embryo exactly opposite the inner depression (Fig. 3.23). The depressions deepen and turn into pockets, *pharyngeal pouches* on the inside and *pharyngeal grooves* on the outside, the former lined with endoderm and the latter with ectoderm. The tissue blocks separating adjacent pouches and grooves are the *pharyngeal arches*. In less advanced vertebrates, a similar development leads to the formation of gills with which the animals breathe: the pouches and grooves grow towards each other like two tunnels that are being dug from opposite sides of a mountain. When they join, they form an opening, the *branchial cleft* (Gk *branchia*, gill), through which water circulates and brings oxygen to the rich network of blood capillaries in the arches. In the human embryo, the grooves and pouches approach each other but do not meet or break through; the embryo therefore never develops gills. The pharyngeal (branchial) grooves, pouches and arches develop into various parts of the human face and throat. The third pharyngeal pouch gives rise to the thymus[7]. At the end of the fifth week of gestation, the endoderm (epithelium) lining the belly side of this pouch begins to grow rapidly, forming a sac-like protrusion into the mesoderm, in the direction of the embryo's hind part (see Fig. 3.23). The growth eventually fills the lumen of the sac with epithelium and, in the sixth week, severs the connection with the gut. The epithelial mass then begins to migrate through the mesenchymal tissue downwards along the primitive gut, with most of the mass concentrated at the leading edge and a thin, elongated portion trailing behind. Sometimes this tail breaks up into small fragments, which then either disappear or persist as isolated thymic nests. In some animals, the migration gives the thymus a rather bizarre form; in birds, for example, the thymus has the appearance of 'corals on a string'. The human thymic primordium stops its migration when it has reached the area of the future breastbone and has slid down under it. There it encounters the primordium that has grown out from the third pharyngeal pouch on the opposite side of the throat. The two primordia appose each other closely, but do not fuse, forming the two lobes of the future thymus. During this time, the primordia consist of epithelial masses without any sign of lymphocytes (Fig. 3.24). The masses become enclosed in connective tissue capsules and compartmentalized by septa, both derived from the surrounding mesenchyme. There is evidence that, in birds at least, this mesenchyme contains cells that originated in the area of the neural crest, and hence are of ectodermal origin. All three germ layers — endoderm, mesoderm and ectoderm—thus contribute to the formation of the thymus. If the neural crest cells are prevented from immigrating into the area of the thymic primordium, the organ fails to develop. Embryologists believe therefore that thymic development depends on a direct interaction between mesenchymal derivatives of the neural crest and the pharyngeal epithelium.

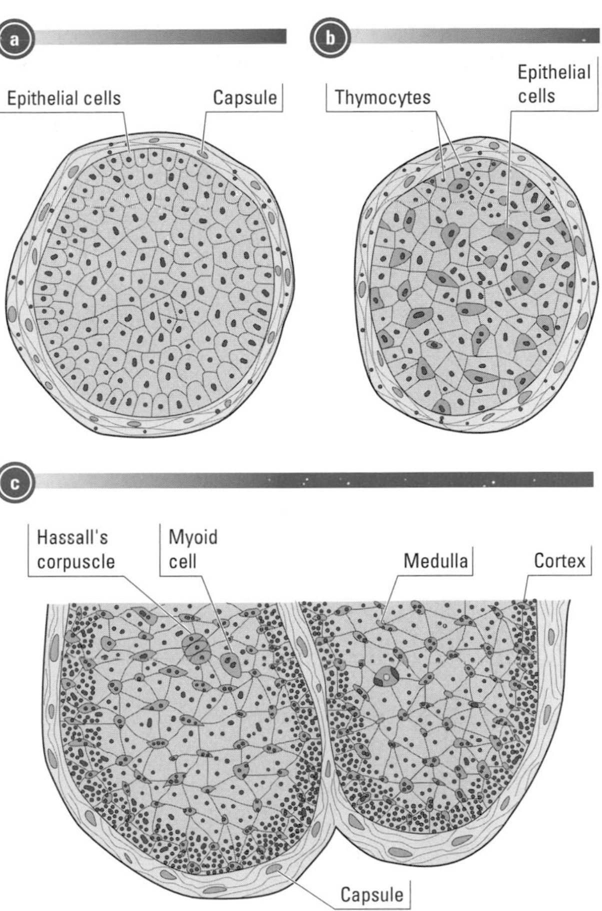

Figure 3.24 Formation of thymus anlage (primordium) during embryogenesis. (a) Epithelial anlage before the immigration of thymocyte precursors. (b) Anlage at the beginning of thymocyte immigration. (c) Differentiation of cortex and medulla. (Based on Hammar (1925), from Corning, H.K. *Lehrbuch der Entwicklungsgeschichte des Menschen*, 2nd edn. J.F. Bergman, Munich.)

At 9–10 weeks of intrauterine life, the first thymocyte precursors begin to arrive in the thymic primordium. They

[6] There are, in fact, five pairs of depressions but the fifth is so poorly developed in human embryos that it is usually considered to be part of the fourth depression.

[7] The development of the human thymus actually begins from the third and fourth pharyngeal pouches but the primordium developing from the fourth pouch becomes embedded in the thyroid and does not contribute to the organization of the definitive thymus.

issue from the yolk sac and the fetal liver, the two haemopoietic organs active at the time (see Chapter 4). The epithelium of the thymic primordium seems to secrete peptides that attract the precursor cells and make them invasive. The interaction of the precursor cells with the primordium's epithelium provides the final stimulus for the completion of thymic development. The first visible consequence of this interaction is the regrouping of the original uniformly distributed lymphocyte precursors into areas of dense and light concentration, the future cortex and medulla of the definitive thymus (see Fig. 3.21). The proliferating precursors force the originally apposed epithelial cells apart, leaving them connected only via cytoplasmic processes and transforming the compact epithelium into a spongework. At 14–15 weeks of gestation, the corticomedullary partitioning of the thymus becomes clearly visible and the primordium is invaded by blood vessels. At 15–16 weeks, the first Hassall's corpuscles appear in the medulla and the thymic architecture resembles that of the neonatal thymus. Studies on birds indicate that the precursor thymocytes are admitted into the developing thymus in waves, alternating with periods in which the thymus is closed to immigration. Whether the thymus continues to admit lymphocyte precursors throughout the life of an individual is not known; however, because thymic activity begins to decline after puberty and mature T cells are long-lived, continuous colonization by large numbers of precursor cells is unlikely.

The thymus reaches its greatest relative weight (with respect to the body) at birth. Absolute thymic weight increases until puberty, after which it declines progressively to 50% or less of its peak value. This age-associated decrease in thymic weight, the *physiological involution* (Latin *involvo*, to roll up) is accompanied by changes in thymic structure: the rate of thymocyte proliferation declines, thymocytes begin to disappear from the cortex, the lobules diminish in size and the septa broaden (Fig. 3.25). Involution may be controlled hormonally because castration slows it down, whereas injection of corticosteroids accelerates it. Occasionally, transient involution may also occur during childhood as a consequence of a stressful accident (e.g. severe burning), infection or corticosteroid treatment (so-called *stress* or *acute involution*).

The thymus is present in all but the most primitive vertebrates: it has not yet been identified in the hagfish and in the lamprey it is nothing more than a mass of lymphoid cells associated with the lining of the pharyngeal pouches. When present, it is derived from the back side of the embryonic gill pouches; only in mammals is it derived from the belly side. Mammals also differ from other vertebrates in that part of their thymus is derived from the skin on the neck of the embryo rather than from the gill endoderm, which is the source of the rest of the organ and of the entire thymus in all other vertebrates.

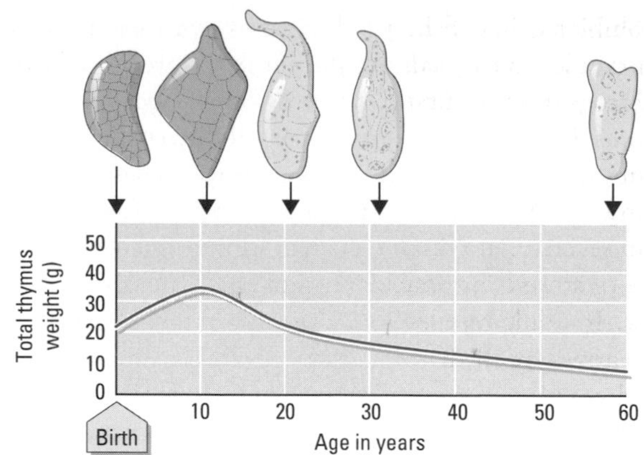

Figure 3.25 Changes in human thymus weight, size and appearance with age (thymic involution). (From Klein, J. (1982) *Immunology: The Science of Self–Nonself Discrimination*. John Wiley & Sons, New York.)

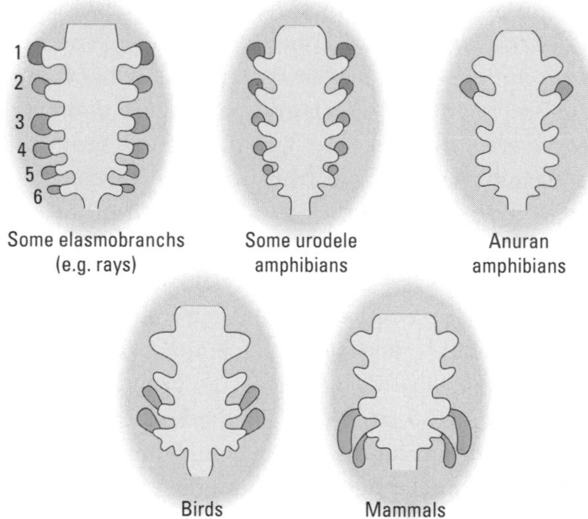

Figure 3.26 Origin of the thymus from pharyngeal pouches in different vertebrate classes. The paired pouches are numbered 1–6. The thymus anlage is darkly coloured. The grey buds are thymic rudiments that eventually disappear without contributing to the formation of the definitive thymus. (From Manning, J.J. & Turner, R.J. (1976) *Comparative Immunobiology*. Halsted, New York.)

The number of gill pouches involved in the development of the thymus varies among the different vertebrate classes (Fig. 3.26). In fish, every gill pouch produces a thymus bud and so the thymus consists of paired, irregular lymphoid masses situated above most of the gill slits. Apodan amphibians, like fish, produce thymic tissue from every embryonic pouch, salamanders from a few thymic buds, and frogs from the first pouch only. Frogs also have a pair of *jugular bodies*, which are thymus-like structures derived from gill pouches (Latin *jugulum*, throat). The thymus of young reptiles and young and adult crocodiles is derived from several embryonic pouches and hence has the appearance of strands of tissue running the length of the animal's neck. In adult reptiles (with the exception of crocodiles), derivatives of all thymic pouches but two degenerate, and the thymus itself then consists of one or two pairs of more compact bodies. The thymus of birds is derived from the second and third embryonic pouches.

Bursa of Fabricius

In birds, the digestive, urinary and reproductive tracts open into a common chamber, the *cloaca* (Latin, sewer). There is a small opening in the chamber's ceiling that leads through a short tunnel to a round or pear-shaped pocket referred to as the *bursa of Fabricius* (Latin *bursa*, purse), after the Italian anatomist and embryologist Hieronymus Fabricius Ab Aquapendente (1537–1619).

In the chicken embryo, the bursa of Fabricius (Fig. 3.27a,b) develops from the endodermal epithelium of the primitive cloaca on the fourth or fifth day of embryogenesis. At that time, cells at one site of the epithelium proliferate, forming a small protrusion that pushes forward along the cloaca. From the floor of this protrusion, finger-like projections grow into the pocket, creating multiple folds or *plicae* (Fig. 3.27c,d). At 11 or 12 days of embryonic development, nodular foci called follicles begin to form from the epithelium lining the pocket's inner surface. The cells within these follicles differentiate into the peripheral cortex and the central medulla, separated by a layer of epithelial cells, including a basement membrane. The epithelium at the corticomedullary junction is a continuation of the epithelial layer lining the pocket. Later in development, epithelial cells of the medulla become stellate (star-shaped) or reticular (net-like) and are surrounded by a rich network of capillaries from the underlying connective tissue. During the seventh or eighth day of embryonic life, lymphocyte precursors begin to migrate from the yolk sac into the bursa. By the tenth day, they enter the epithelium by passing through the basement membrane, proliferate in the medulla of the developing follicles and then enter the cortex, again passing through the basement membrane. The immigration of lymphocyte precursors transforms the original epithelial nodule into a lymphoid follicle. The number of lymphocytes in the follicles increases rapidly, partly because of the immigration of new lymphocyte precursors, but mainly as a result of repeated divisions of the lymphocytes already residing in the bursa. The mean generation time of follicular lymphocytes is 7–9 hours.

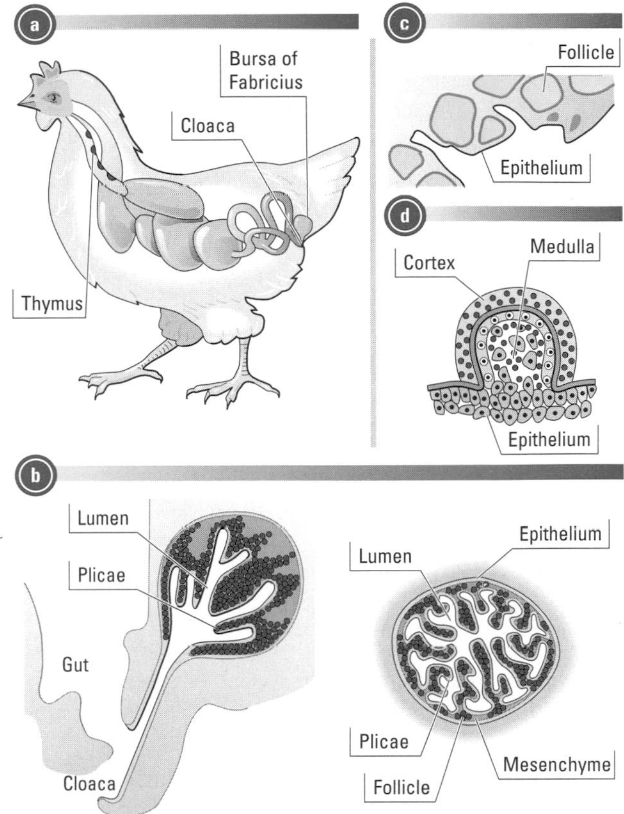

Figure 3.27 Bursa of Fabricius. (a) Location in the bird's body. (b) Section through the cloacal region. (c) Portion of plical epithelium with follicles. (d) Lymphoid follicle. (Modified from Klein, J. (1982) *Immunology: The Science of Self–Nonself Discrimination*. John Wiley & Sons, New York.)

During their residence in the follicles, the precursors transform into mature cells that leave the bursa as *bursa-derived* or *B lymphocytes* (B cells). The emigrating B lymphocytes are carried by the bloodstream to peripheral lymphoid organs, primarily the spleen. The bursa of Fabricius undergoes age-dependent physiological involution: in the domestic fowl[8], bursal activity begins to decline at about 7–13 weeks after hatching, when the birds become sexually mature, and the organ gradually diminishes in size. Involution can also be induced artificially by injecting androgenic hormones into the birds. Injection of hormones into the eggs early in embryonic life arrests bursal development almost entirely.

[8] The bird described by immunologists as a 'chicken' is a domestic form of a species that taxonomists refer to as 'jungle fowl'. We therefore use the more accurate description 'domestic fowl' in this book.

Further reading

Balinsky, B.I. (1975) *An Introduction to Embryology*, 4th edn. W.B. Saunders, Philadelphia, PA.

Crouse, D.A., Turpen, J.B. & Sharp, J.G. (1985) Thymic non-lymphoid cells. *Survey of Immunologic Research*, **4**, 120–134.

DiFiore, M.S.H., Mancini, R.E. & De Robertis, G.D.P. (1977) *New Atlas of Histology*. Lea & Febiger, Philadelphia, PA.

Fawcett, D.W. (1994) *Bloom and Fawcett: A Textbook of Histology*, 12th edn. Chapman & Hall, New York.

Fujita, T., Tanaka, K. & Tokunaga, J. (1981) *SEM Atlas of Cells and Tissues*. Igaku-Shoin, Tokyo.

Glick, B. (1985) The ontogeny and microenvironment of the avian thymus and bursa of Fabricius: contribution of specialized cells to the avian immune response. *Advances in Veterinary Science and Comparative Medicine*, **30**, 67–90.

Gross, J.A. & Flye, M.W. (1993) *The Thymus. Regulator of Cellular Immunity*. R.G. Landes Co., Austin, TX.

Junqueira, L.C., Cameiro, J. & Contopoulos, A. (1977) *Basic Histology*. Lange, Los Altos, CA.

Kampmeier, O.F. (1969) *Evolution and Comparative Morphology of the Lymphatic System*. Thomas, Springfield, IL.

Kessel, R.G. & Kardon, R.H. (1979) *Tissues and Organs: A Text-Atlas of Scanning Electron Microscopy*. W.H. Freeman, San Francisco, CA.

Krstić, R.V. (1984) *Illustrated Encyclopedia of Human Histology*. Springer-Verlag, Berlin.

Krstić, R.V. (1991) *Human Microscopic Anatomy: An Atlas for Students of Medicine and Biology*. Springer-Verlag, Berlin.

Langman, J. (1975) *Medical Embryology*, 3rd edn. Williams & Wilkins, Baltimore, MD.

Ritter, M.A. & Crispe, I.N. (1992) *The Thymus*. IRL Press, Oxford.

Scollay, R. (1983) Intrathymic events in the differentiation of T lymphocytes: a continuing enigma. *Immunology Today*, **4**, 282–286.

Wang, H. (1972) *An Outline of Human Embryology*. Williams & Wilkins, Baltimore, MD.

Weiss, L. (1972) *The Cells and Tissues of the Immune System: Structure, Functions, Interactions*. Prentice-Hall, Englewood Cliffs, NJ.

Yoffey, J.M. & Courtice, F.C. (1970) *Lymphatics, Lymph and the Lymphomyeloid Complex*. Academic Press, London.

Zapata, A.G. & Cooper, E.L. *The Immune System: Comparative Histophysiology*. John Wiley & Sons, Chichester.

chapter 4 Blood cells in vertebrate immunity

From stem cells to progenitor cells

At any point in life, an adult human being possesses some 10^{12} lymphocytes. Of these, 10^9 die every day so that if they were not continually being replenished from a stock, we would all run out of lymphocytes in approximately 3 years. The stock does not consist of lymphocytes, however, because the body simply does not have the capacity to store all the cells it will ever need. Instead the stock comprises a few cells only, each capable of producing thousands of lymphocytes without depleting itself. The stockpile is called the *haemopoietic stem cell compartment* (Greek *haima*, blood; *poiésis*, production) because it produces not only lymphocytes but also all other cells of the blood: the erythrocytes, platelets, granulocytes and monocytes.

The first haemopoietic stem cells of a human embryo appear in the third week of development in the wall of a structure called the *secondary yolk sac*: 'secondary' because it supersedes an earlier primary structure and 'yolk sac' because it is a bag containing nutrients for the early embryo just like the yolk in a bird's egg. The yolk sac wall is made of two germ layers, the mesoderm and the endoderm, but these are not the layers that form the actual embryo; rather, they are outside the embryo proper and are therefore called *extraembryonic*. Between the layer of the extraembryonic endoderm and the layer of the extraembryonic (splanchnopleuric) mesoderm is a loose tissue of star-shaped cells, the *mesenchyme*, and it is from these cells that the first elements of the blood form (Fig. 4.1). The origin of the mesenchymal cells is uncertain. In amphibians, commitment of two blastomeres to form primitive haematopoietic progenitors is demonstrable as early as in a 32-cell embryo. The commitment is revealed by the expression of a suite of haemopoietic transcription factors, including zink finger proteins GATA-1 and GATA-2. In mammals, too, cells are apparently commited to haemopoiesis prior to its establishment in the yolk sac, but the precise location of these progenitors has not been determined.

In the yolk sac wall, some of the mesenchymal cells lose their projections and aggregate into clumps, the *blood islands*. Cells inside the island become rounder and enlarge into erythroblasts, the primitive red blood cells. Cells on the outside flatten out and interconnect, forming small bags and short tubes containing fluid and erythroblasts. The individual tubes begin to fuse together to form the primitive blood vessels, which eventually connect the yolk sac with the heart in the embryo proper and with the maternal tissue of the uterine wall.

In the second month, the site of blood formation gradually shifts from the yolk sac to the fetal liver which has been colonized by a separate population of neural crest-derived stem cells (Fig. 4.2). It is at this time that the first lymphocytes (and also other cells) appear in the blood. In the third month, some blood formation also takes place in the spleen, although far less intensely than in the liver. The fetal spleen is apparently seeded by haemopoietic stem cells from the liver. In the fifth month, the stem cells finally settle down in the bone marrow, where they remain for the rest of the indi-

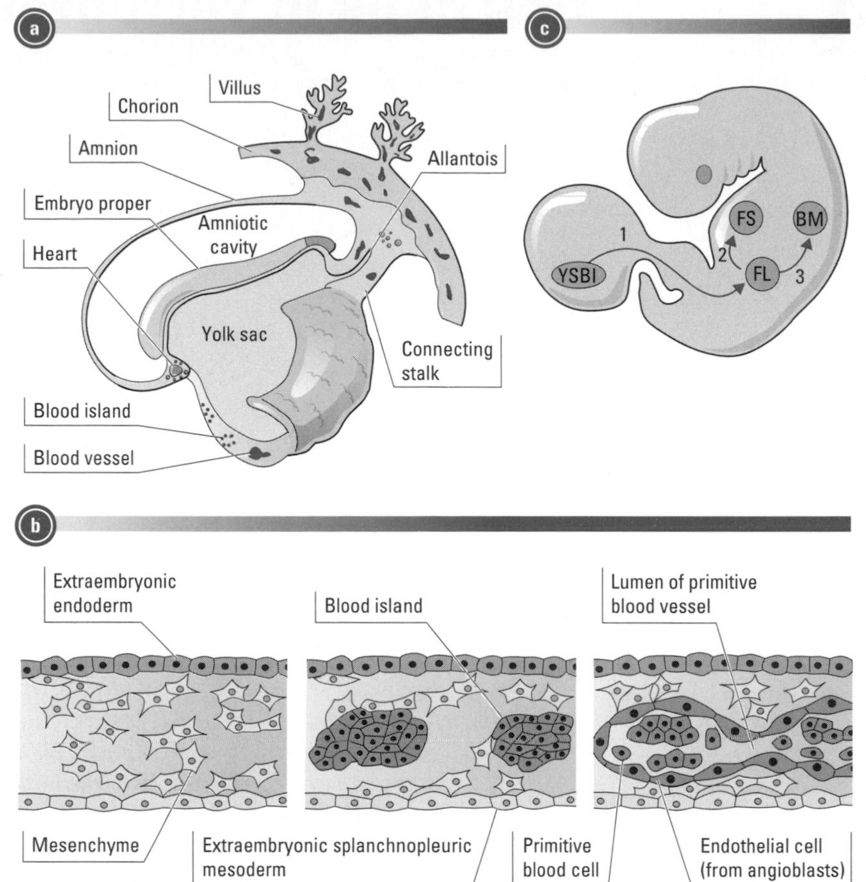

Figure 4.1 Blood and blood vessel formation in the human embryo. (a) Formation of blood islands and primitive blood vessels in the wall of the yolk sac, the connecting stalk and the chorion of a 19-day-old embryo. (Chorion is the outermost of the fetal membranes, formed from the extraembryonic somatopleuric mesoderm and the overlying trophoblast.) The drawing shows a cross-section through the embryo as well as part of the yolk sac rippled with the bulging blood islands. (b) Successive stages (from left to right) of blood vessel formation in the yolk sac wall. (c) Presumed pathways of haemopoietic stem cell migration (indicated by arrows); numbers specify order of migratory movements. BM, bone marrow; FL, fetal liver; FS, fetal spleen; YSBI, yolk sac blood islands. (b, Modified from Langman, J. (1975) *Medical Embryology*, 3rd edn. Williams & Wilkins, Baltimore.)

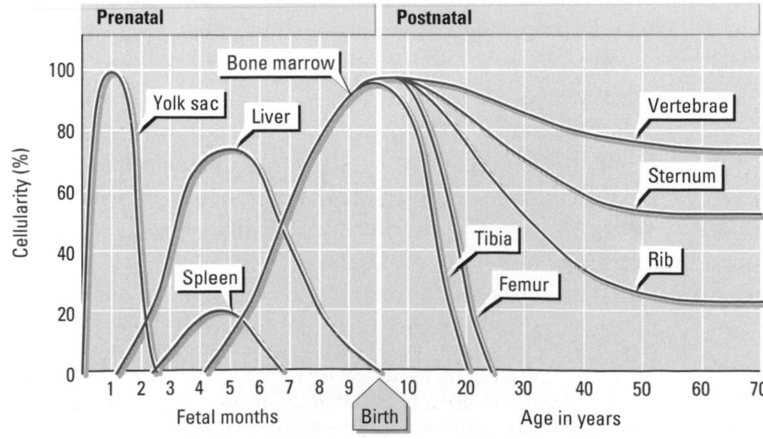

Figure 4.2 Blood formation at different sites in the human body during prenatal and postnatal development. (Modified from Erslev, A.J. & Weiss, L. (1986) In *Hematology*, 3rd edn (Eds W.J. Williams *et al.*). McGraw-Hill, New York.)

vidual's life. Blood formation in human liver and spleen ceases just before birth, but in mice, for example, it apparently continues at a low level in the spleen even in adult animals.

In the bone marrow, haemopoietic stem cells divide periodically with long intervals between individual divisions. The daughter cells either return to the *stem cell pool* (the stem cells have *renewed* themselves or *self-renewed*) or become *committed* to differentiation. The process of differentiation is a long one and involves several cell generations. It ends with the emergence of the mature blood cell, which lives for a while, performing its function, and then dies

If we designate the original stem cell *S*, the committed cells C_1, C_2, C_3, etc., the progenitor cell committed to the formation of a particular blood cell, say erythrocyte, *P*, and the mature cell *M*, we can depict the differentiation process schematically thus:

$$S \rightarrow C_1 \rightarrow C_2 \rightarrow C_3 \rightarrow \ldots \rightarrow P \rightarrow \ldots \rightarrow M$$

In this scheme, C_1 is different from *S*, C_2 is different from C_1, C_3 is different from C_2, and so on, all the way to the mature cell. The difference between the cells is that they express different genes and the progression is like an unravelling computer program. It is irreversible in that *S* can give rise to C_1 but C_1 cannot give rise to *S*; C_1 can give rise to C_2 but C_2 cannot generate C_1 and so on, towards the mature cell which has no option but to die. There are two principal views on how the progression takes place.

One view is that all the committed cells have one choice only: to give rise to the next member of the series by cell division. The only option open to C_1 is to differentiate into C_2, the only option open to C_2 is to turn into C_3, and so on. The other view, now favoured by many cell biologists and supported by most experimental evidence, regards blood cell differentiation as a gradual loss of 'stemness' (the ability of self-renewal). Here, the early *C* cells can choose between two options: they can differentiate into the next member of the series or they can renew themselves. Thus, C_1 does not need to turn immediately into C_2; it can, just like the *S* cell, produce identical copies of itself for a while (produce more C_1 cells), and only later may some of its progeny differentiate further. Unlike the *S* cells, however, the C_1 cells do not enter the quiescent G_0 phase of the cell cycle between divisions (Fig. 4.3); instead, one division is immediately followed by the next. Also, unlike the *S* cell, the C_1 cell's ability to renew itself is limited. For all we know, the *S* cells can go on renewing themselves throughout the entire lifespan of an individual. Not so the committed cells. They can only withstand a finite number of self-renewing cycles and their self-renewing capacity decreases with the progression towards the mature state. For example, if C_1 can go through 50 self-renewing cycles, C_2 can go through 25, C_3 through 12, and so on (these figures are arbitrary; the actual numbers are not known). In this example, the C_7 cell, obviously, can no longer self-renew but can only differentiate into C_8, and the same applies to all the cells that follow C_7 in the series. If we define a stem cell as a cell capable of producing copies of itself, then obviously not only *S* but also C_1–C_6 in our example are stem cells[1].

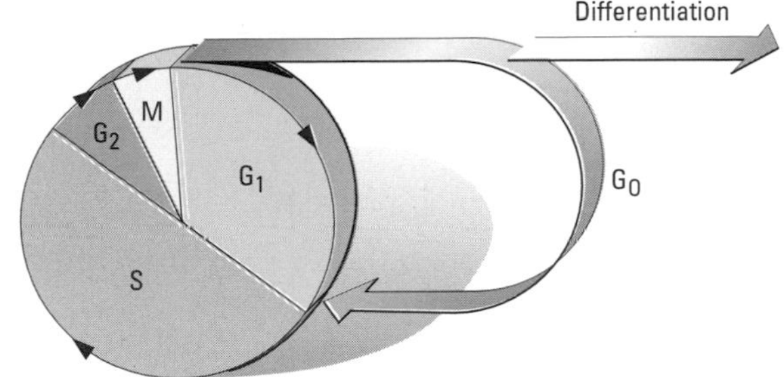

Figure 4.3 Cell cycle of a stem cell. G_0, resting or quiescent phase; S, synthetic phase (DNA is synthesized and replicated); G_2, second gap phase (the period between the completion of DNA synthesis and the next, M phase); M, mitotic phase (the period of cell division); G_1, first gap phase (the period between the completion of cell division and the start of DNA synthesis).

The individual steps in the progression from *S* via *C* and *P* to *M* remain largely unidentified. At some point, the progression begins to channel itself into distinct *cell lineages*, each lineage representing a sequence of cells tied together by a direct ancestor–descendant relationship. There are at least eight such lineages named after the mature cells with which they terminate: erythrocytic, megakaryocytic, monocytic, neutrophil, eosinophil, basophil, B lymphocytic and T lymphocytic (Fig. 4.4). Where the lineages split in the progression and what form the splitting takes is controversial. There is some evidence to suggest that the progression first splits into two lineages, lymphocytic and myelocytic, and that these then split further, the former into B and T lymphocytic and the latter into the remaining six lineages; however, this view is not universally accepted.

Most of the names of the intermediates in the progression reflect the assay used for their identification. Assays for haemopoietic stem cells fall into two categories: *in vivo* assays involving live animals and *in vitro* assays carried out in cell culture. In an *in vivo* assay an animal is *irradiated* by

[1] Some cell biologists regard the multiplication of *C* cells as proliferation rather than self-renewal and prefer to reserve the term 'stem cells' for the *S* cells. The essential difference between *S* and *C* cells is that the former can sustain haemopoiesis for the entire life of an individual, whereas the latter can do so for a limited period of time only.

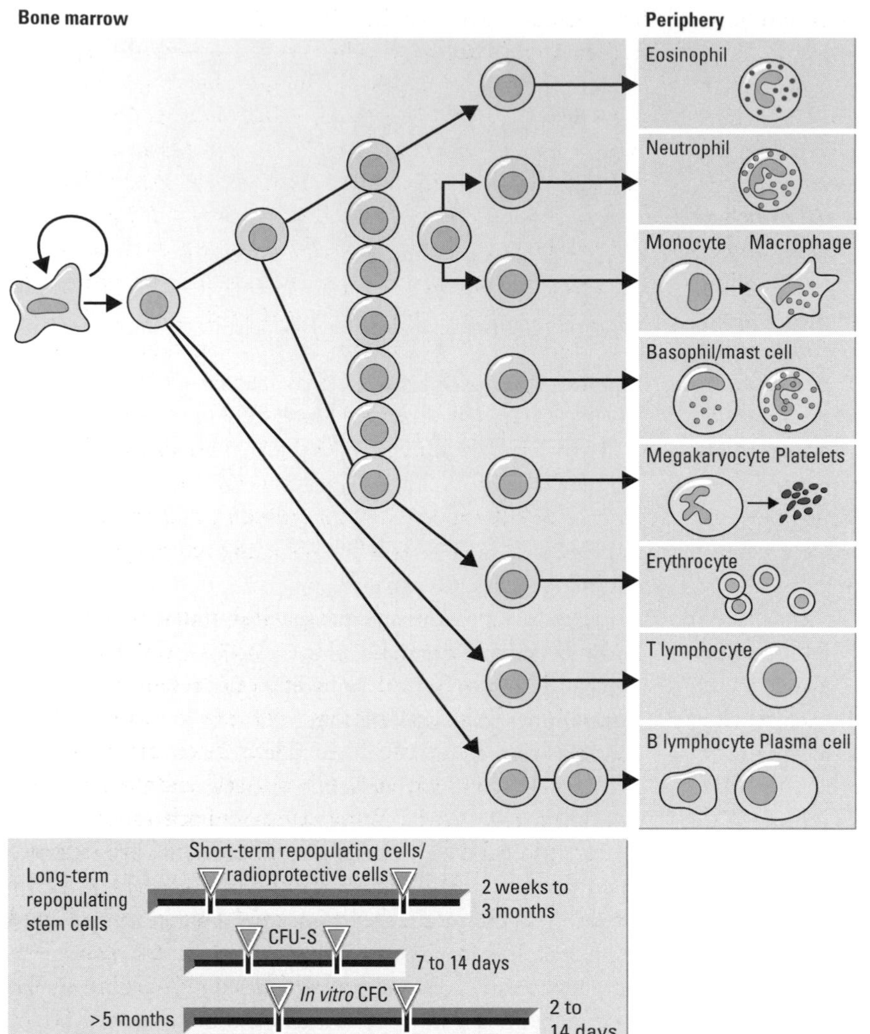

Figure 4.4 Haemopoietic progression: the origin of blood cells from haemopoietic stem cells. Because of uncertainties regarding the interrelationships among the individual pathways, no details of the progression are shown. Functional characteristics of the cell populations as measured by the various assays are given at the bottom of the figure. The times given apply to the mouse. 'Periphery' refers to the blood circulation and tissues other than bone marrow. The curved arrow indicates self-renewal. CFU-S, colony forming unit-spleen; CFC, colony forming cell. (Modified from Keller, G. (1992) *Current Opinion in Immunology*, **4**, 133.)

exposure to ionizing radiation (e.g. X-rays or γ-rays) at a dose that kills the radiosensitive haemopoietic stem cells without seriously damaging most of the other somatic cells. In the absence of haemopoietic stem cells, the animal dies (the radiation dose is said to be *lethal*) when its supply of differentiated blood cells runs out, which happens within a few weeks after irradiation. However, the animal can be saved if a suspension of bone marrow cells (or some other source of haemopoietic stem cells) from a genetically identical individual is introduced (*transplanted*) into its blood. The bone marrow cells settle in the spleen and bone cavities and begin to repopulate the spaces vacated by the dying cells of the haemopoietic compartments. If the transplant manages to produce sufficient numbers of mature blood cells before the recipient's supply is exhausted, it will provide protection from radiation death. Procedures relying on the protective power of the transplanted haemopoietic cells are therefore referred to as *radioprotection assays*.

Experiments have shown that when bone marrow is separated by physical means into *S*-enriched and *C*(*P*)-enriched fractions and these are then inoculated into lethally irradiated mice, the *S*-enriched fraction alone fails to protect the recipient from radiation death. In this case, the recipient's supply of mature blood cells runs out before the stem cells manage to produce new generations of mature cells. The *C*(*P*)-enriched fraction, on the other hand, protects the irradiated recipient, but only for a short time because after all the transplanted *C* and *P* cells of the graft have differentiated into mature cells, there are no *S* cells to produce new *C* cells. Only the combination of *S* and *C*(*P*) fractions provides long-lasting protection: the *C*(*P*) cells protect the recipient until the time at which the *S* cells take over the production of blood cells. The inoculated *C*(*P*) fraction thus provides short-term and the *S* fraction long-term protection of the recipient.

In another *in vivo* assay, bone marrow cells are inoculated into lethally irradiated mice but in low numbers; they thus populate the recipient's spleen only sparsely, forming discrete *colonies* that can be examined on histological sections. The composition of the colonies, each of which is derived from a single cell (the *colony forming unit-spleen* or *CFU-S*) varies depending on the position of the founding cell in the haemopoietic progression and the time at which the spleens were examined after the inoculation. Thus a colony can be founded by a pre-CFU-S, the *S* stem cell itself; a late CFU-S, a *C* cell at various stages of commitment; or an early CFU-S, a *P* cell committed to a particular lineage (see Fig. 4.4).

In vitro assays involve the growth of bone marrow cells in culture and are either long or short term. In *short-term culture*, bone marrow cells are suspended in a semi-solid medium, such as agar or methylcellulose, and plated on a *feeder layer* of embryonic fibroblasts in a culture dish. Individual stem cells form discrete colonies of proliferating and differentiating cells that grow for 10–14 days, reach a size of 50–2000 cells and then degenerate. The cells of the feeder layer produce factors necessary for the growth of the colonies (*colony-stimulating factors* or CSFs), which accumulate in the medium. The feeder cells can be replaced by a *conditioned medium* in the form of a supernatant from a culture of embryonic fibroblasts grown without the bone marrow cells. In *long-term culture*, the function of the fibroblasts is fulfilled by a bone marrow-derived adherent cell population. A bone marrow placed into a culture dish without a feeder layer loses most of its haemopoietic cells within 1–3 weeks but retains certain stromal elements, including endothelial cells, giant fat-containing cells and macrophages (see Chapter 5 for explanation and details), which grow in multiple layers at the bottom of the dish. If the culture is then recharged with fresh bone marrow, it supports the growth of haemopoietic cells for weeks or even months. Each colony is again presumed to have been founded by a single colony-forming unit in a different stage of commitment which determines the colony's composition. The names of the presumed founders reflect this interpretation: *CFU-GEMM* (or *CFU-Mix*) differentiates into granulocytes, erythrocytes, monocytes and megakaryocytes, a mixture of which are found in the colony; *CFU-GM* produces granulocytes (basophils and neutrophils) and monocytes; *CFU-Mega* gives rise to megakaryocytes; and so on. The erythrocytic lineage is founded by a cell that gives rise to large clusters or 'bursts' and hence is referred to as *burst-forming unit-erythroid* or *BFU-E*.

In the later stages of the haemopoietic progression, the intermediate cells can be identified by their appearance. For example, the neutrophil lineage passes through the following morphologically distinguishable stages (Fig. 4.5): *myeloblast* (cell with a large, round nucleus and scanty cytoplasm); *promyelocyte* (cell with cytoplasmic granules that stain blue or violet with standard dyes used in haematological preparations; not shown in Fig. 4.5); *myelocyte* (cell with clumped chromatin, the mass of the relaxed chromosomes of the interphase, in the nucleus and prominent granules in the cytoplasm); *metamyelocyte* (cell with coarsely clumped chromatin in the bean-shaped nucleus; not shown in Fig. 4.5); *band (stab) cell* (cell with a typically curved, U-shaped nucleus whose lobes are connected by thick bands; not shown in Fig. 4.5); and *neutrophil* (cell with nucleus fragmented into several oval or sausage-shaped lobes connected by thin threads, and characteristic granules in the cytoplasm that have no preference for either acidic or basic dyes).

The entire haemopoietic progression is dependent on the presence of *haemopoietic growth factors* (HGFs). These were initially discovered as substances present in the conditioned medium and required for the growth of bone marrow cells in culture, i.e. CSFs. They are produced by non-haemopoietic cells (fibroblasts, endothelial cells, monocytes, activated T lymphocytes and others) but act on the haemopoietic cells at different stages in the progression. At a given stage, the target cell expresses an *HGF receptor* (HGF-R) on its surface that binds the factor specifically and then passes a signal into the interior of the cell. Two hypotheses have been put forward to explain the indispensability of the factors: one claims that the action of HGFs commits a haemopoietic cell to take the next step in the progression; according to the other, the entire programme responsible for the progression is 'wired into' the haemopoietic cell and the factors merely keep the cells alive so that they are able to realize the programme. Since there is experimental evidence supporting both views, some of the factors may indeed incite the cells to take the next step in the progression while others prevent them from committing suicide. Different factors act in distinct stages of the progression. The late-acting factors are relatively lineage specific in that each of them participates in the terminal divisions of a particular maturation pathway. They include *erythropoietin* (EPO), which is active in the erythrocytic lineage; *granulocyte colony-stimulating factor* (G-CSF), which is necessary for granulocyte differentiation; *thrombopoietin* (TPO), whose targets are cells of the megakaryocytic lineage; *monocyte colony-stimulating factor* (M-CSF), which participates in the differentiation along the monocytic pathway; *interleukin (IL)-15*, an essential factor in T lymphocyte differentiation; and *IL-5*, which is

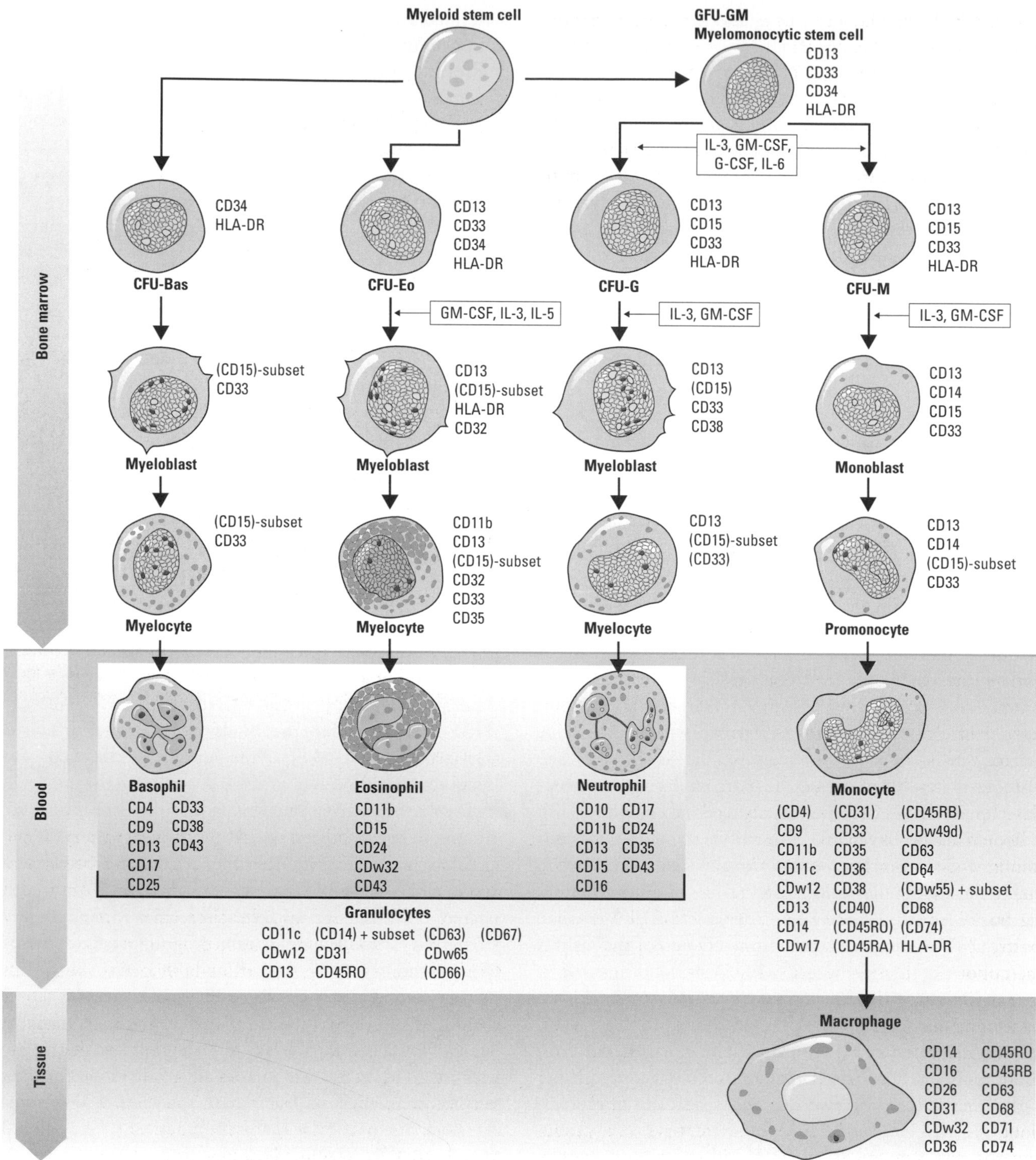

Figure 4.5 The myeloblastoid cell lineages, their molecular markers and growth factors (boxed). The promyelocyte, metamyelocyte and band cells are omitted for simplicity. CD, cluster of differentiation, is a generic term for cell surface markers; HLA-DR is one type of human major histocompatibility complex molecules.

involved in B lymphocyte and eosinophil differentiation. Factors involved in the proliferation of more primitive cells in the progression (the cells of the *C* compartment) affect the division of several cell lineages; they include *IL-3*, *IL-4*, *IL-7* and *IL-9*, and the *granulocyte macrophage colony-stimulating factor* (GM-CSF). Finally, there are factors that act on the primitive stem (*S*) cells, either by forcing them to leave the G_0 phase and enter the cell division phase, or by rendering them responsive to later-acting HGFs. Three such factors have been described: *IL-1*, *IL-6* and *stem cell factor* (SCF). The first two, however, are quite promiscuous in their choice of targets and their physiological role in haemopoiesis is therefore questionable. SCF is less promiscuous in its action but it is not restricted to haemopoietic stem cells either.

Experiments with long-term bone marrow cultures have demonstrated that a special microenvironment is necessary for full realization of the haemopoietic progression. In mammals, a *haemopoietic microenvironment* is provided primarily by the stromal tissue of the bone marrow. Bone marrow, the tissue that fills the cavities of some of the bones, comprises two types: red and yellow. The *red bone marrow* derives its colour from the abundance of erythrocytes and their precursors, while the *yellow bone marrow* owes its hue to the presence of numerous adipose (fat) cells. The red marrow produces blood cells, whereas the yellow marrow is haemopoietically inactive, although it can convert into blood-forming tissue in stress situations. In a human newborn, all the marrow is red; in an adult, red marrow is restricted to the breastbone, vertebrae, ribs, clavicles and bones of the pelvis and skull.

Bone marrow, like many other soft organs, has two basic components: parenchyma and stroma. Parenchyma is the functional part of the organ, whereas stroma is the supporting framework (the Greek word *stroma* literally means a mattress). The functional part of the bone marrow is the haemopoietic tissue; the supporting part consists of a sponge-like maze of reticular as well as other cells, blood vessels and nerves. Blood is supplied to the bone marrow by the *nutrient artery*, which in long bones enters the marrow about midshaft and then branches out into two ('left' and 'right') *central longitudinal arteries* (Fig. 4.6). These run along the bone's longitudinal axis, sending out shoots towards the marrow's periphery. The smaller arteries branch out further into arterial capillaries which then become veins, but a special kind of vein, richly branched and with walls consisting of a single layer of cells resting on the basement membrane. Because of these characteristics, the veins are referred to as *venous sinuses*. They carry blood back towards the marrow's centre via the *radial veins*, which empty into the *central longitudinal vein* (*sinus*)

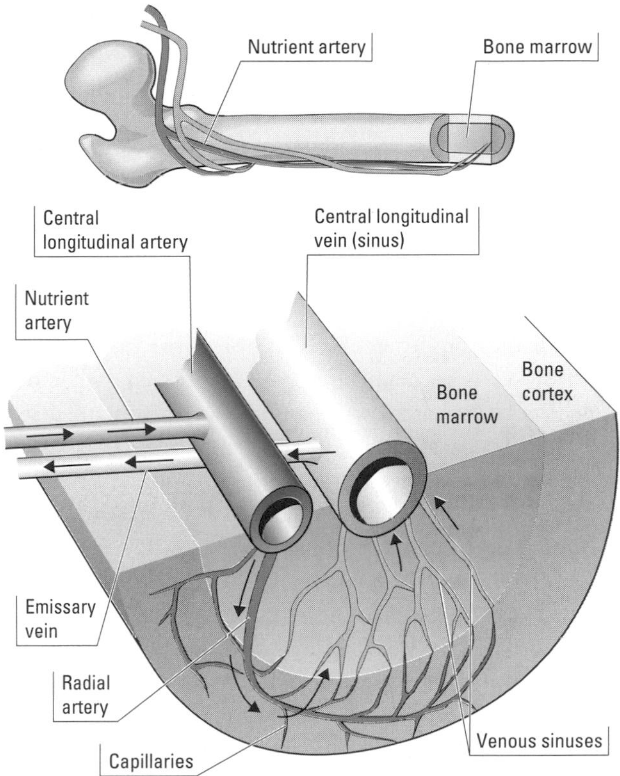

Figure 4.6 Blood supply to a long bone and its marrow. Arrows indicate the direction of blood flow. Haemopoiesis occurs in the stroma between the venous sinuses. (Based on *Journal of NIH Research*, 6, 96, 1994.)

running parallel with the central longitudinal artery. Where blood from the nutrient artery enters the bone, blood from the longitudinal vein leaves it via a connection to the *emissary vein*, which runs parallel to the nutrient artery.

The blood vessels are enmeshed by the *reticular framework* consisting mainly of irregularly shaped reticular cells, interconnected via their numerous processes and reticular fibres that are associated with the cells and often enveloped by them. The intercellular spaces of the framework are filled with a ground substance, the *extracellular matrix*, in which the haemopoietic cells are embedded. Both the reticular cells and the glycoproteins of the extracellular matrix are apparently necessary for haemopoiesis. The reticular cells produce some of the HGFs and the matrix proteins assist in the interaction of the factors with the haemopoietic cells. While some of the factors are secreted into fluids bathing the haemopoietic cells, others may remain membrane bound and require direct interaction between the HGF on the reticular cell and the receptor on the target haemopoietic cell. Alternatively, the released HGFs may bind to the extracellular matrix proteins and then interact with the receptors on the target cells.

In mammals, the initial stages of blood formation occur entirely in the haemopoietic tissue outside the blood vessels. To enter the circulatory system, newly formed cells must therefore pass through the sinus wall. This passage is an active process of 'burrowing', in which the cell must first make a hole in the basement membrane, push aside the cells of the sinus wall and then squeeze through the tunnel thus formed into the sinus.

Visualizing the different cell types in the haemopoietic progression has been a problem. As mentioned earlier, only the cells in the terminal stages of the progression are distinguishable by classical histological methods, whereas the remaining cells can be separated roughly into two fractions only, according to their size and density. The earliest cells of the progression have the appearance of what immunologists call the *small lymphocyte*, a round cell in which the nucleus takes up most of the volume and the cytoplasm is limited to a thin rim around it, whereas the cells of the intermediate stage have the appearance of a *blast*, a large cell with abundant cytoplasm. A more precise distinction of the early and intermediate cells proved to be difficult by these methods. Investigators have therefore put much effort into the discovery of *molecular markers*, molecules that serve to identify a particular cell type (see Fig. 4.5). Most of the markers are cell-surface molecules detectable by their reaction with specific antibodies. They have been assigned a variety of acronyms that will be explained when the respective marker is given closer attention. A number of markers have been described for some of the cells of the haemopoietic progression, especially the cells of the T and B lymphocytic lineage, and these will be mentioned in the next chapter. The marker constellations of other cells are less defined and more controversial. In particular, a controversy still rages in regard to the early cells. It has been claimed that the pluripotential[2], self-renewing stem cells of the mouse are identified by the combination of markers Thy-1^{lo}Lin$^-$Sca-1^+ (where Thy-1^{lo} stands for low expression of glycoproteins otherwise expressed at a high level in thymocytes and T lymphocytes; Lin$^-$ indicates the absence of lineage markers CD4, CD8, Mac-1 (CD11b), Gr-1 and CD45; and Sca-1^+ indicates the presence of the stem cell antigen-1) but this is disputed by some investigators. Human stem cells are believed to be characterized by the combination of markers CD34$^+$, MHC-DR$^-$, Lin$^-$ and CD38$^+$.

In the rest of this chapter, we describe the mature blood cells (with the exception of lymphocytes, which will be dealt with in the next chapter) together with a few cells of uncertain origin. All the blood cells are, in one way or another, involved in immunity, but lymphocytes play the leading part, especially in the adaptive response. For this reason, more attention will be given to them than to the other cells.

Mature cells

Of the blood cells produced by an adult mammal, only the T lymphocytes differentiate in part outside the bone marrow. The remaining cells go through the haemopoietic progression in the bone marrow and enter the circulation as mature or nearly mature cells: erythrocytes (red blood cells; Figs 4.7 & 4.8), platelets and leucocytes (white blood cells). Leucocytes are divided into two families, mononuclear and polymorphonuclear. *Mononuclear leucocytes* have a large, round nucleus and clear cytoplasm; they are the monocytes and lymphocytes. *Polymorphonuclear (PMN) leucocytes* or *polymorphs* have an oddly shaped nucleus (Greek *poly*, many; *morphos*, shape, hence 'polymorphonuclear' refers to a 'nucleus of many shapes') and highly granulated cytoplasm; because of the latter feature they are also called *granulocytes*. They are the neutrophils, eosinophils and basophils but since the first of these three cell types is present in the blood in vastly greater numbers than the other two, the terms 'polymorphs' and 'granulocytes' are often used as synonyms for neutrophils. Lymphocytes and neutrophils are the dominant leucocytes of normal blood; all other leucocytes are present in much lower numbers.

Platelets

While in the bone marrow, the megakaryocyte enlarges and its chromosomes multiply but the cell itself does not divide. The cytoplasm of the megakaryocyte ('cell with a huge nucleus') then fragments into some 4000 pieces, each of which surrounds itself with a membrane and enters the bloodstream as a *platelet* (*thrombocyte*; from Greek *thrombos*, clot of blood; *kytos*, cell; Fig. 4.9a). Mammalian platelets are therefore cells without nuclei; platelets of other vertebrates are nucleated.

The characteristic plate shape of thrombocytes is imposed on them by the tension of an internal triple hula-hoop (see Fig. 4.8). The hoop, the *marginal bundle*, consists of a single rope of microtubules wound three times around the circumference of the cell. Another peculiarity of the platelet is that it is permeated through and through by a

[2] The *S* cell and possibly some of the C cells have the potential to give rise to all the different blood cells, i.e. they are pluripotent. The *P* cell, on the other hand, can differentiate into one cell type only, i.e. it is unipotent.

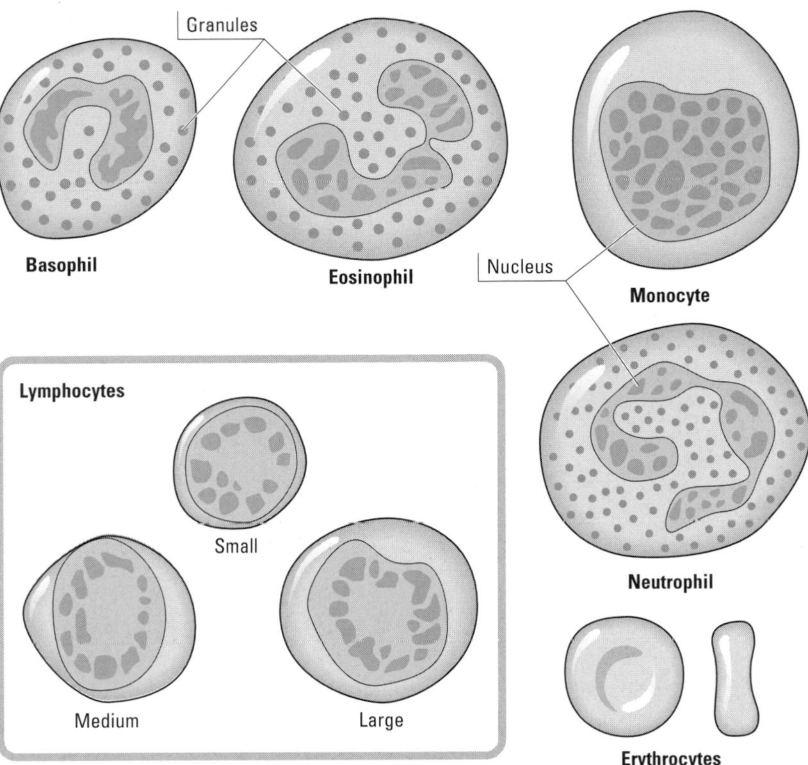

Figure 4.7 Blood cell gallery I: cells as seen in blood smears, stained with Giemsa or some other similar stain and observed with the aid of a light microscope. The colours shown are not those actually seen on a smear.

labyrinth of channels and conduits that give the cell a sponge-like appearance. Like sponges, platelets also soak up constituents of the plasma and occasionally squeeze them out again. On stained blood preparations, the peripheral part of a platelet is transparent, whereas the more central parts are dense because they contain small membrane-bound vesicles or granules. These are of two basic kinds, *dense granules (bodies)* and *α granules*. The former are homogeneous, filled with material that does not allow electrons of an electron microscope to pass through and therefore appears dense. The latter are heterogeneous, varying in size and shape. The two types differ also in their content. The dense granules contain various nucleotide phosphates (ADP, ATP, GDP, GTP, i.e. adenosine diphosphate and triphosphate, guanosine diphosphate and triphosphate, respectively), pyrophosphates and orthophosphates, calcium cations and serotonin. The α granules are of two subtypes: true α granules and acid hydrolase-containing vesicles. The *true α granules* contain an assortment of substances, some of which are present only in platelets (platelet factor 4, β-thromboglobulin), while others are also present in the plasma (fibrinogen and some of the clotting factors). The *acid hydrolase-containing vesicles* resemble lysosomes in that they carry enzymes capable of degrading materials into their basic constituents and act at a pH of 4.5–5.0. Platelets also contain *peroxisomes* with enzymes for inactivation of hydrogen peroxide.

The function of platelets is to plug holes in blood vessels and to help stop bleeding. The damaged inner surface (endothelium) of a punctured blood vessel activates the resting platelets. As the flying saucers of the platelets descend on the damaged site and develop false feet (pseudopodia; Fig. 4.9b), one almost expects to see little green men march out. Instead, however, the saucers *aggregate* around the leak and in each of them the marginal bundle begins to constrict, hoarding the granules in the centre of the cell. The granules then fuse one by one with the membranes of the internal labyrinth and release their content into the channels, from which it is then squeezed out to the exterior of the cell. Once this *release reaction* is completed, the granules disappear for the most part from the cell (the platelets have *degranulated*) and the microtubulin of the marginal bundle depolymerizes. Some of the granule constituents are described in Chapters 11 and 21.

Neutrophils

The terms 'neutrophil', 'eosinophil' and 'basophil' were introduced by the German bacteriologist and immunologist Paul Ehrlich (1854–1915) at the end of the nineteenth century. Ehrlich, realizing how difficult it was to see any-

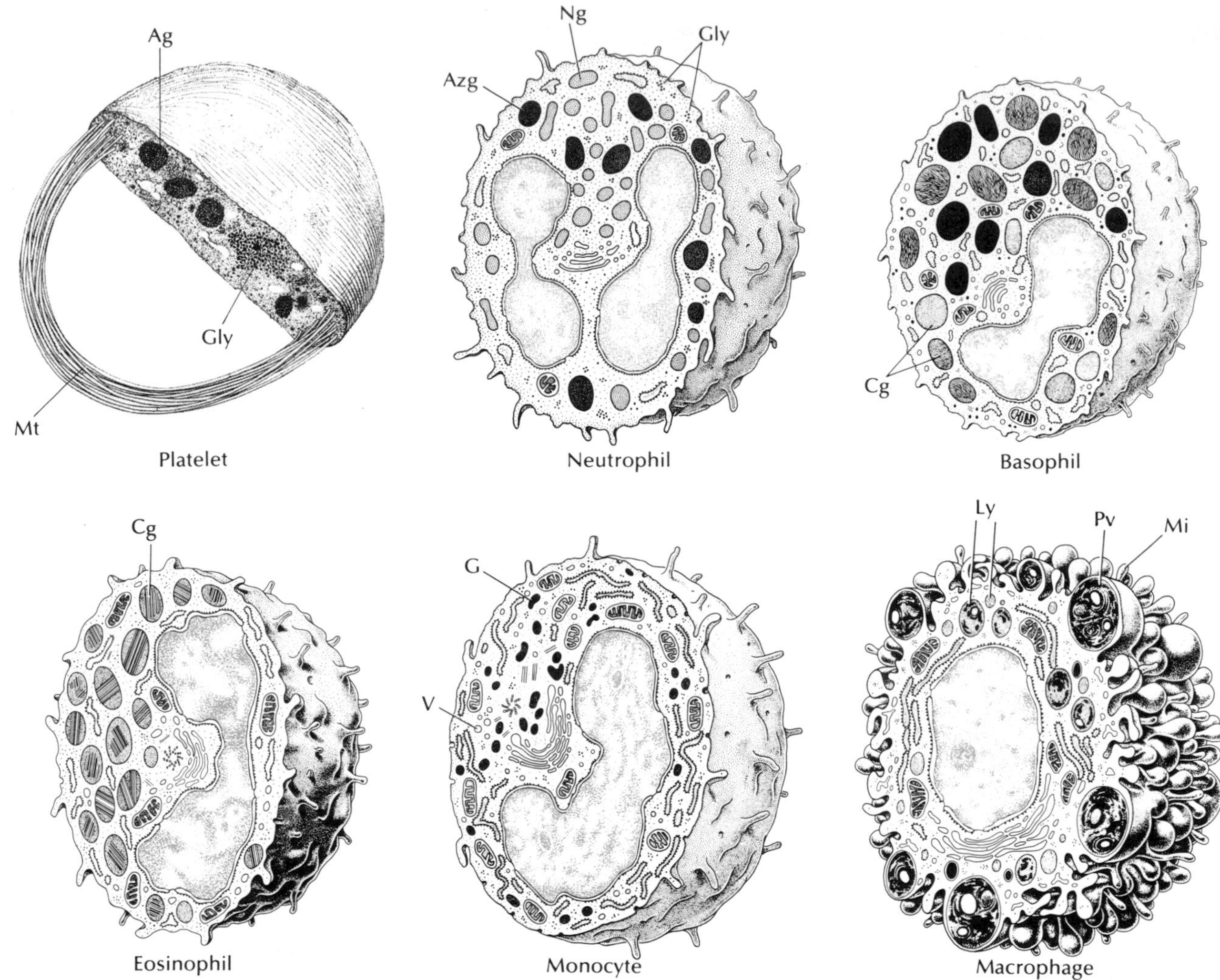

Figure 4.8 Blood cell gallery II: cells as seen with the aid of transmission and scanning electron microscope. Lymphocytes are omitted because they are shown separately in Chapter 5. Ag, alpha granule; Azg, azurophilic granule; Cg, crystalloid granule; G, granule; Gly, glycogen particles; Ly, lysosome; Mi, microvillus; Mt, microtubules encircling the platelet; Ng, neutrophilic granule; Pv, phagocytic vacuole; V, vesicle. (Platelet based on *Melloni's Illustrated Medical Dictionary* (1979) Williams & Wilkins, Baltimore; remaining drawings modified from Krstić, R.V. (1978) *Die Gewebe des Menschen und der Säugetiere*. Springer-Verlag, Berlin.)

thing inside a cell, decided to attach dyes to the cellular constituents in a way similar to that used in dyeing textiles. Since the composition of the constituents varies widely, it is to be expected that some of them will be negatively charged and will therefore interact with positively charged (*acidic*) dyes, while others will be positively charged and will bind negatively charged *basic* dyes. The former constituents will be *acidophilic*, while the latter will be *basophilic*. A third category of constituents may be expected to be both positively and negatively charged, binding both acidic and basic dyes; these constituents will be *neutrophilic*. Since the basic and acidic dyes differ in colour, various cell components will stain differently, and it will be easier to distinguish them.

A common way of *differentially staining* blood cells is to collect a drop of blood from a fingertip or earlobe on a microscope slide, spread it into a thin film with another slide, air-dry the film, stain it—for example with the Giemsa stain — and wash and air-dry it again. The Giemsa stain, named after the German chemist and bacteriologist Gustav Giemsa (1867–1948), is a mixture of positively charged (cationic, basic) methylene blue and negatively charged (anionic, acidic) red eosin (Greek *éos*, dawn; Fig. 4.10). The combination of methylene blue and red eosin stains the cytoplasm blue to grey, the nuclei dark purple and the granules either purple, blue or red. Cells with purple-, blue- or red-staining granules are the neutrophils, basophils and eosinophils, respectively.

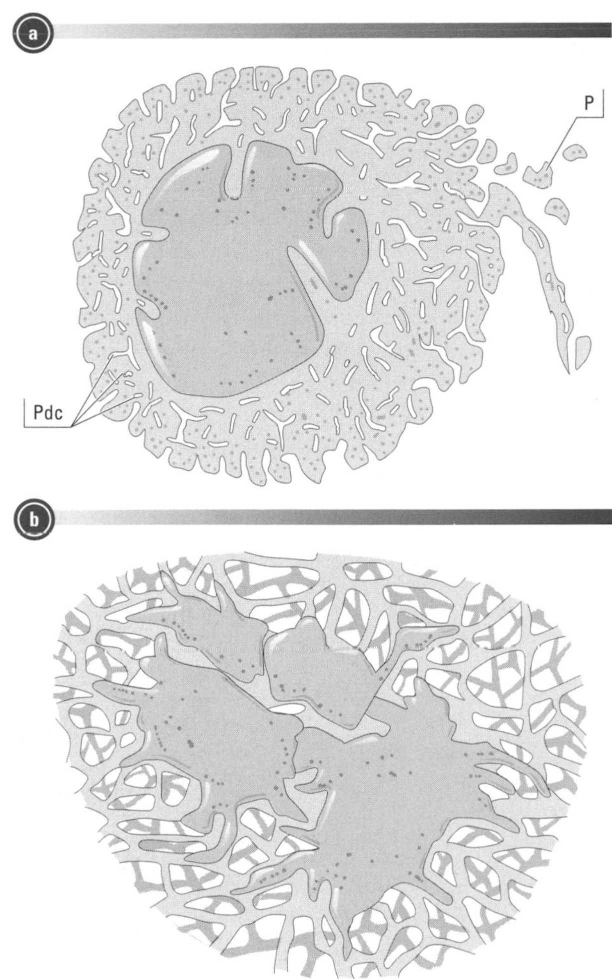

Figure 4.9 Origin of platelets from a megakaryocyte (a) and morphological transformation of activated platelets (b). In (a) the giant megakaryocyte with very large lobulated nucleus develops numerous channels demarcating the future platelets (Pdc). The cell eventually fragments and releases some 2500 platelets (P). In (b) platelets with pseudopodia are shown descending on the damaged wall of a blood vessel. (a, Based on Krstić, R.V. (1984) *Illustrated Encyclopedia of Human Histology*. Springer-Verlag, Berlin.)

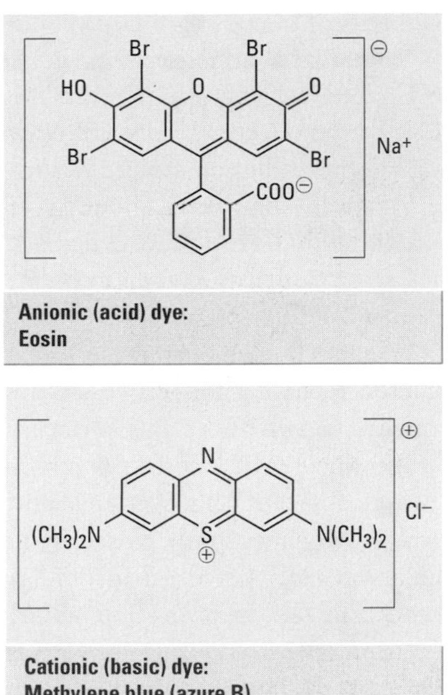

Figure 4.10 Formulas of anionic and cationic dyes used for staining blood cell smears. After the removal of Na^+, the methylene blue has a negative charge and can bind to positively charged amino acid side-chains in proteins, for example. After the removal of Cl^-, the eosin has a positive charge and can bind to negatively charged amino acid side-chains in proteins.

In blood films, the mature neutrophils can be recognized according to two features: a nucleus that is segmented into two to five oval or sausage-shaped lobes, connected by thin filaments; and purple-staining granules (see Fig. 4.7). Neutrophils contain two types of granule, *primary* and *secondary* (see Fig. 4.8). The names refer to the fact that the primary granules appear first and the secondary granules somewhat later during the development of the cells (in the promyelocyte and myelocyte stages, respectively). The primary granules are also called *azurophilic* because of their propensity to interact with blue azure dyes. The secondary granules were called 'specific' by Ehrlich because they characterize (are specific for) the neutrophilic lineage; they are the ones that bind acidic and basic dyes equally well and hence stain greyish-purple. The primary granules are smaller than the secondary ones and are in the minority (three-quarters of the granules are of the specific type). The primary granules are, in fact, lysosomes rich in hydrolases, lysozyme, myeloperoxidase and cationic proteins. The secondary granules contain, in addition to lysozyme, lactoferrin (a protein originally found in milk and carrying an iron-containing haem group), collagenase (a collagen-cleaving enzyme) and vitamin B_{12}-binding protein. (For further details of some of these constituents, see Chapters 11 & 21.) The plasma membrane of a neutrophil contains receptors capable of binding immunoglobulin (Fc receptors; see Chapter 8) and complement (see Chapter 12), as well as β-adrenergic and insulin receptors.

Upon release from their cradle in the bone marrow, the neutrophils enter the bloodstream, where they tumble along with other cells for 6–10 hours. When they reach the capillaries, they bump their way through the heavy traffic towards the outermost zone of the flowing blood and move along in a relatively clear area of the plasma (*margination*). As they hit the blood vessel wall here and there, they get a foothold in the slimy lining of the postcapillary venules and momentarily come to rest. The adherence of neutrophils to the endothelial cells of the postcapillary venule is mediated by a set of specialized adhesion molecules; these are described in Chapter 9. The initial reversible interaction with molecules of the selectin family is followed by more stable binding to other adhesion molecules such as ICAM-1 (see Chapter 9). At any one time, about two-thirds of the neutrophils in the blood are found clinging to the vessel walls. As they settle down, they turn into small amoebas: they stretch out false feet (pseudopodia) and then slowly drag the rest of their bodies over these feet, much like a caterpillar tractor, repeating this process again and again, and thus crawling slowly over the surface. They crawl about three times their own length in a minute, searching for the sites where adjacent cells overlap slightly forming a sort of flap valve, which is tightly closed by fluid pressure and intercellular 'cement'. Once a neutrophil finds this cell junction, it sends a finger-like projection into it, forces open the valve by pushing the two cells slightly apart and begins to squeeze through the gap and the underlying basement membrane. In this process of *diapedesis* (which literally means 'the act of leaping across') the lobulation of the nucleus proves to be an advantage because it provides flexibility that a cell with a round nucleus would not have. As the neutrophil oozes out on to the other side of the wall, the valve closes up again behind it so that no fluid escapes from the blood vessel. Whether the neutrophil opens the valve by brute force alone or whether it also dissolves the cement enzymatically is still a matter of debate among cell biologists.

Once it has reached the other side of the wall, the neutrophil continues its crawl through the tissues. In particular it infiltrates tissues that are in contact with the outside world, i.e. mucous membranes and the skin. It persists in these tissues for about 1–2 days and then dies and is either removed or passes to the outside world with the material expelled from the respiratory and intestinal tracts. The normal daily toll amounts to half a cupful of packed neutrophils, but this loss is continuously compensated for by the daily production of some 100 billion neutrophils in the bone marrow. The purpose of the tissue crawl is to find foreign objects. If that happens, the neutrophil swallows the object by the process of phagocytosis and releases the contents of the granules on it (*degranulation*). The active substances in the granules then either degrade the object right down to the basic constituents of living matter or, if this is impossible, the neutrophil dies of indigestion.

Eosinophils

The two characteristic features of an eosinophil are the nucleus divided into two tear-shaped lobes and large secondary (secretory) granules with affinity for acid stains (see Figs 4.7 & 4.8). Like neutrophils, eosinophils have Fc and complement receptors on their surfaces, but in addition they also have H_1 and H_2 histamine receptors as well as other receptors not borne by neutrophils. In the centre of the secondary granule, embedded in a surrounding matrix, sits a crystal composed of repeating subunits of the *major basic protein* (MBP). The crystal is electron-dense so that on electron micrographs the granules have a dark core. The granule matrix contains *eosinophil cationic protein* (ECP), *eosinophil-derived neurotoxin* (EDN) and a number of enzymes. Further enzymes are present in the primary granules (lysosomes), which the eosinophil has in common with the neutrophil. (The granule constituents are described in Chapters 11 & 21.)

Mature eosinophils released into the bloodstream from the bone marrow head straight for the connective tissues at sites similar to those that also attract neutrophils. They stay in the blood for about 13 hours and then exit into the tissues, where they live for a few days longer than neutrophils. Their main function is to spill the content of their granules onto larger parasites. They are, however, also capable of phagocytosis.

Basophils

The nucleus of a basophil is irregularly shaped but without the sharply distinct lobes found in other granulocytes, and the granules in the cytoplasm react with basic dyes that stain them dark purplish blue (see Figs 4.7 & 4.8). The internal structure of the granules varies, depending on the histological treatment; sometimes it appears to be crystalloid, but at other times it reveals concentric lamellar structures that look like scrolls of parchment; occasionally, it may even seem to be uniformly dense. The granules contain large amounts of heparin and histamine, as well as numerous enzymes such as decarboxylase, histidine dehydrogenase and diaphorase (lipoamide dehydrogenase; see Chapters 11 & 21). In contrast to neutrophils and eosinophils, basophils usually do not contain peroxidase in their granules. Heparin has many anionic, uniformly spaced sulphate groups that bind molecules of cationic dyes, such as toluidine blue, electrostatically (see Chapter 11). The aggregated toluidine blue molecules absorb light at a lower wavelength than the non-aggregated molecules and so appear red rather than blue. This change in the colour of a dye after it binds to tissue components is termed *metachromasia* (Greek *meta*, after; *chrōma*, colour). Basophils are the rarest of all the blood cells; they are largely absent from tissues under physiological conditions. Their lifespan in circulation is less than 2 weeks. They express receptors for a special class of immunoglobulin molecules (IgE; see Chapter 8). Basophils resemble mast cells, which will be described shortly, and the two cell types have similar functions but are not different stages of the same lineage.

Monocytes and macrophages

While erythrocytes and platelets hardly qualify as cells and granulocytes, with their oddly shaped shrunken nuclei, give the impression of tottering on the grave's edge, monocytes and lymphocytes are very healthy in appearance and, indeed, can live for months or even years. The monocyte is the largest of all the blood cells, measuring about 15 μm in diameter (see Fig. 4.7). It has a kidney-shaped nucleus that occupies approximately half of the cell volume, the depression in the nucleus being caused by the centrosome located in it. The chromatin is arranged in a characteristic 'raked' pattern of fine parallel strands (see Fig. 4.8). The cytoplasm, which stains greyish-blue with Giemsa, contains a variable number of fine, pink or purple-staining granules. Often the granules are so numerous that they give the cytoplasm a pink hue. The surface of a monocyte is ruffled like a bloodhound's face. The ruffling reduces repulsive forces between the monocyte and other cells or surfaces and provides surplus membrane necessary for locomotion and phagocytosis. When isolated and placed in a culture vessel, monocytes adhere to and spread over the glass surface. In the flattened monocyte, the nucleus and the granules are in the centre while the periphery contains a clear cytoplasm. The edges of the attached monocytes undulate like the 'wings' of a stingray. When it is on the move, the monocyte assumes a hand-mirror shape with the 'handle' (*uropod*) trailing behind the body (*protopod*; Fig. 4.11). The surfaces of monocytes are studded with receptors for the Fc region of immunoglobulin molecules and for complement factors, as well as with molecules used for adherence to platelets, lymphocytes, endothelial cells and extracellular matrix (see Chapter 21).

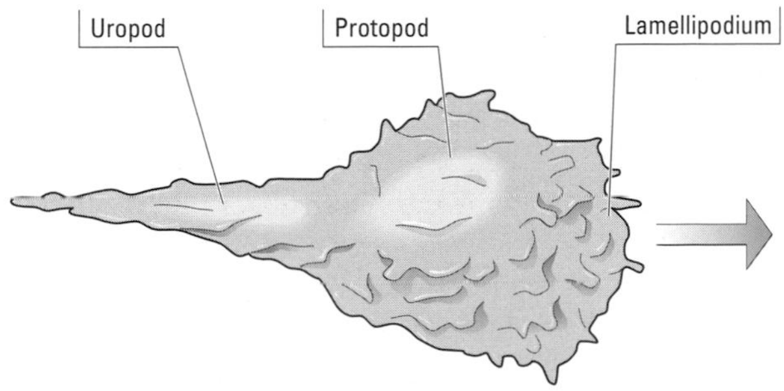

Figure 4.11 Monocyte in motion. The front moves forwards (arrow) like a wave towards the beach and then turns backwards as it hits the 'sand'.

In the embryo, monocytes are among the first blood cells to appear in the yolk sac. In an adult individual, monocytes leave the bone marrow in a relatively immature stage and then stay in the blood for about 3 days. The total number of monocytes in human blood is approximately 1.7×10^9 cells or about 1–6% of all blood leucocytes. Only about 1% of the circulating cells proliferate but they are all capable of phagocytosis.

Some of the monocytes leave the blood randomly at different sites, while others adhere to the walls of the sinuses in organs such as liver, spleen, lymph node, pituitary gland and adrenal gland. The sinus-lining populations interact with the underlying endothelial cells and are ideally poised to stop any pathogens that may have invaded these organs. The monocytes that leave the circulation marginate, adhere to the slimy inner surface of the capillary and postcapillary venule with the help of adhesion molecules, and scrabble around until they find the junction of two endothelial cells (see Chapters 9 & 21). They then squeeze through by diapedesis, in the same way as neutrophils. Monocytes are leaving the circulation all the time; however, their emigration is markedly enhanced in response to tissue injury or infection. On the other side of the capillary, the monocytes transform into *macrophages*. They swell to five to ten times their original size, heighten their phagocytic capacity, increase the content of hydrolytic enzymes in their lysosomes, increase the number of mitochondria to supply more energy and enlarge their Golgi apparatus to produce more lysosomes.

Once in the tissues, the macrophages have two options: they either take up residence in the tissue or they turn into wandering cells. How they make the choice is not known. Macrophages that opt for settling down send out small branches (dendrites) by which they affix themselves in the particular place, i.e. they become *fixed macrophages*. However, their residence is not completely permanent. When the need arises, as for example in the case of a nearby infection, they lift their anchors and set sail for another outpost. In different parts of the body, the fixed macrophages are often given alternative names. In the connective tissues under the skin or around muscles they are called *histiocytes* ('tissue cells'), in the spleen *littoral cells*, in the liver *Kupffer cells*, in the brain *microglial cells*, in the kidney *mesangial cells*, in the lungs *alveolar macrophages* and in the erythropoietic islands of the bone marrow *nurse cells*. The resident macrophages retain their ability to proliferate.

The wandering or *free macrophages* crawl incessantly through tissues (mainly connective tissues) looking for something to devour. They are scattered all over the body and they respond to stimuli such as infection or even food consumption. If you happen to be munching a chocolate bar while you are reading this book, then at this very moment several million macrophages are leaving the lymph nodes in the walls of your intestine to enter the tract and help unload the cargo.

Free macrophages are large cells, 25–50 μm in diameter, with long processes called *lamellipodia*[3] and numerous finger-like projections (*microvilli*) on the surface. Like monocytes, macrophages have a propensity to adhere to and spread over glass surfaces. When a *vital stain* (i.e. a dye that stains living cells) such as trypan blue is injected into an animal, it is taken up by the macrophages and sequestered into their granules, which then stand out as deeply stained. Macrophages have two populations of granules. The first population is made up of modified lysosomes, analogous to the azurophilic granules in neutrophils. These granules contain many hydrolytic enzymes that are used for the digestion of material taken up by phagocytosis (see Chapters 15 & 21). The second population is characterized by the absence of the enzyme alkaline phosphatase. Like neutrophils and monocytes, macrophages express a variety of receptors on the cell surface (Fc and complement receptors, among others) that help them to ingest microorganisms.

Macrophages are cells with an insatiable appetite for particles, foreign or self. True to their name, these 'big eaters' swallow and digest the ingested particles by releasing the contents of lysosomes on to them, and what they cannot digest they regurgitate (see Chapter 15 for further details). Unlike neutrophils, which die when satiated with ingested material, macrophages keep on ingesting, digesting and regurgitating. Sometimes, when the ingested particles prove impossible to digest (as for example in the case of the bacterium that causes tuberculosis), several macrophages fuse together to form *giant cells* that trap the offender (see Chapter 21).

Macrophages, however, are also the body's scavengers. They devour diseased or battered erythrocytes, exhausted neutrophils and pieces of dead cells. Macrophages manufacture and secrete a large assortment of biologically active compounds that mediate and regulate a number of reactions participating in the body's defence (see Chapters 11 & 21). Macrophages also initiate specific immune responses by taking up foreign proteins, degrading them into peptides and presenting some of the peptides to the T lymphocytes (see Chapters 6 & 16). Finally, when activated, macrophages can kill some tumour as well as other cells.

Together with monocytes, macrophages, free or fixed, form a dense network poised to capture any 'fish' that has slipped through the nets of the other trapping mechanisms. The network is referred to as the *mononuclear phagocyte system* (MPS) or the *reticuloendothelial system* (RES). The current concept of the RES, however, differs from the original one. Researchers once believed that all cells that stained with vital dyes acquired the dyes by phagocytosis. When they injected a vital dye into an animal, they found that, in addition to fixed macrophages, free macrophages and monocytes, the reticular cells of the lymphoid tissue and the endothelial cells of the vascular system were also stained. They therefore assumed that these last two cell types were also phagocytic and that they were developmentally related to the monocytes and macrophages. Hence researchers included all these cells in the reticuloendothelial system. We now know, however, that the reticular and endothelial cells are incapable of phagocytosis and are unrelated to monocytes and macrophages. There is therefore no longer any reason to call the system 'reticuloendothelial', but the name persists. Today's RES consists of monocytes and macrophages; the exclusion of neutrophils from the RES is illogical, but then so is the term 'reticuloendothelial system'.

Cells with uncertain affinities

The cells described thus far (and the lymphocytes to be described in the next chapter) have two characteristics in common: first, they are all derived from a common haemopoietic stem cell in the bone marrow; and second, they spend a significant portion of their career in the bloodstream and hence qualify as 'blood cells'. The two cell types described next share at least one of these characteristics with the blood cells: the *mast cells* do not circulate with the blood in any significant numbers but they may be derived from the same progenitor as granulocytes; and the *dendritic cells* are present in the blood and perhaps even share a haemopoietic stem cell with the other blood cells.

Mast cells

While comparing blood smears and tissue sections, Paul Ehrlich noticed cells in the latter that resembled basophils, yet were clearly distinct from them. Because the cells were particularly abundant in tissues of well-fed animals, he called them *Mastzellen* (German *Mast* means 'fattening material'). Mast cells resemble basophils in more than one

[3] Lamellipodium (Latin *lamella*, a thin leaf; Greek *pous*, foot) is a sheet-like extension of cytoplasm that forms transient adhesions with cell substrate.

way. Like basophils, mast cells stain with basic dyes such as toluidine blue, whose colour they then change (they display metachromasia). The staining is caused by cytoplasmic granules with a content similar to that of basophil granules, and dominated by heparin and histamines (Fig. 4.12). Like basophils, mast cells express cell surface receptors for IgE molecules and degranulate when activated by IgE binding. The degranulation releases potent chemical mediators implicated in a wide spectrum of immunological processes (see Chapters 11 & 21). The important differences between these two cell types are summarized in Table 4.1. These differences clearly establish that mast cells are not simply a variant of basophils. While basophils mature in the bone marrow, circulate in the blood and migrate into the tissues, mast cells mature outside the bone marrow and the blood. The mast cell progenitor, which may be derived from the same stem cell as all the blood cells, leaves the bone marrow early during its differentiation, enters the bloodstream and then invades the connective tissue, where it matures. Even after their maturation, some mast cells retain an extensive proliferation potential. Their lifespan is believed to range from 8 to 18 days.

In rodents, there are at least two subsets (types) of mast cells, connective-tissue type and mucosal type. *Connective-tissue type mast cells* (CTMC) are present in the skin, peritoneal cavity, lymphoid organs and lungs. They are particularly abundant around large and small blood vessels. They contain heparin, store large amounts of histamine and exhibit little or no dependence on T-lymphocyte-derived factors. *Mucosal-type mast cells* (MMC) are prominent in the mucosal layer of the digestive tract. They lack heparin, contain small quantities of histamine and are exquisitely sensitive to T-lymphocyte regulation. The two mast cell types can probably interchange ('transdifferentiate'), their phenotypes being determined by the microenvironment in which their final differentiation occurs. Mast cells play an important part in host defence against intestinal worm infection and dermal tick infection, as well as in wound healing and allergic diseases (see Chapters 21 & 23).

Dendritic cells

As the name implies, the main feature of dendritic cells are the long, branched, cytoplasmic processes (Greek *dendron*, tree; Fig. 4.13). In the tissues there are many unrelated cells with this appearance, and here's the rub: How does one tell them apart? At present, dendritic cells are most reliably identified by their function, less reliably by their molecular markers and least reliably by their morphology. Their function is to capture foreign proteins, process them and, while doing this, migrate to local lymphoid tissue where there are large numbers of T lymphocytes. In this tissue, the dendritic cells engage the T lymphocytes, adhere to them and activate them, thus initiating a local immune response. Although other cells, particularly monocytes, macrophages and B lymphocytes, can also stimulate T lymphocytes in this way, dendritic cells are the best at this by far (see Chapter 16). Their 'phenotype' (the combination of molecular markers they carry on their surfaces) is an adaptation to this function: dendritic cells express a variety of adhesion molecules

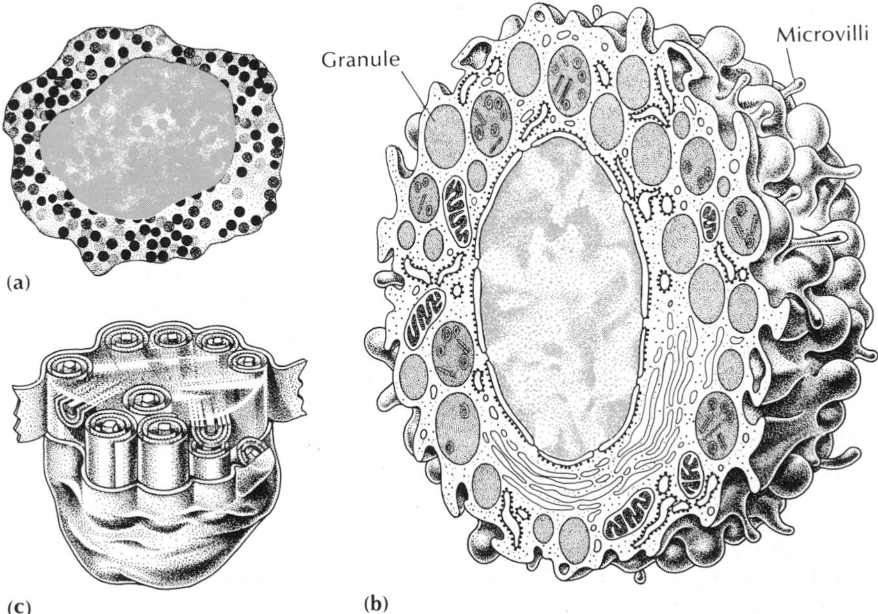

Figure 4.12 Mast cells viewed with the aid of a light (a) and electron microscope (b). (c) Section through a granule. (a, Modified from Bessis, M. (1977) *Blood Smears Reinterpreted*. Springer International, Berlin; b and c, from Krstić, R.V. (1978) *Die Gewebe des Menschen und der Säugetiere*. Springer-Verlag, Berlin.)

Table 4.1 Comparison of basophil and mast cell characteristics.

Characteristic	Basophil	Mast cell
Distribution	Blood	Connective tissue, mucosa
Size (diameter)	10–12 μm	20–30 μm
Glycogen aggregates	Yes	No
Cell surface	Short, blunt microvilli	Thin, elongated folds
Nucleus	Bilobed	Unsegmented
Granules	Few, large (1.5 μm)	Many, small (0.5 μm)
Chloroacetate esterase reaction	Negative	Positive
Chromatin condensed on the periphery of the nucleus	Yes	No
Mitotic activity	No	Yes

necessary for the interaction with T lymphocytes as well as MHC molecules required for the presentation of peptides to the T-cell receptors; one of their most characteristic markers is CD83. In contrast to monocytes and macrophages, dendritic cells lack or express only low levels of receptors for complement factors and immunoglobulins, have a low content of certain enzymes, such as non-specific esterases and acid phosphatases, and are poor at phagocytosis but good at endocytosis.

In humans, dendritic cells have been found in every organ of the body with the exception of the brain and the cornea. Although normally present in low numbers, they form an extensive network that pervades the entire body. In some organs and tissues they bear different names and immunologists are still debating whether they are all of the same type, variants of one basic type or different cells. In the skin, they are called *Langerhans' cells* after the German histologist Paul Langerhans (1847–1888); they are not to be confused with islet cells of the pancreas, also discovered by Langerhans. Langerhans' cells form a three-dimensional network in the epidermis but some can also be found in the dermis. They are intimately associated with nerve endings and were initially thought to be part of the nervous system. A characteristic feature of Langerhans' cells is the presence of *Birbeck granules* in their cytoplasm, which are membrane-bound bodies that resemble a tennis racquet with a characteristically striated 'handle' on cross-section (see Fig. 4.13). Their granules are formed by protrusions from the Golgi apparatus but their content and function are unknown.

Some of the Langerhans' cells, in particular those that have come into contact with foreign matter, migrate into the skin-draining lymphatic vessels and assume the morphology of *veiled cells* characterized, as the name indicates, by the development of numerous extensions in the form of flaps or 'veils'. Their origin is revealed in some of them by the persistence of rudimentary Birbeck granules. The cells are then brought, via afferent lymphatics, into the local

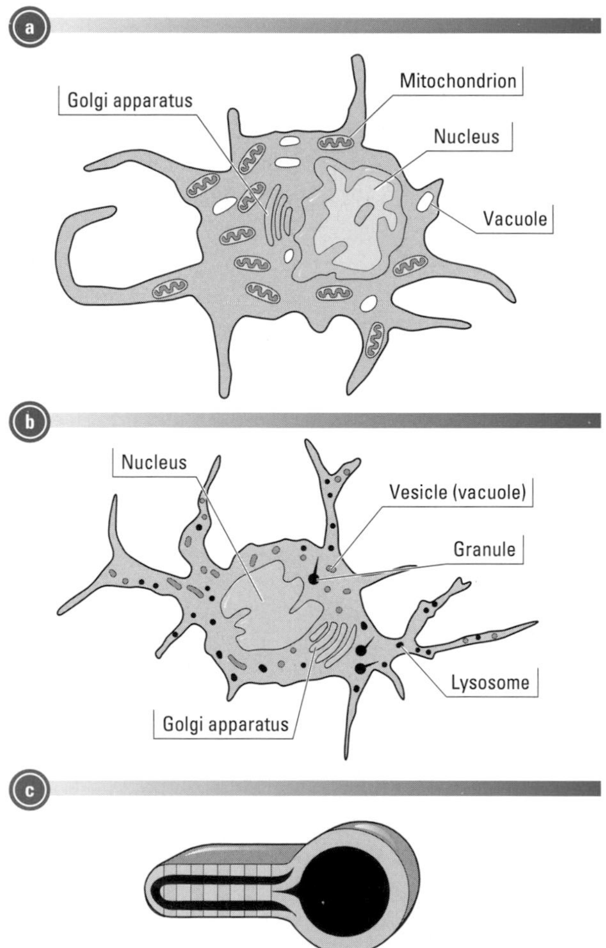

Figure 4.13 Dendritic (a) and Langerhans' (b) cells observed with the aid of an electron microscope. A characteristic of the Langerhans' cell is the Birbeck granule (c), which is disc-shaped and expanded at one end into a vesicle. On sections, the disc portion shows characteristic striation.

lymph nodes, where they settle down in the interfollicular lymphoid tissue of the cortex, lose their Birbeck granules and become *interdigitating cells* ('interdigitation' in histology refers to the formation of cell processes that extend towards and between similar processes of neighbouring cells, like fingers of one hand that are pushed between the fingers of the other.)

The interdigitating dendritic cells must be distinguished from *follicular dendritic cells* (FDC) of the lymph node. Although both are termed 'dendritic' on account of their dendritic morphology, they are two very different cell types. Like the interdigitating dendritic cells, follicular dendritic cells bind foreign matter but do not process it as 'true' dendritic cells do. Instead, they keep it on their surface and transport it to places where it can be picked up and processed by other cells, especially B lymphocytes. The two dendritic cell types are probably of different origin. The FDC are not derived from the bone marrow.

Not only in the skin but also in other organs and tissues, dendritic cells can be organized into meshwork that fills the spaces or *interstices* of these organs. They are therefore summarily referred to as *interstitial dendritic cells.* Particularly rich meshworks of interstitial dendritic cells can be found in the mucosa, the liver and the lungs. Under the influence of the local microenvironment, the characteristics of the cells in these organs may vary somewhat. And, of course, dendritic cells are abundant in all lymphoid organs. *Lymphoid dendritic cells* may again differ somewhat in their properties from the interstitial cells and between the different lymphoid organs. It is now believed, however, that all these variable cells are derived from a common progenitor cell in the bone marrow that might be related to the progenitor of the myeloid cells. After maturation in the bone marrow, the newly formed dendritic cells enter the bloodstream, circulate for an unspecified period of time and then enter the various tissues, where they may develop tissue-specific characteristics.

Further reading

Abrahamson, J.S. & Wheeler, J.G. (eds) (1993) *The Neutrophil.* IRL Press, Oxford.

Bazan, J.F. (1990) Haemopoietic receptors and helical cytokines. *Immunology Today*, **11**, 350–354.

Bessis, M. (1977) *Blood Smears Reinterpreted.* Springer International, Berlin.

Beutler, E. *et al.* (eds) (1995) *Williams Hematology*, 5th edn. MacGraw-Hill, New York.

D'Andrea, A.D. (1994) Hematopoietic growth factors and the regulation of differentiative decisions. *Current Opinion in Cell Biology*, **6**, 804–808.

Dexter, T.M. & Spooncer, E. (1987) Growth and differentiation in the hemopoietic system. *Annual Reviews in Cell Biology*, **3**, 423–441.

Dexter, T.M., Garland, J.M. & Testa, N.G. (eds) (1990) *Colony-stimulating Factors. Molecular and Cellular Biology.* Marcel Dekker, New York.

Dzierzak, E. & Medvinsky, A. (1995) Mouse embryonic hematopoiesis. *Trends in Genetics*, **11**, 359–366.

Galli, S.J., Dvorak, A.M. & Dvorak, H.F. (1984) Basophils and mast cells: morphologic insights into their biology, secretory patterns, and function. *Progress in Allergy*, **34**, 1–141.

Gleich, G.J. & Adolphson, C.R. (1986) The eosinophilic leukocyte: structure and function. *Advances in Immunology*, **39**, 177–253.

Golde, D.W. & Gasson, J.C. (1988) Hormones that stimulate the growth of blood cells. *Scientific American*, July, 34–42.

Hoffman, R. *et al.* (eds) (1995) *Hematology: Basic Principles and Practice*, 2nd edn. Churchill Livingstone, New York.

Jandl, J.H. (ed) (1995) *Blood: Textbook of Hematology*, 2nd edn. Little, Brown, Boston, MA.

Keller, G. (1992) Hemopoietic stem cells. *Current Opinion in Immunology*, **4**, 133–139.

Metcalf, D. (1984) *Hemopoietic Colony Stimulating Factors.* Elsevier, Amsterdam.

Metcalf, D. (1992) Hemopoietic regulators. *Trends in Biochemical Science*, **17**, 286–289.

Peschle, C. (1987) *Normal and Neoplastic Blood Cells: From Genes to Therapy.* Annals of the New York Academy of Sciences, New York.

Spry, C.J.F. (1988) *Eosinophils.* Oxford University Press, Oxford.

Uchida, N., Fleming, W.H., Alpern, E.J. & Weissman, I.L. (1993) Heterogeneity of hematopoietic stem cells. *Current Opinion in Immunology*, **5**, 177–184.

Van Furth, R. (1980) *Mononuclear Phagocytes: Functional Aspects.* Martinus Nijhoff, The Hague.

Van Furth, R. (1992) *Mononuclear Phagocytes: Biology of Monocytes and Macrophages.* Kluwer Academic Publishers, Dordrecht, The Netherlands.

Whetton, A.D. & Dexter, T.M. (1993) Influence of growth factors and substrates on differentiation of haemopoietic stem cells. *Current Opinion in Cell Biology*, **5**, 1044–1049.

Williams, D. & Nathan, D.G. (eds) (1991) The molecular biology of hematopoiesis. *Seminars in Hematology*, **28** (2), 114–176.

Williams, L.A., Egner, W. & Hart, D.N.J. (1994) Isolation and function of human dendritic cells. *International Review of Cytology*, **153**, 41–103.

chapter 5 Lymphocytes

What is a lymphocyte?

Morphologically, lymphocytes are a rather undistinguished bunch. They are small cells, usually no larger than 5 μm in diameter when alive and free, although when they are flattened on glass, as in blood smears, they measure between 8 and 12 μm in diameter. Only a small number of blood lymphocytes (< 2%) are larger in size, constituting the population of *intermediate* and *large lymphocytes* (see Fig. 4.7). A conspicuous feature of the *small lymphocytes* is that the round, slightly indented nucleus occupies some 90% of the cell volume. The nuclear chromatin is densely packed in coarse, heavily staining masses, which is a feature characteristic of cells with very low gene activity. The thin rim of agranular cytoplasm contains many free ribosomes (which give it a light blue hue on Giemsa-stained preparations), but almost no endoplasmic reticulum and only a poorly developed Golgi system.

On scanning electron micrographs, lymphocytes resemble chestnuts, with small finger-like projections (microvilli) extending from their surfaces (Fig. 5.1). In contrast to monocytes and macrophages, lymphocytes do not display any folds, ridges or ruffled membranes. The number of microvilli depends not only on the functional state of the cell but also on its handling by the scientist; under certain circumstances, some lymphocytes may appear almost bald. Like monocytes, lymphocytes move actively through tissues by pushing their bodies (protopods) forwards and dragging their 'feet' (uropods) behind them (see Fig. 4.11).

In the blood, lymphocytes are, after neutrophils, the most numerous white blood cells, representing from 20 to 45% of all leucocytes. One microlitre of human blood contains some 2500 lymphocytes and the adult human body contains approximately 10^{12} lymphocytes. Only a small fraction of this large number, however, has any semblance of permanence; most lymphocytes are ephemeral appearances with some 10^{9} lymphocytes being generated by the bone marrow per day and about the same number dying every day, largely in the lymphoid tissues.

Lymphocyte heterogeneity

Under the microscope, all lymphocytes look alike, differing only in size, number of cell-surface microvilli and other physiologically variable features; yet under this surface of morphological homogeneity is hidden a whole universe of amazing heterogeneity. First, the lymphocytes fall into three large *sets*, the T, B and natural killer (NK) cells. The NK cells constitute a special category that has only recently been demonstrated definitively to constitute a lymphocyte set. We will therefore leave their description until the end of the chapter and focus first on T and B cells. The T and B sets are split into *subsets* defined by a variety of criteria. Finally, each subset is a mosaic of *clones*, each clone expressing a receptor specific for a different antigenic epitope.

Lymphocyte sets

How can we distinguish these cells from one another when, morphologically, they all look the same? The answer lies in the magic word 'marker'. Most of the markers that differentiate lymphocyte sets, subsets, sub-subsets and clones have

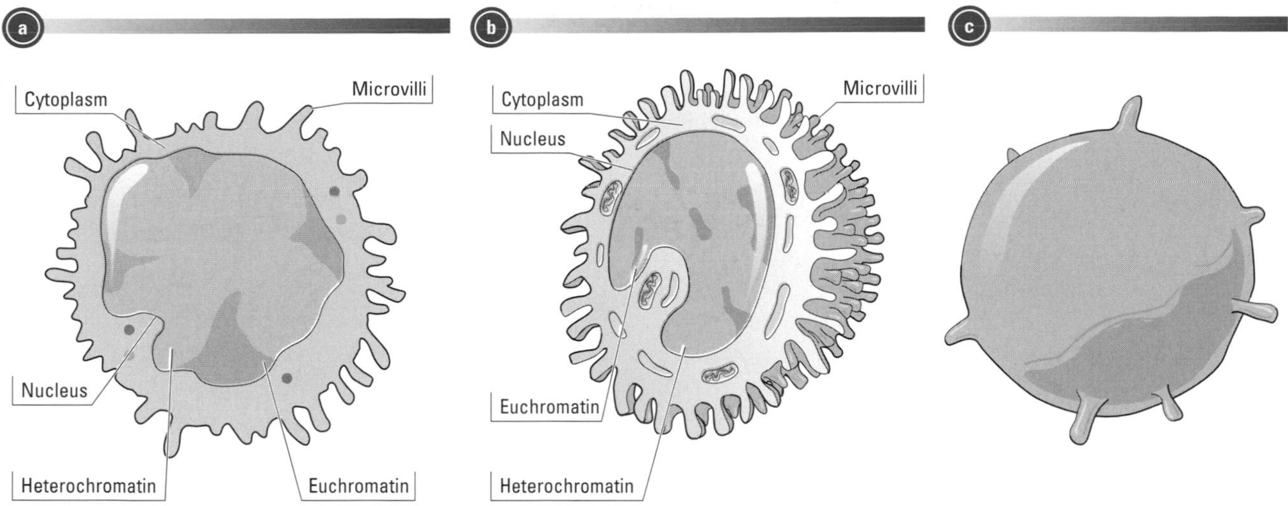

Figure 5.1 Lymphocyte viewed with the aid of a light microscope (a) and an electron microscope (b, c). Two functional states of lymphocyte surface are shown: (b) with microvilli and (c) smooth.

been identified with the help of antibodies (Table 5.1). In humans, such antibodies are raised almost exclusively by immunizing other species, usually the mouse or rabbit, against human lymphocytes (i.e. by *xenogeneic immunization*). In animals, some of the antibodies are produced by the immunization of a given individual with lymphocytes of another individual of the same species (i.e. by *allogeneic immunization*). These immunizations take advantage of differences in the cell-surface molecules between species (*xenoantigens*) or between individuals of the same species (*alloantigens*). The antigens identified in the individual laboratories are first given a working designation, which can be anything that tickles the fancy of the particular investigator. Later, they are assigned an official name according to certain rules set by nomenclature committees. In humans, the antibodies are submitted to the International Workshop on Leukocyte Differentiation Antigens, which meets periodically to compare the submitted reagents. Antibodies that satisfy the specified criteria for the definition of a new antigen are officially recognized and the identified antigen is assigned the CD symbol, which means neither 'certificate of deposit' nor 'corps diplomatique' but *cluster of differentiation* (read 'a group of antibodies that react with the same antigen'), and is then given the next available serial number. The known CD antigens are listed in Appendix 3. In the mouse, antigens expressed exclusively or predominantly on lymphocytes are designated by the symbol Ly, combined with a serial number. Some 40 Ly antigens, controlled by different genes, have been described and designated Ly1 to Ly40. For historical reasons, an additional seven antigens, expressed predominantly on B lymphocytes, are designated

Table 5.1 Markers distinguishing human T and B lymphocytes.

		Expression on cells	
Marker	Function	T	B
TCR	Antigen receptor	+	–
BCR	Antigen receptor	–	+
CD2	Adhesion receptor (SRBC R)	+	–
CD3	Part of TCR complex	+	–
CD4	MHCII co-receptor HIV receptor	(+)	(–)
CD5	Adhesion/signalling receptor (CD72R)	+	(+)
CD6	Adhesion receptor (?)	+	–
CD8	MHCI co-receptor	(+)	–
CD19	Part of the CR2 complex	–	+
CD20	Ca^{2+} channel	–	+
CD21	CR2, EBV receptor adhesion receptor (binds CD23)	–	(+)
CD22	Adhesion receptor (lectin)	–	(+)
CD32	FcγRII	–	+
CD49c	Component of the laminin receptor (CD49c/CD29 or VLA-3)	–	+
CD72	Adhesion receptor (CD5)	–	+
CD79α,β	Parts of BCR complex	–	+
CD80	Ligand of CD28	–	+
CD121a	IL-1 receptor	+	–

BCR, B-cell receptor; CD, cluster of differentiation; CR, complement receptor; EBV, Epstein–Barr virus; HIV, human immunodeficiency virus; IL, interleukin; MHCI (II), major histocompatibility complex class I (II); R, receptor; SRBC, sheep red blood cells; TCR, T-cell receptor; VLA, very late antigen; (+) indicates expression on a lymphocyte subset.

Lyb2 to Lyb8; and one antigen expressed predominantly on thymocytes is designated Thy1 (the human homologue of Thy1 is CDw90). Individual Ly epitopes (determinants) are designated by Arabic numerals separated from the antigen symbol by a period (e.g. Ly1.1, Ly1.2, Ly2.1, etc.). Alleles are referred to by lower case letter superscripts (e.g. *Ly1^a*, *Ly1^b*, *Ly2^a*, etc.). However, whenever an Ly antigen is shown to be a mouse homologue of a human CD antigen, the Ly symbol is changed to mCD.

There are at least five CD antigens that are expressed on nearly all *human T lymphocytes* but are absent on most other cells, including B lymphocytes: CD2, CD3, CD6, CD7 and CDw121a. The most convenient marker of *mouse T lymphocytes* is the *thymus 1* or *Thy1 antigen*. It occurs in two forms: Thy1.1 controlled by the *Thy1^a* allele and Thy1.2 controlled by the *Thy1^b* allele, which differ by a single amino acid. Genetically pure mouse strains express either one or the other of the two forms. The antigen is also expressed on brain cells and on a few other cells as well. Interestingly, its human homologue (CDw90) is expressed on brain cells but not on lymphocytes.

Table 5.2 Organ distribution of human T and B lymphocytes.

	% Lymphocytes	
Organ	T	B
Thymus	>99	<0.5
Lymph node	75	25
Spleen	33	66
Blood	55–75	15–30
Bone marrow	5	>75

Most of the *human B lymphocytes* express the CD19, CD20, CD49c, CD72, CD79α, β and CD80 antigens, which are not expressed on T lymphocytes or other cells. The proportions of T and B cells in different human organs are given in Table 5.2.

Lymphocyte subsets

T lymphocytes can be divided into subsets according to the constitution as well as specificity of their antigen receptors, the markers they express and the function they carry out (Fig. 5.2). According to the *composition of the T-cell receptor* (TCR), T lymphocytes fall into two categories, α:β T cells and γ:δ T cells, the former expressing receptors composed of α and β polypeptide chains and the latter of γ and δ chains (see Chapter 7). The α, β, γ and δ chains are encoded in separate genes. In the mature T lymphocyte pool, α:β T cells constitute the majority and γ:δ T cells the minority.

The *specificity of the α:β TCR* distinguishes T lymphocytes into those that recognize peptides presented by class I major histocompatibility complex (MHC) molecules (they are said to be *class I restricted*), and those that recognize peptides presented by class II MHC molecules (they are said to be *class II restricted*). The γ:δ T cells can also recognize the antigen alone, without the participation of MHC molecules. Mature human α:β T lymphocytes fall into two main subsets defined by the *CD4* and *CD8* molecules, $CD4^+CD8^-$ and $CD4^-CD8^+$, which constitute about 60% and 40% of the cells, respectively. In addition, mouse α:β T lymphocytes consist of a minor subset of $CD4^-CD8^-$ cells, which in humans is still poorly defined.

Based on their *function*, α:β T lymphocytes can be divided into at least two subsets, helper T cells and

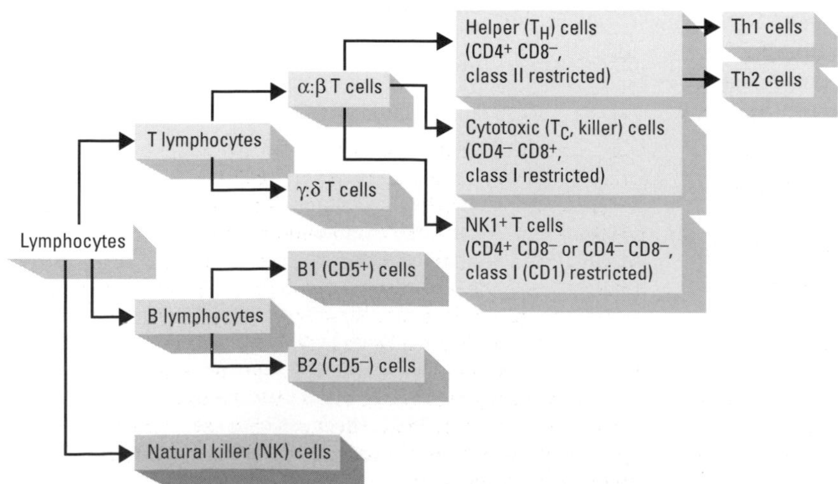

Figure 5.2 Classification of human lymphocytes. T_H lymphocytes can also be class I restricted and $CD4^-CD8^+$; T_C lymphocytes can also be class II restricted and $CD4^+CD8^-$.

cytotoxic T cells. *Helper T (T_H) cells* are so designated because, upon activation, they secrete a number of *cytokines* that control and coordinate other cells participating in the ongoing immune response (see Chapter 10). The *cytotoxic T (T_C) cells*, when activated, acquire the capacity to lyse target cells carrying antigens recognized by their TCR. Although T_C cells may also secrete certain lymphokines, they do so to a lesser extent than T_H cells.

The relationship between the T-lymphocyte subsets defined by these criteria is complex but the rule of thumb is this: in the $\alpha:\beta$ T-cell subset the $CD4^+CD8^-$ cells are the T_H lymphocytes that recognize the antigen in the context of class II MHC molecules, while the $CD4^-CD8^+$ cells are the T_C lymphocytes that recognize the antigen in the context of class I MHC molecules (see Fig. 5.2).

The T_H subset is divided further into two sub-subsets, T_H1 and T_H2, according to a functional criterion (the molecules secreted by the cells upon stimulation). The *T_H1 cells* produce interleukin (IL)-2, interferon-γ (IFN-γ) and tumour necrosis factor-β (TNF-β)[1]. The *T_H2 cells* produce IL-4, IL-5, IL-6, IL-10 and IL-13. Both cells also produce other cytokines such as IL-3 and granulocyte macrophage colony-stimulating factor (GM-CSF). It is believed that T_H1 and T_H2 cells arise as a result of antigenic stimulation from precursor pT_H cells. There is also at least one other sub-subset, the *T_H0 cells,* which is capable of producing IL-2, IFN-γ and IL-4, as well as other cytokines; the *pT_H cells* produce IL-2, but not IFN-γ or IL-4. The relationship of T_H0 cells to T_H1 and T_H2 cells is controversial. In humans, the T_H0, T_H1 and T_H2 subsets are not well defined.

There are several exceptions to the rule of thumb, one of them being the set of *NK1+ T lymphocytes*, which has thus far been studied extensively only in mice. NK1 is a surface molecule of the NK cells that neither develop in the thymus nor express TCRs. The NK1+ T cells, by contrast, mature in the thymus (although perhaps not all of them) and express the $\alpha:\beta$ TCR. They are either $CD4^+CD8^-$ or $CD4^-CD8^-$. Like NK cells they have cytotoxic functions, but unlike NK cells they can only interact with target cells that express MHC class I molecules (some of them are therefore class I-restricted $CD4^+$ cytotoxic cells). The class I molecules are, however, of a special kind, differing in several properties from the classical MHC molecules (see the section on CD1 in Chapter 6 and Table 21.5 in Chapter 21). NK1+ T cells have the potential of secreting IL-4, IL-5, IL-10 and IFN-γ.

[1] *Interleukins* are cytokines secreted by lymphocytes, usually in response to stimulation. Cytokines are soluble molecules that act on other cells, influencing their growth and differentiation. *Interferons* are cytokines that induce cells to resist virus replication. *Tumour necrosis factors* are cytokines that, under certain circumstances, kill tumour cells. (For details of these cytokines see Chapter 10.)

They have been detected in the thymus and some non-lymphoid organs, in particular the liver, in which they constitute 40–50% of all lymphocytes; they also occur at a relatively high frequency in the bone marrow.

The *B lymphocytes* are divided into two subsets, B1 and B2 cells, by the presence or absence of the CD5 protein on their surfaces. The human CD5 (formerly Ly1 in the mouse) is primarily a T-cell antigen, but it is also expressed on a small subset of B lymphocytes, the $CD5^+$ or *B1 cells*, which

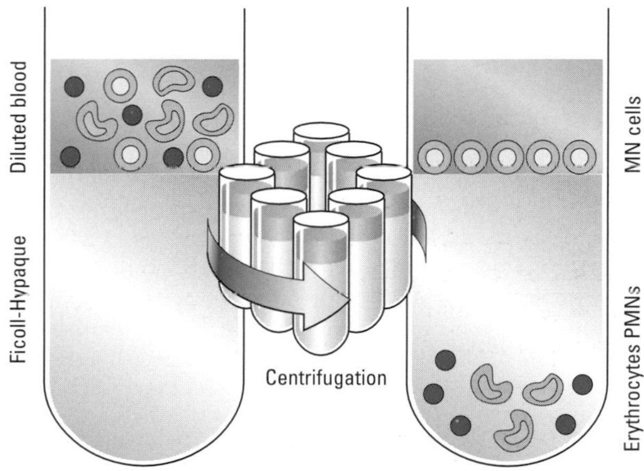

Figure 5.3 Isolation of human lymphocytes (and monocytes) by density centrifugation. A sample of peripheral blood (i.e. blood flowing through the vessels remote from the heart) that has been prevented from clotting by the addition of an anticoagulant (such as calcium disodium ethylenediaminetetraacetic acid, EDTA) and diluted appropriately with balanced salt solution is layered (without intermixing) over a column of Ficoll-Hypaque with sodium diatrizoate in a centrifuge tube. Ficoll is a synthetic, high molecular mass (M_r 400 000), extensively branched polymer of the disaccharide sucrose and epichlorohydrin, which is readily soluble in water. Sodium diatrizoate (M_r 635) is the sodium salt of 3,5-diacetamido-2,4,6-triiodobenzoic acid whose function is to provide optimal density and osmolarity:

COONa
I I
H_3C-C-N N-C-CH_3
O H I H O

Commercially available mixtures of the two compounds are manufactured under the trade names Ficoll-Paque or Ficoll-Hypaque (Pharmacia LKB). On centrifugation (typically at 400 *g* for 30–40 min) cells in the blood sample sediment towards the blood–Ficoll interface, where erythrocytes, on contact with Ficoll, aggregate and sink to the bottom of the tube. Polymorphonuclear (PMN) cells (granulocytes) also sediment through to the bottom of the Ficoll layer because of their density, whereas lymphocytes, monocytes (mononuclear or MN cells) and platelets, which do not have a density high enough to enter the Ficoll layer, accumulate at the interface, where they can be collected. Approximately 95% of the cells in the collected fraction are mononuclear leucocytes.

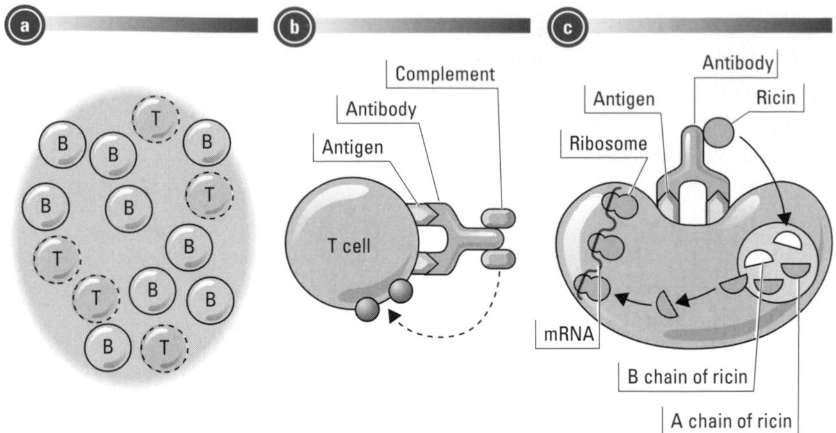

Figure 5.4 (a and b) Separation of T and B lymphocytes by complement-mediated cytotoxicity. Suspension of T and B lymphocytes is incubated together with complement and antibodies specific for a cell-surface antigen expressed on the former but not on the latter cells. (a) T lymphocytes are killed, B lymphocytes survive. (b) Antibody binds specifically to the antigen on the surface of a T lymphocyte and activates complement proteins, which then puncture the cell's plasma membrane. (c) Killing of cells by an immunotoxin, a hybrid molecule consisting of an antibody and a plant toxin, such as ricin, contained in an extract of castor beans. The molecule of ricin consists of two polypeptide chains: an A chain that is responsible for the toxin effect and a B chain that functions as a lectin with specificity for galactose-containing glycoproteins or glycolipids. After binding to a cell via the B chain, the ricin molecule is taken up by endocytosis, the two chains separate and the A chain enters the cytoplasm where it enzymatically inactivates the EF2-binding portion of the 60S ribosomal subunit. By preventing the binding of the elongation factor-2 to the ribosome, the A chain inhibits intracellular protein synthesis and thus kills the cell (see Chapter 6). To prepare an immunotoxin, the disulphide bond linking the A and B chains is cleaved and the isolated A chains are covalently attached to the antibody molecules. The antibody in the immunotoxin binds specifically to its corresponding cell-surface antigen and the complex is taken up by the cell; once inside the cell, the A chain escapes into the cytoplasm, thereby killing the cell. In the absence of the B chain, however, the killing is rather inefficient. An alternative method for constructing an immunotoxin is therefore to attach the entire ricin molecule to the antibody and to prevent the B chain from binding the immunotoxin to undesired cells by blocking its binding site with galactose.

are characterized by the expression of one type of cell-surface immunoglobulin (IgM) and virtual absence of another (IgD) (see Chapter 8). The CD5 protein is a receptor that binds the B-lymphocyte molecule CD72 (formerly Lyb2 in the mouse); it has been suggested that the binding promotes interaction between B cells. B1 cells of mice lacking the *CD5* gene are much more easily induced to proliferate as a result of signals received via that surface IgM than B1 cells of mice carrying the gene. The CD5 protein is therefore thought to act as a negative regulator of the IgM-induced growth signals. The CD72 molecule is expressed on all B lymphocytes. The $CD5^+$ B cells may arise from different progenitor cells than the $CD5^-$ cells and the two subsets seem to recognize different types of antigen (see Chapter 17 for further information). The $CD5^+$ lymphocytes dominate in the B-cell population of the peritoneal cavity[2] but they are rare in the spleen and lymph nodes. The majority of B lymphocytes are $CD5^-$ (the *B2 cells*).

[2] The peritoneum is the transparent membrane lining the abdominal cavity. The peritoneal cavity is the space between the peritoneum covering the abdominal walls and the peritoneum covering the viscera.

Additional heterogeneity of both B and T lymphocytes is a reflection of distinctive stages in their differentiation. These stages, often characterized by a specific combination of markers, are described later in this chapter.

Superimposed on the set and subset heterogeneity of lymphocytes is the *clonal heterogeneity*, which rests on the diversity of the antigen receptors, i.e. the TCR of T lymphocytes and the B-cell receptor (BCR) of B lymphocytes. The antigen receptors determine the *specificity* of individual lymphocytes, i.e. their ability to recognize and respond to particular antigens.

Methods of lymphocyte identification and separation

It is in the nature of the scientific method to take things apart and put them together again. To learn how lymphocytes behave under defined circumstances, it is necessary to separate them from other cells and to work with relatively pure populations. Immunologists working with animals have a ready source of lymphocytes in the lymphoid organs, especially lymph nodes. Although a cell suspension obtained by teasing out a lymph node is a far cry from a pure lymphocyte population, its lymphocyte content is sufficiently high for use in some types of experiments; if not, purification must follow. Human immunologists must satisfy themselves with palatine tonsils or, more commonly, with blood samples. To enrich them in lymphocytes, the samples are subjected to *density centrifugation* (Fig. 5.3). The method exploits the fact that blood cells differ in their density (weight relative to volume). Hence, when they are placed on the surface of a liquid of a specific density, those with density greater than that of the fluid will sink to the bottom of the tube when spun in a centrifuge, whereas those with lower density will gather at the liquid's surface. In this manner, lymphocytes and monocytes (mononuclear cells) can be separated from the rest of the blood cells.

A cell suspension enriched in lymphocytes can be separated into T- and B-cell populations and these into their subsets by one of several methods: immunocytotoxicity, (immuno)adhesion, rosetting, immunomagnetic beads or flow cytometry. *Immunocytotoxicity* is a method based on a principle exploited supremely well by many totalitarian governments, a principle of eliminating undesirable elements so that only the preferred ones are left. If B cells are required, all the T cells are killed and the remainder is harvested (Fig. 5.4a), whereas if T cells are needed all the B cells are obliterated. The hired killer, in this case, is complement, a system of proteins that assemble on the plasma membrane to form a tunnel connecting the outside with the inside of the cell (see Chapter 12). A cell with a punctured plasma membrane is like a leaky boat: it fills with water and dissolves (the cell is *lysed*). The creation of the tunnel is initiated by an antibody, which binds to a molecule on the cell's surface and then activates the first component of the complement system (Fig. 5.4b). To isolate T cells by this method one must therefore have an antibody that binds to a cell-surface antigen present on all B but not T lymphocytes, and to separate B cells one must have an antibody with just the opposite specificity. Some of the CD-specific antibodies are eminently suitable for this purpose. It is also possible to attach a toxin to the antibody by chemical means and thus to produce an *immunotoxin*, which then kills the cells without the participation of complement (Fig. 5.4c).

In the *nylon-wool separation method* (Fig. 5.5), a wad of artificial wool is packed into a syringe barrel and a suspension of lymphocytes is percolated through the jungle of threads. Because B lymphocytes, as well as most phagocytic cells and all dead cells, stick to the threads in greater numbers than T lymphocytes, the T cells that come out of the syringe are 95–98% pure.

In the *immunoadhesion method* the same idea is applied,

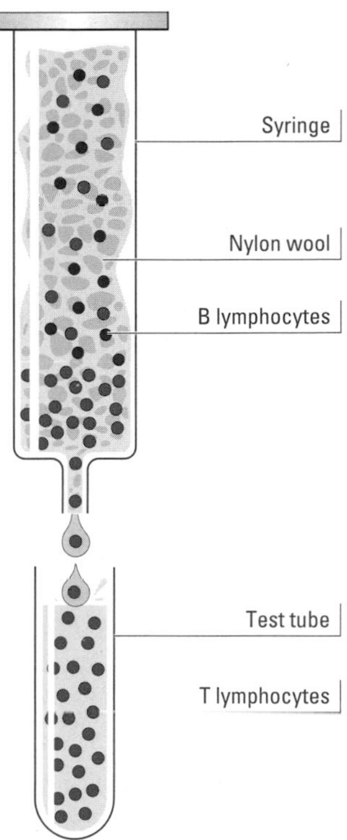

Figure 5.5 Separation of T and B lymphocytes by passing a cell suspension through a column of nylon wool. B lymphocytes adhere to the wool while T lymphocytes pass through.

except that instead of relying on some poorly defined 'stickiness' to nylon fibres, the surface of solid beads are coated with antibodies specific for either B or T lymphocytes. The beads are made of cross-linked dextran (Sephadex), agarose (Sepharose), polyacrylamide or glass. Although the antibodies stick non-specifically to the beads, a cleaner separation is achieved by attaching them chemically by their tails (Fig. 5.6a). The antibodies, like trapeze artists, then have their 'hands' free to grab the antigens on the cells that pass through the column of beads. The method is designed primarily for collecting cells that have passed through the column and for separating them from those that are retained. If the retained cells are to be collected, they must be unfastened by a change of pH to release the grasp of antigens by the antibodies. A variation of column immunoadhesion is the *panning* method (Fig. 5.6b). If you have ever been struck by 'gold fever', and that possibility is remote, you may know that 'panning' means 'to wash gravel in a pan, searching for gold'. The gold that immunologists seek is a pure lymphocyte set or subset and their pan is the Petri dish. When the dish is coated with appropriate antibodies, only cells carrying the corresponding antigen stick to it and the free cells can be removed by decantation.

In the *rosetting technique*, human lymphocytes are mixed

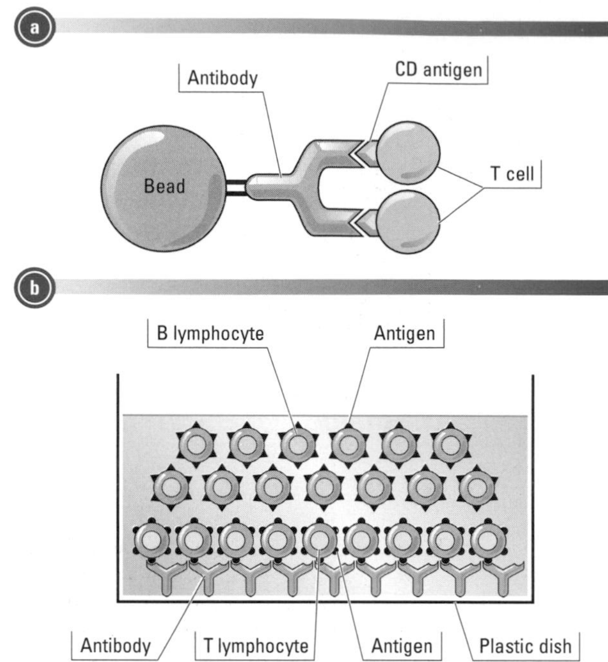

Figure 5.6 Separation of T and B lymphocytes on a column of antibodies coupled to beads (a) and by 'panning' (b). Antibodies specific for a T-lymphocyte antigen are attached to the surface of the bead or to a plastic dish. Only T lymphocytes bind to these antibodies; B lymphocytes pass through the column (a) or remain in suspension and can be poured off (decanted) from the dish (b). The beads, antibodies and cells as depicted are not drawn to scale. For the sake of simplicity, each cell is shown to bind one antibody only.

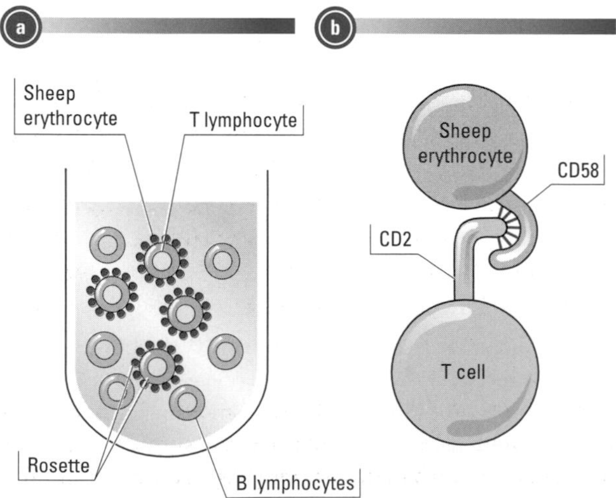

Figure 5.7 Separation of T and B lymphocytes by the rosetting technique. Sheep erythrocytes mixed with human lymphocytes bind to T cells but not to B cells, forming rosettes with the former (a); these can be removed from the cell suspension by centrifugation. The binding occurs between the CD2 molecule (the E-receptor) of the T cells and a CD58 molecule of the erythrocytes (b). The cells are not drawn to scale.

with sheep erythrocytes and the resulting miniature roses or *rosettes* (single lymphocytes surrounded by erythrocytes; Fig. 5.7) are separated from the rest of the suspension by centrifugation. The erythrocytes in the rosettes are then lysed and the lymphocytes recovered.

Immunomagnetic methods exploit the principle of immunoadhesion with a twist: the antibody-coated beads are made of a paramagnetic material[3]. Cells bearing the antigen recognized by the antibodies bind to the beads and can be separated from cells not bearing the antigen by holding the beads in place with a strong magnetic force while pouring off (decanting) the suspension (Fig. 5.8).

Flow cytometry is a technique for measuring and characterizing cells flowing individually through an aperture, where they are exposed to light or electric current. The cell properties are determined by their effects on the light beam (absorbance, reflection or emission of light of another wavelength) or by electrical transmission. The method can be used to identify cells in a mixture (*analytical flow cytometry*) or to separate different cell types from one another (*sorting*). A widely used instrument for cell separation is the *fluorescence-activated cell sorter* (FACS) (Fig. 5.9).

Development of T lymphocytes

The T-lymphocytic lineage is conceived in the bone marrow (fetal liver) and the T lymphocytes are raised and educated in the thymus. In the bone marrow (fetal liver), the same stem cell that gives rise to other blood cells also spawns the progenitor of the T lymphocyte, the founder of the T-lymphocytic lineage. The progenitor enters the bloodstream, which delivers it to the thymus and the rest of the development, all the way to the mature T lymphocyte, occurs in this organ. The mature T cell leaves the thymus by re-entering the bloodstream and spends the rest of its career circulating

[3] Any moving electric charge is surrounded by a magnetic field. The net magnetic effect of an atom with its elementary moving electric charges depends on the distribution and spin of its electrons. Materials can be divided into three groups according to their net magnetic effects: ferromagnetic, paramagnetic and diamagnetic. *Ferromagnetic materials*, from which magnets are made, contain domains in which the dipoles of the atoms are oriented in the same direction. The magnetic dipoles of all these atoms can easily be aligned when placed in a magnetic field and the materials themselves then become the source of strong, durable magnetic fields. *Paramagnetic materials* also consist of atoms that show a net magnetic effect, but these are not organized into domains. The dipoles of these atoms do become slightly aligned with an external field and the materials thus become magnetic but the magnetism quickly disappears after the removal of the field, when the atoms return to their original, unaligned orientation. Atoms of *diamagnetic materials* display a net magnetic effect only when placed in an external magnetic field and then it *opposes* that of the external field.

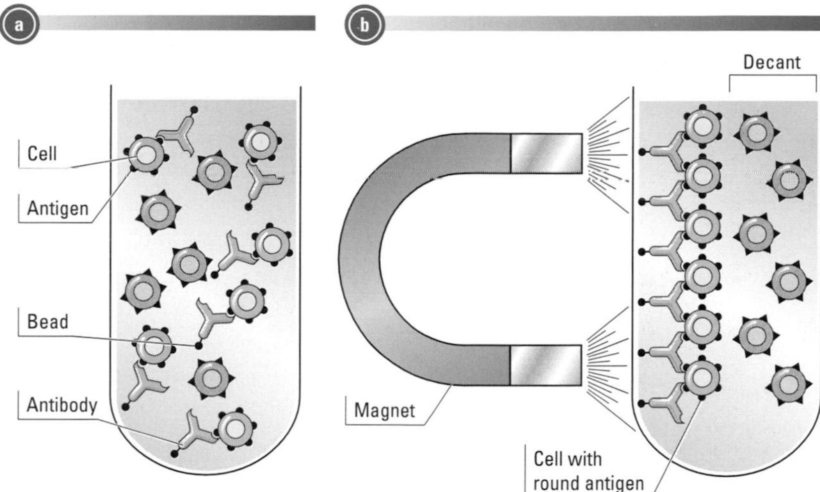

Figure 5.8 Immunomagnetic method of lymphocyte separation. (a) A lymphocyte suspension containing two types of cells distinguished by surface antigens (round or spiked symbols) is mixed with antibodies specific for the 'round' antigens. The antibodies, which have paramagnetic beads attached to them, bind to one of the two cell types. (b) The force of a strong magnetic field magnetizes the beads and pulls them to the wall of the tube, together with the attached antibody and the bound cell; the cells remaining in the suspension can then be poured off. Removal of the magnet releases the cells from the wall of the tube into the suspension, where they can be separated from the antibodies (and the beads) by a treatment that disrupts antigen–antibody interactions. The method thus involves both positive selection (antibody binding to the cells with the 'round' antigen) and negative selection (the absence of antibody binding to the cells with the 'spiked' antigen). The beads are produced by continuous *in situ* formation of iron oxides and hydroxides such as maghemite, γF_2O_3, inside the pores of highly porous polymeric spheres of the same size, typically between 2 and 5 μm. The process leads to the production of very small grains of oxides evenly distributed throughout the whole volume of the bead. At the end of the procedure, the pores of the beads are filled with polymeric material. The beads must not display even the slightest magnetic effect after exposure to a magnetic field because in the process of attaching antibodies to their surfaces they are repeatedly isolated by the use of a magnet, washed and then redispersed and any remaining magnetism would interfere with their redispersion. For this reason, paramagnetic rather than ferromagnetic material is used for the production of the beads (the former loses its magnetic properties quickly after removal of the magnetic field, but the latter does not). For simplicity, only one antibody molecule is shown to bind to each cell; in reality, many antibodies are involved. The beads, antibodies and cells are not drawn to scale.

through the body; it can apparently re-enter the thymus only when activated.

The function of the mature T lymphocyte is to recognize MHC-bound peptides and, if these are of non-self origin, to initiate the adaptive immune response. The most important event in the development of the T lymphocyte, and one that establishes the cell's identity, is therefore the assembly of the molecule capable of recognizing MHC-bound peptides, the TCR. The assembly occurs in two main steps: first, genetic information necessary for the synthesis of the TCR polypeptide chains is brought together by rearranging appropriate DNA segments; and second, two different chains are united into heterodimers; accessory molecules such as CD3 are added to the heterodimers and the entire complex is expressed on the cell surface. We will describe the process in detail in Chapter 7, but to accurately depict T-lymphocyte development a brief preview must be provided.

There are four chains to the TCR, α, β, γ and δ, which can assemble in two combinations (α:β) and (γ:δ). Their expression on the cell surface identifies the α:β T cells and the γ:δ T cells. Each polypeptide chain can be differentiated into three (α and γ) or four (β and δ) parts: V–J–C or V–D–J–C (the meaning of these symbols is explained in Chapter 7). Each of these parts is encoded in a separate DNA segment and the widely separated segments are brought together (*rearranged*) on the chromosome before a transcript that can be translated into a complete TCR chain is produced.

The chains are synthesized in the cytoplasm independently of each other. To reach the cell surface, they must associate either with their partner (β with α and γ with δ) or its surrogate (the β chain can associate with the so-called *pre-TCR alpha* or *pTCRα* chain, which is encoded in a distinct gene and is not directly related to any of the four TCR chains). They must also associate with another complex molecule, CD3, which is involved in signal transmission. On the cell surface, the α:β TCR heterodimers are co-expressed with their *co-receptors*, the CD4 or CD8 mole-

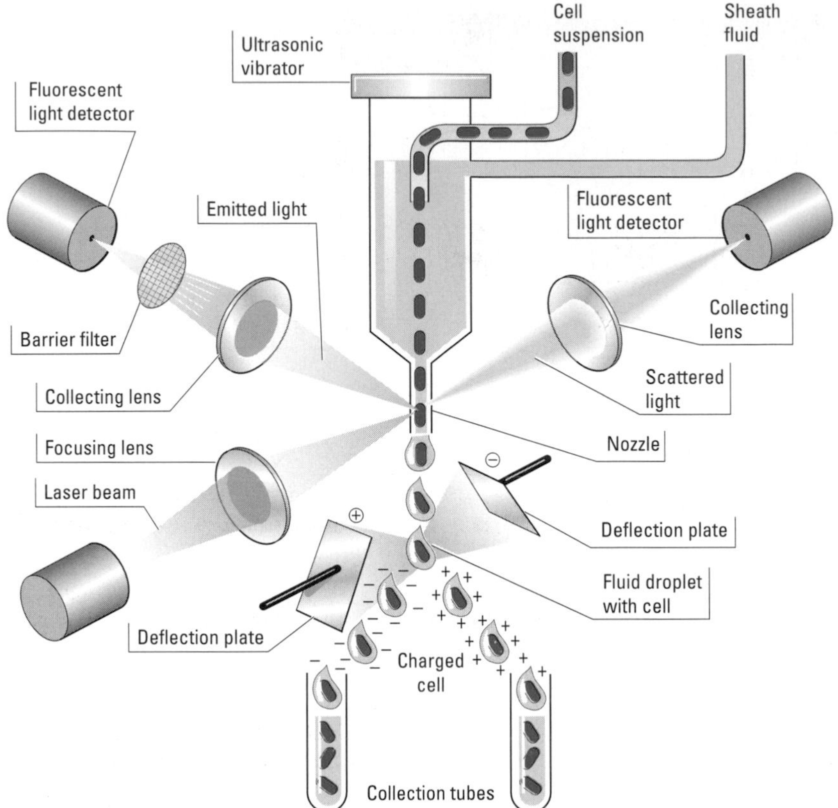

Figure 5.9 Cell sorting in the fluorescence-activated cell sorter (FACS). A suspension of cells is allowed to react with antibodies that are specific for particular molecules on the surface of one of the cell types in the mixture. The antibody has a fluorochrome attached to it. The suspension is then mixed with a buffer (sheath fluid) and droplets, each containing a single cell, are generated by ultrasonic vibrations in a nozzle. The droplets pass one by one through a laser beam, a beam of high-intensity light of a particular wavelength. As the beam hits the cell, two things happen. The fluorochrome molecules absorb the light but emit light of another wavelength (pink). The emitted light is focused by collecting lenses on a barrier filter, which only allow light of a certain wavelength to pass through. Light detectors (photomultipliers) placed behind the barrier filter can then record whether light of a given wavelength has been emitted from the cell and passed through the filter. At the same time, however, because of the cell curvature and surface unevenness, the light of the laser beam hits the cell at different angles and in turn is reflected from the cell at different angles, i.e. it is scattered. The character of the light scatter depends on the cell's size and density: the larger and denser the cell, the more light it scatters. The degree of light scatter is estimated by measuring light rays reaching the photomultipliers at two different angles in relation to the laser beam: a low angle (a forward scatter) and a right or obtuse angle (side scatter). The computer then uses these two estimates to determine the size and density of the cell. Based on this information and information regarding the emission of the fluorescent light, the computer checks whether the cell meets certain criteria for a particular cell type and, depending on the outcome, sends a signal to impart a certain electric charge to the droplet. As the droplets pass through an electric field generated by the deflection plates, they are sorted according to their charge and collected in tubes.

cules. The co-receptors recognize the invariant part of the MHC molecule and participate in signal transmission that follows this recognition. The γ:δ TCR heterodimers function without the CD4 and CD8 co-receptors.

Once expressed on the cell surface, the TCR becomes capable of binding its ligand. There is, however, a fundamental difference in the way the α:β TCR and the γ:δ TCR recognize their ligands and in the type of ligands they recognize. The α:β TCR recognizes peptides bound to the MHC molecule, together with part of the MHC molecule. The γ:δ TCR, on the other hand, may not be involved in MHC recognition at all; it may recognize its ligands independently of MHC.

The progression from progenitor cell to mature T lymphocyte involves sequential activation or inactivation of groups of genes and the corresponding expression or suppression of their products. Several of these genes (proteins) have been identified but the function of only some of them in this progression is known. They can all, however, be used as markers for differentiating individual stages. Besides the

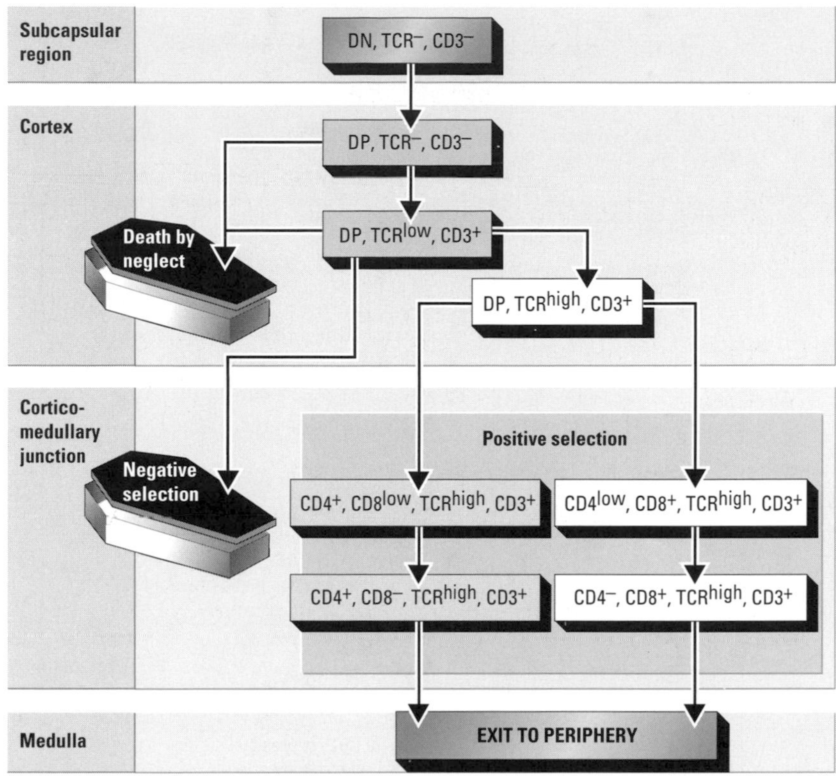

Figure 5.10 Thymocyte (α:β T-cell) development in the thymus. DN, double negative (CD4−CD8−); DP, double positive (CD4+CD8+); CD, cluster of differentiation; TCR, T-cell receptor.

genes controlling the different TCR chains and the chains of the co-receptors (CD4, CD8), there are genes involved in the regulation of cell growth (*protooncogenes*[4] such as *Lck*, *ZAP70* and *Fyn*); genes specifying enzymes necessary for the rearrangement of TCR DNA segments (*RAG1* and *RAG2*) or their further diversification (*terminal deoxynucleotidyltransferase* or *TdT*; see Chapter 7); *receptors for cytokines* (such as the IL-2 receptor, the α chain of which is also referred to as CD25); and *adhesion molecules* (such as CD2 and CD44; see Chapter 9).

[4] When defective, protooncogenes become *oncogenes* that can cause cells to grow continuously and to form tumours, hence their name (Greek *onkos*, mass, bulk, tumour). Some of the oncogenes were originally identified by their presence in tumour-causing retroviruses, which occasionally pick up the genes when they integrate into host cell DNA. The cellular (proto) and viral (mutated, abnormal) oncogenes are designated as c-*onc* and v-*onc*, respectively. Many of the oncogene designations are derived from the names of the corresponding retroviruses. One group of oncogenes, the *receptor protein tyrosine kinase* or *R–PTK* family, codes for cell-surface molecules that convert extracellular signals into intracellular ones: the activated receptors transfer the terminal phosphate group from adenosine triphosphate (ATP) to the hydroxyl group on the tyrosine residue of a particular intracellular protein and thus initiate a signal-transfer chain reaction; see Chapter 10.

After this preview, we now proceed with the description of T-cell development (Figs 5.10 and 5.11). The progenitor cells that arrive in the thymus from the fetal liver or bone marrow via the blood lack most of the cell-surface molecules that characterize mature T lymphocytes and their *TCR* genes have an unrearranged configuration. Their differentiation potential is uncertain. If they are taken out of the thymus, they give rise to lymphocytes and to NK cells (more of which later), but to none of the myeloid cell types. It is not known whether they are a mixture of progenitors of these cells or whether a single progenitor has the potential to differentiate into different types. Interestingly, however, cells that give rise only to T lymphocytes have been isolated from the fetal blood. At some stage therefore the differentiation programme must become restricted to the T-lymphocytic lineage, but whether cells arriving in the thymus have reached this stage remains an open question.

Once in the thymus, the progenitor cells interact with the stromal tissue and are thereby stimulated to divide repeatedly (to proliferate). It has been estimated that in the thymus of a young adult mouse, approximately 50 million new cells arise through division each day. Since the number of cells in the thymus remains constant (*c.* 1–2 × 10^8) and since only 1 million cells leave the thymus daily, 98% of the

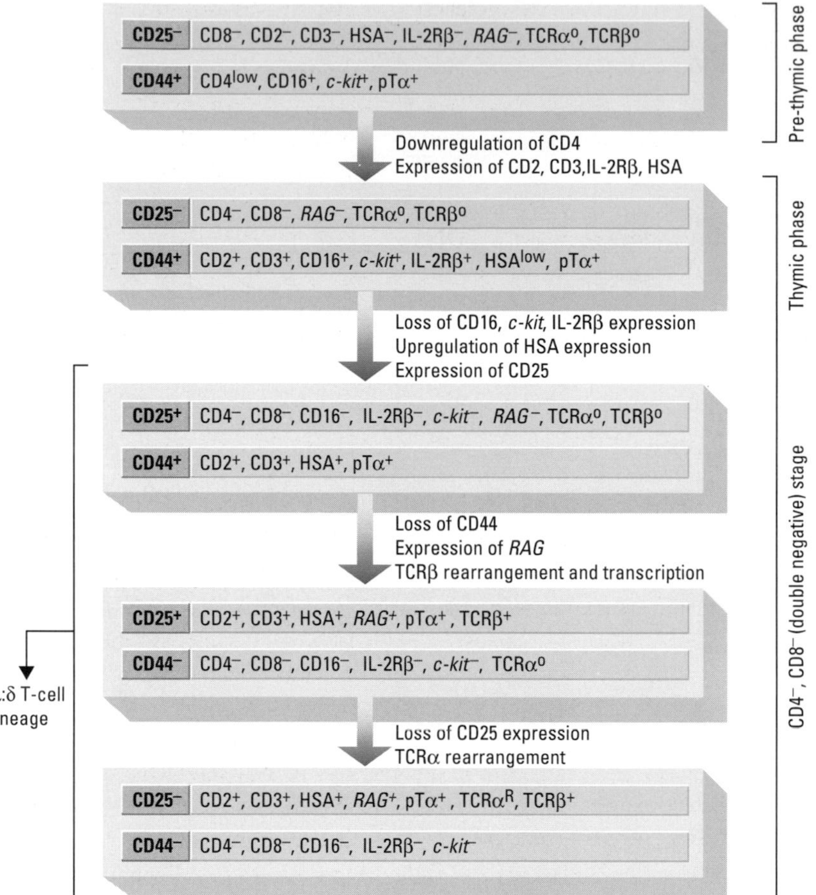

Figure 5.11 The early thymic phase of mouse T-lymphocytic progression. Each large rectangle represents a distinct stage characterized by the markers listed within it. The most important markers are highlighted. CD, cluster of differentiation; HSA, heat-stable antigen (the mouse homologue of human CD24); IL, interleukin; R, receptor; *RAG*, recombination activating gene; pT, pre-T-cell receptor; TCR, T-cell receptor. Superscripts: R, rearranged; 0, not rearranged, not expressed; +, expressed; –, not expressed.

newly generated cells must die each day. With such a massive demise of cells, one would surely expect to see signs of decay in the thymus, such as areas of necrosis, but nothing of this sort is discernible. The death of the cells apparently occurs under highly organized, impeccable conditions; neither damage to the surrounding tissue nor debris is left behind. Each cell is believed to be programmed to die if it is not specifically instructed to carry on. Such genetically programmed cell death or *apoptosis* (from the Greek meaning 'the shedding of leaves in autumn') is not restricted to cells in the thymus, but might be a feature of all cells in every organism. Several of the genes participating in the programme have been identified and isolated; most are highly conserved across a wide range of animal groups. A cell undergoing apoptosis first produces the enzymes needed to destroy itself, then shrinks, condenses its nucleus and cleaves its DNA into small fragments by its own endonucleases. The cell then usually fragments into membrane-bound apoptotic bodies, which are rapidly engulfed and digested by neighbouring cells. There is thus no leakage of potentially dangerous contents from the dying cell and damage to other cells is avoided.

Of the markers used to discern individual stages of the T-lymphocytic progression, four have proved to be particularly useful: CD4, CD8, CD25 and CD44. The cells arriving in the thymus express the CD4 molecule at a low level but the expression is quickly *downregulated* (reduced by regulatory mechanisms to a level at which it cannot be detected by standard methods) so that the proliferating cells are of the CD4⁻CD8⁻ phenotype. Another sign that the cell and its progeny are undergoing the 'rites of passage' is the expression of CD2 and, in the mouse, the Thy1 molecule on their surfaces. From this point onwards, these two molecules remain expressed throughout the entire lifespans of all the cells and their progenies in the lineage. They characterize cells of the lineage influenced by the thymic microenvironment, the *thymocytes,* but are also retained by those cells that leave the thymus as mature T lymphocytes, and furthermore they are expressed by T lymphocytes that developed extrathymically.

The separation of the lineages leading to the γ:δ and α:β T cells occurs at some point in this double-negative (DN) stage. In both lineages, the *TCR* genes rearrange and attempt to produce functional proteins (see Chapter 7). If they succeed, the assembled TCR chains, together with the chains of the CD3 complex, appear on the cell surface. In the γ:δ lineage, the *CD4* and *CD8* genes remain silent during the entire γ:δ T-cell differentiation process and the mature γ:δ T cells therefore remain double negative. The mature γ:δ T cells leave the thymus apparently without undergoing selection of any kind. In the thymus of a young adult or an adult individual, only a small minority of progenitor cells reaching the thymus differentiates into γ:δ T cells; the majority becomes α:β T cells. In an embryo just the opposite happens. In the mouse, which has been used extensively as a model in T-cell developmental studies, progenitor cells arrive in the thymus at 11 days of gestation (the mouse's gestation period lasts 20–21 days) and for several days afterwards virtually all progenitors differentiate along the γ:δ pathway (Fig. 5.12). Only at about 16 days of gestation does the differentiation begin to shift towards α:β T-cell production.

A summary of the α:β differentiation pathway appears in Fig. 5.10; the markers expresed at the various differentiation stages are listed in Fig. 5.11. As the T-cell progenitors enter the thymus in the subcapsular region, they lack CD4 and CD8 molecules on their surface (they are DN) and express neither the TCR nor the CD3 molecule so that their surface phenotype is DN, TCR$^-$, CD3$^-$. From the subcapsular region the cells (their progeny) descend ever deeper into the cortex and then enter, through the corticomedullary junction, the medulla from which, if all went well on the way, they exit into the bloodstream. Along this route, the cells transform from T-cell progenitors into thymocytes and these ultimately into mature T lymphocytes. The transformation is marked by profound changes in the cell's behaviour and phenotype, both reflecting changes in the activities of the encoding genes. Already in the subcapsular region, the cells begin to divide mitotically and continue to proliferate as they then enter the cortex. Simultaneously, they activate their *CD4* and *CD8* genes and express the CD4 and CD8 molecules on their surfaces, thus becoming double positive (DP), their phenotype changing from DN, TCR$^-$, CD3$^-$ to DP, TCR$^-$, CD3$^-$. During their proliferation they also begin to rearrange their *TCR* genes and when they succeed in producing an expressible combination of α and β chains they display them, together with the CD3 chains, at a low level on their surfaces. The phenotype of the thymocytes in this stage thus becomes DP, TCR^{low}, CD3$^+$. Cells that fail to produce expressible TCR carry on with the rest of their programme, which stipulates self-destruction. However, even cells that have succeeded in reaching the DP, TCR^{low}, CD3$^+$ stage are not saved from the Grim Reaper. To stay alive and continue their development, their TCRs must engage MHC molecules primarily on thymic (cortical) epithelial cells, and possibly also on other cells. The number

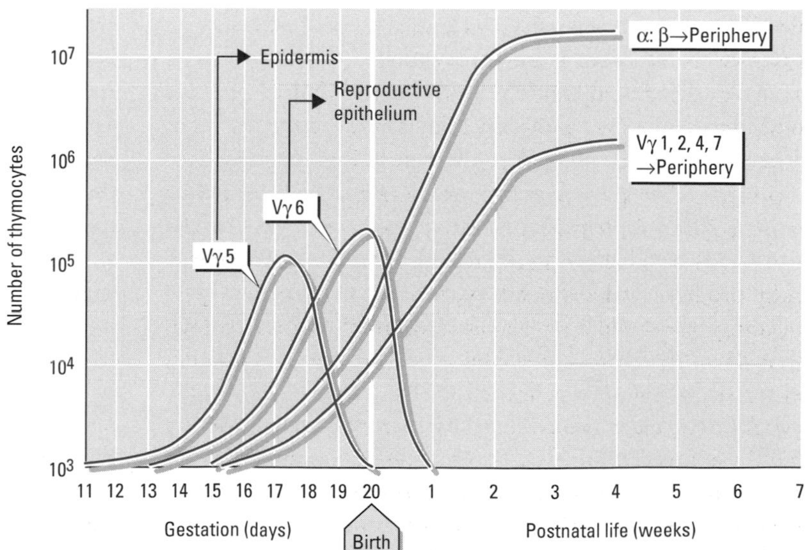

Figure 5.12 Emergence of γ:δ (Vγ5; Vγ6; Vγ1,2,4,7) and α:β T cells in the thymus of a mouse embryo and a newborn mouse. Arrows indicate target organs of migration.

of different MHC molecules expressed by an individual is small, however, and most thymocytes find themselves without matching MHC molecules for their TCRs; these cells, too, will succumb to programmed cell death. The majority of thymocytes will therefore die within 3–4 days after their last division because they have failed to find matching ligands for their receptors (i.e. *death by neglect*); only cells that have specifically engaged their TCRs with corresponding MHC molecules on epithelial cells will differentiate further. They increase the level of TCR expression and thus enter the DP, TCR^{high}, $CD3^{+}$ stage.

What happens next is controversial: two hypotheses have been put forward to explain how further differentiation may proceed. According to the *instructive hypothesis*, the specificity of the TCR determines which class of MHC molecule the thymocyte will engage. If the receptors happen to bind a class I molecule, the CD8 co-receptor binds to the relatively invariant part of the MHC molecule and a signal is sent into the cell's interior to shut down the synthesis of the CD4 molecules. The thymocyte then passes (via a $CD4^{low}CD^{high}$ intermediate) to the *single-positive* (SP) stage $CD4^{-}CD8^{+}$. If, on the other hand, the TCR happens to bind a class II molecule, the opposite happens and the cells pass (via the $CD4^{high}CD8^{low}$ intermediate) to the $CD4^{+}CD8^{-}$ SP stage. According to the *stochastic hypothesis*, the transition from DP to SP thymocyte occurs in two steps. In the first (stochastic) step, the thymocyte randomly downregulates one of the two genes, either *CD4* or *CD8*, producing $CD4^{low}CD8^{high}$ or $CD4^{high}CD8^{low}$ cells, respectively. In the second (selective) step, the thymocyte tries to bind the co-receptor to the MHC molecule that is bound to its TCR. If the TCR is bound to a class I molecule and the thymocyte by chance has downregulated the CD4 molecule, the co-receptor will be able to bind the MHC molecule and differentiation will proceed to the $CD4^{-}CD8^{+}$ stage. If, on the other hand, the thymocyte happened to downregulate the CD8 molecule, further maturation will not be possible and the thymocyte again dies by neglect. Similar but contrary outcomes are possible in the case of thymocytes whose TCRs have engaged MHC class II molecules. As some experiments support the instructive and others the stochastic hypothesis, a third explanation combining features of both has been proposed. It suggests that the DP thymocyte whose TCR is engaged with the appropriate MHC molecule downregulates either CD4 or CD8 at random. When it is in the transitional $CD4^{low}CD8^{high}$ or $CD4^{high}CD8^{low}$ stage, it then checks its TCR specificity again on another MHC-positive cell. If the receptor–co-receptor specificities match it will proceed to the next stage, but if it downregulated the wrong co-receptor the thymocyte will die by neglect. This process, in which the engagement of the TCR with MHC molecules saves the thymocyte from programmed cell death and enables it to differentiate further, constitutes *positive selection*. It is carried over several stages of the differentiation pathways and probably involves interaction of the thymocyte with different stromal cells.

In the preceding description MHC molecules were discussed as if they were recognized by the thymocyte's TCR alone without the involvement of peptides, and indeed some hypotheses of T-cell development do postulate the recognition of 'empty' MHC molecules in certain differentiation stages. Evidence is now accumulating, however, which invalidates such claims. Whenever thymocytes interact with MHC molecules via their TCRs, they always appear to recognize the peptide–MHC assembly, just like mature $\alpha{:}\beta$ T lymphocytes. Moreover, the peptides bound to thymic MHC molecules by no means seem to be special, again contrary to the postulate of another series of hypotheses. Although some of the MHC-bound peptides found in the thymus are largely, but not exclusively, restricted to this organ, others are derived from ubiquitous proteins brought into the thymus with the blood. The suggestion that MHC molecules present one set of peptides to immature T cells and an entirely different set to mature T cells is not supported by experimental evidence.

These observations present a prodigious enigma. How can the same or very similar sets of ligands interacting with the same sets of TCRs lead to dramatically different outcomes, depending on the circumstances, i.e. differentiation of immature T cells in the thymus and no response of mature T lymphocytes in the periphery? A number of explanations have been put forward but of these only one is consistent with most of the available data, the *avidity (affinity) hypothesis*. Affinity, you will recall, is the strength of single-ligand binding to a single receptor. Often, however, when two molecules interact and nearly always when two cells interact, the binding involves more than one ligand and one receptor site or more than one ligand–receptor pair. The total strength of binding involving multiple sites or multiple ligand–receptor pairs is the *avidity* of the interaction. Since the total strength of interaction will obviously depend on the number of participating ligand–receptor pairs, avidity will be influenced by the density of the receptors on the cell surface. The principal assumption of the avidity/affinity hypothesis is that different strengths of binding can be translated into different signals. Some immunologists believe that the affinity of the interaction between the TCR and the peptide–MHC assembly is the decisive factor, but an ever-increasing number of researchers are now convinced that avidity rather than affinity determines the fate of a differentiating thymocyte. Not a single TCR–peptide–MHC interaction alone but the total of all interactions, together with interactions involving the co-receptors, the density of the TCRs on the thymocyte, the concentration of the MHC molecules on the stromal cells and perhaps other factors all conspire in generating different signals. There appear to exist certain thresholds of avidity which, when crossed, qualitatively change the response of a cell. If there is no interaction or only an extremely weak interaction that fleetingly engages the TCR with the peptide–MHC ligand, no life-saving signals are generated and the thymocyte commits programmed suicide (death by neglect). If the avidity of the interaction is strong enough to keep the cells together for more than just a fleeting moment, but below a certain threshold, differentiation signals are generated (*positive selection*). Finally if the avidity is strong and above the threshold, the thymocyte is again left to its fate which stipulates programmed cell death (*negative selection*).

It is still a matter of controversy whether positive and negative selection occur more or less simultaneously and actually represent two sides of the same coin (weak interaction → positive selection, strong interaction → negative selection) or whether they follow each other and, if so, in what order. Available evidence indicates, however, a considerable overlap between the two. The physical setting for the overlap is believed to be provided by the distribution of the different cell types in the thymus. It was mentioned earlier that the differentiating thymocyte migrates directionally in the thymus, first from the subcapsular region via the cortex into the corticomedullary junction and then into the medulla. On its way it encounters different cell types, not only thymocytes but also stromal cells (cortical thymic epithelial cells, macrophages, dendritic cells and possibly other 'professional' antigen-presenting cells (APCs)). The interaction with different cells influences the response of the thymocyte to the signals it receives. The physical setting may provide an avidity gradient for the interactions. In the outer regions of the cortex, conditions exist for lowest-avidity interactions mainly because the density of TCRs on the DP, TCR^{low}, $CD3^{+}$ thymocytes is low. As the cells enter the deeper regions of the cortex and the TCR density on their surfaces increases, higher-avidity interactions become possible. By the time the thymocyte reaches the corticomedullary junction, it also reaches the *avidity threshold*. Any interaction stronger than the avidity threshold generates signals leading to apoptosis; the cells undergo negative selection. The corticomedullary junction and the medulla contain significant numbers of professional APCs such as macrophages and dendritic cells which, because of their ability to present peptide–MHC ligands efficiently, provide conditions for high-avidity interactions and thus for negative selection. This conclusion is supported by experiments that demonstrate the ability of a negatively selecting ligand to induce positive selection in the absence of professional APCs.

The avidity hypothesis also makes two additional assumptions. First, a positively selected T cell driven by a particular ligand loses its ability to respond to that ligand (*desensitization*), while retaining its ability to respond to other ligands. Second, the relative avidity of interaction required for positive selection is lower than that needed for the triggering of mature T lymphocytes. Experimental evidence supporting both assumptions has been reported. Experiments have also revealed one unexpected feature of the interactions. It appears that the specificity of the TCR is influenced by the encounter with a particular ligand. It has been demonstrated that thymocytes possessing the same TCR (in terms of amino acid sequence) but positively selected by different ligands have a different reactivity.

To summarize: the current concept of $\alpha:\beta$ T-cell development in the thymus envisages each thymocyte expressing a different TCR generated by the rearrangement of the encoding genes. Thymocytes that fail to come up with an expressible TCR or thymocytes that express a TCR for which the individual does not possess any matching peptide–MHC ligands die by neglect. Thymocytes with TCRs that find a matching ligand on the thymic epithelial cells undergo positive selection: the interaction of their TCRs with the corresponding ligands saves them from programmed cell death. The interactions are at first of low avidity, but as the cells intrude deeper into the cortex and the density of TCRs on their surfaces increases the avidity of the interactions rises. Up to a certain avidity threshold, the interaction always saves the thymocytes from apoptosis, allows them to develop further and at the same time makes them unresponsive to ligands binding to them with the same (or lower) avidity as the positively selecting ligand. In the deep cortex, the corticomedullary junction and parts of the medulla, conditions exist for high-avidity interactions between TCRs and their ligands presented by professional APCs. Thymocytes that interact with APCs with a strength above the avidity threshold are instructed to commit suicide – they are weeded out by negative selection. Those that interact with avidity below the threshold are allowed to mature and to move into the periphery.

Mature peripheral T lymphocytes are not activated by self-peptide–self-MHC molecules because they have been desensitized to the level of avidity with which these ligands interact with their TCRs. There are, however, certain peptides in the periphery that the developing T cells did not have the opportunity to encounter in the thymus. If these ligands bind with avidity at or below the avidity that desensitized the developing T cells, they will not activate the mature T lymphocytes. However, even if they bind with a higher affinity than the desensitizing avidity, they will not necessarily activate the T cells either because the avidity level required for activation in the periphery is set higher than the threshold level for positive selection. If the avidity exceeds even this level, the T cells will be prevented from responding by other mechanisms (see Chapter 20). By contrast, if the mature T lymphocytes encounter foreign peptide bound to self-MHC molecules, they will not be compelled to commit suicide even though the avidity of the interaction exceeds the threshold level; instead, they will be activated by the interaction. This outcome is the result of a change in the programme that occurred at the completion of the selection phase of T-cell development. The change consists of re-routing signals generated by high-avidity interactions from a pathway leading to apoptosis to a pathway leading to lymphocyte activation. In this manner, T lymphocytes learn how to ignore self and respond to non-self.

The distribution of individual cell types in the thymus is summarized in Table 5.3. Most of the cells in the medulla appear to be mature T lymphocytes. They could either be cells awaiting exportation into the blood circulation or T lymphocytes that the thymus holds back for its own protection.

The majority, but not all, of the T lymphocytes found outside the thymus are graduates of the thymic school. A minority appears to have developed extrathymically, although even their maturation may have been influenced indirectly by thymus-derived cells or factors. The evidence for extrathymic development is fairly strong for a sublineage of γ:δ T cells residing in the gut epithelia but controversial for other γ:δ T lymphocytes and for all α:β T cells. The γ:δ T cells of the gut epithelia are characterized by the expression of TCR derived from a particular set of *V*-gene segments and by the expression of CD8α homodimers rather than CD8αβ heterodimers. They appear in the gut prior to the colonization of the thymus by bone marrow-derived progenitor cells. Other γ:δ T cells believed to have differentiated extrathymically are found in the lungs and the liver.

Evidence for extrathymic development of α:β T cells in the gut and the liver has been reported by some investigators but is contested by others. The CD4CD8 phenotypes

Table 5.3 Distribution of cell types in the thymus of a young-adult mouse.

Co-receptor expression			
CD4	CD8	Cell type	Percentage
–	–	Immature progenitor cells	3
–	–	γ:δ TCR-expressing cells	1
–	–	α:β TCR-expressing cells	2
–	+	Immature	1
+	+	Immature	78
+	–	Mature	10
–	+	Mature	5

CD, cluster of differentiation; TCR, T-cell receptor.

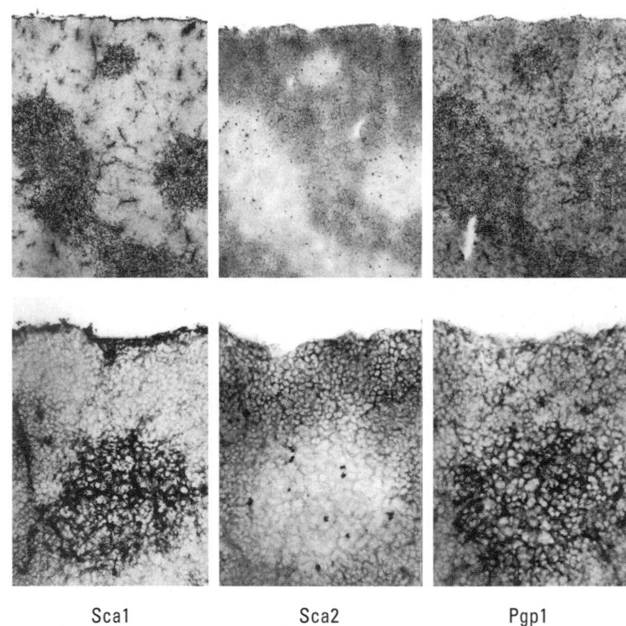

Figure 5.13 Expression of Sca1, Sca2 and CD44 (Pgp1) molecules on cells of the mouse thymus: an example illustrating the use of immunohistochemical methods in the study of thymocyte maturation. Whole thymus extirpated from a mouse is snap-frozen by being dipped into dry ice (solid CO_2) and then cut into thin sections using a cryostat (a refrigerated mechanical device for cutting frozen, unfixed tissue samples). The sections are incubated with mouse antibodies specifically reacting with the Sca1, Sca2 and CD44 molecules, then with rat antibodies reacting with the mouse antibodies and labelled with biotin and finally with horseradish peroxidase–avidin complex (the principle of this technique is described in Chapter 14). The stain becomes visible if amino-9-ethylcarbazole is used as a substrate (dark spots). The sections show that Sca1 is expressed nearly confluently in the subcapsular and medullary regions of the thymus, whereas in the cortex its expression is limited to blood vessels and connective tissue. Sca2 expression is the reverse of Sca1: no staining of the medulla, but strong staining of the cortical regions. The labelled CD44 antibodies stain the medulla and the cortex in a dendritic pattern, but do not stain the subcapsular region. Top and bottom rows, magnifications 10× and 40×, respectively. Sca, stem-cell antigen. (From Spangrude, G. J. *et al.* (1988) *Journal of Immunology*, **141**, 3697–3707.)

of these controversial cells are: CD4+CD8(αβ)−, CD4−CD8(αβ)+, CD4−CD8(αβ)− (these three types are indistinguishable from cells found in the thymus), CD4+CD8(αα)+ and CD4−CD8(αα)+ (these two types are unique to the intestinal epithelium).

Methods for the study of T-cell development

The thymus, as pointed out earlier, is a very sequestered, very secretive place. How can immunologists possibly find out what is going on in this secluded abode? The simplest but also the least informative way is to make *histological sections* of the thymus at different stages of its development and to highlight the cells expressing a particular marker using tagged reagents that bind specifically to this marker (e.g. fluorescein-labelled antibodies; Fig. 5.13). The branch of immunology in which histological (cytological) methods are combined with immunological methods based on the use of labelled reagents (usually antibodies) is referred to as *immunohistochemistry* or *immunocytochemistry*.

It is also possible to remove an embryonic thymus just after it has been seeded by haemopoietic precursors or cells and grow it for a limited period in an *organ culture in vitro* (Fig. 5.14). The advantage of the method is that the culture is easily accessible to experimental manipulation.

Much has been learned about the function of the thymus from *radiation chimeras*. To the ancient Greeks, a chimera was a mythical, fire-breathing monster whose anatomical features were a blend of lion, she-goat and serpent (Fig. 5.15). To a biologist, a chimera is an organism consisting of two or more genetically distinct cell types that is produced as a result of mutation, transplantation or the fusion of different embryos. To an immunologist, a radiation chimera is an animal produced by destroying the haemopoietic and lymphoid tissue with ionizing radiation and then replacing it by tissue (usually bone marrow or fetal liver cells) from another individual (Fig. 5.16). By varying the genotype of the host and the graft, an immunologist can

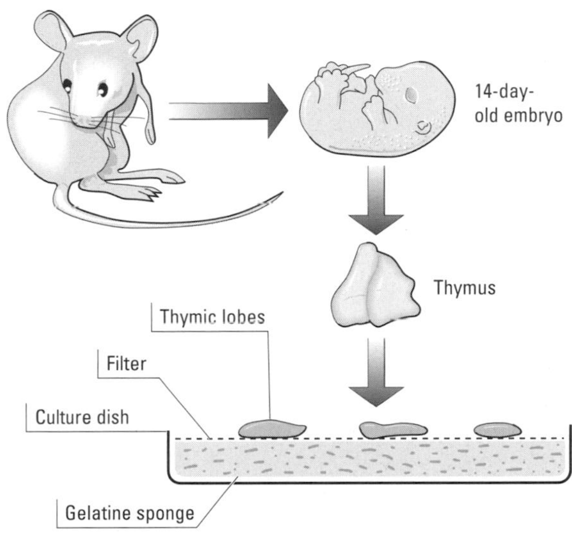

Figure 5.14 *In vitro* thymus culture. The thymus is removed from a 14-day-old embryo and individual lobes are placed on a polycarbonate filter that is laid on a gelatine sponge soaked with a culture medium in a Petri dish. The organ can be kept in culture for about 2–3 weeks, during which time the thymocytes continue to divide and the lobes grow in size.

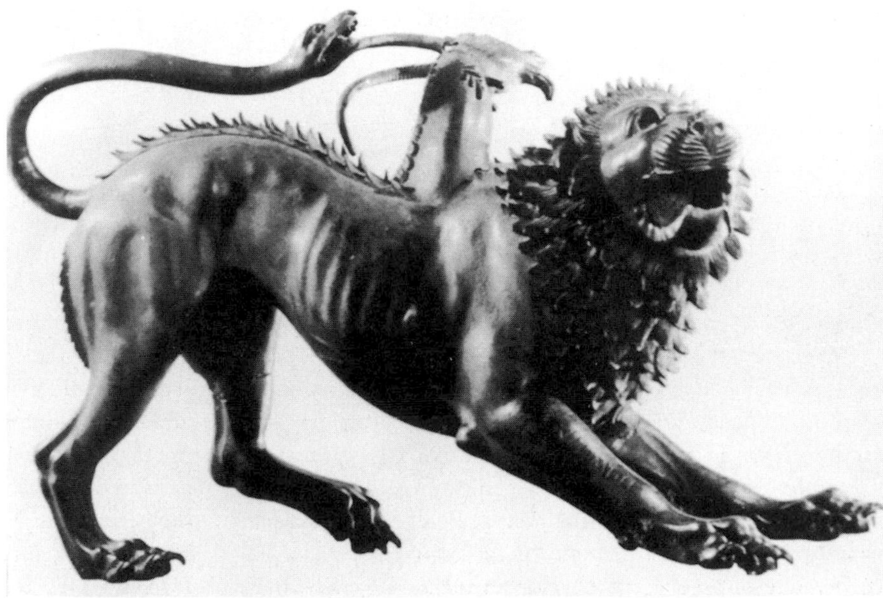

Figure 5.15 The Chimera. Etruscan Bronze. Archaeological Museum, Florence.

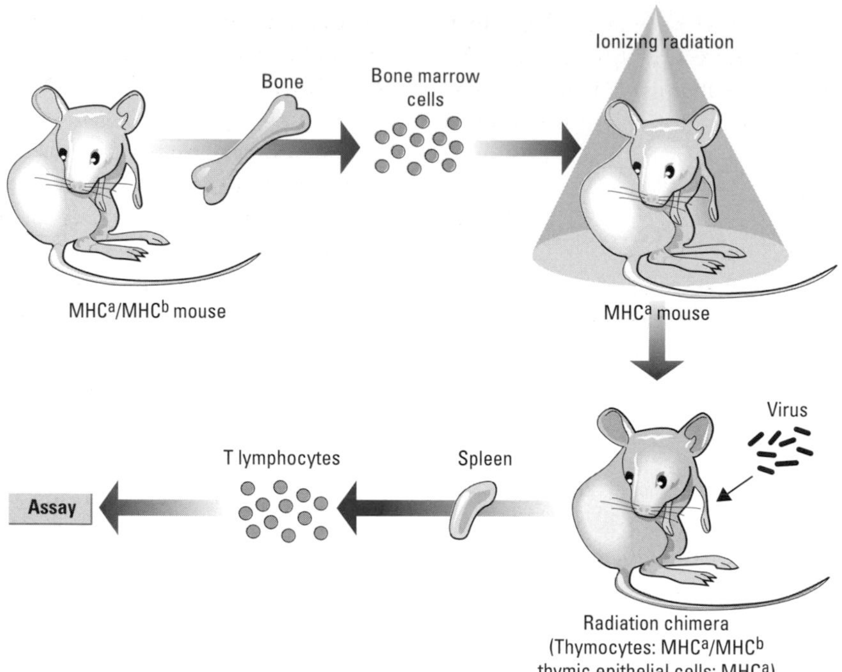

Figure 5.16 Immune response of a radiation chimera. Bone marrow cells from an adult mouse of a strain expressing two different alleles at class I *MHC* loci (MHC^a and MHC^b) are inoculated into a lethally irradiated adult mouse of a strain expressing only MHC^a class I genes. In the irradiated recipient all MHC^a lymphoid cells die as a consequence of the radiation effects but are replaced by MHC^a/MHC^b lymphocytes, which differentiate from the inoculated bone marrow cells. The thymic epithelial cells and other stromal cells which are more radioresistant than lymphoid cells survive the radiation exposure and remain MHC^a. Consequently, the differentiating MHC^a/MHC^b thymocytes encounter only MHC^a but not MHC^b molecules on the thymic epithelial cells. When fully established 6–24 weeks after irradiation, the chimeras receive a dose of a virus to which they respond by producing cytotoxic T lymphocytes specific for the virus-infected target cells. When the T lymphocytes are isolated from the spleen of the infected mouse, they can be shown to kill virus-infected MHC^a but not virus-infected MHC^b target cells. This result is interpreted as indicating that the MHC^a/MHC^b thymocytes of the chimera have undergone positive selection on the MHC^a epithelial cells of the thymus during which only thymocytes capable of recognizing peptide–MHC^a molecules have been saved from programmed cell death. A modified version of this experiment shows that thymocytes also undergo negative selection. If MHC^a/MHC^b bone marrow cells are inoculated into the lethally irradiated MHC^a recipient and a piece of skin from an MHC^b donor is later grafted onto the chimera, the graft is not destroyed (non-chimeric MHC^a mice would promptly reject an MHC^b skin graft; see Chapter 24). This result suggests that T lymphocytes capable of recognizing MHC^b molecules and attacking MHC^b-bearing cells have been removed from the repertoire of the chimeric mouse, presumably during the negative selection phase in the thymus, when they encountered molecules of the dendritic cells and macrophages derived from the inoculated MHC^a/MHC^b bone marrow cells.

study the effect of varied genetic environments on cell development. Bone marrow transplantation can be combined with the removal of the thymus (*thymectomy*) and its replacement by an organ from another individual (*thymic chimeras*).

Experimental conditions that come closest to physiological conditions have been achieved by applying some of the methods of genetic engineering. Two approaches in particular have proved to be highly informative in the study of T-lymphocyte development: transgenic animals and knockout mice. In a *transgenic animal*, a foreign gene (*transgene*) is integrated into the genome of the recipient at such an early stage of embryonic development that all cells of the adult organism, including the germ cells, will carry it (Fig. 5.17). The transgene inserts itself into the host cell DNA randomly; one has no control over the site of integration. The expression of the transgene can, however, be controlled so that it occurs only in certain tissues (e.g. in the pancreas if the transgene is combined with the regulatory region of the insulin gene) or at a specific time (e.g. upon addition of zinc to the water supply if the transgene bears the regulatory region of the metallothionein gene, which is activated by zinc). Because the transgene is also present in the germ cells, the progeny of a transgenic animal is transgenic, too. A number of transgenic strains of mice carrying foreign TCR, MHC, immunoglobulin and CD genes, as well as genes coding for antigens, have been developed and used in the study of lymphocyte (both T and B) differentiation. Their advantage is that physiologically they are entirely normal except for the presence of the foreign transgene.

The surest way of finding out a gene's function is to inactivate it or, in laboratory jargon, to 'knock it out' and then study the consequences. Until recently, immunologists have relied on nature to inactivate genes for them but since the rate at which any one gene will be silenced by mutation is approximately 10^{-9} per generation and the odds that the mutated gene is the one under scrutiny are between 1 : 40 000 and 1 : 100 000, the number of immunologically important genes inactivated in this way is small. The rate (but not the odds) can be increased somewhat by the exposure of an animal to mutagens, substances or factors that cause mutation to occur at higher frequencies than normal, but the chance of obtaining the right mutation is remote. In the last decade, however, methods have become available that allow an investigator to target a particular gene for inactivation. *Gene targeting techniques* sprang out of conventional gene transfer methods but differ from them in that the introduced gene does not integrate randomly into the recipient's chromosomes; it 'homes' to the site at which the DNA sequence is to a large degree identical to its own—the introduced (replacement) gene and the resident (target) gene are genetically *homologous*. The two genes align with each other by matching their sequences, break at their ends, and swap positions in a process termed *homologous recombination* (Fig. 5.18). As a result of the swap, the locus originally occupied by the target gene is now occupied, in one of the two homologous chromosomes, by the replacement gene. If the latter has been manipulated, before its introduction into the cell, in such a way that it is incapable of producing a functional protein, the cell will now contain one functional and one inactive gene at a particular locus. The cell can then be introduced into an embryo in which it will contribute to development. If its contribution includes the germ line, the replacement gene can be transmitted to the offspring and by judicial breeding, *knock-out animals* can be obtained in which both copies of the gene at a given locus are inactive. If such an animal lives, the effects of the absence of a functional gene at this locus can be deduced.

In some of the most recent versions of the targeted gene replacement procedure, it is possible to produce animals in which the gene is inactivated in certain tissues only (Fig. 5.19). This modification enables an investigator to study the effects of gene inactivation on a defined tissue even in the case of those genes that would otherwise kill the embryo at an early stage because they are required in another tissue as well.

Knock-out mice have been created for many of the immunologically important genes (*MHC* class I and II, *CD4*, *CD8*, *Ig*, *IL-2*, *IL-4*). Surprisingly, the effects of most of these gene inactivations are relatively minor. For example, mice without functional class I genes lack CD4$^-$CD8$^+$ T lymphocytes, yet they survive even when exposed to a variety of viruses. These results must surely mean that the immune system is highly resilient in that it possesses numerous back-up and stand-in systems to take over whenever a failure occurs in one of its components. They also demonstrate that even in vertebrates, non-adaptive immunity has remained an important defence mechanism.

B-lymphocyte development

The cradle of mammalian B lymphocytes is the blood and placenta of an embryo, the liver and the omentum (the double-layer membrane connecting various abdominal organs with one another) of a fetus, and the bone marrow of a newborn and an adult. In mice, B-lymphocyte development takes place in the fetal liver in one wave and ceases shortly after birth, when it is taken over by the bone marrow. In the latter organ, it continues throughout life, although the number of B lymphocytes produced decreases gradually with age. B lymphocytes produced by the fetus and newborn differ from those produced in bone marrow in some of the molecular markers. In particular, the former do not express the *TdT* gene during their development and consequently do not insert additional nucleotides between *D* and *J* or *V* and *D* segments of the rearranging BCR genes (see Chapter 8). They are therefore somewhat less diverse than bone marrow-produced B lymphocytes.

In an adult mouse or human, most but not all of the maturation phase of B-lymphocyte development takes place in the bone marrow. The immature cells are then exported into the blood circulation and presumably delivered to the spleen. There they are either selected to enter the pool of long-lived, recirculating (mature) B cells, or they die. It has been estimated that about 2×10^7 immature B cells enter the spleen each day and that of these, 2×10^6 cells enter the pool of mature B cells. B-lymphocyte development, like that of all other haemopoietic cells, is governed by sets of genes activated in a certain programmed order. Only some of these genes have been identified: genes coding for the BCR and its surrogates and co-receptor molecules; genes involved in BCR rearrangement; genes encoding transcription factors; genes controlling surface receptors for cell–cell interactions; genes for programmed cell death; and genes coding for proteins involved in signalling. Only the first of these gene sets is uniquely expressed during B lym-

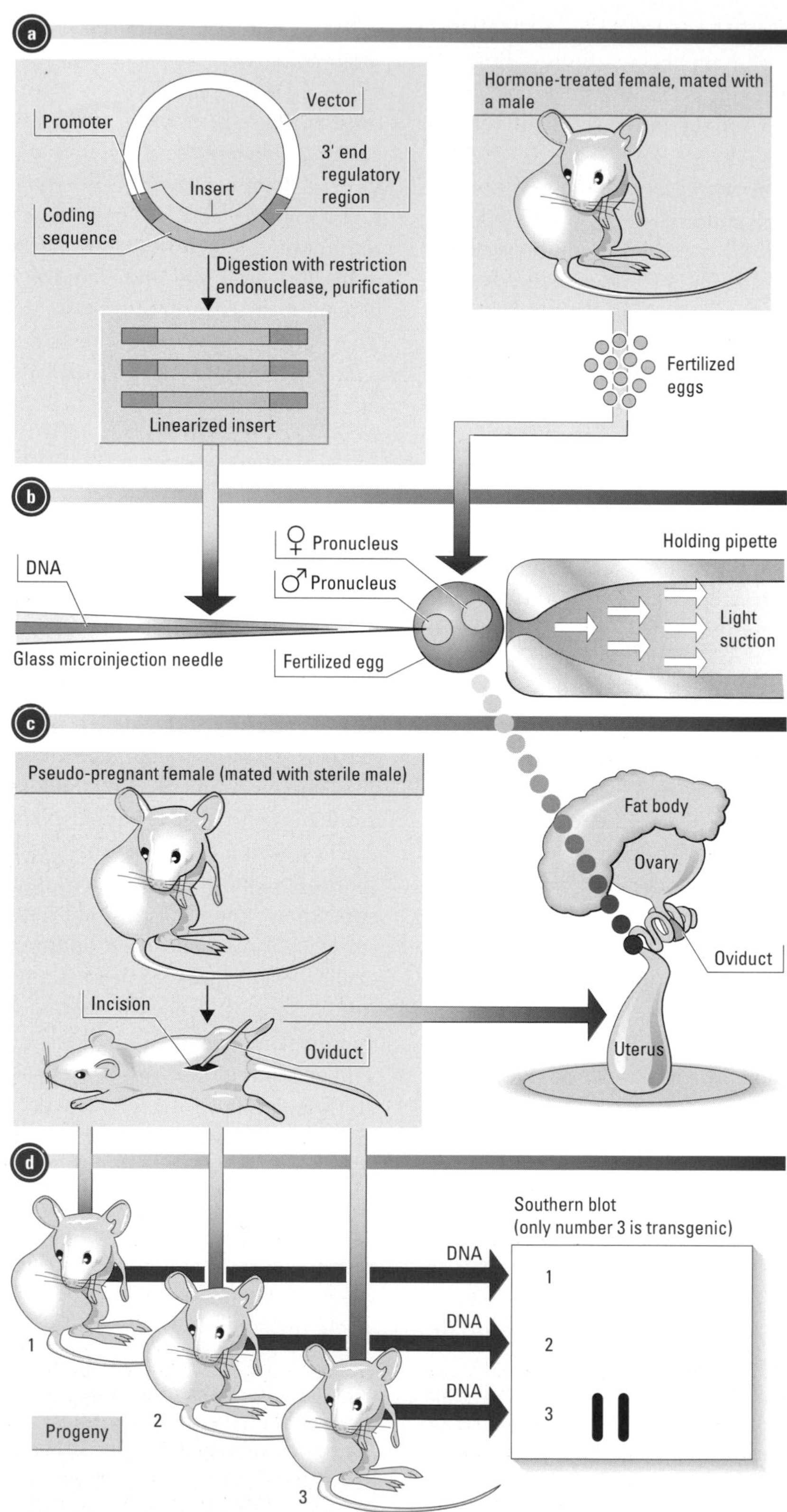

Figure 5.17 Production of transgenic mice. The procedure consists of several steps, which are diagrammed from top to bottom of the figure. (a) Cloning of the gene. The gene to be transferred is isolated from the genome (i.e. the complete gene complement of an organism) of the donor (another individual of the same species or a different species), together with its own

phopoiesis; the others also participate in the differentiation of other cell types.

The BCR consists of four polypeptide chains, two identical heavy (H) and two identical light (L) chains. The mammalian H chains are encoded in one cluster of genes, the L chains in two. Each cluster consists of multiple DNA segments *V*, *J* and *C*; the H-chain gene cluster has, in addition, several *D* segments. Although in the initial stages of their activation the clusters can be transcribed into RNA in the form in which they are arranged in the germ-line cells, in the later stages rearrangement of the DNA segments is indispensable for transcription (see Chapter 8). Rearrangement takes place in two stages in the H-chain cluster (D_H to J_H and then V_H to D_HJ_H) and in one stage in the L-chain clusters (V_L to J_L). The *BCR* genes are also referred to as *immunoglobulin* (*Ig*) genes.

Although the *BCR* genes are activated in the early stages of B-lymphocyte development, in its mature form the receptor does not appear on the cell surface until much later. The expression of mature BCR is preceded, however, by the appearance of forerunner receptors (pre-BCR), which bear certain similarities to the former but are encoded in different genes. Because the polypeptides of the forerunners substitute for the definitive ones, they are referred to as *surrogate H and L chains*. The nature of the surrogate H chain has not yet been defined; it is believed that at least two glycoproteins (gp) contribute to its assembly, gp130 and gp35–65 (the numbers stand for the estimated molecular

---

Figure 5.17 (*Continued.*)
regulatory region (*promoter*; see also Fig. 7.14) located 5′ to (upstream from) the coding part, and regions necessary for the processing of its transcript (mRNA) located 3′ to (downstream from) the coding sequence. Alternatively, the gene's own promoter is replaced by a promoter from another gene that will ensure transcription of the transgene in a different tissue or at a different rate than the gene's own promoter. For manipulation during its isolation and multiplication *in vitro*, the foreign DNA is inserted into a cloning *vector*, a DNA molecule capable of autonomous replication in a host (usually bacterial) cell. The vector can be derived from either a bacterial plasmid, (bacterio)phage or a *cosmid*, an artificially constructed hybrid structure containing elements of a phage (cohesive ends, hence the name) and a plasmid. Before use, however, the vector is digested with a specific *restriction endonuclease*, an enzyme that attacks nucleotides at the vector–insert junction, and if the construct was originally in a circular form, the insert is now linearized. The DNA (the gene) is purified and diluted so that several hundred copies of the gene are present in 1 pl of the solution; it is then ready for the injection. (b) Production of fertilized eggs and microinjection. In the meantime, fertilized egg cells (*oocytes*) are obtained by treating females with sex hormones (to induce superovulation), mating them with males and flushing the egg cells out of the oviduct shortly after fertilization. The sticky cumulus cells surrounding the egg cell are removed by digestion with the enzyme hyaluronidase. An egg cell is grasped by a holding pipette and held fast by light suction. It is oriented in such a way that the *pronuclei* (the nuclei of the egg or sperm before their fusion into a single zygote nucleus) are visible, and a fine injection pipette (glass needle) filled with the DNA solution at its tip is inserted into it. For insertion, the pipette must pierce the *zona pellucida* (the thick, extracellular glycoprotein matrix surrounding the egg cell), the oocyte's plasma membrane and the membrane of the pronucleus, and deliver 1 or 2 pl of the DNA solution into the pronucleus. After injection, the eggs are transferred into a culture and maintained until they can be implanted into a surrogate mother. In the culture, the zygotes are sometimes allowed to develop into embryos for up to several days. (c) Embryo transfer. To obtain surrogate mothers, the oestrous cycle of the egg donor and recipient must be synchronized by mating the recipient with a vasectomized (sterile) male. The recipient's oviducts are then exposed surgically, 10–15 microinjected embryos are transferred into each and the pregnancy of the surrogate mother is allowed to proceed all the way to birth. (d) Detection of integration. Since not all gene transfers are successful (the success rate is only 10–30%), each individual must be tested to ascertain whether the foreign DNA has indeed been incorporated into the host chromosome. The tests can be carried out in a variety of ways, the most common of which are Southern blotting and amplification by polymerase chain reaction (PCR). In the *Southern blotting technique*, a DNA sample is isolated from the transgenic animal, fragmented by digestion with restriction endonucleases and the strands of the DNA double helix are disengaged by heating, separated by electrophoresis in an agarose gel and transferred to a nitrocellulose filter (or other binding matrix). The filter is then incubated with a solution containing a single-stranded, labelled *DNA probe* that is complementary to part of the transgene. Binding (*hybridization*) of the probe is ascertained by visualization of the label. (The PCR technique is described in Fig. 7.27.) Integration does not, however, guarantee expression of the transgene, which must therefore be tested separately, for example with antibodies specific for the protein product of the transgene. If integration has occurred, only one copy of the transgene per genome is usually found; on rare occasions, two or more copies are incorporated at different places. Sometimes, multiple copies integrate in tandem at one place. The integration appears to occur at random and if a gene homologous to the transgene is carried by the recipient it is hardly ever the target of insertion. The mechanism by which the transgene integrates is poorly understood. It seems that the transferred (*transfected*) piece of DNA binds (becomes *ligated*) end to end into a double-stranded break appearing by chance in one of the recipient cell's chromosomes. No homology between the transferred piece and the DNA at the breakpoint site seems to be required and for this reason the process is referred to as *non-homologous recombination*. The unintegrated DNA is rapidly lost by degradation and dilution during cell division because it lacks signals enabling it to replicate autonomously. The transferred pieces often interact with each other and may rearrange during this process.

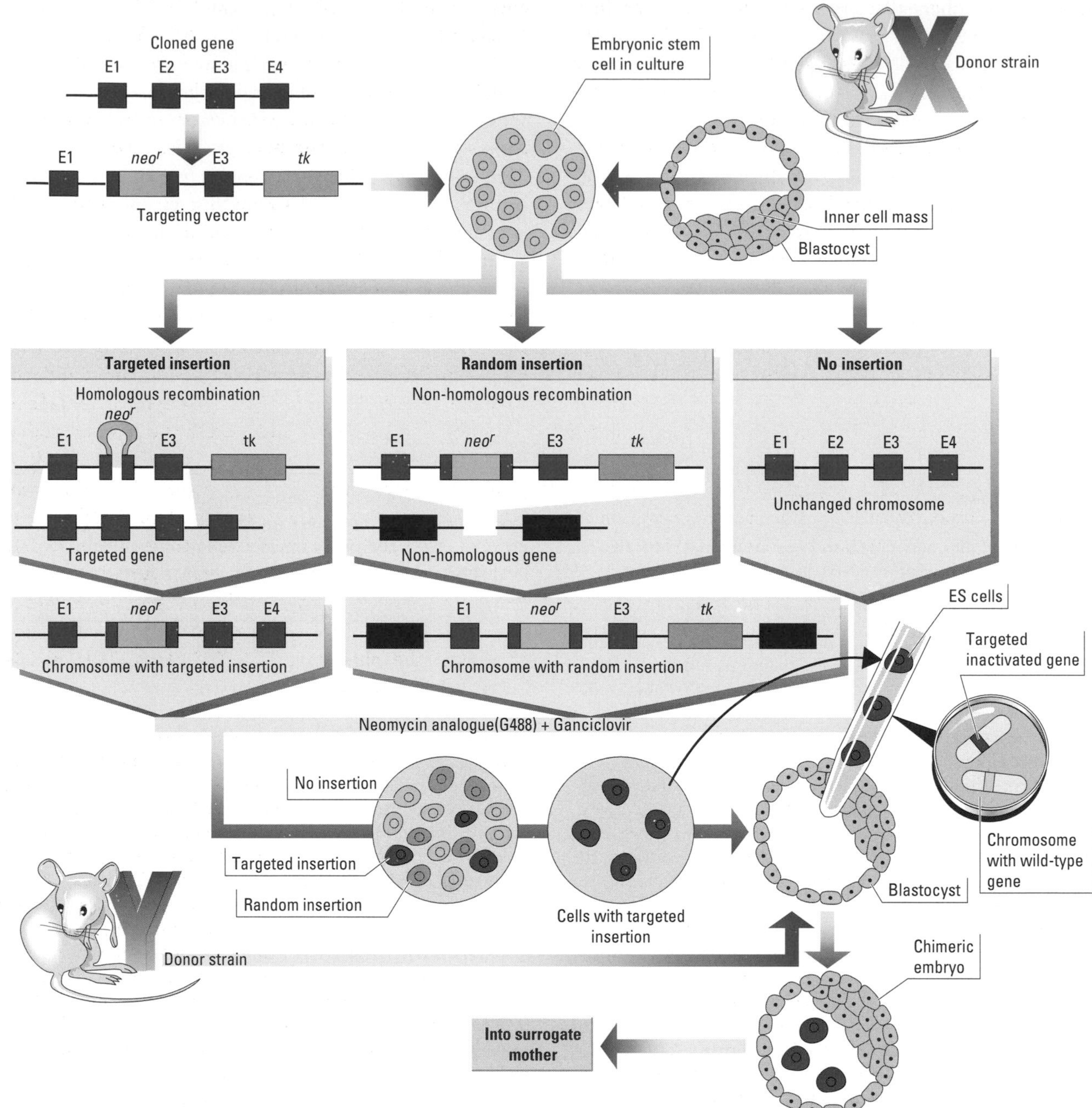

Figure 5.18 Targeted gene replacement and the production of 'knock-out' mice. The procedure is carried out in two phases, *in vitro* and *in vivo*. In the *in vitro* phase, a gene (let us call it a 'replacement gene') is isolated and cloned by standard techniques and two other genes are inserted into it, *neo*^{r} and *tk*. The *neo*^{r} gene is derived from bacteria in which it confers resistance to the antibiotic neomycin. The antibiotic inhibits translation of mRNA into proteins; a related drug, G418, has a similar effect in mammalian cells. The *tk* gene, which is derived from the herpes simplex virus, encodes the enzyme thymidine kinase which catalyses the conversion of the nucleotide thymidine into thymidine monophosphate (TMP). The *neo*^{r} gene is inserted into the middle of the replacement gene's coding sequence, whereas the *tk* gene is appended to one end of the replacement gene. Both the *neo*^{r} and the *tk* genes carry their own promoters and are therefore regulated independently of the replacement gene. The DNA segment containing the replacement gene–*neo*^{r}–*tk* construct (the *targeting vector*) is then introduced by one of several means into the nuclei of embryonic stem (ES) cells grown *in vitro*. The ES cells are derived from the *inner cell mass* of an early mouse embryo (blastocyst); they have been adapted to growth in culture but have retained their full differentiation potential. Any ES cell, when introduced into a blastocyst, can give rise to any cell type, including germ cells. Three situations can occur following the introduction. First, the introduced DNA fails to integrate into the recipient cell's chromosomes. Second, the introduced DNA

masses of these glycoproteins). The surrogate L chain is encoded in two genes, *VPREB* (V_{preB}) and λ*5* (*IGLL*). The *VPREB* gene encodes a protein called ι (iota), the λ*5* gene a protein termed ω (omega). The two proteins associate non-covalently to form the surrogate L chain.

Both the pre-BCR and the BCR are associated with two other types of polypeptide chains, Igα (CD79α) and Igβ (CD79β), encoded in the *MB1* (also written as *mb-1*) and *B29* genes, respectively. The association is non-covalent and the Igα and Igβ chains are believed to function as signal transduction molecules. Each pre-BCR and BCR seems to be associated with two identical α and two identical β chains.

The serial activation of the *pre-BCR*, *BCR* and other genes can be used to divide B-cell development into five stages: proB cell, preB cell I, preB cell II, immature B cell and mature B cell (Fig. 5.20 & Table 5.4). In the *progenitor (pro) B-cell stage* of the mouse, the progeny of haemopoietic stem cells shows, for the first time, a clear commitment towards differentiation along the B-lymphocytic lineage. The proB cells express CD19, a component of the B cell co-receptor complex, the membrane-bound receptor tyrosine kinase c-kit, the heavily glycosylated sialoglycoprotein CD43 (a possible ligand of the cell adhesion molecule ICAM-1; see Chapter 9), the surrogate L (SL) chain encoded in the *VPRB* (V_{preB}) and *IGLL* (λ_5) gene (see Chapter 8), the glycoproteins gp130/gp35–65 associated with the SL chain on the surface and the TdT, RAG1 and RAG2 proteins in the nucleus (see Fig. 5.20 & Table 5.4). None of the *Ig* genes are rearranged yet but portions of some of them are transcribed into RNA. The cells can be grown in tissue culture on stromal cells in the presence of IL-3 and IL-7. Similar cells seem to exist in humans also but they have not been fully characterized as yet.

The hallmark of the mouse *precursor (pre) B-I cell stage* is the $D \rightarrow J_H$ rearrangement of gene segments at the H chain-encoding locus on both chromosomes; the L chain-encoding locus remains unrearranged. The preB-I cells continue to express CD19 (this molecule will remain expressed during the entire differentiation pathway), c-kit, CD43 and the SL/gp130/gp35–65 complex on the surface and the TdT, as well as RAG1 and RAG2 proteins in the nucleus. Like the proB cells, they can be grown in tissue culture on stromal cells and in the presence of IL-3 and IL-7. When transplanted into lightly irradiated mice bearing a genetic defect that blocks B-cell differentiation, the cells will reconstitute peripheral B-cell compartments for as long as half a year. In humans, cells presumably equivalent to the mouse preB-I cells have the phenotype SL$^+$, CD10$^+$, CD19$^+$, CD34$^+$, TdT$^+$, RAG1$^+$, RAG2$^+$.

Figure 5.18 (*Continued.*)
integrates randomly into a chromosome by non-homologous recombination (by the same process on which the production of transgenic animals is based). Third, the replacement gene finds its homologue on the chromosome, aligns with it (looping out the non-homologous part represented by the *neo*^{r} insert) and then recombines: breaks occur at corresponding positions at the ends of the replacement and target genes and both exchange their position. The result of this *homologous recombination* is the replacement of a wild-type gene by a gene disrupted by *neo*^{r} in one of the ES cell's chromosomes; the *tk* gene is lost during this process as shown. The frequency of the three situations declines in the order in which they are listed. Most cells do not integrate the introduced DNA at all; of those that do, most insert it randomly into their chromosomes; and only very few cells undergo targeted gene replacement (the ratio of non-homologous to homologous insertions is between 10 000 : 1 and 1000 : 1). Obviously, if one had no way of selecting the cells that have undergone insertion by homologous recombination, the search for them would be all but futile. To select the cells in which targeted gene replacement has occurred, the transfected ES cells are placed into a medium containing two drugs, the neomycin analogue G418 and ganciclovir. G418 kills all cells not carrying the *neo*^{r} gene, i.e. all cells with no insert. Ganciclovir is a thymidine analogue which, if incorporated into the DNA by the viral thymidine kinase instead of thymidine, kills the cell; it therefore eliminates all cells with random insertions. The only cells left after selection are those with targeted insertion: the *neo*^{r} gene protects them from the lethal effects of G418 and the absence of the *tk* gene (which they lost during the process of homologous recombination) protects them from the effects of ganciclovir. (The ES cells contain the *tk* gene but the enzyme it controls is much less effective in incorporating ganciclovir into DNA than its viral counterpart.) These cells are then transferred into blastocysts in the second, *in vivo* phase of the procedure, and the embryos are grown to term in surrogate mothers, just as in the transgenic animal procedure (see Fig. 5.17). To find out whether the transfer has been successful, blastocysts are used from a mouse strain with a coat colour differing from that of the strain from which the ES cells were derived. Because the introduced ES cell is only one of several pluripotential cells in the blastocyst, it contributes to part of the developing embryo only, so that the adult is a chimera in which cells and tissues of different origin intermix (the intermixing of coat colour-producing cells, for example, is revealed by a striped or patchy appearance of the mice). The ES cells may or may not contribute to the formation of the germ line; only if they do contribute can the replaced gene be transmitted to the progeny. In the chimera, the ES cell-derived cells carry the replacement gene in one chromosome only, while the homologous chromosome carries the original, wild-type gene (the cells are *heterozygous*). If the replacement gene is transmitted to the progeny, however, *homozygotes* can be obtained by appropriate mating. They are the true 'knock-out' mice because, here, both copies of the studied gene are rendered non-functional by the presence of the *neo*^{r} gene insert in their coding sequence. They provide the opportunity to test the importance of the studied gene for survival of the animal and the functions in which it is involved. E, exon.

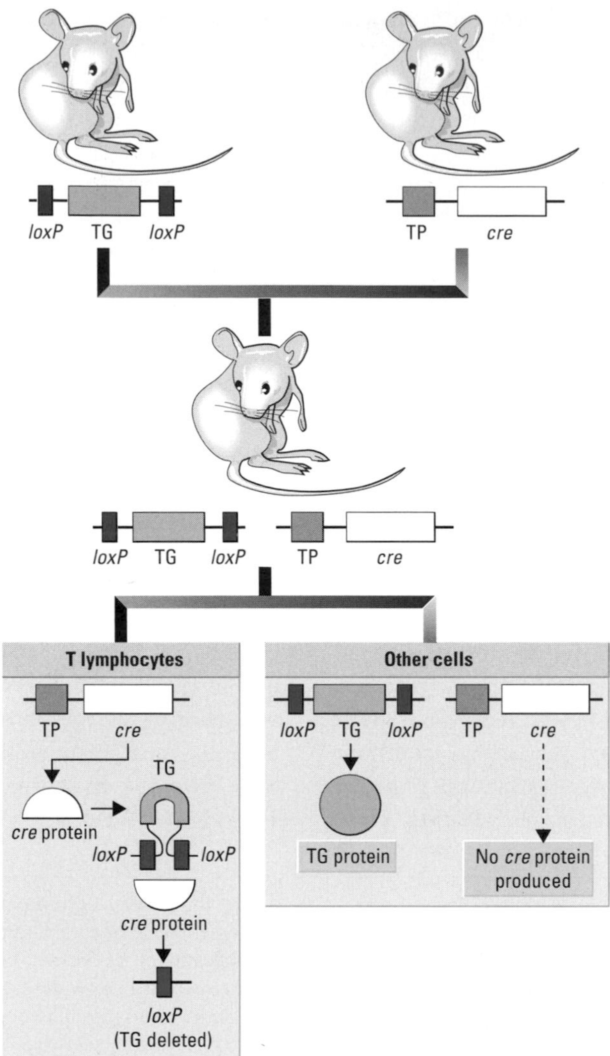

Figure 5.19 Tissue-specific inactivation of a gene in 'knock-out' mice. The bacteriophage P1, which infects and multiplies in the bacterium *Escherichia coli*, replicates its DNA in such a way that several genomes are arranged in a single string in tandem (they are *concatenated*). The string is then cleaved into individual genomes by a special form of recombination. Each genome has a site termed *loxP* at both its ends (for *lo*cus of crossing over, *x*, of phage, *P1*), which is less than 40 base pairs (bp) long and consists of two 13-bp inverted repeats separated by an 8-bp spacer. A protein encoded in the phage gene *cre* (from *c*auses *re*combination) binds to these *loxP* sites: to one *loxP* site at the end of one genome and to another *loxP* site at the beginning of the adjacent genome. The binding brings the two sites together and the enzyme then excises the entire sequence between them, thus separating the two genomes. This property of the *loxP–cre* system is utilized for achieving tissue-specific gene inactivation as depicted in this figure. The method requires the production of two types of mice: one in which the target gene has been replaced by a gene flanked by the *loxP* sequences (this replacement must be achieved in embryonic stem cells and these must then be introduced into an embryo following the procedure summarized in Fig. 5.18); and another in which the *cre* gene, spliced to a regulatory region responsible for tissue-specific expression, has been inserted at a random site into the genome (these are standard transgenic mice produced by the method described in Fig. 5.17). Neither of the two types is adversely affected by the transfer. In the former, the replaced gene functions normally because there is no cre protein produced to act on the *loxP* sites; in the latter, there are no *loxP* sites on which the cre protein could act. However, when the two types are mated and the two elements of the *loxP–cre* system find themselves in the same cell of the hybrid, the system becomes potentially functional. This potential is realized only in those cells that produce factors capable of activating the regulatory region of the transgene. Thus, if the regulatory region binds factors produced by T lymphocytes, the *cre* gene is activated in these cells and the protein it produces acts on the two *loxP* sites that flank the target gene. As a result of this action, the target gene is excised and if the *loxP* elements are present on both homologous chromosomes a knock-out situation arises in which the T cells alone lack the target gene. TG, studied target gene; TP, T cell-specific promoter (regulatory region).

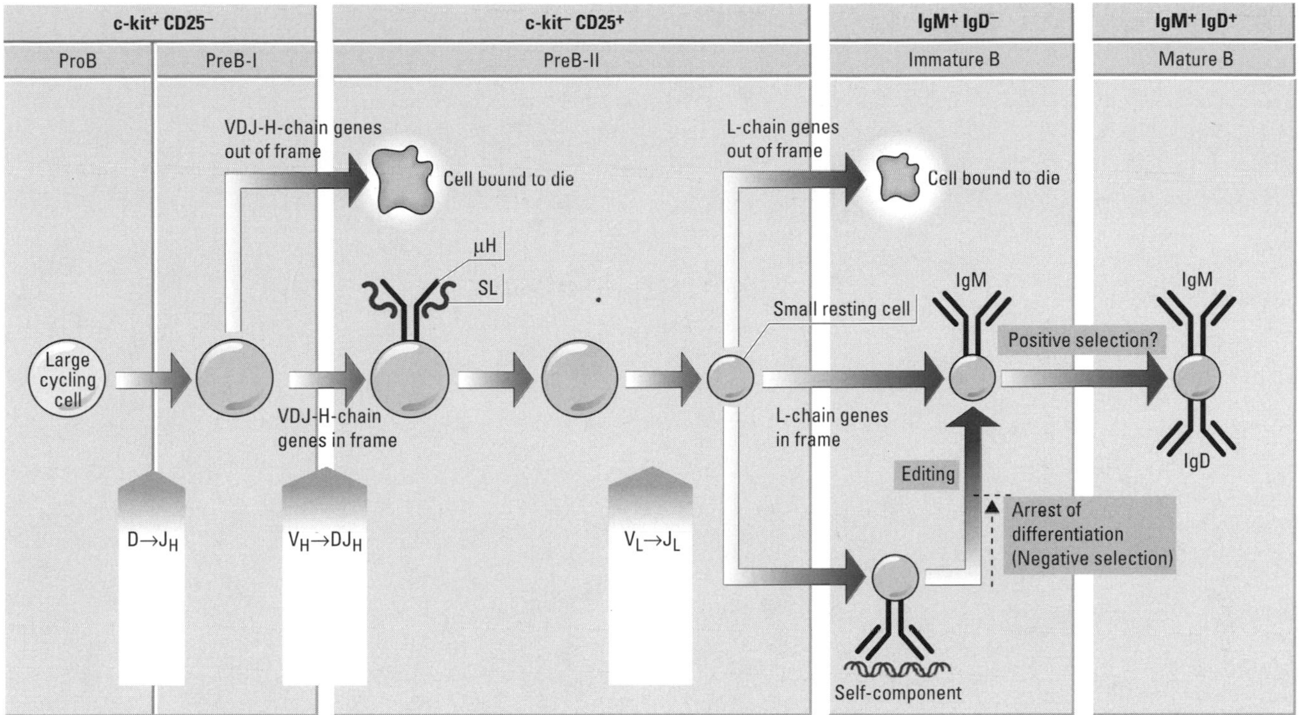

Figure 5.20 Cellular stages and molecular markers of B-cell development in humans and mice. CD, cluster of differentiation; $D \rightarrow J_H$, $V_H \rightarrow DJ_H$, heavy-chain gene rearrangements; Ig, immunoglobulin; μH, μ-type heavy chain; SL, surrogate light (chain); *V*, *D*, *J*, segments of *Ig* genes; $V_L \rightarrow J_L$, light-chain gene rearrangements. (Modified from Rolink, A. *et al.* (1995) *Immunologist*, 7, 125.)

The *precursor B-II cell stage* can be divided (in the mouse at least) into three substages: the large cycling preB-II cells type 1, the larger cycling preB-II cells type 2 and the small resting preB-II cells. The expression 'cycling cell' refers to cells that are repeatedly taken through the mitotic cycle (they proliferate), in contrast to resting cells which remain in the G_0 phase of the cycle. The *large cycling preB-II type I cells* engage in two-step rearrangements of their H chain-encoding loci: $D \rightarrow J_H$ and $V_H \rightarrow DJ_H$. If the rearrangement is successful (*productive*) and can be used to produce a functional protein (the μH chain), further rearrangements are discontinued. The μH chain is expressed on the cell's surface in association with the SL chain, a combination referred to as the *pre-B receptor*. The expression of preB receptors is required for the selection of cells with productively rearranged H-chain genes, for proliferative expansion during the transition from preB-I to preB-II cells, as well as for shutting down the rearrangement machinery on both chromosomes and guaranteeing that of the H chain-encoding loci on the two chromosomes only one remains expressed (*allelic exclusion*; see Chapter 8). The L chain-encoding loci remain unrearranged and inactive at this stage. The mouse large preB-II type I cells no longer express c-kit, TdT, RAG1, RAG2 and they have downregulated the expression of CD43. They are the first cells of the B-lymphocytic lineage to express the CD25 cell-surface marker (the α chain of the IL-2 receptor), although it is not clear to what purpose. The cells can no longer be cloned on stromal cells in the presence of IL-3 or IL-7. Comparable human preB cells have lost the expression of CD34 and TdT, but they remain CD10+ and CD19+.

The mouse *large cycling preB-II type 2 cells* have a similar phenotype to that of the type 1 cells, except that they have switched off the SL chain-encoding genes and turned on the *RAG1* and *RAG2* genes again. The two *RAG* genes are transcribed into RNA, but no RAG proteins are as yet produced. The type 2 cells also show the first signs of activity at the L chain-encoding loci: although the genes have not yet rearranged, they are transcribed into RNA at low levels.

In the *small resting preB-II cell stage*, the cycling has come to a halt and the size of the cells has been reduced to that of a small lymphocyte. By the time the cells have reached this stage, a large proportion of them are found to have rearranged their L chain-encoding loci, although it is not yet clear whether the $V_L \rightarrow J_L$ rearrangements are productive because the L chains do not appear on the cell surface at this early stage. The mouse preB-II are also the first cells of the B-lymphocytic lineage to express CD40 (a

Table 5.4 Markers of B-cell development in mice and humans. (Modified from Rolink, A. *et al.* (1995) *Immunologist*, 7, 125.)

Marker	ProB/preB-I	Large preB-II type 1	Large preB-II type 2	Small preB-II	Immature B	Mature B
Mouse						
CD19	+	+	+	+	+	+
c-kit	+	–	–	–	–	–
CD43	+	+/–	–	–	–	–
CD44	+	+	+	+	?	?
CD45	+	+	+	+	+	+
SL chain	+ (associated with gp35–65/gp130)	+ (μH)	–	–	–	–
CD25	–	+	+	+	+/–	–
CD40	–	–	–	+	+	+
TdT	+	–	–	–	–	–
μH chain protein	–	+	+	+	+	+
H chain RNA	+	+	+	+	+	+
L chain RNA	–	–	+	+	+	+
RAG1, RAG2 RNA	+	–	+/–	+	+	–
Human						
CD34	+	–	–	–	–	–
CD19	+	+	+	+	+	+
CD10	+	+	+	+	+	–
SL chain	+ (association unknown)	+ (μH)	–	–	–	–
CD40	–	–	–	+	+	+
TdT	+	–	–	–	–	–
μH chain protein	–	+	+	+	+	+
RAG1 RNA	+	?	?	+	+	–

CD, cluster of differentiation; c-kit, product of a protooncogene coding for protein *ki*nase (tyrosine); gp, glycoprotein; H, heavy; L, light; *RAG*, recombination activating genes; SL, surrogate light; TdT, terminal deoxynucleotidyltransferase.

molecule that binds hyaluronic acid and thus mediates cell adhesion), but to what purpose is again not clear. The *RAG1* and *RAG2* genes are used at this stage to produce not only RNA but also proteins which then participate in secondary L-chain gene rearrangements. The phenotype of the corresponding human cells is CD34⁻, CD10⁺, CD19⁺, CD40⁺, TdT⁻, SL⁻, μH⁺ (cytoplasmic protein), RAG1⁺, RAG2⁺ (both at the RNA level).

In the *immature B-cell stage*, the rearranging L chain-encoding genes are tested to determine the expressibility of their products. If the products have the properties of an L chain capable of association with the μH chain, the H_2L_2 tetramer is inserted into the membrane and expressed on the cell surface as the BCR of the mIgM type (*m* for membrane and *M* for μ; the designation sIgM, where *s* stands for surface, is sometimes used instead of mIgM). The immature B cells continue to express RAG1 and RAG2 proteins, presumably for participation in additional L-chain gene rearrangements, if these prove necessary (see below). They cease to express the CD25 molecule but continue expressing the CD19 and CD40 molecules. Unlike mature B lymphocytes, immature B cells do not respond by proliferation and maturation into immunoglobulin-secreting cells when exposed to antigen or mitogen. Instead, interaction of the cell-surface BCR with self molecules in the bone marrow arrests further differentiation into mature mIgM⁺ B cells. Such cells are then left to commit suicide. Before this happens, however, it is possible that the immature B cells get another chance to rearrange their L chain-encoding genes and so succeed in producing a combination of H and L chains that does not bind self components. Such *L-chain editing* might be the reason why the *RAG1* and *RAG2* genes remain expressed during the immature B-cell stage. The elimination of self-reactive cells in the bone marrow is a form of *negative selection*. In contrast to negative selection in the thymus, however, it does not require the participation of MHC molecules because the BCR, unlike the TCR, recognizes antigenic molecules alone.

All progenitor, precursor and immature B cells in the bone marrow are short-lived; their half-life appears to be between 1 and 4 days. Most of the cells die in the bone marrow and only about 2–5% of the immature mIg⁺ B cells are selected every day to leave the bone marrow and become *mature B lymphocytes*. How the cells are selected for transition from the immature to the mature type is not known. There are two alternative hypotheses explaining the positive selection: first, a homeostatic mechanism picks immature cells randomly, without regard for the BCR specificity of their surfaces; and second, unidentified antigens choose cells for maturation according to their BCR specificity. The transition from immature to mature B cells is marked by the expression of another type of BCR, the IgD molecule, in which the μH chains have been replaced by δ (delta) chains. The surface phenotype of the *mature B cells* is therefore mIgM+, mIgD+. The mature cells also express a number of other markers in which they differ from immature B cells (see Chapter 17). The cells are sensitive to antigens and mitogens, both of which stimulate their proliferation and further differentiation into immunoglobulin-secreting cells, the former specifically, the latter non-specifically. The early mature B cells may still be short-lived; if stimulated, they may proliferate and differentiate into IgM-secreting cells without help from T lymphocytes, without further diversification of their *Ig* genes by somatic hypermutations (see Chapter 8) and without establishment of B-cell memory. Later, mature B cells emerge whose stimulation, with the help of T lymphocytes, leads to the production of B cells that secrete other types of immunoglobulins, diversify their *Ig* genes by somatic hypermutation and differentiate into long-lived memory B cells. The T cell-independent and T cell-dependent mature B cells can be distinguished not only functionally but also by a set of characteristic markers.

An important driving force of B-cell development is the interaction with stromal cells of the bone marrow. Numerous interactions involving a variety of adhesion molecules (see Chapter 9) probably take place, but of these only a handful have been identified (Fig. 5.21). One of the earliest adhesion molecules expressed on the cells of the B-lymphocytic lineage is CD44, which binds to the hyaluronate on stromal cells. Hyaluronate is a major polysaccharide of the connective tissue consisting of alternating D-glucuronic acid and *N*-acetylglucosamine residues. The CD44–hyaluronate interaction may not send any signals to the proB cell itself, but it does enable other interactions to take place, particularly that between c-kit (CD117) on the proB cell and stem cell factor (SCF, a membrane-bound form of a cytokine) on the stromal cell. The c-kit–SCF interaction leads to the expression of the c-kit tyrosine kinase activity, which is used by the cell to generate other signals. Some of these may lead to the expression of the receptor for IL-7, a cytokine produced by the stromal cells. The signals generated from the interaction of IL-7 with its receptors, together with signals generated by other interactions, provide stimuli for cell division and thus extensive proliferation of the differentiating proB and preB cells. The limiting factor restraining proliferation might be the extent to which the surface of stromal cells is available for contact with proB and preB cells. Surface contact would seem necessary for

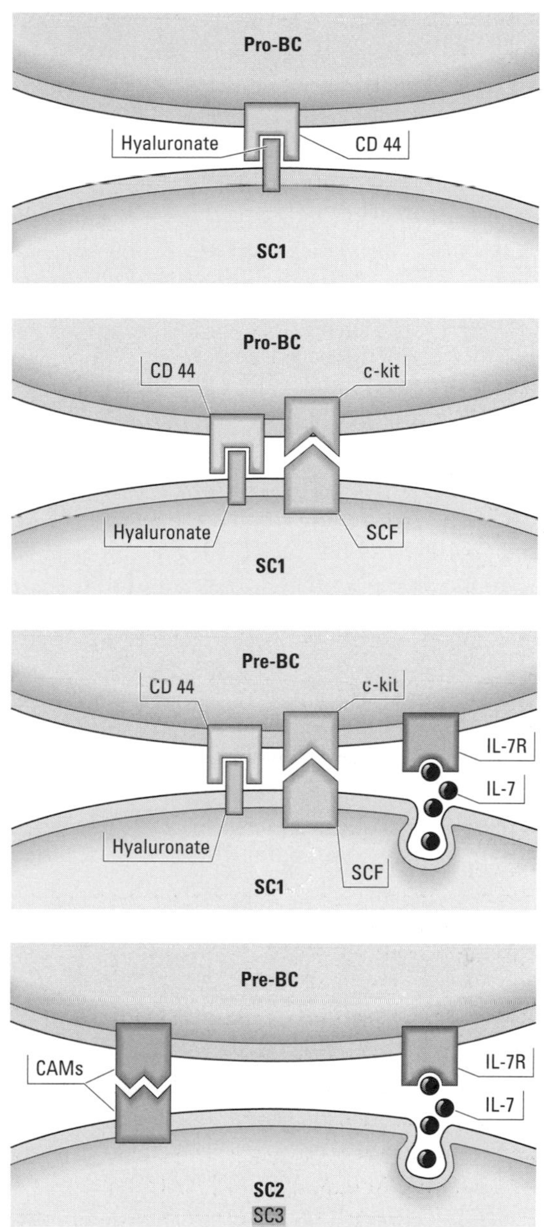

Figure 5.21 Some of the interactions between developing B cells (BC) and stromal cells (SC) in the bone marrow. CAM, cell-adhesion molecule; CD, cluster of differentiation (molecule); IL-7, interleukin-7; IL-7R, receptor for interleukin-7; SCF, stem cell factor.

proliferation to take place but as there is only so much of it available, only the proB and preB cells attached to the stromal cells can divide, while their progeny embarks on further differentiation. This does not mean that in subsequent stages contact with stromal cells is no longer necessary. It probably is, but it may involve different stromal cell types and cell-adhesion molecules. Indeed, morphological studies seem to suggest that B cells in various stages of differentiation occupy different regions of the bone marrow (Fig. 5.22).

In the bone marrow of a young adult mouse, the proB compartment consists of 1×10^6 cells, the preB-I compartment 2×10^6 cells, the preB-II compartment 7×10^7 cells and the compartment of immature B lymphocytes 2×10^7 cells. The compartment of mature B lymphocytes in the entire mouse contains approximately 5×10^8 B2 ($CD5^-$) cells and 5×10^6 B1 ($CD5^+$) cells. The greatest expansion of the B lymphocytic pool therefore occurs in the mature B-cell compartment and is driven by the encounter with antigen.

It is not known at what stage the B1 and B2 cell paths diverge. It has been suggested that the two subsets might be the products of distinct lineages derived from different progenitor cells. The foregoing description of the progression applies to the B2-cell lineage.

There are many obvious parallels between the differentiation of B and T lymphocytes. Although encoded in distinct genes, the BCR and TCR are assembled in similar ways that include the use of surrogate chains before the expression of the real receptor, rearrangement of the encoding gene segments prior to full expression and the use of the same genes (*RAG*, *TdT*) to accomplish the rearrangement and diversify the receptors. The genetic programme that unfolds during the progression, too, seems to be very similar in the two lineages. There is good correspondence between the main developmental stages, the progression seems to pass through analogous switch-points and some of the genes involved in differentiation are again shared by the two differentiating pathways. Finally, both lineages involve stages in which positive and negative selection of the differentiating cells takes place. All these similarities strongly suggest that the two lineages have a common evolutionary origin and that at one stage in the evolution of the vertebrate immune system only one lineage existed that was neither T nor B but an ancestor of the two. Whether this stage has been retained in any of the extant animal taxa is a question that begs an answer.

Evolution

Our knowledge of lymphopoiesis in vertebrates other than *mammals* and birds is fragmentary. Mammals, particularly

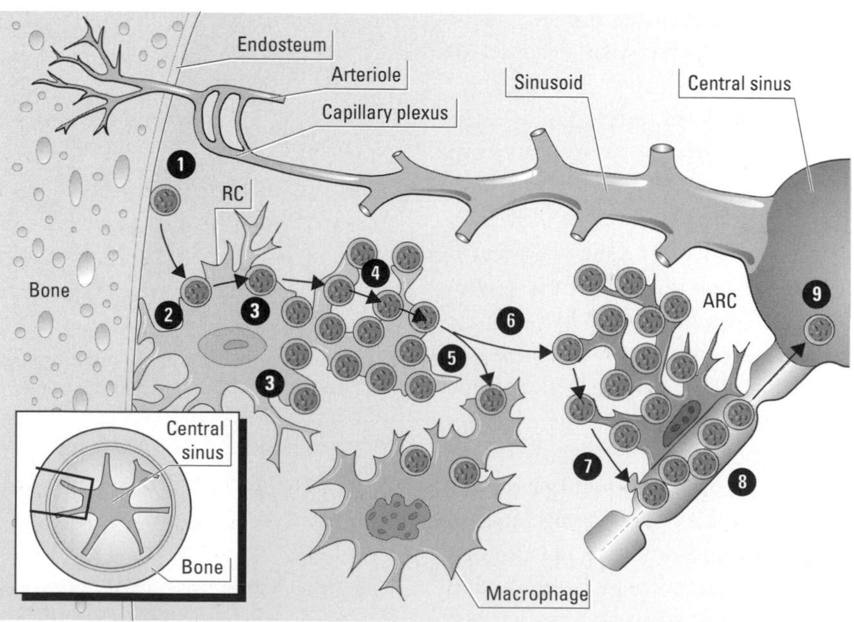

Figure 5.22 Interactions between developing B cells (successive stages indicated by numbers from 1 to 9) and the stroma (ARC, adventitial reticular cells; RC, reticular cells) of the bone marrow. The figure shows a transverse section of a femoral marrow (insert) with an arteriole leading to a capillary plexus near the endosteum (the membrane lining bone cavities), draining into a wide sinusoid and then to a large central sinus. (From Jacobson, K. & Osmond, D.G. (1990) *European Journal of Immunology*, **20**, 2395–2404.)

the mouse, have been studied extensively for the obvious relevance of such studies for human health. In *birds*, T lymphopoiesis takes place in the thymus, as in other vertebrates, but the entire B lymphopoiesis occurs not in the bone marrow but in the bursa of Fabricius, an organ unknown in any other vertebrate class. The bursa develops early in embryonic life and, subsequently, the entire B-cell development proceeds in this organ and the generation of the B-cell repertoire is completed before hatching (in contrast to mammals, in which B lymphopoiesis continues throughout life). How the birds came to this anomaly is not known. It is not because of a lack of bone marrow, which they not only possess but also use to produce all other blood cells as do other vertebrates. Perhaps an investigation of lymphopoiesis in reptiles, crocodiles in particular, the closest living relatives of birds, will shed some light on this interesting conundrum.

In *reptiles*, the dominant site of haemopoiesis is the bone marrow, with the spleen playing a variable part in this process, but the site of lymphopoiesis remains unknown. Some *amphibians* (the anurans, represented by frogs) use bone marrow and spleen for haemopoiesis, including B-lymphopoiesis; other amphibians use spleen, liver and intestinal submucosa. All *jawed fish* generate their blood cells in a primitive kidney (pronephros), spleen (or at least spleen-like tissue) and intestinal wall; only few fish have haemopoietic foci associated with some of their head bones. *Jawless fish* produce blood cells in the pronephros and in unorganized haemopoietic foci in the anterior foregut wall, a tissue interpreted by some investigators as representing the primitive spleen. Information about lymphopoiesis in any of the fish groups is virtually non-existent.

Natural killer cells

To an immunologist, 'natural' is everything that shows an immediate response independent of a prior encounter with the substance stimulating this response. *NK cells* are therefore cells that lyse other cells (targets) almost immediately upon mixing, within 4 hours to be precise. They thus differ from cytotoxic T lymphocytes, which also kill their targets but only after several days of exposure to stimulating cells either *in vivo* or *in vitro*. NK cells, again in contrast to T_C cells, do not require the presence of MHC molecules on target cell surfaces for killing to occur; in fact, the presence of certain class I molecules *inhibits* the cytotoxic activity of NK cells.

Most NK cells have the morphology of what histologists call *large granular lymphocytes* (LGL), which are lymphoid cells with a low nuclear-to-cytoplasmic ratio, indented nucleus and azurophilic granules in the cytoplasm (here

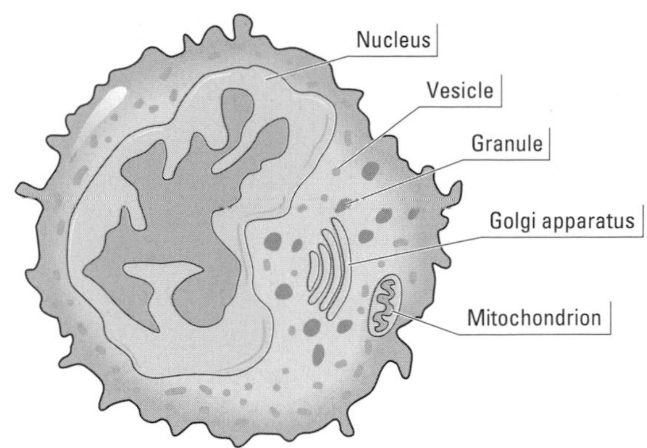

Figure 5.23 Large granular lymphocyte (natural killer cell) viewed with the aid of an electron microscope.

'large' means 'larger than typical (small) lymphocytes'; Fig. 5.23). This morphology is, however, not restricted to NK cells; some resting T cells and activated T_C cells can also be classified morphologically as LGL.

Human NK cells are identified as lymphocytes by the $CD3^-$, $CD16^+$, $CD56^+$ combination of markers, mouse NK cells by the combination $CD3^-$, $NK1.1^+$. The absence of the CD3 complex of chains distinguishes NK cells from T lymphocytes. NK cells may express one of the CD3 chains (zeta, ζ) in association with the CD16 molecule and they contain other CD3 components in the cytoplasm, but they never insert the entire complex into their membranes as T lymphocytes do. The CD16 (FcγRIII) molecules are often used to separate NK cells from other lymphocytes because they are otherwise present only on neutrophils and macrophages. CD56 is a form of neural cell adhesion molecule (NCAM). A further distinction between NK cells and other lymphocytes is in the receptors via which they are activated. NK cells express neither the TCR nor the BCR on their surfaces, although they may accumulate intracellularly truncated, non-functional transcripts of TCR β- and δ-encoding genes. They also do not productively rearrange their *TCR* or *BCR* genes and develop normally in mice in which the *RAG1* and *RAG2* genes have been knocked out. Because, however, they do not kill cells indiscriminately, they must have receptors by which they identify their targets; these are described in Chapter 7.

NK cells constitute only a small fraction of lymphocytes circulating in the bloodstream (approximately 5–10% of all human mononuclear cells). They are rare in the spleen and virtually absent in the thymus and lymph nodes. NK cells presumably mature outside the thymus but their maturation pathway has not been elucidated. Certain T-cell subpopulations also express NK cell markers (CD16, CD56, NK cell receptors) and exhibit NK cell-like activities.

Further reading

T lymphocytes

Allison, J.P. (1993) γδ T-cell development. *Current Opinion in Immunology*, **5**, 241–246.

Arnold, B., Schönrich, G. & Hämmerling, G.J. (1992) Extrathymic T-cell selection. *Current Opinion in Immunology*, **4**, 166–170.

Godfrey, D.I. & Zlotnik, A. (1993) Control points in early T-cell development. *Immunology Today*, **14**, 547–553.

Guy-Grand, D. & Vassalli, P. (1993) Gut intraepithelial T lymphocytes. *Current Opinion in Immunology*, **5**, 247–252.

Haas, W. & Tonegawa, S. (1992) Development and selection of γδ T cells. *Current Opinion in Immunology*, **4**, 147–155.

Kisielow, P. & von Boehmer, H. (1995) Development and selection of T cells: facts and puzzles. *Advances in Immunology*, **58**, 87–209.

Kruisbeek, A.M. (1993) Development of αβ T cells. *Current Opinion in Immunology*, **5**, 227–234.

Pardoll, D. & Carrera, A. (1992) Thymic selection. *Current Opinion in Immunology*, **4**, 162–165.

Shortman, K. (1992) Cellular aspects of early T-cell development. *Current Opinion in Immunology*, **4**, 140–146.

Methods

Baringa, M. (1994) Knockout mice: round two. *Science*, **265**, 26–28.

Capecchi, M.R. (1989) Altering the genome by homologous recombination. *Science*, **244**, 1288–1292.

Capecchi, M.R. (1994) Targeted gene replacement. *Scientific American*, March, 34–41.

Joyner, A.L. (ed.) (1993) *Gene Targeting. A Practical Approach*. IRL Press, Oxford.

Melton, D.W. (1994) Gene targeting in the mouse. *BioEssays*, **16**, 633–638.

Murphy, D. & Carter, D.A. (eds) (1993) *Transgenesis Techniques. Principles and Protocols*. Humana Press, Totowa, NJ.

Sedivy, J.M. & Joyner, A.L. (1992) *Gene Targeting*. W.H. Freeman, New York.

Shapiro, H.M. (1988) *Practical Flow Cytometry*, 2nd edn. Alan R. Liss, New York.

B lymphocytes

Burrows, P.D. & Cooper, M.D. (1993) B-cell development in man. *Current Opinion in Immunology*, **5**, 201–206.

Chen, J. & Alt, F.W. (1993) Gene rearrangement and B-cell development. *Current Opinion in Immunology*, **5**, 194–200.

DuPasquier, L. (1993) Phylogeny of B-cell development. *Current Opinion in Immunology*, **5**, 185–193.

Hagman, J. & Grosschedl, R. (1994) Regulation of gene expression at early stages of B-cell differentiation. *Current Opinion in Immunology*, **6**, 222–230.

Landreth, K.S. (1993) B lymphocyte generation as a developmental process. In *Developmental Immunology* (Eds E.L. Cooper & E. Nisbet-Brown), pp. 238–273. Oxford University Press, Oxford.

Law, C.-L. & Clark, E.A. (1994) Cell–cell interactions that regulate the development of B-lineage cells. *Current Opinion in Immunology*, **6**, 238–247.

Linette, G.P. & Korsmeyer, S.J. (1994) Differentiation and cell death: lessons from the immune system. *Current Opinion in Cell Biology*, **6**, 809–815.

Melchers, F., Karasuyama, H., Haasner, D. *et al.* (1993) The surrogate light chain in B-cell development. *Immunology Today*, **14**, 60–68.

Melchers, F., Haasner, D., Grawunder, U. *et al.* (1994) Roles of IgH and L chains and of surrogate H and L chains in the development of cells of the B lymphocyte lineage. *Annual Review of Immunology*, **12**, 209–225.

Rajewsky, K. (1992) Early and late B-cell development in the mouse. *Current Opinion in Immunology*, **4**, 171–176.

Rolink, A. & Melchers, F. (1993) Generation and regeneration of cells of the B-lymphocyte lineage. *Current Opinion in Immunology*, **5**, 207–217.

Rolink, A. & Melchers, F. (1993) B lymphopoiesis in the mouse. *Advances in Immunology*, **53**, 123–156.

Rolink, A., Andersson, J., Ghia, P. *et al.* (1995) B-cell development in mouse and man. *Immunologist*, **3**, 125–151.

Roth, P.E. & DeFranco, A.L. (1995) Intrinsic checkpoints for lineage progression. *Current Biology*, **5**, 349–352.

Weill, J.-C. & Reynaud, C.-A. (1992) Early B-cell development in chickens, sheep and rabbits. *Current Opinion in Immunology*, **4**, 177–180.

Weissman, I.L. (1994) Developmental switches in the immune system. *Cell*, **76**, 207–218.

Natural killer cells

Lanier, L.L. & Phillips, J.H. (1992) Natural killer cells. *Current Opinion in Immunology*, **4**, 38–42.

Seminars in Immunology (1995) Vol. 7 (entire volume).

Yokoyama, W.M. (1995) Natural killer cell receptors. *Current Opinion in Immunology*, **7**, 110–120.

Yokoyama, W.M. (1995) Natural killer cell receptors specific for major histocompatibility complex class I molecules. *Proceedings of the National Academy of Sciences USA*, **92**, 3081–3085.

chapter 6 Major histocompatibility complex molecules and their relatives

From the vantage point of defence, parasites fall into two categories: extracellular and intracellular. *Extracellular parasites* may enter the body, but not the cells. They live among the cells, taking nutrients from and releasing substances into the body fluids. Most eukaryotic parasites, bacteria and fungi lead this kind of existence. *Intracellular parasites*, on the other hand, enter the host's cells and spend a large part of their life cycle there. They include all the viruses, some bacteria and a few eukaryotic parasites. A cell, however, is not a homogeneous entity: it is partitioned into a number of compartments, each of which has a somewhat different microenvironment. It is therefore very significant in which of the compartments the intracellular parasite lodges. Moreover, the extracellular parasites, although normally subsisting on the outside, come in contact with some of the intracellular compartments. This happens when phagocytic cells, in their role of the body's defenders, engulf some of the extracellular parasites or their products.

The two principal cellular compartments are the *cytosol*, the non-particulate part of the cytoplasm, and the *vesicular compartment*, the particulate part (Fig. 6.1). Viruses and some other intracellular parasites ultimately always end up in the cytosol; the remaining intracellular parasites and the extracellular parasites or their products land in the vesicular compartment. Parasites in these two compartments are handled differently by the host's adaptive immune system, and the molecules that distinguish initially whether a foreign molecule (antigen) comes from the cytosol or the vesicular compartment are controlled by a set of genes summarily referred to as the *major histocompatibility complex* (*MHC*, or *Mhc*). To grasp the difference in the handling of antigens in the two compartments, let us consider in outline the two situations—one exemplified by virus entry into a cell and the other by the uptake of bacterial matter.

Handling of foreign substances by cells

In both situations, the first step is the interaction of the particle (virus or bacterial matter) with the host cell's plasma membrane. This interaction involves molecules in the plasma membrane (*receptors*) and molecules on the surface

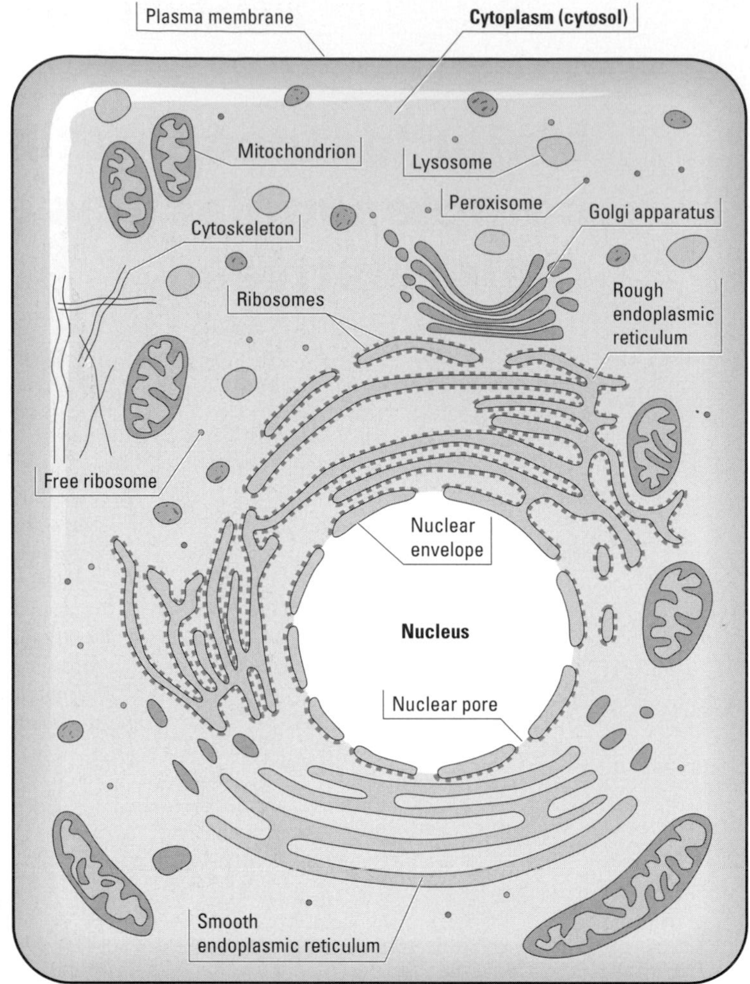

Figure 6.1 Compartments of an animal cell. Bounded by the plasma membrane, a eukaryotic cell consists of a nucleus and cytoplasm. The *plasma membrane* is a glycoprotein-containing lipid bilayer (a structure consisting of two sheets of lipid) that defines the interface between the cell's inner (intracellular) and outer (extracellular) environment. It is permeable to certain gases but not to most other molecules, which can cross the membrane at specialized 'gates' constructed from transporter proteins. The *nucleus* is a double membrane-bounded structure that contains most of the cell's genetic material organized into *chromatin* and during cell division into *chromosomes*, see Fig. 6.8. The *nuclear envelope* is interrupted at intervals by large *nuclear pores* through which the nucleus communicates with the rest of the cell. The pores are highly selective in letting molecules in and out of the nucleus: only molecules containing certain signal sequences can cross it. The *cytoplasm* is the region of the cell lying outside the nucleus. It consists of the cytosol and the vesicular compartment. The *cytosol*, the soluble portion of the cytoplasm, contains the *cytoskeleton* (the network of three kinds of fibres: microtubules, microfilaments and intermediate filaments) and small particles such as free *ribosomes* (structures made of RNA and protein subunits and critically involved in protein synthesis). The cytoskeleton gives the cell its shape and its mobility. The *vesicular compartment* is a system of internal membranes that encloses specific regions from the rest of the cytoplasm and thus defines a collection of subcellular membrane-limited structures or *organelles* (in this sense, the nucleus is the largest organelle). The cytoplasmic organelles include endoplasmic reticulum, Golgi apparatus, mitochondria, lysosomes and peroxisomes. The *endoplasmic reticulum* (ER) is a system of membrane-enclosed spaces used for the synthesis and transport of certain molecules within the cell. It consists of a series of interconnected flattened discs (cisternae), which are of two types, rough and smooth. In the *rough endoplasmic reticulum* (RER), the membranes are studded on their cytosolic faces with ribosomes, which in the electron microscope give them a coarse appearance. The membranes with their ribosomes are involved in the synthesis, processing and transport of proteins destined for the plasma membrane, certain organelles or for secretion. (Proteins destined to remain in the cytosol are synthesized on free ribosomes.) The *smooth endoplasmic reticulum* (SER), which lacks ribosomes, is involved in the synthesis of steroids. The *Golgi apparatus*, named after the Italian histologist Camillo Golgi (1843–1926), is a system of membranes organized into a stashed array (like a stack of plates in a kitchen). Different membranes of the stack contain different sets of enzymes that catalyse the addition of sugars to proteins and lipids; the resulting glycoproteins and glycolipids are then directed by the membranes to appropriate places in the cell. The *mitochondria* are self-replicating organelles bounded by two membranes, outer and inner, and involved in the production of cellular energy in the form of adenosine triphosphate (ATP) by oxidation of small molecules. The *lysosomes* are organelles containing hydrolytic enzymes that degrade many proteins, nucleic acids, lipids and other materials taken up by a cell. (Hydrolytic enzymes use water to break down a substrate.) The *peroxisomes* are organelles that contain oxidative enzymes (i.e. enzymes that catalyse reactions in which electrons are removed from a substrate) used in the metabolism of substances such as hydrogen peroxide.

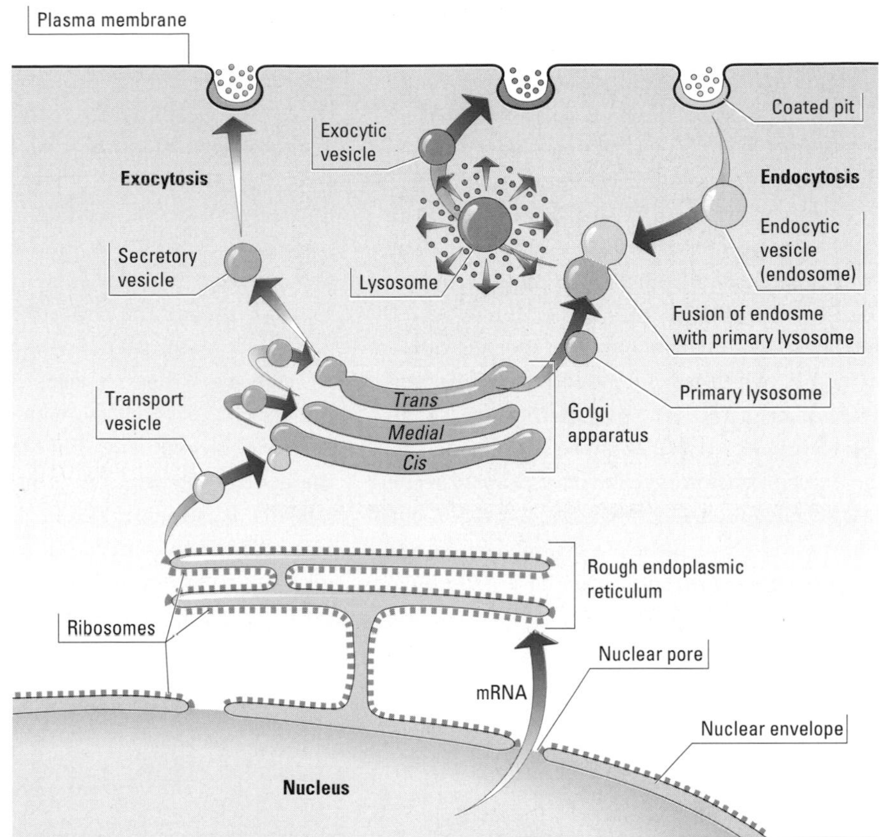

Figure 6.2 The vesicular compartment of a cell. An internal system of membranes is used to import material into the cell and export molecules to the external milieu, as well as to synthesize molecules and to deliver them to different places. Messenger RNA (mRNA) synthesized on the DNA template in the nucleus leaves this organelle through the pores in the nuclear envelope and in the cytoplasm attaches to ribosomes on the surface of the rough endoplasmic reticulum (RER). Proteins translated from the mRNA enter the lumen of the RER and are partially glycosylated (adorned by sugar residues) and the resulting *glycoproteins* are sequestered into *transport vesicles*, which continuously pinch off from the edges of the membranes. The transport vesicles migrate to the *cis* (forming) face of the Golgi apparatus and fuse with its membranes. In the Golgi apparatus, the proteins are further glycosylated by different sets of enzymes residing on the individual leaves. The delivery of glycoproteins from one leaf to the next is probably achieved with the help of another set of transport vesicles. After they have passed through the medial face and reached the *trans* (maturing) face of the Golgi apparatus, the glycoproteins are collected in a *secretory (exocytic) vesicle* that delivers them to the plasma membrane. The fusion of the secretory vesicle with the plasma membrane either integrates the glycoproteins into the latter (if they are membrane bound) or releases them into the extracellular environment (if they are in a free form). The process by which material from the cell's interior is delivered to the cell surface is referred to as *exocytosis*. The reverse of exocytosis is *endocytosis*, a process by which material from the cell's exterior is delivered into the cell. (*Phagocytosis* is a form of endocytosis, i.e. an uptake of particulate material by a cell. An uptake of fluid material is referred to as *pinocytosis*). Endocytosis is facilitated by the interaction of the extracellular material with molecules on the cell surface, the *receptors* in the plasma membrane. The complexes of the material (ligands) with the receptors gather in circumscribed concave areas on the cell surface, which often have a proteinaceous coat on their cytoplasmic side (*coated pits*). The depressions deepen and a spherical, membrane-bounded structure, a *vesicle*, pinches off from the cell surface with the extracellular material inside. The vesicles then lose their coat (if they had one) and become *endosomes*. Their further fate depends on circumstances, but often endosomes fuse with *primary lysosomes*, another set of vesicles that continually bud off from the *trans* face of the Golgi apparatus. Primary lysosomes contain over 40 different digestive enzymes, which they gathered in the Golgi apparatus. The fusion of endosomes with primary lysosomes results in mature *lysosomes* in which the digestive enzymes break down the proteins, nucleic acids and lipids taken up by the endocytic vesicle. The digestion is facilitated by the mildly acidic environment in the lysosome. Some of the digestion products pass through the lysosomal membrane into the cytosol and are reused. The indigestible contents of the lysosome are returned to the extracellular environment by exocytosis. Before this happens, the receptors are segregated into another vesicle and are reused after they have been exocytically returned to the plasma membrane.

of the parasite or its derivative (*anti-receptors*, *ligands*) and it is followed invariably by a membrane-mediated uptake of the foreign matter. An uptake (and discharge) of fluids, soluble molecules and particulate material are a part of normal cell physiology (Fig. 6.2). Cells continually interiorize material from the extracellular environment and exteriorize substances from their interior. The interiorization or *endocytosis* involves a progressive invagination and eventual pinching off of a region of the plasma membrane and thus the formation of an *endocytic vesicle*. (Here *vesicle* means a spherical particle in which a lipid bilayer surrounds a fluid-filled space.) Newly formed endocytic vesicles interact with other vesicles in the cell, part with some of the receptors, return to the cell surface and fuse with the plasma membrane. The exteriorization or *exocytosis* is the reverse of endocytosis: a vesicle pinched off from the internal membranes of a cell migrates towards the plasma membrane and fuses with it, releasing its contents into the extracellular environment.

There are several ways by which viruses enter a cell (Fig. 6.3). Non-enveloped viruses (those that protect their genetic material by a protein coat or *capsid* but that lack a lipid envelope) either leave their coat at the port of entry (i.e. at the plasma membrane, as does, for example, the polio virus) or are taken up into endocytic vesicles and then uncoated inside the cell (e.g. reoviruses). Enveloped viruses (i.e. those that have a lipid membrane in addition to the protein coat) enter cells by fusing their envelope with the host cell membrane either directly on the cell surface (e.g. herpes virus) or after having been taken up into endocytic vesicles (e.g. influenza virus). The uncoating (the release of the genetic material from the capsid) can also occur by a variety of mechanisms, but the end result is always the same: the genetic material lands in the cytosol, usually near the nucleus. It is then taken up by the nucleus, where it replicates. The new material is transcribed into mRNA which migrates to the cytoplasm, where it is translated into viral proteins and these then assemble into new viral particles.

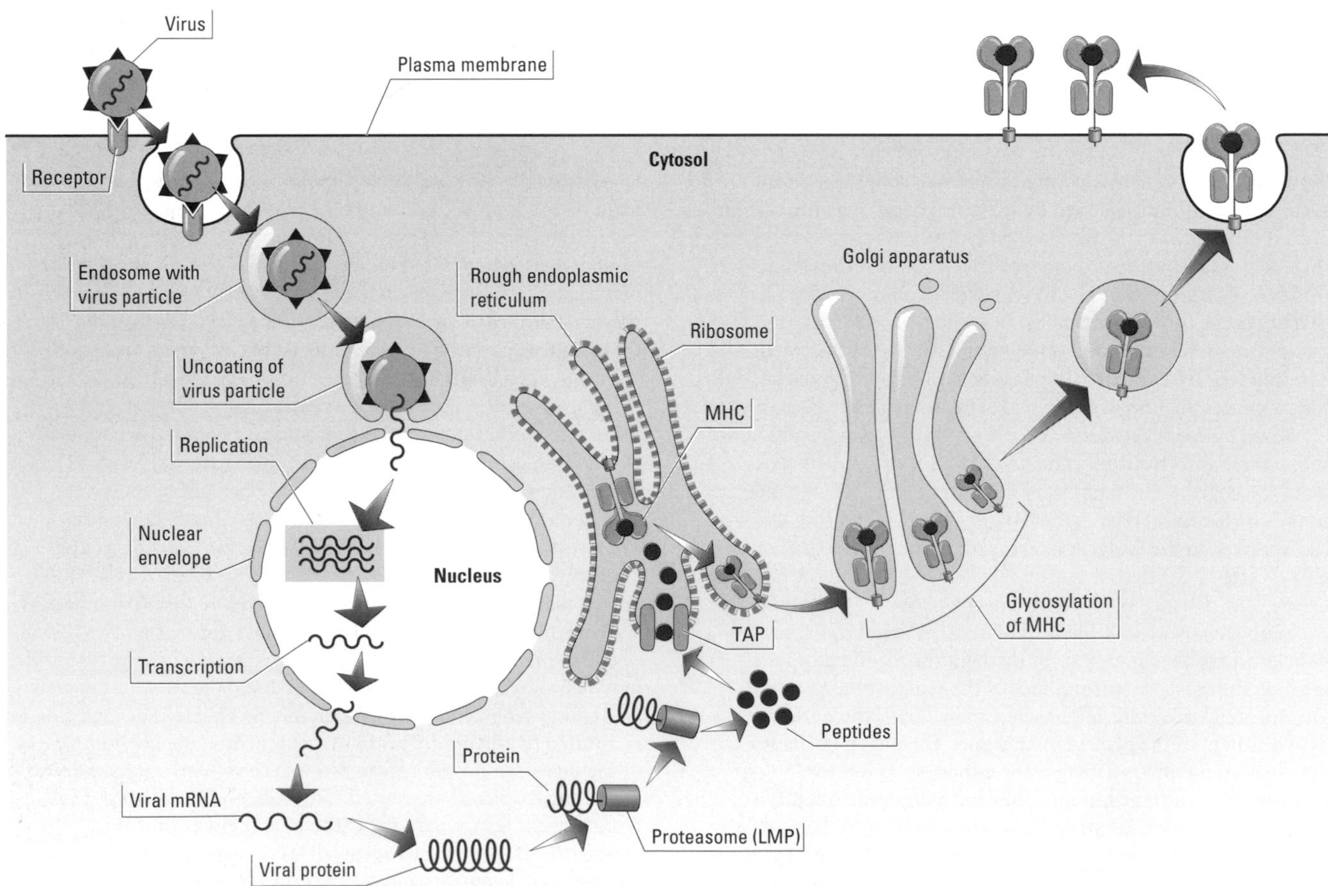

Figure 6.3 The endogenous (cytosolic) pathway of antigen processing and presentation via the major histocompatibility complex (MHC) class I molecules. Explanation in the text: follow the arrows starting from the upper left-hand corner. LMP, low molecular mass protein; TAP, transporter associated with antigen processing.

The adaptive immune system notices the presence of the virus at the stage at which viral proteins appear in large amounts in the cytosol (see Fig. 6.3). Floating in the cytosol are complex proteins termed *proteasomes*, whose function is to cut long polypeptide chains into short *peptides*. Proteasomes do not distinguish between self and non-self proteins and normally act on the cell's own proteins that have, for one reason or another, been marked for disposal. In an infected cell, however, proteasomes also slice viral proteins into peptides. The various peptides are then transported across the membranes of the rough endoplasmic reticulum (RER). The transport is effected by a set of specialized protein structures residing in the RER membrane, the *peptide transporters*. On the luminal side of the membrane, the peptides are loaded onto one of two classes of MHC molecules, the *class I MHC molecules*. A cell possesses different types of proteasomes and a variety of peptide transporters. Those involved in the generation of peptides destined to be loaded onto class I MHC molecules are referred to as *low molecular weight (mass) proteins* or *large multifunctional proteases* (both abbreviated as LMP) and *transporters associated with antigen processing* (TAP, a member of a family of ATP-binding cassette (ABC) transporters; the meaning of these designations will become clear later). The MHC class I molecules consist of two polypeptide chains, the membrane-anchored α and the non-anchored β polypeptides. The chains are synthesized separately on the luminal surface of the RER and when they come together to form a dimer, the peptides are loaded onto them, into a specialized groove formed by the α chain.

The loaded MHC class I molecules are then transported, via the Golgi apparatus and with the help of transport and exocytic vesicles (see Fig. 6.2), to the cell surface where they are integrated into the plasma membrane. The cell's surface is thus studded by MHC class I molecules complexed with peptides. In an uninfected cell, the molecules are loaded with self peptides; in an infected cell, many of them bear non-self (viral) peptides. The adaptive immune system has learned to ignore the MHC–self-peptide complexes and to respond to the non-self-peptide–MHC assemblies. The latter are recognized by the T-cell receptors (TCRs) of the CD8+ T lymphocytes and this recognition activates the T cells (Fig. 6.4). The activated cells divide and some of their progeny differentiates into lymphocytes capable of killing cells that display the same peptide on their class I MHC molecules. These cytotoxic T (T_C) lymphocytes thus target cells infected with the virus and then eliminate them, along with the parasite.

The generation of peptides from antigenic proteins is referred to as *antigen processing*; the display of the MHC–peptide complexes at the cell surface is termed *antigen presentation*; and the cells that carry out the latter are known as *antigen-presenting cells (APC)*. We discuss the entire process of combating intracellular parasites in greater detail in Chapter 21, and return to the MHC class I, LMP and TAP molecules later in this chapter. Here, we must first describe the response to parasites processed in the vesicular compartment.

Consider a protein that has been released from a bacterium lodged in an extracellular space (Fig. 6.5a). The protein binds to a receptor on the host cell surface and is interiorized by endocytosis (see Fig. 6.2). The resulting *early endosome* fuses with primary lysosomes from the Golgi apparatus (see Fig. 6.2) and the bacterial protein is broken down into peptides by the lysosomal enzymes in the resulting *late endosome*. What happens next is still under intensive investigation, but it appears that another, highly

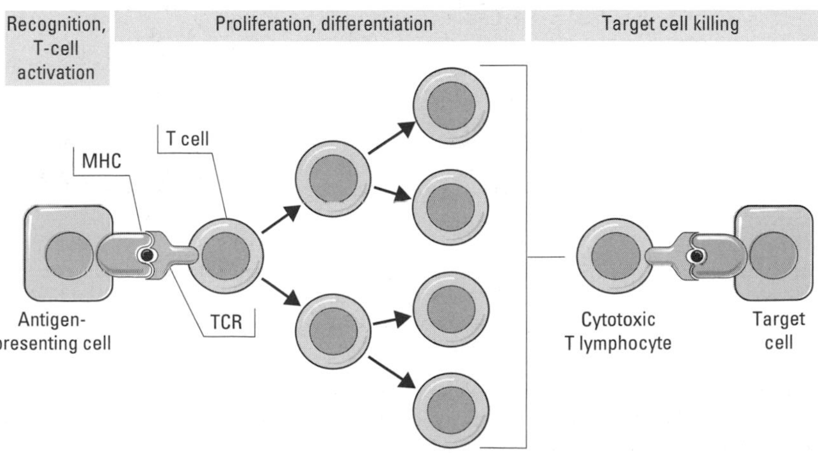

Figure 6.4 Cellular immune response initiated when the T-cell receptor of T lymphocytes recognizes peptide bound to the MHC class I molecule on the antigen-presenting cell. Explanation in the text.

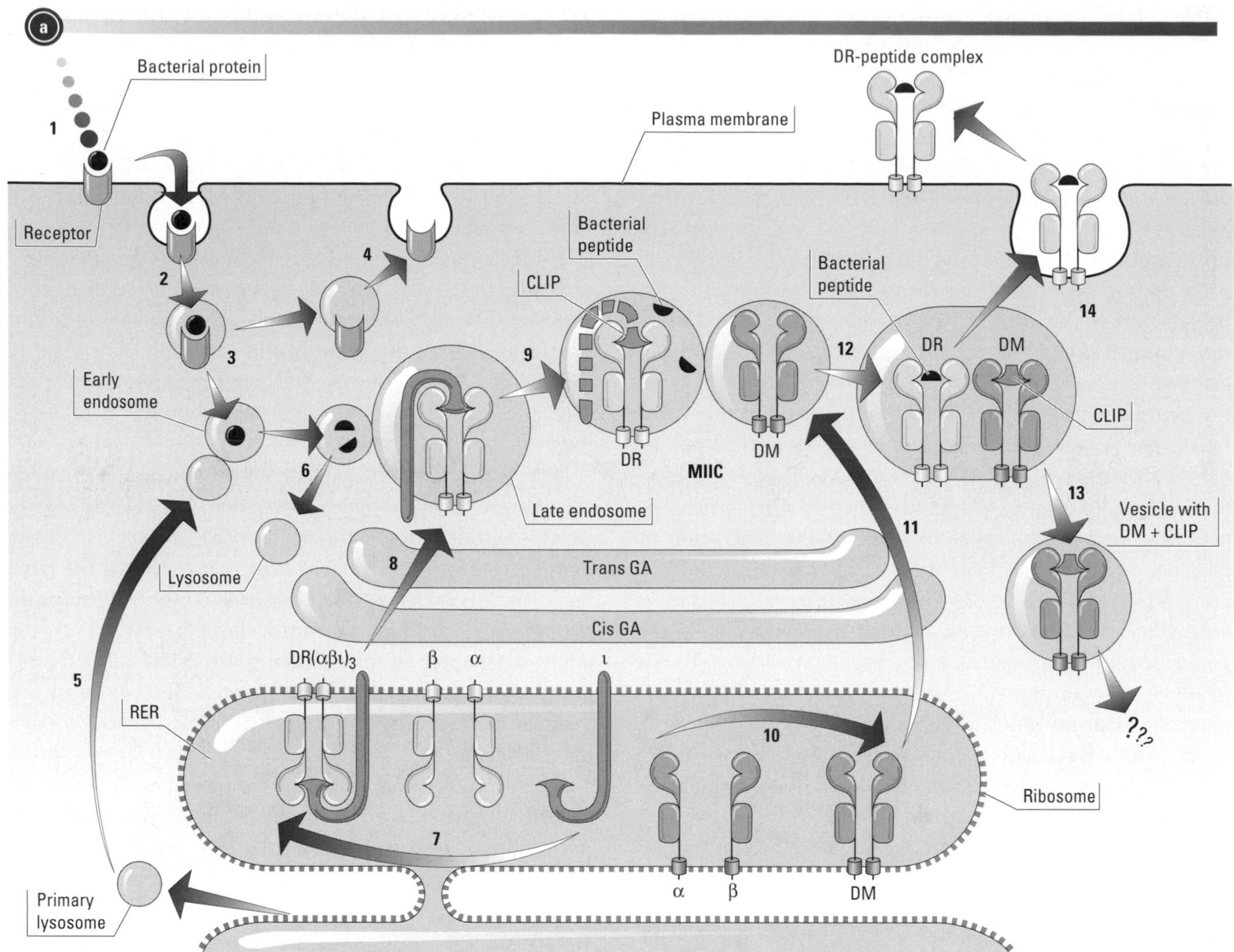

Figure 6.5 (a) Exogenous (vesicular) pathway of antigen processing and presentation via the MHC class II molecules. The individual steps are as follows. 1. Bacterial protein binds to a receptor on the surface of an antigen-processing cell. 2. The receptor–protein complex is interiorized by endocytosis. 3. In the endocytic vesicle, the protein is released from the receptor. 4. The receptor is recycled back to the cell surface by exocytosis. 5. Primary lysosomes bud from the rough endoplasmic reticulum (RER) and fuse with the endocytic vesicle forming an early endosome. 6. In the latter, the bacterial protein is degraded into peptides, the indigestible parts are segregated into the lysosome and the remainder of the endosome fuses with another vesicle that contains MHC class II (HLA-DR) molecules. 7. The two chains (α, β) of the DR molecule are synthesized separately on the membranes of the RER; they then associate with each other and with the invariant chain (ι) also synthesized in the RER. 8. The complex of 3α, 3β and 3ι chains is passed (via transport vesicles, which are not shown) through the Golgi apparatus (GA) and then delivered (via another transport vesicle, which is also not shown) to the peptide-containing endosome. 9. In the late endosome, the invariant chain is degraded, but one part of it, the class II-associated invariant chain peptide (CLIP), remains bound to the α:β heterodimer in the MHC class II compartment (MIIC). 10. In the meantime, the α and β chains of the HLA-DM molecule are synthesized in the RER and (11) delivered via the Golgi apparatus to the MIIC. 12. The DM molecules release CLIP from the DR molecule and the latter binds the bacterial peptide. 13. The DM–CLIP complexes are segregated into separate vesicles whose fate is unknown. 14. The DR–peptide complexes are delivered to the cell surface by exocytosis. (b) Loading of peptides (PT) onto MHC class II molecules. Follow arrows starting from the lower right-hand corner (solid arrows indicate molecular interactions, broken arrows transport between compartments). In the rough endoplasmic reticulum, newly synthesized α and β chains associate transiently with binding protein (BiP) and calnexin and with the invariant chain (Ii), 3α, 3β and 3Ii chains, forming a nonameric complex $(\alpha\beta)_3\mathrm{Ii}_3$. BiP and calnexin dissociate and the nonamer is delivered to the Golgi apparatus. Some nonamers are delivered to the cell surface and then rapidly internalized into endosomes. Most nonamers, however, are delivered directly from the Golgi apparatus (the *trans*-Golgi network) into a specialized endosomal peptide-loading compartment, the MHC class II compartment or MIIC. The delivery is steered by at least two leucine-based sequence motifs in the cytoplasmic region of the Ii

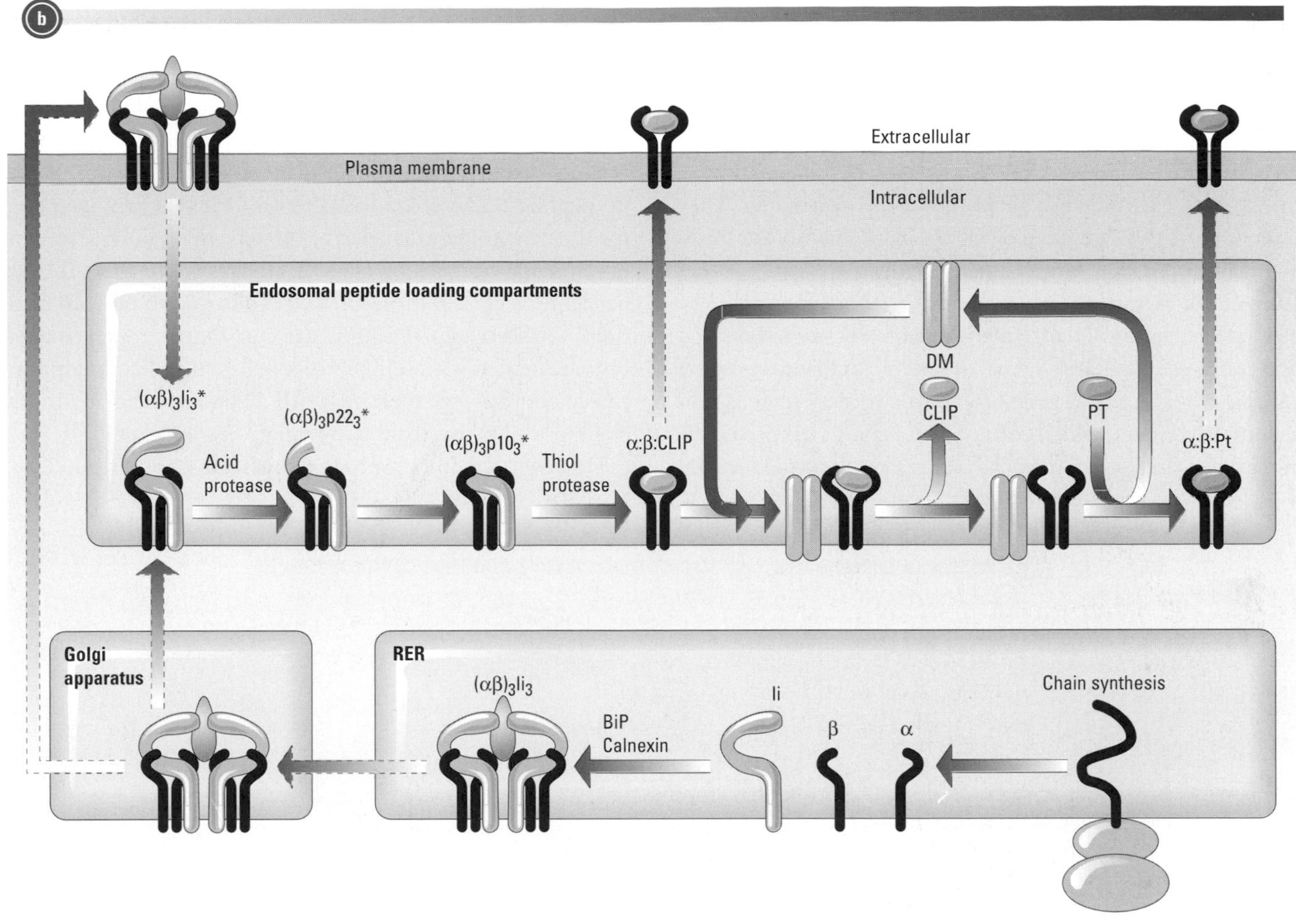

Figure 6.5 (*Continued.*)
chains. In the MIIC, the invariant chain is stepwise proteolytically degraded. First, acid (aspartic) proteases cleave the chain to M_r 22 000 intermediates (p22) and M_r 10 000 intermediates (p10); then thiol proteases such as cathepsin B cleave p10 to class II-associated invariant chain peptide or CLIP. (In this part of the figure, only three chains of the nonamer are depicted for the sake of simplicity.) CLIP, which is derived from residues spanning positions 81–104 of the Ii chains and is 20–24 residues long, remains bound to the groove of the class II molecules, each α:β heterodimer bearing one CLIP. The proteolysis is possible because this part of the Ii chain has an extended, disordered form easily accessible to the proteolytic enzymes. With the completion of the proteolysis, the nonamer falls apart and only α:β heterodimers whose grooves are occupied by CLIPs remain. Some of the α:β–CLIP complexes are delivered to the cell surface, but the majority of the complexes remain in the MIIC and exchange CLIP for peptides (PT) generated in lysosomes from proteins (self and non-self) brought into the cell from the cell exterior. The exchange is facilitated by the DM molecules which associate transiently with the α:β–CLIP complex. DM molecules enhance the dissociation of CLIP from the complex and thus enable the exogenously derived peptides to take their place. The nature of the interaction of CLIP and of the exogenously derived peptides with the groove is very similar: the peptides are stretched out and some of their side-chains are inserted into the pockets in the groove's wall; these will be described later in this chapter. The spontaneous dissociation of CLIP from the groove is usually slow (the rate, however, varies among different class II allelic products) and the DM molecule speeds it up by an unknown mechanism. Once the exogenously derived peptide is loaded into the groove, the DM molecule dissociates itself from the complex and is reused for loading peptides onto other α:β heterodimers. The loaded peptides are then delivered to the cell surface by an unknown route (they may be transported along the endocytic pathway, the MIIC may directly fuse with the plasma membrane or the molecules may be transported by vesicles such as those used for recycling of molecules). Modes of peptide loading different from those just described apparently also exist. Some peptides are loaded independently of the Ii chains (other proteins may bind to the α:β heterodimers instead of the Ii chains and are subsequently cleaved) and independently of the DM molecules, probably during recycling of class II molecules. From some class II molecules, CLIP apparently dissociates spontaneously and fast enough to make DM-mediated enhancement superfluous. DM molecules can apparently also act on the intermediate complexes before the final α:β–CLIP complexes are produced. The molecules enhance not only the dissociation of CLIP but also of certain other peptides (e.g. those derived from the myelin basic protein). (From Busch, R. & Mellins, E.D. (1996) *Current Opinion in Immunology*, 8, 51.)

specialized set of vesicles brings MHC molecules into the endosome. These molecules are of a different class than the class I molecules participating in the cytotoxic pathway; they are referred to as *class II MHC molecules*. Like the class I molecules, the class II molecules are synthesized on the membranes of the RER as two polypeptide chains, α and β, both of which are anchored in the membrane. They assemble on the luminal side of the RER membranes into α:β heterodimers, which then associate with another polypeptide termed the *invariant chain* (Ii or ι for iota). The Ii chain is structurally unrelated to the MHC molecules and its encoding gene is not part of the chromosomal region occupied by the *MHC* gene. The α:β:ι trimers then assemble into nonamers, which contain three chains of each of the three kinds (in Fig. 6.5 only the trimers are depicted for simplicity). The class II α:β dimers have, like the class I α chain, a groove that can bind peptides, but in the α:β:ι trimers (nonamers) the groove is blocked by the invariant chain. In contrast to the class I molecules, which are loaded with peptides at the time of their assemblage, the class II molecules are for a while prevented by the invariant chain from taking up peptides. There is a good reason for this arrangement, for the foreign peptides derived from extracellular proteins never reach the site of class II synthesis and assemblage; hence if the class II molecules were allowed to take up peptides as the α and β chains are put together they would become loaded with self peptides before they had an opportunity to pick up their non-self peptides. The invariant chain prevents this from happening.

However, the invariant chain also has another function.

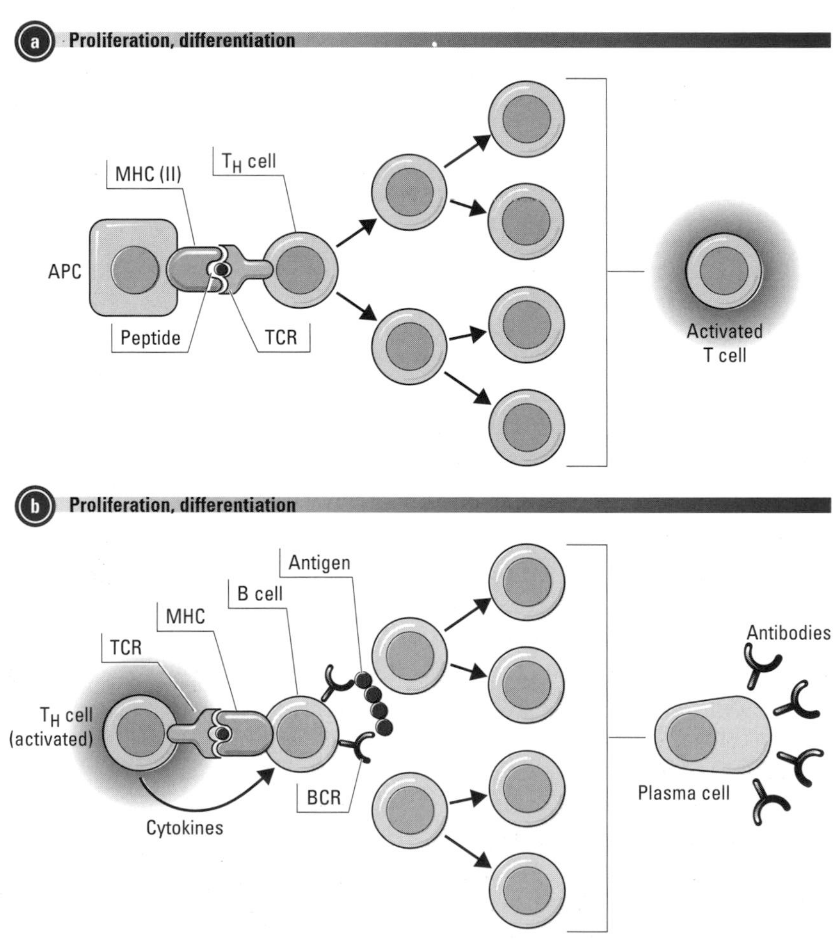

Figure 6.6 Humoral immune response. (a) A peptide bound to MHC class II molecules on an antigen-presenting cell (APC) is recognized by the T-cell receptor (TCR) on a helper T (T_H) lymphocyte (CD4+) which is thereby activated. (b) The activated T_H cell recognizes the same peptide bound to the MHC class II molecule on a B lymphocyte (the peptide has been produced by processing in the B cell after the latter has bound a bacterial protein via its B-cell receptor, BCR, and interiorized it). At the same time, antigen (bacterial protein) cross-links the BCRs on the B lymphocyte and thus generates a signal which, together with a cytokine stimulus from the activated T_H cell, in turn activates the B cell. After proliferation, the B cell differentiates into an antibody-secreting plasma cell.

It contains a signal that segregates the $\alpha:\beta:\iota$ complexes into specialized vesicles termed the *MHC class II compartment* (MIIC). This segregation happens after the complexes have been delivered by transport vesicles from the RER to the *trans*-face of the Golgi apparatus. In the MIIC vesicles that have budded off from the Golgi apparatus, all of the invariant chain is enzymatically degraded except for one peptide, which remains complexed to the peptide-binding groove of the $\alpha:\beta$ dimer. This *class II-associated invariant chain peptide* (CLIP) thus continues to prevent the class II molecules from taking up other peptides. The degradation of the invariant chain breaks up the nonamers so that in the MIIC the class II molecules are now in the form of $\alpha:\beta$ dimers complexed with the CLIP.

The MIIC vesicles then fuse with the late endosomes and it is here that the two limbs of the vesicular pathway meet: the endosomes with the broken-down peptides of the bacterial proteins and the class II molecules with binding sites for the peptides still blocked by CLIP. Exactly how the CLIP is removed is still uncertain but it is clear that the removal requires the participation of yet another set of molecules, probably delivered to the endosome by another set of vesicles. They are the *DM molecules*, which are related to the class II molecules in that they, too, consist of α and β chains with a structure similar to that of the classical class II α and β chains. The DM $\alpha:\beta$ dimers, however, are not associated with invariant chains and unlike classical $\alpha:\beta$ dimers they are not destined for expression on the cell surface. The interaction between classical class II and DM molecules leads to the release of CLIP from the former; perhaps the conditions in the MIIC are such that they favour the binding of CLIP to DM rather than to classical class II molecules. The vacated groove of the classical class II molecules is then immediately loaded with the peptides present in the MIIC. The loaded class II molecules are sequestered into specialized exocytic vesicles that bring the molecules to the surface and integrate them into the plasma membrane. The unused foreign material is sequestered into lysosomes and the DM molecules are possibly recycled.

The events are more complex than we have described them (for additional information, see Fig. 6.5b) and many of the complexities are still unresolved. In particular, it is still controversial in which compartment the loading of the peptides onto the class II molecules occurs. There may, in fact, be several compartments that can carry out this function. Also unclear is the origin, the mode of action and the fate of the DM molecules.

At the cell surface, the peptides complexed with the class II molecules are recognized by TCRs on the $CD4^{+}$ T lymphocytes (helper T cells, T_H; Fig. 6.6). The recognition event is translated into a signal that activates the T lymphocytes and induces them to proliferate and differentiate. The activated cells secrete soluble substances (cytokines) that act on other cells, among which are also B lymphocytes. Mature B lymphocytes bind antigens via their *B-cell (immunoglobulin) receptors* (BCRs), but this binding does not require the participation of MHC molecules and it is not restricted to processed peptide. Some of the antigen bound by the BCR is internalized, processed by the B cell and the resulting peptides are presented in association with class II molecules on the cell surface. The class II MHC–peptide assemblies of the B lymphocyte are recognized by the T_H cells activated by the recognition of the same assembly. This interaction results in the secretion of cytokines by the latter and these then provide the second signal to the B cell (the first signal resulting from the binding of the antigen by the BCR). The delivery of the two signals activates the B lymphocyte, the cell divides and some of the progeny sets on a course towards terminal differentiation into plasma cells, which secrete a soluble version of the BCR, the *antibodies*. Their presence in the extracellular fluids makes the antibodies a highly suitable tool for dealing with extracellular parasites. The requirement for

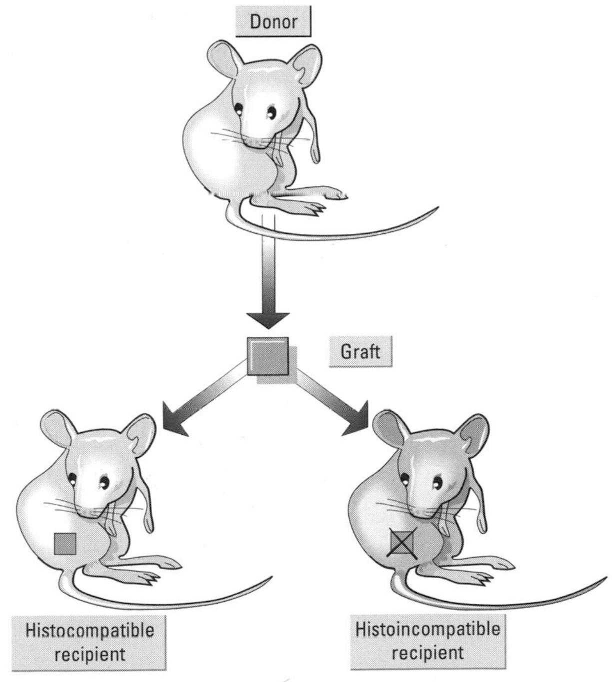

Figure 6.7 The concept of histocompatibility. A graft (e.g. a piece of skin) transferred (transplanted) from a donor onto a genetically identical recipient heals in and survives for the lifetime of the recipient lives. A similar graft is destroyed (rejected) by the host's immune system if it is transplanted onto a genetically disparate recipient. The immune response is elicited by histocompatibility antigens controlled by histocompatibility genes.

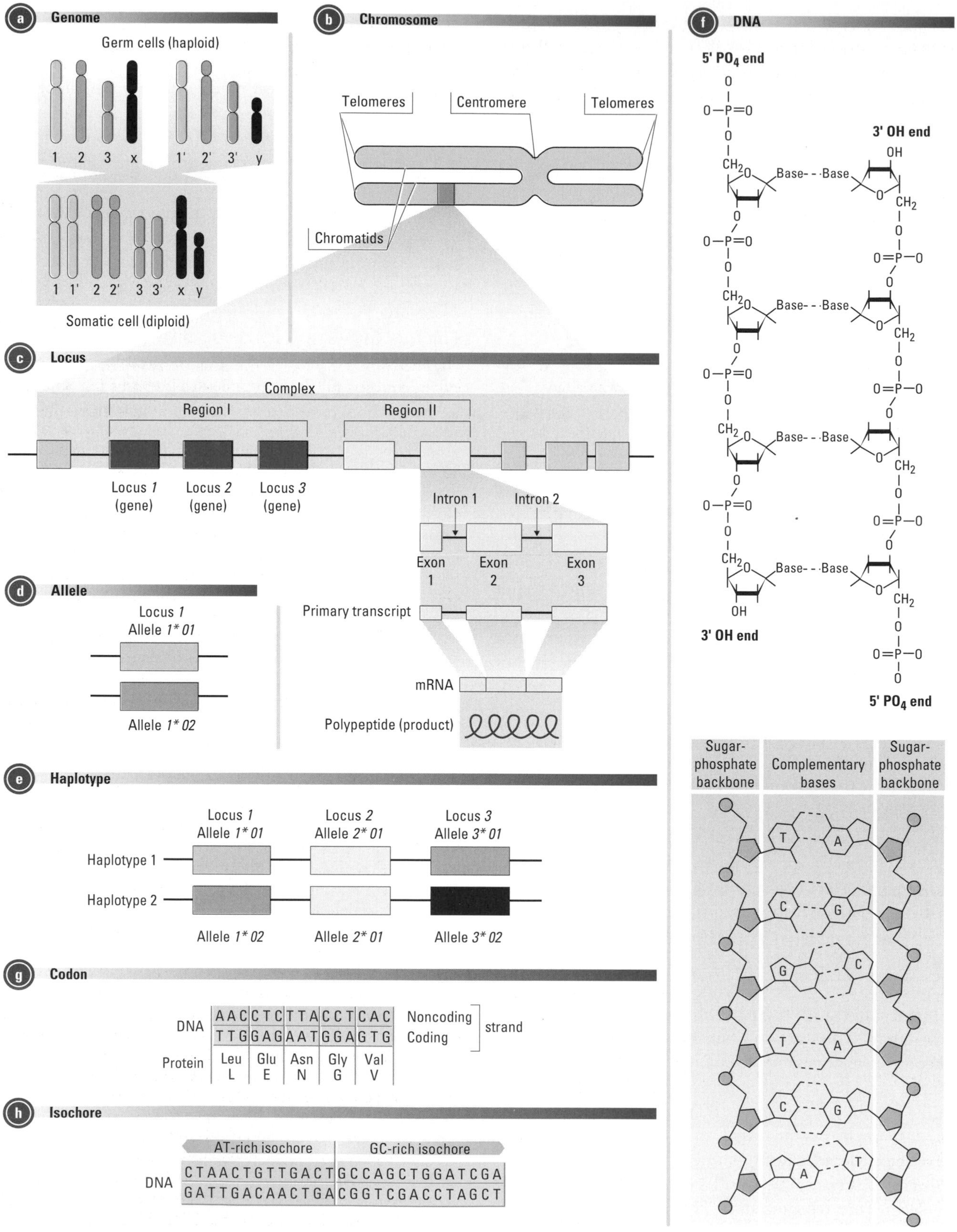

a Genome

Germ cells (haploid)

1 2 3 x 1' 2' 3' y

1 1' 2 2' 3 3' x y

Somatic cell (diploid)

b Chromosome

Telomeres

Centromere

Telomeres

Chromatids

c Locus

Complex

Region I

Region II

Locus *1* (gene)

Locus *2* (gene)

Locus *3* (gene)

Intron 1

Intron 2

Exon 1

Exon 2

Exon 3

Primary transcript

mRNA

Polypeptide (product)

d Allele

Locus *1*
Allele *1* 01*

Allele *1* 02*

e Haplotype

	Locus *1*	Locus *2*	Locus *3*
	Allele *1* 01*	Allele *2* 01*	Allele *3* 01*
Haplotype 1			
Haplotype 2			
	Allele *1* 02*	Allele *2* 01*	Allele *3* 02*

f DNA

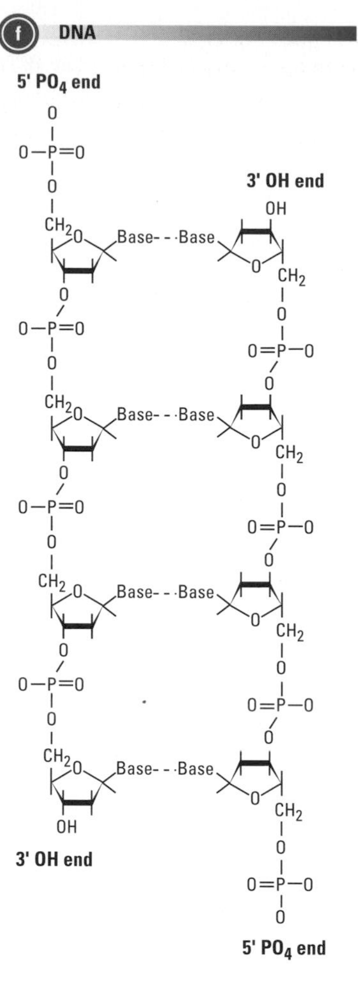

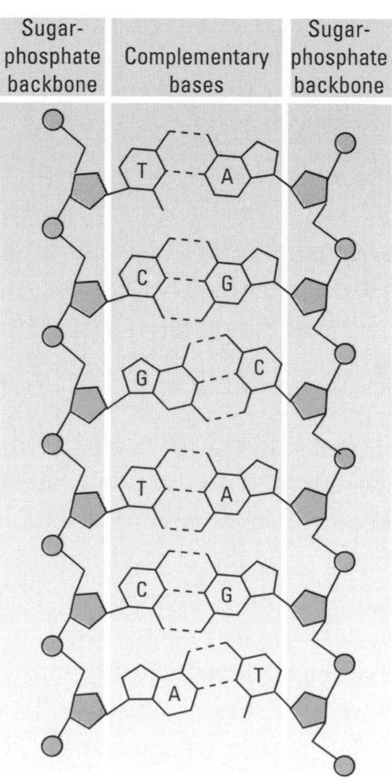

g Codon

DNA	AAC	CTC	TTA	CCT	CAC	Noncoding	strand
	TTG	GAG	AAT	GGA	GTG	Coding	
Protein	Leu L	Glu E	Asn N	Gly G	Val V		

h Isochore

	AT-rich isochore	GC-rich isochore
DNA	CTAACTGTTGACT	GCCAGCTGGATCGA
	GATTGACAACTGA	CGGTCGACCTAGCT

interaction between T and B lymphocytes in the form described assures that the antibodies the B cells will ultimately secrete will be directed against the same antigen (although not necessarily the same part of the antigenic molecule) that has stimulated the T lymphocytes. It thus guarantees the specificity of the immune response.

As in the case of the class I-mediated pathway, the events leading to the degradation of foreign proteins and the gen-

Figure 6.8 (*Opposite*.) Genetic terminology. (a) The total nuclear DNA of a *germ cell* such as the spermatozoon or the oocyte constitutes the *genome*; all other *(somatic) cells* of a multicellular organism have double the amount of DNA compared to the germ cells, i.e. they are *diploid*, while the germ cells are *haploid*. The genome is partitioned into *chromosomes*, which in germ cells form a single set, whereas in diploid cells they are present in two sets so that each chromosome has a partner or *homologous chromosome*. In the haploid germ cell, chromosomes thus occur singly, whereas in diploid cells they exist in pairs, where the members of each pair are very similar to each other but usually not identical. Each species has a fixed number of chromosome pairs distinguishable by their length and morphology. Humans have 23 pairs of chromosomes, which are numbered from the longest (chromosome 1) to the shortest (chromosome 22); chromosome pair 23 comprises the sex chromosomes X and Y; pairs 1–22 are the *autosomes*. (b) After the completion of DNA synthesis in the S phase of the cell cycle, each chromosome of a somatic cell consists of two DNA duplexes held together at a site termed the *centromere* (the chromosome ends are the *telomeres*). As the cell enters the mitotic stage and prepares for cell division, the duplexes, together with the associated proteins (the *chromatin fibres*), begin to condense into sausage-shaped structures, the *chromatids*. Each chromosome of the mitotic stage thus consists of two *sister chromatids* joined by the centromere. The condensation reaches its maximum in the *metaphase* when the chromosomes assemble in the equatorial plane of the mitotic spindle awaiting segregation to the spindle's poles. (c) Researchers often focus on a particular stretch of the DNA sequence, which is then referred to as a *locus* (or a 'nuon' in a recently proposed terminology; *nuon* is 'any stretch of nucleic acid sequence that may be identifiable by any criterion'). In this book, we concentrate on loci that are copied (*transcribed*) into RNA (the *primary transcript*), that carry out specific functions in the life of the organism and that include information necessary for the regulation of transcription (in particular the so-called *promoter sequences*). We refer to such DNA stretches as *genes*. In virtually all the genes we consider, the *primary transcript* is processed into a shorter version (the *messenger* or *mRNA*) by excision of parts of the sequence, and parts of the mRNA are *translated* into a protein. The process by which a gene is transcribed into a primary transcript, which is then processed into mRNA, which is then translated into a protein, will be referred to as *expression of a gene*. The parts of the gene retained in the mRNA are the *exons* (short for 'expressed part of a gene'), while those parts removed (*spliced out*) from the primary transcript are the *introns* (short for 'intervening sequence'). A gene that has lost its function is a *pseudogene*. In the translation process, nucleotide triplets (*codons*) of the nucleotide sequence specify individual amino acids in the protein sequence. The gene is said to *code for* a protein and the protein is said to be *encoded* in the gene. (d) Genes occupying corresponding positions on homologous chromosomes constitute *alleles* which can be identical or may differ in their sequence to some extent. (e) The constellation of alleles at two or more loci of a single chromosome is the *haplotype*. A cluster of related loci on a chromosome is a *gene complex* which can be divided into *regions* such that genes within a region are more related to one another than they are to genes in other regions. The standard practice in genetics is to print gene (allele, haplotype) symbols in italics and protein symbols in roman type. Another rule of genetic nomenclature is to avoid using Greek letters in gene symbols; such letters are reserved for polypeptide chains of proteins. Both these practices will be adhered to in this book. Moreover, wherever standardized nomenclature has been agreed upon, it too will be used even when it is not universally accepted by immunologists. (f) Each of the two strands of the *deoxyribonucleic acid* (DNA) molecule consists of a linear array (sequence) of *nucleotides*, each nucleotide consisting of a *nitrogenous base*, the sugar deoxyribose and a phosphate group, PO_4. The alternating phosphate and sugar units form the backbone of the strand; the bases determine its sequence. The four bases are adenine (A), guanine (G), thymine (T) and cytosine (C), the first two being purine and the last two pyrimidine derivatives. The two strands are held together by the pairing of G of one strand with C of the other strand and of A with T (*complementary pairing*). The carbon and nitrogen atoms in the ring structure of the bases are numbered 1, 2, 3, etc., whereas the carbon atoms of the sugar are numbered 1′, 2′, 3′, etc. In the sugar–phosphate backbone, the phosphate groups connect the 3′ carbon of one deoxyribose with the 5′ carbon of the next. As a result of this linkage, each strand has a free phosphate group attached to the 5′ carbon of the deoxyribose at one end and a free hydroxyl (OH) group attached to the 3′ carbon at the other end. The termini of the strand are therefore referred to as the *5′ end* (read 'five prime') and the *3′ end* (read 'three prime'), respectively. By convention, nucleotides are always read in the $5' \rightarrow 3'$ direction. By another convention, the direction towards the 5′ end from any given point in the sequence is referred to as *upstream* and the opposite direction as *downstream*. (g) In the DNA molecule, only one of the two strands contains information for the assembly of a particular polypeptide. The information is *encoded in* the nucleotide sequence of this strand, in such a manner that each amino acid is specified by one nucleotide triplet (*codon*). The names of the 20 amino acids that occur in proteins are abbreviated either to three letters or one letter (L or Leu, leucine; E or Glu, glutamic acid; N or Asn, asparagine; G or Gly, glycine; V or Val, valine; for a complete list of abbreviations, see Appendix 1). (h) The DNA molecule is a linear mosaic of regions with low GC content alternating with regions of high GC content; the regions are termed *isochores*. The *GC content* is expressed as a percentage of G + C nucleotides in a 'window' containing a certain number of nucleotides. Here, the GC content of the AT-rich isochore is 5/13 = 0.38 or 38%; the GC content of the GC-rich isochore is 9/14 = 0.64 or 64%.

eration of peptides suitable for complexation with MHC class II molecules are referred to as *antigen processing* and the display of the class II–peptide complexes at the cell surface for recognition by CD4+ T lymphocytes as *antigen presentation*. The MHC molecules and the molecules required for antigen processing and presentation will be described in this chapter; the TCR and BCR in the next two chapters; the cytokines and other molecules involved in the interaction between T and B lymphocytes in Chapters 9 and 10; and the responses, schematically and simplistically summarized in Figs 6.4 and 6.6, are discussed in detail in Chapters 16 and 17. However, before we delve into the description of the MHC, we must explain how the complex came to its name.

A patch of tissue taken from one individual and transplanted to another is destroyed by the recipient's immune system because the cells in the donor tissue express molecules on their surfaces that are different from those expressed by the recipient. The molecules act as antigens and as such stimulate the recipient's lymphocytes (Fig. 6.7). The antigens thus determine whether the tissue will be immunologically compatible with the recipient, i.e. they act as *histocompatibility antigens*, encoded in *histocompatibility genes*. The speed with which the transplanted tissue is destroyed depends on the particular histocompatibility antigens by which the donor and the recipient differ. Most of the antigens are weak (*minor*) in that, when acting singly, they only stimulate a delayed and slow tissue destruction. There is, however, one set of antigens that elicits rapid destruction and thus has a major effect on tissue compatibility. These are the major histocompatibility antigens encoded in a set of clustered loci, the *major histocompatibility complex*. MHC antigens are not related in any way to the minor histocompatibility antigens. The latter are a mixed bag of proteins that have only two things in common: they are expressed on the cell surface and their peptides are loaded onto MHC molecules (for further details, see Chapter 24).

MHC is a generic name; in some species, the MHC has an additional name that in most cases consists of the species' name and the words 'lymphocyte (leucocyte) antigen'. Thus, human MHC is the *human leucocyte antigen* (HLA), cattle MHC is the *bovine leucocyte antigen* (BoLA), pig MHC is the *swine leucocyte antigen* (SLA), and so on. In some species, however, other names are used for historical reasons. The mouse MHC, for example, is called *histocompatibility 2* (H2, previously H-2) because the histocompatibility genes were numbered in the order of discovery, *H1*, *H2*, *H3*, etc., and *H2* happened to be one of the first to have been identified. (Actually, it was the very first *H* locus and the very first MHC recognized but, for reasons that would take too long to explain, it was thought to be second.) The rat MHC is the *Rat1* or *RT1* (like Airforce-1; note the modesty of rat MHC researchers!). The MHC of the domestic fowl is referred to as the *B complex* because it was originally identified as one of several blood group loci, which were designated sequentially by capital letters. In many species, the complex is designated by an abbreviation of the scientific genus and species name and *Mhc*. For example, the MHC of the chimpanzee, ***Pan troglodytes***, is *Patr-Mhc*, that of the orang-utan, ***Pongo pygmaeus***, is *Popy-Mhc* and so on.

Genomic organization

The human *MHC* resides on the short arm of *chromosome 6* in the band 6p21.3 (Figs 6.8 & 6.9). It takes up at least 4 million nucleotide pairs (base pairs or 4×10^6 bp, which equals 4000 kilobase pairs or 4×10^3 kb, which equals 4 megabase pairs or 4 Mb). It is rather arbitrarily divided into three *regions* designated I, II and III, which together contain more than 120 loci (Fig. 6.10). The *class I region* on the telomeric side of the complexes spans 2 Mb and contains at least 25 but perhaps as many as 50 loci (new loci are being added to the growing list as the study of this region progresses). The *class II* region on the centromeric side spans 0.8 Mb and contains 34 loci. The *class III* region in the middle of the complex spans 2.2 Mb and contains at least 63 loci. Thus, the gene densities in the human *MHC* are one gene per 20 kb, 40 kb and 15 kb in the class I, II and III regions, respectively. In the entire complex, less than 10% of the DNA sequence is potentially translatable into protein and more than 90% has no known function. At the level of the DNA sequence, the human *MHC* can be divided into two parts or *isochores* (see Fig. 6.8) differing in their GC contents. The border between the two isochores falls approximately between the class II and class III regions, the class II region being characterized by a low (<50%) and the class III and class I regions by a high (>50%) GC content. Thus in the coding sequences of the class III and class I regions, the third nucleotide (base) of each codon has a higher chance of being G or C than being A or T.

The three *MHC* regions contain three types of genes. One type comprises the *MHC genes proper*, which encode proteins with the potential of presenting peptides to the TCRs. Some of these genes may have subsequently lost this function but their structure indicates that they once had at least the potential for it. The second type comprises *non-MHC genes with immune functions*. The structure of the proteins encoded in these genes is very different from that of the MHC proteins proper and there is no indication of any direct evolutionary relationship between the two types, but

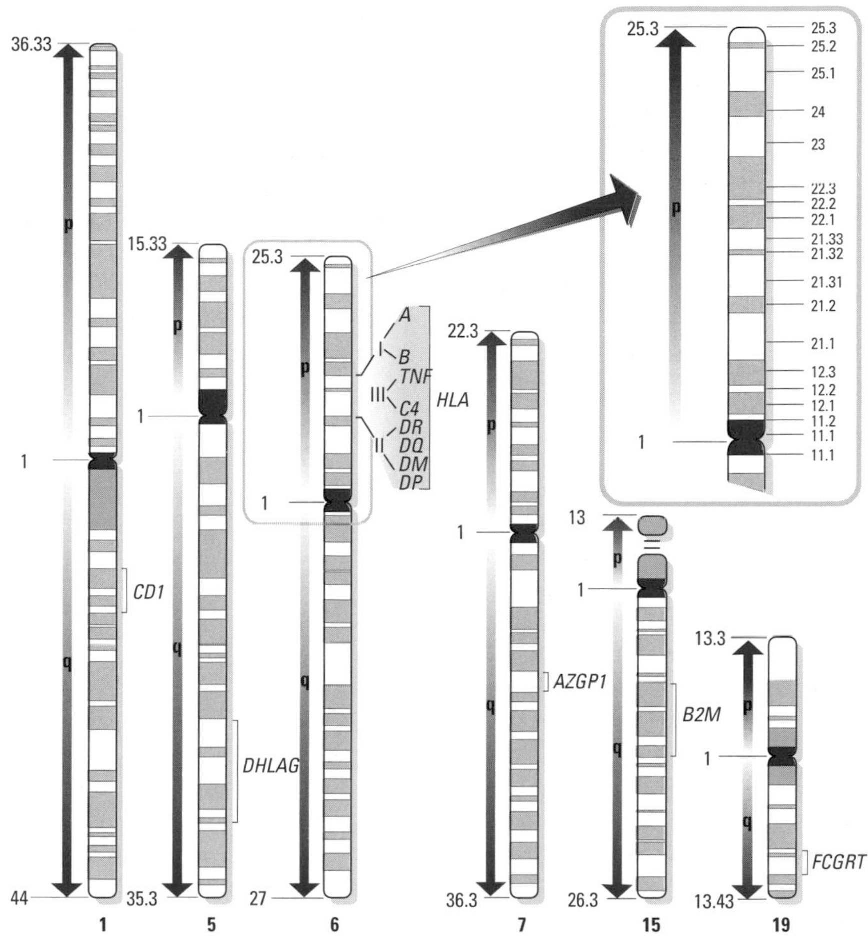

Figure 6.9 Location of the *MHC* and *MHC*-like genes on the human chromosomes. When treated briefly with the proteolytic enzyme trypsin and stained with the Giemsa reagent, *metaphase chromosomes* reveal a pattern of alternating dark and light bands, i.e. they become *banded*. The pattern (the number and width of the bands) distinguishes the individual chromosome pairs (within each pair the two chromosomes normally show the same pattern) and thus can be used for their identification. Metaphase chromosomes are numbered, according to their relative length, from 1 to 22 (the autosomes); the sex chromosomes are designated X and Y. To facilitate communication between gene mappers (those investigators who strive to determine the position of the individual genes on the chromosomes), a reference system that can be compared to mapping coordinates has been designed for each chromosome. The centromere divides the chromosome into two arms, the short p and the long q arm (for *petit* and *queue*, respectively). Each arm is then divided into sections (1, 2, 3, etc.), each of the sections into subsections (11, 12, 13, 21, 22, etc.), each subsection into sub-subsections (11.1, 11.2, 11.3, 21.1) and so on, according to the need. The numbering on each arm always proceeds in the direction from the centromere to the end of the chromosome (the telomere). The sections, subsections and sub-subsections largely reflect the gradual increase in resolution of the banding pattern as the technique improves over the years. Using this reference system, the position on the chromosome can be specified. For example, the position of the *HLA* complex is given as 6p21.3 which means 'chromosome 6, short arm, section 2, subsection 1, sub-subsection 3'. *AZGP1*, Zn-α_2 glycoprotein 1; *B2M*, β_2-microglobulin; *CD1*, cluster of differentiation 1; *DHLAG*, major histocompatibility complex, class II gamma polypeptide, the invariant chain; FCGRT, Fc receptor, IgG, α-chain transporter; *HLA*, human leucocyte antigen. These *MHC*-like genes are discussed later in this chapter. In these diagrams only one chromatid of each chromosome is shown and the constriction indicates the position of the centromere. The chromosome number is given below each chromosome.

the proteins carry out immunological functions and this fact alone is enough for some immunologists to consider the two types to be functionally related. The ties that have been proposed to exist between the two types of proteins, however, often strain one's imagination. The third type comprises genes that even the most fantasy-endowed immunologists have to concede have nothing to do with immunity. This third type, which outnumbers the first two types in the human *MHC*, is concentrated in the class III region but scattered loci with non-immune functions occur also in

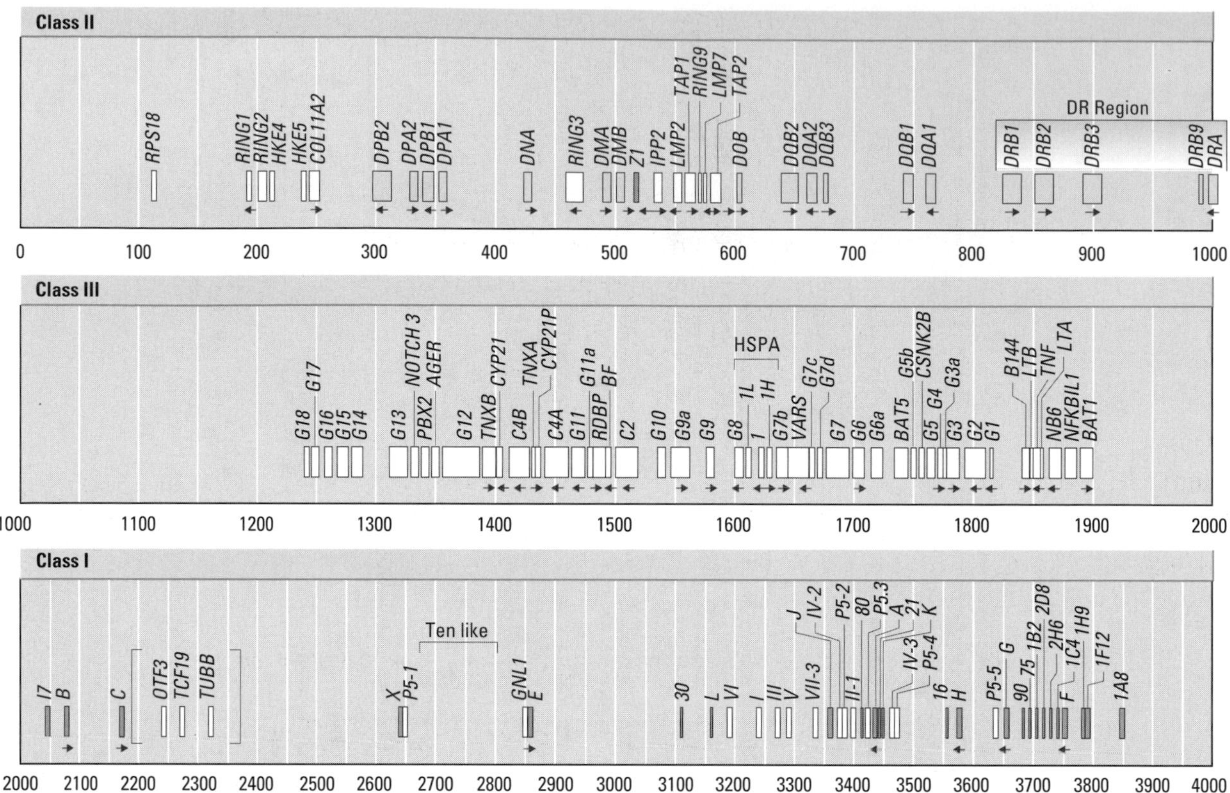

Figure 6.10 Physical map of the human *MHC*. Rectangles indicate loci and arrows their transcriptional orientation (where it is known). The scales are in kilobase pairs (kb). The width of the rectangles indicates approximately the length of the sequence occupied by the loci. The *MHC* (*HLA*) loci proper are indicated by closed rectangles (class I and class II loci are differentiated by shading); all other loci are indicated by open rectangles. The map is contiguous (the order is: centromere . . . class II. . . class III. . . class I. . . telomere), but here, for logistic reasons, it is divided into three sections representing the three regions. *AGER*, advanced glycosylation end product-specific receptor; *B144*, B144 protein (expressed in B cells); *BAT*, HLA-B-associated transcript; *BF*, complement factor B; *C2*, complement component 2; *C4A(B)*, complement component 4A (B); *COL11A2*, collagen, type XI, alpha-2; *CREBL1*, cAMP responsive element binding protein-like 1; *CSNK2B*, cassein kinase 2, beta; *CYP21 (P)*, cytochrome P450, subfamily XXI (pseudogene); *G*, gene; *GNL1*, guanine nucleotide binding protein-like 1; *HKE*, human homologue of mouse *H2K* end gene; *HSP70A1* (L, H), heat-shock protein, M_r 70,000, No. 1 (like, homologous); *IPP2*, inhibitor of the protein phosphatase type 2; *LMP*, large multifunctional protease; *LTA(B)*, lymphotoxin, alpha (beta); *NB6*, meaning not specified; *NFKBIL1*, nuclear factor kappa light chain gene enhancer in B cells inhibitor-like 1; *NOTCH3*, homologue of *Drosophila* gene responsible for 'notched wings' mutation; *OTF3*, octamer binding transcription factor 3; *PBX2*, pre-B-cell leukaemia transcription factor 2; *RDBP*, RNA-binding protein (codes for dipeptide repeat of arginine or R and aspartic acid or D); *RING*, 'really interesting gene'; *RPS18*, ribosomal protein S18; *RXRB*, retinoid X receptor beta; *TAP*, transporter, ABC; *TCF19*, transcription factor 19; *TNF*, tumour necrosis factor; *TNX*, tenascin X; *TUBB*, tubulin, beta; *VARS*, valyl-tRNA synthetase. (Based on the MHCDB database; see Newell, W.R., Trowsdale, J. & Beck, S. (1994) *Immunogenetics*, **40**, 109.)

the class I and class II regions. Human *MHC* genes proper occur only in the class I and class II regions. There have been various speculations as to how this situation may have arisen but these can be resolved only when the *MHC* organization in other vertebrates becomes known. The limited data available thus far (Fig. 6.11) paint a picture of tremendous upheavals in organization during evolution of the *MHC*. Although many placental mammals have their *MHC* organized similarly to humans, others differ considerably from the human prototype. Even individuals of the same species (and this includes humans, as we shall learn shortly) may differ in the number and arrangement of the *MHC* genes they carry. Some associations are indeed the same as those found in the human *MHC*, but in birds or in bony fish the *MHC* genes proper are interspersed with other genes that are not part of the human *MHC* and the *MHC* genes proper are scattered over the genome. These observations cast doubts on efforts to ascribe significance to the conservation of gene neighbourhoods. Just because the same two genes are neighbours in the human and in the frog does not

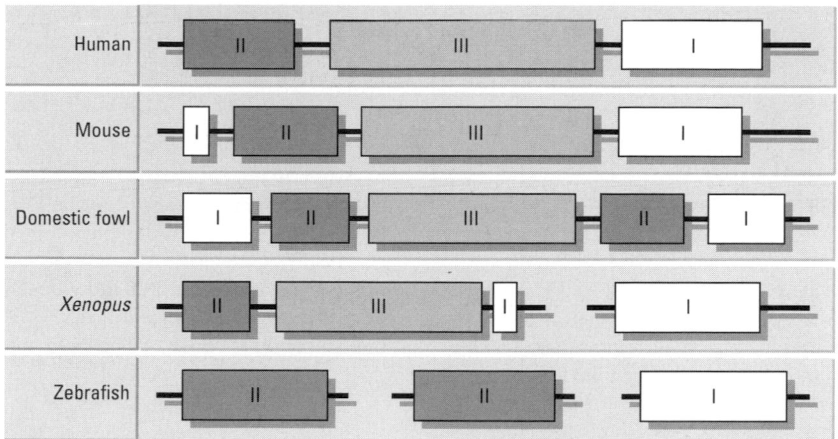

Figure 6.11 Organization of the *MHC* in mammals (human, mouse), birds (domestic fowl), amphibians (the clawed toad, *Xenopus laevis*) and bony fish (the zebrafish, *Danio rerio*). Here, the three regions are represented as blocks of loci. Each unit indicates a separate chromosome so that, for example, in the zebrafish the *MHC* is distributed over three different chromosomes (in this species, class III loci flanking the *MHC* genes are omitted).

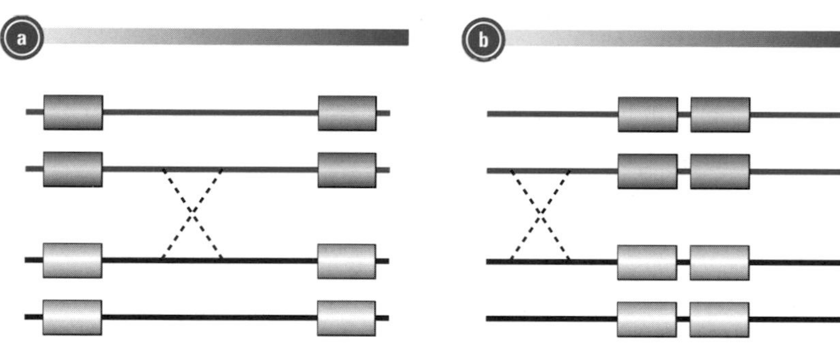

Figure 6.12 The principle of genetic mapping. When two loci (rectangles) reside on the same chromosome, there is a preponderance of parental combinations among the progeny, whereas when they are on different chromosomes, parental- and recombinant-type progenies appear with equal frequencies. The reason for the former situation is that the genes on the same chromosome are inherited together, unless they are separated by *crossing-over* (dotted lines). *Recombination* would separate genes in every meiosis if they were on the opposite ends of the chromosome (a) because normally at least one crossing-over occurs per chromosome per meiosis. Genes less than this distance apart (b) will not always exchange places (recombine) and thus there will be instances when the products of meiosis carry only parental gene combinations: the genes will show a tendency to be inherited together or *linked*. How strong the *linkage* is depends on how often the two genes recombine by crossing-over. The probability of crossing-over between two loci depends on the physical distance between them: the greater the distance, the higher the chance of crossing-over in the particular interval. A measure of linkage is the *recombination frequency* (f), which is obtained by dividing the number of recombinants by the total number of progeny tested. The relationship between distance and recombination frequency also allows geneticists to *map* genes. Consider as an example three genes, A, B and C, and their respective alleles, a, b and c. Because genes furthest apart have the highest probability of crossing-over occurring between them, they give the highest frequency of recombination. Hence, if we find in an appropriately designed cross that the recombination frequency between A and C is higher than that between A and B or between B and C, we can conclude that the gene order is $A \ldots B \ldots C$. This relationship can be depicted by constructing a *genetic (linkage) map*. Distances on the genetic map are expressed in *map units* or *centimorgans* (*cM*), where 1 map unit equals 1% of recombination (i.e. recombination frequency multiplied by 100); 1 cM is one-hundredth of a morgan so that 1 M equals 100% of recombination. Thomas Hunt Morgan, after whom the measurement was named, was an American geneticist (1866–1945).

mean that this association is required for their functions. There are many examples of clearly unrelated genes remaining neighbours throughout the entire course of vertebrate evolution.

There are two principal ways of determining the order of genes in a chromosomal segment like the *MHC*; in other words, of constructing a *map* of the segment. One way relies solely on methods of classical genetics (Fig. 6.12) and

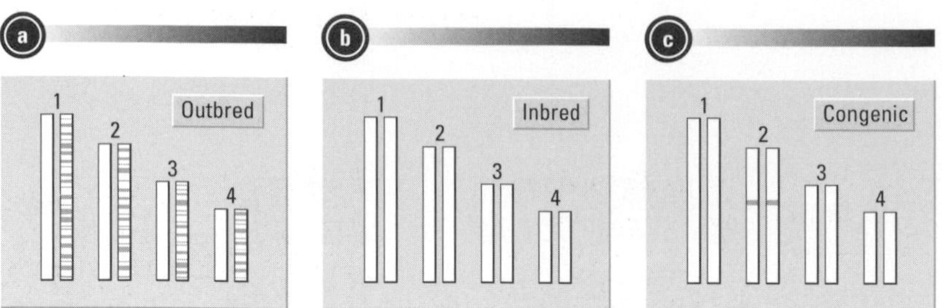

Figure 6.13 Outbred, inbred and congenic strains. A hypothetical organism with only four chromosome pairs (1–4) is shown. In each pair one chromosome is taken as a standard (open bar) to which the other chromosome is compared: where differences in DNA sequence occur, a stripe is drawn. In an *outbred* individual (a) there are many such differences between the homologous chromosome (the individual is heterozygous at many loci). These differences occur at different loci in the various individuals so that no two individuals are genetically the same. In an *inbred* individual (b) the two chromosomes in each pair have an identical DNA sequence, at least in theory, and all the individuals are genetically identical. A *congenic* individual (c) is also inbred, but it differs from another inbred individual at a single locus (indicated by a grey stripe in chromosome 2). Collections of individuals of these three types constitute outbred, inbred and congenic *strains*.

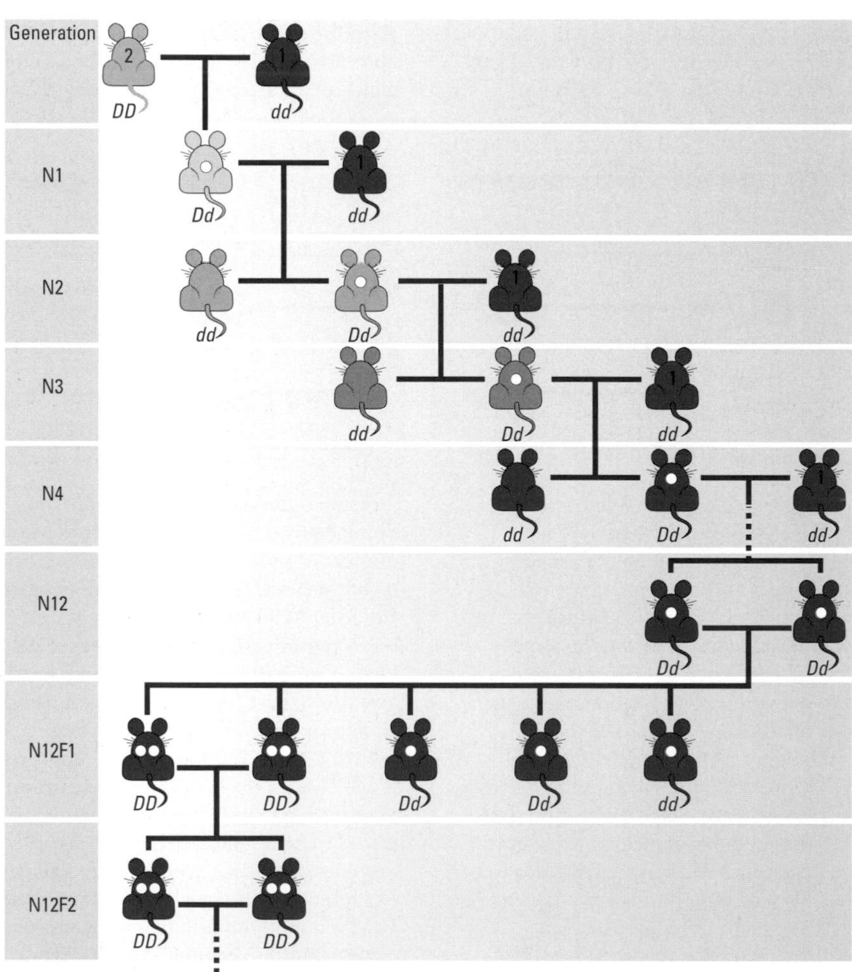

Figure 6.14 Production of a congenic strain. The process begins with mating of two mouse strains, 1 and 2, one of which is inbred (strain 1), while the other need not be. Strain 2 carries an allele (*D*) at a particular locus which one wants to introduce into strain 1 (to replace the *d* allele in this strain). The progeny of this mating (N1 generation) is typed, an individual carrying the *D* allele is selected, and mated with a strain 1 individual. The process is repeated in the N2 and all subsequent generations, always mating the D^+ individual with a strain 1 individual. After 12 generations, *D*/*d* heterozygous individuals are mated together and from the resulting *DD* homozygotes a strain is established that, theoretically, has all the genes of strain 1 except for the *D* gene (the white dot in the mouse symbol) which comes from strain 2. The effect of the repeated mating to strain 1 in each N generation is the introduction of more and more strain 1 genes into the strain that is being developed.

results in a *genetic map* (also referred to as *linkage map* because it is based on *linkage* of genes, i.e. the tendency of genes on the same chromosome to be inherited together) in which distances are expressed in units of recombination (*centimorgan*, cM). The other utilizes methods of molecular genetics and leads to a *physical map* in which distances are measured in numbers of nucleotide pairs. Methods of classical genetics have been used most successfully in the house mouse in which their application has been greatly facilitated by the availability of inbred, congenic and *H2* recombinant strains. *Inbred strains* (Fig. 6.13) are collections of genetically identical or nearly identical individuals produced by repeated matings of close relatives. Their use largely eliminates genetic variability, which might otherwise influence the outcome of an experiment and make its interpretation difficult. *Congenic strains* (Fig. 6.14) are groups of inbred strains that are genetically identical or nearly identical except for one chromosomal segment. (Strains that differ at one locus only are referred to as *co-isogenic*.) They have proved to be indispensable in studies testing the effect of the *MHC* on immune response, disease susceptibility and various other traits. Finally, *H2 recombinant strains* (Fig. 6.15), which can be either outbred, inbred or congenic, are established from individuals in which recombination took place within the *H2* complex. They have provided a virtually unlimited supply of individuals carrying a reshuffled *MHC* and have thus been instrumental in placing genes into specific *MHC* regions. Although molecular biological methods have supplanted these three tools of classical genetics in some areas of immunological research, in certain other areas progress would be slowed down considerably without them. After all, molecular biology's high level of sophistication is useless if a gene encoding a given trait has not been isolated (*cloned*). However, to clone a gene responsible for a specific phenotype, one must use organisms expressing this phenotype. The correlation of a phenotype with a particular short region of the genome from which the controlling gene can then be isolated is tremendously facilitated by the availability of inbred, congenic and *MHC* recombinant strains.

The molecular methods include *pulsed-field gel electrophoresis* (PFGE) (Fig. 6.16) and analyses based on the use of *phage clones* (Fig. 6.17), *cosmid clones* (Fig. 6.18) and *yeast artificial chromosomes* (YACs; Fig. 6.18). To cover the entire region, multiple overlapping clones must be obtained and analysed by the method of *chromosome walking* (Fig. 6.19). Most recently, *DNA sequencing* of the entire *MHC* region has been added to this list. In spite of all the methodological advances, physical mapping over megabase distances is not a trivial task and so the availability of detailed maps of the human and mouse *MHC*,

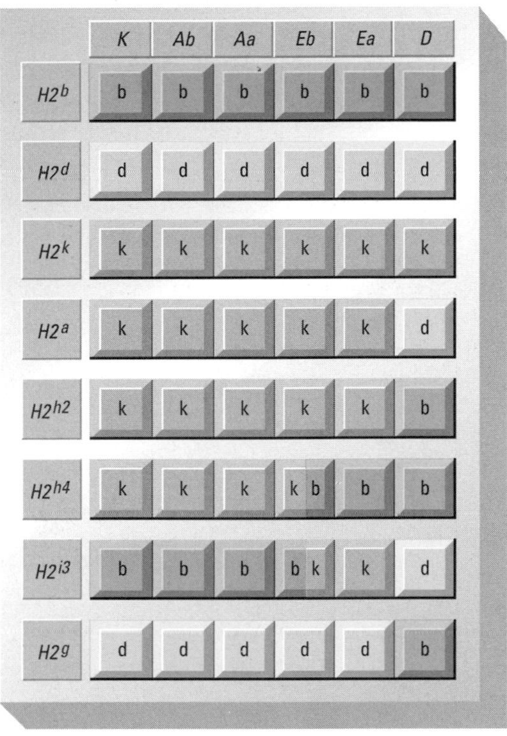

Figure 6.15 *H2* recombinant haplotypes of inbred mouse strains. The first three haplotypes listed ($H2^b$, $H2^d$ and $H2^k$) are not related to one another in a known way. The next five haplotypes, on the other hand, are derived from the first three by genetic recombination. The $H2^a$ haplotype, for example, is derived from $H2^k$ and $H2^d$. The crossing-over occurred between *Ea* and *D* loci in such a way that the recombinant haplotype received the K^k, Ab^k, Aa^k, Eb^k and Ea^k alleles from $H2^k$ and the D^d allele from $H2^d$.

together with sequencing of over one-third of the human *MHC*, must be regarded as considerable achievements. There is a good correspondence between genetic and physical maps of the human and mouse *MHC* (1 cM corresponding roughly to 1 Mb of human DNA), even though it is known that the probability of recombination is not evenly distributed over the segment. In the mouse *MHC* in particular, there are sites in the *H2* complex in which recombination occurs frequently (the so-called *hotspots*) and others in which it is rare.

The mapping process has not been completed for the *MHC* of any one species but it has progressed furthest in the human (*HLA*) and mouse (*H2*) complexes. A summary of what has thus far been learned about the three *HLA* regions follows. In the *HLA class I region* (see Fig. 6.10), *MHC* loci proper (the class I loci) are interspersed with unrelated loci of no known immunological function. The latter include loci coding for tubulin β chain, GTP-binding protein, octamer-binding transcription factor and others. Of the

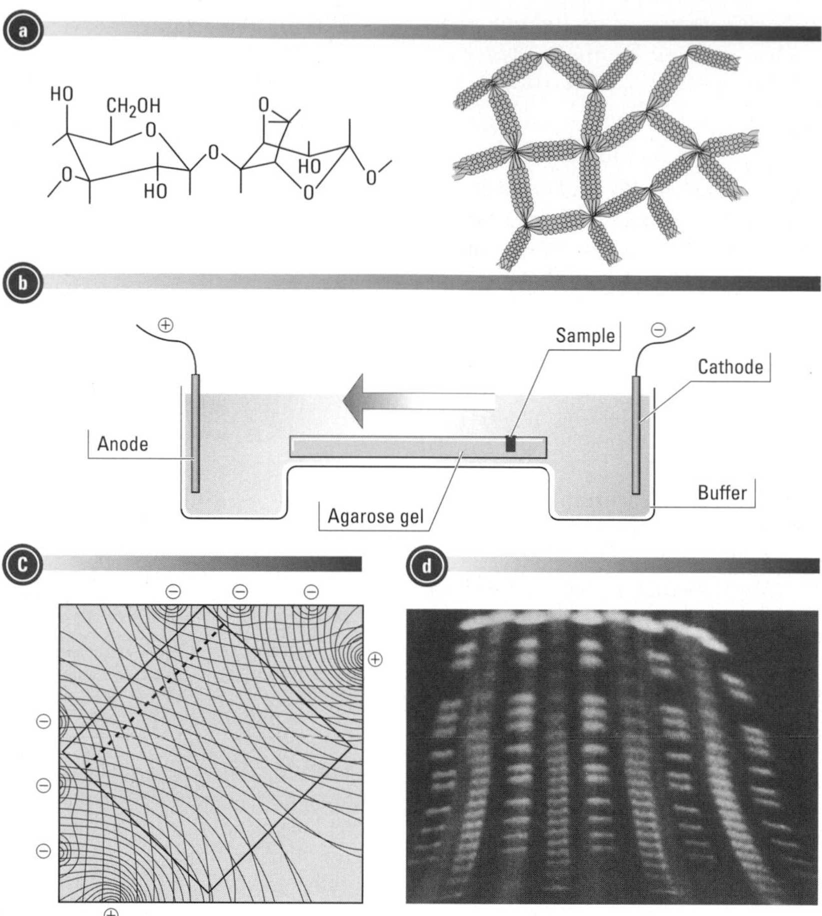

Figure 6.16 Principle of the pulsed-field gel electrophoresis (PFGE) technique. *Agarose* (a) is a polysaccharide obtained from red seaweed. The basic sugar units (left) form long chains (polymers), which cross-link into a three-dimensional mesh (right). When mixed with warm buffer, agarose dissolves but on cooling forms a semi-solid *gel* which can be used as a supporting medium for the separation of protein or DNA molecules. Melted agarose can be poured onto a glass plate, samples introduced into slabs in the solidified gel and the gel placed into a chamber filled with buffer (b). Introduction of an electric current starts the protein or DNA molecules moving in the direction of the current or opposite to it. In this conventional *electrophoresis*, however, all DNA molecules larger than 50 kb migrate with the same mobility and hence molecules of different sizes do not separate from one another. To achieve separation of large DNA molecules, an electrophoretic apparatus is used in which the direction of the electric current can be alternated in short intervals (*pulses*) (c). The DNA molecules are first allowed to migrate one way, during which time they stretch out lengthwise in the direction of the electric field. The current is then stopped for a short time and subsequently started again but at a different angle (e.g. 90°) to the first direction. During the stoppage interval the molecules begin to relax—to coil back—the longer molecules relaxing slower and to a lesser extent than the shorter ones (the relaxation time also depends, however, on the size of the pores in the gel). Consequently, larger molecules need more time to reorient themselves than the smaller ones when the current is reintroduced in a new direction and separation according to size occurs. The technique allows the separation of molecules of up to 10 million base pairs in length. Groups of molecules of similar size form bands in the gel that can be visualized after staining with ethidium bromide (d). This agent intercalates between individual nucleotides of a DNA strand and fluoresces when irradiated with ultraviolet light. The samples for PFGE must be prepared in a special way so as not to break down the large molecules into small fragments. Whole cells are embedded in a block of low-melting point agarose, the block is placed in a buffer containing enzymes that cut the DNA into long pieces, and after incubation, the whole block is inserted into a slot in the agarose gel for electrophoretic separation of the molecular fragments. (Modified from Westermeier, R. (1993) *Electrophoresis in Practice*. VCH, Weinheim.)

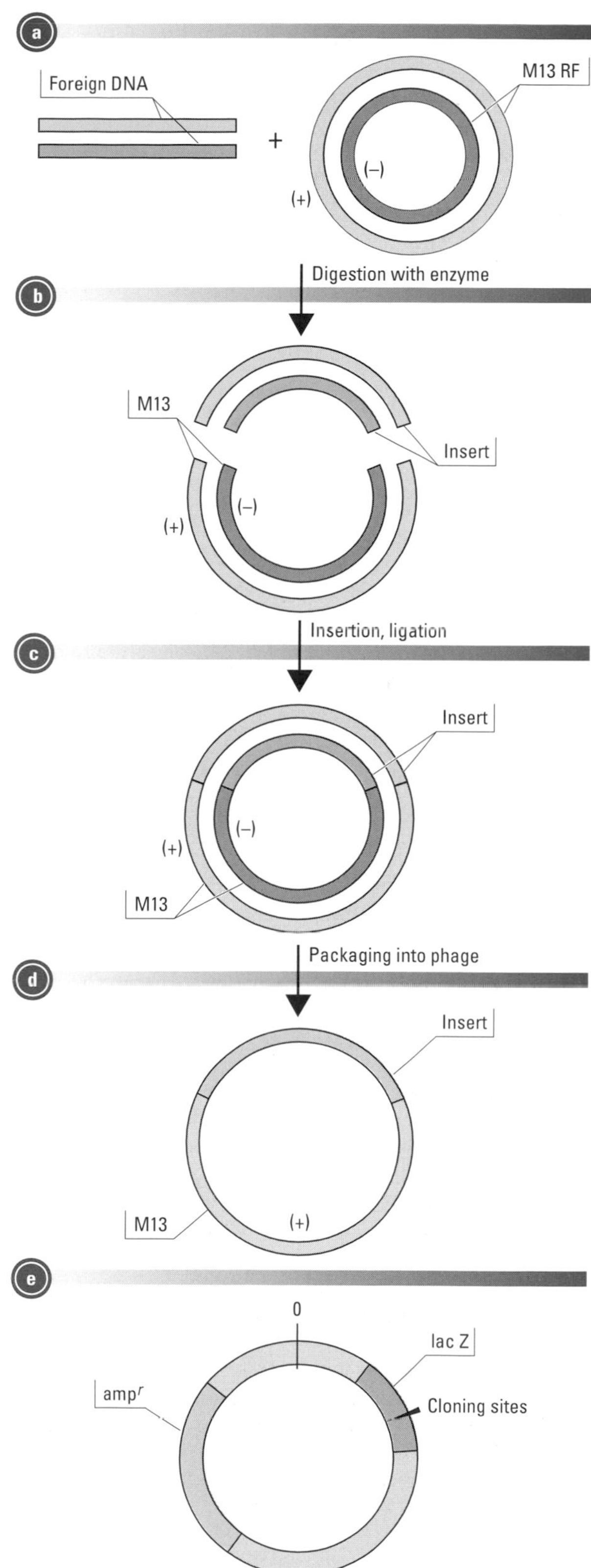

Figure 6.17 Vectors used for cloning small DNA molecules. The isolation of a particular DNA fragment (its separation from all other fragments and its multiplication at will) is referred to as *cloning*. To isolate it, the fragment must be inserted into a suitable *cloning vector*, which is also a DNA fragment but one capable of replication. When the vector replicates in a suitable host cell, it also replicates the *insert*. Small inserts can be placed into (a) the bacteriophage *M13* (<2 kb) or (b) into a *plasmid* (<10 kb). M13 is a single-stranded phage, but when it reproduces it goes through a transient double-stranded *replicative form* (RF). Only one of the two strands (+) is packaged into new phage coats; the other (–) is not. To use it for cloning, the RF is isolated, the circular DNA is cut open with an appropriate enzyme (a), the insert is ligated to the ends (b), the circle resealed and transferred into bacteria (c). In the bacteria, the RF with the insert replicates and the new DNA molecules are packaged into phage particles that retard the growth of the host cells (d). When the RF-bearing bacteria are plated on the top of an agarose layer, colonies of the infected (transformed) bacteria become visible as plaques distinguishable from the background because of their retarded growth. *Plasmids* (e) are small, circular DNA molecules present in some bacteria and carrying, for example, genes for resistance to antibiotics. They replicate independently of the bacterial chromosome. To serve as vectors, they must be engineered: some parts must be cut out and others introduced from various sources. A large selection of plasmid vectors is now available commercially. In the one depicted in (e), the three essential parts are the site at which replication originates (*O*), the *lac Z* gene derived from *Escherichia coli* and the ampicillin resistance (*amp^r*) gene. The *lac Z* gene itself is modified in such a way that its non-essential part has been replaced by an artificial sequence containing several sites recognized by different enzymes that cut double-stranded DNA molecules. One of these sites is used to cut the plasmid vector open and to insert the cloned fragment into the *lac Z* gene. The intact *lac Z* gene produces the enzyme β-galactosidase, which cleaves the sugar galactose; it also acts on another artificial substrate which, when cleaved, turns blue. When the *lac Z* gene is interrupted by the insert, it becomes non-functional and no blue colour is therefore produced. This system serves to distinguish plasmids with and without inserts. The plasmid DNA is introduced into *E. coli* bacteria that are ampicillin sensitive and carry a defective *lac Z* gene, and the transformed bacteria are spread on plates containing the antibiotic ampicillin. Bacteria that did not take up the plasmid vector are killed by the antibiotic, whereas transformed bacteria grow and form colonies owing to the presence of the *amp^r* gene in the plasmid. Bacteria containing vectors into which the insert failed to incorporate produce β-galactosidase specified by the *lac Z* gene and their colonies turn blue when the appropriate substrate is added to the medium. Colonies of bacteria containing vectors with inserts, on the other hand, remain white because the *lac Z* gene has been inactivated by the insertion. Using this method, bacterial colonies in cells containing the vector with the insert can be identified and isolated. This selection system has also been applied to the M13 vector for an increased efficiency of cloning.

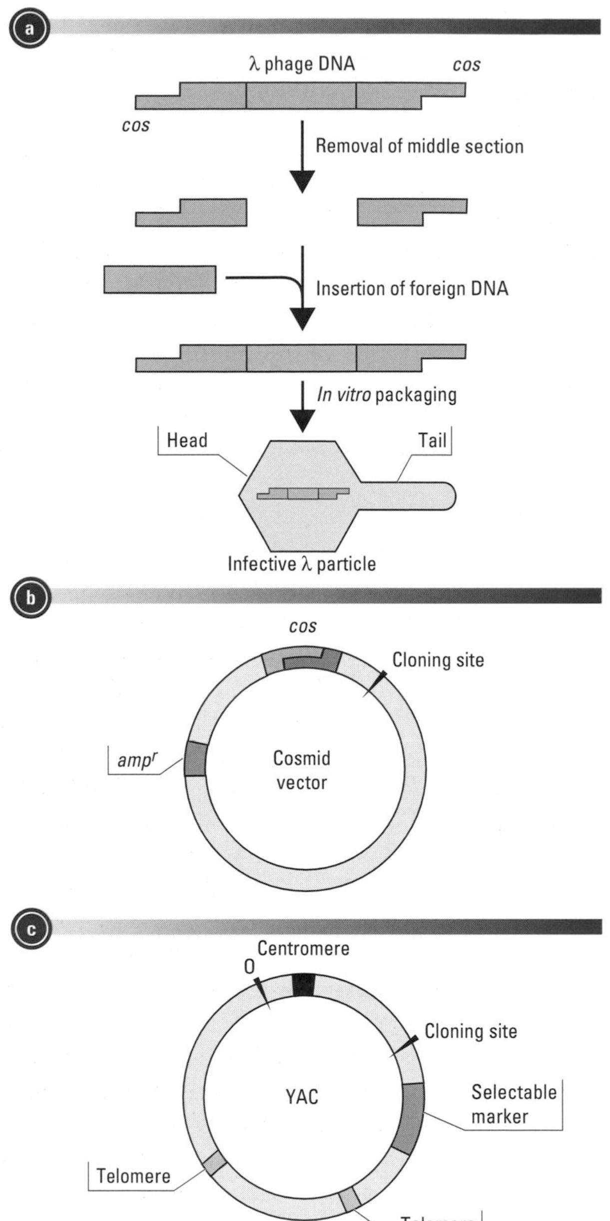

Figure 6.18 Vectors used for cloning of medium-size and large DNA molecules. Plasmids with inserts larger than 7–10 kb tend to lose their foreign DNA and this makes plasmid vectors unsuitable for cloning larger DNA fragments. Medium-size DNA fragments (range between 15 and 20 kb) can be cloned in a vector obtained from the bacteriophage λ (lambda). (a) The middle portion of this phage's linear DNA is not needed for its replication and so can be cut out by appropriate enzymes and replaced by an insert. If the insert is about 15–20 kb long, the size of the vector with the insert is about 45 kb, which is in the range accepted by the phage's heads (smaller or larger DNA segments are rejected). The vector plus insert DNA can be introduced *in vitro* into empty phage heads (*in vitro* packaging) produced by mutant phages and the particles can then be completed by the addition of phage tails. The complete phages can be used to infect bacteria. The phage attaches to the bacterial surface by its tail, injects its DNA content into the cell and the double-stranded linear DNA then circularizes through the binding of short, single-stranded, overhanging regions at both ends (*cohesive* or *cos sites*). The circular DNA replicates and the new phage particles lyse the infected bacteria, forming clear plaques on the bacterial lawn. The phages with the inserts can be picked from the plaques. (b) DNA molecules up to 45 kb in length can be cloned in *cosmids*, which are plasmids derived from bacteria with λ phage *cos* ends added to them so that they can be circularized in a phage. The plasmid also contains a gene for resistance to ampicillin (*ampʳ*) or to some other antibiotic that is used for selection. In all other respects (packaging, infection, etc.), cosmids are handled like λ phages. Because the plasmid is much shorter than λ DNA, it can carry long inserts and still be in the size range accepted by the phage heads (the *cos* sequences are all that is required for acceptance). (c) Very large DNA molecules (> 100 kb) can be cloned in *yeast artificial chromosomes* or *YACs*. The YAC vector contains a centromere necessary for segregation of the chromosomes during mitosis, telomeres necessary for sealing the chromosome's ends, the origin of replication (*O*) and a selectable marker, all derived from a yeast chromosome. It also contains a cloning site through which the circular DNA can be opened and the long foreign DNA inserted into the circle. When introduced into a yeast cell, the YAC behaves as if it were one of the yeast's chromosomes, i.e. it replicates and its copies segregate into daughter cells. Cells carrying the YAC can be isolated via the selectable marker.

HLA class I loci, eight are known to be occupied by expressed genes (*HLA-A*, *-B*, *-C*, *-E*, *-F*, *-G*, *MICA* and *MICB*), four by full-length pseudogenes (*HLA-H*, *-J*, *-K* and *-L*), four by truncated pseudogenes (*HLA-75*, *-16*, *-80* and *-90*) and three by gene fragments (*HLA-17*, *-21* and *-30*). The expressed genes fall into two categories, class Ia and class Ib. The proteins encoded in the *class Ia (classical) genes* are known to bind peptides and present them to T lymphocytes, are expressed on the surface of most somatic cells but at particularly high levels in lymphoid cells and exist in human populations in many versions (*alleles*). If the proteins encoded in the *class Ib (non-classical) genes* present peptides to T lymphocytes at all, they do so for a restricted spectrum of peptides only and perhaps to a restricted subset of T cells; their expression in different tissues is different from that of class Ia molecules; and they exist in a small number of variants only. *HLA-A* and *-B* are considered to be *bona fide* class Ia loci, whereas *HLA-E*, *-F* and *-G* are typical class Ib loci. The *HLA-C* locus falls somewhere between the class Ia and class Ib categories in that the ability of the protein it encodes to present peptides under physiological conditions has yet to be

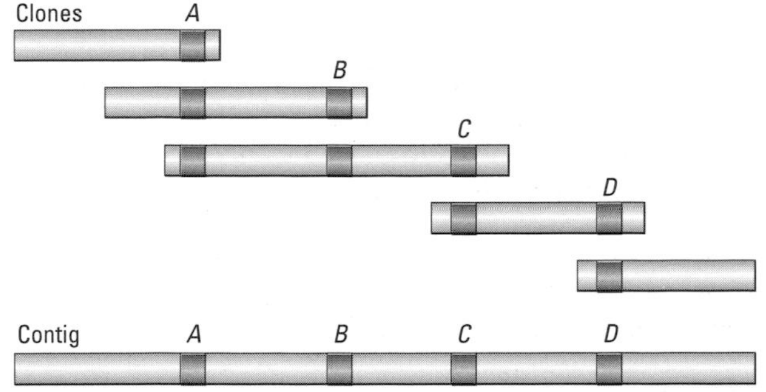

Figure 6.19 The principle of chromosome walking. A single clone, even if inserted in a YAC, covers only a short segment of a chromosome. To extend this segment over a longer region, a technique termed *chromosome walking* is used. The initial clone is cut enzymatically into smaller pieces and pieces located near the end of the clone and free of highly repetitive sequences are isolated by cloning (*subcloning*) in a plasmid vector. The insert (*A*) is then used to screen a collection of DNA fragments in vectors (clones in a *library*) that presumably cover the entire genome of an organism. Clones containing sequences identical to the insert *A* (identity is established by DNA–DNA hybridization) are identified and characterized and those that extend beyond the original clone are selected. A new short fragment *B* is isolated from near the end of this set of clones by subcloning and the entire procedure is repeated. In this way, a series of overlapping clones is obtained, each covering only a short segment but all together extending over a longer contiguous region of the genomic DNA (*contig*) as if one were 'walking' along the chromosome from a starting point in one or both directions.

demonstrated, its expression is lower and the number of alleles present at appreciable frequencies in populations smaller than that of the *HLA-A* and *-B* loci. The *M*HC class *I c*hain-related *A* and *B* (*MICA* and *MICB*) loci have been singled out from the class Ib category mainly because they appear somewhat older than the other loci in that category.

The classification into class Ia and Ib categories is probably too simplistic. In reality, the class I loci may form an array ranging from *HLA-B*, which appears to be functionally most active and has the largest number of alleles; to the less active but still fully functional *HLA-A* locus; then to *HLA-C*, which may be functionally phasing out; onto the *HLA-E*, *-F*, *-G* loci, which may have retained some remnants of previous functionality or may have been specialized to present only certain peptides and other ligands (in the mouse some of the class Ib proteins have apparently been specialized to present formylated peptides encoded in genes of the mitochondrial DNA; see Chapter 21); and over recently inactivated pseudogenes and truncated pseudogenes to gene fragments. This continuum might reflect the dynamic birth and death process of *MHC* loci, which has apparently characterized the evolution of the *MHC* since its inception. The process itself might in turn reflect an effort on the part of the organism to strike a balance between expressing too many and too few *MHC* loci, both extremes being disadvantageous for the species (this point is dealt with later). Some of the genes in the continuum may occasionally assume new functions altogether, as has probably been the case with the *CD1*, *FCGRT* and *AZGP1* genes, which are similar to class I genes but not part of the *MHC* (they, too, are described later). Some immunologists believe that the *HLA-G* gene might be in the process of assuming a new function connected with tissue compatibility between the fetus and the mother (the gene is expressed in embryonic and placental tissues, which do not express any other *MHC* genes). There is, however, very little evidence to support such speculations.

The *HLA class II region* contains 11 class II genes, four genes involved in processing of proteins into peptides that are loaded onto class I molecules (the *LMP2* and *LMP7* genes coding for subunits of a proteasome as well as *TAP1* and *TAP2* genes coding for ABC transporter proteins), one class I pseudogene (*HLA-Z1*), at least two genes coding for proteins not involved in immunity and several as yet unidentified pseudogenes (see Fig. 6.10). The class II genes, summarily referred to as *HLA-D*, fall into five families: *DP*, *DN*, *DM*, *DO*, *DQ* and *DR*. (The *DN* and *DO* loci were originally thought to represent different families but were later shown to belong to the same family; the official change in the designation of one of the loci is overdue.) In each family, there are two types of loci, *A* and *B*, which encode α and β polypeptide chains, respectively. Each class II molecule is an α:β heterodimer, whereby the two chains always come from the same family (i.e. DPα associates with DPβ, DMα with DMβ and so on). Chains from different families normally do not associate into heterodimers (the association of DNα with DOβ is an indication that the corresponding *DNA* and *DOB* genes are in fact members of the same family). If multiple genes are present in a given family, they are distinguished by Arabic numerals so that the full names of the genes are *DPA1*, *DPA2*, *DPB1*, *DQA1* and so on.

In all gene families except *DR* the number of loci in humans (and also in many other primates) is the same. With regard to the *DR* family, all humans have one *DRA* locus but they differ in the number of *DRB* loci per chromosome, which can range from two to five (Fig. 6.20). There are altogether nine known *DRB* loci, of which *HLA-DRB1* is definitely functional and *-DRB5* is probably functional; if *-DRB3* and *-DRB4* are functional at all then only to a limited extent, while the rest (*-DRB2*, *-DRB6*, *-DRB7*, *-DRB8*) are pseudogenes; *-DRB9* is a gene fragment. The different numbers and combinations of *DRB* genes define various *HLA-DR haplotypes*, which fall into five main

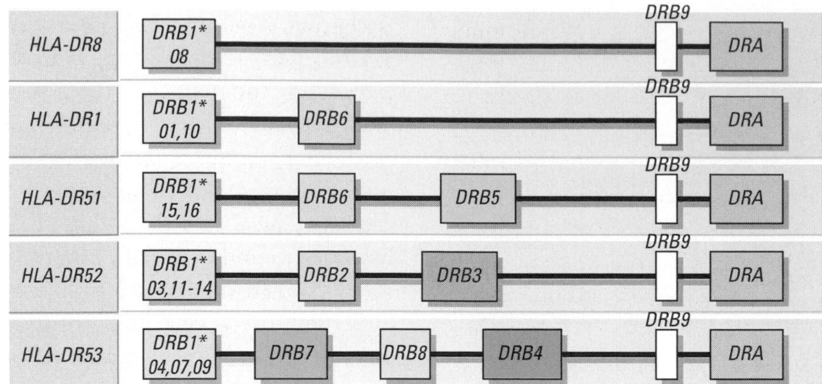

Figure 6.20 Human *DR* haplotypes. *DRB1–DRB9* are different loci. *DRB2*, *DRB6*, *DRB7* and *DRB8* loci are occupied by pseudogenes; *DRB9* is a gene fragment. Loci shared by different haplotypes (*DRB1* and *DRB6*) are occupied by different alleles. In each haplotype group, variant haplotypes are distinguished by the presence of different alleles at the various loci. All haplotypes share one invariant *DRA* locus.

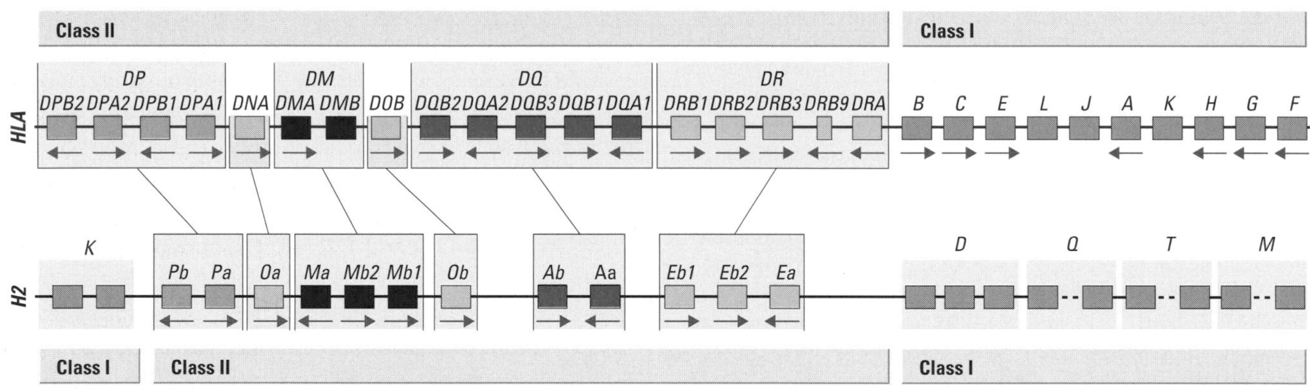

Figure 6.21 Simplified maps of human (*HLA*) and mouse (*H2*) class I and class II regions. In the *HLA* map, all the class II loci proper are listed (of the *DR3* haplotype); of the class I loci proper, only those that have received an official designation are listed. In the *H2* map, only the class II loci are listed by names. Correspondence between groups of loci are indicated by connecting lines. There is no correspondence between the human and mouse class I loci. The order of loci corresponds to reality; the distances between loci and their sizes do not. Arrows indicate transcriptional orientation.

groups (Fig. 6.20). Many other *DR* haplotype groups exist in non-human primates. For easier orientation, simplified maps of human class II and class I regions are given in Fig. 6.21.

The *class III region* does not contain any *MHC* genes proper. It does, however, contain several genes that are involved in immunity, in addition to many that are not (see Fig. 6.10). In the first category are genes coding for the complement components C4, C2 and factor B (see Chapter 12), as well as genes specifying tumour necrosis factor and lymphotoxin (see Chapter 10). The class III loci that are not known to be involved in immunity include loci coding for steroid 21-hydroxylase, valyl-tRNA synthetase, heat shock protein and others.

Gene structure

As has already been explained, there are two classes of *MHC* genes proper and in each class there are two types of genes, one coding for the α and the other for the β polypeptide. In the *HLA* system, the class II genes are designated by three capital letters and a series of numbers. The first letter (*D*) identifies a gene (locus) as class II, the second letter specifies which family it belongs to (*M*, *N/O*, *P*, *Q* or *R*) and the third letter indicates the gene type (*A* for α, *B* for β). The first number following these three letters specifies the locus and the remaining numerals the allele. The locus and allele designations are separated by an asterisk (*) and in the allelic designations the first two digits indicate major alleles, whereas the following two or more digits indicate minor variants of these alleles. Unfortunately, *HLA* class I nomenclature follows somewhat different rules. If *D* stands for class II, all other letters of the alphabet are reserved for the class I genes and are used to designate different loci. The alleles are then designated by numbers as in the case of class II genes. In the mouse *H2* system, some letters are used to designate class I loci (*D*, *K*, *L*, *M*, *Q*, *T*) while others refer to class II loci (*A*, *E*, *O*, *P*) and the type of loci are distinguished by small letters (*Aa*, *Ab*, *Ea*, *Eb* and so on; here mouse *A* corresponds to human *Q* and mouse *E* is homologous to human *R*). Alleles are designated by small superscript letters (Ab^b, Ab^k, Eb^d and so on) and *H2* haplotypes by a combination of letters and numbers ($H2^a$, $H2^b$, $H2^d$, $H2^{i5}$ and so on). For most other vertebrates, the rules for a unified nomenclature require the *Mhc* symbol (consisting of genus and species name abbreviation) to be followed by *U* (class I, for *unus*) or *D* (class II, for *duo*), then by family designations (*A*, *B*, *C*, etc.) and then by gene type designation (*A* for α and *B* for β); allelic designations are modelled on the *HLA* system.

Both the class I and class II genes are split into *exons* and *introns*; the entire gene except for its controlling region is transcribed into RNA but the introns are then removed during the processing of the primary transcript. The exon–intron organization of the *MHC* class I genes is remarkably similar in the various vertebrate species. Moreover, there is a good correspondence between exons of the genes and the domains they code for (Fig. 6.22). (A protein *domain* is a region of the molecule characterized by certain structural and functional features that distinguish it from other regions of the same molecule.) Each *class IA gene* consists of six or seven exons (E1 through E7). *Exon 1* encompasses the *5′ untranslated (5′UT) region* and the stretch of DNA coding for the *signal (leader) peptide (sequence)*. The 5′UT region is transcribed into an RNA sequence that becomes part of the mRNA but is not translated into a protein. The signal peptide is responsible for the passage of a protein through a membrane during protein synthesis in the RER; after it has fulfilled this function it is clipped off and so does not appear in the mature protein (see also Chapter 7). *Exons 2, 3* and *4* code for three domains termed α1, α2 and α3, respectively. The α1 and α2 domains contain the collection of sites that bind peptides produced by the processing of other proteins; they are therefore termed *peptide-binding domains*. The α3 domain has a characteristic structure first described for immunoglobulin molecules (see Chapter 8) and hence is referred to as *immunoglobulin-like domain*. *Exon 5* codes for the *connecting peptide* and the *transmembrane region*. The former constitutes a bridge between the α3 domain and the transmembrane region; the latter anchors the α chain in the membrane. The α1, α2 and α3 domains, together with the connecting peptide, form the chain's extracellular part. The last one or two exons (*E6* and *E7*) code for the *cytoplasmic region* (tail), which extends the α chain a short distance into the cell's interior, and for the 3′ untranslated (3′UT) region.

The *class IB gene* deviates from other class I genes in that it is not part of the *MHC* (in humans it resides on chromosome 15) and that the protein it specifies is not anchored in the membrane. In fact, the protein was first described in a free form as one of the components of vertebrate blood plasma and termed *β_2-microglobulin* (β_2m); its involvement with the MHC class I molecules was recognized only later. Nonetheless, the intimate association of β_2m with the class Iα chains justifies regarding it as the β chain of the class I molecules and regarding the controlling region on chromosome 15 as a class I locus. The *B2M* gene consists of four exons, the first of which encompasses the 5′UT region and, in addition, specifies the first few amino acid residues of the protein; the second exon specifies the bulk of the protein sequence; the third exon codes for the last few residues of the protein and part of the 3′UT region; and the fourth exon encompasses the rest of the 3′UT region. The mature protein is composed of a single immunoglobulin-like domain (see Fig. 6.22).

There is some variation in class II gene organization among the vertebrates but, in general, in mammals the *A* genes consist of five and the *B* genes of six exons. In both gene types, exon 1 encompasses the 5′UT region and the sequence coding for the signal peptide; exon 2 specifies the α1 (*A* genes) or the β1 (*B* genes) domain, with both domains of the two chains contributing jointly to the peptide-binding region (PBR) of the class II molecule; exon 3 specifies an immunoglobulin-like domain (either α2 or β2); and the remaining exons code for the connecting peptide, the transmembrane region, the cytoplasmic tail and the 3′UT region (Fig. 6.23).

Gene expression and its regulation

As we have already indicated, the *class Ia genes* are expressed on most adult somatic cells. Exceptions include neurons, cells of the exocrine pancreas, myocardial cells, sperm cells at certain stages of development and certain cells of the placenta. Class I molecules are also absent on the surfaces of unfertilized eggs and on cells of early embryos. Of the adult somatic cells, lymphocytes, both B and T, express the highest levels of class Ia molecules, while all other cells express varying but generally lower levels. The expression can be changed both upwards (*upregulated*) or

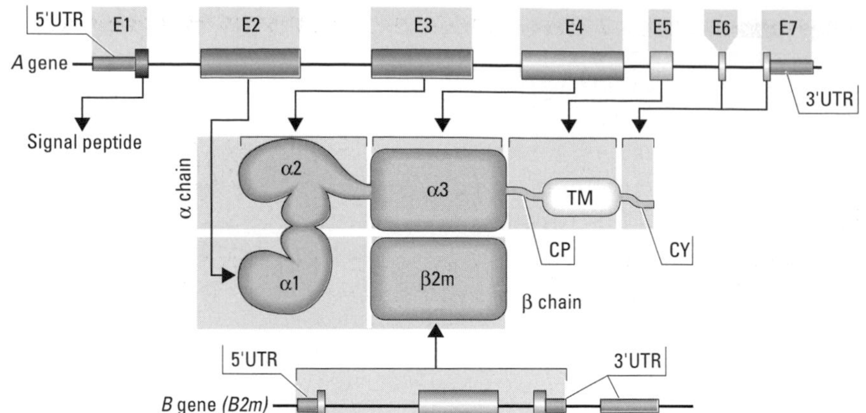

Figure 6.22 Correspondence between exons of genes and domains of proteins in the class I *MHC* system. CP, connecting peptide; CY, cytoplasmic tail; E, exon; TM, transmembrane region; UTR, untranslated region.

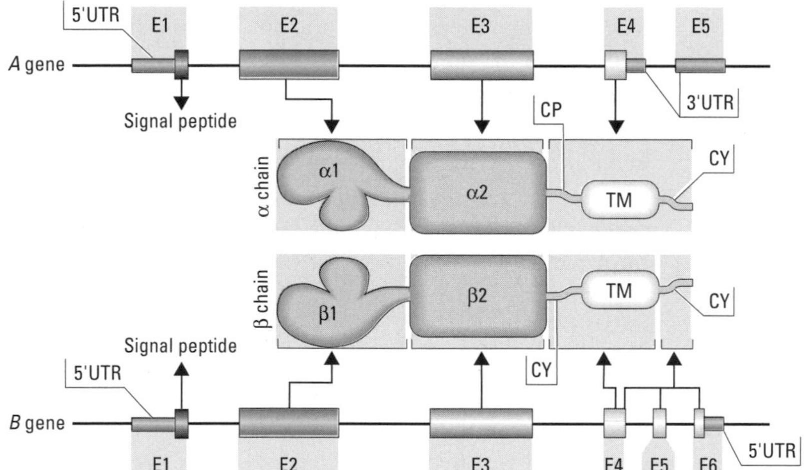

Figure 6.23 Correspondence between exons of genes and domains of proteins in the class II *MHC* system. CP, connecting peptide; CY, cytoplasmic tail; E, exon; TM, transmembrane region; UTR, untranslated region.

downwards (*downregulated*) by a variety of factors such as viral infection and various cytokines (e.g. interferons).

The expression of class Ia genes is regulated by sequences upstream of the coding part. The short sequences called *motifs* or *boxes* (the sequences are highly conserved and are therefore usually highlighted by rectangular enclosures in figures and tables) are the sites that bind proteins involved in the initiation of transcription of DNA into RNA. The proteins, generally referred to as *transcription factors* or *nuclear factors* (because they are found in the nucleus), either accelerate or slow down transcription. They come under a variety of names that are compressed into often exotic-sounding abbreviations. Some of the factors are gene-specific or cell-specific, while others act on many different genes in different cell types. Their general mechanism of action is considered in the next chapter; here we merely enumerate the motifs and the proteins that bind to them in so far as they are known to influence *MHC* gene transcription.

The region that regulates gene transcription lies upstream of the site at which transcription begins (the *transcription initiation site*), although some regulatory motifs may also be located in other parts of the gene, for example the introns. The upstream *regulatory region* can be divided loosely into two parts, the promoter and the enhancers. The *promoter* operates over a short distance (in mammalian class I genes it is located some 35 bp upstream of the transcription initiation site), is always located 5′ to the gene and operates only when in the correct orientation. It contains two motifs common to many genes, the *TATA box* and the *CCAAT box*. These two boxes determine the site at which transcription will begin (see Chapter 7). The *enhancers* operate over distances of several kilobases, independently of orientation and location 5′ or 3′ to the gene. They regulate the activity of the promoter (see Chapter 7). The same sequence motif may be used by many different genes in various cell types; it can also be repeated within the same gene; and it can appear in both the promoter and enhancer regions.

The three main parts of the *MHC* class I enhancer

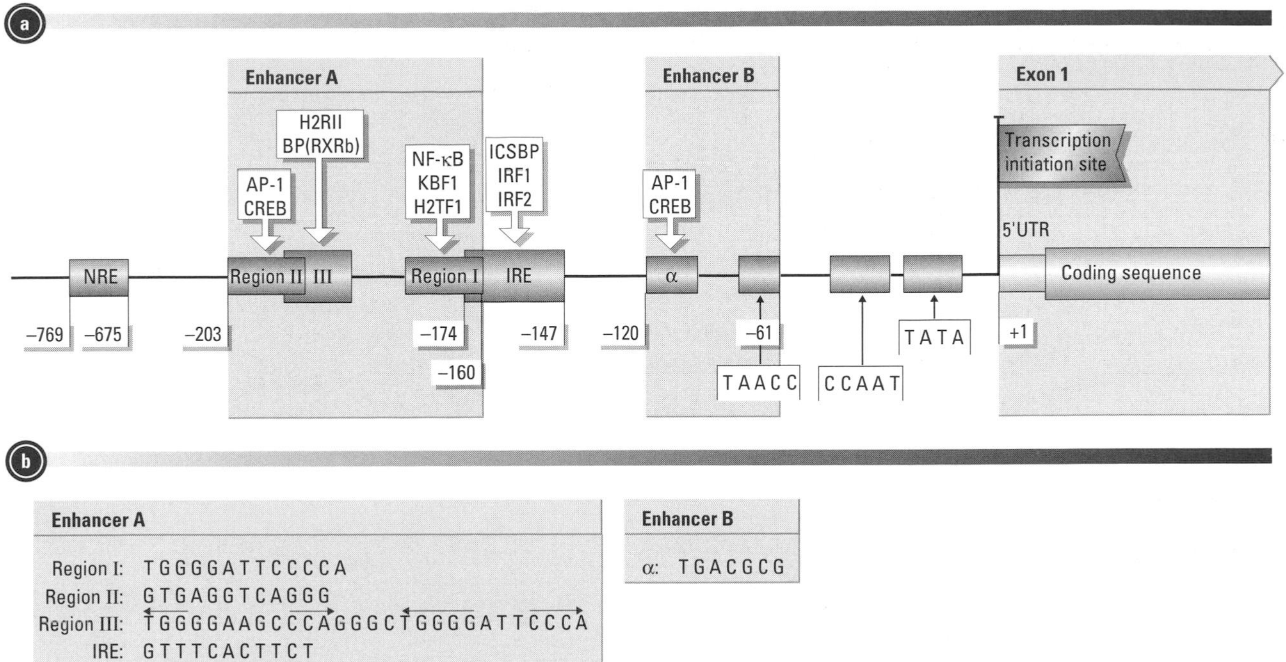

Figure 6.24 The regulatory region of *MHC* class I genes. (a) Location of the individual sequence motifs (red boxes) upstream from the transcription initiation site. The various proteins known to bind to these motifs are indicated by the arrow-associated symbols. The negative numbers indicate the distances (in numbers of nucleotides) from the transcription initiation site, which is assigned the number +1. (b) Sequences of individual motifs. Region III contains two palindromes (indicated by arrows). AP1, activation protein 1; CREB, cAMP response element binding factor; H2RIIBP, *H2* region II binding protein; H2TF1, *H2* transcription factor 1; ICSBP, interferon consensus sequence binding protein; IRE, interferon responding element; IRF, interferon regulatory factor; KBF1, K^b factor 1; NF-κB, nuclear factor kappa B; NRE, negative regulatory element; RXRb, HLA-DRAX region box; UTR, untranslated region.

segment are enhancer A, interferon response element and enhancer B (Fig. 6.24). Further upstream of this main segment is believed to be a region that suppresses class I gene expression, the negative regulatory element (NRE). Of the three, *enhancer A* (also referred to as *class I regulatory element*, CRE) has the strongest influence on class I gene expression. It is divided further into three regions, of which regions II and III partially overlap. *Region I* binds factors present in tissues that express high levels of class I molecules; these factors are absent in brain cells and fetal tissues, which normally do not express class I molecules. *Regions II and III* bind transcription factors irrespective of class I expression. The *interferon response element* (IRE), which contains short motifs called the *interferon consensus sequence* (ICS) and *interferon responding sequence* (IRS), is used by cells in which the expression of class I molecules can be increased by treatment with interferon. The treatment results in the production of nuclear factors that bind to the IRE. *Enhancer B* has a relatively weak influence on class I gene expression. Its main sequence motif is referred to as α. The transcription factors known to bind to the various enhancer elements are listed in Fig. 6.24.

The expression of *MHC* class II genes is more restricted than that of class I genes. In most species, class II molecules are found on mature B lymphocytes (but not B-progenitor cells and plasma cells), activated (but not resting) T lymphocytes, macrophages, dendritic cells and thymic epithelium. Most other cells are class II negative but some of them can be induced to express class II molecules after treatment with cytokines (in particular interferon) and certain other agents. A large number of external stimuli are known to have an influence on the level of class II gene expression, either upregulating or downregulating it.

The regulatory elements controlling the expression of class II genes have been best characterized in the case of the *HLA-DRA* locus (Fig. 6.25). They have been mapped to the segment upstream of the transcription initiation site (here the entire segment is often referred to as the promoter) and to the first intron of the *DRA* gene. The upstream regulatory region can be divided into two parts, proximal and

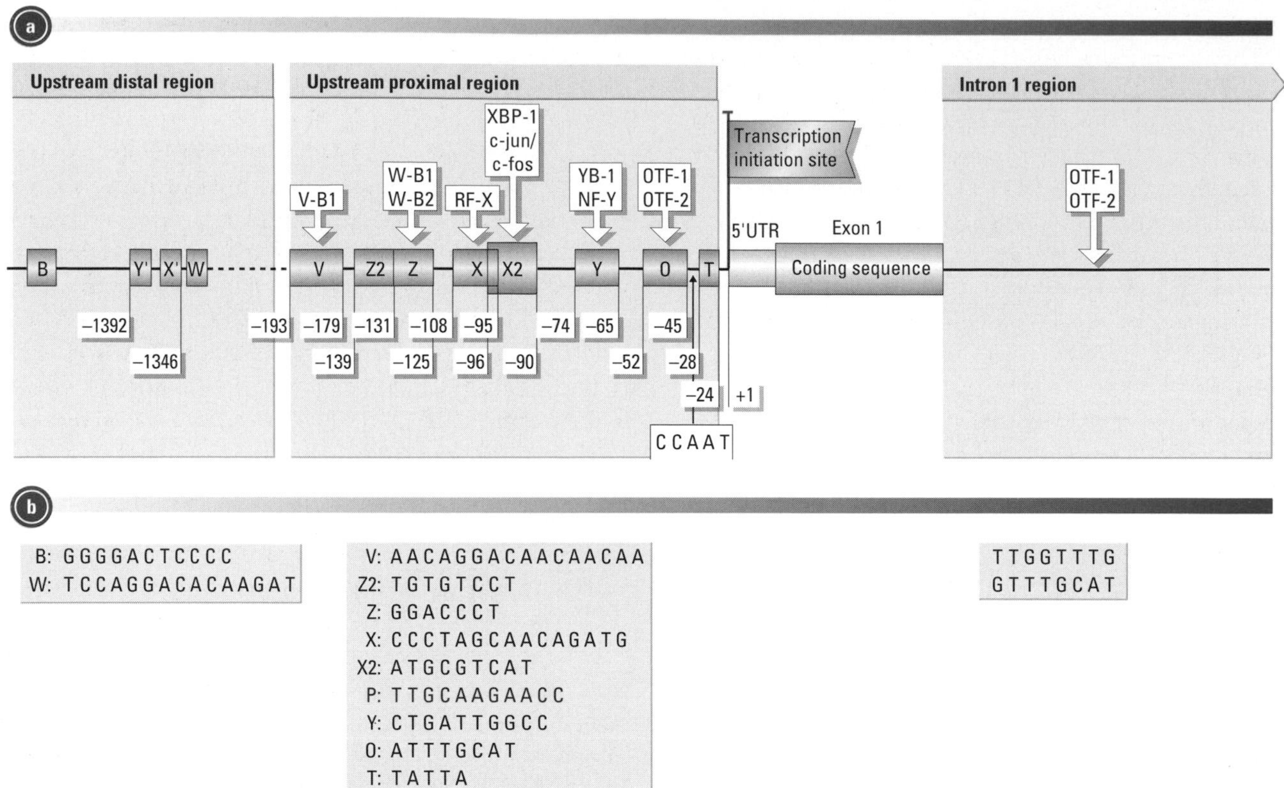

Figure 6.25 The regulatory region of *MHC* class II genes (**a**). The location of individual sequence motifs (red boxes) upstream from the transcription initiation site and in intron 1. The various proteins known to bind to these motifs are indicated by the arrow-associated symbols. The negative numbers indicate the distances (in numbers of nucleotides) from the transcription initiation site, which is assigned the number +1. (b) Sequences of individual motifs. c-fos, cellular homologue of a viral oncogene isolated from Finkel–Biskis–Jinkins murine osteogenic sarcoma virus; c-jun, cellular homologue of a viral oncogene first isolated from the avian sarcoma virus 17 (from *ju-nana*, which means 17 in Japanese); NF-Y, **n**uclear **f**actor **Y** (binding); OTF-1 and -2, **o**ctamer **t**ranscription **f**actor 1 and 2; RF-X, **r**egulatory **f**actor binding to the **X** box; UTR, untranslated region; V-B1, **V**-**b**inding 1; W-B1 and 2, **W**(Z)-**b**inding 1 and 2; XBP, **X**-**b**inding **p**rotein; YB-1, **Y**-**b**inding 1.

distal (relative to the transcription initiation site). The *proximal region* is necessary but not sufficient for the constitutive expression of class II genes in B lymphocytes and the enhancement of this basal expression by the action of interferon γ (IFN-γ). It contains, in addition to the TATA and CCAAT boxes, a series of sequence motifs referred to by various letters of the alphabet (O, Y, X, X2, P, Z and V). The *TATA box* is present in all the class II genes but plays only a minor part in their expression, whereas the *CCAAT* box is present in only some of the genes. Immediately upstream of the TATA box is the *octamer* (O) sequence, which consists of eight nucleotides and is also found in many other genes, including the immunoglobulin genes (see Chapter 8). The *Y box* has the sequence 5′-CTGATTGGCC-3′; the complementary sequence to this is GACTAACCGG, of which the middle part (TAACC) is an inversion of the CCAAT box sequence. The *X box* consists of two partially overlapping motifs, X and X2, which bind different transcription factors. The X2 box, however, is present in only some class II genes. The *Z box* also goes under at least three other names (W, S and H), all of which refer to the same element. The reason for this confusion is that unlike the other boxes, which are highly conserved among various class II genes, the sequence of the Z box varies and so has been given different designations in different genes. It contains at least two sequence motifs, which have been referred to as Z or SRV2 (GGACCC) and Z2 or SRV1 (GGACAC, where SRV stands for Servenius, the investigator who, with his co-workers, was the first to note the sequences). Between the X and Z boxes is a stretch rich in pyrimidine nucleotides (T and C), the *pyrimidine tract element* or the *P box*. It does not appear to bind any transcription factors but exerts weak transcription-enhancing activity by influencing the binding of proteins to the X box. The *V box* acts as a weak suppresser of transcription. It contains motifs with sequence similarity to the Z and X boxes.

The *distal upstream elements* are still not well characterized. They are responsible for the constitutive expression of class II genes in B lymphocytes but their function appears to depend on the activity of the proximal elements. The region contains several motifs resembling the X and Y boxes in their sequences, as well as at least two other motifs, the *B motif* and the *W box*; the latter should not be confused with the W (= Z) box of the proximal region.

The *first intron* of the *HLA-DRA* gene contains another seven elements believed to be involved in gene regulation (see Fig. 6.25): TOPO II, O, CTE, another TOPO II, NMAR, Ig switch and CTE. The two *TOPO II elements* represent potential attachment sites for the enzyme topoisomerase II, which is involved in changing the geometry of the chromatin fibres during activation (see Chapter 7). The *octamer (O) sequence* (GTTTGCAT) is similar to that found in the promoter region. The *NMAR* (*nuclear matrix-associated region*) represents sequences thought to be involved in the interaction between the chromatin fibres and the scaffolding of the nuclear matrix (see Chapter 7). The presence in the class II gene intron of sequences implicated in *immunoglobulin isotype switching* $(TGGGGG)_4$ is a mystery (see Chapter 8). The *CTE* (*core transcriptional enhancer*) element contains sequences TTGTGGTTTGG, TTGGTTTG and GTGTGTTTG, which are similar to SV40 and polyoma viral enhancers. The transcription factors that bind to the various regulatory elements of the class II genes are listed in Fig. 6.25.

Gene polymorphism

Genes are subject to change, i.e. they mutate. *Mutations* alter the sequence of the gene; they usually occur because of errors during DNA replication. Mutations in the non-coding regions and approximately one-third of the mutations in the coding regions do not change the amino acid sequence of the encoded protein. The latter are termed *synonymous mutations* in contrast to *non-synonymous mutations*, which do change the amino acid sequence. Synonymous mutations occur because the genetic code is *degenerate*, which means that the same amino acid can be specified by more than one codon. Mutations are rare and random events so that it is not possible to predict precisely when and where in the genome they will occur. It is, however, possible to give the probability with which a mutation will occur in a given unit of genetic information. A measure of this probability is the *mutation rate*, the frequency of mutations per unit of time (generation, year). Mutation rates may vary from gene to gene.

Mutations can take place in both the cells of the germ line and in somatic cells. Somatic mutations persist only in the lineage derived from the cell in which the mutation occurred; they are lost with the demise of the individual. *Germ-cell mutations* may be passed onto the progeny if the cells bearing the mutations participate in fertilization and the creation of a new individual. Although billions of germ cells are produced during the lifetime of an individual, only a tiny fraction is selected for fertilization and the probability that these will bear the mutation is very low. Most mutations are therefore never registered — they perish shortly after they have arisen. Even in the tiny fraction of mutations that are passed onto the progeny, the overwhelming majority has no effect on the evolution of the population comprising a species. To have an effect, a mutation would have to reach a certain frequency, which most mutations do not. A mutation may disappear either because its bearers do not reproduce or, if they do, the germ cell bearing the mutation is by chance not chosen to found the next generation. As long as the mutant allele represents a tiny minority in the totality of genes (the *gene pool*), it leads a precarious existence in the sense that it can be lost by chance from the pool at any time. Only when it reaches a certain appreciable frequency does its chance for persisting longer in the population improve and only then does it play a part in evolution; 'appreciable' is regarded as a frequency of 0.01 or 1%. Any allele with a frequency of <0.01 is regarded as a *rare variant*, whereas an allele with a frequency of ≥ 0.01 (but <1) is considered to constitute *polymorphism*. Hence, not all alleles found in a population contribute to the polymorphism of a gene and unless the frequency of an allele is known to be $\geq 1\%$ it should not be included in the polymorphism of a locus. 'Polymorphism' means 'many forms'; the opposite of polymorphism is *monomorphism*, the presence of only one form (allele) at a given locus in a population; the presence of a few alleles constitutes *oligomorphism*.

A polymorphic allele can end its existence in a population in one of two ways (Fig. 6.26): its frequency may either drop to zero and the allele may disappear from the population or it may continue rising until it reaches the frequency of 1 or 100%. In the latter case, it replaces all other alleles that may have been present in the population and its frequency stops fluctuating, i.e. the allele (mutation) becomes *fixed*. The great majority of mutations suffer the former fate (a loss from the population) and only from time to time does one of them manage to break through and advance towards fixation. Although it is not possible to predict exactly which mutation (allele) will become fixed, how long it will take for the 'chosen' mutation to reach the fixation frequency and how frequently mutant alleles will break away and proceed to fixation, formulas for calculating the *probabilities* of all these events are available (see Fig. 6.26). Thus, the probability that a given mutation becomes fixed is $1/(2N_e)$, where N_e

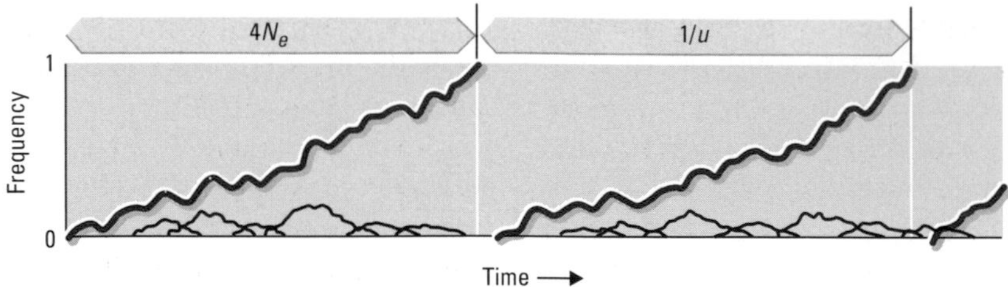

Figure 6.26 Fate of neutral mutations in a gene pool. Each wavy line represents the gradual changes in the frequency of a newly arisen mutation. Most mutations are lost from the pool shortly after they have arisen without attaining appreciable frequencies. Occasionally, however, a mutation manages to break away from this 'background' fluctuation noise and to increase in frequency until it becomes fixed (achieves frequency of 1). The average time it needs for this is $4N_e$, where N_e is the number of breeding individuals in the population. A population of N_e diploid individuals has $2N_e$ genes at each autosomal locus. All the genes have the same probability of becoming fixed, which is $p = 1/(2N_e)$. If the mutation rate of the genes is u per gene per generation, then the fixation (substitution) rate is $K = 2up$. Substituting for p gives

$$K = 2N_e u \frac{1}{2N_e} = u:$$

the substitution rate is equal to the mutation rate. A substitution rate of u means that one substitution occurs per u generations so that the average interval between two fixations is $1/u$ generations. (Based on Kimura, M. (1983) *The Neutral Theory of Molecular Evolution*. Cambridge University Press, Cambridge.)

is the *effective population size* or roughly the number of breeding individuals in a population. The average time it takes for a mutation to become fixed is $4N_e$ generations and the frequency with which fixations occur (the *fixation rate*) equals the mutation rate. If, for example, the effective population size of a species is $N_e = 10^4$, then the probability of fixation for any one mutation is $1/(2\times10^4) = 5\times10^{-5}$, the time needed for fixation of a mutation is 4×10^4 generations and if the mutation rate is 10^{-9} per site per year, this also will be the rate with which mutations will become fixed.

A common way of estimating the frequency of fixations is based on the comparison of sequences of homologous loci in two different species whose divergence time is known from the fossil record. An alignment of the sequences reveals the fixations as differences in nucleotides at certain sites. The differences constitute *substitutions* of original nucleotides by other nucleotides in one or both species. Instead of fixation rate, one can also speak of *substitution rate*, K, which is defined as the number of substitutions per site per unit of time. Furthermore, since the accumulation of differences between sequences in the two species constitutes evolution, the fixation rate represents also a form of *evolutionary rate*. Because the frequency of fixation may be different for synonymous and non-synonymous substitutions, it is convenient to differentiate between the *synonymous substitution rate*, K_S and *non-synonymous substitution rate*, K_N. The number of differences between two genes prorated per one site is termed the *genetic distance*, d, and is usually calculated separately for synonymous (d_S) and non-synonymous (d_N) differences.

An example may help readers to grasp the meaning of the various terms. Consider the nucleotide sequence of a gene at a particular locus from species A and another sequence of a gene at a homologous locus from species B. Align the two sequences so that identical nucleotides occupy corresponding *sites*, and identify the differences (*nucleotide substitutions*). Suppose you find two differences between the two coding sequences, each of which is 300 nucleotides long. Then the *genetic distance* between the two genes is d = 2/300 or 0.007 so that in each gene there are 0.003 substitutions per site. Assume further that one of the substitutions is synonymous and the other non-synonymous and that of the 300 sites 70 are synonymous. The synonymous and non-synonymous distances are then $d_S = 1/70$ or 0.014 and d_N = 1/230 or 0.004. If the divergence time of the two species is 2 million years (my), the total substitution rate is $K = 2/300/(4\times10^6) = 1.67\times10^{-9}$ per site per year, the synonymous substitution rate is $K_S = 1/70/(4\times10^6) = 3.6\times10^{-9}$ per synonymous site per year and the non-synonymous substitution rate is $K_N = 1/230/(4\times10^6) = 1.1\times10^{-9}$ per non-synonymous site per year. (The reason for using the value of 4×10^6 is that substitutions had 2 my from the ancestor to species A and another 2 my from the same ancestor to species B to accumulate.)

If the alleles at a polymorphic locus are equivalent in their effect on the reproductive success of an individual (i.e. they are *neutral*), their fate in the population is determined by chance (the probability of sampling) and their behaviour in the gene pool represents *random genetic drift* (their frequencies drift randomly like a cork bobbing on the surface of a swimming pool). If, on the other hand, the possession of one of the alleles imparts a reproductive advantage or disadvantage to an individual (i.e. the allele is either *advantageous* or *disadvantageous*), its fate is influenced, in addition to random genetic drift, by *selection*, either *positive* (in the case of an advantageous allele) or *negative* (in the case of a disadvantageous allele). Positive selection accelerates the progress of an allele towards fixation, negative selection accelerates the loss of an allele. The formulas for probability of fixation, fixation time and fixation frequency introduced earlier all apply to *neutral* mutations only; for alleles under selection, a different set of formulas must be used.

There is nothing unusual about a gene being polymorphic. If one could sequence all the genes of all the individuals in a human population, one would probably find that most if not all loci are polymorphic, if not in their coding sequence, then at least in their introns. The reason we devote an entire section to the polymorphism of the *MHC* loci is that it is special, different from the polymorphism of all other loci. *MHC* polymorphism is notable in two respects: its extent and its nature. The usual situation with polymorphic loci is that there are one or two alleles that occur at high frequencies and a few additional alleles which occur at much lower frequencies. Some of the *MHC* loci (for example the class Ib loci or the human class II loci *HLA-DRB3* or *-DRB4*) also display this type of polymorphism. However, polymorphism of the *MHC* loci that are known or thought to be most actively involved in peptide presentation has a different character: There are large numbers of alleles at each locus and many of them occur at similar frequencies (i.e. there is no one dominating allele). At the latest count, 59, 118 and 36 alleles have been registered at the *HLA-A*, *-B* and *-C* loci, respectively; for the *HLA-DRB1*, *-DQA1*, *-DQB1*, *-DPB1* and *-DPA1* loci the numbers are 168, 19, 30, 73 and 8, respectively. While a few of these alleles may represent rare variants, most are known to occur at appreciable frequencies. Moreover, new alleles are still being described and only very few human populations have been *HLA*-typed adequately.

The second distinctive feature of *MHC* polymorphism is the large genetic distance between some of the alleles. Whereas the distances between alleles at most loci are almost always less than 0.01, the distances between some of the alleles at most polymorphic *MHC* loci are more than 10 times higher. While at non-*MHC* loci whole alleles usually do not differ by more than one or a few substitutions, at polymorphic *MHC* loci single exons of two alleles may differ by as many as 36 substitutions (Fig. 6.27). There are, of course, also pairs of *MHC* alleles that differ by one substitution only, but most allelic pairs lie between these two extremes. A plot of frequency against the number of substitutions in pairwise allelic comparisons results in a normal curve with pairs differing by 10–20 substitutions being most frequent (Fig. 6.27). This distribution of distances undoubtedly reflects the age distribution of alleles (more about this point later).

Variability within an *MHC* locus is distributed very unevenly. Most of it is concentrated in exon 2 of the class II loci and exons 2 and 3 of the class I loci. Furthermore, within these exons variability is mostly concentrated in certain sites, while the remaining sites are largely invariant. Because the variability is believed to have functional significance, it is important to evaluate how much of the nucleotide diversity translates into protein differences. A commonly used way of expressing protein variability is the *Wu–Kabat plot*, named after the American immunologists Tai Te Wu and Elvin A. Kabat. These two researchers gave *variability* quantitative meaning by defining it as the number of different amino acid residues observed at a given protein position divided by the frequency of the most common amino acid at that position. By plotting variability thus defined against amino acid residue number, proper weight is given to amino acids represented at different frequencies at a given position in the protein sample. Variability plots of class I α1 and α2 domains and of the class II β1 domain (Fig. 6.28) identify several positions as highly variable. Significantly, these same positions, as will be explained later in this chapter, form the PBR of the MHC molecule.

What might be the reason for the difference between the polymorphism of the *MHC* and non-*MHC* loci? An obvious answer may seem to be: the substitution rate. If the *MHC* substitution rate were 10 times faster than that of other loci, this would explain both the presence of many alleles in the population and the large genetic distances between some of the alleles. However, this explanation had to be abandoned when it became clear that there is nothing unusual about the substitution rates of the *MHC* genes. The non-synonymous substitution rate of the PBR in the *MHC* genes is 5.9×10^{-9} per non-synonymous site per year; the synonymous substitution rate is 1.18×10^{-9} per synonymous site per year. Both values are within the range formed by the substitution rates of non-*MHC* genes. Since in mammals synonymous substitutions are selectively neutral, the rate of synonymous substitutions is expected to equal the rate of synonymous mutations. It follows, therefore, that the mutation rate at the *MHC* loci is low and hence that there must be another reason for the uniqueness of the *MHC* polymorphism. This reason was revealed when *MHC* sequences from different species became available and could be compared. It was then noticed that, for example, some human *MHC* alleles were more similar to certain chimpanzee or gorilla alleles than they were to other human alleles (Fig. 6.29). When phylogenetic trees of alleles at

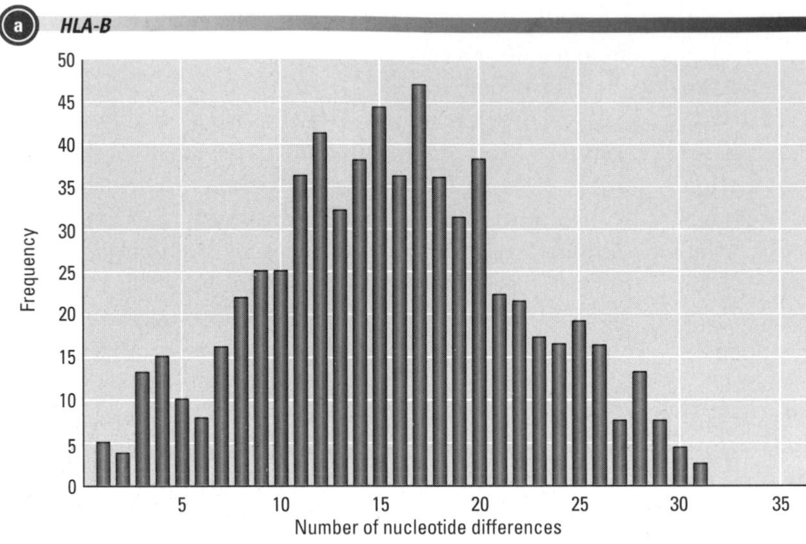

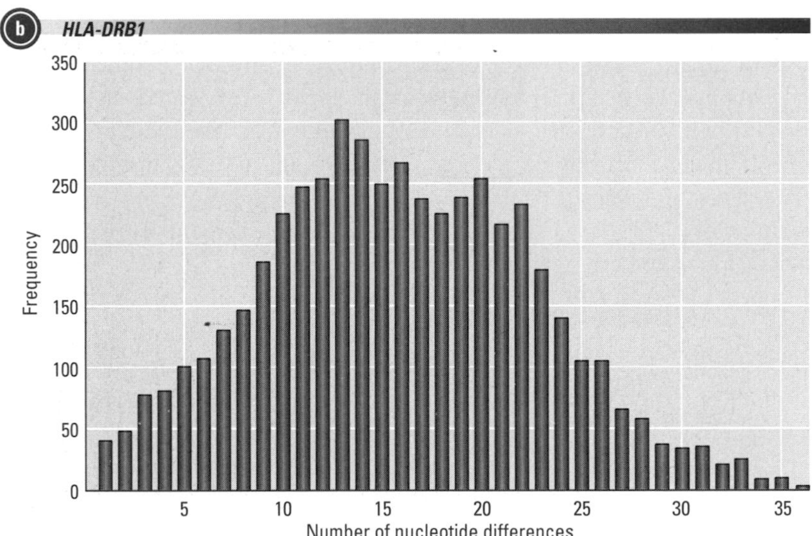

Figure 6.27 Distribution of numbers of nucleotide differences in pairwise comparison of *HLA-B* and *-DRB1* alleles (exon 2 only). The sequences of exon 2 of the known alleles at these loci were aligned, each sequence compared with all other sequences and differences counted in each combination. The *y* axis gives the number of combinations having the number of differences indicated on the *x* axis. The comparisons involved 37 *HLA-B* sequences ($37 \times 36 = 1332$ combinations) and 101 *HLA-DRB1* sequences ($101 \times 100 = 10\,100$ combinations). (Courtesy of Colm O'hUigin.)

homologous loci were generated, the alleles did not segregate into clusters according to the species of origin, but rather were intermingled (Fig. 6.30). The intermixing of alleles from different species indicated that some of the alleles arose before the species diverged from one another, i.e. that their ancestors were already present as polymorphisms in the common ancestor of the species. In groups of closely related species (e.g. the cichlid fishes in the Great Lakes of East Africa or Darwin's finches on the Galápagos Islands) one actually finds identical alleles in different species. In more distantly related species (such as humans, chimpanzee and gorilla, which diverged approximately 4.5 my ago), identical alleles are no longer present, but alleles of one species differing from alleles of another species in one or very few substitutions only are common. In even more distantly related species (e.g. humans and orang-utan or gibbon, which diverged 13–16 my ago), the distances between the alleles are greater still but the interspecific affinities are nevertheless clearly recognizable. Since alleles are defined as variants at a given locus of a given species, it is more appropriate to refer to the related genes in interspecies comparisons as *allelic lineages*. Comparison of *MHC* sequences from various primates has revealed that some of the allelic lineages now represented in humans go back all the way to the ancestors of apes and Old World monkeys, which lived some 20–30 my ago. When one traces the lineages backwards in time, they appear to coalesce gradually into fewer and fewer lineages until only one, the ancestor of all the extant alleles, is left (Fig. 6.31). The coalescence process is akin to showing a movie in reverse. In reality, the process was one of *divergence* rather than coalescence. All alleles now present in the human population

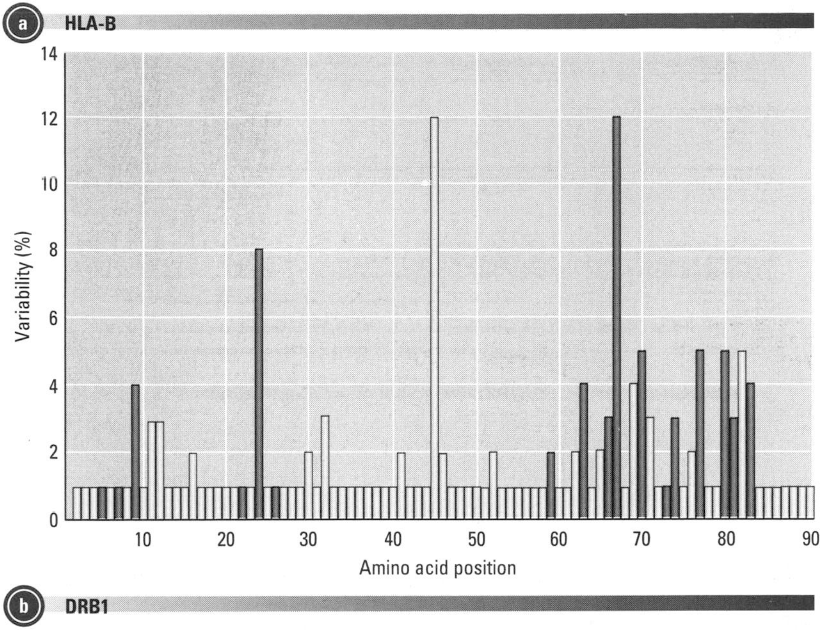

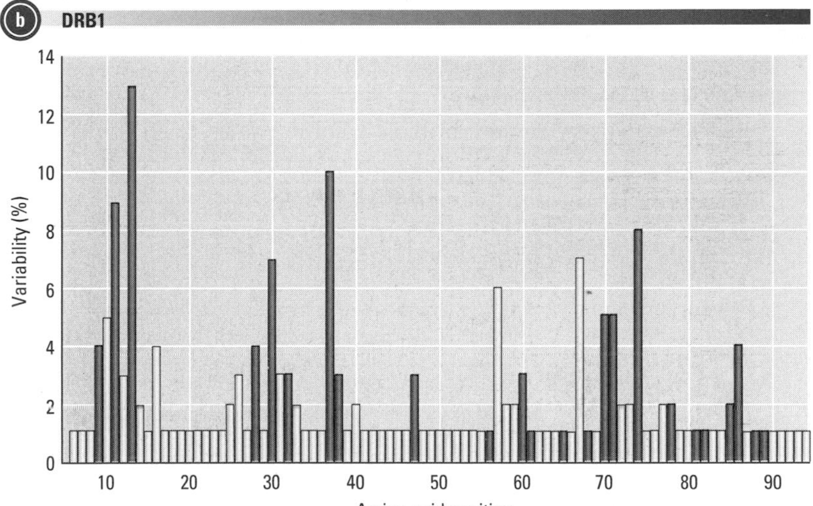

Figure 6.28 Wu–Kabat variability plot of HLA-B and -DRB1 amino acid sequences (α1 and β1 domains, respectively). Positions contributing to the peptide-binding region are highlighted. (Courtesy of Colm O'hUigin.)

began as a single gene whose progeny gradually accumulated substitutions and thus diverged into lineages along the lines of descent. As some of the lineages were lost during the process, the gaps between the surviving lineages gradually increased. This process occurred over many millions of years during which time species came and went, whereas the allelic lineages persisted by being passed on from ancestral to emerging species. The evolution of the allelic lineages thus transcends the evolution of species, i.e. it is *trans-specific* in character. It is this trans-specific mode of evolution that is responsible for uniqueness of the *MHC* polymorphism. Since alleles at non-*MHC* loci begin to diverge mostly *after* the divergence of a species, they have time to accumulate only very few differences during the 2–3 my of the species' lifespan. The *MHC* alleles, on the other hand, have had a much longer time to accumulate differences and that is why the genetic distances between them can be so large. Polymorphisms at different *MHC* loci have apparently been founded at different times in the past: The lineages at the *HLA-DRB1* locus go back to 20–30 my ago; those at the *HLA-A* locus to a 'mere' 5–10 my ago; and alleles at the class Ib loci may have arisen after the emergence of *Homo sapiens* less than 1 my ago.

The trans-specific nature of *MHC* evolution accounts for the difference between *MHC* and non-*MHC* polymorphism but it does not explain why the two types of loci evolve so differently. This explanation must be sought in the principles that underlie the emergence of new mutations. We mentioned earlier that the ultimate fate of a new mutation is either extinction or fixation. A neutral mutation does not persist as a polymorphism longer than, on average, $4N_e$ generations. Since, however, the *MHC* alleles have persisted

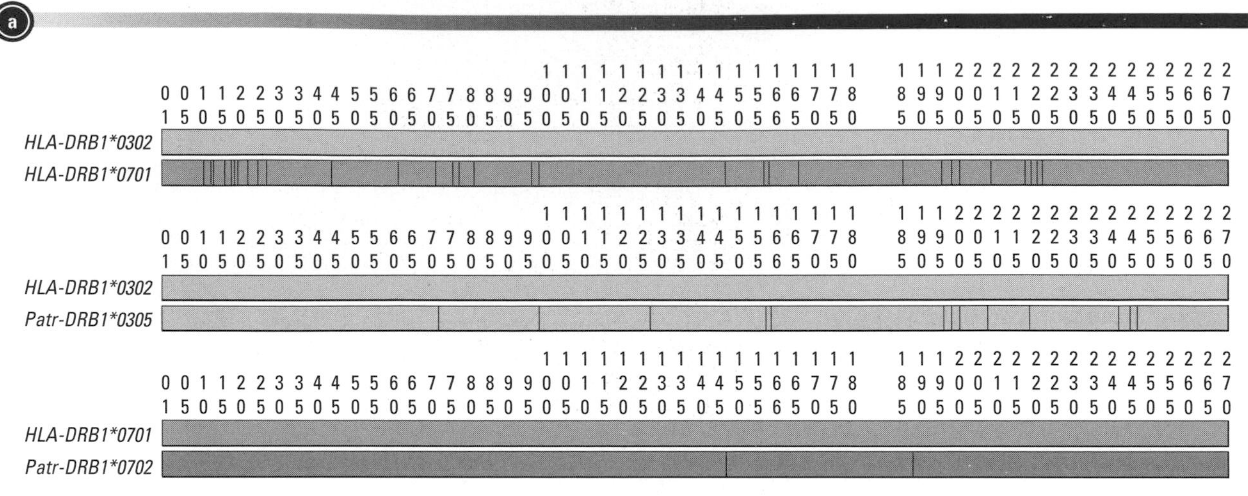

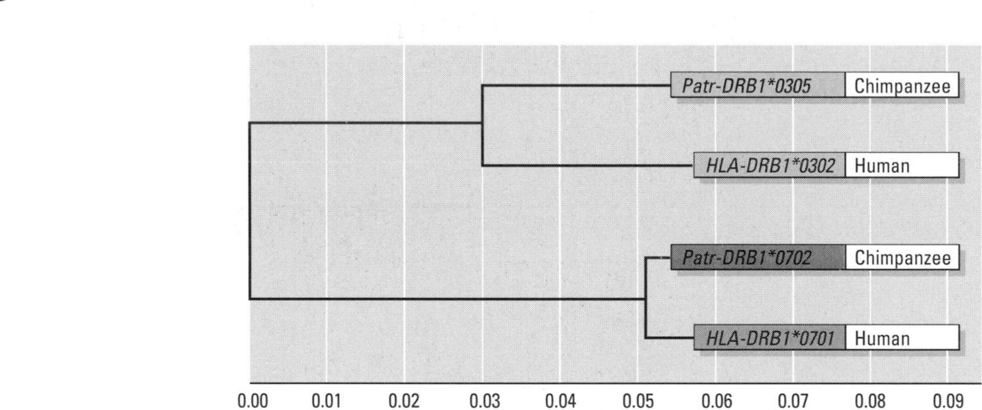

Figure 6.29 Trans-species character of *MHC* polymorphism. (a) Comparison of two human (*HLA*) and two chimpanzee (*Patr*) *MHC-DRB1* exon 2 nucleotide sequences. In each pair, the upper bar is used as a standard; differences from this standard are indicated in the lower bar by vertical lines. Numbers above the bar indicate nucleotide sites. (b) Phylogenetic tree (*dendrogram*) of the four genes from (a). The tree reflects the degree to which individual sequences are related to one another and hence, by extension, their possible divergence from one another during evolution. Here, relatedness of two sequences is assessed by the *genetic distance*, which is basically the number of positions at which the sequences differ divided by the total number of positions compared. The smaller the distance, the more closely related the two sequences are. There are several ways (algorithms) by which genetic distances can be used to construct phylogenetic trees (and there are also methods for constructing dendrograms without using genetic distances). The one commonly used, the *neighbour-joining method* (which was also used to construct dendrograms in this figure), is based on the following principle: in preparation for tree construction, sequences are aligned and genetic distances for all possible pairwise combinations are calculated and arranged into a distance matrix. In the neighbour-joining method, the pair giving the shortest overall length is chosen. It is then considered as a single entity and a new matrix is produced for all the pairwise combinations. A new pair is then found that gives the shortest overall length and this pair is then joined to the pair chosen in the first round of calculations. The procedure is repeated in this manner until all pairs are joined and a dendrogram with a particular topology is obtained. (From Klein, J., Takahata, N. & Ayala, F.J. (1993) *Scientific American*, **269**, 78.)

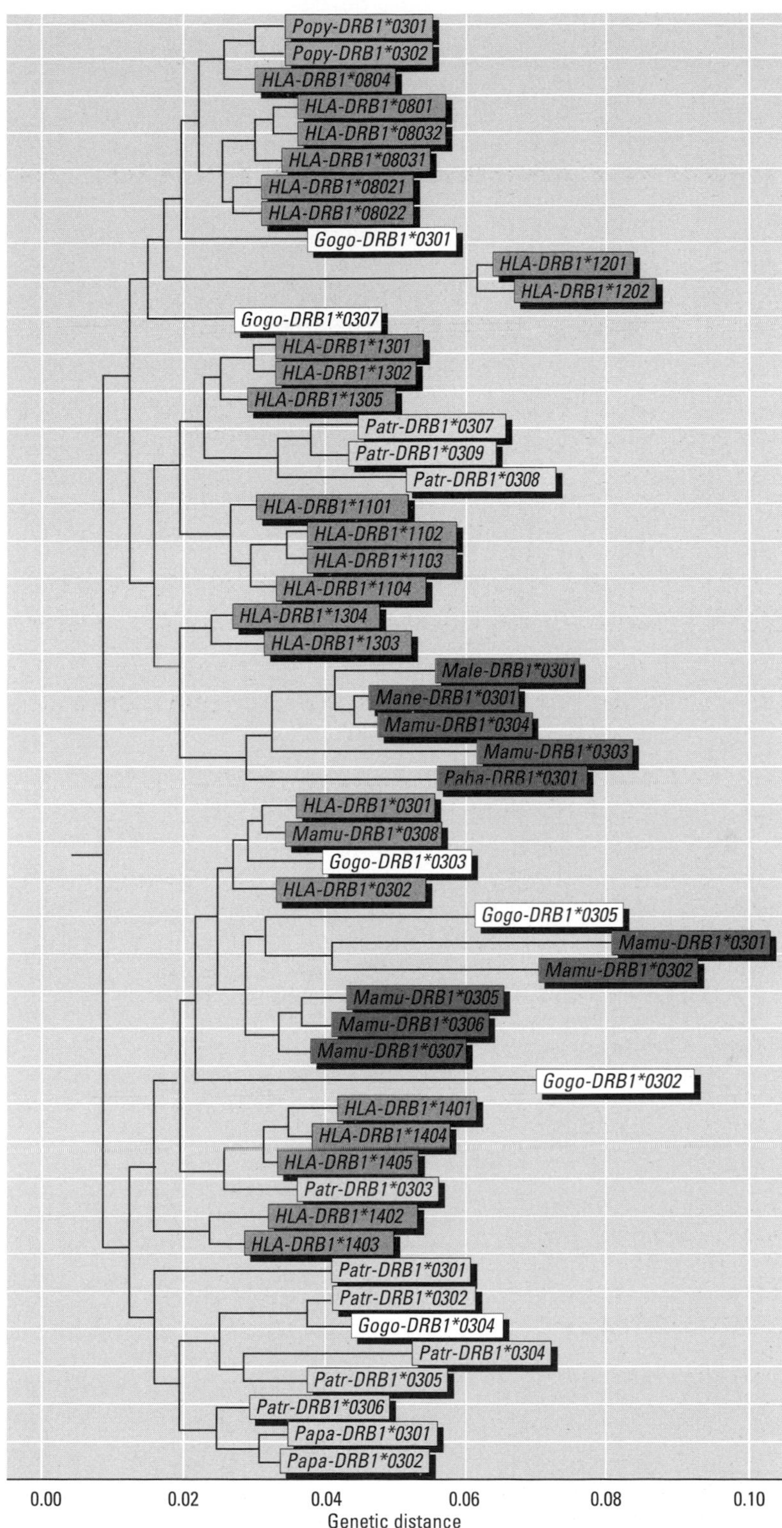

Figure 6.30 Phylogenetic tree of *Mhc-DRB1* alleles showing the intermingling of genes from different primate species. The tree was constructed by the neighbour-joining method (see Fig. 6.29) using exon 2 nucleotide sequences. *Gogo*, gorilla (***Gorilla gorilla***); *HLA*, human; *Male*, drill (***Mandrillus leucophaeus***); *Mamu*, rhesus macaque (***Macaca mulatta***); *Mane*, pigtail macaque (***Macaca nemestrina***); *Paha*, hamadryas baboon (***Papio hamadryas***); *Papa*, pygmy chimpanzee (***Pan paniscus***); *Patr*, chimpanzee (***Pan troglodytes***); *Popy*, orang-utan (***Pongo pygmaeus***). *Mamu*, *Mane*, *Male* and *Paha* are Old World monkeys; the rest are apes. (Courtesy of Colm O'hUigin.)

much longer than this they obviously cannot be neutral. Evidence that their evolution is influenced by natural selection is indeed available. As has already been explained, synonymous changes do not alter the amino acid sequence of a protein and are therefore largely unaffected by selection. Most non-synonymous changes, on the other hand, are deleterious because meddling with the amino acid sequence usually reduces or totally obliterates the functionality of a protein. They are therefore eliminated by negative or *purifying selection*, and in a gene in which these two types of change occur the proportion of synonymous substitutions is greater than the proportion of non-synonymous substitutions ($d_S > d_N$). Most genes that have been analysed do indeed show a preponderance of synonymous over non-synonymous substitutions. However, in certain parts of the polymorphic *MHC* genes the opposite is true: in the part coding for the PBR, non-synonymous substitutions occur more frequently than synonymous ($d_N > d_S$; Fig. 6.32), while in the rest of the gene, as in most other genes, $d_S > d_N$. This preferential accumulation of non-synonymous substitutions must be the result of *positive selection*, which favours diversification of the PBR.

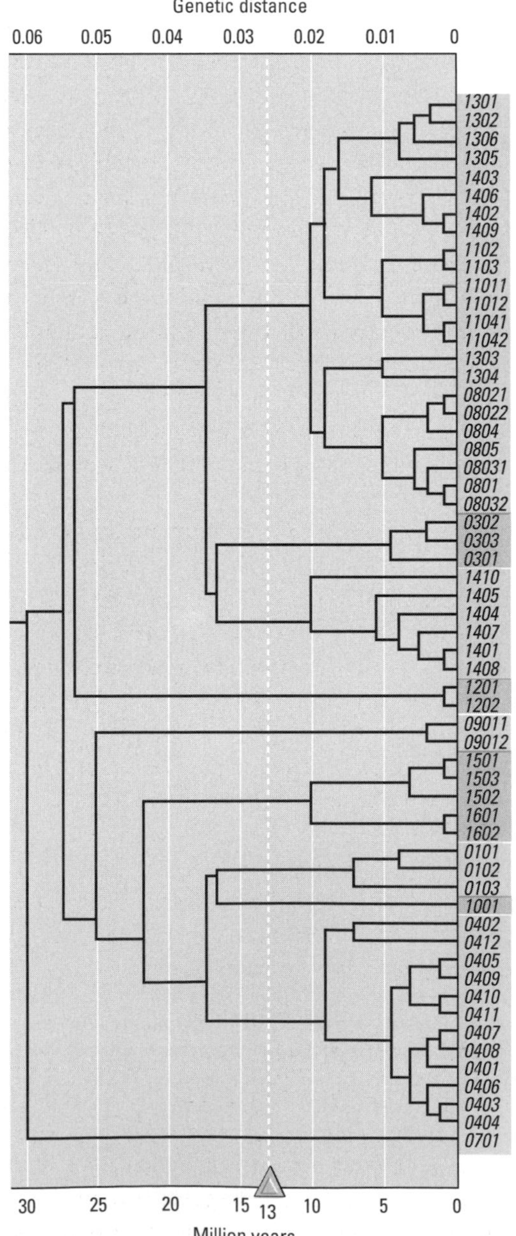

Figure 6.31 Coalescence of *Mhc-DRB*1 allelic lineages. Sequences of 58 *HLA-DRB1* alleles (exon 2) present in the human population were used to construct a phylogenetic tree by the unweighted pair-group method with arithmetic means (UPGMA). In this method, distances are calculated for all pairs of *operational taxonomic units* (*OTUs*, here sequences in pairwise comparisons) and the pair with the shortest distance is identified and used to draw the first branch of the tree. This pair is now considered as a single OTU and used to calculate a new distance matrix and the new pair separated by the shortest distance is used to draw another branch of the tree. The process is thus repeated until all the OTUs are connected and the tree thus completed. The UPGMA is more suitable than the neighbour-joining method in situations in which not only genetic distance scale (top) but also time scale (bottom) is desired. The extant alleles are indicated by the numbers on the extreme right; their grouping reflects the coalescence (divergence) process in relation to time. Thus, for example, the alleles **1301* and **1302* diverged from a common ancestor ~ 2 my ago; this ancestor diverged from **1306* about 4 my ago and so on. At 13 my (broken line), the time of separation of African and Asian great apes, all the extant alleles coalesce into nine lineages. In other words, the groups of extant alleles differentiated by the sequence of pink and grey blocks diverged 13 my ago. (Courtesy of Colm O'hUigin.)

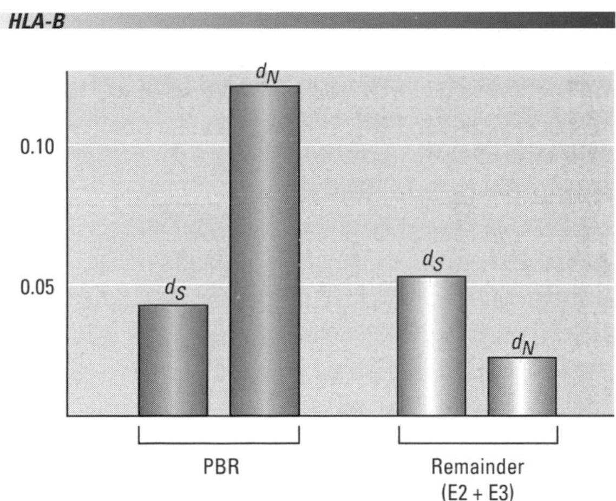

Figure 6.32 Numbers of synonymous (d_S) and non-synonymous (d_N) nucleotide substitutions per 100 sites in the peptide-binding region (PBR) and the remainder of exons 2 and 3 of the *HLA-B* locus. The numbers were calculated from pairwise comparisons of 88 *HLA-B* allelic sequences. (From Hughes, A.L. & Hughes, M.K. (1995) *Immunogenetics*, **42**, 233.)

Natural selection can be quantified by measuring *fitness* (w), the relative survival and reproductive success (contribution to future generations) of an individual. By convention, the allele that provides an individual with the highest survival and the greatest reproductive success is assigned the fitness value of $w = 1$. Compared with the fittest allele, all other alleles in the population have, by definition, lower fitness by a factor referred to as the *selection coefficient*, s (so that $w = 1 - s$). Hence the selection coefficient is a quantitative measure of the reduction in fitness in comparison with the fittest allele, a measure of selective disadvantage ($s = 1 - w$). The selection coefficient of the polymorphic *MHC* loci has been estimated to be $s < 0.01$. This means that fewer than 1% of *MHC* homozygotes (individuals carrying identical alleles at *MHC* loci on both chromosomes) die or are disadvantaged in comparison to heterozygotes. Whether the effect of natural selection on *MHC* genes varies with time is unclear. However, many examples of *MHC* monomorphic populations and species persisting without any apparent handicaps are known. On the other hand, the persistence of allelic lineages over many millions of years is an indication of the lasting influence of positive selection. The simultaneous persistence of many alleles is an indication that, in the long run at least, selection does not favour one allele over all others but rather diversification into a large number of variants. This type of selection is termed *balancing* because the various alleles remain in the population in a state of balance against loss and fixation, a state of *balancing polymorphism*. The diversification of the persisting alleles is achieved by the gradual accumulation of nucleotide changes at different sites. These changes are not 'substitutions' as defined earlier because they do not achieve fixation; instead they persist in the population at polymorphic frequencies and are therefore more appropriately termed *incorporations*.

Because balancing selection influences the PBR only, and because the PBR's function is to capture and present peptides derived from parasites, it is believed that parasites are the actual agent of selection. In very simplistic terms, the more diversified the PBR, the lower the chance that a parasite-derived peptide may not be bound by the MHC molecules and hence that the parasite may escape detection by the adaptive immune system of the host.

The actual nature of the selection process is controversial. The two competing hypotheses are referred to as overdominance selection and frequency-dependent selection. *Overdominance* is a condition in which the heterozygote manifests a trait more extremely than does either homozygote. In the context of selection, overdominance (*heterozygous advantage*) refers to a situation in which the fitness of the heterozygote is greater than that of either homozygote. The term *frequency-dependent selection* has many meanings; the one usually used in the context of *MHC* genes refers to a situation in which an allele is at a relative selective advantage when rare; as its frequency increases, its selective advantage wanes. No experimental data are available to enable one to choose unambiguously between these two hypotheses.

MHC alleles diversify primarily by mutations. To what degree other mechanisms contribute to further diversification is uncertain. The fact that alignments of sequences from a large number of alleles have an often patchy appearance with stretches (*motifs*) of similar sequence appearing in various combinations in different alleles has been interpreted as evidence for frequent exchanges (*gene conversions*) of short segments between alleles. An alternative explanation of this phenomenon is that the motifs arise independently in different genes as a result of *convergent evolution*—by repeated mutations and selection for certain combinations of amino acid residues in the encoded proteins. The restriction of the motifs to the PBR is consistent with this interpretation.

MHC genes in populations

Animals live in interbreeding groups occupying defined regions, i.e. in *populations*. All genes in a given population constitute a *gene pool* in which each gene occurs with a certain frequency. To calculate the *gene frequency*, we count how many times a given gene (allele) occurs in a sample population and then divide this number by the total number of genes (alleles) at a given locus in this sample. For example, if we find that in a sample of 100 individuals, there are 80 *AA*, 18 *Aa* and 2 *aa* individuals, the frequency of the *A* gene is 178/200 = 0.89. (The total number of *A* genes in the sample is $2 \times 80 + 18 = 178$; the total number of genes, *A* and *a*, is $2 \times 100 = 200$.) The frequencies of some of the *HLA* genes are given in Table 6.1.

The laws governing the combination of genes in a population are not unlike those determining the probabilities of gene encounter in two pools of gametes. If the frequencies of the *A* and *a* genes in the sperm pool of a given male were p and q, respectively, and the frequencies of the *A* and *a* genes in the egg pool of a female were the same, the probabilities of the genes meeting in a zygote would then be:

		Egg	
		p	q
Sperm	p	p^2	pq
	q	pq	q^2

In other words, the probabilities for the three possible combinations would be p^2AA, $2pqAa$ and q^2aa. If the individuals in a population mate randomly, this simple relationship must also apply to them so that in this population there will be p^2AA, $2pqAa$ and q^2aa individuals. A population in which frequencies of homozygotes and heterozygotes approach the frequencies predicted by this *Hardy–Weinberg law* is said to be in *genetic equilibrium*. The law makes two important predictions. First, after one genera-

Table 6.1 Frequencies of alleles at the *HLA-A* and *-B* loci in different populations. (From Baur, M.B. *et al.* (1984). In *Histocompatibility Testing* (Eds E.D. Albert *et al.*). Springer-Verlag, Berlin.)

Allele	Caucasoids	Mongoloids	Negroids	Allele	Caucasoids	Mongoloids	Negroids
A1	14.2	1.0	8.1	*Bw41*	0.9	0.1	2.3
A2	28.9	28.1	17.5	*Bw42*	0.2	0.5	5.8
A3	13.2	1.5	6.7	*B44*	12.3	6.0	7.7
A11	6.3	11.7	1.9	*B45*	0.4	0.1	2.3
A23	1.4	0.1	8.0	*Bw46*	0.1	3.6	0
A24	10.3	31.4	4.8	*Bw47*	0.2	0.4	0
A25	2.4	0	0	*Bw48*	0	1.6	0
A26	3.2	7.2	4.5	*B49*	1.8	0.3	2.3
A28	4.7	2.1	9.9	*Bw50*	1.1	0.3	0.6
A29	2.9	5.2	1.6	*B51*	6.2	7.8	1.9
A30	3.5	2.3	11.0	*Bw52*	2.0	7.3	0.6
A31	2.9	5.2	1.6	*Bw53*	0.5	0.3	6.7
A32	3.9	0.4	2.3	*Bw54*	0.1	6.7	0
Aw33	1.4	6.0	3.9	*Bw55*	1.6	2.1	0
Aw34	0.1	0.3	5.1	*Bw56*	1.1	1.5	0.3
Aw36	0.1	0.1	3.2	*Bw57*	2.9	0.7	2.9
Aw43	0	0	1.3	*Bw58*	0	1.2	0
Aw66	0.2	0.5	0.3	*Bw60*	3.8	6.5	2.3
AX	0.4	1.7	5.0	*Bw61*	2.1	11.7	1.5
Sample size*	2163	976	311	*Bw62*	6.1	9.6	2.6
				Bw63	0.7	0	1.9
B7	11.5	4.7	12.1	*Bw64*	1.1	0	1.3
B8	9.6	0.2	5.5	*Bw65*	2.6	0.2	1.6
B13	2.9	3.8	1.6	*Bw67*	0	0.1	0
B18	5.5	0.3	4.2	*Bw71*	0.1	0.4	0.8
B27	3.4	1.6	1.9	*Bw72*	0.3	0.5	7.1
B35	10.5	10.2	7.1	*Bw73*	0.1	0.2	0
B37	1.6	0.6	1.3	*BX*	0.4	1.6	1.3
B38	2.5	0.7	1.6	Sample size*	2132	968	311
B39	2.0	0.4	0				

* Number of haplotypes counted.
X, unidentified allele ('blank').

tion the two alleles *A* and *a* will be present in frequencies $p^2AA:2pqAa:q^2aa$. Second, these frequencies will not change in subsequent generations and the population will remain in equilibrium.

Thus far we have considered a single locus with two alleles. Let us now consider two loci, each with two alleles, *A*, *a*, *B* and *b*, with frequencies *p*, *q*, *r* and *s*, respectively, where $p + q = 1$ and $r + s = 1$. The genes can be arranged in four combinations, *AB*, *Ab*, *aB* and *ab*, with frequencies x_1, x_2, x_3 and x_4, respectively, where $x_1 + x_2 + x_3 + x_4 = 1$, $p = x_1 + x_2$, $q = x_3 + x_4$, $r = x_1 + x_3$ and $s = x_2 + x_4$. The population will be in equilibrium with respect to the *A* and *B* genes when $x_2x_3 = x_1x_4$ or $x_2x_3 - x_1x_4 = 0$. If the latter product is not zero but instead some other value *D* or Δ (delta), the population is in momentary *disequilibrium*. Given time, it will eventually approach equilibrium by gradually decreasing the value of *D*. The speed of the approach to equilibrium will depend on whether the two loci are linked or not and, if they are, how close the linkage is. The closer the linkage, the stronger the *linkage disequilibrium* and the longer the process towards equilibrium. The existence of linkage disequilibrium in a population may indicate either that a particular *MHC* haplotype has recently been introduced into the population and there has not been enough time to attain equilibrium or that the particular combination of alleles is favoured by selection. Linkage disequilibrium is therefore an important parameter characterizing a population. Certain combinations of *HLA* genes have indeed been found to be present in disequilibrium in certain human populations and this fact has been used to make inferences about the origin of these populations and about human migrations. A striking manifestation of linkage disequilibrium are the *ancestral haplotypes*, the same combinations of alleles at *MHC* loci found among unrelated individuals in various populations. Ancestral haplotypes are believed to have been present in the founding stocks of these populations and to have remained untouched by recombination up to the present. The length of these haplotypes (the number of loci included in the linkage disequilibrium) varies, but in some instances it extends over much of the *MHC*.

MHC molecules

The product of each of the *MHC* genes is a *polypeptide chain* (a long sequence of amino acid residues), which combines with a polypeptide produced by another locus to form a *heterodimer*. After the addition of carbohydrate chains and complexation with peptides, the *MHC glycoprotein* is expressed on the cell surface. The two polypeptide chains of the heterodimer are held together by *non-covalent bonds* (Fig. 6.33). Neighbouring amino acid residues in the polypeptide chain are hooked up by the *peptide bond* (Fig. 6.34a), which is an example of a *covalent bond*. If even numbers of cysteine residues are present in the polypeptide chain, they can form pairs linked by another form of covalent bond, the *disulphide bond* or *bridge* (Fig. 6.34b). The cysteine residues participating in the disulphide bond formation can be separated by a large number of other amino acid residues, but they come together by looping out the intervening sequence.

The linear sequence of the amino acid residues in the polypeptide constitutes the protein's *primary structure* (Fig. 6.35). The local spatial arrangement of the polypeptide's backbone atoms (the *main chain*) without regard to the conformation of the side-chains is the *secondary structure*; it is maintained by non-covalent bonds between amino acid residues a short distance apart. The secondary structure rests on a few basic motifs such as the α-helix, β-strand and β-pleated sheet (Fig. 6.35). The folds assemble into higher order configuration, the *domains* of the *tertiary structure* (see Figs 6.22 & 6.23) and the domains of the two chains in the heterodimer arrange into a higher order still, the *quaternary structure*. The higher orders of structure are revealed by *X-ray diffraction analysis* (Fig. 6.36) of suitable protein crystals.

As has already been mentioned, each MHC molecule, class I or class II, consists of two different chains, α and β. The class I α chains are glycoproteins with relative molecular mass (M_r) of approximately 44 000 and the polypeptide chain is approximately 350 amino acid residues long. The class I β chain, the β_2m, is a soluble protein with an M_r of 11 500 and length of 99 amino acid residues. The class II α and β chains are both glycoproteins, the former having an M_r of 31 000–34 000, the latter of 26 000–29 000. The length of the α chain ranges from 229 to 233 amino acid residues, that of the β chain from 255 to 238 residues, depending on the controlling locus. Both the class I and class II molecules have an extracellular part, membrane-spanning part and a cytoplasmic (intracellular) part (see Figs 6.23 & 6.24). They can also be viewed as comprising three structural modules: the peptide-binding, the immunoglobulin-like and the membrane-anchoring modules (Fig. 6.37). Each module consists of domains and regions. The description of the modules and domains follows.

The *peptide-binding module* consists of two peptide-binding domains, which in class I molecules are contributed by a single polypeptide chain (α) and in class II molecules by two chains (α and β). The domains are designated α1 and α2 in class I molecules or α1 and β1 in class II molecules. The module has the appearance of a deep *groove* (cleft)

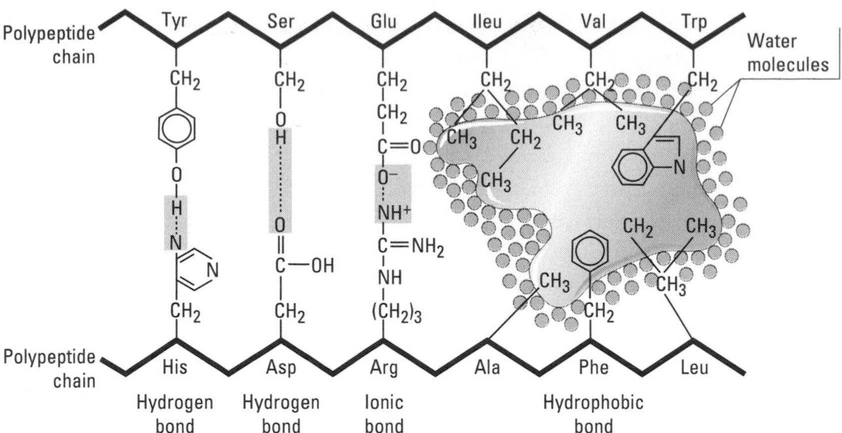

Figure 6.33 Examples of non-covalent bonds. In the *hydrogen bond*, a hydrogen atom forms a link between two strongly electron-negative atoms (here between O and N in one example or between two O atoms in another). Only O, N and F atoms are sufficiently electronegative to take part in hydrogen bonding. In the *ionic bond* (in proteins often referred to as *salt bridge*), one or more electrons from one atom shift to another atom, and the resulting positive and negative ions attract each other electrostatically. In the *hydrophobic bond*, in contrast to the previous two types of non-covalent bonds, there is no actual link between the atomic groups involved. Instead, atoms, groups of atoms or molecules are forced to adhere to one another just as two oil droplets are compelled to fuse into a larger drop in water. Because of the polarization of its molecules, water is a highly cohesive substance. A non-polarized (non-charged) molecule placed in water takes up space and separates water molecules, creating an energetically unfavourable situation. When two non-polarized molecules are placed in water, they take up twice the space and the situation becomes even less favourable. To improve this condition, water molecules push the two non-polar molecules together so that they occupy as little space as possible. Hence, non-polar molecules stay together not because they form bonds between each other, but because they are driven together by the tendency of water to retain its cohesiveness.

between two parallel ridges (Fig. 6.38). The groove is approximately 30 Å long and 12 Å wide in the middle. [One angstrom, Å, named after the Swedish physicist, Anders J. Ångström) is equal to 10^{-10} of a metre]. The bottom (floor) of the groove is formed by a single β-pleated sheet consisting of eight antiparallel β-strands, four strands contributed by one domain (α1 in class I and class II molecules) and another four by the other domain (α2 in class I molecules and β1 in class II molecules). The two ridges are formed by two α-helices, again contributed by different domains. The grooves of the class I and class II molecules differ at their ends. The groove of the class I molecules tapers off at both ends to a width of about 5Å and is then closed completely by bulky amino acid side-chains contributed, for example, by tyrosine and tryptophan, which act like boulders blocking the entrance to and exit from a canyon. The groove of the class II molecules, on the other hand, is open at both ends because of structural reorganizations in these regions in which the terminal two turns of the α-helix have been replaced by extended structures (so that the α-helices of class II molecules are shorter than those of class I molecules) and the bulky residues have been replaced by ones with small side-chains. The α2 domain of the class I molecules and the β1 domain of the class II molecules contain two cysteine residues approximately 60 residues apart that are linked covalently by the disulphide bond. This bond, together with a series of salt-bridges and hydrogen bonds, stabilizes the domains.

Each of the ellipsoidal *immunoglobulin-like domains* (α3 and β_2m in class I molecules, α2 and β2 in class II molecules) resembles, as the name implies, the constant domain of the heavy chain in immunoglobulin molecules (see Chapter 8). The characteristic structure shared by these domains is termed the *immunoglobulin fold*. It is described in detail in Chapter 8; here it is sufficient to say that in MHC molecules the fold consists of seven antiparallel β-strands organized into two β-pleated sheets apposed to each other like the faces of a sandwich. One sheet consists of three and the other of four β-strands and the individual strands are interconnected by loops (Fig. 6.39). The sheets are held together by hydrophobic interactions and by a disulphide bond between two cysteine residues spaced approximately 60 amino acid residues apart in the primary structure but brought together by the folding. In class I molecules, the β-strands of the two sheets in the α3 domain run perpendicular to the β-strands of the β_2m. The two domains face each other by parts of the four-stranded sheets (the first two strands of β_2m facing the fourth and fifth β-strands of the α3 domain). The two faces interact mostly via hydrogen bonds, the two domains (α3 and β_2m) being held together

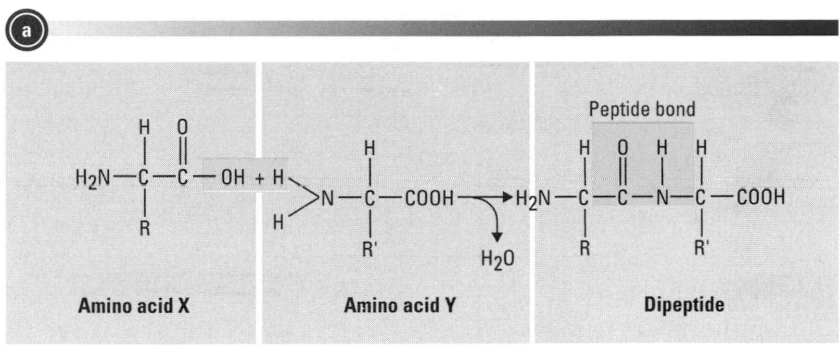

Figure 6.34 Two types of covalent bonds commonly occurring in proteins. In a covalent bond, two adjacent atoms share one or more electron pairs in their outermost energy levels (orbitals) and the sharing provides each atom with a stable octet of electrons in these levels. In the *peptide bond* (a) two amino acids conjoin by the union of the carboxyl (COOH) group of one with the amino (NH_2) group of the other, eliminating one water molecule. The *disulphide bond* (b) is formed by the oxidation and joining of two cysteines into a disulphide, termed cystine. One-half of the cystine molecule, corresponding to one cysteine residue, is sometimes referred to as half-cystine. R, side-chain.

exclusively by non-covalent bonds. The β_2m also interacts with the underside of the eight-stranded β-sheet of the α1 and α2 domains and in addition there is a small area of contact between the α3 and α1–α2 domains. In terms of an overall structure, the α1 and α2 domains form the top of the molecule, the β_2m is located under the centre of the top and the α3 domain under the lower left corner of the peptide-binding module (see Fig. 6.37). Each of the domains is approximately 90–100 amino acid residues long (in the HLA-A molecule the domains take up these amino acid positions: α1, 1–90; α2, 92–182; α3, 183–270; and β_2m, 1–99).

In the class II molecules, the α2 and β2 domains correspond to the β_2m and α3 domains, respectively. The packing of the class II domains resembles that of the class I domain except that the β2 of class II is offset relative to α3 of class I by about 15° (see Fig. 6.37), presumably to allow the two chains to interact with each other by non-covalent, mostly hydrogen bonds; these bonds hold the α and β chains together. In contrast to class I molecules, which remain α:β heterodimers throughout their life cycles, the class II α:β heterodimers apparently assemble, with the participation of the invariant chain, into higher order polymers. The class II chains first form dimers and then dimers of the dimers (Fig. 6.40). These higher-order associations, too, are mediated exclusively by non-covalent bonds. The class II α1 and β1 domains range in length from 84 to 96 residues depending on the species and the controlling gene family; the α2 and β2 domains are usually each 94 residues long. The human DR α chain has two carbohydrate moieties, one linked to the asparagine residue at position 78 in the α1 domain and the other to the asparagine residue at position 118 in the α2 domain. The DR β chain has a single carbohydrate moiety attached to the asparagine residue at position 19 in the β1 domain.

The *membrane-anchoring module* consists of the connecting peptide, the transmembrane region and the cytoplasmic tail. The *connecting peptide* is a stretch of about a dozen largely hydrophilic amino acid residues. It extends from the C-terminus of the α3 domain in the class I molecule and the C-termini of the α2 and β2 domains in the class II molecules to the amino acid residue with which the polypeptide chain enters the lipid bilayer. Connecting peptides are probably straight segments of the chains, accessible to protein-cleaving enzymes such as papain. This accessibility has enabled investigators to obtain soluble forms of the extracellular part of the MHC molecules, particularly class I molecules, for structural analysis.

The *transmembrane region* spans the lipid bilayer of the plasma membrane. The inside of the bilayer is highly hydrophobic and to cross it a protein segment must contain mostly hydrophobic amino acid residues and must, in addition, be arranged in such a way that the polar groups of any hydrophilic residues present interact with each other; unengaged groups would disturb the structure of the membrane. The transmembrane region of the MHC polypeptide chains fulfils these requirements. It consists of 19–26 largely hydrophobic residues and it seems to form several turns of the α-helix in which polar residues of one chain (in the case of class II molecules) face polar residues of the other chain (Fig. 6.41). These interactions probably help to keep the chains of the heterodimer together.

As the chains enter the plasma membrane or exit from it on the cytoplasmic side, they probably interact with the

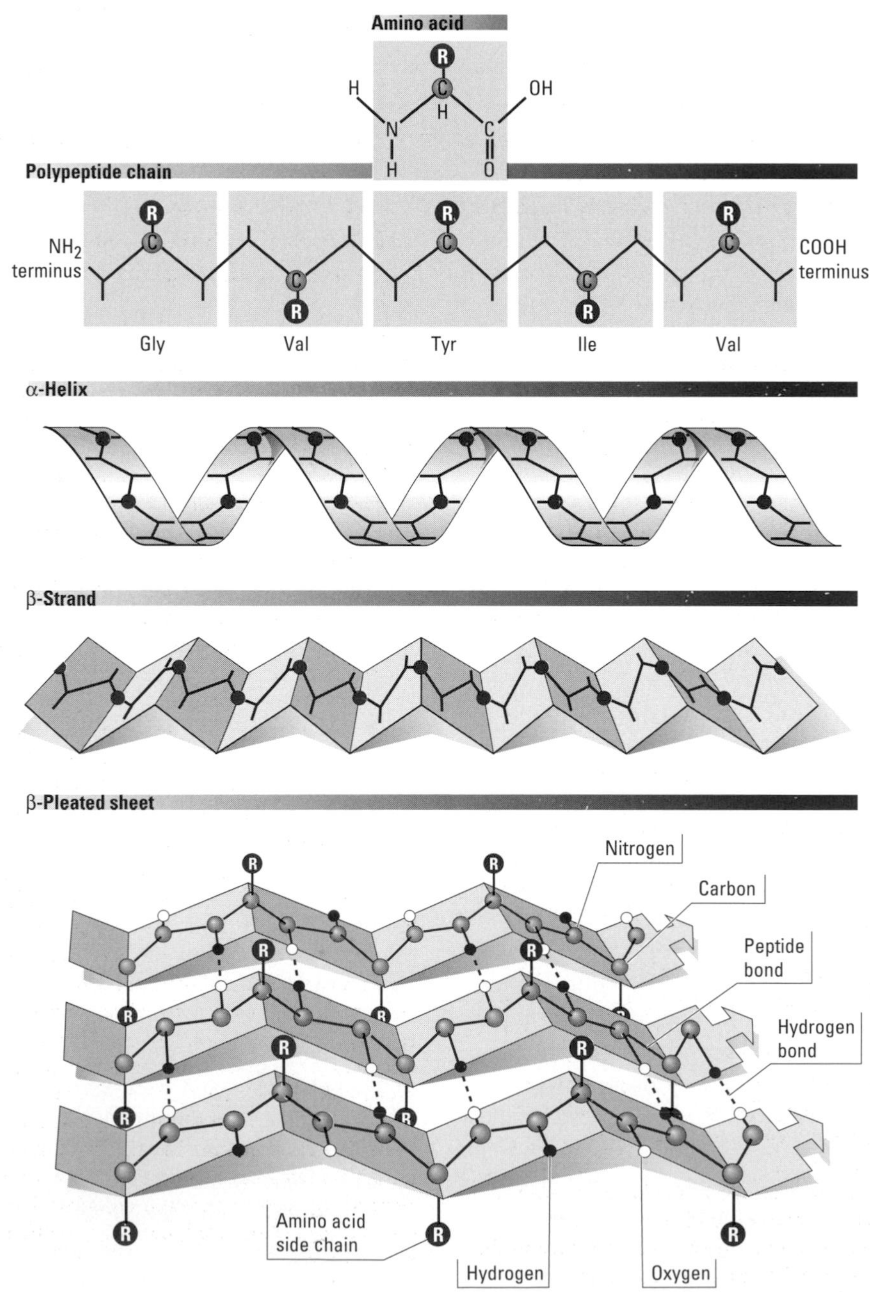

negatively charged phosphate groups of the phospholipids in the bilayer. Positively charged residues (e.g. arginine) are indeed found at these positions in the polypeptide chains. The electrostatic interaction anchors the polypeptide chains in the phospholipid bilayer.

The *cytoplasmic tail* ranges in length from a few amino acid residues to two dozen or so. It usually contains the sequence Ser-Asp/Glu-X-Ser-Leu (where X is any amino acid residue), which can potentially be recognized by the enzyme *protein kinase* C (PKC). The enzyme catalyses the attachment of a phosphate group, $-PO_4^{2-}$, to the serine and thus *phosphorylates* it. Phosphorylation of a protein facilitates its interaction with microtubules and microfilaments of the intracellular cytoskeleton and often serves as an intermediate step in signal transmission from the cell's exterior to its interior. Whether the cytoplasmic tails of MHC proteins are indeed phosphorylated *in vivo* and if so what function, if any, the phosphorylation serves is uncertain.

Glycosylation (the addition of carbohydrate moieties to a protein) of the MHC polypeptides takes place in three stages: first, a core oligosaccharide is synthesized on one of the lipids (dolichol) of the membrane; second, the oligosaccharide is transferred from the lipid to the protein and trimmed; and third, the oligosaccharide is processed (modified) by the removal of some and addition of other sugar units (Fig. 6.42). The first two stages take place on the membranes of the endoplasmic reticulum and the third stage in the Golgi apparatus. The membranes of these organelles contain batteries of *glycosyl transferases*, enzymes that catalyse the addition of sugar units to the growing oligosaccharide chain (*glycan*). The enzymes are controlled by genes that are not part of the *MHC* and that do not specialize in glycosylation of MHC protein but rather work on all proteins synthesized in the RER and destined for export to the cell surface. The synthesis of the *core oligosaccharide* begins with the attachment of a phosphate group (phosphorylation) to dolichol, followed by the attachment of the first sugar residue, *N*-acetylglucosamine, to the phosphate group. The reaction is catalysed by the enzyme *N*-acetylglucosamine transferase, which has specificity for both the phosphorylated lipid and the activated (nucleotide) form of *N*-acetylglucosamine (UDP-

---

Figure 6.35 (*Opposite.*) Principles of protein structure. Proteins are linear chains of amino acid residues. Each *amino acid* has an *amino* (NH_2) and *carboxyl* (COOH) *group*, as well as a hydrogen atom and a *side-chain* (R, for radical) attached to a single carbon atom (C_α). The side-chains differentiate the 20 amino acids that normally occur in proteins. The union of the carboxyl group of one amino acid with the amino group of another amino acid, accompanied by the elimination of a water molecule, results in a *dipeptide*, in which the two amino acid *residues* (they are no longer complete amino acid molecules) are linked by the *peptide bond*

$$\begin{array}{cc} \mathrm{O} & \mathrm{H} \\ \| & | \\ -\mathrm{C}- & \mathrm{N}- \end{array}$$

(see Fig. 6.34a). The attachment of additional amino acids (always via peptide bonds) results in the formation of a tripeptide, tetrapeptide, pentapeptide and ultimately *polypeptide*. The peptides always have a free amino group at one end (the *amino* or *N- terminus*) and a free carboxyl group at the other (the *carboxyl* or *C-terminus*). Because protein synthesis proceeds from the N- to the C-terminus, this is also the order in which the sequence of the amino acid residues of a protein is given. The *backbone* of the polypeptide chain is formed by the repeating trio of atoms $(C\text{-}C\text{-}N)_n$. The sequence of amino acid residues (the *primary structure*) determines the conformation of the protein. Three levels of protein structure are recognized above the primary structure: secondary, tertiary and quaternary. The *secondary structure* comprises regions in which successive residues are spatially arranged in a certain characteristic way in terms of distances between atoms, angles formed by covalent bonds and distribution of non-covalent bonds. There are a few basic types of such regions, of which the two most common ones, the α-helix and the β-strand (the Greek letters have the same function as in the designations 'first' and 'second' type), are depicted here. In the *α-helix* the backbone of the polypeptide chain is arranged like a corkscrew. It is coiled and each loop is situated at the same distance from the preceding one. There are 3.6 amino acid residues for every turn of the screw and each carbonyl (C═O) group of the helix forms a hydrogen bond with the fourth NH group in the direction towards the C-terminus. All side-chains project from the axis of the helix. In a *β-strand*, the polypeptide chain zig-zags and is more extended than in the α-helix. In a protein, often two or more β-strands arrange themselves next to each other in a single plane and form a *β-pleated sheet* so named because it resembles a pleated skirt. Here, alternate side-chains point in opposite directions from the sheet. The arrangement is stabilized by hydrogen bonds (see Fig. 6.33) between the neighbouring strands, which can run either *parallel* or *antiparallel* (as shown here) to each other. (Two strands both oriented in the same N- to C-terminus direction are considered parallel; those oriented in opposite directions are antiparallel.) The strands in each sheet are connected by *loops* that have a more variable structure than either α-helices or β-strands. The loop structure depends on their amino acid sequence and their position in the protein. Generally, loops are on the surface of a protein whereas α-helices and β-strands can be inside. The β-pleated sheets are elements of the *tertiary structure*, which refers to the packing of elements of the secondary structure into compact units or *domains*. An example of a tertiary structure is given in Fig. 6.37. The arrangement of the protein domains consisting of two or more chains is referred to as the *quaternary structure* (see Fig. 6.40). Proteins consisting of two, three or four polypeptide chains are referred to as dimers, trimers and tetramers, respectively. Proteins composed of two identical chains are *homodimers*; those composed of two different chains are *heterodimers*.

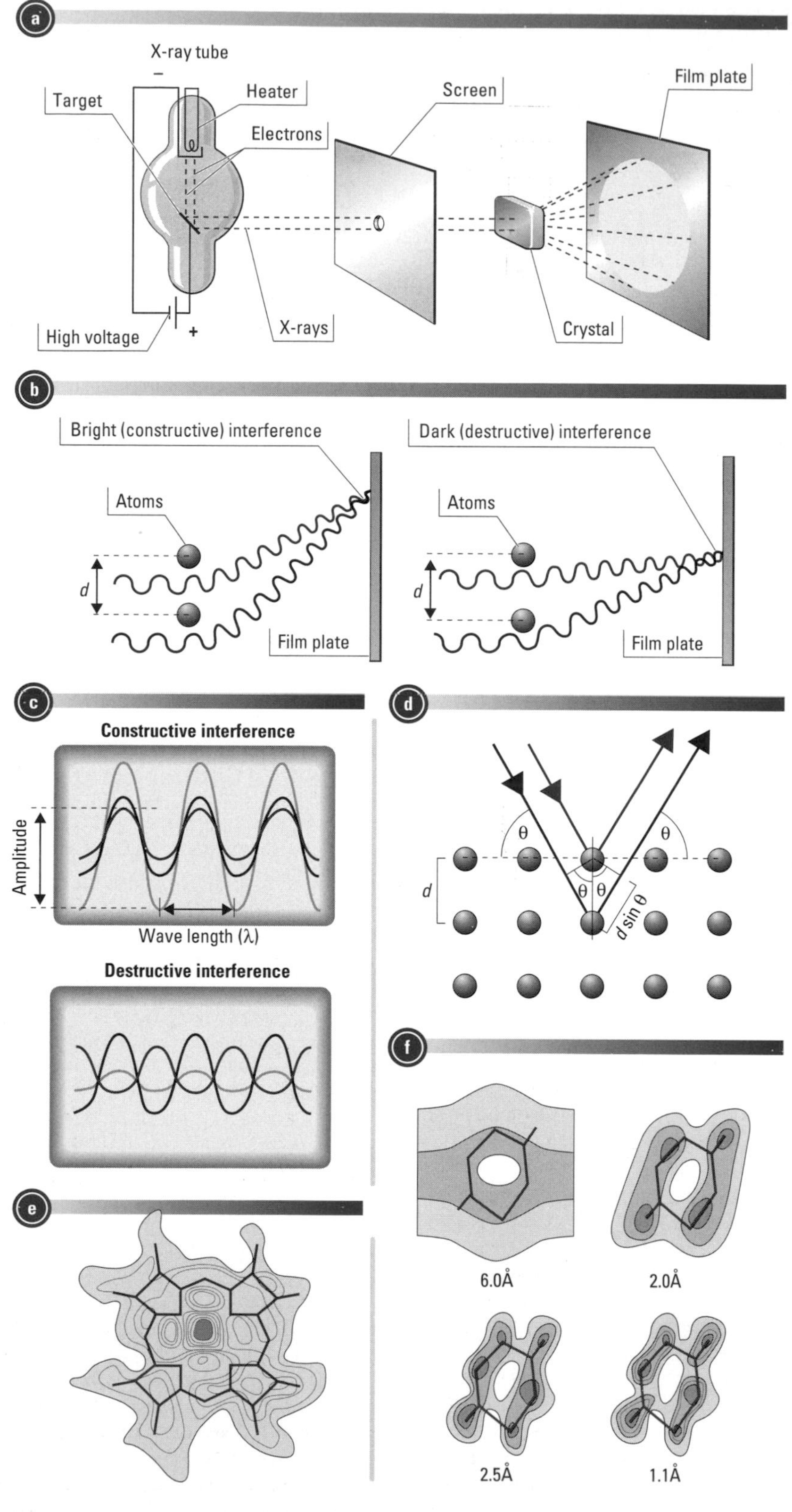
a
X-ray tube
Target
Heater
Electrons
Screen
Film plate
Crystal
X-rays
High voltage
b
Bright (constructive) interference
Dark (destructive) interference
Atoms
d
Film plate
c
Constructive interference
Amplitude
Wave length (λ)
Destructive interference
d
θ
d sin θ
e
f
6.0Å
2.0Å
2.5Å
1.1Å

GlcNAc). Once the GlcNAc residue is linked to the lipid, another enzyme catalyses the addition of a second GlcNAc residue, then another enzyme the addition of a mannose residue, and so on, until the core oligosaccharide is fully assembled. Upon the emergence of the glycosylation site from the RER membrane, the glycan is transferred from the lipid to the protein. It is then trimmed, first of three glucose residues and subsequently of four mannose residues. In the Golgi apparatus additional mannose residues are removed from the trimmed core and other sugars are added to it in their stead. This process converts the oligosaccharide chain from the original *high mannose type* to the *complex type* (Fig. 6.43). The fully glycosylated protein then leaves the Golgi apparatus and integrates into the plasma membrane. Some oligosaccharides of the MHC molecules seem to participate in the interaction between the molecules and certain receptors on natural killer cells (see Chapter 7).

MHC molecules as antigens

As a consequence of *MHC* gene polymorphism, individuals differ in their MHC molecules. To the immune system of an individual A with type A MHC molecules, type B MHC molecules of individual B are as foreign as molecules of a bacterium or a virus. An individual A has therefore the potential to respond immunologically to MHC type B molecules. This potential is, however, realized only in two situations. The first occurs when the immune system of an MHC type A mother encounters cells of her MHC type B fetus, as sometimes happens during delivery. The second situation is that in which cells, tissues or organs of individual A (donor) are artificially grafted onto individual B (recipient). In both situations, the MHC molecules act as antigens that stimulate immune response. These types of antigens that differentiate individuals of the same species are termed *alloantigens* (in contrast to *xenoantigens* that differentiate different

Figure 6.36 (*Opposite.*) The principle of X-ray diffraction analysis. A prerequisite for the analysis is the availability of crystallized protein. A *crystal* is an ordered, three-dimensional lattice formed by repeated points (ions, atoms, molecules). To study the arrangements of the points in a crystal lattice, X-rays produced by the electron bombardment of a metal target in an X-ray tube are passed through a filter and the resulting monochromatic (single wavelength) beam is focused on the crystal (a). The rays, which have a wavelength of approximately the same order as the distances between neighbouring points, penetrate the crystal and travel through it until they encounter one of the points of the lattice. The encounter results in the wave bending around the point (*diffraction*), the degree of which depends on the wavelength of the ray and the size of the point (b). Waves diffracted by the same or different points interact and the result of this interaction depends on the *phase* they are in and the distance they have travelled from the bending point. In waves in the same phase, the peaks and troughs coincide and are added together to give a wave of greater amplitude (*constructive interference*; c); on the film plate behind the screen they produce a brighter spot than either of the waves alone. In waves in a different phase, the peaks of one wave coincide with the troughs of the other and so they partly cancel each other out, giving a wave of lower amplitude (*destructive interference*; c); the resulting spot on the film plate is dimmer than that produced by each wave alone. The result is a characteristic constellation of bright and dim spots on the photographic plate, the *diffraction pattern*. The position of the spots of differing intensities in the diffraction pattern depends on the distance d between the points in the crystal, the wavelength λ (lambda) and the angle θ (theta) between the ray before and after bending (d). The relationship between all three parameters is given by Bragg's equation: $2d \sin \theta = \lambda$. Because of the dependence on θ, by changing the angle at which the X-ray beam hits the lattice (by rotating the crystal) and registering the angle of the incoming rays at which bright spots of constructive interference appear in the diffraction pattern, the distances between the points in the crystal lattice can be calculated. Since there are many point-to-point distances in the crystal, large numbers of spots are found at many different angles, each of which satisfies Bragg's equation. The abstract image can be transformed into a real one by a set of equations and complex calculations carried out by a computer. The calculations provide information about the density of electrons at the individual points in the crystal, which in turn identify the points as individual atoms or ions. The electron density distribution in a single plane is traced by contour lines on a transparent sheet in the same way that altitude contour lines are drawn on geological survey maps (*electron-density maps*; e). By stacking sheets representing different sections on top of each other, one produces a three-dimensional image of the crystal. Theoretically, one should be able to deduce the position of every atom in the molecule and thus the protein's primary structure from the best X-ray diffraction pictures; in practice, however, the analysis is so complex that knowing the amino acid sequence of a protein beforehand makes the determination of tertiary structure a considerably easier task. Since proteins produce very complex X-ray diffraction patterns, the analysis is carried out stepwise. First, only spots with certain intensities are chosen and a rough model of the molecule is constructed. Then additional spots are taken into account and more details are added to the model. Finally, all the spots are considered and the position of each atom in the molecule is determined. The quality of the electron density depends on how well ordered the crystals are. Improvement of crystal quality leads to an increasing *resolution* of the diffraction data (greater amount of detail seen; f). Resolution is measured in angstrom (Å) units. In (e), the red lines indicate the haem structure of a myoglobin molecule, the red dot the central iron atom. In (f), the red outlines indicate diketopiperazine structure at different resolution levels. (e, After Kendrew, J.C. *et al.* (1960) *Nature*, **185**, 434; f, after Hodgkin, D.C. (1960) *Nature*, **188**, 445.)

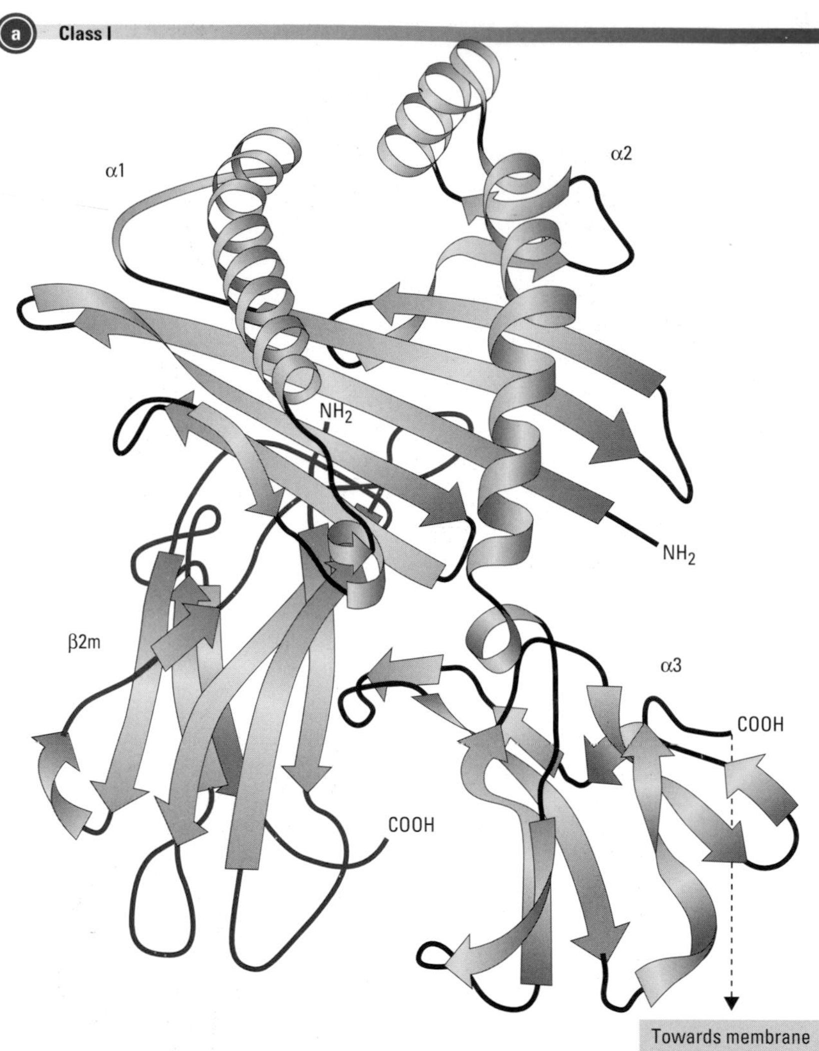

Figure 6.37 Three-dimensional structure of class I (a) and class II (b) MHC heterodimers (ribbon models): side view. Only the extracellular parts of the two molecules (for which X-ray crystallography data are available) are shown. The site of papain cleavage in the class I molecule is indicated. β-strands are indicated by wide arrows, loops by connecting narrow lines. (a, Based on Bjorkman, P.J. *et al.* (1987) *Nature*, **329**, 506; b, based on data of Brown, J.H. *et al.* (1993) *Nature*, **364**, 33.)

species). MHC alloantigens of a graft can be recognized either by T lymphocytes alone or by both T and B lymphocytes. The recognition leads to cellular and humoral immune responses. Both responses can be measured by a variety of techniques, referred to collectively as *histogenetic* (those based on T-lymphocyte activation) and *serological* (those based on the production of antibodies in the serum and other body fluids). The two most commonly used histogenetic methods of MHC detection are mixed lymphocyte reaction (MLR) and cell-mediated lymphocytotoxicity (CML; both are described in Chapter 24).

The *HLA* class II loci were originally defined by MLR; only later were serological methods used. The first histogenetically defined *HLA* class II locus was originally referred to as *HLA-D* because the first three letters of the alphabet had already been used to denote class I loci. The first serologically defined class II locus was subsequently termed *HLA-DR* for 'D-related', because its precise relationship to the histogenetically defined locus was unclear. Later, when it was found that multiple families of class II loci existed, these were designated *DP*, *DQ* and *DR*. Most of the antigens controlled by the *DP* loci were recognized by a form of MLR called the PLT test (see Chapter 24); antigens controlled by other loci were identified by the MLR and by serological methods.

To detect an antigen serologically, an antibody must be found that recognizes it specifically. Standard immunization procedures produce *polyclonal antibodies*, a mixture of antibodies specific for different parts of the same molecule or for different molecules. Techniques are also available for producing *monoclonal antibodies* specific for one part of an antigenic molecule only (see Chapter 8).

The sources of human polyclonal antibodies are the sera of multiply transfused patients, multiparous women and

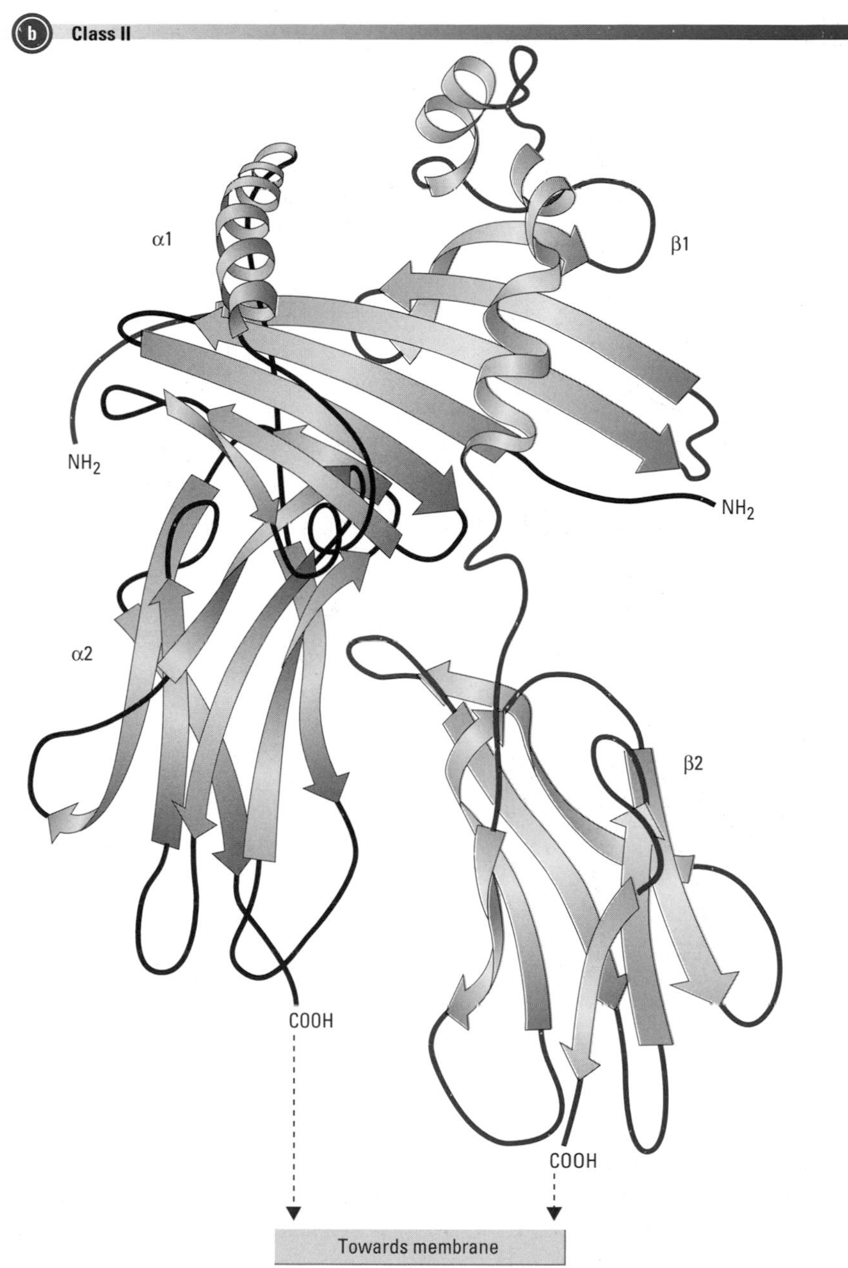

Figure 6.37 *Continued.*

volunteers who have been immunized by skin grafting. In animals, polyclonal antibodies are obtained by repeated inoculation of lymphoid cells in the peritoneal cavity of the recipient followed by bleeding at the proper time after the injection. The preferred mode of immunization is between *Mhc*-disparate individuals of the same species resulting in the production of allogeneic antibodies or *alloantibodies*. Xenogeneic antibodies or *xenoantibodies* produced by immunizations between different species are less desirable. Most monoclonal antibodies used in the study of mouse MHC antigens are derived from allogeneic immunizations. Virtually all HLA-specific monoclonal antibodies are derived from xenogeneic immunizations, usually mouse anti-human. A reliable method for the large-scale production of human HLA-specific monoclonal antibodies has not been developed as yet (see Chapter 8).

Antibodies bind via their combining sites to small areas on the surface of MHC molecules, the *epitopes*. Although many antigens carry more than one epitope, MHC molecules are particularly rich in them. A single molecule may bind dozens of different antibodies, not all at the same time of course. The epitopes are scattered over the surface of the

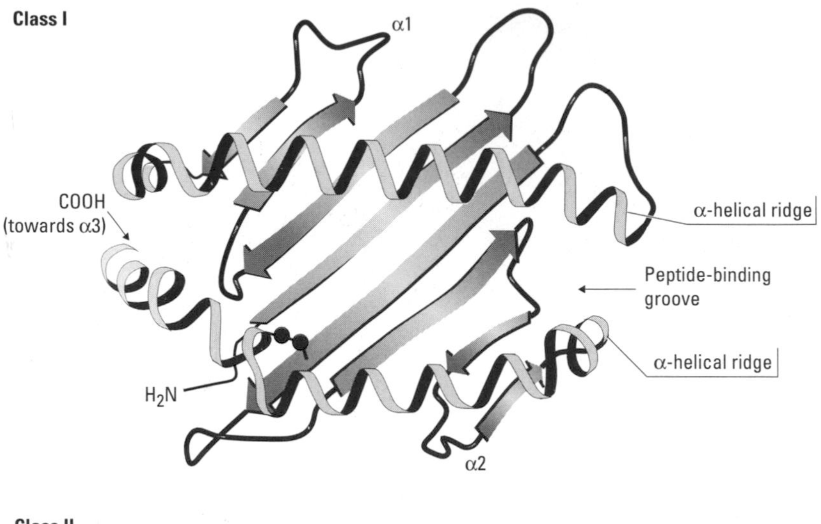

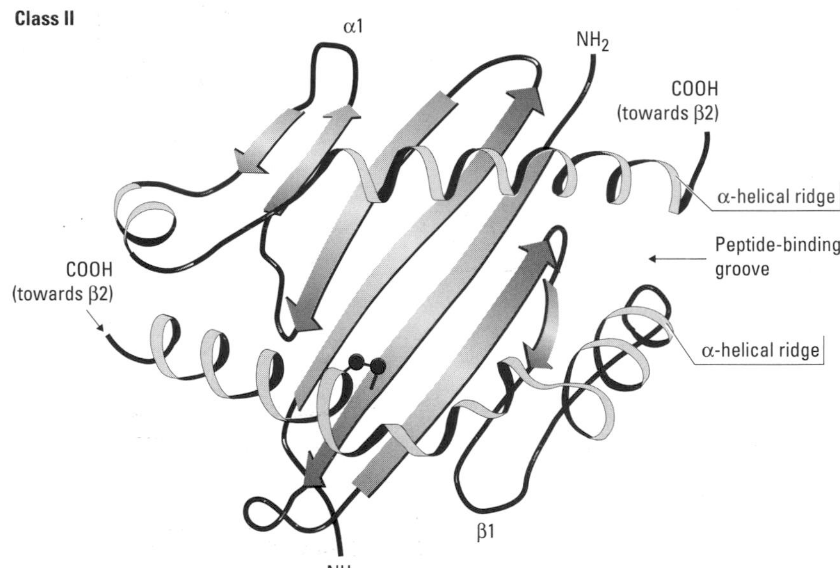

Figure 6.38 Three-dimensional structure of the class I and class II peptide-binding modules: view from the top. These ribbon-type models basically trace the backbone and not the side-chains of the polypeptide. The end-blockages of the groove in the class I module are therefore not visible. Filled circles represent disulphide-bonded cysteine residues; β-strands are indicated by wide arrows, loops by connecting narrow lines. (Class I is based on Bjorkman, P.J. *et al.* (1987) *Nature*, **329**, 506; class II is based on data of Brown, J.H. *et al.* (1993) *Nature*, **364**, 33.)

MHC molecule, but some of them at least are clustered into discrete *antigenic sites*. Several antigenic sites have been identified on some of the well-known MHC molecules; most of them reside on the surface of the class I α1 and α2 domains and class II β1 and α1 domains. Some epitopes may also span two adjacent domains.

Some epitopes are shared between different MHC molecules while others are more or less restricted to a particular molecule. The former are called *public* and the latter *private* epitopes. MHC molecules of different individuals can therefore be distinguished serologically in two ways: by the particular combination of public epitopes and by their unique private epitopes. For example, an MHC molecule A may be characterized by the combination of epitopes 2, 5, 7 and 18; molecule B by the combination 1, 5, 6, 11 and 18; molecule C by the combination 1, 6, 7, 12, 19 and so on, where each of these epitopes is present in at least two molecules, but the combination of epitopes is unique. Molecules A, B and C, however, may also be characterized by epitopes 3, 9 and 15, respectively, which occur only in the particular molecule and in no other.

HLA serologists originally did not bother defining public epitopes and concentrated instead on finding the most restricted epitopes approaching the status of the private epitopes. H2 serologists, on the other hand, tried to be as comprehensive as they could in defining the antigenic profile of individual H2 molecules, registering both private and public epitopes. However, the difference between the serological definition of HLA and H2 molecules lies merely in the degree of thoroughness rather than in principle. Most of the HLA antigens now officially recognized are not truly private; each is shared by more than one distinct molecule, although the number of these molecules may be low and they may be related. In addition, monoclonal antibodies

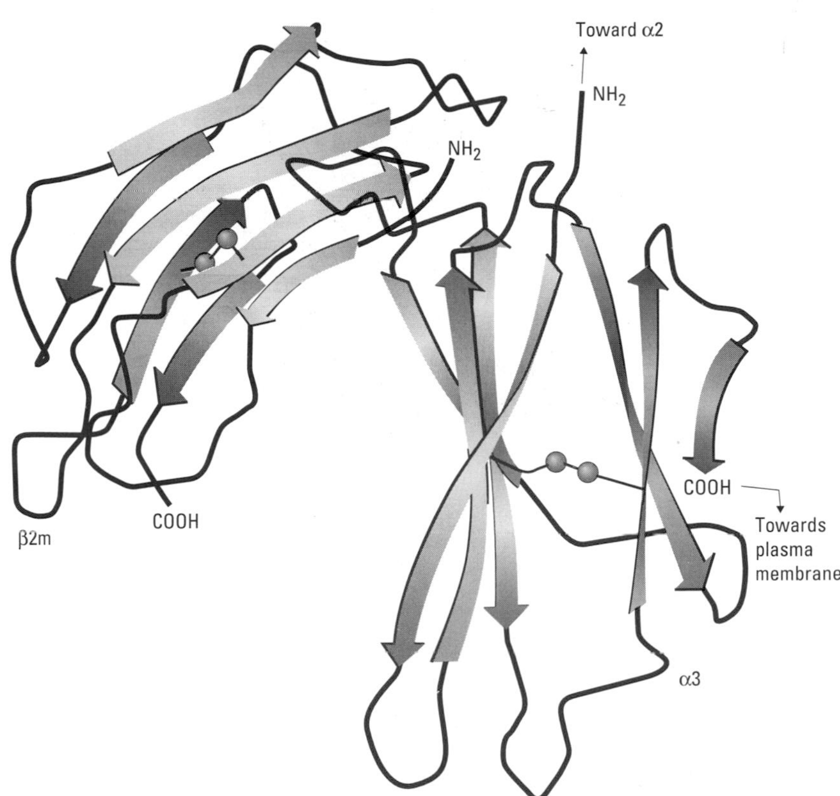

Figure 6.39 Three-dimensional structure of the class I immunoglobulin-like module (α3 and β_2m domains; ribbon model). Each domain contains two β-pleated sheets: the β-strands (arrows) of the two sheets are differentiated by shading; the connecting lines represent the loops; and the filled circles disulphide-bonded cysteine residues. (Based on Bjorkman, P.J. *et al.* (1987) *Nature*, **329**, 506.)

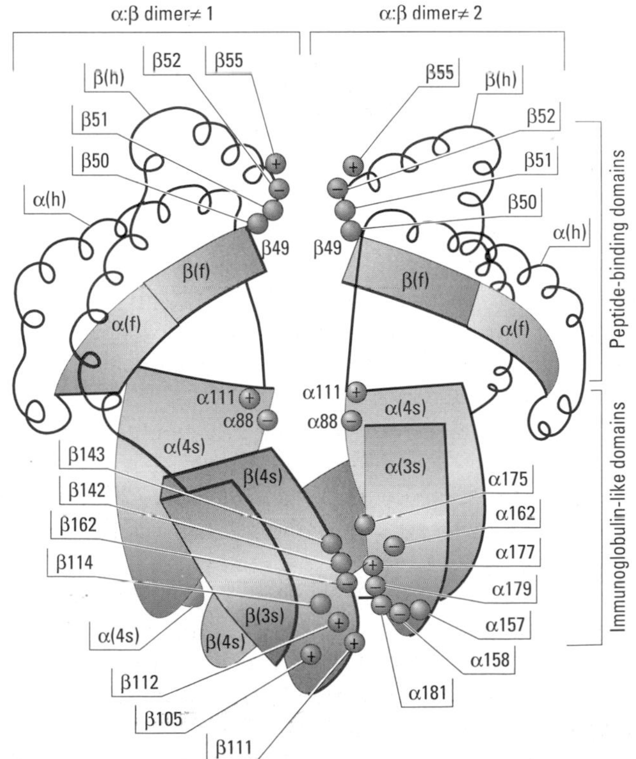

Figure 6.40 Diagrammatic representation of the three-dimensional structure of a class II tetramer ('dimer of a dimer'). h, α-helix; f, floor of the peptide-binding groove; 3s, 4s, three- or four-stranded β-sheet of the immunoglobulin-like domain; α, β, α and β chains, respectively. Amino acid residues making contacts between the dimers in the HLA-DRB1 molecule are indicated by circles and numbers (only one interface is shown); + and – signals indicate positively or negatively charged residues. (Modified from Brown, J.H. *et al.* (1993) *Nature*, **364**, 33.)

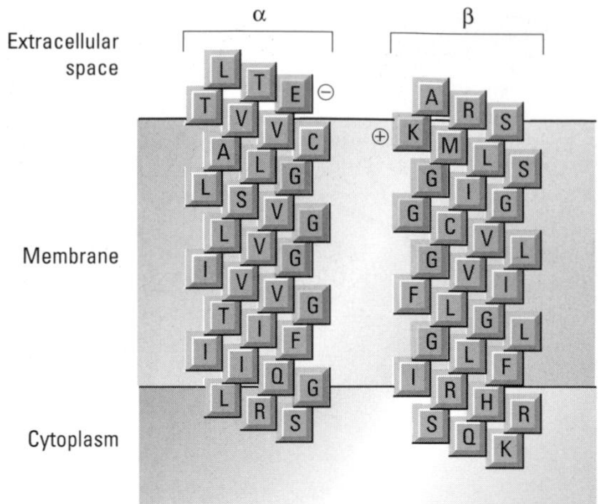

Figure 6.41 Two-dimensional representation of the transmembrane regions of mouse class II α and β chains. Letters indicate amino acid residues in the international single-letter code (see Appendix 1). They are arranged in such a way as to suggest turns of an α-helix. + and – indicate positively and negatively charged residues, respectively. The conserved glycine residues at the presumed interface of the two chains are highlighted. (From Cosson, P. & Bonifacino, J.S. (1992) *Science*, **258**, 659.)

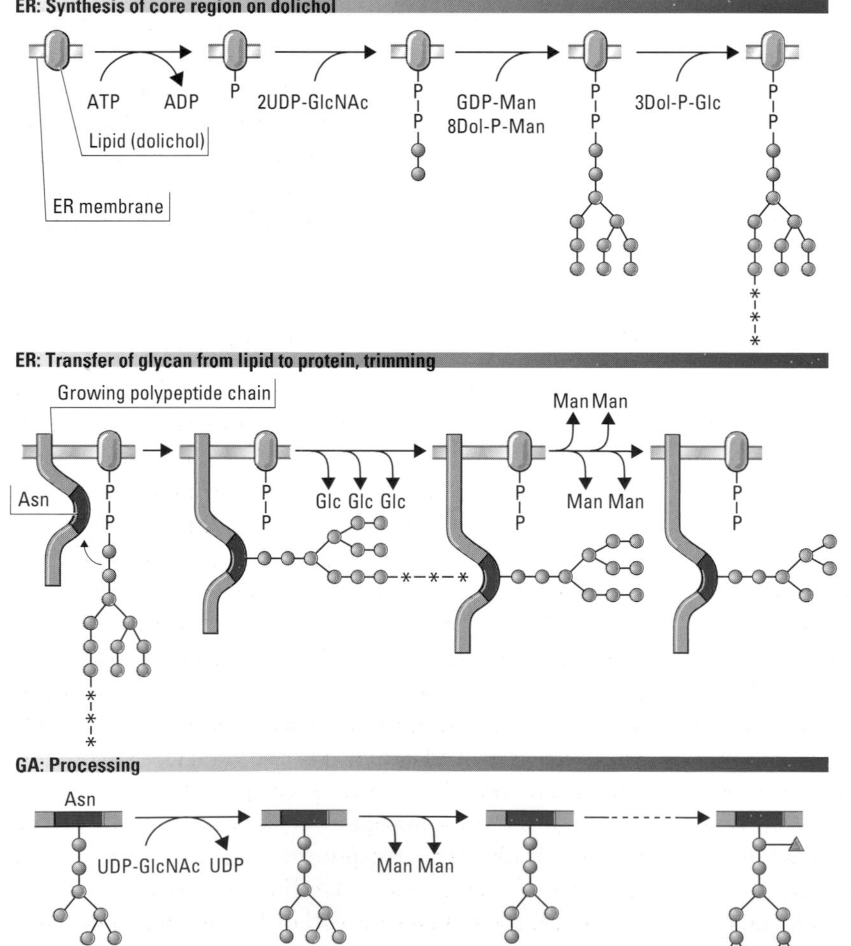

Figure 6.42 Biosynthesis and processing of oligosaccharides of the type attached to MHC polypeptide chains. ADP, adenosine diphosphate; ATP, adenosine triphosphate; ER, endoplasmic reticulum; GA, Golgi apparatus; GDP, guanosine diphosphate; P, phosphate; UDP, uridine diphosphate; ●, GlcNAc (*N*-acetylglucosamine); ●, Man (mannose); *, Glu (glucose); ●, Gal (galactose); ▲, Fuc (fucose); ■, NANA (sialic acid).

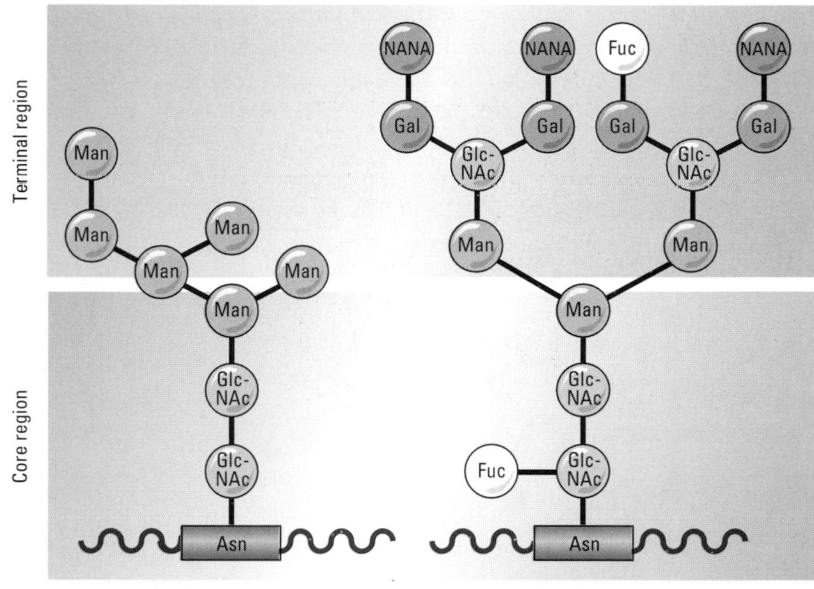

Figure 6.43 Two types of oligosaccharides linked to MHC polypeptides. Asn, asparagine; Fuc, fucose; Gal, galactose; GlcNAc, *N*-acetylglucosamine; Man, mannose; NANA, sialic acid.

recognizing widely distributed public epitopes are now also available. In the H2 system, on the other hand, several of the public epitopes have a rather limited distribution and actually resemble the 'private' epitopes recognized by HLA researchers. Finally, the division of epitopes into public and private is merely an artificial and operational one. 'Artificial' because there is no qualitative difference between the two (the private epitopes are merely one extreme of an apparently continuous range), and 'operational' because often what today is classified as a private epitope can tomorrow, when new individuals are included in the analysis, be split into two epitopes, at least one of which is shared by two distinct molecules and hence qualifies as public. MHC serology has thus been in a constant state of flux, with epitopes being continuously split and reclassified and with new epitopes emerging.

The serological definition of HLA molecules is the result of an intense international collaboration between the *HLA-typing laboratories* in many countries of the world. The collaboration consists of exchanging reagents, standardizing the techniques of tissue typing, standardizing nomenclature and sharing knowledge. The HLA typists meet every 3 or 4 years at *Histocompatibility Testing Workshops* to compare results obtained in the interim and to designate new epitopes ('antigens'), genes and gene families. Some antigens are first given tentative 'workshop' (abbreviated 'w') designations and only later, when their existence is firmly established, is the 'w' prefix dropped. Even established antigens may disappear from official lists as the years go by, because they are split into two or more antigens as new reagents become available. Originally, the major impetus for HLA typing was the prospect of matching donors and recipients for organ transplantation. To this was added later the quest for genes that influence susceptibility to certain diseases and that have been shown to be linked to the *HLA* complex. The HLA antigens have, however, also become useful markers for studying the origin and migration patterns of human populations.

The peptide–MHC assemblage

The function of MHC molecules is to bind peptides that could potentially be recognized by antigen-specific receptors on T lymphocytes. Whether MHC molecules are also involved in other functions is not known but it would not be surprising if they were because many proteins carry out more than one function. Various auxiliary functions have been suggested for the *MHC* but unambiguous evidence for their authenticity has thus far not been provided.

Because of their peptide-binding function, MHC molecules can be regarded as receptors, but they are receptors of a special kind. At least three features distinguish MHC receptors from other receptors: dependence of MHC expression on the presence of peptides; stability of peptide–MHC assemblages; and relative promiscuity in binding. While other receptors are unoccupied by ligands for most of their lifespan, MHC molecules associate with peptides early in their career (class I molecules immediately after their synthesis in the RER and class II molecules after the removal of the surrogate peptide provided by the invariant chain in the endosomal compartment) and remain complexed for their entire tenure on the cell surface. In fact, if for some reason they fail to acquire a suitable peptide, their career is shortened and most of them even fail to reach the cell surface.

Like other receptor–ligand complexes, the peptide–MHC assemblages are in a dynamic state in which the two components continually associate, dissociate and then reassociate again. However, while other receptor–ligand complexes are in a state of equilibrium in which the association–dissociation rates are equal, in the peptide–MHC assemblages the dissociation rate is slower than the association rate. Consequently, the peptide–MHC assemblages are extremely stable under physiological conditions. This feature is essential for the function of MHC molecules, which is effected on the cell surface in an environment virtually devoid of suitable free peptides. Such an environment would normally favour rapid dissociation of the complexes, not giving the MHC molecules enough time to carry out their function. The stability of the assemblages thus assures that the MHC molecules retain the peptides long enough for T lymphocytes to recognize them.

Finally, while most receptors are highly selective (monogamic) as to which ligands they bind, each MHC molecule is capable of binding hundreds, perhaps thousands, of different peptides, which often have little in common in terms of their sequence, and each peptide can be bound by several different MHC molecules. Yet MHC receptors are not non-specific: each molecule binds a certain set of peptides and does not bind many other peptides. The sets bound by different MHC molecules may overlap, but they are nevertheless distinct. Class I- and class II-binding peptides are of different origin, the former being generated in the cytosol and the latter in the vesicular compartment. However, the main factor responsible for the differences in peptide binding by different MHC molecules is the polymorphism of their encoding loci. Each allele specifies a somewhat different binding region of the molecule and thus a distinct, albeit wide, spectrum of peptides the molecule will be able to bind.

Information about peptides bound to MHC molecules has been obtained by four principal methods. In one, proteins are digested by enzymes or by other means and the resulting peptides are incubated at high concentration with cells expressing MHC molecules on their surfaces. As the bound peptides slowly dissociate from the MHC molecules, they are replaced by those surrounding the cell, but only if the free peptides fit into the binding groove. Individual peptides can thus be tested one by one and the MHC molecules to which they bind can be established for each one. In the second method, MHC molecules are isolated biochemically from the cells, purified and denatured so as to release the bound peptides. The latter are then purified, sequenced and their identity determined. In the third method, the identity of the bound peptide is determined by X-ray diffraction analysis of the crystallized MHC protein. The fourth method is based on the use of a phage display library, which is described in Chapter 8 (see Fig. 8.50). In this technique, random oligonucleotide sequences are translated into peptides which are displayed on the surfaces of phage proteins and 'empty' MHC molecules produced in insect cells are tested for their ability to bind some of the peptides.

To bind, a peptide must fit into the binding groove of the MHC molecule. It must stretch out, assume an extended β-strand configuration and then wedge itself into the groove. For the sake of clarity, it is convenient to imagine atoms participating in the formation of the groove as small balls arranged in space in a certain way characteristic of the particular compound, as in the *space-filling models* of molecules. (In reality, of course, an atom is not a solid sphere but largely an empty space pervaded by an electromagnetic field.) A space-filling model of the peptide-binding module (Fig. 6.44) reveals that the surface with which the peptides interact is not at all smooth and flat, which might have been the impression gained by the depiction in Fig. 6.38, but rather highly irregular, with many bumps and ridges. To understand the difference between the depictions in Figs 6.38 and 6.44, we must remind ourselves of the two principal elements of (poly)peptide structure: the main chain and the side-chains. The *main chain* (backbone) is a highly regular structure of repeating units (*residues*), each unit consisting of a central C_α atom attached to an amino (N—H) and a carbonyl group (C=O):

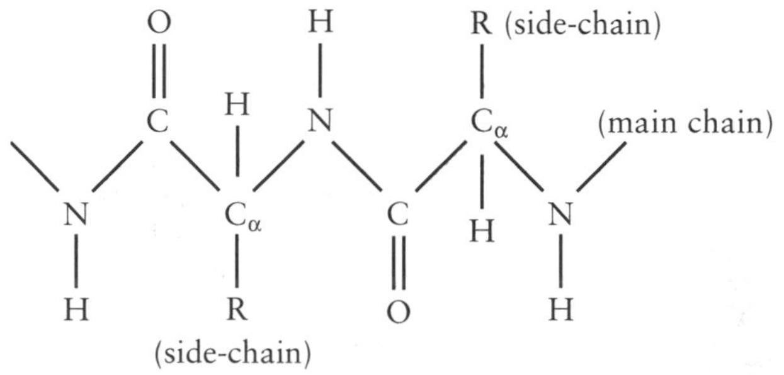

```
            O         H          R (side-chain)
            ‖         |          |
            C    H    N          Cα        (main chain)
  \       /   \  |  /   \      / | \      /
     N          Cα        C      H    N
     |          |         ‖           |
     H          R         O           H
            (side-chain)
```

The peptide can then assume the α-helical, β-strand or some other configuration. The depiction in Fig. 6.38 is that of a main-chain structure. The *side-chains* (R) attached to the carbon atoms of the main chain are highly diverse; they identify individual amino acid residues. Since they project from the main chains of the groove's floor and the α-helical ridges into the groove, they are responsible for the irregularity of the surface seen in Fig. 6.44. They are also responsible

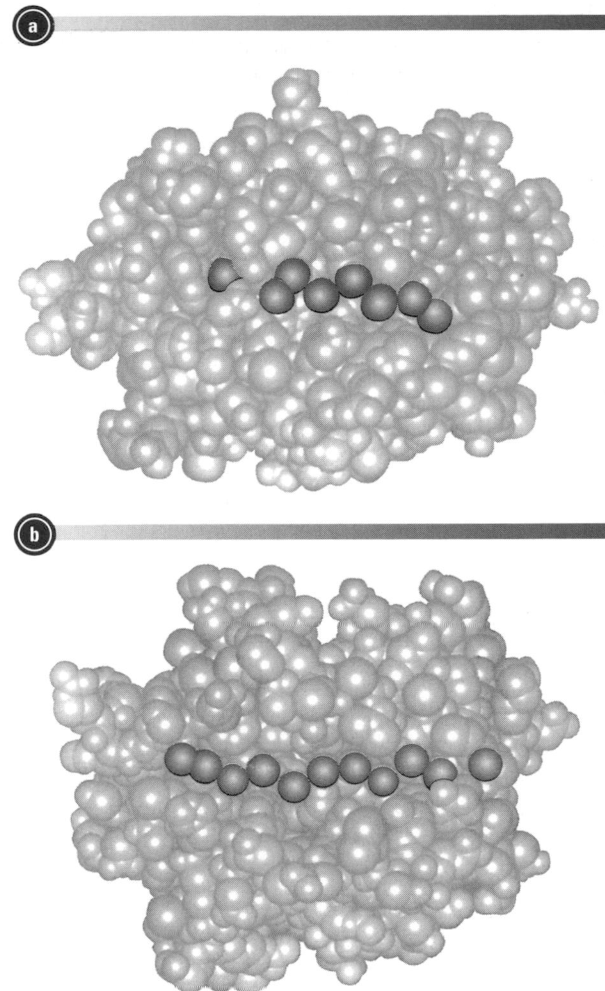

Figure 6.44 Space-filling models of the MHC peptide-binding groove occupied by a peptide (view from the top). (a) Complex of class I molecule and peptide. (b) Complex of class II molecule and peptide. Red spheres, peptide atoms; grey spheres, atoms of the MHC molecule. (From Germain, R. (1994) *Cell*, 76, 287.)

for the differences between the groove surfaces of MHC molecules controlled by different alleles of a given locus. The alleles have different nucleotide sequences which translate into differences in amino acid sequences, and variation in amino acid residues means that different side-chains will be projecting into the peptide-binding groove. The differences in the groove's surface topography in turn determine which peptides will fit into the furrow.

A characteristic feature of the groove's topography is a series of *pockets* or circumscribed areas in which the groove's main cavity extends towards the interior of the molecule (caves in the walls of the canyon, to return to our earlier metaphor). It is primarily the peptide's interaction with these pockets that determines whether the peptide will be stably bound by the MHC molecule. The interaction can, in principle, take place between side-chains forming the pocket of the MHC molecule and the main chain of the peptide that fits into this pocket, or the side-chains of the MHC molecule and the side-chain of the peptide. The former is relatively independent of the peptide's sequence, whereas the latter is strictly sequence dependent. The peptide's side-chains must, of course, in both cases fit into the pockets and so the peptide must possess specific *anchor residues* at positions juxtaposed to the pockets, but where side-chain to main-chain interactions are involved the requirements for a specific residue are relaxed. As long as the side-chains forming the pocket are able to interact with polar atoms of the peptide's main chain it does not matter much which side-chain the peptide has at the particular position. The relative sequence independence of the side-chain to main-chain interactions is responsible for the promiscuity of peptide binding; the sequence dependence of the side-chain to side-chain interactions sets limits on this promiscuity and accounts for the differences in peptide-binding capabilities of molecules controlled by different alleles at *MHC* loci. A manifestation of this restriction is that peptides must possess a certain *motif* (must have certain amino acid residues at certain positions; Tables 6.2 and 6.3) to be able to bind to a particular MHC molecule characterized by specific residues in the PBR. In human class I molecules, the PBR positions are 5, 7, 9, 22, 24, 26, 59, 63, 66, 67, 70, 73, 74, 75, 77, 80, 81 and 84 in the α1 domain and 95, 97, 99, 114, 116, 143, 146, 147, 152, 155, 156, 159, 163, 167 and 171 in the α2 domain; in class II (DRB1) molecules, the sites are 7, 9, 11, 22, 24, 26, 31, 32, 43, 51, 53, 54, 55, 58, 62, 65, 68, 69, 72 and 76 in the α1 domain and residues 9, 11, 13, 28, 30, 32, 37, 38, 47, 56, 60, 61, 65, 70, 71, 78, 81, 82, 85, 86, 88 and 89 in the β1 domain.

Since the groove of class I molecules is closed at both ends, the length of the peptide it can accommodate and bind efficiently is limited to nine amino acid residues; slightly longer or shorter peptides do bind, but less efficiently. This length variation is made possible by the nature of the binding: in the class I groove, peptides are fastened primarily by their ends (residues 1, 2, 8 and 9 of a nonamer) to the ends of the groove and remain relatively free in their middle part. Most bound peptides, in fact, form a bulge approximately one-third of the way from the terminus by lifting their main chain up from the groove's floor (Fig. 6.45). Slightly longer and shorter peptides can therefore be accommodated by varying the extent of the bulging: shorter peptides assume a more extended conformation, whereas longer peptides just buckle up higher. Because of its exposed position, the bulge is believed to be recognized preferentially by the TCR.

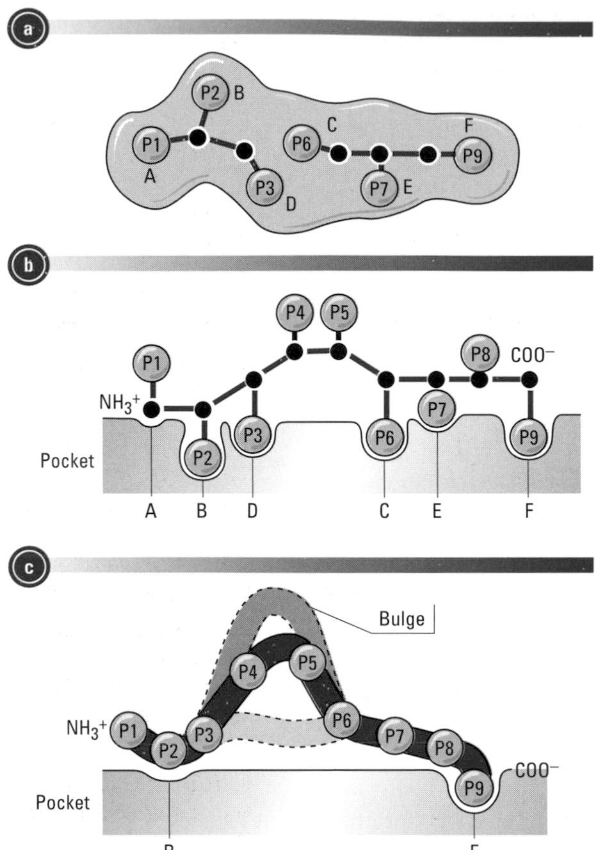

Figure 6.45 Peptide interaction with class I molecules. View of the groove from the top (a) and from the side (b). A–F, binding pockets in the class I molecule; P1–P9, side-chains of amino acid residues in the peptide (main chain carbon atoms are indicated by closed circles). The P1, P4 and P5 side-chains of the peptide point towards the solvent ('up') and are therefore likely to be recognized by the T-cell receptor. The side-chains of P2, P3, P6 and P9 face the groove and are accommodated in the corresponding pockets; they are therefore not available for recognition by the T-cell receptor. The amino (NH_3^+) and carboxyl (COO^-) groups of the peptide interact with the residues lining pockets A and F, respectively. Peptides of different length can be accommodated in the groove by assuming either extended or bulged-out conformation (c). In (a), the bulged-out residues (P4 and P5) are not shown, so the peptide appears interrupted. (a and b, Based on Matsumara, M. *et al.* (1992) *Science*, 257, 927; c, based on Parham, P. (1992) *Nature*, **460**, 300.)

The fastening of the peptides to the ends of the class I groove is mediated by bonds between highly conserved amino acid residues and the charged and polar main-chain atoms of the peptide. In the HLA molecules, Tyr 7 of the β-sheet, Tyr 59 of the α-helix in the α1 domain, as well as Tyr 159 and Tyr 171 of the α-helix in the α2 domain, form a network of hydrogen bonds at the peptide's N-terminus (residues 1 and 2). Similarly, Tyr 84 of the α-helix in the α1 domain, as well as Thr 143, Lys 146 and Trp 147 of the α-helix in the α2 domain form another network of hydrogen bonds at the peptide's C-terminus (residues 8 and 9). These two networks link together the α-helices and the β-sheet at both ends of the groove and thus not only hold the peptide in the groove but also stabilize the three-dimensional structure of the MHC molecule. Without these bonds (i.e. without the peptide in the groove), the class I molecule is highly unstable. Because the stereochemical arrangement of the main-chain atoms relative to the side-chains is different at the two ends of the peptide, there is a *polarity* to the peptide binding: the peptide fits into the groove only with its N-terminus oriented towards the Tyr 7, Tyr 59, Tyr 159 and Tyr 171 cluster of MHC residues and its C-terminus oriented towards the Tyr 84, Thr 143, Lys 146 and Trp 147 cluster.

Six pockets have been identified in the grooves of human class I molecules (pockets A–F). Of these, those that interact with the second (P2) and last (P9) residues of the peptide are most important for anchoring of the peptide. Hence P2 and P9, the latter in particular, are the primary anchors. The remaining pockets provide the surface for the side-chain to side-chain interactions with the secondary anchors. The *A pocket* interacts with the NH_3^+ group at the N-terminus of the peptide (see Fig. 6.45). Because this group is part of the main chain, these interactions are the same for all peptides. The side-chain of the P1 residue points towards the solvent ('up') and thus has no special pocket to fit into. The *F pocket* interacts in part with the $-COO^-$ group of the C-terminus and in part with the side-chain of the ultimate residue of the peptide. The former is a side-chain to main-chain interaction and hence constant; the latter a side-chain to side-chain interaction and hence variable, sequence dependent. The side-chain of the peptide's last residue always points into the pocket ('down'); the side-chain of the penultimate residue always points towards the solvent ('up') and is therefore often exposed. The *B pocket* is always present but is sometimes deep and sometimes shallow. In the former case, it is considered to be one of the main pockets; in the latter case the main pocket function is taken over by the pocket that accommodates residue 6 of the peptide. The side-chains of the peptide's residues 2 and 3, as well as 6 or 7, usually point into the MHC molecule ('down') and are therefore considered to be strong anchors (see Fig. 6.45). Side-chains of the peptide's residues 4 and 5, on the other hand, have a strong tendency to point towards the solvent ('up') and therefore presumably contact the TCR molecule. Hence the main anchors of peptides bound to class I molecules are residues 2 or 6 and 8 (in octamers) or 9 (in nonamers). The side-chains of these residues are buried in the pockets and make contacts over a large surface area.

Table 6.2 Peptides found associated with human class I MHC molecules.

Molecule	Peptide	Source
HLA-A1	Y T S **D** Y F I S **Y**	Ets-1
	Y L **D** D P D L K **Y**	Cytosine methyl transferase
	I A **D** M G H L K **Y**	Nuclear factor
	S *T* **D** H I P I L **Y**	Fructose-6-amino transferase
	D *S* **D** G S F F L **Y**	Human IgG_4 279–287
	A *T* **D** F K F A M **Y**	Cyclin type D
	Y *T* A V V P L V **Y**	Human J-chain 102–110
	Y *T* **D** Y G G L I F N S **Y**	Cytochrome *c* oxidase
HLA-A2.1	L **L** D V P T A A **V**	IP-30 signal sequence
	S **L** L P A I V E **L**	Protein phosphate 2A
	Y **L** L P A I V E **I**	ATP-dependent RNA helicase
	M **V** D G T L L L **L**	HLA-E signal sequence
	Y **M** N G T M S Q **V**	Tyrosinase
	M **L** L S V P L L **L** G	Calreticulin signal sequence
	L **L** L D V P T A A **V**	IP-30 signal sequence
	L **L** L D V P T A A V Q **A**	IP-30 signal sequence
	V **L** F R G G P R G **L** **L** **A** **V** **A**	SSRα signal sequence
HLA-A11	S **V** L N L V I V **K**	Ribosomal protein S6
	K **V** V N P L F E **K**	Ribosomal protein L7A
	R **T** Q N V L G E **K**	Ribosomal protein S3
	A **S** F D K A K L **K**	Thymosin B-10
	A **T** A G D G X X E L R **K**	Prohibitin
HLA-A24	K **Y** P N E F F L **L**	Protein phosphatase 1
	Y **Y** E E Q H P E **L**	NK/T-cell activation protein
	A **Y** V H M V T H **F**	Unknown
	V **Y** X K H P V S **X**	Unknown
HLA-A68.1	D **V** F R D P A L **K**	Ribosomal 60S homologue
	K **T** G G P I Y K **R**	Influenza NP 91–99
	T **V** F D A K R L I G **R**	HSP70 protein B/HSP70
HLA-B7	A **P** **R** T V A L T **A**	HLA-DP signal sequence
	A **P** **R** T L V L L **L**	HLA-A2.1 signal sequence
	A **P** **R** P P P K P **M**	Ribosomal S26 protein
	S **P** **R** Y I F T M **L**	Topoisomerase II
	R **P** K S N I V L **L**	CD20
	L *V* *M* *A* *P* *R* T V **L**	HLA-B7 signal sequence
	A **P** **R** T V A L T A **L**	HLA-DP signal sequence
	A A S K E R S G V S **L**	Histone H1
HLA-B27	R **R** I K E I V K **K**	HSP89α
	G **R** I D K P I L **K**	Ribosomal protein
	R **R** S K E I T V **R**	ATP-dependent RNA helicase
	R **R** V K E V V K **k**	HSP89β
	R **R** Y Q K S T E **L**	Histone H3.3

The sequence of the peptides is given in the international single-letter code (see Appendix 1). Residues in bold are at the main anchor positions; residues in italics are at auxiliary positions. Lower-case residues are probable assignments. X, Leu or Ile.
ATP, adenosine triphosphate; CD, cluster of differentiation; HLA, human leucocyte antigen; HSP, heat-shock protein; Ets-1, *E*-*t*wenty-*s*ix-1 (oncogene discovered in the E26 retrovirus); IP, interferon-regulated protein; MHC, major histocompatibility complex; NK, natural killer; NP, nucleoprotein; SSR, signal sequence receptor.

Table 6.3 Peptides found associated with human class II (DRB) MHC molecules.

Molecule	Peptide	Source
DRB1*0101	I P A D **L** R I **I** S **A** N G C K V D N S	(N$^+$/K$^+$) ATPase
	S D **W** R F **L** R **G** Y H Q Y A	HLA-A2
	R V E **Y** H F **L** S P Y V S P K E S P	Transferrin receptor
	Y K H T **L** N Q **I** D S V K V W P R R P	Bovine fetuin
	A I L E **F** R A **M** A Q F S R K T D	Self peptide SP3
DRB1*0401	V D D T Q **F** V R F D **S** D A A S Q R M E P R A	HLA-A2
	V D D T Q **F** V R F D **S** D A A S P R G E P R A	HLA-Cw9
	L R S **W** T A **A** D **T** A A Q I T Q R K W E A	HLA-Cw9
	D L S S **W** T A **A** D **T** A A Q I T Q R K W E A	HLA-Bw62
	G S L **F** V Y N I **T** T N K Y K A F L D K Q	VLA-4
	A E A L E R M **F** L S F P **T** T K T	Bovine haemoglobin
DRB1*1101	I D F **Y** T S **I** T **R** A R F E E	Human HSP (HSP70/HSC70)
	C P A G **Y** T C N V **K** A R S C E K	Human granulin D
	V N H **F** I A E F **K** R K H K K D	Human HSCP
	M R **Y** F H T S V S R P G R G E P	HLA-Bw61
	K H K V **Y** A C E V T H Q G L S	Human Ig κ-chain

VLA, very late antigen. For explanations and other abbreviations, see Table 6.2.

In contrast to the class I groove, the groove of class II molecules is open at both ends. It can therefore accommodate longer peptides by allowing them to project out of the furrow (Fig. 6.46). The peptides bound to class II molecules range in length from 13 to 18 amino acid residues. Because the $-NH_3^+$ and $-COO^-$ groups at the peptide termini lie outside the groove, there are no strong charges for side-chain to main-chain interactions at the ends of the class II groove. Another difference between class I and II peptide binding is the lack of a peptide bulge in the middle of the class II groove. Class II-bound peptides are generally more flattened out in the groove than class I-bound peptides. The main reason for this is that in the class II groove the conserved residues that form side-chain to main-chain bonds (some residues also form main-chain to main-chain bonds) are not concentrated at the ends of the groove but rather are distributed along the cleft. In the DRB1 molecules, the conserved residues are Asn 62, Asn 69 and Arg 76 in the α chain as well as Trp 61, His 81 and Asn 82 in the β chain. Most of the class II pockets appear to be involved in interactions with the anchor residues. The pockets in the groove of class II molecules are generally shallower than those in class I molecules. Four pockets are usually dominant: two at the ends and two in the middle; they correspond to the class I pockets that bind peptide residues 2, 9 (or 8), 5 and 7. The class II peptide-binding motifs are generally more variable than those of class I molecules (see Table 6.3).

The range of peptides a particular MHC molecule can

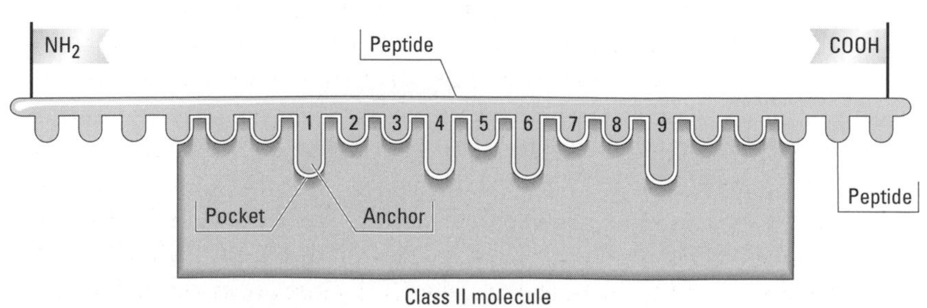

Figure 6.46 Diagrammatic representation of peptide interaction with MHC class II molecules. 1–9, amino acid residues of peptide.

bind is wide but not unlimited. It can therefore happen that an individual has a constellation of MHC molecules, none of which will bind a particular peptide to the extent sufficient for the stimulation of an immune response. In the early days of MHC studies, it was noted that certain inbred strains of animals, especially the mouse, failed to respond to specific, usually relatively simple, antigens to which other strains responded well. Crosses between the non-responder (low responder) and responder (high responder) strains revealed that the ability to respond was often controlled by a single *immune response (Ir) gene* that mapped into the class II region of the species' *MHC*. However, the true identity of the *Ir* genes remained a mystery for some time.

An important clue to the resolution of the *Ir* gene puzzle was the observation that T lymphocytes obtained from animals infected with a particular virus were able to kill other cells infected with the same virus, but only if the target cells shared with the T_C cells certain class I MHC molecules (see Chapter 5). The immune response to the virus seemed to be restricted by the MHC type of the infected cells and the *MHC restriction* was found to resemble the *Ir* gene effect in the sense that in both situations the MHC influenced the immune response in a decisive manner. Because the *Ir* genes co-mapped with the class II genes and the MHC restriction involved class I genes, a possible explanation was that the underlying mechanism of *Ir* gene control was the same as that of MHC restriction. We now know that this is indeed the case. MHC restriction ensues because the TCR is unable to recognize an antigen unless it is presented by an MHC molecule in the form of an MHC-bound peptide. We know also that one of the reasons an individual fails to respond to an otherwise antigenic peptide is that the peptide does not fit into the MHC groove.

The failure of peptides to bind to MHC molecules is, however, not the only reason for non-responsiveness. In some cases, apparently, an individual can be a non-responder to a peptide because the latter resembles a component in the individual's body and because T lymphocytes potentially capable of recognizing this component have been eliminated to avoid a self-directed immunological attack (see Chapters 5 & 25). The non-responsiveness is thus in this case caused by a *blind spot* (a 'hole') in the T-cell repertoire.

MHC and disease association

Given the involvement of the *MHC* in the initiation of the immune response, it could perhaps have been expected that certain diseases caused by immunological dysfunctions would be found associated with the complex. Moreover, given the presence in the *MHC* of genes that do not have an immunological function, it could also be expected that the occurrence of some non-immunological diseases would also be controlled by this chromosomal region. Both these expectations have been borne out by studies of humans and animals. In patients with certain diseases, particular *HLA* alleles have been found to occur more frequently than they do in groups of healthy individuals. In other words, the diseases are associated with certain *HLA* alleles. Only in one case is the association almost absolute: virtually all patients with *narcolepsy* (a disease characterized by a sudden, uncontrollable compulsion to sleep during waking hours) have the *HLA-DRB1*02* allele. (There are, of course, plenty of individuals who have the *HLA-DRB1*02* allele and do not suffer from narcolepsy.) All other *HLA*–disease associations are of a statistical nature, some of them being stronger than others. For example, *ankylosing spondylitis*, a disease characterized by inflammation and stiffening of the vertebrae, ossification of the spinal ligaments and ensuing spinal deformities, occurs in Caucasians with a frequency of 0.5–4 per 1000 males and 0.05–0.5 per 1000 females. Approximately 90% of the Caucasians afflicted with this disease carry the *HLA-B*27* allele. Since the allele is present in only 9% of healthy individuals, its frequency in patients with ankylosing spondylitis is increased 10 times so that individuals carrying the *B*27* allele are clearly more susceptible to the disease than individuals carrying other *HLA* alleles. In this case, the association between *HLA* and the disease is indisputable and apparent even in a small sample of patients. In other cases, however, the association may be so weak that very large groups of patients must be tested to prove its statistical significance. For example, *Hodgkin's disease*, characterized by the neoplastic transformation of B lymphocytes in a specific stage of their development, occurs with a frequency of about 4 in 100 000. About 40% of patients with this disease carry the *HLA-A*01* allele in comparison to about 32% in a control population.

The firmly established *HLA*–disease associations are listed in Table 6.4. Many other associations have been reported, but they are all so weak that their significance is questionable. The associations may change as the *HLA* region becomes better defined. For example, myasthenia gravis, a chronic disease characterized by muscular weakness that may progress to paralysis, was originally found to be associated with *HLA-B*08* but later a much stronger association with *HLA-DRB1*03* was recognized (the two alleles often occur together in a haplotype). Although the diseases in Table 6.4 are a mixed bag, a number of them have certain features in common. With the exception of juvenile diabetes, they are all rare, occur after the age of reproduction and have little or no effect on viability or fertility. In most cases, the *HLA* genes are associated with sus-

Table 6.4 Association between HLA and disease. (Courtesy of A. Svejgaard.)

Disease	HLA marker	Frequency (%) Patients	Frequency (%) Controls	Relative risk	Aetiological (preventive) fraction
Rheumatological disorders					
Ankylosing spondylitis	B27	90	9	87.4	0.89
Reactive arthropathy including Reiter's disease	B27	79	9	37.0	0.77
Acute iridocyclitis	B27	52	9	10.4	0.47
Rheumatoid arthritis	DR4	69	34	4.2	0.53
Juvenile chronic arthritis	B27	25	9	3.2	0.17
Pauciarticular early-onset juvenile chronic	DRB1*11	55	25	3.8	0.41
arthritis	DRB1*08	38	7	9.9	0.34
	DPB1*				
Behçet's disease	B51	29	10	3.8	0.21
Systemic lupus erythematosus (SLE)	DR3	66	25	5.8	0.55
	B8	48	25	2.8	
Organ-specific autoimmune endocrine diseases					
Insulin-dependent diabetes mellitus (IDDM)	DR3	52	25	3.3	0.36
	DQB1*0201	66	45	2.4	
	DR4	77	34	6.4	0.65
	DQB1*0302	60	14	9.5	0.54
	DR2	7	28	0.19	(0.23)
	DRB1*1501				
	DRB5*0101				
	DQB1*0602	3	17	0.15	(0.15)
Idiopathic Addison's disease	DR3	67	25	6.3	0.56
Graves' disease	DR3	55	25	3.7	0.40
Hashimoto's thyroiditis	DR11	28	11	3.2	0.19
Postpartum thyroiditis	DR4	73	34	5.3	0.59
Other organ-specific autoimmune disorders					
Coeliac disease	DR3	78	25	10.8	0.71
	DQB1*0201				
	DQA1*0501				
	DR7, 11	0–44	1–4	6–10	0.04–0.10
	DR7, DQB1*0201				
	DR11, DQA1*0501				
Dermatitis herpetiformis	DR3	84	25	15.9	0.79
Sicca syndrome	DR3	76	25	9.7	0.68
Myasthenia gravis	DR3	45	25	2.5	0.27
	B8	53	25	3.4	
Idiopathic membranous nephropathy	DR3	80	25	12.0	0.73
Goodpasture's syndrome	DR2	86	28	15.9	0.81
Multiple sclerosis	DR2	61	28	4.1	0.46
	DRB1*1501				
	DRB5*0101				
	DQB1*0602				
Optic neuritis	DR2	48	28	2.4	0.28
Narcolepsy	DR2	99	28	169	0.98
Pemphigus vulgaris (Jewish population)	DR4	87	32	14.4	0.81
Pernicious anaemia	DR5	40	11	5.4	0.33
Alopecia areata	DR4 and DR5				
	DQB1*0301	65	23	6.1	0.54
Psoriasis vulgaris	Cw6	87	33	13.3	0.81
Birdshot retinochoroidopathy	A29		8	109	
Subacute thyroiditis	B35	70	15	13.7	0.65

(Continued on p. 143.)

Table 6.4 (*Continued.*)

Disease	HLA marker	Frequency (%) Patients	Controls	Relative risk	Aetiological (preventive) fraction
Infections					
Lepromatous leprosy	DR2				
Severe malaria	B53	17	25	0.61	
Other immune disorders					
Immunization against HPA-1a platelet-specific alloantigen	DR3 DR52	97	25	113.0	0.96
IgA deficiency	DR3	50	25	3.0	0.33
Also associated with DR7					
C2 deficiency	Associated with the *A25, B18, DR2* haplotype				
C4 deficiency	Associated with the *B8, DR3* haplotype				
Malignancies					
Hodgkin's lymphoma	A1	40	32	1.4	0.12
Acute lymphatic leukaemia	A2	62	53	1.4	0.18
Non-immune disorders					
21-hydroxylase deficiency	B47	6	0.4	15.4	0.05
Idiopathic haemochromatosis	A3	76	28	8.8	0.67

Explanations: in HLA marker column, symbols with asterisks indicate alleles; symbols without asterisks indicate serologically defined antigens. For every disease, the markers showing the strongest associations are given. In many cases in which it is difficult to decide whether HLA-DR or DQ markers are responsible for the association both markers are given.

The strength of HLA–disease association is calculated from 2 × 2 tables:

	Number of individuals Marker present	Marker absent
Patients	*a*	*b*
Controls	*c*	*d*

Frequency of marker in patients: $fp = \frac{a}{a+b}$

Frequency of marker in controls: $fc = \frac{c}{c+d}$

Absolute risk: $AR = F\left(\frac{fp}{fc}\right)$

Relative risk: $RR = \frac{ad}{bc}$

Aetiological fraction: $AF = \left(\frac{RR-1}{RR}\right)$

Preventive fraction: $PF = \frac{(1-RR)}{RR(1-fp)+fp}$

F, Lifetime risk in the general population.

Relative risk (*RR*) indicates how many times more frequently a disease occurs in individuals with the HLA marker compared with the frequency of the disease in individuals without this marker. For positive association (i.e. when the HLA marker is more frequent in patients than in the control sample), *RR* is >1.0; for negative associations it is <1.0; and when there is no association, *RR* = 1.

An *aetiological fraction* (*AF*) indicates how much the HLA marker in question 'contributes' to the disease at the population level. It can be estimated for positive associations only, in which case it can range from zero (no association) to 1.0 (absolute association). For negative associations, a *preventive fraction* (*PF*) can be estimated.

Table 6.4 (*Continued.*)

Example:

	No. of individuals (%) HLA-B27-positive	HLA-B27-negative	Total
Patients with ankylosing spondylitis	108 (90%)	12	120
Controls	311 (9.4%)	2990	3301
Total	419	3002	3421

$RR = (108)(2990)/(12)(311) = 86.5$
$AR = (0.003)(0.90/0.0094) = 0.0286$
$EF = [(86.5 - 1)/86.5](0.90) = 0.89$, i.e. 89%

ceptibility rather than resistance to the disease and the associations are often with genes that are found at a relatively high frequency in the population. Several of the diseases have an autoimmune character: they are characterized by the presence of antibodies or T lymphocytes specific for self components. Many of the diseases affect joints (ankylosing spondylitis, Reiter's syndrome, rheumatoid arthritis, systemic lupus erythematosus, sicca syndrome), endocrine glands (Graves' disease and thyroiditis affect the thyroid gland) or skin (Behçet's disease, psoriasis, dermatitis herpetiformis, pemphigus).

For only one of the diseases in Table 6.4 is the cause known. *Congenital adrenal hyperplasia*, which is associated with *HLA-B*47*, is caused by a mutation in the gene coding for the enzyme 21-hydroxylase, one of the enzymes involved in biosynthesis of corticosteroids. This defect leads to an overgrowth of the adrenal gland and excessive secretion of adrenal hormones. The gene for the enzyme happens to be located within the *HLA* complex. The reason for the association is that the mutation that inactivated the 21-hydroxylase gene apparently occurred in an individual carrying the *HLA-B*47* allele and was then passed onto the progeny, together with this allele. Many of the patients with this form of adrenal hyperplasia are probably descendants of this mutant individual. The causes of the other diseases are listed in Table 6.4; the reasons for their association with *HLA* are, however, not known. At least some of the diseases may not involve the *HLA* genes themselves but rather, as is the case with congenital adrenal hyperplasia, result from the defect in an as yet unidentified gene in the *HLA* complex. However, evidence for the involvement of *HLA* genes themselves is accumulating. It has been demonstrated, for example, that pathological conditions resembling ankylosing spondylitis develop in some mice and rats into which the *HLA-B*27* gene has been artificially introduced. There is also suggestive evidence that two of several genes controlling susceptibility to insulin-dependent diabetes mellitus (IDDM) are those specifying the HLA-DQ molecules. According to one hypothesis, individuals with Arg 52 in both of their DQ α chains and lacking Asp 57 in both of their DQ β chains have the highest susceptibility to IDDM.

Several suggestions have been made as to how the *HLA* genes might be involved in disease susceptibility. According to the *mimicry hypothesis*, antigens carried by a particular pathogen may resemble a certain HLA allomorph (product of an allelic gene). As the individual carrying this allomorph is unresponsive to it, it is susceptible to the disease caused by the pathogen. For example, one of the antigens of *Klebsiella* is believed by some investigators to resemble HLA-B27 and the pathogen is thought to be responsible for initiating the process leading to ankylosing spondylitis. According to the *receptor hypothesis*, HLA molecules function as, or are required for the expression of, receptors for pathogens, hormones or drugs. For example, some researchers speculate that patients with coeliac disease (a disease characterized by an intolerance to gluten, a protein present in wheat, rye, oats and barley) possess a receptor for gluten and that *HLA-B*08*, with which the disease is associated, is required for the expression of this receptor. According to the *Ir-gene hypothesis*, the association between *HLA* and disease arises because certain individuals are unresponsive to certain critical epitopes of those pathogens that are presumably responsible for the disease. Finally, according to the *altered-self hypothesis*, the agent responsible for the disease alters molecules of the patient's body, which are then regarded as foreign by the body's immune system and consequently become the target of an immune attack. It is possible that all five of these proposed explanations apply, each to different diseases. It is also possible, however, that none of them applies and that the correct explanation has still to be put forward.

Conspicuously underrepresented in Table 6.4 are infectious diseases. Since the function of MHC molecules is the presentation of parasite-derived peptides, one might have expected that infectious diseases would dominate the list: whenever an MHC molecule fails to present a parasite-derived peptide, its bearer (lacking other MHC molecules capable of presenting the peptide) should become susceptible to this parasite. Yet, there are only two infectious diseases on the list in Table 6.4 and even their association with the *HLA* complex is open to doubt. The association of *HLA-DR2* with *lepromatous leprosy*, a severe form of infection by *Mycobacterium leprae* that spreads uncontrolled by the immune system, is relatively weak. (Here, 'DR2' stands for serologically defined antigen controlled by the *HLA-DRB1* locus.) And the association of HLA-B53 (again an antigen designation) with protection against *Plasmodium falciparum*, the protozoan that causes a severe form of malaria, has been observed in some African populations but could not be confirmed in others. The reasons for this general lack of association between *HLA* and infectious diseases are unclear. One possibility is that selection has eliminated susceptible alleles from the human population and that the alleles now present in the population provide an equal degree of protection. Another possibility is that the antigens presented by the agents of infectious diseases are very complex and that the infected individual is always able to respond to at least some of their antigenic components. One could also argue that most infectious diseases do not show association with *HLA* because their causative agents have become so destructive that the MHC-based immune system can no longer deal with them efficiently. But these are all speculations; the fact is that we do not know why the MHC appears to have so remarkably little influence on susceptibility to infectious diseases.

Defects in *MHC* gene expression

This brings us to the following question: how important is the *MHC* in the life of an individual? The answer should come from the study of individuals that either lack the *MHC* altogether or fail to express some or all of the *MHC* genes. It is probably significant that, to this day, not one single individual has been found, either among humans or among other mammals, that lacks MHC molecules completely. This fact suggests that MHC-negative individuals do not survive far beyond birth. Supporting this conclusion is the discovery that a *partial* deficiency in the expression of MHC molecules is accompanied by severe immunological defects. The deficiency is referred to as the *bare lymphocyte syndrome* (BLS) and it exists in three forms: *type I BLS* affects MHC class I molecules only, *type II BLS* affects MHC class II molecules only and *type III BLS* affects both class I and class II molecules. Patients with BLS often have normal numbers of lymphocytes, although the representation of T lymphocyte subsets can be reduced dramatically. The lymphocytes respond normally to mitogens but are unable to respond to antigenic stimulation and consequently the patients suffer from recurrent viral and bacterial infections. If bone marrow transplantation is not carried out, the patients die at an early age. Of the three forms, the best studied is type II BLS, which leads to the reduction or absence of HLA-DP, -DQ, -DR and -DM molecules on cell surfaces and to a reduction in the number of $CD4^+$ T lymphocytes. In extreme cases, no class II proteins and no mRNA can be demonstrated in the patient's cells even though the class II genes are not defective. The potential functionality of the class II genes can be shown by fusion of the patient's B lymphocytes with B cells of a healthy individual. The fusion activates the MHC class II genes derived from the patient and normal expression of class II molecules follows. This observation indicates that the gene defect in BLS patients is in a *trans*-acting factor (i.e. a gene on one chromosome acting on genes on another chromosome). Segregation analysis has indeed confirmed that the defective gene is not part of the *MHC*. Fusion of B cells derived from two different patients sometimes restores the expression of class II molecules and sometimes does not. In the former case, *gene complementation* is said to occur: since the defective gene in the two patients presumably lies at two different loci, the gene that is defective in one cell is complemented by a functional gene in the other and vice versa. At least four complementation groups could be defined by this test and the defective genes in three of the groups were tentatively identified. One is the *class II transactivator gene (CIITA)*, which codes for a nuclear protein required for class II expression. It is believed to act as a co-activator in the class II gene transcription machinery (see Chapter 8). BLS patients of this complementation group have mutations that lead to faulty splicing of the RNA transcribed from this gene. The second gene codes for the *regulatory factor X5 (RFX5) protein*, which is known to bind to the X box of the class II gene promoter. BLS patients of this complementation group have mutations in this gene that shorten the length of the produced proteins or cause faulty splicing. In the absence of a functional RFX5 protein, the entire class II gene promoter region remains unoccupied and no RNA is transcribed from the gene. The third gene is still poorly characterized. It presumably codes for a protein with an M_r of 36 000 (*p36*), which may form heterodimers with the RFX5 protein.

Experiments with animals, however, tell a somewhat different story than those with HLA-deficient humans. As was discussed in Chapter 5, methods are now available that allow inactivation of genes at will (see Figs 5.18 & 5.19) and the production of individuals that lack the proteins controlled by these genes. The application of these methods has yielded MHC-deficient mice, either class I or class II deficient, and the mating of the two yielded animals deficient in both classes. The mouse is particularly suitable for this type of experiment because certain mouse strains have only two expressed class II genes, *H2-Aa* and *H2-Ab*, which correspond to the *HLA-DQA* and *-DQB* genes respectively. Class II-deficient mice can therefore be produced by inactivating these two genes. Class I-deficient mice can be obtained by inactivating a single gene, *B2m*. Since all class I molecules use the same β chain, which is controlled by the *B2m* locus, and since the β chain is necessary for normal expression of the class I molecules on the cell surface, a *B2m* knock-out mouse should lack class I as well as class I-related molecules on the surfaces of its cells.

As it turns out, class I-deficient mice do not lack cell-surface class I molecules entirely, but the level of expression of these molecules is greatly diminished. The cells apparently express some class I α chains without β chains, but complexed with peptides. Furthermore, these rudimentary class I molecules seem to be functional in at least some experimental situations. Despite this low level 'leakage' in class I molecule expression, the *B2m*-negative mice are profoundly, but again not absolutely, deficient in CD8+ T lymphocytes. Somewhat surprisingly (in view of the T-cell deficiency), the *B2m*-negative mice do not uniformly succumb to infections by intracellular parasites. Their sensitivity to viral infections varies dramatically, depending on the virus and the conditions. For example, they are highly sensitive to an infection by the lymphocytic choriomeningitis virus, show the same sensitivity as control mice to the Sendai or vaccinia viruses and deal efficiently with influenza virus of low virulence under conditions of mild infection (but not with viruses of high virulence and under conditions of severe infection). Similarly, the *B2m*-negative mice are sensitive to *Mycobacterium tuberculosis* and *Trypanosoma cruzi* but are resistant to *Leishmania major* (the last two being protozoal parasites).

The class II-deficient mice have a greatly reduced but detectable level of CD4+ T cells in both the thymus and the peripheral organs. The origin of the remaining CD4+ T cells (about 5% of the level seen in control mice) is enigmatic. One possibility is that the mice express a low level of class II molecules that are controlled by genes other than *H2-A* (for example, the homologue of the *HLA-DO* gene). The decrease in CD4+ cells is accompanied by an increase in the number of CD8+ T cells. The B lymphocyte compartment seems to be largely unaffected by the absence of class II molecules. The B-cell responses that do not require participation of T_H cells are unaffected in these mice, as are T_C-cell responses.

Mice deficient in both class I and class II molecules have greatly reduced numbers of both CD4+ and CD8+ T lymphocytes. But much like their singly deficient counterparts, they are fertile and survive for many months when maintained in a sterile environment. These results may come as a surprise, in particular in view of the severity of BLS in humans. They presumably indicate, however, that the immune system is very plastic and has several compensatory mechanisms at its disposal: when some of the mechanisms are abrogated, others take over and substitute for them to some degree at least. The results probably also point to differences among species in the degree of effectiveness of the compensatory mechanisms: in some species (e.g. mouse) the compensation is efficient enough to assure survival of the individual under less taxing conditions, whereas in others (e.g. humans) it is less efficient and the consequences of MHC deficiency are more dramatic.

Class I-related molecules

In addition to the MHC class I molecules, there is a group of class I-related or class I-like glycoproteins that is controlled by genes located outside of the *MHC*. Each of the glycoproteins has the basic structure of a class I molecule in that it consists of an α chain associated (with one exception) with the β_2m chain, which is encoded in the same *B2M* gene as the β_2m of class I molecules. The α chain has the characteristic domain structure of a class I α chain and the encoding gene, too, is organized like a class I gene. The class I-like genes are clearly evolutionarily related to the class I genes proper, from which they apparently diverged at different times. At least one of the class I-related molecules is known to have assumed a new function, different from that of the class I molecules. The function of the other class I-related molecules is uncertain. The molecules include CD1, FCGRT, Zn-α_2-glycoprotein and human cytomegalovirus glycoprotein.

CD1

Among the first monoclonal antibodies produced by the newly developed technique of fusing tumour cells with immune B lymphocytes (see Chapter 8) was one set that reacted with human cortical (but not medullary) thymocytes and certain leucocytes. When later the CD nomenclature was introduced for antigens defined by groups (clusters) of monoclonal antibodies with similar reactivities and differentiating different cell types ('clusters of differentiation'), the thymocyte antigens defined by these first antibodies were given the designation CD1. The CD1 antigens are cell-surface glycoproteins consisting of an α chain complexed with β_2m. The α chain is controlled by a family of loci that vary in number among the different species. In humans, there are five non-polymorphic loci, *CD1A–CD1E*, all located in a single region of about 200 kb on chromosome 1 (Fig. 6.47).

Although all the loci are transcribed, only a small fraction of the transcripts is processed in the standard way. Some of the other transcripts are either spliced only partially or spliced in alternative ways to produce two or more mature mRNAs from the same primary transcript. Splicing of some of the transcript removes the exons coding for the transmembrane region of the α chain and the chain is then either secreted or retained in the cell, instead of being displayed on the cell surface. Finally, some of the transcripts are translated in alternative reading frames. Whether there is any functional significance to this variation in expression, which may differ from tissue to tissue, is not known.

The *CD1D* gene is the most divergent of the five human genes; the remaining four genes are more closely related to one another in terms of sequence similarity. In the mouse, only the *CD1D* homologues appear to be present; the other genes have apparently been deleted from the mouse genome. The *CD1D* gene also differs from the other *CD1* genes in its tissue expression: it is strongly expressed mainly on the cells of the gastrointestinal epithelium, while the *CD1A*, *B*, *C* and *E* genes are expressed on APCs such as Langerhans and dendritic cells and on B lymphocytes. The *CD1A*, *B*, *C* and *E* genes may have diverged from the *CD1D* gene functionally as well. Evidence has been provided that the CD1D molecules bind peptide just like class I molecules and presumably present them to a specialized subset of T lymphocytes. The CD1A group of molecules, on the other hand, has been shown to bind lipids such as mycolic acid, and glycolipids such as lipoarabinomannans, which occur in the cell walls of mycobacteria (*M. tuberculosis* and *M. leprae*; see Chapter 21). The lipids are apparently generated by processing in the endocytic compartment, but without the participation of DM or TAP molecules. The processing may therefore involve as yet unidentified molecules. The lipids are believed to bind to the CD1 equivalent of the peptide-binding groove and to be recognized by selected T lymphocytes including $CD4^-CD8^-$ cells. The high content of hydrophobic residues in the groove equivalent may be an adaptation to lipid binding. It has been suggested that CD1 molecules and the T-cell subset that recognizes them carry out a specialized immune function focused on a restricted set of pathogens.

FCGRT

Immunoglobulin molecules, as discussed in Chapter 8, can be divided functionally into two parts: Fab, which binds the antigen; and Fc, which is bound by various receptors (*Fc receptors*) on different cell types. The latter binding is the first step in a process that leads to the execution of various functions, for example phagocytosis. One of the receptors, originally discovered on the epithelial cells of the small intestine in neonatal rats, binds one class of immunoglobulin molecules (IgG) from a mother's milk and transports them across the epithelial cells; it is therefore referred to as *FCGRT* (Fc receptor, IgG, α-chain transporter). The transport involves endocytosis of the IgG–FCGRT complexes into endosomal vesicles, at the luminal surface of the epithelium, migration of the vesicles to the other surface, exocytosis and release of the IgG from the FCGRT (this *transcytosis* is described in more detail in Chapter 8). The transport supplies the newborn with maternal antibodies until it is able to generate its own in sufficient quantities. Similar receptors have also been found in other mammals and in birds. In humans, FCGRT in the placenta presumably transfers maternal IgG molecules to the fetus. Several other Fc receptors have been described (see Chapter 8), but they are not related to FCGRT.

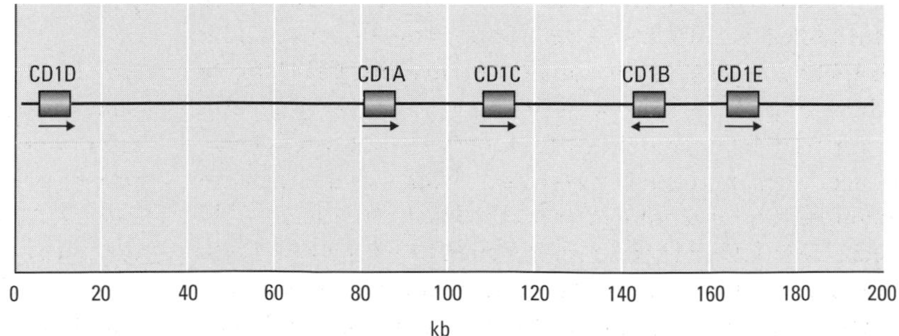

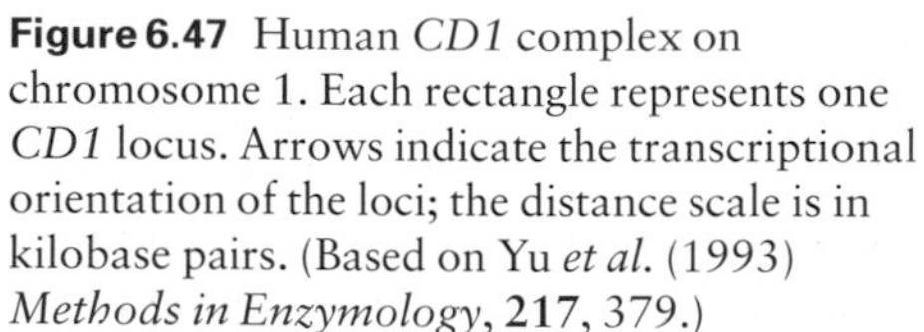
Figure 6.47 Human *CD1* complex on chromosome 1. Each rectangle represents one *CD1* locus. Arrows indicate the transcriptional orientation of the loci; the distance scale is in kilobase pairs. (Based on Yu *et al.* (1993) *Methods in Enzymology*, **217**, 379.)

In the species thus far studied, FCGRT is an α:β heterodimer in which the β chain is controlled by the β_2m locus. The α chain, a polypeptide similar to the α chain of class I molecules, is encoded in the *FCGRT* locus on human chromosome 19. The similarity is in the sequence, in the organization of the polypeptide into domains, in the tertiary structure and in the exon–intron organization of the encoding gene.

The three-dimensional structure of the FCGRT α3 domain closely matches that of the class I α3 domain. The structure of the FCGRT α1 and α2 domains resembles that of the class I peptide-binding module, but with some important differences (Fig. 6.48). As in class I molecules, the FCGRT α1 and α2 domains form a single β-sheet topped by two α-helices, one provided by the α1 and the other by the α2 domain. But the α-helix of the α2 domain has a proline instead of the usual valine at position 162, which kinks the chain approximately in the middle. As a result of the kink, the 40 N-terminal residues of the α2 helix, the preceding short helix (residues 133–147) and the two outermost β-strands of the α2 sheet (residues 127–132) are translocated and block the groove. The α-helices are also much closer together than in class I molecules and the groove is thus narrower. The structure of the pockets, too, has been altered to such an extent that interaction with peptides is all but impossible. FCGRT-bound peptides have, indeed, not been found.

All this indicates that the FCGRT has lost its peptide-binding function and acquired a new function—to bind the Fc part of the IgG molecule. This binding does not involve the groove but rather the side of the FCGRT molecule. Specifically, the sides of the α1, α2 and β_2m domains of FCGRT interact with the sides of the C_H2 and C_H3 domains of IgG (Fig. 6.49; see Chapter 8). The groove may, however, participate in FCGRT function in that by binding ions or some other small molecules at a certain pH it may trigger a conformational change that leads to the release of the IgG molecule from the complex. In crystals, FCGRT occurs as a dimer of the heterodimer (see Fig. 6.48).

Zn-α_2-glycoprotein

The addition of zinc ions to blood plasma precipitates a protein that in an electric field migrates in the α_2 region (see Chapter 8) and contains about 18% carbohydrate, the *Zn-α_2-glycoprotein* (Zn-α_2-gp). The human Zn-α_2-gp consists of a single polypeptide chain controlled by the *AZGP1* locus on chromosome 7 (region 7q22.1–7q22; see Fig. 6.9). The *AZGP1* locus consists of four exons, which are homologous to the first four exons of the class I α chain-encoding genes. Exon 4 of the *AZGP1* gene ends with a stop codon and the sequence that follows it has no significant similarity to any part of an *MHC* gene. Similarly, the 5′UT region of the *AZGP1* gene lacks the regulatory elements found in class I genes. The mature Zn-α_2-gp therefore presumably consists of three domains corresponding to the α1, α2 and α3 domains of the class I molecule; it lacks the transmembrane and the cytoplasmic regions, which is why it is found

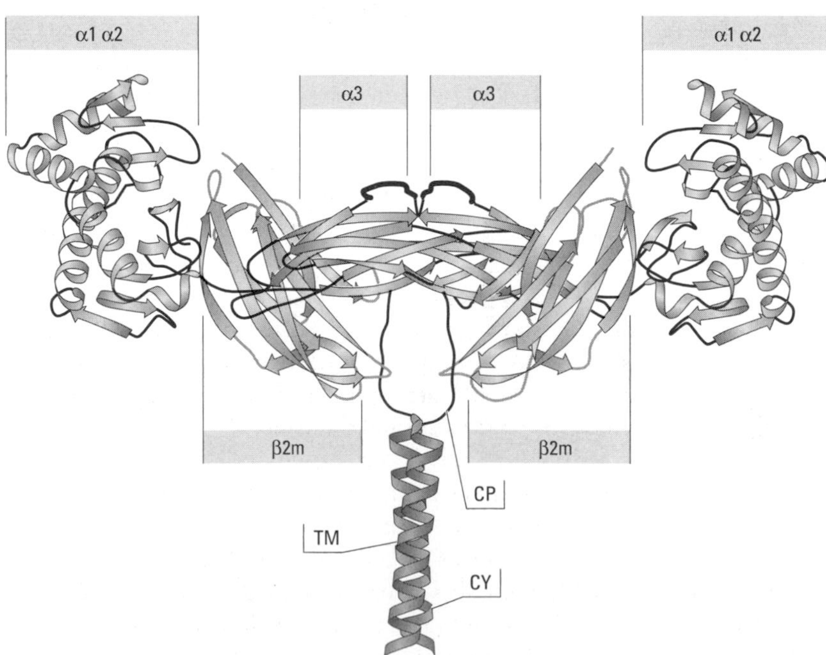

Figure 6.48 Three-dimensional structure of the FCGRT dimer of heterodimers (side view; ribbon model). The connecting peptide (CP), transmembrane region (TM) and cytoplasmic tail (CY) are modelled; the rest is based on X-ray crystallographic data. α chains are grey, β_2-microglobulin pink and disulphide bonds red; the rest of the symbols are as in Fig. 6.37. (Based on data of Burmeister, W.P. *et al.* (1994) *Nature*, **372**, 336.)

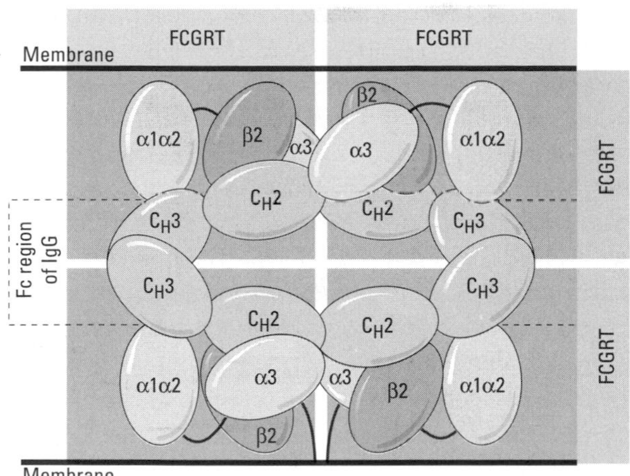

Figure 6.49 Postulated interaction between FCGRT and IgG molecules on the surface of an intestinal epithelial cell. Four FCGRT molecules are shown to interact with two IgG molecules (of which only the Fc regions are shown; the arrangement of Fab regions in this structure is unclear). The two membranes of a single cell surface could be provided by adjacent, finger-like projections (microvilli) of different cells. C_H2 and C_H3 are domains in the IgG Fc region. (Slightly modified from Burmeister, W.P., Huber, A. H. & Bjorkman, P.J. (1994) *Nature*, 372, 379.)

in a soluble form in the plasma. There is no evidence available to indicate that it associates with β_2m. The human genome contains, in addition to the *AZGP1* locus, at least one *AZGP* pseudogene. The functional gene appears to be non-polymorphic. The function of Zn-α_2-gp is not known. In addition to plasma, the glycoprotein is also present in other body fluids, including seminal plasma, sweat, saliva, urine and cerebrospinal fluid. It has been speculated that Zn-α_2-gp may bind and transport some invariant substances in the plasma.

Human cytomegalovirus glycoproteins

Cytomegaloviruses are among the largest members of the herpes virus family and among the largest animal viruses altogether. They are widely distributed among mammals and are usually species specific. The *human cytomegalovirus (HCMV)* is restricted to the human species in which it is very widely distributed; almost everybody is infected by it. It is transmitted through person-to-person contacts with saliva, urine, vaginal excretions, seminal fluid, breast milk and blood. It is usually not highly pathogenic, causing mononucleosis-like syndromes in adults (fever, malaise and sore throat accompanied by greater than normal number of mononuclear leucocytes in the blood) but in infants intravaginal infection can damage the central nervous system and cause birth defects. In immunosuppressed patients it can cause hepatitis, pneumonia and gastrointestinal diseases, often characterized by a pathological enlargement of cells in the liver, lungs and kidney (hence the name of the virus). Following the primary infection of otherwise healthy adults, the virus becomes latent in the leucocytes and can cause chronic or recurrent infections. The virus particle consists of a core and an envelope. The core contains long (240 kb) double-stranded DNA enclosed in a capsid of viral proteins. The envelope is a lipid bilayer containing some 30 different virus-encoded proteins.

It has been discovered that one of the envelope proteins binds β_2m from the blood plasma. The viral gene encoding this protein (HCMV-H301) has been cloned and sequenced and shown to have significant sequence similarity to a class I *MHC* gene. The *HCMV-H301* gene contains the entire coding sequence of a class I gene but has no introns. It encodes an α chain-like protein that is integrated into the viral envelope via its transmembrane region with the α1, α2 and α3 domains on the outside of the virus particle. The α3 domain apparently associates with β_2m from the blood. The HCMV-H301 protein is believed to facilitate the entry of the virus into a cell: once the β_2m-coated virus particles come in contact with a target cell, an exchange of virus-bound β_2m with HLA-bound β_2m is thought to take place and trigger internalization of the virus by receptor-mediated endocytosis. The virus is thought to have acquired the gene by integrating into its genome a DNA produced by reverse transcription of a class I mRNA.

Evolution of the *MHC* genes

MHC genes have been found in all vertebrate classes except the oldest, the jawless fishes (Agnatha or Cyclostomata). The latter arose more than 500 my ago and were once a highly diversified and widespread group but have since been reduced to two families, the lampreys (Petromyzontidae, some 30 recognized species in nine genera) and hagfishes (Myxinidae, some 20 species in six genera). The jawed fishes (Gnathostomata) diverged from the jawless fishes some 450 my ago; the lampreys separated from the hagfishes about 500 my ago. *MHC* genes are thus at least 450 my old. All attempts to find *MHC* genes in the agnathans have failed and the same is true also, as we learn later, for the TCR and immunoglobulin genes. Whether this means that jawless fishes lack all these genes or whether their *MHC* (*TCR*, *Ig*) genes are so different from those of other vertebrates that they have not been detected by the available methods remains undecided. There is no reason to expect that *MHC* genes will ever be found in invertebrates.

The *MHC* genes of the various gnathostomes are remarkably similar in their organization, their regulation, the distribution of polymorphism and other features. The higher order of structure of the proteins encoded in these genes, and by implication the function of the proteins, is presumably also the same in different vertebrates. All gnathostomes studied thus far have the two, and only these two, *MHC* classes, I and II. This is a very different situation from that of the TCR and immunoglobulins, which evolved disparate classes with somewhat dissimilar functions in different vertebrates (see Chapters 7 & 8). The organization of the chromosomal region occupied by the *MHC* genes, on the other hand, varies considerably from taxon to taxon (see Fig. 6.9). Not only do different class III genes become part of the *MHC* in the different taxa, but also the class I and II genes themselves are subject to a high turnover rate. New genes are continually created by gene duplication and old ones are deleted from the region. The *MHC* region thus interminably expands and contracts with time like the bellows of an accordion. This dynamism in *MHC* evolution may occur in response to changing demands on the system. The complex is thus in a constant state of flux with some genes in various stages of inactivation and others at different levels of functionality.

The origin of *MHC* genes can only be speculated upon. The three modules of the MHC molecules differ from one another so much in their structure that an assumption of their independent origin is probably justified. Assemblage of new molecules from prefabricated modules seems to be common in the evolution of proteins. At its basis is the shuffling of exons in the genome, an evolutionary process in which old genes, in particular spare copies of duplicated genes, are taken apart and their exons used to create new genes. *Exon shuffling* has been used by experimentalists to graft parts of one gene onto a portion of another (Fig. 6.50) in attempts to gain information about the function of the different regions. In evolution, exon shuffling, made possible by the correspondence between exons and domains, provides material for selection to come up with new combinations of functional properties.

However, the sources of the three MHC modules remain unidentified. Immunoglobulin-like domains are widely distributed among a variety of proteins (see Chapter 8), any one of which could have been the donor of the MHC immunoglobulin-like domains. (The immunoglobulin-like domains are present in invertebrates, so they must be older than the MHC which is presumably restricted to vertebrates.) Domains similar to those of the membrane-anchoring module have also been found in a variety of unrelated proteins and they may have arisen independently several times in evolution. The peptide-binding module, on the other hand, has thus far been found only in MHC molecules, although similar but not necessarily related struc-

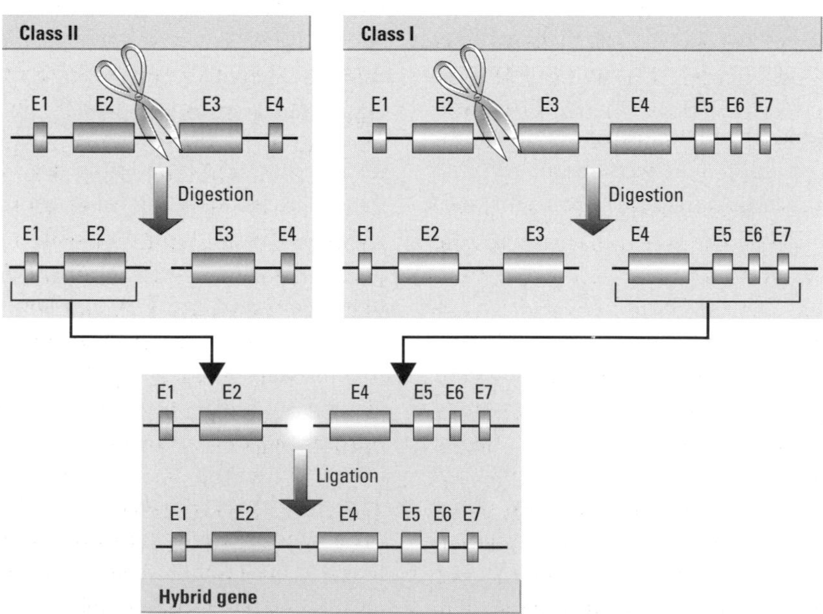

Figure 6.50 Experimental exon shuffling: the generation of a class I/class II hybrid. To produce the hybrid gene, the class I and class II genes are isolated (separated by gene-cloning techniques), each is exposed to a suitable restriction endonuclease that cuts the gene at the desired position, the fragments are separated by gel electrophoresis and the 5′ half of one gene (class II) is joined with the 3′ half of the other gene (class I). The hybrid gene is cloned and inserted into the genome of a suitable cell to produce hybrid class I/class II molecules. E, exon.

tures exist in proteins of the *interleukin-8* family and the *endothelial cell protein receptor* (ECPR) of the coagulation pathway (see Chapter 21). A similar structure is also suspected to be present in the group of *heat-shock proteins*. One purely hypothetical scheme of *MHC* gene and protein assemblage is depicted in Fig. 6.51. The order in which the class I, II, *A* and *B* genes emerged is controversial.

The neighbouring genes in the midst of which the class I and class II loci emerged became the class III loci. It seems unlikely that the original constellation of loci (the primordial *MHC*) has remained unaltered during subsequent evolution. Some class III loci were probably moved to other chromosomes (as were also some class I loci) and loci from other chromosomes may have been moved into the complex. It will therefore be difficult to reconstruct the constellation of loci in the primordial *MHC*. There are some loci, however, that seem to have been associated with the *MHC* right from its inception. A remarkable correspondence has been noticed between the composition of human non-class I, non-class II *MHC* loci on chromosome 6 and that of a cluster of loci on chromosome 9. The *MHC*-associated loci *TAP1/TAP2*, *LMP2/LMP7*, *HSP70-hom/HSPA1/HSPAL* and *C4* have their homologues (ATP-binding cassette-2, proteasome beta-8 and -9, glucose-related protein M_r 78 000 and C5, respectively) on chromosome 9. It appears therefore that the corresponding regions on chromosomes 6 and 9 arose by duplication from an ancestral region that contained the ancestors of the *TAP*, *LMP*, *HSP* and *C4* loci. Whether the class I and class II loci arose from any of the loci in the ancestral segment or whether they were assembled on another chromosome and then invaded the segment, after its duplication, remains an open question.

The human class Ia and Ib genes emerged after the divergence of primates and rodents, and this is also true for the mouse class Ia and Ib genes. Human and mouse class I genes thus derive from different ancestral genes (Fig. 6.52). The one exception appears to be the group represented by the *MICA* gene, which may have emerged before mammalian radiation. Human class II genes, on the other hand, are much older, having diverged before the radiation of placental mammals and some of them perhaps before the separation of placentals from marsupials (Fig. 6.53). However, the mammalian class II genes apparently arose from a common ancestor after the separation of reptiles (and birds) from mammals. Only the *DM* loci may be older still and antedate the divergence of the major tetrapod groups. The class I-related genes seem to be of unequal age. The oldest might be the *CD1* genes although, contrary to claims by some immunologists, their emergence postdates the separation of class I and II genes and may actually postdate the divergence of amphibians. The *FCGRT* gene may have arisen before the divergence of reptiles (birds) and mammals, while the *AZPG1* gene might be a mammalian invention (see Fig. 6.52). The age of the *HCMV-H301* gene is difficult to estimate because viruses evolve at rates very different from those of vertebrates.

Accessory molecules to MHC molecule assembly

Assemblage of class I and class II molecules

This chapter ends where it began, with a note about the biosynthesis of MHC molecules. This time, however, the focus is not on the class I and II polypeptides themselves, but rather on the molecules participating in their folding and assemblage. As the class I or class II polypeptide chain emerges from the assemblage line on the membranes of the endoplasmic reticulum, it is met, like all other nascent polypeptide chains, by a party of *molecular chaperones*. A chaperone, as you know, is a 'person, especially an older or married woman, who accompanies young unmarried people in public or is present at their parties, dances, etc. for the sake of propriety or good form'. A molecular chaperone is a protein that binds to an unfolded chain of another protein to prevent any illicit interactions. Molecular chaperones recognize features of a protein structure on the nascent chain and by associating with them prevent the formation of knots that would interfere with appropriate folding. They also prevent nascent peptides from forming aggregates with other proteins prematurely. The chaperones thus drive the emerging polypeptide chain to fold in a proper way, although they themselves do not impose a structure on the synthesized protein. As the correct fold emerges, the molecular chaperones dissociate themselves from the protein so that mature, fully folded proteins are not accompanied by chaperones. Molecular chaperones were originally identified as proteins whose synthesis in cells is induced by a rapid rise in temperature, the *heat-shock proteins* (HSPs). Temperature shock results in denaturation (unfolding) of proteins and the HSPs prevent the protein assuming an irreversibly denatured configuration. The HSPs also assist emerging polypeptide chains in attaining a proper folding. The many genes controlling HSPs fall into several families distinguished primarily by the molecular mass of the encoded molecules. The three main families are HSP60, HSP70 and HSP90. Genes coding for members of the HSP70 family are part of the *MHC*, at least in mammals and amphibians.

In mouse cells, the emerging class I α chains associate with the molecular chaperone *calnexin*, a calcium-binding protein residing in the membrane of the endoplasmic reticulum, and then with *TAP*, of which more later. Calnexin and TAP dissociate from the class I α:β heterodimers after they have been loaded with peptides. In human cells, nascent class I α chains are found associated with either calnexin or another molecular chaperone, the *binding protein* (BiP), a member of the HSP70 family. Both chaperones dissociate from the α chain after this has become associated with β_2m but before the acquisition of peptides, and the class I heterodimer then associates with TAP. It is believed that TAP (together with calnexin in mouse cells) regulates the intracellular transport of the newly synthesized class I molecules. The species difference in class I protein assemblage is attributed to differences in the α-chain sequence. Calnexin is believed to interact with the α chain in two steps. In the initial step, it binds to the carbohydrate moiety as soon as this has become attached to the α chain. In the second step, the two components brought together by the initial binding interact via their protein parts. Chaperones other than calnexin and BiP may also associate with nascent α chains, but these are still poorly characterized. They appear to be members of the HSP90 family.

The assemblage of class II molecules occurs in two stages that take place in different cellular compartments, the first stage in the endoplasmic reticulum and the second in the acidic endosomal compartment. The class II α chains

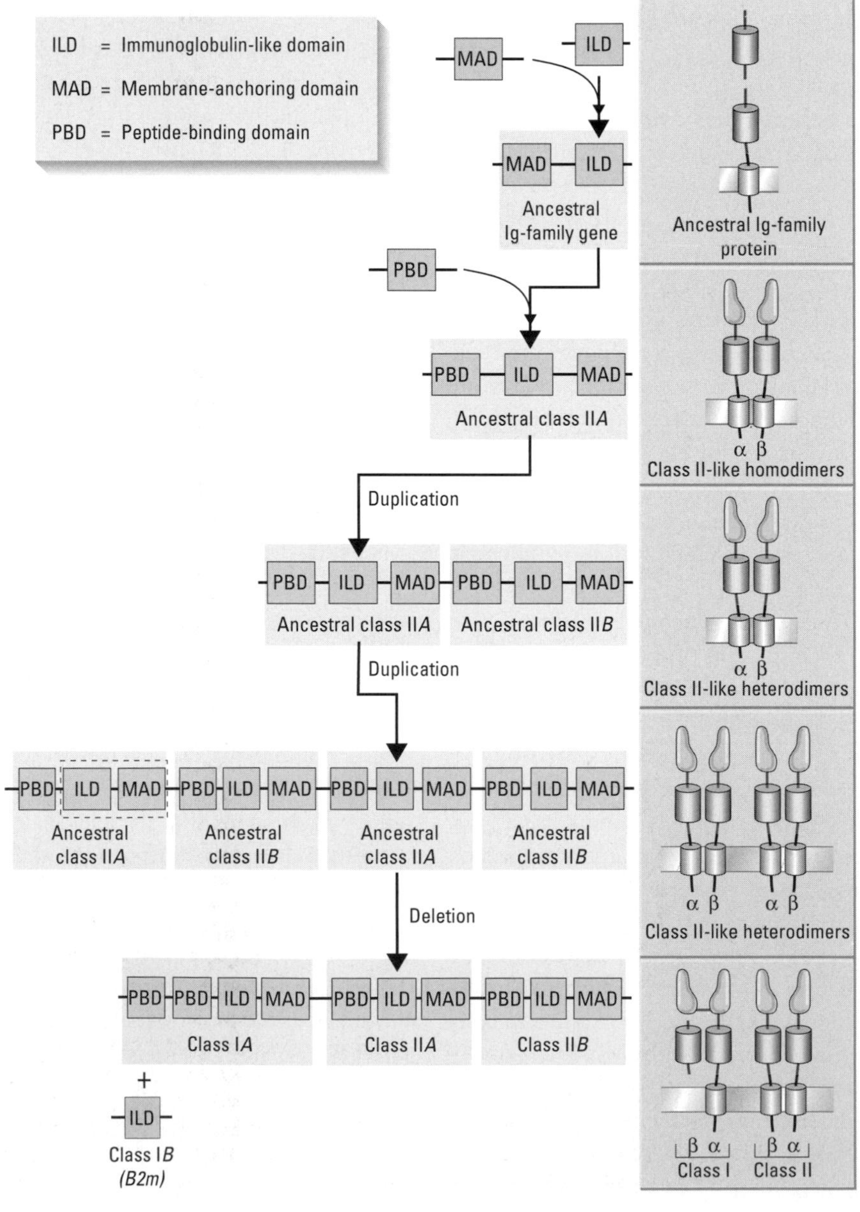

apparently associate first with the β chains and the α:β heterodimers then associate with preassembled trimers of the invariant chain thus creating α:β:ι nonamers. In this assemblage, the invariant chain has the function of a chaperone (it also has other functions, as mentioned earlier). Several other chaperones have been found associated with class II chains in the endoplasmic reticulum, including calnexin and BiP, but it is not clear in which order they associate with the chains and which of these associations occur under physiological conditions in which cell types.

There are three important accessory molecules that are essential in the assemblage of MHC molecules and which therefore deserve closer scrutiny: the proteasomes, which generate peptides for loading on the assembling class I molecules; the transporters, which deliver the peptides into the lumen of the endoplasmic reticulum for loading; and the invariant chain, which targets the class II molecules into the endosomal compartment, prevents peptides from binding to the class II molecules prematurely and acts as a molecular chaperone to promote the egress of the newly synthesized class II α:β heterodimers. The description of these three molecules follows.

Proteasomes

Cells degrade proteins in lysosomes and in the cytosol. Lysosomes contain a collection of *proteolytic enzymes (proteases)*, each of which has a relatively simple subunit structure and a single active (catalytic) site. There are three principal types of these proteases, depending on whether they catalyse peptide bond cleavage on the carboxyl side of a basic, hydrophobic or acidic amino acid residue. They are referred to as trypsin-like, chymotrypsin-like and peptidylglutamyl-peptide hydrolase-like proteases, respectively. The degradation of proteins in the cytosol is carried out by *proteasomes* or particles (bodies) with proteolytic activity. In contrast to lysosomal proteases, proteasomes consist of a large number of subunits, each proteasome has multiple catalytic sites (they are also referred to as *multicatalytic protease complexes*) and each has all three of the basic types of proteolytic activities so that they degrade a wide range of proteins.

Eukaryotic cells contain very large proteasomes that are referred to as 26S particles according to their sedimentation properties during ultracentrifugation (where S is the Svedberg unit). Each 26S particle, which has an M_r of 2 million, consists of two 19S and one 20S particle that can also exist independently of each other (Fig. 6.54). The 19S particle is composed of multiple subunits, some of which are related in sequence to certain transcription factors. The particle binds adenosine triphosphate (ATP) and enzymatically cleaves off one phosphate from it, thus releasing some of the energy stored in the phosphate bonds. The subunits involved in this process are members of a family of ATPases,

Figure 6.51 (*Opposite.*) Postulated origin of *MHC* genes and proteins. Early on in *MHC* evolution, an exon encoding a soluble immunoglobulin-like domain (ILD; perhaps resembling β_2-microglobulin, β_2m) was joined by a membrane-anchoring domain (MAD) exon, thus producing a prototypic membrane-anchored member of the immunoglobulin superfamily. An exon coding for a domain with the MHC fold (PBD, peptide-binding domain) and derived from another gene family was then added to the gene and an ancestral class II-like gene was generated. The added element consisted of a single PBD exon; had it consisted of two PBD exons, then a primitive class I gene would have been generated first. However, the derivation of a class II from a class I gene would require more steps than a derivation the other way around. It is assumed that the ancestral class II gene was of the *A* variety (coding for the α chain), because in phylogenetic trees constructed from MHC-ILD sequences, class II α chains are usually seen to diverge first, followed by class II β chains and then by class I α chains. The undifferentiated ancestral class II α chains formed homodimers in the plasma membranes and their grooves assumed the function of presenting foreign peptides to CD4+ T lymphocytes. The resulting immune response led to the production of immunoglobulin-based antibodies. This scheme requires MHC molecules, T-cell receptors and immunoglobulins to have emerged simultaneously during evolution. After subsequent duplication of the ancestral class I *A* gene, the second copy began to evolve towards a class II *B* gene encoding class II β chains. In the plasma membrane, homodimers were gradually replaced by α:β heterodimers, which were selectively advantageous because they provided a greater potential for peptide-binding region (PBR) variability. After subsequent duplication of the two-gene segment, and deletion of two exons, an ancestral class I *A* (α-chain-encoding) gene emerged in which two PBD exons became associated with single ILD and MAD exons. For steric reasons, the class I α chains probably could not form homodimers or heterodimers with class II chains, but they acquired β_2m, the product of a separate gene (*B2M*) and by then already present in the body fluids and used for other purposes. The non-covalent association with β_2m enabled the class I α chains to reach the cell surface and thus become functional immediately. The origin of the *B2M* gene remains a mystery. At least some phylogenetic trees show β_2m separating from class II α after the separation of the latter from class II β and class I α. However, this scheme would leave the ancestral class I α chains without β_2m for a long evolutionary period, and hence unexpressed and non-functional. It is unlikely that class I *A* genes could survive such a period intact, and it is therefore more probable that *B2M* diverged from class II *A* before the divergence of class II *B* and class I *A* from class II *A* genes. (From Klein, J. & O'hUigin, C. (1993) *Current Opinion in Genetics and Development*, 3, 923.)

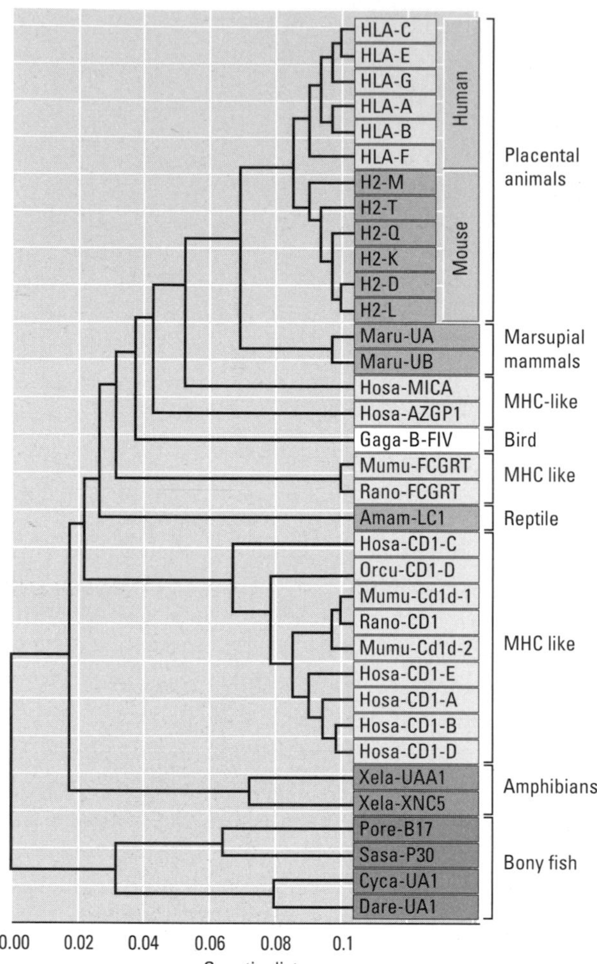

Figure 6.52 Phylogenetic tree of class I MHC proteins. The tree was obtained by using the neighbour-joining algorithm. Aman, *Amieva amieva* (Amieva lizard); AZGP1, Zn-α_2-glycoprotein 1; Cyca, *Cyprinus carpio* (carp); CD, cluster of differentiation; Dare, *Danio rerio* (zebrafish); FCGRT, Fc receptor, IgG, α-chain transporter; Gaga, *Gallus gallus* (domestic fowl); HLA, human leucocyte antigen; Hosa, *Homo sapiens* (human); H2, histocompatibility 2; Maru, *Macropus rufogriseus* (red-necked wallaby); MICA, MHC class I chain-related A; Mumu, *Mus musculus* (house mouse); Orcu, *Oryctolagus cuniculus* (European rabbit); Pore, *Poecilia reticulata* (guppy); Rano, *Rattus norvegicus* (brown rat); Sasa, *Salmo salar* (Atlantic salmon); Xela, *Xenopus laevis* (clawed toad). (Courtesy of Colm O'hUigin.)

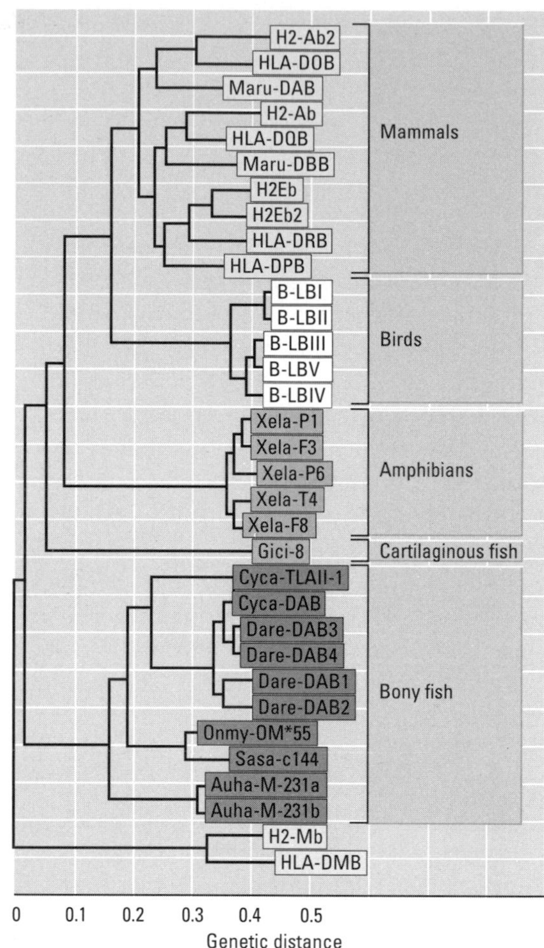

Figure 6.53 Phylogenetic tree of class II β MHC proteins. The tree was obtained by using the neighbour-joining algorithm. Auha, *Aulonocara hansbaenschi* (cichlid fish from Lake Victoria); B, B complex of domestic fowl; Cyca, *Cyprinus carpio* (carp); Dare, *Danio rerio* (zebrafish); Gici, *Ginglymostoma cirratum* (nurse shark); HLA, human leucocyte antigen; H2, histocompatibility 2 (mouse); Maru, *Macropus rufogriseus* (red-necked wallaby); Onmy, *Oncorhynchus mykiss* (rainbow trout); Sasa, *Salmo salar* (Atlantic salmon); Xela, *Xenopus laevis* (clawed toad). (Modified from Kasahara, M. *et al.* (1995) *Transplantation Immunology*, 3, 1.)

which are widely distributed in prokaryotes and eukaryotes. At least five different ATPase subunits have been found in the 19S particle. The 20S particle consists of 28 subunits that can be arranged into two groups, α (A) and β (B), on the basis of sequence similarity. The subunits are arranged into four stashed rings, each ring containing seven subunits (Fig. 6.55a). One 20S particle contains up to 14 different species of subunits, the α-subunits forming the two outer and the β-subunits the two inner rings. Each subunit has the same tertiary structure forming a sandwich of two β-stranded sheets, rimmed by several α-helices. Constrictions of the ring, lined by hydrophilic residues, delineate three chambers in the cylinder (Fig. 6.55b). All 14 catalytic sites of the 20S particle are located in the central chamber, on the ends of the β-subunits. The particle has up to five different protein-degrading activities.

Abnormal or damaged proteins, as well as various regulators that have fulfilled their function and whose extended persistence in the cytosol or nucleus would disturb the cellu-

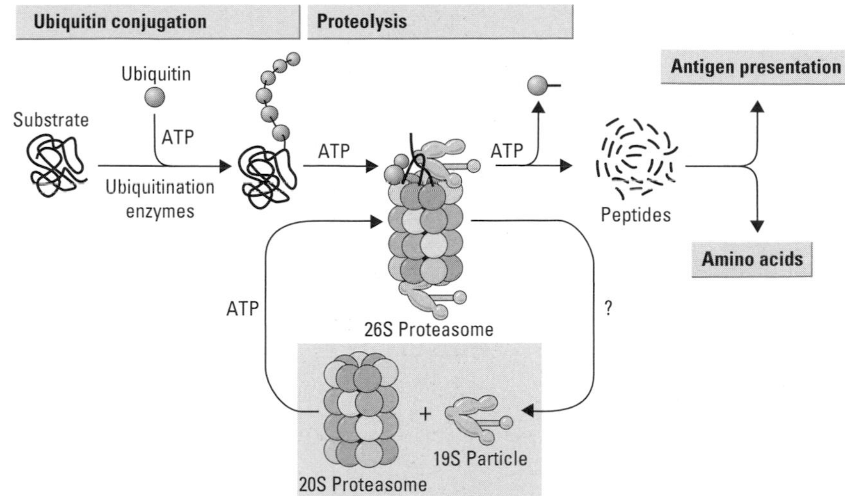

Figure 6.54 The protein degradation pathway in the cytosol. Description in the text. (Slightly modified from Goldberg, A.L. (1995) *Science*, **268**, 522.)

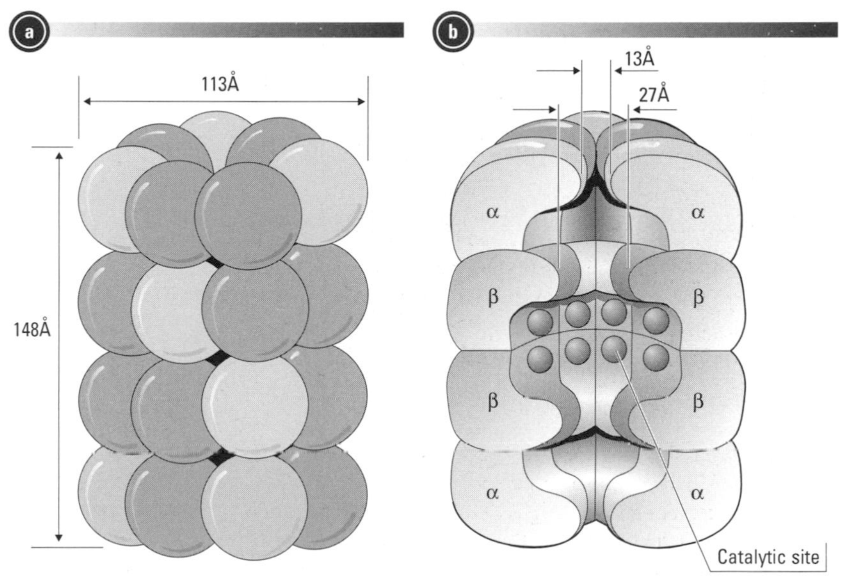

Figure 6.55 The structure of the proteasome: the 20S particle. (a) Complete particle of 28 subunits arranged into four rings with seven subunits per ring. (b) View into the interior of the particle showing the four constrictions and the three chambers. (a, From Rivett, A.J. (1993) *Biochemical Journal*, **291**, 1; b, from Weissman, J.S., Sigler, P.B. & Horwich, A.L. (1995) *Science*, **268**, 523.)

lar mechanics, are marked for degradation by the attachment to them of multiple molecules of a special protein, which because of its wide distribution is called *ubiquitin* (see Fig. 6.54). The marked protein is taken up by the 19S particle (the 'mouth') of the proteasome. The particle unfolds the protein in a chaperone-like manner and threads the polypeptide through the narrow constriction into the antechamber of the 20S particle. These activities require energy, which is provided by the cleavage of ATP catalysed by the ATPases of the 19S particle. The unfolded polypeptide chain may be stored in the antechamber and slowly fed through the second narrow constriction into the central chamber with the catalytic sites. In the central chamber, the polypeptide is cut into fragments four to nine residues long, which are then released through the third and fourth constrictions by an unknown mechanism. The narrowness of the constriction and the location of the chamber with the catalytic sites deep in the particle prevent most proteins from entering the proteasome. To get into the proteasome, proteins must be marked by ubiquitin, unfolded by the 19S particle and then threaded through the narrow openings. These mechanisms thus safeguard useful proteins from premature degradation.

The α-subunits of the 20S particle are encoded in genes at seven loci, the β-subunits in genes at 10 loci: the proteasome alpha (*PSMA*) and proteasome beta (*PSMB*) loci, respectively. Of the 10 *PSMB* loci six form pairs, each pair derived by duplication from an ancestral gene. The pairs are *PSMB5–PSMB8*, *PSMB6–PSMB9* and *PSMB7–PSMB10*. The *PSMB8* and *PSMB9* loci are also known under the names *low molecular mass proteins*, *LMP7* and *LMP2*, respectively; these are the two loci found in the class II region of the *MHC*. The *PSMB10* gene is on human chromosome 9 and the other *PSMB* and *PSMA* loci are on other chromosomes. The expression of the *PSMB8*, *PSMB9* and *PSMB10* loci requires induction by IFN-γ; the expression of the other loci does not. After IFN-γ induction, the subunit encoded in the *PSMB8*, *PSMB9* and *PSMB10* loci replace the β-subunits encoded in the *PSMB6*, *PSMB7* and *PSMB8* loci. The replacement changes the type of peptides produced by the proteasome.

The modified proteasome cleaves preferentially peptide bonds after hydrophobic residues and thus produces mostly peptides with hydrophobic or basic C termini that are then transported into the lumen of the endoplasmic reticulum for loading onto class I molecules. Peptides that are not transported into the endoplasmic reticulum are degraded further into individual amino acids by exopeptidases in the cytosol.

Transporters associated with antigen processing

The lipid bilayer of the endoplasmic reticulum is impermeable to compounds such as the peptides generated by proteasomes. To enter the lumen of the endoplasmic reticulum where they can bind to the class I molecules, the peptides must be ferried across the membrane by specialized *transporters associated with antigen processing*. The transporters are members of a large superfamily of proteins (over 50 members at the last count) distributed widely among both prokaryotes and eukaryotes. Each member possesses two conserved domains, the so-called *ATP-binding cassette*, by which it can bind ATP and cleave off phosphate from it to release energy. In addition, each *ABC transporter* has a transmembrane domain composed of an α-helix that crosses the membrane not once but five to six times. The ABC transporters ferry a variety of compounds across membranes: ions, amino acids, sugars, vitamins and peptides.

Vertebrate ABC transporters fall into four groups: P-glycoproteins (Pgp), which pump out drugs from cells and mediate multiple drug resistance; cystic fibrosis transmembrane conductance regulators (CFTR), which transport ions (the disease cystic fibrosis is caused by a mutation in the human *CFTR* gene); peroxisomal membrane proteins (PMP), which specialize in transport across membranes of the cellular organelle, the peroxisome; and TAP. Pgp and TAP are more related to each other than to the other transporter groups and might have been transferred into the nuclear genome from mitochondrial DNA.

Each TAP unit consists of two non-covalently associated subunits, TAP1 and TAP2, encoded in closely related but non-identical genes in the *MHC* class II region. In humans, the *TAP* genes are closely linked to the *LMP* genes, the order being *LMP2*...*TAP1*...*LMP7*...*TAP2* (see Fig. 6.10). They are believed to have arisen by gene duplication from a single ancestral gene. In other transporters, the genes encoding the two subunits are believed to be of inde-

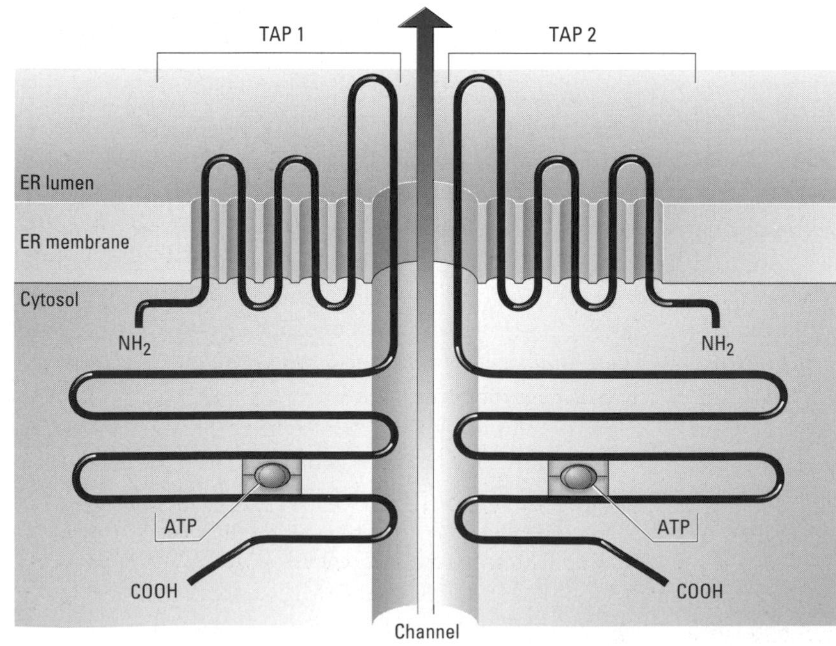

Figure 6.56 Hypothetical structure of the TAP molecule consisting of two subunits, TAP1 and TAP2. Slightly modified from Momburg, F., Neefjes, J.J. & Hämmerling, G.J. (1995) *Current Opinion in Immunology*, **6**, 32.

pendent origin. Each of the human *TAP* genes has 11 exons and 10 introns. The ATP-binding domain of each TAP subunit is on the cytosolic side of the endoplasmic reticulum and the TAP1 and TAP2 subunits form a channel by which the peptides traverse the endoplasmic reticulum membrane (Fig. 6.56). The close association of TAP with class I molecules in the endoplasmic reticulum membrane apparently facilitates loading of the peptides. In cells deficient in TAP function, peptide loading is drastically reduced and class I molecules that reach the cell surface without the peptides are highly unstable. The defect can be corrected by the introduction of functional *TAP* genes into these cells.

Not all the peptides generated by proteasomes are transported by TAP. Thus, mouse TAP preferentially transport peptides with hydrophobic C termini, whereas the human homologues transport peptides with both hydrophobic and hydrophilic C termini. (Human class I molecules have a correspondingly broader range in their ability to accommodate peptides with different C termini.) In the rat, two *TAP* alleles code for transporters that ferry different sets of peptides across the endoplasmic reticulum membrane: the TAP specified by the so-called *cim*[a] allele transports peptides with both hydrophobic and hydrophilic C termini, whereas the protein specified by the *cim*[b] allele transports preferentially peptides with hydrophilic C termini. In general, however, *TAP* genes show very limited polymorphism and hence provide only limited potential for varying the repertoire of delivered peptides. Although the TAP channel apparently sets a limit also on the length of the peptides that can cross it, peptides longer than can be accommodated by class I molecules are transported into the endoplasmic reticulum lumen. These are then either trimmed further in the endoplasmic reticulum or recycled to the proteasomes for additional trimming.

The invariant chain

The dependence of class II molecules on the invariant chain (Ii) is manifested most dramatically in mice in which both Ii alleles have been inactivated by methods of genetic engineering (see Chapter 5, Fig. 5.18). In the absence of Ii chains, very few class II molecules reach the cell surface. They accumulate instead in the endoplasmic reticulum, and the molecules that do arrive at the cell surface are conformationally altered and unstable because of a lack of stabilizing peptides.

The Ii chain is an integral membrane glycoprotein encoded in a single gene (*DHLAG*), which in humans is located on chromosome 5. The chain exists in several forms that differ in length and are produced from the same gene

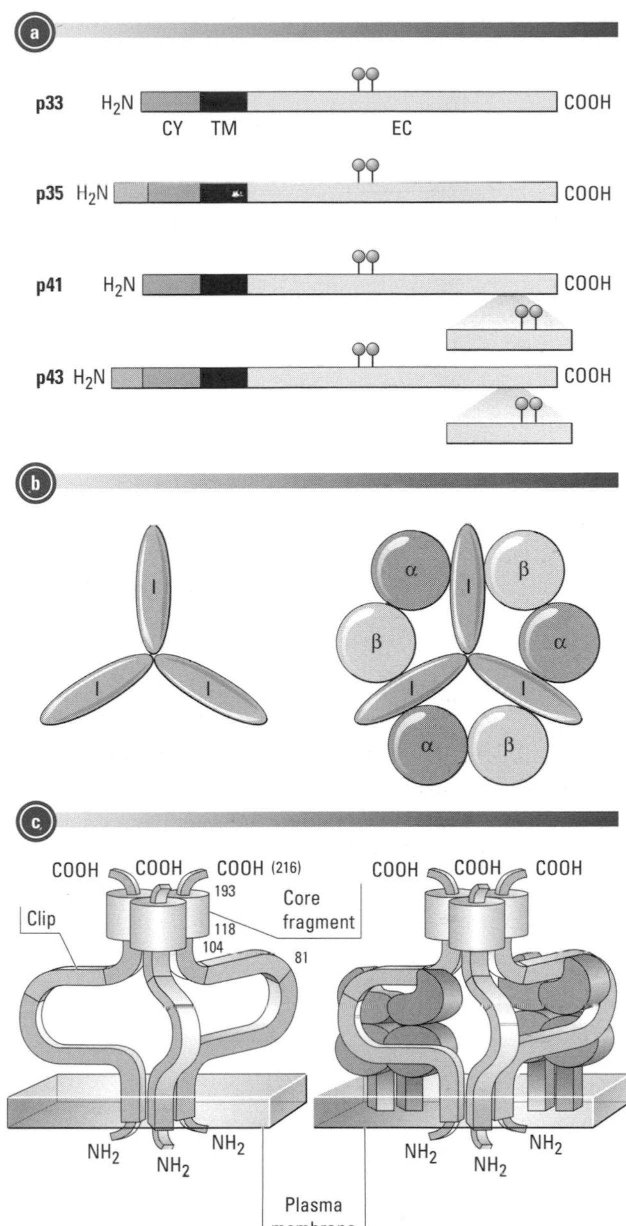

Figure 6.57 The invariant chain (Ii). (a) Four different forms of the chain: p35 results from initiation of translation from a site upstream from that used to produce p33; p41 results from the use of an extra exon that is not used in the production of p33 or p35; the extra exon codes for a segment of additional 64 amino acid residues that bears two extra carbohydrate moieties; p43 results from the use of both the upstream translation initiation site and of the extra exon. CY, cytoplasmic region; EC, extracellular region; TM, transmembrane region. (b) The Ii trimer (left) and class II–Ii nonamer. I, invariant chain; α, β, chains of the class II heterodimer. (From Cresswell, P. (1992) *Current Opinion in Immunology*, 4, 87.) (c) Models of the Ii chain trimer and the MHC class II-Ii chain complex. (From Cresswell, P. (1996) *Cell*, 84, 505.)

by differential processing of the primary transcript (Fig. 6.57). In humans, the main forms are p33, p35, p41 and p43 (p for protein, numbers for molecular mass), each of which has two carbohydrate moieties attached to the polypeptide chain. A small fraction of Ii chains also acquires chondroitin sulphate side-chains. The p33, the major form, has a transmembrane region of 26 largely hydrophobic amino acid residues, an N-terminus of 30 residues on the cytosolic side of the endoplasmic reticulum and a C-terminal part of 160 residues projecting into the lumen of the endoplasmic reticulum. The intraluminal part apparently assumes an extended conformation so that it can reach the PBR of the class II molecule. The two carbohydrate moieties are N-linked to the intraluminal part of the chain.

After their synthesis, three Ii chains associate to form a trimer, which then binds three class II α:β heterodimers to form a nonamer (Fig. 6.57). The association between the Ii chain and the class II molecule involves amino acid residues 81–104 of the former (these are the residues that form the CLIP) and the PBR of the latter. The Ii chains of the trimer interact with one another in transmembrane and C-terminal regions. The complex that forms in the endoplasmic reticulum is passed via the Golgi apparatus into the endosomal compartment, where the Ii chain is degraded and the CLIP is replaced by endosomally generated peptides, with the help of the DM molecules (see Fig. 6.5b). The class II molecules then appear on the cell surface without the Ii chain.

Further reading

Bendelac, A. (1995) CD1: presenting unusual antigens to unusual T lymphocytes. *Science*, **269**, 185–186.

Benham, A., Tulp, A. & Neefjes, J. (1995) Synthesis and assembly of MHC–peptide complexes. *Immunology Today*, **16**, 359–362.

Benoist, C. & Mathis, D. (1990) Regulation of major histocompatibility complex class II genes: X, Y and other letters of the alphabet. *Annual Review of Immunology*, **8**, 681–715.

Bijlmakers, M.-J. & Ploegh, H.L. (1993) Putting together an MHC class I molecule. *Current Opinion in Immunology*, **5**, 21–26.

Bjorkman, P.J. & Parham, P. (1990) Structure, function, and diversity of class I major histocompatibility complex molecules. *Annual Review of Immunology*, **59**, 253–288.

Blumberg, R.S., Gerdes, D., Chott, A., Porcelli, S.A. & Balk, S.P. (1995) Structure and function of the CD1 family of MHC-like cell surface proteins. *Immunological Reviews*, **147**, 5–108.

Bouteiller, P.L. (1994) HLA class I chromosomal region, genes, and products: facts and questions. *Critical Reviews in Immunology*, **14**, 89–129.

Busch, R. & Mellins, E.D. (1996) Developing and shedding inhibitions: how MHC class II molecules reach maturity. *Current Opinion in Immunology*, **8**, 51–58.

Ciechanover, A. (1994) The ubiquitin–proteasome proteolytic pathway. *Cell*, **79**, 13–21.

Cogswell, J.P., Zeleznik-Le, N. & Ting, J.P.-Y. (1991) Transcriptional regulation of the HLA-DRA gene. *Critical Reviews in Immunology*, **11**, 87–112.

Cresswell, P. (1992) Chemistry and functional role of the invariant chain. *Current Opinion in Immunology*, **4**, 87–92.

Engelhard, V.H. (1994) How cells process antigens. *Scientific American*, August, 44–51.

Germain, R.N. (1994) MHC-dependent antigen processing and peptide presentation: providing ligands for T lymphocyte activation. *Cell*, **76**, 287–299.

Glimcher, L.H. & Kara, C.J. (1992) Sequences and factors: a guide to MHC class II transcription. *Annual Review of Immunology*, **10**, 13–49.

Goldberg, A.L. (1995) Functions of the proteasome: the lysis at the end of the tunnel. *Science*, **268**, 522–523.

Grusby, M.J. & Glimcher, L.H. (1995) Immune responses in MHC class II-deficient mice. *Annual Review of Immunology*, **13**, 417–435.

Halloran, P.F. & Madrenas, J. (1990) Regulation of MHC transcription. *Transplantation*, **50**, 725–738.

Hansen, J.A. & Nelson, J.L. (1990) Autoimmune diseases and HLA. *Critical Reviews in Immunology*, **10**, 307–328.

Higgins, C.F. (1993) Introduction: the ABC transporter channel superfamily—an overview. *Seminars in Cell Biology*, **4**, 1–5.

Howard, J.C. (1995) Supply and transport of peptides presented by class I MHC molecules. *Current Opinion in Immunology*, **7**, 69–76.

Hughes, A.L. (1991) Evolutionary origin and diversification of the mammalian CD1 antigen genes. *Molecular Biology and Evolution*, **8**, 185–201.

Hughes, A.L. (1995) Origin and evolution of HLA class I pseudogenes. *Molecular Biology and Evolution*, **12**, 247–258.

Hughes, A.L. & Hughes, M.K. (1995) Natural selection on the peptide-binding regions of major histocompatibility complex molecules. *Immunogenetics*, **42**, 233–243.

Kasahara, M., Flajnik, M.F., Ishibashi, T. & Natori, T. (1995) Evolution of the major histocompatibility complex: a current overview. *Transplant Immunology*, **3**, 1–20.

Klein, J. (1986) *Natural History of the Major Histocompatibility Complex*. John Wiley & Sons, New York.

Klein, J. & O'hUigin, C. (1993) Composite origin of major histocompatibility complex genes. *Current Opinion in Genetics and Development*, **3**, 923–930.

Klein, J. & O'hUigin, C. (1994) The conundrum of nonclassical major histocompatibility complex genes. *Proceedings of the National Academy of Sciences USA*, **91**, 6251–6252.

Klein, J., Satta, Y., O'hUigin, C. & Takahata, N. (1993) The molecular descent of the major histocompatibility complex. *Annual Review of Immunology*, **11**, 269–295.

Kostyu, D.D. (1991) The HLA gene complex and genetic susceptibility to disease. *Current Opinion in Genetics and Development*, **1**, 40–47.

Lechler, R. (ed.) (1994) *HLA and Disease*. Academic Press, London.

Madden, D.R. (1995) The three-dimensional structure of peptide–MHC complexes. *Annual Review of Immunology*, **13**, 587–622.

Margulies, D.H. (1992) Peptides tailored to perfection? *Current Biology*, **2**, 211–213.

Neefjes, J.J. & Ploegh, H.L. (1992) Intracellular transport of MHC class II molecules. *Immunology Today*, **13**, 179–184.

Neefjes, J.J. & Momburg, F. (1993) Cell biology of antigen presentation. *Current Opinion in Immunology*, **5**, 27–34.

Nepom, G.T. & Erlich, H. (1991) MHC class II molecules and autoimmunity. *Annual Review of Immunology*, **9**, 493–525.

Peters, J.-M. (1994) Proteasomes: protein degradation mechanism of the cell. *Trends in Biochemical Sciences*, **19**, 377–382.

Porcelli, S.A. (1995) The CD1 family: a third lineage of antigen-presenting molecules. *Advances in Immunology*, **59**, 1–98.

Rammensee, H.-G. (1995) Chemistry of peptides associated with MHC class I and class II molecules. *Current Opinion in Immunology*, **7**, 85–96.

Rammensee, H.-G., Falk, K. & Rötzschke, O. (1993) MHC molecules as peptide receptors. *Current Opinion in Immunology*, **5**, 35–44.

Rivett, A.J. (1993) Proteasomes: multicatalytic proteinase complexes. *Biochemical Journal*, **291**, 1–10.

Rothbard, J.B. (1994) One size fits all. *Current Biology*, **4**, 653–655.

Singer, D.S. & Maguire, J.E. (1990) Regulation of the expression of class I MHC genes. *Critical Reviews in Immunology*, **10**, 235–257.

Srivastava, R., Ram, B.P. & Tyle, P. (1991) *Immunogenetics of the Major Histocompatibility Complex*. VCH Publishers, New York.

Stroynowski, I. & Forman, J. (1995) Novel molecules related to MHC antigens. *Current Opinion in Immunology*, **7**, 97–102.

Ting, J. P.-Y. & Baldwin, A.S. (1993) Regulation of MHC gene expression. *Current Opinion in Immunology*, **5**, 8–16.

Touraine, J.L., Marseglia, G.L., Betuel, H., Souillet, G. & Gebuhrer, L. (1992) The bare lymphocyte syndrome. *Bone Marrow Transplantation*, **9**, 54–56.

Trowsdale, J. (1995) 'Both man & bird & beast': comparative organization of MHC genes. *Immunogenetics*, **41**, 1–17.

Van Bleek, G.M. & Nathenson, S.G. (1992) Presentation of antigenic peptides by MHC class I molecules. *Trends in Cell Biology*, **2**, 202–207.

Williams, D.B. & Watts, T.H. (1995) Molecular chaperones in antigen presentation. *Current Opinion in Immunology*, **7**, 77–84.

Wlodawer, A. (1995) Proteasome: a complex protease with a new fold and a distinct mechanism. *Structure*, **3**, 417–420.

chapter 7 The T-cell and natural killer cell receptors

The function of the T-cell receptor (TCR) is to recognize foreign substances (antigens) and to translate the recognition into a signal that activates the T lymphocyte. Each T cell expresses approximately 50 000 TCR molecules on its surface but every one of these has the same specificity: they all recognize one particular kind of antigen. Different T lymphocytes express TCRs of different specificities so that the entire pool has the potential of recognizing all foreign antigens. Because of the nature of its ligand, the TCR is sometimes referred to as *antigen-specific receptor*. In addition to the antigen, the TCR also recognizes the MHC molecule presenting the antigen on the surface of an *antigen-presenting cell*. Assisting the receptor proper are the co-receptor and accessory molecules. *Co-receptor molecules* are cell-surface glycoproteins that increase the sensitivity of the antigen receptor by binding to the same ligand as the receptor but at a different site and by participating in signalling for activation. *Accessory molecules* are molecules stably associated with the receptor and often involved in transmission of the signal from the cell surface to the cell's interior. Finally, the expression of the TCR during T-cell development is preceded by the appearance of *surrogate chains*, which associate with one of the chains of the receptor proper before the definitive receptor is assembled.

The TCR proper

The TCR on the cell surface is a protein decorated with carbohydrate chains; it is encoded in DNA regions (*genes*) of chromosomes housed in the cell nucleus. The pathway leading from the gene in the nucleus to the protein on the cell surface is, with one important exception, similar to the pathway commonly observed in most human genes (Fig. 7.1). The portion of the chromosome in which the *TCR* genes reside is first *opened up* (made accessible) to regulatory proteins, the genes themselves are *activated*, and one strand of each gene is then copied (*transcribed*) into a single strand of RNA (*primary transcript*). The copying process encompasses both the *exons* and the *introns* but the latter are subsequently removed (*spliced out*) and the resulting *messenger RNA* (mRNA) is moved from the nucleus to the cytoplasm. There it is used as a template for the assembly of amino acid residues, i.e. it is *translated* into the polypeptide. Upon association with other polypeptides, the complex anchored in the membrane is delivered to the cell surface, where it is displayed in the appropriate orientation. The *TCR* gene is split into three (*V*, *J*, *C*) or four (*V*, *D*, *J*, *C*) segments separated by intervening sequences that can often be quite long (the *V* and *C* segments are, in addition, split into exons and introns). For transcription to occur, the dispersed segments must be brought together—the gene has to be *rearranged*. (Partial transcription, however, can occur from an unrearranged gene.) The rearrangement takes place in the developing T cell, but normally in no other cell. The *TCR* genes thus exist in two configurations: an *unrearranged configuration* found in germ cells (and somatic cells other than T lymphocytes) and a *rearranged configuration* found in somatic T cells.

TCR genes

The human *TCR* genes occupy three regions (loci) on two different chromosome pairs (Fig. 7.2). The loci are designated *TCRA/D*, *TCRB* and *TCRG* (corresponding to the Greek letters α, δ, β and γ)[1]. The first of these three loci is actually a composite of two: the *TCRD* locus inserted into the middle of the *TCRA* locus. When referring to individual segments, abbreviations can be used in the form V_A, J_A, C_A, V_B, D_B, etc., where each index letter indicates the particular chromosomal locus (e.g. V_A is the *V* segment of the *TCRA* locus). Similar rules also apply to the mouse *TCR* locus designations, except that in this species only the first letter of the symbol is capitalized (i.e. *Tcra*, *Tcrb*, etc.). The human *TCRB* and *TCRG* loci occupy distinct regions on different arms of chromosome 7 (the position of the former is given as 7q35, that of the latter as 7p15; see Fig. 7.2). The *TCRA/D* loci are located on the long arm of chromosome 14, their position being 14q11.2. Six V_B segments have also been found on the short arm of human chromosome 9, where they have apparently been translocated from chromosome 7, probably in a single event. They do not contribute to the formation of TCR molecules on the cell surface and hence are referred to as *orphons*[2].

Two of the four *TCR* loci (*A* and *G*) contain three types of gene segments (*V*, *J* and *C*) and the other two (*B* and *D*) contain four (*V*, *D*, *J* and *C*). Each *V* segment consists of two exons (see Fig. 7.1): the first exon specifies approximately 12 (the exact number depends on the type of the gene) amino acid residues of the *signal* (*leader*) *peptide*, which does not appear in the mature protein, and the second exon codes for a few additional residues of the leader peptide, as well as about 90 residues constituting the N-terminal part of the mature protein. The *D* and *J* segments are typically 12–18 and 55–65 base (nucleotide) pairs (bp) long, respectively. The *C* segment consists of four exons, only the first three of which are translated into protein; the fourth exon constitutes the *3′ untranslated (UT) region*, which contains signals necessary for processing the mRNA.

Each *TCR* locus contains one or two *C* segments, two or three *D* segments (in the case of *TCRB* and *TCRD* loci; the *D* segments are absent in the *TCRA* and *TCRG* loci) and a few to several dozen *J* and *V* segments (Table 7.1). The basic arrangement of the clusters of gene segments in the human *TCR* regions is *V*...(*D*)...*J*...*C* (Fig. 7.3) but the *TCRA* locus has *TCRD* segments inserted between the V_A and the J_A clusters so that here the order is $V_A \ldots V_D \ldots D_D \ldots J_D \ldots C_D \ldots J_A \ldots C_A$. (The arrangement is further complicated by the fact that one of the V_D segments has been taken out of the V_D cluster and placed, in an inverted orientation, between the C_D and J_A segments; see Fig. 7.3.) At the *TCRB* locus, the D_B–J_B–C_B region has been duplicated so that the $V_B \ldots D_B \ldots J_B \ldots C_B$ set is followed by another $D_B \ldots J_B \ldots C_B$ set. Finally, in the *TCRG* region, the J_G and C_G segments have also been duplicated so that the $V_G \ldots J_G \ldots C_G$ set is followed by another $J_G \ldots C_G$ set. Similar organizations of the *TCR* regions are also found in the mouse and therefore the changes responsible for the departure from the basic *V*...(*D*)...*J*...*C* arrangement must have occurred before the ancestors of humans and the mouse went their own ways, which took place between 60 and 80 million years (my) ago. Although a segment is missing here and there in the one or the other species and some segments have been duplicated, there is generally a good correspondence between human and mouse segments. They are said to be *orthologous*, having diverged at the same time as the human and mouse ancestors. There is thus a high degree of conservation in the organization of the *TCR* loci in the human and the mouse. However, not all the

Table 7.1 Number of gene segments in human and mouse *TCR* loci.

	Number of segments (human/mouse)			
Locus	*V*	*D*	*J*	*C*
TCRA	45/100	0	61/50	1/1
TCRB	75/25	2/2	13/12	2/2
TCRD	4/10	3/2	4/2	1/1
TCRG	14/7	0	5/3	2/4

TCR, T-cell receptor.

[1] These are official designations promulgated by the International Union of Immunological Societies (IUIS Subcommittee on Nomenclature). Some authors, however, still designate the loci by Greek letters (i.e. TCRα, TCRβ, TCRγ, TCRδ) even though this usage is *not* sanctioned by the committee. Greek letters may be used to designate proteins but not genes.

[2] In molecular biology, orphons are any genes separated from a tandem multigene family and transposed to a new position. They are usually non-functional and gradually accumulate so many mutations that their origin ultimately becomes indeterminable.

corresponding segments are functional in both species. Some of the segments contain premature stop codons or further defects that render them unusable and classify them as *pseudogenes*. Selective inactivation of *TCR* gene segments may reflect an adaptation to the different needs of the two species.

The individual segments in each of the *V*, *D* or *J* clusters differ in their nucleotide sequence. A quantitative measure of the difference between two sequences is the parameter termed *percent similarity* (referred to by some immunologists as 'percent homology' but this is incorrect because 'homology' cannot be quantitated). To obtain percent similarity, two sequences are *aligned*, i.e. placed one under the other so that identical residues occupy the same positions.

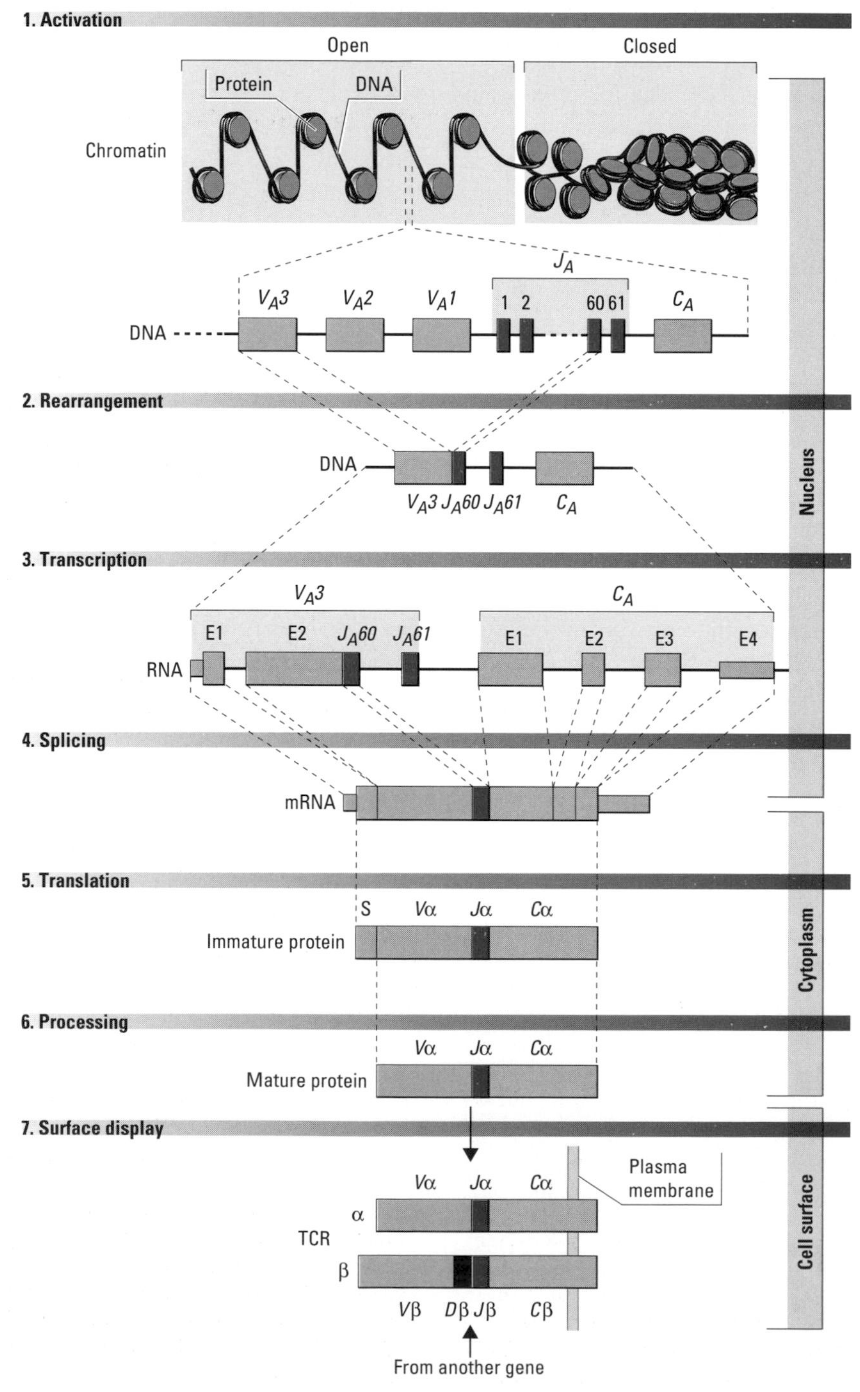

The sites at which the two sequences share the same residue are then counted and the number obtained is divided by the total number of sites compared and multiplied by 100. Comparisons of this sort have revealed that some *V* segments of a given *TCR* locus are more similar to each other than they are to the rest of the segments. The segments can be grouped into *families* in which the members of a given family are more similar to one another than they are to any member of any other family. The explanation for the various degrees of similarity undoubtedly lies in the origin of the *V* segments. Each family must have arisen from a single ancestral segment, presumably by repeated duplication. Immediately after the duplication, the segments were all identical but, with time, they began to diverge from one another as they each accumulated different mutations. However, because the individual families arose from different ancestral segments that already differed in their sequences, the diverging members of a given family have remained more similar to one another than to segments in other families. (The ancestral segments, of course, were in turn derived from a single ancestor.) At the human *TCRA* locus, the 45 *V* segments fall into 32 families; at the *TCRB* locus, the 52 functional (a total of 75) segments fall into 34 families; at the *TCRD* locus, each of the ten[3] *V* segments represents a separate family; and at the *TCRG* locus, the 14 *V* segments fall into seven families (one family of eight segments, the remaining six families containing one segment each). Because most of the human *V*-segment families have their counterparts in the mouse, they too must have been established before the divergence of human and mouse ancestors more than 60–80 my ago.

[3] Figure 7.3 shows only 3 + 1 V_D segments; the remaining V_D segments are presumed to be located somewhere in the V_A region. We know of their existence only because they are expressed in γ:δ T lymphocytes.

The four human *TCR* loci occupy regions ranging in length from 150 to 500 kb of DNA. The combined length of the four *TCR* loci is approximately 1 Mb. The total number of base pairs in the haploid human genome is estimated at 3000 Mb; the *TCR* thus takes up more than just a negligible proportion of human DNA.

Activation of *TCR* genes

The inside of a nucleus resembles an attic in a large apartment block where several parties are simultaneously drying their laundry. The area is criss-crossed by clothes-lines that are supported by props and hang in loops under the weight of the pegged, wet linen. In the nucleus, the clothes-line is the DNA double helix; the linen, the coding sequences; the intervals of unoccupied line, the non-coding segments; the pegs, the nucleosomes; and the props, the scaffold of the nuclear matrix (Fig. 7.4a). Each *nucleosome* is a group of four pairs of proteins (histones) held together by two turns of the DNA double helix and a fifth histone. Nucleosomes are distributed along the double helix at more or less regular intervals approximately 60 bp long. The DNA double helix, together with the nucleosomes, constitutes the *chromatin fibre*, which in an inactive state is coiled into a *solenoid* (resembling the coil of wire into which a movable core is drawn), and in which the individual nucleosomes are

Figure 7.1 (*Opposite.*) The pathway from the *TCR* gene to the TCR protein (from top to bottom). 1. *Activation of the TCR chromosomal region.* The chromatin (the basic fibre comprising the chromosome and consisting of one long DNA molecule associated with many proteins) in the *TCR* region (here the *TCRA* region) undergoes changes that make it more accessible to a variety of regulatory proteins. One of these changes is loosening of the tight coil into which the chromatin is otherwise compacted: the transition from 'closed' to 'open' chromatin. The enlarged section below the picture of the chromatin depicts the germ-line arrangement of the gene segments in the *TCRA* region (only a few of the V_A and J_A segments are shown and the *TCRD* region residing between V_A1 and J_A1 is omitted altogether). 2. *DNA rearrangement (recombination).* One of the V_A segments (here V_A3) is moved next to one of the J_A segments (here J_A60) and the two are fused together into a single hybrid *VJ* segment. The DNA between these two segments (here encompassing V_A2, V_A1, the entire *TCRD* complex, and segments J_A1–J_A59) is deleted from the chromosome. The enlarged diagram of the rearranged part below shows the exon (E)–intron organization of the V_A and C_A segments. 3. *Transcription.* This enlarged section also indicates the part of the DNA that is transcribed into the RNA molecule. The resulting transcript thus encompasses the entire region from exon 1 of V_A3 to the end of exon 4 of C_A. 4. *Splicing.* All intervening sequences are excised from the transcript and the exons are spliced together as indicated by the broken lines. The resulting mRNA is transferred from the nucleus into the cytoplasm. 5. *Translation.* The mRNA is used as a template for the assembly of a polypeptide chain from amino acids. Translation begins at a certain distance from the 5′ end of the mRNA (5′ untranslated region) and proceeds towards the 3′ end, always three nucleotides (codon) specifying one amino acid residue at a time. The 3′ end of the mRNA remains untranslated (3′ untranslated region; here corresponding to exon 4 as indicated by a narrow box). An immature α chain of the TCR is thus produced. 6. *Processing.* The first 20 or so amino acid residues of the immature chain, the signal peptide, are clipped off and a few other changes are made to produce the mature α chain. 7. *Cell-surface expression.* The α chain combines with the β chain that is produced along a similar pathway by the *TCRB* chromosomal region and the complex is displayed on the cell surface as the mature TCR. S, signal peptide.

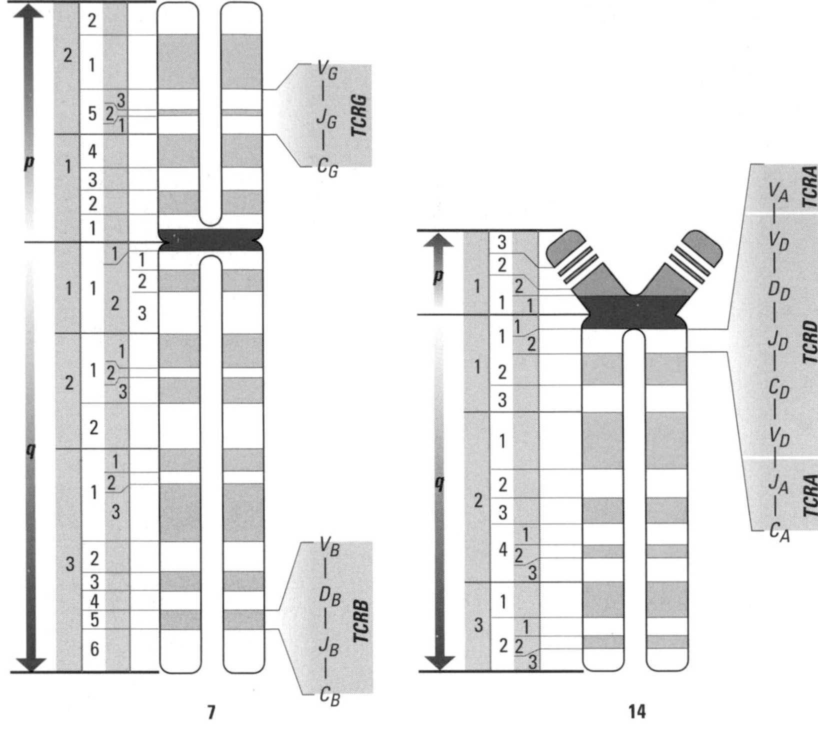

Figure 7.2 The position of TCR complexes on human chromosomes 7 and 14. Note that the orientation of the complexes in respect to the centromere is still not known. For explanation of the numbering system see Fig. 6.9.

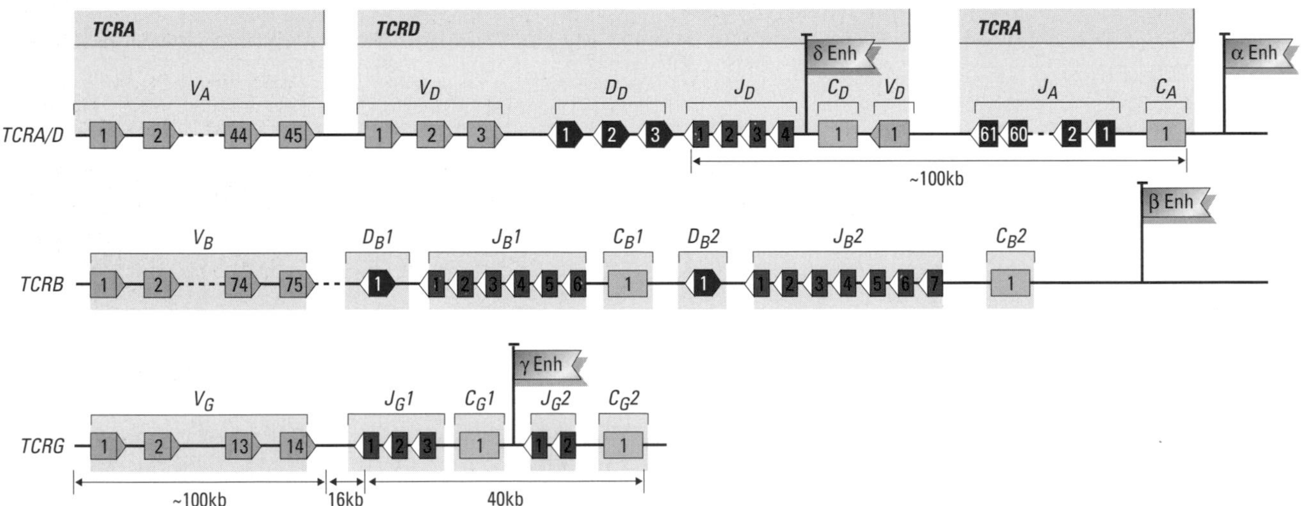

Figure 7.3 Organization of human TCR loci. Rectangles represent individual gene segments, triangles recombination signals (described later in this chapter). The 12-bp spacer recombination signals are indicated by open triangles, the 23-bp spacer signals by closed triangles. Interconnecting lines represent intervening sequences. Dotted lines indicate that the segments between the bordering numbers are not shown. The position of the enhancer (*Enh*) regions described later in the chapter is also shown. Brackets above the gene segments indicate groupings into clusters; double-headed arrows provide an estimate of distances in kilobase pairs.

closely packed together (Fig. 7.4b; see also Fig. 7.1). The loops that hang between two adjacent *matrix association regions* (MAR, the 'props') are some 50–100 kb long. The chromatin fibre is attached to the matrix by proteins.

The chromatin, as just described, is functionally inert. It doubles each time before the cell divides, but otherwise shows little activity. The chromatin of a *TCR* locus begins to change at some point after the progenitor cell has committed itself to the T-lymphocytic lineage. One of the signs of commitment is the production of soluble factors that can bind to a specific region of the DNA in the *TCR* locus. The factors are tissue specific in that they are only produced in cells committed to differentiation into lymphocytes. Indeed, they themselves may have been produced in response to other factors, which have been produced in response to other factors still, and so on. This chain of events may reflect the way differentiation proceeds in general.

The attachment of the soluble factors is possibly a signal for the unwinding (*gyration*) of the chromatin coil to begin. The unwinding can only take place when the coil is fixed to a swivel point, i.e. the proteins affixed to the nuclear matrix. The unwinding of the solenoid, probably combined with other changes, opens the tightly packed chromatin by forcing it to assume a 'string-of-beads' configuration (Fig. 7.4c) and thus makes it accessible to a variety of proteins. The *open chromatin* has two special characteristics. The first of these is an increased sensitivity to digestion with *deoxyribonuclease I* (DNase I, an enzyme that degrades DNA), a result of heightened accessibility of DNA. Within the sensitive region there are shorter regions that are hypersensitive to DNase I digestion. These exquisitely sensitive sites are digested first when the region is exposed to DNase.

The second characteristic of open chromatin is *hypomethylation*. Methylation is the addition of a methyl group, $-CH_3$, to a compound. Of the four bases in the DNA molecule, only one, cytosine, can be methylated by the attachment of the methyl group to the C-5 atom. Methylation, which converts cytosine into 5-methylcytosine (metC), has no effect on the formation of hydrogen bonds between methylcytosine and guanine and so the informational content of the DNA molecule remains the same. In eukaryotic DNA, methylated cytosines are always located next to guanine residues on the same strand. The proportion of the CpG dinucleotides is therefore an indication of the degree to which a given DNA molecule can be methylated. A high content of CpG dinucleotides can indicate high methylation and vice versa. In mammals, 50–75% of all the CpG dinucleotides are methylated.

Methyl groups are added to cytosines in selected CpG dinucleotides after DNA replication of the newly synthesized chain. The addition is catalysed by the enzyme methylase, which apparently acts only on the DNA in which one of the two strands is methylated already:

```
 Met                  Met                   Met
  |                    |                     |
-C—G—              —C—G—                 —C—G—
 ⋮  ⋮   Replication   ⋮  ⋮    Methylation    ⋮  ⋮
-G—C—  ——————————>  —G—C—  ——————————>   —G—C—
    |                                        |
   Met                                      Met
```

DNA methylation is believed to be one way of regulating gene activity, perhaps through the alteration of protein–DNA interactions. Functionally active genes are usually less methylated than their inactive counterparts. Demethylation (the removal of methyl groups) turns the gene on, methylation turns it off. The demethylation of

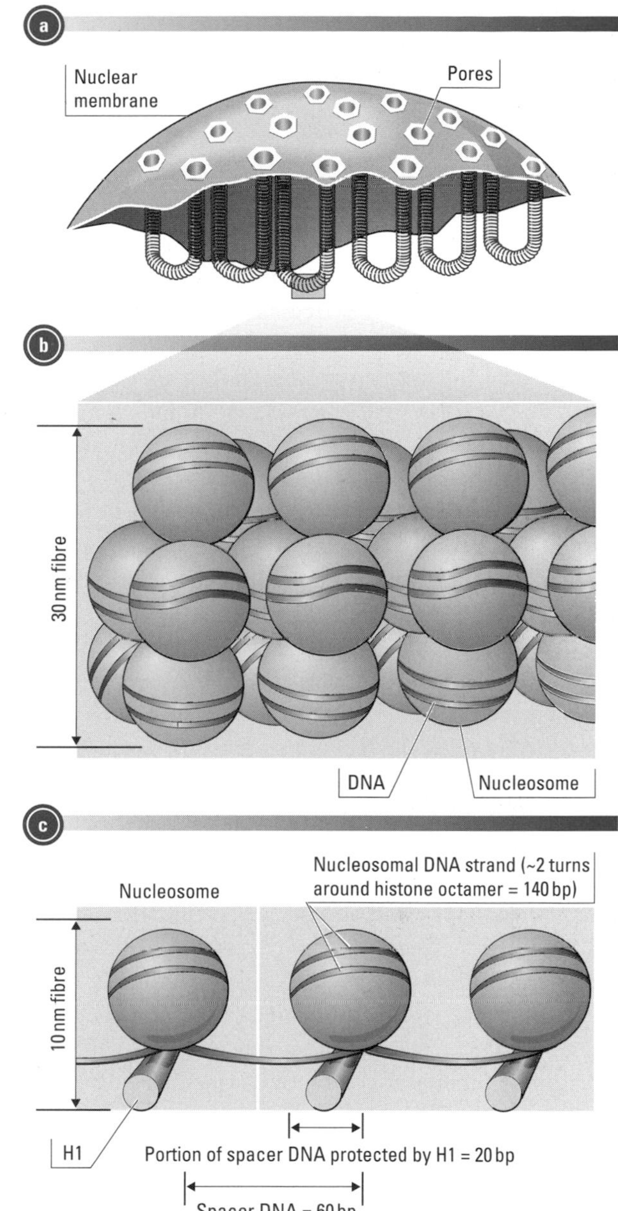

Figure 7.4 Organization of chromatin fibres in the nucleus. (a) Part of a nuclear membrane with tightly coiled chromatin loops hanging from its inner surface and attached via components of the nuclear matrix. (b) Enlarged section of the tightly coiled chromatin fibre (indicated by a rectangle in (a)). (c) Extended (active) chromatin showing the beads-on-a-string configuration of nucleosomes. It is from such a chromatin fibre that RNA is transcribed. H1, histone 1.

sequences in the chromosomal regions occupied by the *TCR* loci is therefore a sign of impending gene activation.

V(D)J joining

The opening of the chromatin allows both transcription of the *TCR* genes and rearrangement of the gene segments, i.e. *V(D)J joining*. Of these two processes, the former begins earlier than the latter but here, for logistical reasons, the *V(D)J* joining process is described first. The joining is a one-step process in the case of the *TCRA* and *TCRG* genes (*V* is joined to *J*) and a two-step process in the case of the *TCRB* and *TCRD* genes (*V* is first joined to *D* and *V–D* is then joined to *J*). The selection of segments for joining from the *V*, (*D*) or *J* clusters is largely random.

The mechanism of the *V(D)J* joining (also referred to as *V(D)J recombination* because of its resemblance to the exchange of genes between homologous meiotic chromosomes) has not yet been elucidated but several important facts have been established already. One of them is the involvement of specialized *joining signals* or *recombination signal sequences* (RSSs) in the process. They are distinct sequences that flank the recombining gene segments—the *V* and *J* segments on one side and the *D* segments on both sides. Each signal consists of three parts: a highly conserved *heptamer* (a sequence of seven nucleotide pairs), a less conserved *nonamer* (a sequence of nine nucleotide pairs) and a non-conserved spacer sequence separating the heptamer from the nonamer (Fig. 7.5). The spacer is either 12 or 23 bp long so that there are two kinds of joining signals: heptamer–12-bp spacer–nonamer or heptamer–23-bp spacer–nonamer. Interestingly, and probably significantly, the length of the spacer corresponds to either one turn (12 bp) or two turns (23 bp) of the DNA double helix. All gene segments of one kind have the same type of joining signals (e.g. all of the human *TCR V*-gene segments are flanked by the 23-bp spacer RSS). The *consensus sequence*[4] of the heptamer is CACAGTG, that of the nonamer ACAAAAACC. The heptamer sequence is imperfectly *palindromic*, which means that it reads almost identically in both directions:

First strand:	$\overrightarrow{\text{CACAGTG}}$
Second strand:	$\overleftarrow{\text{GTGTCAC}}$

The nonamer is an A/T-rich sequence:

First strand:	ACACAAACC
Second strand:	TGTGTTTGG

Each *V* gene segment has an RSS at its 3′ end; each *D* segment has RSSs at both ends; and each *J* segment has an RSS at its 5′ end. The consensus heptamer and nonamer sequences provide the most efficient recombination signals. Naturally occurring RSSs that deviate from the consensus are less efficient and efficiency variation may be one of the factors controlling the frequency with which individual gene segments are involved in the rearrangement. As far as is known, no sequences other than the RSS are required for *V(D)J* recombination to occur.

The process probably begins by the attachment of specific proteins to certain DNA sequences (presumably RSSs) flanking randomly selected gene segments, for example one *V* and one *J* segment in the case of *TCRA* or *TCRG* genes. The attachment of other proteins to these sites then follows until the complete *recombination machinery* is assembled. Only three of these proteins have been identified, two of which are probably the first two proteins to take up their positions on the RSSs of the DNA. The two are controlled by the *recombination activating genes 1* and *2* or *RAG1* and *RAG2*. The third protein, RAG cohort protein 1 or RCH1, interacts specifically with the RAG1 components and thus enhances the efficiency of the recombination process. It shows sequence similarity to certain nuclear envelope-associated proteins of yeasts. The *RAG1* and *RAG2* genes are so different in their sequences that they must be of independent origin, yet in all vertebrates thus far studied they are located next to each other, separated by only 10–12 kb of intervening sequence. This observation, combined with the fact that their entire coding sequence is compacted into a single exon, has led to the speculation that they might be of viral or fungal origin and that their inser-

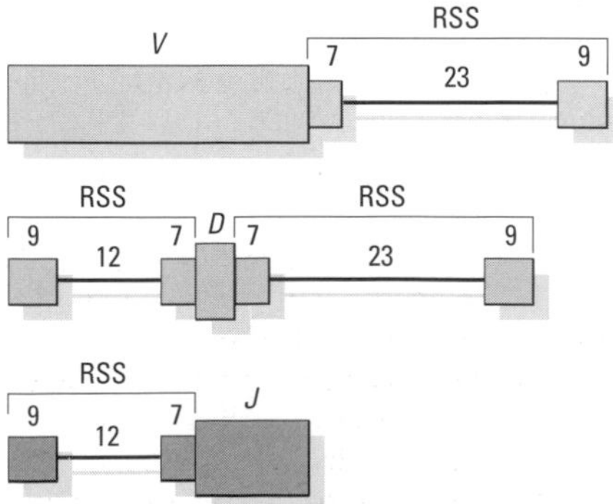

Figure 7.5 Schematic depiction of recombination signal sequences (RSS) flanking the *V*, *D* and *J* segments of human *TCR* genes. 7, heptamer; 9, nonamer; 12 and 23, one-turn and two-turn spacer, respectively.

[4] By consensus sequence, molecular biologists understand an imaginary sequence in which each site is occupied by the nucleotide or amino acid residue found most frequently at that site when many actual sequences of a given group are compared.

tion into the chromosomes of ancestral vertebrates was one of the crucial events in the evolution of the *V(D)J* recombination system. The sequences of the two RAG proteins are highly conserved among the various vertebrate classes. Mice in which *RAG1* and *RAG2* genes have been knocked out by targeted recombination do not rearrange their *TCR* and *BCR* genes and *RAG1* and *RAG2* are the only genes that need to be introduced into fibroblasts to initiate rearrangements. Furthermore, RAG-mediated recombination can be induced in artificial substrates that contain the RSSs. Efficient joining of *TCR* gene segments requires one of the segments to be flanked by a 12-bp spacer RSS and the other by a 23-bp spacer RSS. This requirement is referred to as the *12/23 rule*.

The proteins attached to the RSSs are believed to bring the two selected gene segments together by looping out the entire intervening sequence. Once the segments are adjacent to each other, one of the proteins of the recombination machinery, perhaps the one encoded in *RAG1*, enzymatically cleaves a single phosphodiester bond between the

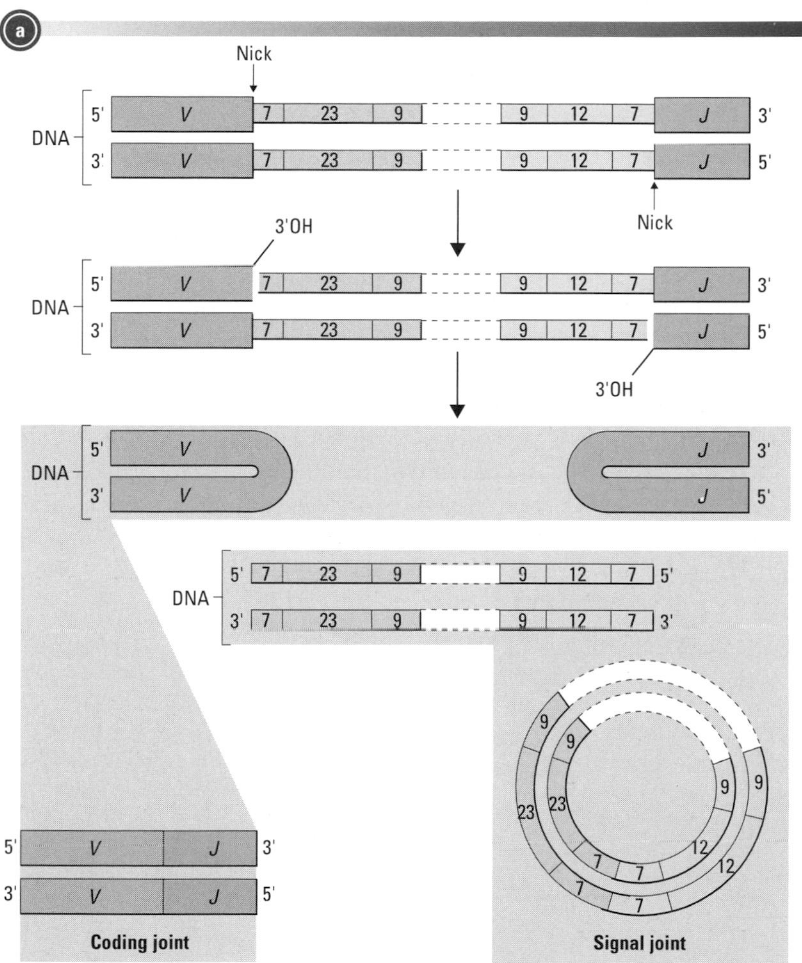

Figure 7.6 Mechanism of *V(D)J* recombination.
(a) Diagrammatic depiction. Bars represent single strands of the DNA double helix, one strand oriented in the 5′ → 3′ and the other in the 3′ → 5′ direction; wide bars are coding segments (*V* and *J*), narrow bars recombination signal sequences (broken lines indicate unspecified intervening sequences). 7, 9, 12 and 23, heptamer, nonamer, 12-bp spacer and 23-bp spacer of the RSS, respectively. (b) Structural changes in the DNA molecule during recombination. The sequence of events is as follows. The *RAG1* product introduces single-stranded cuts (nicks) at the border between the coding segments and RSSs (here one nick between the V segment and the RSS on one strand and another between the RSS and the *J* segment on the complementary strand). The cuts break the phosphodiester bonds in the strands and expose a free 3′-OH group at each site. The hydroxyl group attacks the phosphodiester bond of the complementary strand and breaks it as well. Simultaneously, in a trans-esterification reaction, new phosphodiester bonds are established between the complementary strands of the coding segments resulting in two hairpin structures. The ends of the RSSs remain free. In subsequent steps, described in detail in Fig. 7.8, the hairpins are resolved and the coding segments are bonded into a coding joint, whereas the RSSs are circularized into a signal joint.

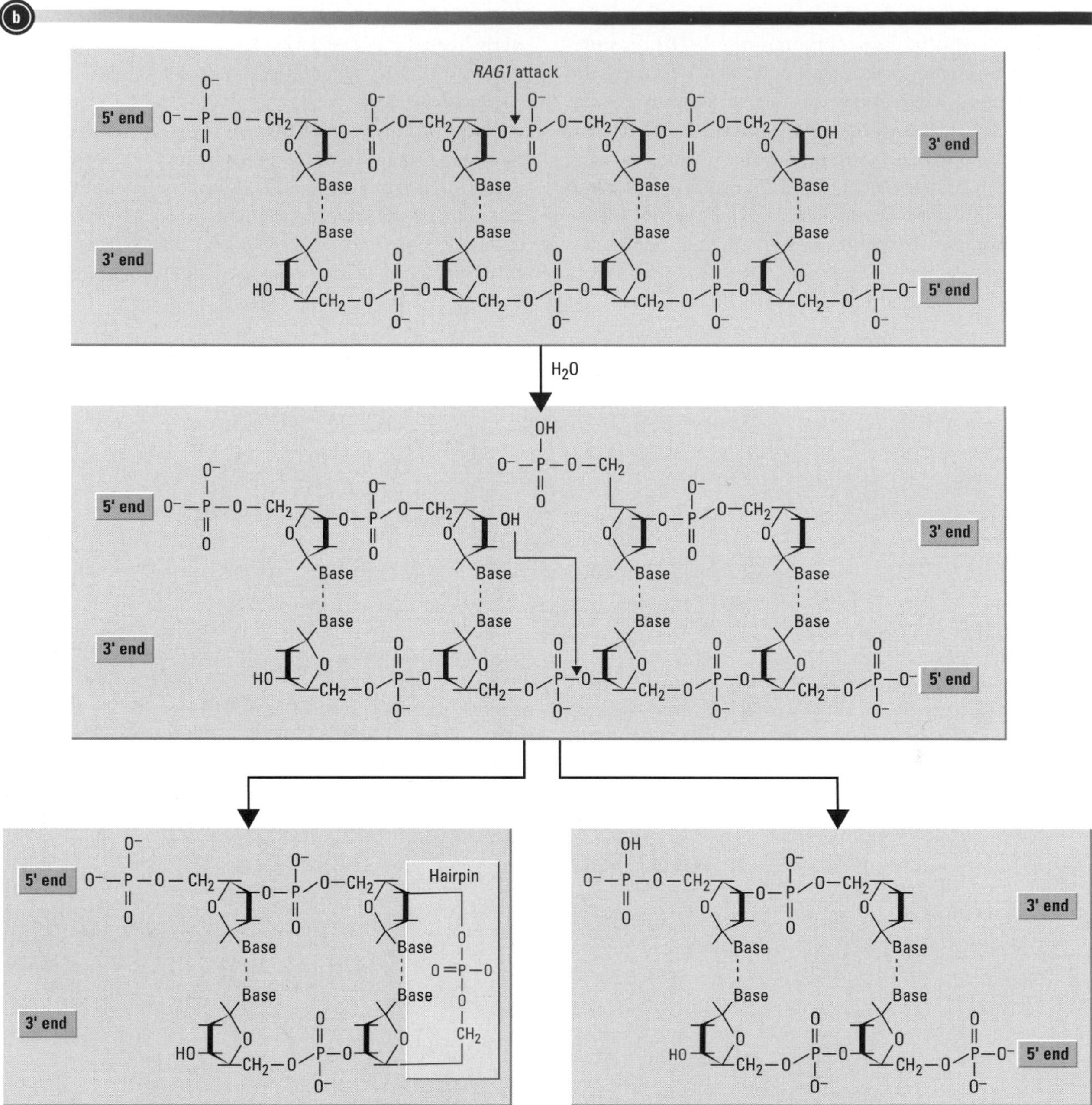

Figure 7.6 *Continued.*

last nucleotide of the coding segment (e.g. the *V* segment) and the first nucleotide of its associated RSS (Fig. 7.6). Simultaneously, it also breaks a single phosphodiester bond on the complementary DNA strand, between the last nucleotide of the RSS and the first nucleotide of the second coding segment (i.e. the *J* segment in Fig. 7.6). At each of these two sites, the enzyme catalyses the addition of a single water molecule to the DNA molecule so that the cleavage generates a free OH group at the 3′ end of the broken strand[5]. This group then reacts with the phosphate of the complementary strand forming a new phosphodiester bond that connects the two strands and gives rise to a *hairpin* structure. The ends of the RSSs remain free. Subsequently, the hairpins of the coding segments are cleaved again and

[5] Similar chemical reactions are used by a variety of transposable elements for integration into chromosomes. This observation supports the contention that the *RAG* genes might be of transposonal origin.

the *V* segment is connected to the *J* segment and this *coding joint* is thus integrated into the chromosome (see below). The heptamer of the 23-bp spacer signal that originally flanked the *V* segment is connected to the heptamer of the 12-bp spacer signal that originally flanked the *J* segment and this *signal joint* is removed from the chromosome (Figs. 7.7 & 7.8). The extrachromosomal, circularized DNA molecule of the signal joint is later degraded and with it the entire intervening sequence between the two heptamers. This form of rearrangement is referred to as *deletional* because it leads to the loss of one section of a chromosome (Fig. 7.9a). An alternative, *inversional rearrangement* occurs in cases in which the recombining segments are in a tail-to-head orientation (Fig. 7.9b). The recombination inverts the *V* segment, giving it the same orientation as the *J* segment. In such cases, the looped-out section is not removed from the chromosome but turned round and reinstated in the opposite direction. The organization of the human *TCR* genes dictates that the majority of rearrangements occur by deletion; inversional rearrangements, however, occasionally occur at the *TCRB* and *TCRD* loci.

Regardless whether the rearrangements are deletional or inversional, the recombinational machinery treats the ends used to form the signal joint differently from those that unite into a coding joint. After the cuts, the ends of both heptamer sequences are blunt, which means that the last nucleotide of one DNA strand is perfectly matched with the last nucleotide of the complementary strand. The recombinational machinery presumably contains an enzyme that recognizes *blunt ends* and then catalyses their joining or *ligation*, here *blunt-end ligation*, via phosphodiester bonds. Because the joining is very precise, no nucleotide is either lost or added at the junction of the two heptamer sequences.

A totally different outcome, however, is observed when the two coding ends (*V* and *J* in our example) are joined together. Here, as explained above, the ends pass through an intermediate stage in which the two complementary strands are covalently bonded into a large hairpin structure. No sooner do the hairpins close than they are opened again by cuts introduced by enzymes in the recombination machinery. If the cuts disrupt the newly formed bond, the original status is restored and the two coding segments are blunt-end ligated just like the signal ends. More commonly than not, however, the strands break between the ultimate and penultimate nucleotides or between adjacent nucleotides further away from the end (see Fig. 7.8). The broken ends are then no longer blunt; instead, one strand is a few nucleotides longer than its complement, so that the ends are now *rugged* or 'sticky' and are therefore handled by enzymes other than those acting on the blunt ends. What follows depends on the particular type of rugged ends created and the particular enzyme targeting them. In the simplest situation, the single-stranded portion serves as a template for the assembly of complementary nucleotides, which are then linked up by one set of enzymes and the ends of the two coding segments are ligated by another (see Fig. 7.8). When that happens, palindromes are created in the joint (see Fig. 7.8) in which nucleotide pairs appear that were not present in the original (pre-recombination) sequence. Because they are part of a palindrome, the extra bases are referred to as *P-nucleotides*. This form of nucleotide addition in recombinant junctions is referred to as *templated* because it is dependent on the use of a single-stranded template at the DNA's end. The recombination machinery, however, also contains two other types of enzymes, one of which trims the ends by attacking either single- or double-stranded DNA molecules. These enzymes delete some of the nucleotides, particularly those that do not match up when the protruding ('sticky') single strands of two molecules begin to form covalent bonds between

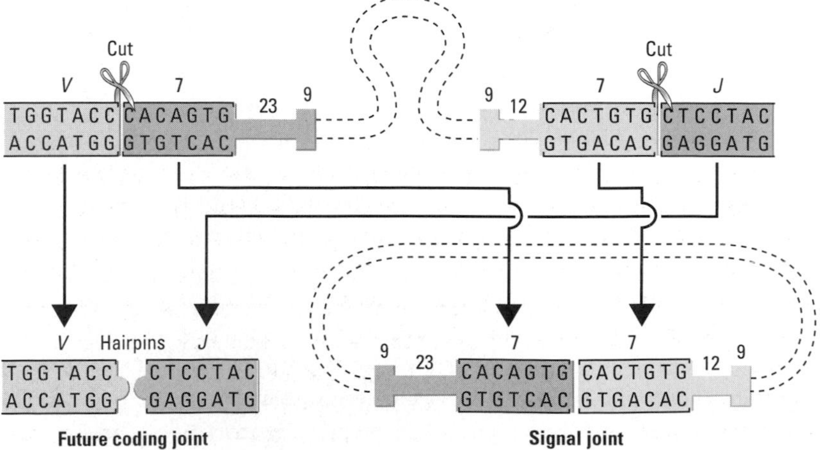

Figure 7.7 Initial stages of *VJ* recombination illustrated on an actual sequence. Blunt-ended joining of the recombination signal sequence (RSS) heptamers, as well as the formation of a circular DNA molecule and a signal joint is shown. The broken lines indicate the sequence intervening between the two gene segments (*V* and *J*). 7, 23 (12) and 9, Heptamer, spacer and nonamer of the RSS, respectively. The formation of the coding joint is depicted in Fig. 7.8.

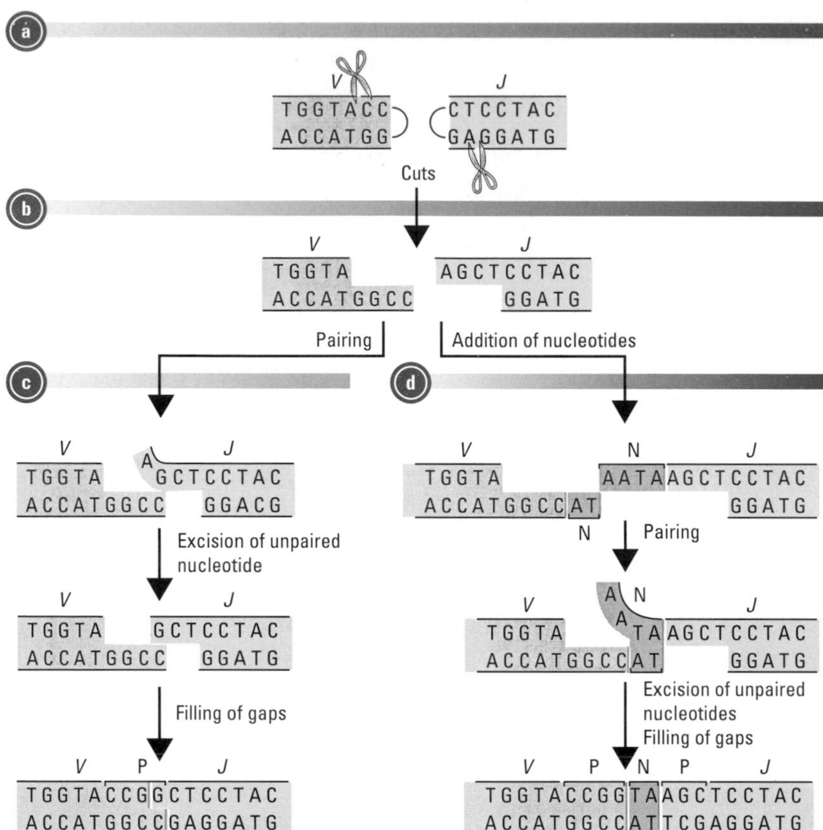

Figure 7.8 The formation of the coding joint. (a) The hairpin ends of the *V* and *J* segments from Fig. 7.7. The loops are cut at the sites indicated by the scissors (only one of several possible combinations of cuts is shown; cuts at other positions would have produced different sequences at the joints). (b) The rugged ('sticky') ends of the *V* and *J* segments resulting from the opening of the hairpin loop. (c) Pairing, excision and gap filling without the addition of new nucleotides by terminal deoxynucleotidyl transferase (TdT). The resulting joint contains a palindromic (P) sequence that was not present in the original (germ-line) *V* and *J* segments. (d) TdT-catalysed addition of nucleotides not templated by the *V* and *J* strands. The non-templated nucleotides (N) and the templated palindromic nucleotides (P) were again not present in the germ-line forms of the *V* and *J* segments. Differences in the number and type of nucleotides added, as well as in the pairing and excision of nucleotides, are responsible for variation at the joint site.

complementary bases. The other type of enzyme is represented by the terminal deoxynucleotidyltransferase (TdT), which is capable of adding nucleotides one by one to the end of a DNA strand without using another strand as a template. The random addition of nucleotides creates the *random type of recombinant junctions* (as opposed to the templated type). The added nucleotides are referred to as *not-templated*, new or *N-nucleotides* (see Fig. 7.8).

The coding junctions, in contrast to the signal junctions, are therefore unpredictable and imprecise, marked both by losses and additions of between one and ten nucleotides. They constitute the basis for the *junctional diversification* of the coding sequences, which is ruled largely by chance: where the breaks occur in the hairpin and what happens to the individual nucleotides of the single strands cannot be predicted. Ultimately, however, complementary pairing of the single strands takes place, the unmatched nucleotides are excised, the gaps are filled and the ends are ligated. The coding segments are thus joined together, but the junctional sequences differ from one another even in those instances in which the starting material in the recombination process was the same. The contrast between the coding and the signal junctions is underscored by experiments on mice bearing two copies of the so-called *scid* mutation, which affects the junctional diversification machinery (see Chapter 26). In *scid* mutants, the formation of coding junctions is drastically reduced, while the formation of signal junctions remains largely unaffected. The gene responsible for the *scid* defect apparently codes for the enzyme *DNA-activated serine/threonine protease kinase* (DNA-PK), a nuclear protein composed of a large (M_r ~ 460 000) catalytic peptide (DNA-PK_{cs}) and a heterodimer (p70/p80) Ku.

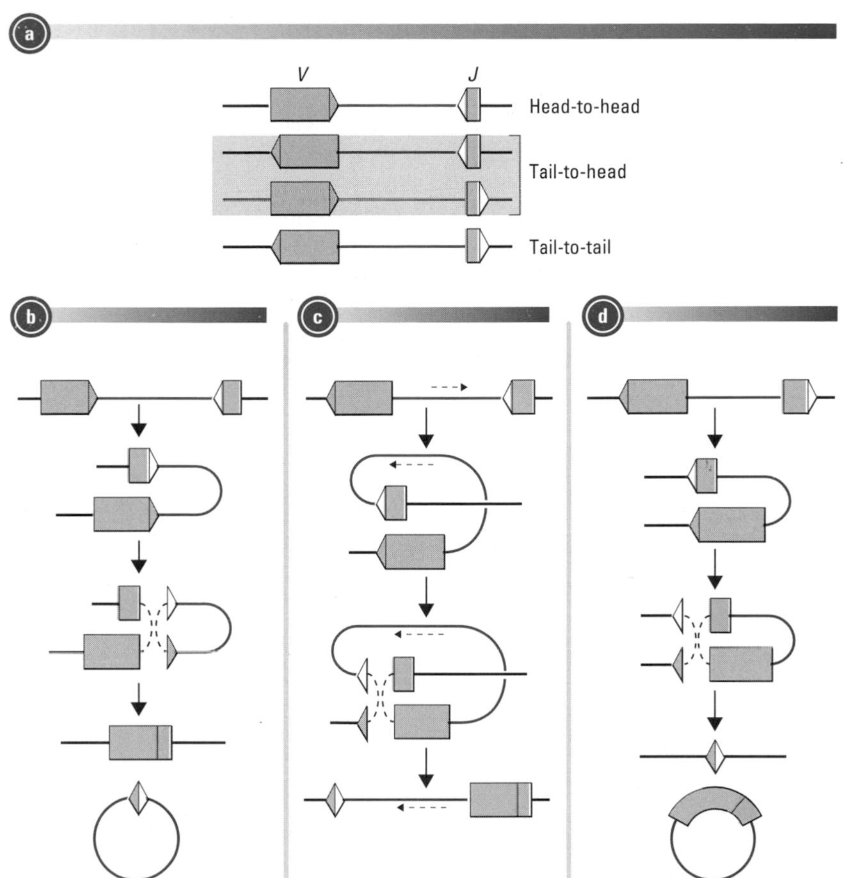

Figure 7.9 (a) Four theoretically possible orientations of two recombination signal sequences (RSSs, triangles) in a *V* and a *J* segment (rectangles) and (b–d) the three theoretically possible types of rearrangement. Both tail-to-head orientations lead to the same type of rearrangement. (b) *Deletional type of rearrangement* resulting from the head-to-head orientation of recombination signals. The two segments come together by a simple looping-out of the intervening sequence and align with each other in the way shown. After double-stranded breaks have separated the segments from their flanking RSSs, the fusion of the RSSs (indicated by the broken line) results in a circular DNA which is thus removed from the chromosome and ultimately lost; the chromosome regains its integrity through the fusion of the *V* and *J* segments (broken line). (c) *Inversional type of rearrangement* resulting from the tail-to-head orientation of the RSSs. The two coding segments come together by an inverted looping-out of the intervening sequence and their RSSs break away from them and fuse with each other (broken line). When the *V* and *J* segments unite, the integrity of the chromosome is restored without the loss of any DNA. The intervening sequence, together with the *V* segment, is reinserted into the chromosome in an inverted orientation (indicated by broken arrows). Most human *TCR* segments have their RSSs in the head-to-head orientation and therefore undergo deletional recombination. Some segments, however, have their RSSs in the tail-to-head orientation and these undergo inversional recombination. (d) *Forbidden deletional rearrangement.* If the RSSs were in the tail-to-tail orientation, the recombination would place the coding segments into the circle excised from the chromosome and the segments would thus be lost. This rearrangement normally does not occur.

The latter binds to free DNA ends and thus targets the DNA-PK_{cs} to the DNA. The enzyme then phosphorylates proteins and thus contributes to the joining of the DNA ends in a manner that has yet to be determined.

In those *TCR* genes that have *D* segments (*TCRD* and *TCRB*), transposition of one of the *D* segments to one of the *J* segments occurs first and is followed by transposition of one of the *V* segments to the fused *DJ* segment. In the *TCR* genes that do not have *D* segments (*TCRA* and *TCRG*), one of the *V* segments is transposed directly to one of the *J* segments.

The recombination process begins shortly after the progenitor (stem) cells have arrived in the thymus, in the double-negative ($CD4^-CD8^-$) stage of thymocyte development. The progenitors differentiate along two different lines. One type of progenitor cells seeds the fetal thymus at approximately 12 days of gestation (it is the first T-cell progenitor to arrive in the thymus) and its *TCR* genes undergo rearrangements during the next day or so. The cells rearrange *TCRD* and *TCRG* genes either simultaneously or the former slightly earlier than the latter, use exclusively one *V*-gene segment at each locus for the rearrangement (*VG3* and *VD1*) and do not undergo junctional diversification. Their progeny therefore is a single clone of cells, all of which express the same γ:δ TCR. The $V_{\gamma}3,V_{\delta}1$ cells appear in the thymus at 14 days of gestation and after maturing migrate exclusively into the skin. Shortly thereafter another monoclonal population of T cells, all expressing the $V_{\gamma}4,V_{\delta}1$ TCR emerges and migrates to the reproductive epithelium (see Fig. 5.12). These two waves of early γ:δ T cells are produced only during the fetal period; their production ceases at birth.

The second type of progenitor cells also appears in the thymus during the fetal period but persists well into adulthood. T cells expressing all other γ:δ and α:β TCRs are derived from these progenitors. They appear first in the fetal thymus at 16–17 days of gestation and then continue to be produced during the postnatal period for as long as the thymus remains functional. The progenitors give rise to both γ:δ and α:β T cells, but the latter numerically come to predominate over the former.

The mechanism by which the two lineages arise from a common progenitor cell remains controversial. Two principal hypotheses have been formulated to explain the relationship between the α:β and γ:δ T-cell lineages. According to one hypothesis, the commitment to one or the other lineage occurs before the *TCR* genes begin to rearrange (pre-rearrangement hypothesis). According to the other hypothesis, lineage commitment is determined by the rearrangement itself (successive rearrangement hypothesis).

In one version of the *pre-rearrangement hypothesis*, the commitment to the γ:δ vs. the α:β lineage is mediated by a *silencer sequence* located in the mouse downstream of the *TCRGC1* gene (the existence of the sequence has been deduced from experiments with transgenic mice but its exact location has yet to be determined). Independently of *TCR* gene rearrangement, progenitor cells are split into two lineages: in one, the silencer machinery remains inactive; in the other, it is activated. *TCRG*, *TCRD* and perhaps also *TCRB* genes rearrange in both lineages but only in the lineage with the silencer switched off is the γ:δ TCR expressed on the surface and this prevents, by a feedback mechanism, the completion of the *TCRB* gene rearrangement and initiation of the *TCRA* rearrangement. In the lineage with the silencer switched on, the assembly of the γ:δ TCR is blocked at the transcription level and hence the cells may proceed to complete TCR gene rearrangement and to initiate the *TCRA* rearrangement.

The latest version of the *successive rearrangement hypothesis* is depicted in Fig. 7.10. The essential tenet of the hypothesis is that thymocytes first attempt to produce functional γ:δ TCR by rearranging their *TCRG* and *TCRD* genes. If they succeed, they become γ:δ T cells; if they fail, they then try to produce functional α:β TCR by rearranging the *TCRA* and *TCRB* genes. If they succeed they become α:β T cells. In the version depicted in Fig. 7.10, the *TCRD* gene rearranges first on one of the two homologous chromosomes, while the *TCRD* gene on the other chromosome remains in a germ-line configuration. The two possible outcomes of the trial are failure (–) or success (+). If the outcome is a failure, the cell tries to rearrange the *TCRD* locus on the homologous chromosome. If it fails again, it will aim at the *TCRB* locus on one of the two chromosomes. If it succeeds, it will attempt to rearrange the *TCRA* locus. Similarly, if the cell, early in the process, succeeds in rearranging the *TCRD* locus, it will proceed with the rearrangement of the *TCRG* locus. If it succeeds, it becomes a γ:δ T cell; if it fails, it will have a go at the *TCRB* and *TCRA* loci; and so on (follow the dichotomies from top to bottom in Fig. 7.10). The available evidence favours the successive rearrangement hypothesis. Consistent with the hypothesis is the observation that in peripheral α:β T cells, the *TCRG* gene is often found to be rearranged in such a way that it could not encode a functional γ chain (the

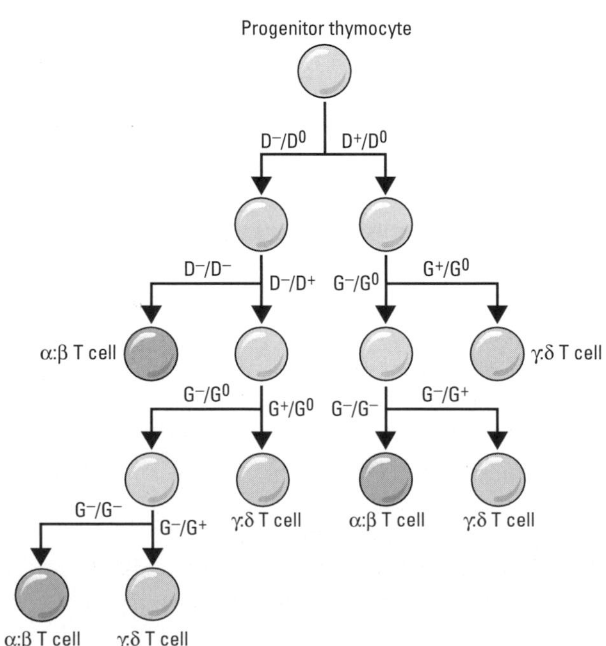

Figure 7.10 Successive rearrangement hypothesis of thymocyte commitment to α:β or γ:δ lineages. *D, TCRD; G, TCRG*; +, productive (functional) rearrangement; –, non-productive (non-functional) rearrangement; 0, absence of rearrangement (germ-line configuration). (Based on Dudley, E. C. *et al.* (1995) *Current Biology*, 5, 659.)

TCRD locus is deleted when the *TCRA* gene rearranges). In γ:δ thymocytes and peripheral T cells, the *TCRB* gene often occurs in partially rearranged ($D \rightarrow J$) form, presumably because some of the *TCRB* rearrangements begin before the *TCRG* rearrangements have been tested for functionality; *TCRA* genes are hardly ever found to be rearranged in these cells.

The success or failure of a rearrangement is decided by the status of the reading frame of the joined segments. Recall that there are three possible ways (*frames*) of reading a nucleotide sequence as a series of triplets (*codons*) and that only one of these (the *in-frame* way) gives a correct transliteration into an amino acid sequence of a protein. The other two (*out-of-frame*) ways, if used, would translate the nucleotide sequence into a protein of entirely different (and hence non-functional) amino acid sequence. Moreover, the out-of-frame ways are likely to run into stop codons earlier than the in-frame reading and thus terminate the translation prematurely. Whenever a nucleotide pair is either inserted into or deleted from a coding sequence of a gene, the reading frame is shifted and from the insertion/deletion (*indel*) site onwards no longer gives a sensical translation (the change is then referred to as *frameshift mutation*). As explained earlier, insertions and deletions of nucleotides are commonplace at the coding junctions of rearranging gene segments. As long as indels involve three nucleotides or multiples of three, the correct reading frame is preserved across the junction. But if the indels consist of one, two, four, five, seven, eight or ten nucleotides, the frame is shifted and the translated protein becomes non-functional. Rearrangements that cause a frameshift are referred to as *non-productive*; those that create in-frame junctions are *productive*. Because many more indels result in out-of-frame than in-frame changes, most rearrangements are of the non-productive type.

If lymphocytes were to express the non-productively rearranged *TCR* genes on their surface, the immune system would be overwhelmed by non-functional cells. To prevent this from happening, each rearrangement is examined for productivity (functionality): the polypeptide chain specified by the rearranged gene is tested for its ability to associate with its partner chains and the complex is checked for its fit in the plasma membrane. (If the sequence changes drastically, the polypeptide fails to fold appropriately, and cannot link up with its partner.)

The rearrangements not only have to be tested for productivity, they must also be stopped as soon as functional chains leave the assembly line. If rearrangement were to continue, a cell would be cluttered with an assortment of receptors on its surface, each specific for a different antigen. The cell and its progeny (the clone) would be oligospecific instead of monospecific and could then be activated by a variety of antigens. A system based on oligospecific lymphocytes might have existed at an early stage in the evolution of adaptive immunity but it must have been extremely inefficient and probably developed later into a monospecific system. The latter requires that *V(D)J* recombinations at a given *TCR* locus are terminated the moment the first productive rearrangement is achieved. Because each *TCR* region is present in the cell in two copies (*alleles*), one on each chromosome of a pair, and because the probability that both rearranging copies would hit upon a productive combination simultaneously is very low, only one of the two alleles is expressed. The phenomenon is referred to as *allelic exclusion* because one of the two alleles is excluded from expression.

The mechanism for achieving allelic exclusion, and termination of *V(D)J* recombination in general, has not been elucidated; it may not be the same for all *TCR* genes. In the α:β lineage, the *TCRB* gene rearranges initially on one chromosome only and if the rearrangement is productive, no further rearrangement takes place on either of the two chromosomes. If it is non-productive, *V(D)J* recombination is attempted on the second chromosome and the rearrangements on both chromosomes then continue until a functional combination of segments is achieved. When that happens, a 'go' signal is given to the *TCRA* gene to proceed with its rearrangements. There are exceptions to this rule, however, which lead to the emergence of cells expressing two types of TCR differing in their β chains.

The *TCRA* genes, on the other hand, do not seem to be subject to any such regulation. Their rearrangement and expression does not prevent further *VJ* recombination. The *VJ* recombination of *TCRA* genes is terminated when the α:β TCR heterodimer on the cell surface binds to a self ligand (self-peptide bound to self-MHC molecule). In this way, the T cell usually ends up with a single α:β TCR on its surface, even though intracellularly it may generate several productively rearranged *TCRA* transcripts: the cells display a phenotypic but not genotypic *TCRA* allelic exclusion. In the γ:δ thymocyte lineage, the *TCRD* gene rearrangement may slightly precede the *TCRG* gene rearrangement but there seems to be a considerable overlap in timing between these two events. It seems therefore, that in this lineage rearrangements stop, presumably by a feedback mechanism, when a functional receptor is expressed on the cell surface.

Transcription of *TCR* genes

To *transcribe* something is to make a written copy of it, for example a speech recorded on magnetic tape. In molecular biology, *transcription* designates a process by which one strand of the double-stranded DNA tape is copied into a single strand of an RNA molecule (Fig. 7.11). The copying process, which is principally the same in *TCR* genes as in most other eukaryotic genes, is carried out by *RNA polymerase*, an enzyme that moves from one end of the coding sequence to the other, temporarily opening the double helix at those sites that it straddles. It then uses one of the two separated DNA strands as a template (*template strand*) for the assembly of complementary ribonucleotides: where the template has a T, G or C, the enzyme places an A, C or G, respectively; where it has an A, it places a U (uracil)-containing nucleotide.

To start its job, the enzyme must take up its position near the beginning of the coding sequence at the transcription *initiation site* (Fig. 7.12) marked by the sequence $N^{C}_{T}A^{CCCC}_{TTTT}$ (where N stands for any of the four nucleotides and $^{C}_{T}$ indicates the presence of either C or T at the particular nucleotide site). The A^{CC}_{TT} in this sequence are the first three nucleotides transcribed. However, the enzyme is

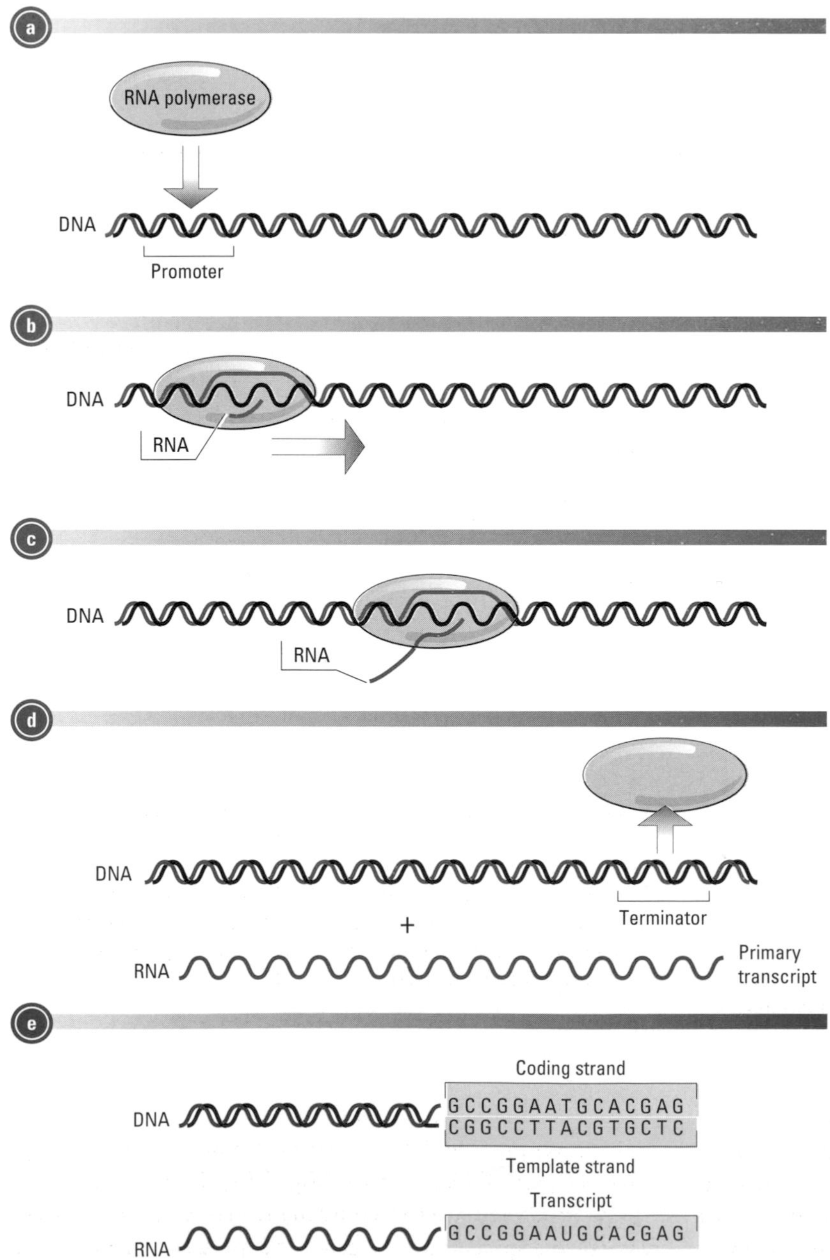

Figure 7.11 Transcription of *TCR* genes. (a) The enzyme RNA polymerase attaches itself to the transcription initiation site in the promoter region of the gene. (b, c) RNA polymerase moves along the gene downstream from the promoter region. At the site at which it is momentarily positioned, the enzyme transiently unwinds a region of the DNA helix and catalyses the attachment of one nucleotide after another to the growing RNA chain. One strand of the unwound DNA serves as a template for the assembly of the ribonucleotides by pairing transiently with their complementary bases. As the 'bubble' progresses, the DNA behind it resumes its double helix configuration and thus displaces the growing RNA strand. (d) When the RNA polymerase reaches the end of the gene, it is dislodged from the DNA double helix. In the meantime, however, other RNA polymerase molecules have attached themselves to the promoter region and are travelling downstream along the gene. (e) Of the two strands of the DNA molecule, one serves as a template for the RNA strand and the latter is therefore identical (except for the replacement of T by U) with the second (coding) DNA strand.

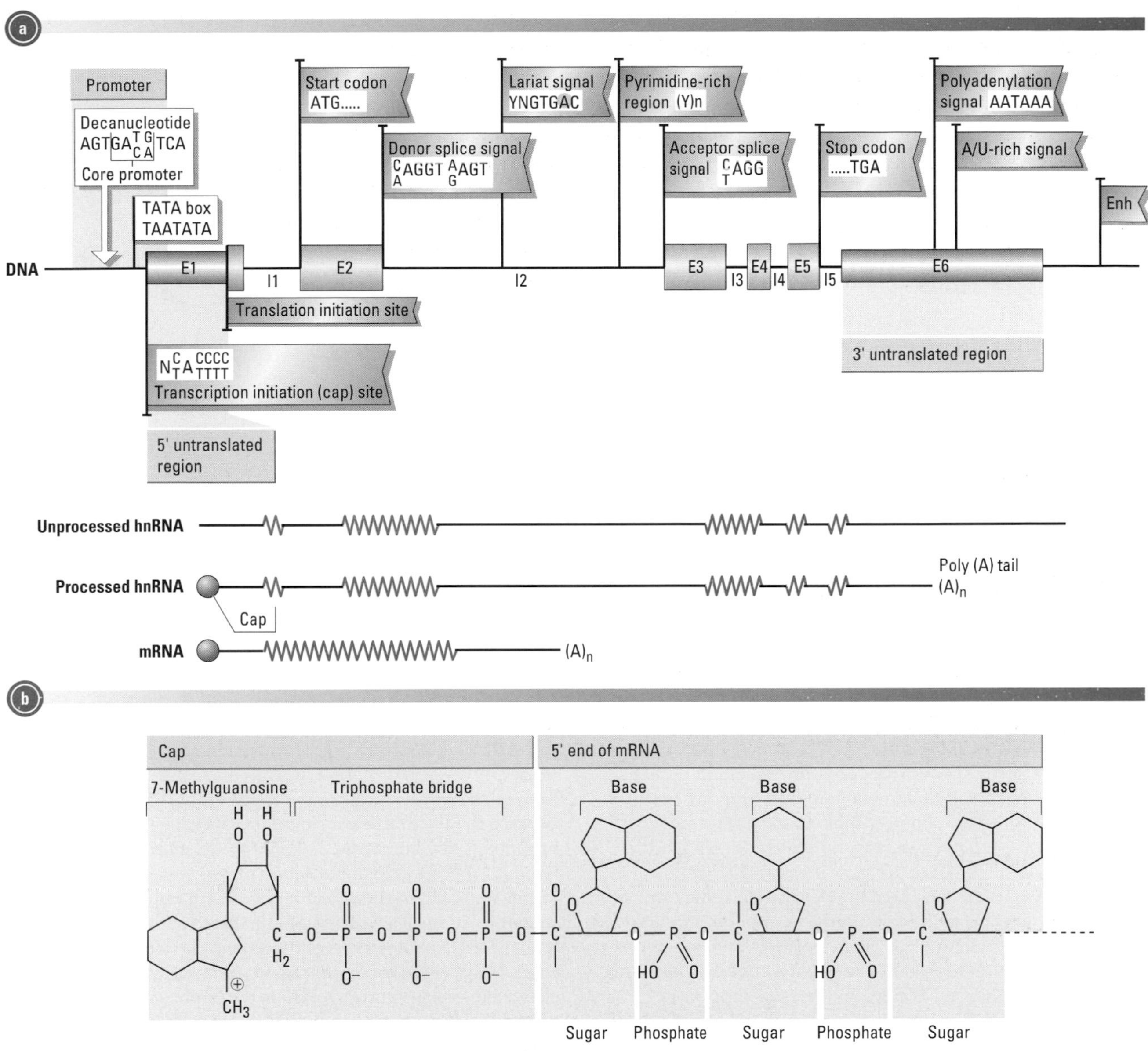

Figure 7.12 (a) Organization of a rearranged *TCR* gene and its transcript. The decanucleotide is the site of transcription factor binding (consensus sequence is given; when two different nucleotides frequently occur at the same site, they are both listed, one above the other); other transcription factors bind to the enhancer (Enh) sequences at the 3′ end of the gene (the sequences are given in Fig. 7.13). The TATA box is the site at which the TATA-box binding protein attaches itself. RNA polymerase begins transcription at the transcription initiation site. Splicing signals are shown only for intron 2; however, similar signals are also found in all other introns. The n in $(A)_n$ usually ranges from 150 to 200 adenosine residues. E, exons; hnRNA, heterogeneous nuclear RNA; I, intron; mRNA, messenger RNA; N, any of the four nucleotides; Y, pyrimidine (C or U). Red regions of the gene and of the transcripts are those that are translated into protein; grey segments represent the untranslated regions. (b) Structure of the 5′ cap at the 5′ end of the processed RNA.

unable to find the initiation site by itself; it must be placed into this position by other proteins, the *transcription factors*. Altogether, some 50 proteins are required to send the RNA polymerase off along the double-stranded track of the coding sequence. Some transcription factors possess specialized regions (domains; Fig. 7.13), by which they are able to recognize and bind to specific short stretches (*motifs* or *boxes*) of DNA sequence (Fig. 7.14). Some of the transcription factors are shared by many genes; others are used only by one gene or by one gene set expressed in a particular

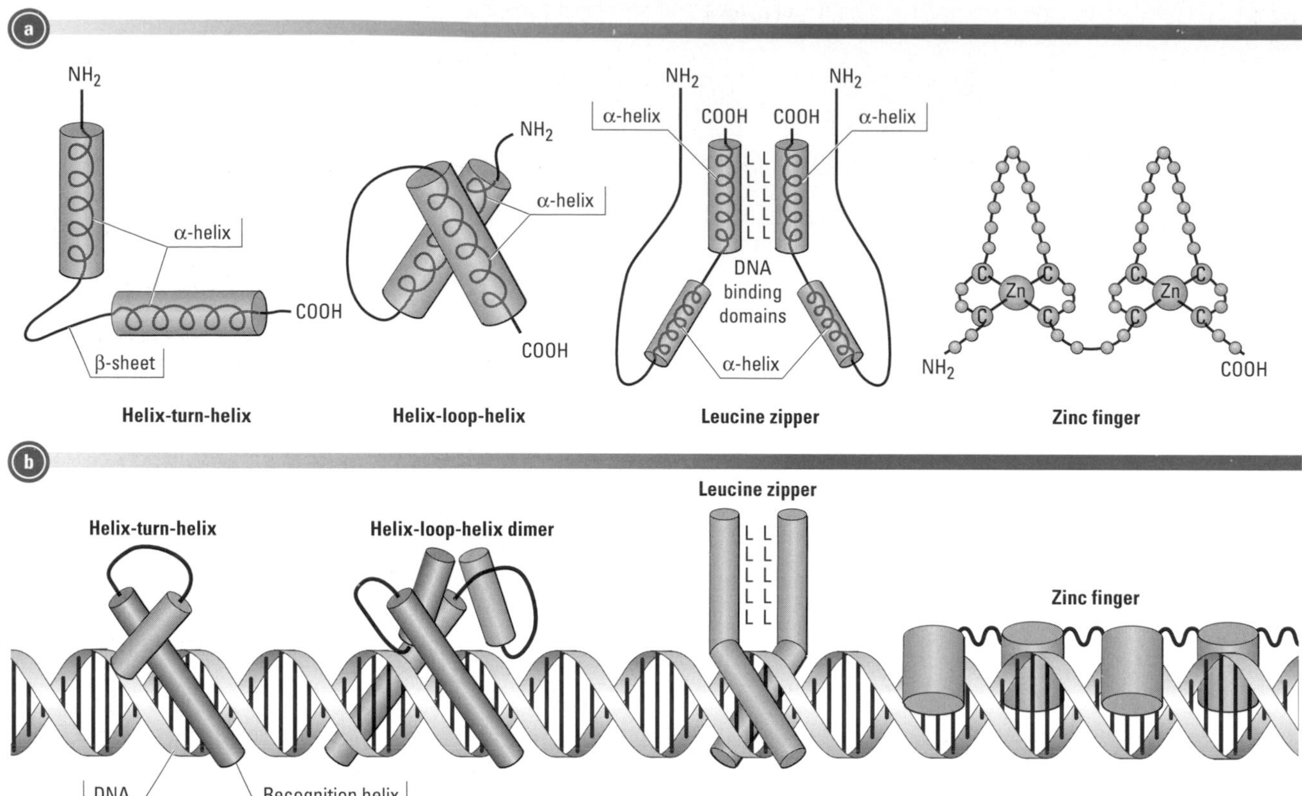

Figure 7.13 Examples of specialized DNA-binding domains in transcription factors. (a) Four types of structural motifs occurring in transcription factors. (b) Interaction of the four motifs with the DNA molecule. *Motif* is a simple combination of a few secondary structure elements (α-helix, β-strand, turn, loop) with a specific geometric arrangement. The *helix–turn–helix (HTH) motif* consists of two α-helices separated by a few (usually four) amino acid residues. The short turn positions the two helices into different planes. One of the two helices fits into the major groove of the DNA molecule and therefore acts as a *recognition helix* that interacts with the DNA nucleotides. In the *helix–loop–helix (HLH) motif* the two α-helices are separated by a flexible loop so that they can be packed into a single plane and interact not only with DNA but also with other protein molecules to form dimers. In the *zinc finger* motif properly spaced cysteines and/or histidines form bonds with a zinc ion (Zn^{2+}). The amino acid residues between the zinc-binding regions loop out into finger-like projections that interact with the DNA molecule. A *leucine zipper motif* is formed by the dimerization of two α-helices, each helix having a stretch of amino acid residues with leucine at every seventh position. The leucine side-chains of one coil snap together with the leucine side-chains of the second coil like the teeth of a zipper. Adjacent to the zipper segment is a stretch of positively charged (basic) residues involved in the binding to a specific region of a DNA molecule. C, cysteine; L, leucine; Zn, zinc.

tissue. The *combinations* of factors vary, however, from gene to gene so that each gene can only be transcribed efficiently when the combination of factors specific for that gene is assembled. Some of the transcription factors involved in the expression of human *TCR* genes are listed in Table 7.2.

The factors comprising the transcription apparatus fall into three categories: basal factors, activators/repressors and co-activators (Fig. 7.15). *Basal factors* take their name from the fact that, in a test tube, the assembly of these proteins enables the RNA polymerase to transcribe the gene it straddles at a basal level. For more efficient transcription, the participation of the activators and co-activators is required. Identical basal factors are generally shared by many genes. One of the basal factors binds to the DNA, specifically to the sequence TATA$^{A}_{T}$A$^{A}_{T}$ – the *TATA box* located upstream from the beginning of the coding sequence. This factor is therefore referred to as the *TATA binding protein* or TBP. The TATA box is part of a regulatory region termed the *core promoter* because it represents the heart of a region that furthers or promotes transcription of a gene. The regulatory sequences in the promoter region are shared by many genes.

Activators/repressors often vary from gene to gene. *Activators* bind to genes at sites known as *enhancers* and, by doing so, determine the specificity of the transcription process because only in their presence does the process run efficiently. Enhancers can be thousands of nucleotides

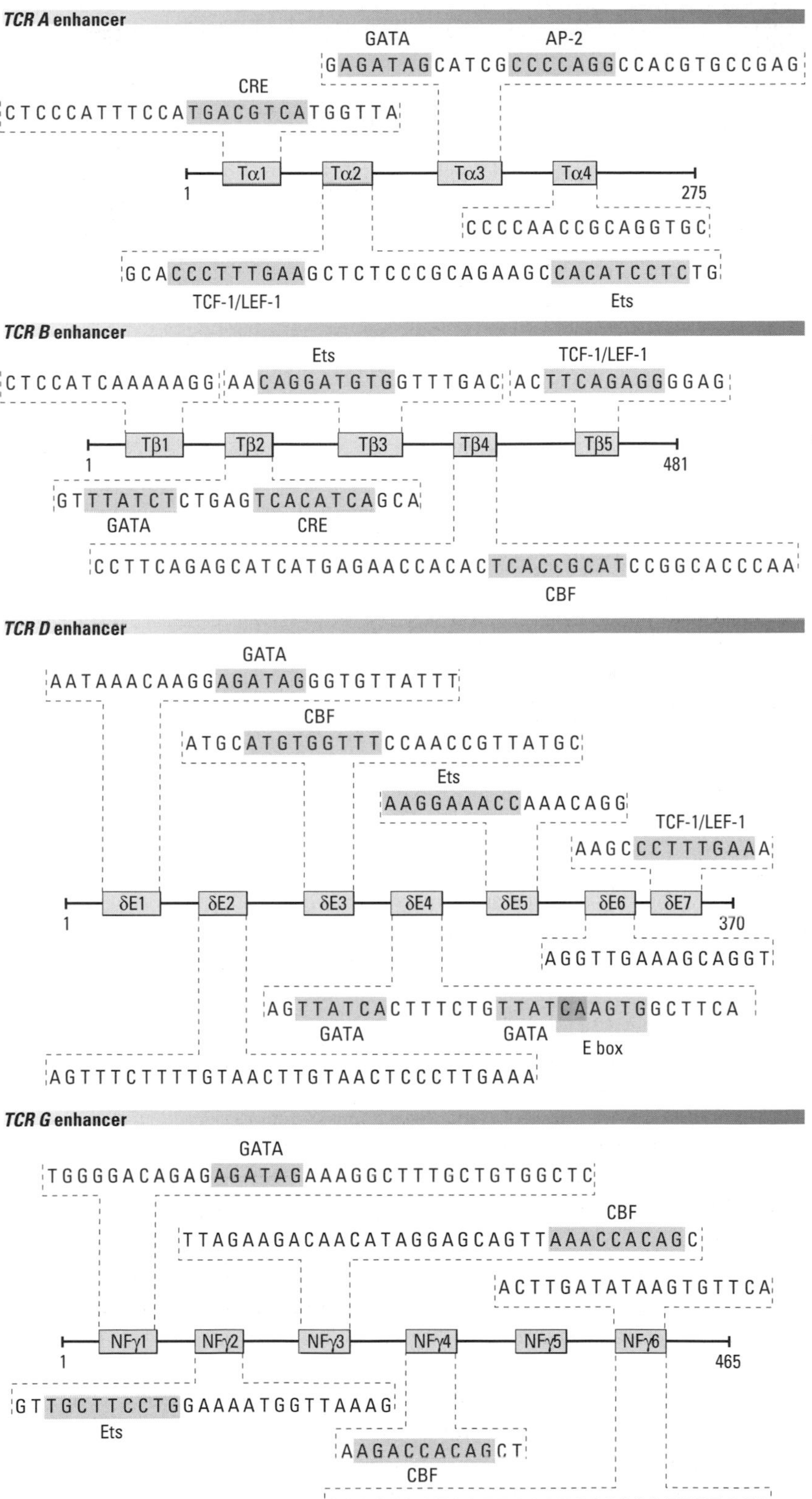

Figure 7.14 Enhancer sequences of human and mouse *TCR* genes. For the location of the enhancer region in each of the *TCR* genes, see Fig. 7.3. The numbers indicate the length of the enhancer region in nucleotide pairs. Only one strand of the DNA double helix is shown. The highly conserved segments of the sequence believed to be critical for interaction with transcription factors are boxed. The designations of the boxes refer to features characterizing either the sequence or the transcription factor that binds to it. AP, activation protein; CBF, core-binding factor; CRE, cyclic AMP-responsive element; Ets, E twenty-six (cellular homologue of a viral oncogene discovered in retrovirus 26); GATA, transcription factor that binds to the sequence WGATAR (where W stands for 'weakly coding bases' A or T, and R for a purine, A or G); LEF, lymphoid-specific protein with enhancer function; TCF, T-cell specific transcription factor. (Slightly modified from Leiden, J. M. (1993) *Annual Review of Immunology*, **11**, 539.)

Table 7.2 Transcriptional factors that regulate *TCR* gene expression. (Modified from Leiden, J.M. (1993) *Annual Review of Immunology*, **11**, 539–570.)

Transcription factor	Target *TCR* gene	Molecular mass (× 10^3)	DNA-binding domain	Recognition sequence	Lineage specificity
CREB		43	Basic domain/leucine zipper		Ubiquitous
CRE-BP1/ATF-2/mXBP	*A, B*	55	Basic domain/leucine zipper	TGACGTCA	Ubiquitous
ATF-4		38	Basic domain/leucine zipper		Ubiquitous
TCF-1	*A, B, D*	30	HMG box		T cells
TCF-1α/LEF-1		53–57	HMG box	${}^{C}_{T}\mathrm{CT}^{C}_{T}\mathrm{T}^{GAA}_{TTT}$	T cells/pre-B cells
Ets-1	*A, B, G, D*	54–60	Basic domain/α helix	${}^{GA}_{CC}\mathrm{GGA}^{T}_{A}\substack{A\\G\\C}{}^{C}_{T}\mathrm{G}$	T cells/B cells
GATA-3	*A, B, D*	47	2Cx zinc fingers	$\substack{A\\T}\mathrm{GATA}\substack{A\\G}$	T cells/kidney/brain
CBF	*B, G, D*	19–40	?	$\substack{C\\T\\A}{}^{T}_{C}\mathrm{G}^{T}_{C}\mathrm{GG}^{TTT}_{CCA}$	Thymus/spleen

ATF, adenovirus transcription factor; CBF, CCAAT box-binding transcription factor; CRE, cyclic-AMP-responsive element; CREB (P), CRE-binding (protein); Ets, E twenty-six (cellular homologue of a viral oncogene discovered in retrovirus 26); GATA, transcription factor that binds to the sequence WGATAR (where W stands for 'weakly bonding bases' A or T, and R for a purine, A or G); HMG, high mobility group; LEF, lymphoid-specific protein with enhancer function; TCF, T-cell specific transcription factor; TCR, T-cell receptor; XBP, X-box binding protein; 2Cx, two cysteine.

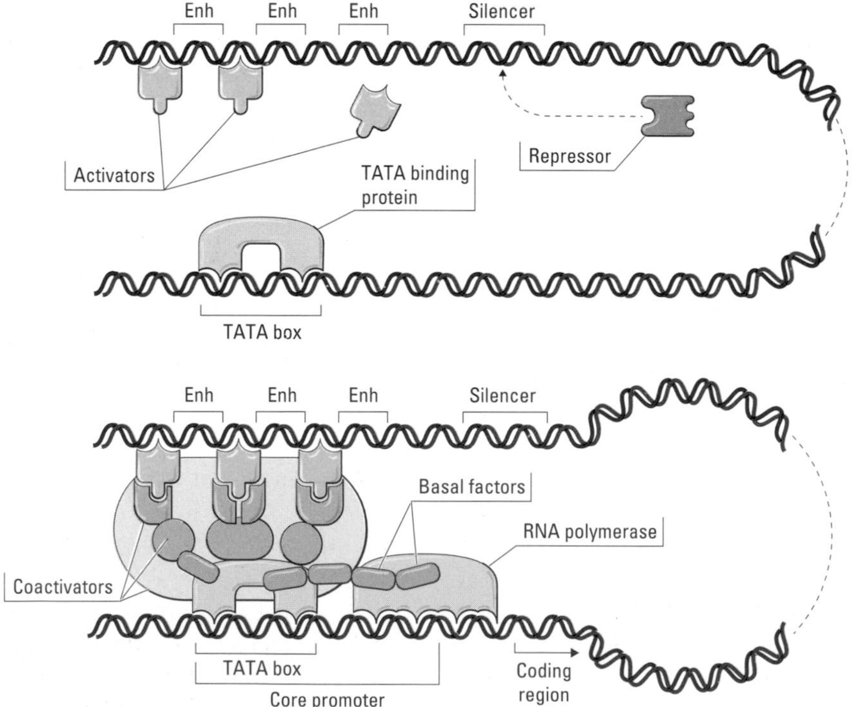

Figure 7.15 Assembly of the transcription apparatus. The entire coding sequence of a *TCR* gene is located between the promoter and enhancer regions. The three types of proteins forming the apparatus (activators/repressors, co-activators and basal factors) are differentiated by degrees of shading. The assembly begins with the attachment of the TATA-binding protein (TBP) to the TATA box of the core promoter region and the attachment of the activators to the enhancer (Enh) sequences (for simplicity only three are shown). It then continues with the assembly of other basal factors around the TBP and the attachment of the co-activators, which bring the activators and basal factors together into a single complex. Once assembled, the apparatus positions the RNA polymerase at the transcription initiation site and transcription of the coding sequence commences. The presence of the silencer in the vicinity of the *TCR* gene is hypothetical.

distant from the initiation site, either upstream or downstream. To be able to take part in the assembly of the transcription apparatus, the enhancer-bound activators must therefore loop-out the DNA between the enhancer and the promoter regions (see Fig. 7.15). The enhancers of the *TCR* genes are generally located downstream from the C segment (see Fig. 7.3); at this position, they are not in danger of being deleted by the rearrangement process.

The task of decelerating transcription or bringing it to a halt entirely when enough mRNA has been manufactured falls to the *repressors*. These proteins bind to specific DNA sequences termed *silencers* and thus apparently interfere with the function of the activators. The activators, and presumably also the repressors, interact with the basal factors via the *co-activators*.

The assembly of the transcription apparatus is probably initiated by the binding of the TBP to the TATA box in the promoter region and by the binding of the activators to the enhancer elements. The co-activators then bring the two assembling complexes together. Once the apparatus is fully assembled and the RNA polymerase is positioned at the transcription initiation site, the enzyme is sent off along the gene like a handcar on a railroad track. Once the first molecule is on its way, the second sets off, and then the third and so on, at a rate determined by the activators. As it rolls along the track, each molecule makes one RNA copy of the template DNA strand, the primary transcript. When it reaches the end of the gene, presumably marked by some as yet unidentified signal sequence, it slides off the DNA double helix and the transcript dislodges from it. During the entire transcription process, the DNA remains wound around the protein components of the nucleosomes and attached to the swivel on the nuclear matrix. The *primary RNA transcript* (*pre-mRNA*) immediately associates with proteins, assuming the appearance of a string of beads. It then joins the pool of *heterogeneous nuclear RNA (hnRNA)*.

While still in the nucleus, the newly synthesized RNA strand is *processed*. Some of the processing reactions (i.e. capping, methylation and polyadenylation) take place before the synthesis is completed, while others (i.e. splicing) occur after transcription (see Fig. 7.12). *Methylation* was described earlier. *Capping* involves the addition of a 7-methylguanosine residue (a 'cap') via a triphosphate bridge to the first nucleotide of the transcript, a reaction catalysed by the enzyme guanyltransferase (see Fig. 7.12b). The enzyme presumably recognizes a specific sequence, the *cap site*, generally YNNNYAYYYYY, where Y is a pyrimidine (C or U) and N is any of the four nucleotides. The function of the cap is to bind the RNA to a ribosome once it reaches the cytoplasm. *Polyadenylation* is the addition of 150–200 adenosine residues (*poly (A) tail*) to the 3′ end of the transcript. The poly (A) tail, however, is not appended to the very end of the primary transcript; a portion of the 3′ segment is clipped off and the tail is added to the newly generated end. Clippage and addition is effected by a complex of proteins assembling at a specific sequence (the *polyadenylation signal*) of the pre-mRNA, slightly upstream from the cleavage site.

In the final processing step, all the introns are removed from the transcript and the exons are joined together in a process resembling *splicing* of magnetic tape during its editing. Splicing is effected by an even larger complex of proteins than polyadenylation and these proteins, too, assemble around specific stretches of sequences at the exon–intron borders and in the intron (the *splicing signals*; see Fig. 7.12).

Translation of TCR transcripts

The processed transcript, mRNA, is delivered into the cytoplasm where its nucleotide sequence is converted into an amino acid sequence, i.e. it is *translated*, with the help of at least two other RNA types (ribosomal and transfer RNA) and a host of different proteins. However, not all of the mRNA sequence is translated; the two ends, the 5′ and 3′ UT regions, do not specify any amino acids. The translated sequence is delineated by the *start codon* AUG and the stop codons UGA, UAA or UGA. The function of the 5′UT region is to assemble the *translation apparatus* in the vicinity of the start signal and to position it correctly; the function of the 3′UT region is less clear, but it is probably associated with the termination of translation and disassembly of the apparatus. The sequence between the start and the stop signals represents an *open reading frame* (ORF) in which the uninterrupted succession of nucleotide triplets (*codons*) specifies the order of amino acids in the encoded polypeptide. The first 20 or so amino acids form the *signal peptide (leader sequence)*. After about 70 amino acids have been linked together on a ribosome, the signal peptide is recognized by the *signal recognition protein* (SRP), which in turn is recognized by a receptor, the *docking protein*, on the endoplasmic reticulum (ER; Fig. 7.16). Assisted by the docking proteins, the signal peptide enters the ER membrane, crosses it and emerges on its luminal surface. As the polypeptide chain grows, it follows the signal peptide and it, too, threads through the ER membrane. Its interaction with the membrane is facilitated by its high content of hydrophobic amino acids. Apart from these characteristics, there are no other common features of the signal peptides of different proteins.

As soon as the entire signal peptide has emerged on the

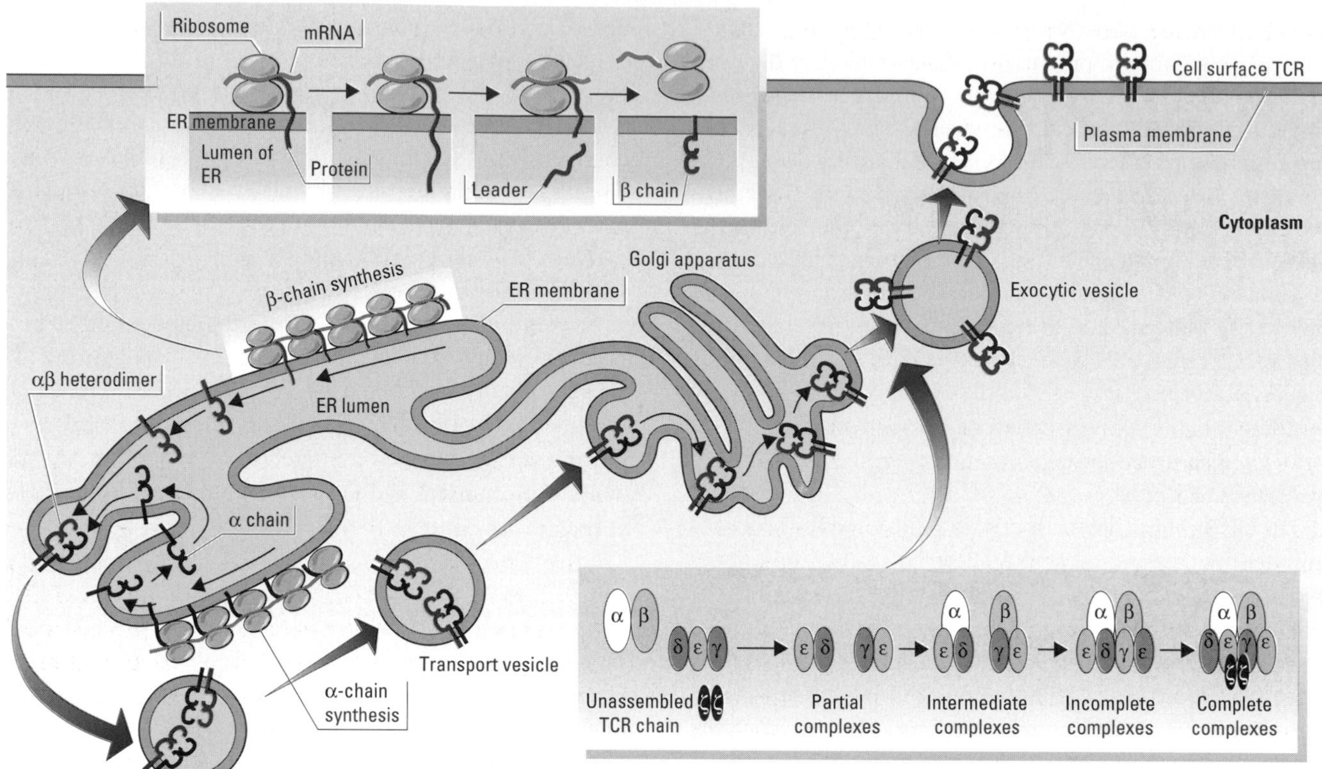

Figure 7.16 Biosynthesis of TCR molecules on membranes of the endoplasmic reticulum (ER). Synthesis of the CD3 complex molecules is not shown for the sake of simplicity; the stages of TCR–CD3 complex assembly are given in the lower inset. The upper inset depicts removal of the signal peptide from the growing polypeptide chain on the luminal side of the ER. In the main figure the arrows indicate the individual stages of biosynthesis, beginning with manufacture of the β chain (upper left) and followed by synthesis of the α chain, dimerization of the two chains, transport of the TCR complex in vesicles to the Golgi apparatus for additional glycosylation and, finally, transport of the fully processed TCR to the cell surface.

luminal side of the ER, it is clipped off by a special *signal protease* residing in the ER membrane (Fig. 7.16 inset). The cleavage site is located at the carboxyl end of a neutral amino acid of the polypeptide chain. The clipped-off signal peptide is then degraded in the lumen of the ER.

As the chain emerges on the luminal side, disulphide bonds form between the cysteine residues. Intramolecular disulphide bonds form while the chain is still growing. The formation of disulphide and other bonds leads to protein folding, which may be one of the forces that pulls the polypeptide through the membrane. Simultaneously, the nascent polypeptide is *glycosylated*: side-chains consisting of three glucose, nine mannose and two *N*-acetylglucosamine residues ($Glc_3Man_9GlcNAc_2$) are attached to emerging asparagine residues (N-linked oligosaccharides) at three to four glycosylation sites. This initial glycosylation is followed immediately by processing of the core oligosaccharides: the stepwise removal of glucose residues by glucosidases in the ER. The partially glycosylated protein threads through the membrane until another segment consisting largely of hydrophobic amino acid residues, the *transmembrane region*, begins to emerge. Once a point is reached at which the transmembrane region spans the ER membrane, the movement stops, presumably because the hydrophobic residues of this region establish a stable interaction with the lipid bilayer and the charged amino acid residues at the end of the transmembrane region anchor the polypeptide. (The retention of TCR β chains is more efficient than that of TCR α chains; the latter often pass into the lumen unhindered and are then degraded.) The transmembrane tunnel is then disassembled. At this stage, the N-terminus and the bulk of the protein are in the lumen, whereas the C-terminus, together with a short tail, are in the cytoplasm outside the ER.

The two TCR chains, α and β in some cells or γ and δ in others, are synthesized separately, as are the accessory chains CD3γ, CD3δ, CD3ε and ζ (these are described later in this chapter). The various chains then associate with one another in the ER membrane in a certain predetermined order (see Fig. 7.16). First, the CD3 chains associate non-covalently into two heterodimers, CD3δε and CD3γε. Second, the TCR α chains associate with the CD3δε dimers and the TCR β chains with the CD3γε dimers, yielding intermediate TCRαCD3δε and TCRβCD3γε protein complexes, respectively. Third, the intermediate complexes associate with each other and disulphide bonds form between the TCR α and β chains, resulting in incomplete TCRαβCD3δεγε complexes. And fourth, the ζ chains form ζζ homodimers, which then associate with the incomplete TCR–CD3 complexes to yield complete TCRαβCD3δεγεζζ complexes. The associations of proteins into complexes are believed to be assisted by at least two molecular chaperone proteins: the *T-cell receptor-associated proteins* (TRAP), which appear to be specific for the CD3γε protein pairs; and *calnexin*, which is capable of interacting with all the TCR–CD3 chains, but not with the ζ chains. Both chaperones dissociate from the TCR–CD3 proteins before their egress from the ER.

Unassembled TCR and CD3 chains are retained within the ER and degraded. Fully or partially assembled TCR–CD3 complexes exit the ER and are delivered, probably in *transport vesicles*, which pinch off from the ER, to the *trans Golgi compartment* (see Fig. 7.16). The partially assembled complexes are then sorted to lysosomes for degradation, whereas the completely assembled complexes are processed further in the Golgi compartment. As the proteins pass through the Golgi apparatus, they are glycosylated further: a variety of additional sugar residues is added to their core oligosaccharides. Other modifications of the TCR complexes may also occur in the Golgi apparatus before the *mature proteins* emerge from it on the *trans* face. The number of N-linked oligosaccharides added to the TCR chain varies: in the human TCR, the α, β and δ polypeptides each contain four, one and two oligosaccharide chains, respectively. The γ chain exists in three versions, γ1, γ2(2*x*) and γ2(3*x*), which have three, four and five glycosylation sites, respectively. The γ1 and γ2 polypeptides have their C regions specified by different gene segments, *TCRGC1* and *TCRGC2*, respectively. The two versions of the γ2 polypeptide, 2*x* and 3*x*, are specified by different alleles of the *C2* segment, which differ in having part of their sequence duplicated (2*x*) or triplicated (3*x*). As a consequence of these changes, the γ2(2*x*) and γ2(3*x*) polypeptides are 16 and 32 amino acid residues longer than the γ1 chain, respectively. In the α:β, as well as in most of the γ:δ heterodimers, the two polypeptides are linked by interchain disulphide bonds near the transmembrane region. Only the γ2(3*x*) version of the γ chains associates with the δ chain non-covalently. The finished products are sorted out from the rest of the membrane-bound molecules, accumulated in circumscribed portions of the *trans* face of the Golgi apparatus and then included in the vesicles budding off from these portions. The vesicles separate from the Golgi apparatus and deliver their cargo of TCR complexes to the plasma membrane nearby. There the membranes of the vesicles fuse with the plasma membrane and the vesicles open (*exocytosis*), thus exposing the TCR complexes to the milieu outside the cell. The complexes have now been delivered and the long odyssey from the gene to the cell surface comes to an end. The synthesis of the TCR γ and δ chains presumably occurs according to the same principle as that of the α and β chains, but the details of this process are not known.

There are, however, certain differences between mature and immature T cells in the way they produce TCR proteins, particularly the TCR α chain. Most of the TCRα protein synthesized in immature CD4+CD8+ thymocytes undergoes rapid degradation, perhaps because of altered processing of one of the oligosaccharide side-chains by the glucosidases in the ER. The half-life of thymocyte TCRα is only 15 min, compared with >75 min in the mature T cell. Because of the rapid degradation, the formation of TCR–CD3 complexes available for transport to the cell surface is severely limited and the cell-surface TCR density is low. The attachment of a ligand to the TCR of the double-positive thymocyte delivers a signal that leads to increased TCR α-chain synthesis compensating for the loss through degradation. The thymocyte then expresses intermediate levels of TCR on its surface. A delivery of a second signal via the engagement of the co-receptor with its ligands is then believed to lead to the stabilization of the TCR α chain and consequently to a further increase in TCR cell-surface density to the level observed in mature T cells.

In the α:β lineage the immature thymocyte also expresses initially a different form of the TCR, the *pre-TCR*, which is not expressed on mature T lymphocytes. The pre-TCR consists of the TCR β chain associated with a *pre-TCR α chain* (pTCRα). The latter will be described in more detail later in this chapter; here it suffices to say that it is encoded in a separate gene expressed during the entire thymocyte development but not in the mature T cell (see also Chapter 5). During *TCRB* recombination, the pTCRα chain may provide means of testing the productivity of rearrangements: β chains incapable of associating with the pTCRα chain are presumably rejected and the recombination continues or, if all options have been exhausted, the cell dies; β chains capable of associating with the pTCRα chain are displayed (together with the accessory proteins) on the cell surface as the pre-TCR. The expression of the pre-TCR and later of the mature TCR are two important checkpoints in the development of the α:β thymocyte at which important decisions are made about the cell's fate (Fig. 7.17). By the time a thymocyte has arrived in its development at check-

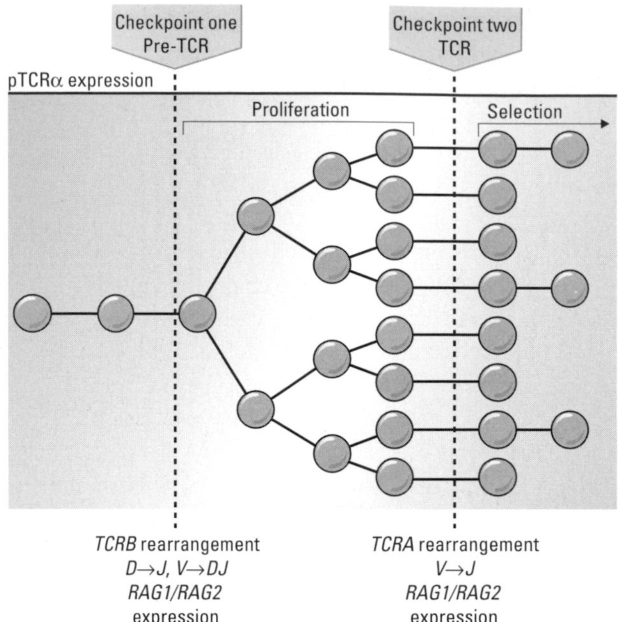

Figure 7.17 The two-checkpoint concept of α:β thymocyte differentiation. Explanation in the text.

point 1, it has activated *RAG1/RAG2* and with them the entire recombination machinery, it has successfully taken the first two steps in the recombination process (it has accomplished the $D_B \rightarrow J_B$ and $V_B \rightarrow DJ_B$ transpositions) and it has expressed the pre-TCR on its surface. At checkpoint 1, the pre-TCR is believed to trigger intense proliferation of the thymocytes and thus their clonal expansion; to downregulate temporarily *RAG1/RAG2*; and to shut off further recombination at the *TCRB* locus. During the period of clonal expansion, TCR recombination is suspended and it is reactivated only when the cells return to a resting state at the end of the period. At this time, *RAG1/RAG2* are upregulated again and the one-step ($V \rightarrow J$) rearrangements at the *TCRA* locus commence. Successful *TCRA* rearrangement and expression of the mature TCR brings the cells to checkpoint 2, at which decisions are made based on the interactions of the TCR with its ligands. During this phase, *RAG1/RAG2* remain active, presumably providing a possibility for α-chain editing of the type observed in the case of immunoglobulin light chains (see Chapter 5). After passing checkpoint 2, the cells shut off the expression of the pTCRα chain and extinguish the expression of *RAG1/RAG2* permanently. A period of selection of the type described in Chapter 5 then follows.

The γ:δ thymocyte lineage presumably passes through similar checkpoints. There is, however, no evidence for the existence of a surrogate TCR chain (the pTCRα associates neither with TCR γ nor δ chains; the expression of *TCRD* and *TCRG* is not clearly separated in time; and the clonal expression in the thymus is apparently much more limited in extent in comparison with the α:β lineage.

Structure of TCR proteins

The rearranged human *TCR* gene has five protein-specifying exons, two in the *V* segment and three in the C segment (Fig. 7.18). Exon 1 of the *V* segment encodes the leader peptide, which does not appear in the mature protein; exon 2 of the *V* segment specifies the variable part of the TCR polypeptide, the *variable (V) domain*. It derives its name from the fact that polypeptide chains encoded in the same locus differ by as much as 40% of their amino acid sequence. Exon 1 of the C segment encodes the *constant (C) domain* of the TCR polypeptide chain, so named because virtually all the chains encoded in the same locus, no matter how much they differ in the V domain, are identical, and when differences do occur they involve less than 5% of amino acid residues. Exon 2 of the *C* segment specifies the *connecting peptide*, which joins the extracellular part of the TCR chain (V + C domains) to the *transmembrane region*. The latter anchors the chain in the plasma membrane and connects it to a short *cytoplasmic tail* on the inside of the cell (Fig. 7.18). In human *TCR* genes, the transmembrane region and the cytoplasmic tail are encoded in one exon but in some other genes they are specified by separate exons.

The V and C domains each contain two invariant cysteine residues between 50 and 80 amino acid residues apart (depending on the domain, chain and species) and located some 20 residues from the ends of the domains (each domain has a length of approximately 110–115 residues). The two cysteines of each domain link up by forming a disulphide bond between their sulphur atoms. The bonding is made possible by looping out the entire intervening sequence and bringing the two cysteine residues close together (Fig. 7.19). The connecting peptide, which is about 15–30 amino acid residues long, normally contains one cysteine residue that forms a disulphide bond with the corresponding cysteine of the partner chain (α with β and γ with δ). This interchain disulphide bond is one of the links holding the two polypeptides of the heterodimers together (Fig. 7.19); the other links occur via non-covalent bonds. In those versions of the human γ chain in which the corresponding region of the C_G segment has been duplicated or triplicated, the connecting peptide assumes a configuration that does not allow the formation of the interchain bond. The γ:δ heterodimers with these versions of the γ chain are therefore not linked by the interchain disulphide bond; they are held together by non-covalent bonds only (Fig. 7.19).

Because crystals of TCR proteins are difficult to produce,

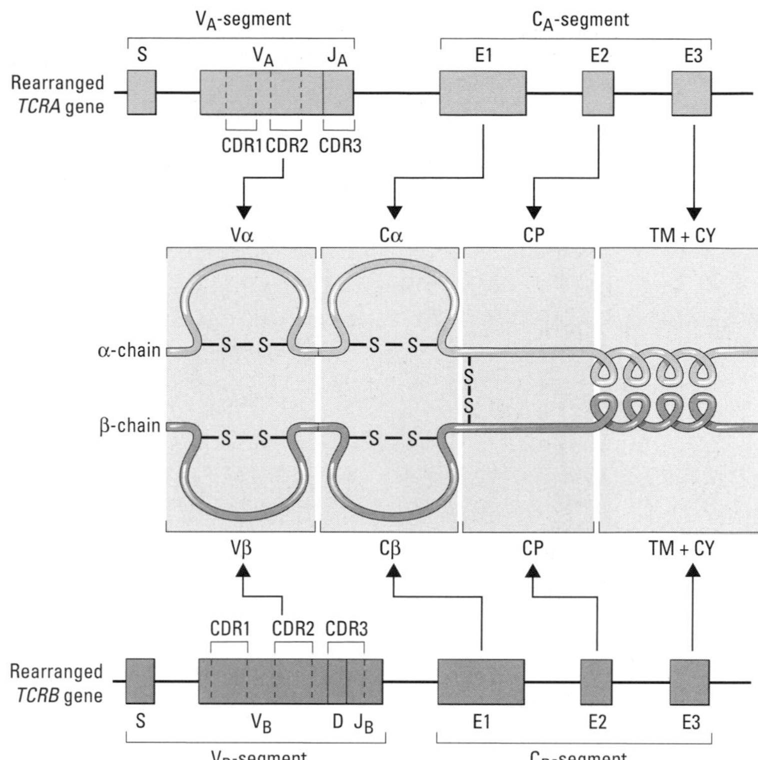

Figure 7.18 Relationship between rearranged *TCRA* and *B* genes and TCR polypeptide α and β chains. E, Exon; CP, connecting peptide; CY, cytoplasmic tail; C, constant region; CDR, complementarity-determining regions (explained later in the text); S, signal peptide; TM, transmembrane region; V, variable region.

the tertiary structure of the TCR has not been fully elucidated as yet. Thus far only crystals of truncated mouse β chains (without α chains, carbohydrates, transmembrane regions and cytoplasmic tails) and of V_α-domain homodimers have been obtained and subjected to X-ray diffraction analysis. The analysis of β-chain crystals has revealed that the organization of the V and C domains is very similar and also closely resembles the organization of the immunoglobulin V and C regions. The basic element of the tertiary structure of both the V_β and C_β domains is a sandwich in which the two bread slices represent the β-pleated sheets (Fig. 7.20). One sheet of the domain is composed of three and the other of four antiparallel β-strands connected by loops. The two sheets are held together by the disulphide bond located approximately in the centre of the domain, and by non-covalent bonds. In the V_β domain, there are additional β-stranded regions that are not part of the β-pleated sheets. If we designate the β-strands of the C_β domain by letters *a–g* in the order in which they follow one another in the polypeptide chain, starting from the N-terminus, we see that strands *a*, *b*, *d* and *e* form one β-pleated sheet, while strands *c*, *f* and *g* form the other (Fig. 7.20). In the V_β domain, there are two β-strands (*c′* and *c″*) inserted between strands *c* and *d*. In this domain, most of the amino acid variability is concentrated in the loops connecting strands *b* and *c*, *c* and *d*, *f* and *g*, as well as *d* and *e*; these loops are the *complementarity-determining regions* (CDR1, CDR2, CDR3) and *hypervariable (HV4) region*, respectively. The term 'complementarity-determining' refers to the widely held view that the amino acid residues in these regions interact, on the principle of complementarity, with the residues of the peptide–MHC assemblages. The loops do indeed all congregate on the very surface of the TCR molecule which comes in contact with the peptide–MHC assemblage. The interaction between the TCR and a viral peptide bound to the HLA-A2 molecule has been elucidated by X-ray crystallography. The study has revealed the relatively flat surface area by which the TCR contacts the MHC/peptide assemblage to be roughly rectangular and to be oriented diagonally to the roughly rectangular peptide-binding region of the class I MHC molecule (Fig. 7.21). The CDR1 of the TCRα chain contacts the N-terminal part of the peptide (residues P1 through P5) and the α-helix of the N-terminal part of the MHC α1 domain. The CDR1 of TCRβ contacts the C-terminal part of the peptide (residue P8) and hovers over (but does not contact) the C-terminal part of the MHC α1 domain. The CDR2 of TCRα does not contact the peptide, but does interact with the α-helix of the C-terminal part of the α2 domain. The CDR2 of TCRβ, surprisingly, contacts neither the peptide nor the N-terminal part of the α2 domain over which it hovers. The CDR3s of the TCRα and

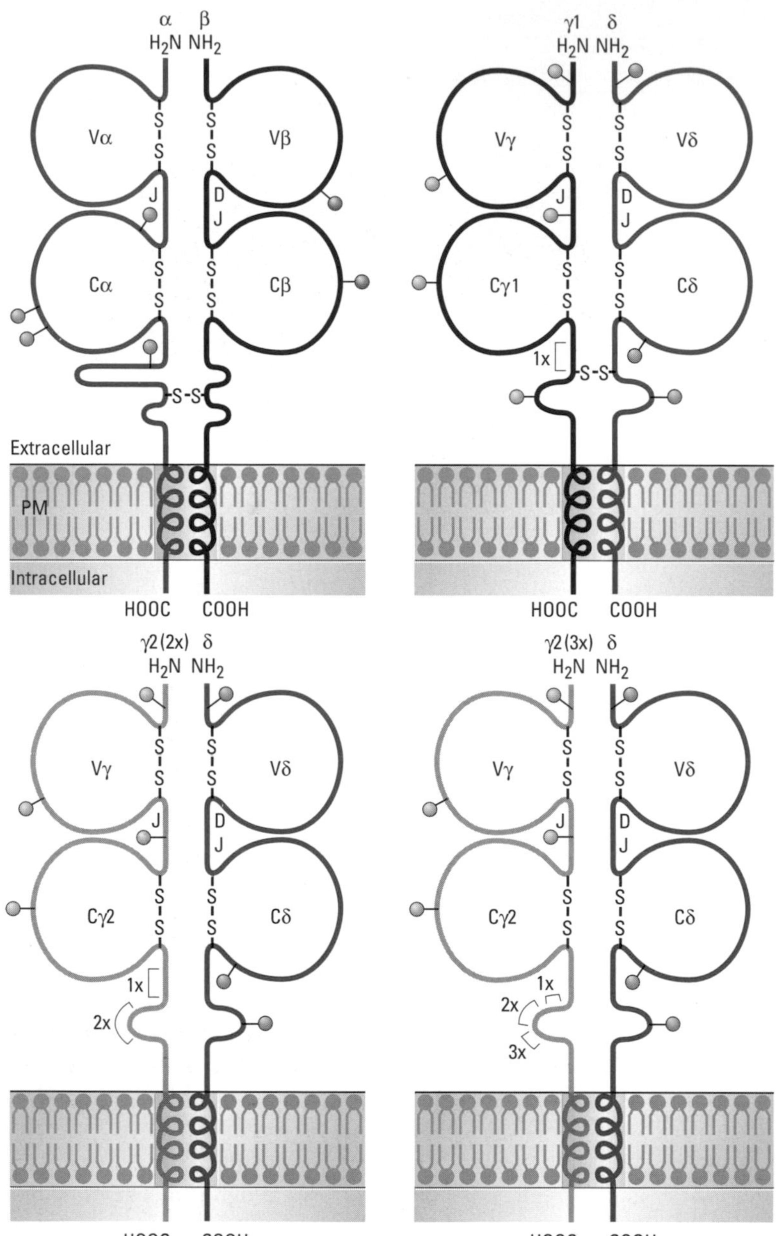

Figure 7.19 Human α:β and γ:δ TCRs, including the forms comprised of three γ-chain variants. The difference between the variants is in the connecting peptide specified by exon 2 of the constant segment in which a short stretch has been duplicated [γ2(2*x*)] or triplicated [γ2(3*x*)]. The added sequence increases the molecular mass of the γ chain from 40 000 (γ1) to 44 000 [γ2(2*x*)] or 55 000 [γ2(3*x*)], and results in the absence of the interchain disulphide bond (S–S). Carbohydrate side-chains are indicated by the symbols ⚬– and ⚬–.

TCRβ chains converge in the centre of the MHC groove, where the gap between them forms a deep pocket into which the peptide residue P5 protrudes. You may recall that it is this residue that arches up out of the groove, while the remaining residues are stretched out within the groove (see Chapter 6). Both CDR3s interact with the P5 residue and, in addition, CDR3 of the TCRβ chain interacts with the P6, P7 and P8 residues. The two CDR3s also contact the α-helix of the MHC molecule — CDR3α the α1 domain, and CDR3β the α2 domain. The extent to which these findings can be generalized remains to be seen. The nature of the interaction between the class II MHC/peptide assemblage and the TCR has not been elucidated. It is believed, however, that the TCRα chain binds to the equivalent of the class I α2 domain, whereas the β chain does not contact the MHC molecule but interacts with the so-called superantigens (see Chapter 13). The superantigens act as a wedge between the TCR and MHC molecule, thus preventing the recognition of the peptide by the TCR, and sidestepping the requirement for specificity in T-cell activation.

The surface of the V_β domain has one region that is predominantly occupied by hydrophobic amino acid residues. This is probably the region that comes in contact with a similar hydrophobic region of the α chain in the α:β

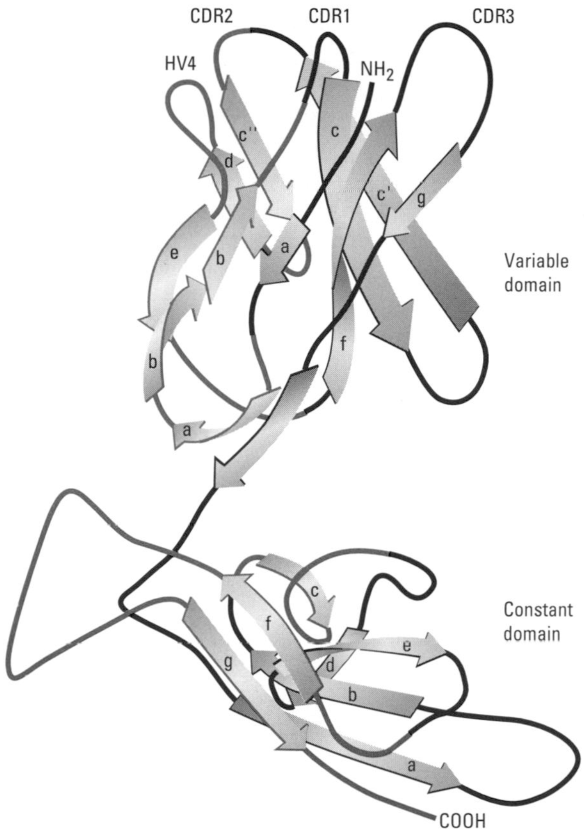

Figure 7.20 Tertiary structure of V_β and C_β TCR domains as deduced from X-ray diffraction analysis: ribbon model. Arrows symbolize β-strands oriented in the N- to C-terminus direction. The two β-pleated sheets of each domain are distinguished by shading. The β-strands of each domain are designated by letters in the order in which they follow each other in the polypeptide chain. (Based on X-ray crystallographic data of Bentley, G. A. *et al.* (1995) *Science*, **267**, 1984.)

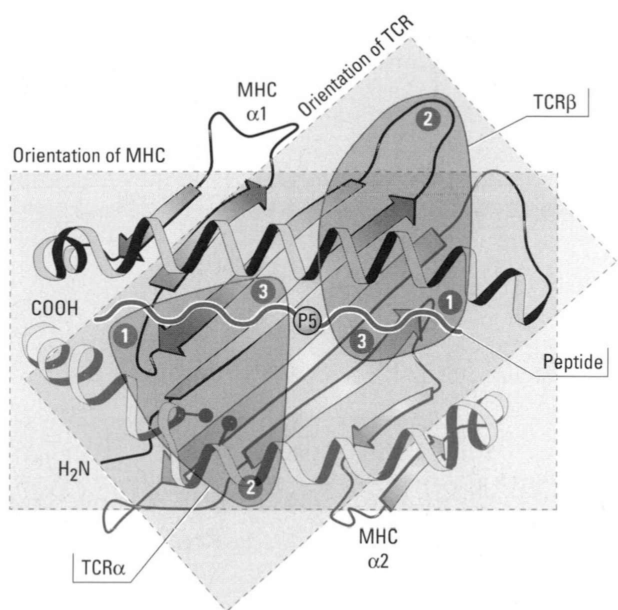

Figure 7.21 Interaction between the TCR and the MHC/peptide assemblage. The peptide-binding groove of the class I MHC molecule occupied by the peptide as seen from the top (see Fig. 6.38). Superimposed upon it is an outline of the TCR binding surface provided by the α and β chains. Approximate positions of the CDR1, CDR2, and CDR3 loops are indicated by the numerals. The mutual orientation of the MHC and TCR molecules is diagrammed by the rectangles. NH_2 and COOH are the amino and carboxyl termini of the MHC α chain; α1 and α2 are the two peptide-binding domains of the MHC class I molecule. (Based on data of D.N. Garboczi *et al.* (1996) *Nature*, **384, 134.**)

heterodimer. The hydrophobic interactions between these two regions (interactions based on the exclusion of water molecules) apparently contribute to the stability of the heterodimer. There is, however, no such hydrophobic region on the surface of the C_β domain; this entire surface is accessible to water molecules. The region of presumed interaction of C_β with C_α has a net negative charge and the interaction may therefore occur largely via salt-bridge formation between oppositely charged residues at the α:β interface.

The interaction between the V_β and C_β domains takes place across extensive, chiefly hydrophobic surfaces provided by highly conserved amino acid residues. In contrast to immunoglobulin molecules in which the V and C domains are connected by a rather flexible hinge (see Chapter 8), in TCR molecules the two domains appear to be in intimate contact with each other, which allows for very little flexibility. This relative structural rigidity may facilitate changes in the shape of TCR molecules, which may occur with their binding to peptide–MHC assemblages; and the transmission of these changes to the CD3 molecules. The interaction between the TCR and CD3 molecules may be mediated by the large protruding loop on the external surface of the C_β domain between β-strands *f* and *g*. The loop contains extra residues at positions 219–232 that are not found in the corresponding region of immunoglobulin molecules.

The V_α domain exists as a homodimer both in solution and in crystals. It is believed that the association of two V_α domains is not an artifact but rather that a similar association of two TCR molecules apposed by their V_α domains takes places also on the T-cell surface. Since MHC dimers are also believed to dimerize (see Chapter 6), it is thought that the interaction with peptide-loaded MHC dimers stabilizes the weak TCR dimers sufficiently to result in receptor activation. The structure of the V_α homodimer resembles that of the immunoglobulin V_LV_H heterodimer (see Chapter 8) with one important difference between the two.

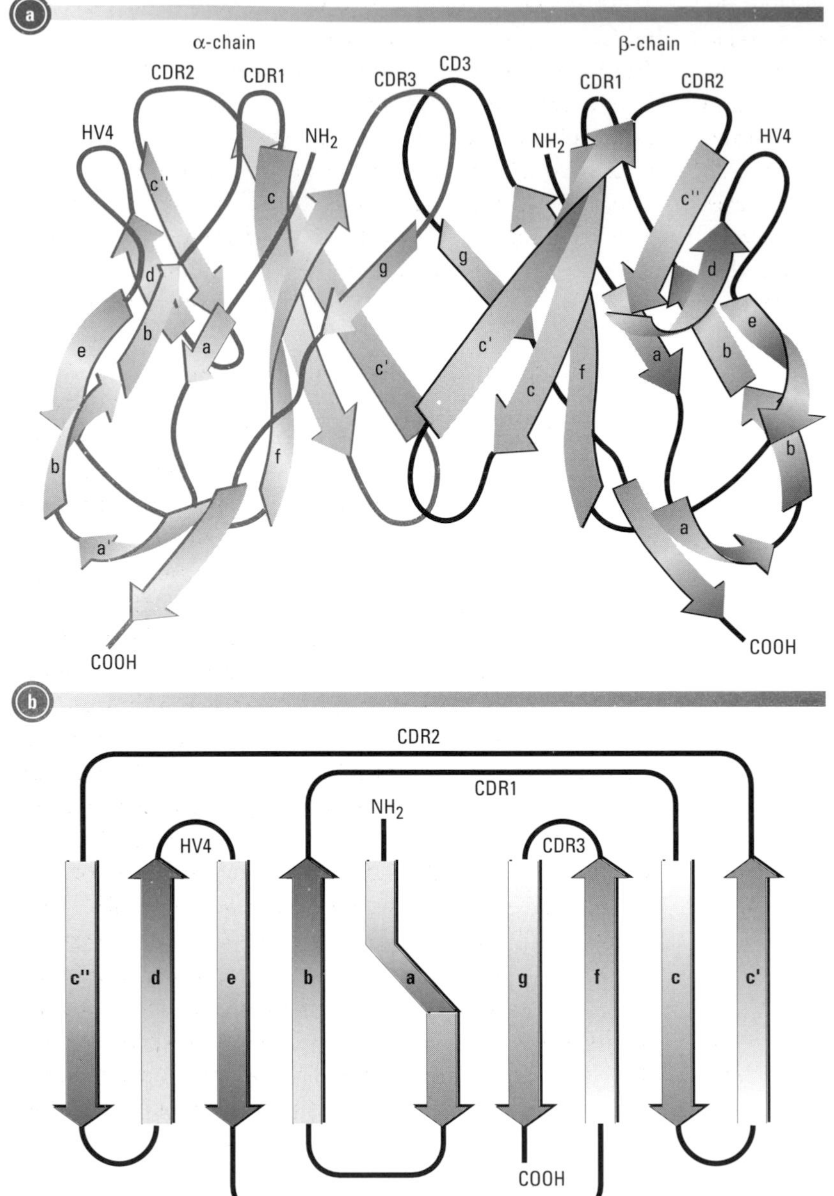

Figure 7.22 Tertiary structure of TCR V_α homodimers. (a) Ribbon model. (b) Diagrammatic representation of folding topology in a single V_α domain. The shading distinguishes the two V_α domains in (a) and the two β-sheets in (b). Arrows symbolize β-strands identified by letters in the order from the N- to the C-terminus. CDR, complementarity-determining region. (Modified from Fields, B. A. *et al.* (1995) *Science*, **270**, 1821.)

In the immunoglobulin V domains (as well as in the TCR V_β domain), the *c″* strand is hydrogen bonded to the *c′* strand in the same β-sheet. In V_α, the *c″* strand is associated with the *d* strand of the adjacent sheet via six backbone-to-backbone hydrogen bonds (Fig. 7.22). The two V_α monomers are held together by numerous van der Waals contacts and 10 hydrogen bonds across the homodimer surface.

The secondary and tertiary structure of the connecting peptide, transmembrane region and cytoplasmic tail of the TCR is not known. In the α:β and γ1:δ TCR, the connecting peptide of the two chains is presumably arranged in such a way as to allow the formation of the interchain disulphide bonds. In the γ2:δ TCR, the structure of the connecting peptide is disturbed to the extent that these bonds can no longer form. The transmembrane region is rich in hydrophobic amino acid residues (leucine, isoleucine, methionine, valine, alanine), as is expected from a peptide buried in the hydrophobic environment of the plasma membrane. Surprisingly, however, it also contains positively charged (basic) residues, in particular lysine. How the charges are accommodated in the hydrophobic milieu is not known but the residues are believed to be involved in the formation of salt bridges with the chains of the CD3 complex. The charged residues near the entrance into, and the exit from, the membrane might help to anchor the polypeptide by interacting with other charged molecules at the interface. Part of the transmembrane region at least seems to assume a helical conformation. The 20–22 amino acid residues of the region could accommodate approximately six α-helical turns but the actual number is probably smaller than that. The length of the cytoplasmic tail varies considerably among the different chains but is generally relatively short, consisting of a few residues only. Whether the tail has any function other than anchoring is unclear.

TCR diversity

The principle of adaptive immunity demands that for every possible peptide, an organism can provide a matching receptor. To fulfil this requirement, mammals, exemplified by *Homo sapiens*, have combined several mechanisms that together produce a receptor repertoire whose size is essentially limited only by the number of lymphocytes in the body. In the case of the TCR these mechanisms include stockpiling of variable gene segments in the genome, combinatorial diversity and junctional diversity.

V-segment stockpile

During their evolution, mammals have stored a significant portion of TCR variability in their genomes in the form of tandem arrays of *V* segments. These arrays are passed from parents to offspring and thus represent a basic variability endowment that each individual expands further using other diversification mechanisms. In humans, the variability endowment consists of some 100 *V* segments (the precise number is not known because new *V* segments are still being discovered and because an unknown proportion of the described *V* segments are non-functional pseudogenes; in addition, individuals may differ in the number of *V* segments they carry at the four loci). The stockpile at each locus can be classified into groups, families and individual members. The four loci (*TCRA*, *TCRB*, *TCRG* and *TCRD*) are known to contain 42, 64, 6 and 6 *V* segments, respectively (not counting orphons but including pseudogenes). The classification into groups and families is based almost exclusively on sequence similarity. By convention, a nucleotide sequence identity of less than 50% is taken as an indication that two segments belong to different groups; a nucleotide sequence identity of greater than 50% but less than 75% assigns two segments to different families; and members of the same family are identical in 75% of their nucleotide sequence or more. TCR families are numbered *V1*, *V2*, *V3* and so on, separately for each locus; members of individual families are numbered *V1S1*, *V1S2*, *V1S3*..., *V2S1*, *V2S3*..., separately for each family. The full designation is then, for example, *TCRAV1S1* (*A* locus, *V1* family, *S1* member of this family, where 'S' stands for 'sequence'). In an alternative, not officially sanctioned nomenclature, segments are designated by Greek letters (e.g. 'Vα1.1'). Some members occur in distinct versions (alleles) and these are distinguished by another row of numbers following an asterisk. The numbers of human TCR groups, families and members are given in Table 7.3; an example of the hierarchical classification appears in Fig. 7.23.

The hierarchy probably reflects the evolution of *V* segments by segment duplication. The first rounds of duplication produced ancestral *AV*, *BV*, *GV* and *DV* segments; subsequent rounds produced ancestors of the groups and families; and the most recent rounds of duplications produced multiple members in some of the families (Fig. 7.23). Most duplications occurred more than 60–80 my ago, before the separation of the major orders of eutherian mammals, as indicated by the comparison of human (as a representative of the primate order) and mouse (as a representative of the rodent order) *V* segments. The degree of relationship between sequences can be expressed in the form of a diagram resembling a tree, a *dendrogram* (Fig. 7.24). A comparison of dendrograms drawn first for sequences of one species (for example the human *TCRBV* segments in Fig. 7.24a) and then for sequences of two species (for example the human and mouse *TCRBV* segments in Fig. 7.24b) show similar branching patterns (*topologies*) and intermingling of segments from both species on the branches. These patterns are consistent with the hypothesis that most of the duplications pre-dated the divergence of primates and rodents; had they occurred after the divergence, all the human *V* segments would be on one

Table 7.3 Human TCR *V* segments.

Locus	Number of Groups	Families	Members
TCRAV	6	32	42
TCRBV	5	34	64
TCRGV	–	6	14
TCRDV	–	3 (6)*	6

* Three *TCRDV* segments appear to be used in the generation of the δ chain exclusively; they are designated *TCRDV101*, *TCRDV102* and *TCRDV103* (numbers above 100 are used to avoid confusion with *TCRAV* segments). Three other segments (*TCRADV6*, *TCRADV17* and *TCRADV21*) have been found to be used in the generation of both the α and the δ chains and there may be more *V* segments in the *TCRA/D* complex used in the same way.

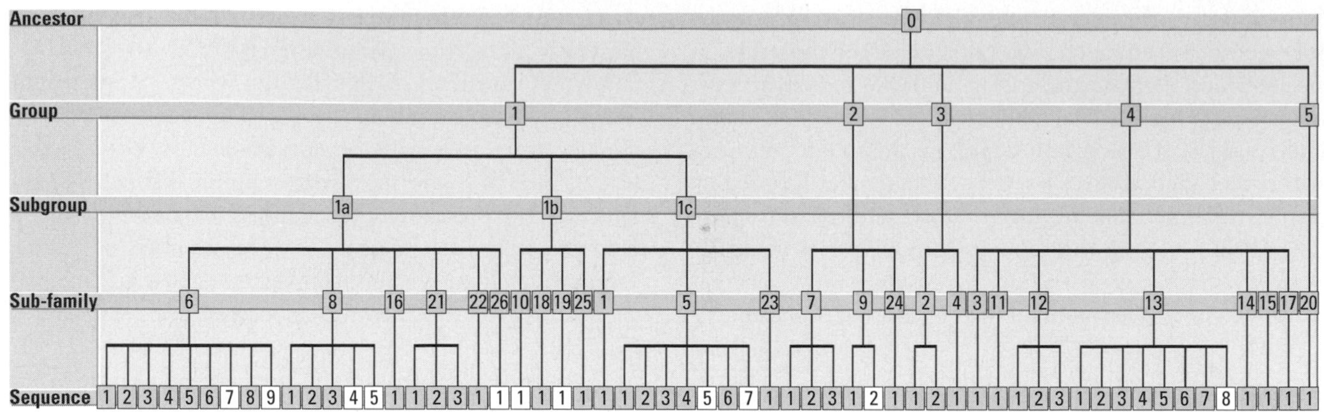

Figure 7.23 Classification of *TCRBV* segments into groups, subgroups, families and individual family members. The hierarchy presumably reflects the origin of extant sequences from a single ancestral sequence by a series of duplications. Closed rectangles in the 'Sequence' row represent segments that are presumably functional; open rectangles indicate known pseudogenes. (Numbering of individual sequences, families, etc. is as used by Arden, B. *et al.* (1995) *Immunogenetics*, **42**, 455.)

branch and all the mouse sequences on another branch of the tree.

Combinatorial diversity

Since the TCR is a heterodimer and both its chains are involved in the recognition of the peptide–MHC assemblage, one chain combined with different versions of the partner chain together produce receptors with different specificities. If we restrict our considerations to differences encoded in the *V* segments, we can calculate how many different α:β and γ:δ receptors can theoretically be created by the combinations of distinct chains. In the case of the human TCR the numbers are $45 \times 48 = 2160$ for the α:β heterodimer and $6 \times 6 = 36$ for the γ:δ heterodimer (counting only functional genes and leaving out pseudogenes, see Table 7.3; the actual numbers of combinations are probably lower than those calculated because some of the *V* segments currently considered to be functional may in fact be pseudogenes). These numbers also give the total scores of possible CDR1 and CDR2 variants that are specified exclusively by the *V* segments. And since presumably the CDR1 and CDR2 interact with the MHC molecule (and not with the peptide), the α:β and γ:δ TCRs can recognize only 2160 and 36 different MHC molecules, respectively. If, on the other hand, we assume that the *D* and *J* segments also contribute to the MHC-recognition sites of the chains, then the number of possible combinations increases correspondingly to $2160 \times 2 \times 61 \times 13 = 3.2 \times 10^6$ combinations for the α:β TCR and $36 \times 3 \times 4 \times 5 = 2160$ combinations for the γ:δ TCR (see Table 7.1).

Let us assume, however, that the CDR1 and CDR2 sites are indeed encoded exclusively in the *V* segments and that the *D* and *J* segments (possibly together with 3′ parts of the *V* segments) encode the CDR3, which interacts exclusively with the MHC-bound peptide. How many peptides would the human TCR then recognize? Ignoring the possible contribution of the *V* segments and considering purely combinatorial possibilities, the estimated number is rather low: $61 \times 2 \times 13 = 1586$ for the α:β TCR and $3 \times 4 \times 5 = 60$ for the γ:δ TCR. The number increases somewhat when one considers that the β chains can be constructed from either one or two (and the δ chain from up to three) *D* segment-encoded peptides. Since a chain containing one *D* segment-encoded peptide will have different binding specificity than a chain containing two or three such peptides, the ability to transcribe and translate more than one *D* segment doubles or triples the number of potential combinations available for peptide recognition. This combinatorial variability, however, is still not enough: the α:β TCRs must be able to differentiate many more than 5000 peptides. The source of this additional variability are the events that take place when the *V* segment joins the *D* (or the *J*) segment and the *V–D* segment joins the *J* segment during TCR gene rearrangement.

Junctional diversity

Earlier in this chapter we learned that after the break at the border between the heptamer of the recombination signal and the *V*, *D* or *J* segment, the coding ends are joined together into a hairpin which then opens up to produce single-stranded sequence stretches at the newly generated ends (see Fig. 7.8). Even if they are not attacked by enzymes,

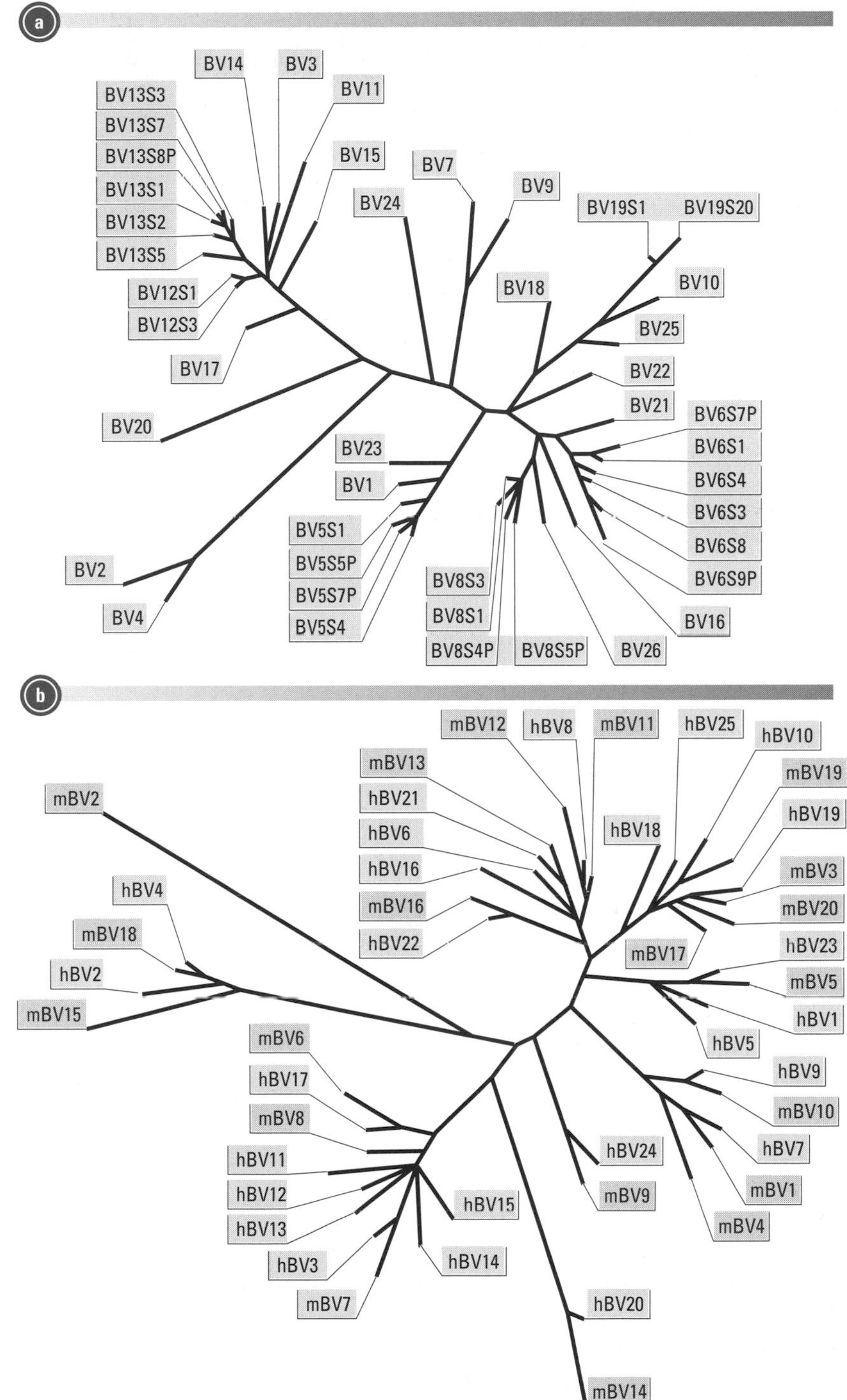

Figure 7.24 Phylogenetic tree (dendrogram) of *TCRBV* sequences. (a) Human *TCRBV* sequences (all known distinct sequences are included). (b) Human (h) and mouse (m) sequences (only one representative sequence of each subfamily is included). In symbols such as *BV8S1*, 'B' stands for β-chain encoding, 'V8' for variable segment subfamily and 'S1' for sequence (member) 1. P, pseudogene. The trees reflect the degree to which individual sequences are related to one another and hence, by extension, their possible divergence from one another during evolution. Dendrograms were constructed by the neighbour-joining method (see Fig. 6.29). (a, From Arden, B. *et al.* (1995) *Immunogenetics*, **42**, 455; b, from Clark, S.P. *et al.* (1995) *Immunogenetics*, **42**, 531.)

the single-stranded sequence stretches template the addition of P-nucleotides absent in the germ-line genes. When an attack by enzymes does occur, some nucleotides of the single-stranded regions are removed and other, non-templated or N-nucleotides are added to the free ends. As both these mechanisms are, for the most part, governed by chance, a different product results from each rearrangement of the same *V*, *D* and *J* segments and thus leads to *junctional diversification*.

The *D* segment provides another source of junctional diversity. Whereas the *V* and *J* segments each have only one ORF (so that if a nucleotide deletion or addition changes the frame, the rearrangement becomes non-productive) in each of the *D* segments all three frames are open. For example, if the original sequence of a *D* segment is:

GGG	ACA	GGG	GGC
Gly	Thr	Gly	Gly

then after the deletion of the first nucleotide the frame shifts and the sequence translates thus:

GGA	CAG	GGG	GC
Gly	Gln	Gly	

(The last two nucleotides may also be deleted, they may form a complete codon if another nucleotide is added to them or they may be read with two nucleotides of the *J* segment from which the first nucleotide has been deleted.) If the first two nucleotides are deleted from one *D* segment, the reading frame shifts further to the right and the remaining sequence reads:

GAC	AGC	GGG	G
Asp	Arg	Gly	

(Here again, the remaining single nucleotide can be either deleted, form a codon with added nucleotides or be read with nucleotides from the *J* segment.)

Because the outcome of the rearrangement at the segmental junctions cannot be predicted, it is also difficult to estimate the extent to which junctional diversification contributes to overall TCR diversity. An educated guess puts the numbers at 10^{11} and 10^{9} different CDR3 sites for the α:β and γ:δ TCR, respectively.

TCR repertoire

Speculating about theoretical possibilities is one thing; finding the actual TCR specificities among lymphocytes is another entirely. One cannot expect all possible TCR variants to be represented among T cells or to occur at the same frequency. Even if there were no influences to bias the selection of individual gene segments for new rearrangements, the effects of positive and negative selection in the thymus and antigen stimulation outside the thymus should be expected to skew the repertoire of mature T cells. To determine which TCR specificities the thymocytes and mature T cells actually possess, immunologists have principally used two kinds of methods, one based on antibodies and the other on molecular probes. In the former, a suspension of T cells with the same TCR specificity is inoculated into an animal, which then produces *antibodies* reacting with this particular type of TCR. By immunizing different animals against various T-cell suspensions, a panel of antibodies can be produced in which each antibody is specific for a different receptor. The antibodies, labelled with a suitable compound for visualization, are then used in one of the assays described in Chapter 14 to determine the number of T cells to which each of the antibodies binds. *Molecular probes* are short nucleotide sequences, each complementary to a variable (unique) part of a given TCR segment. In its single-stranded form, the probe can be tested for its ability to find a complementary strand in a pool of transcripts isolated from thymocytes or T lymphocytes. The binding can be revealed in different ways, for example by the *polymerase chain reaction* (PCR) or by the RNase protection assay. The principle of PCR, a method used frequently for various purposes in immunology as well as in many other fields of study, is explained in Fig. 7.25. In the *RNase protection assay*, the bound probe protects the transcript from degradation by the enzyme ribonuclease T1, which digests single-stranded RNA molecules and thus all those transcripts that have not found a guardian probe. (The enzyme also digests the unbound probe.) The probe–transcript hybrids that remain after RNase treatment can be identified according to their size when separated by electrophoresis in a polyacrylamide gel. None of these methods allows the investigator to determine the TCR specificity of each of the many millions of T lymphocytes in every single individual. By necessity, the observations are therefore restricted to a small number of individuals selected from a large population and hence are associated with a substantial error range. It is therefore hardly surprising that the results of the individual studies are sometimes contradictory.

A priori, one might expect to find different repertoires in individuals bearing disparate MHC molecules and also in helper T (T_H) lymphocytes as compared to cytotoxic T (T_C) lymphocytes: in the former because of the MHC's intimate involvement in shaping the T-cell repertoire; in the latter because of the close association between MHC class II and CD4 molecules (which earmark the T_H cells) on the one hand and MHC class I and CD8 molecules (characterizing the T_C cells) on the other. Yet, even these influences have proved difficult to demonstrate. No influence of *MHC* gene types on the T-cell repertoire could be found in randomly selected, unrelated persons. In studies carried out on large families, however, *MHC*-identical siblings had more similar distribution patterns of V_B-segment frequencies than *MHC*-disparate siblings; yet, at the same time, no evidence for *MHC*-affected usage of V_A segments could be found. Similarly, an indication that CD4+ T cells preferentially use certain *V* segments, while CD8+ cells use different ones has been obtained in some studies but not in others. Evidence for intrinsic rearrangement preferences, which may override MHC- or CD4/CD8-dependent influences, has also been reported: in one study of human thymocytes, as few as

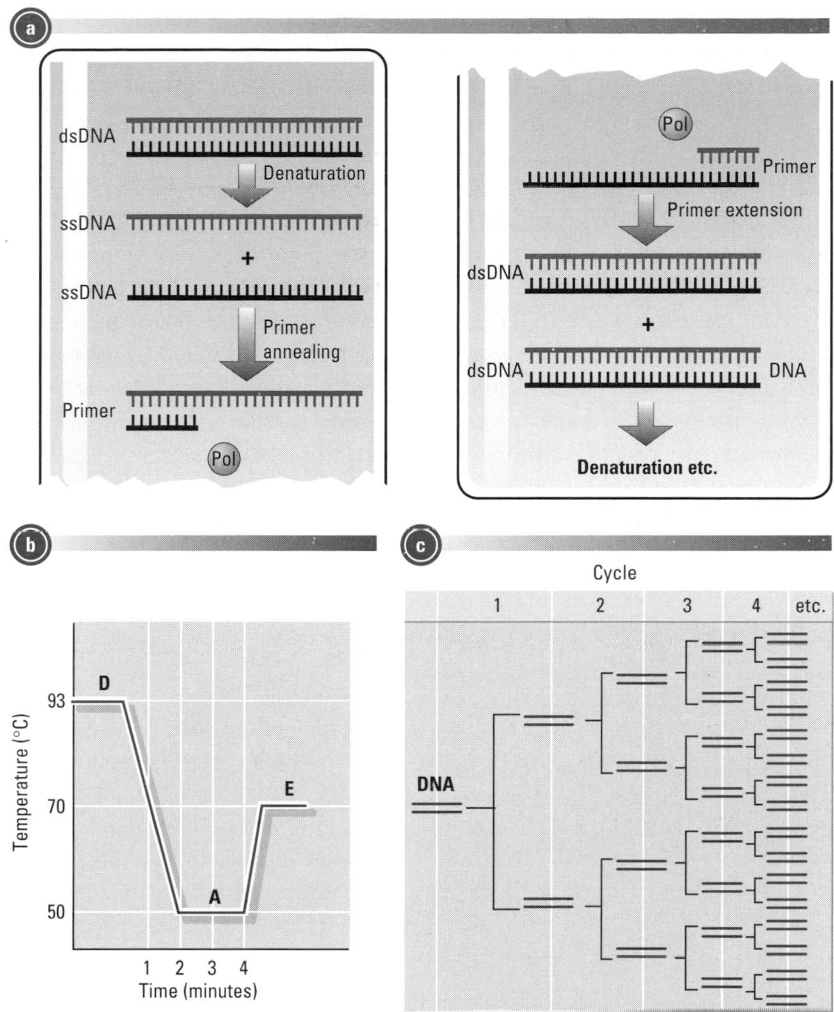

Figure 7.25 Principle of the polymerase chain reaction (PCR). (a, b) A solution containing double-stranded DNA (dsDNA) molecules, two primers (short stretches of nucleotides, one complementary to a DNA segment of one strand, the other to a segment on the opposite strand, usually less than 1000 nucleotides 'downstream' from the first), the four types of nucleotides from which DNA molecules are synthesized in the form of deoxynucleoside triphosphates, and heat-resistant DNA polymerase (pol; an enzyme necessary for DNA synthesis) is heated to 93 °C. This is the temperature at which the bonds holding the two DNA strands together break and the single strands (ssDNA) separate from each other (*denaturation*, D). The temperature is then reduced to approximately 50 °C, a condition at which the primers (but not the separated DNA strands) find and establish bonds with their complementary sites (*primer annealing*, A). In the third step, the temperature is raised to 70 °C, an optimum for the activity of *Taq* DNA polymerase, an enzyme isolated from the hot-spring bacterium, *Thermus aquaticus*. The enzyme attaches to the primer and then moves along the ssDNA template, adding one complementary nucleotide after another, all the way to the end of the strand (*primer extension*, E). Because the same thing happens on the second strand, two identical dsDNA molecules are produced. The 70 °C temperature is too high for DNA polymerases of most other organisms to function but not high enough to denature the DNA molecules. After completion of the first cycle of the reaction, in the next cycle the temperature is raised again to 93 °C and the steps are repeated. This reaction cycle is repeated 30 times or more in a special machine capable of achieving rapid temperature changes (*thermocycler*). (c) The number of copies of DNA molecules increases rapidly from cycle to cycle as if by chain reaction: the original single molecule produces two molecules, which produce four molecules, which produce eight molecules and so on, until the reaction mixture runs out of ingredients. Thirty reaction cycles produce 3×10^{10} copies of the target sequence.

seven *V* segments from different families were found to contribute to almost half the TCR β-chain repertoire. In general, however, the observed bias in the TCR repertoire has, with one exception, been relatively minor. The exception is the effect of the Mls antigens on the T-cell repertoire in the mouse.

Certain viruses have the ability to insert their genetic material (after it has been converted from single-stranded RNA to double-stranded DNA) into the chromosomes of the host cell. If such an insertion occurs in a germ cell that is then used in the creation of a new individual, these *retroviral genes* can be passed on from generation to generation as if they were the host's own genes. Many, if not all, mammalian species have different retroviral genes integrated at various places in their chromosomes and some of the genes encode molecules that are expressed on the surfaces of the host's cells. In the mouse, for example, genes derived from the mammary tumour virus (a virus capable of causing a form of 'breast' cancer in this species) encode glycoproteins on the surface of lymphocytes and these molecules are then capable of stimulating lymphocytes from individuals that either lack them altogether or express their variants. Because of this capability, the glycoproteins have been termed *Mls antigens* (for *M*ixed *l*ymphocyte *s*timulation).

The Mls molecules associate with one particular type of mouse MHC class II molecule (the H2E molecules) and thus complexed then interact with the β chain of the α:β TCR (although they can also interact with the TCR even if they are not complexed with the class II molecules). The Mls–TCR interaction does not involve the peptide- and MHC-recognizing regions of the TCR; it may involve the HV4 region in a different manner from the typical MHC–peptide–TCR interaction. In all these characteristics, Mls molecules resemble the *superantigens* of certain microorganisms (see Chapter 13). Each Mls molecule has affinity for a certain type of the TCR β chain, irrespective of the chain's peptide- or MHC-binding specificity. Thus, for example, the molecule encoded in the *Mls^a* gene binds to all β chains specified by segments of the *BV6*, *BV8* and *BV9* families. During T-cell maturation any thymocyte expressing a β chain specified by segments from these families is induced to undergo apoptosis and all these cells are deleted from the T-cell repertoire. Since the *BV6* family has seven functional members, each of which can occur in many variants produced by the rearrangement process, the deletion of so many specificities creates a large 'hole' (figuratively speaking) in the T-cell repertoire. It is believed that because of the 'hole' or *blind spot* in the repertoire of receptors, the immune system of the affected individuals may not be able to 'see' (recognize) certain peptide–MHC combinations.

Evolution

TCRB genes have been cloned from representatives of cartilaginous fishes (sharks), bony fishes (trout), amphibians (clawed toad), birds (domestic fowl) and of course mammals (several species). *TCRA* genes are known to be present in mammals and birds. This distribution, along with other observations, makes it very likely that all jawed vertebrates possess *TCR* genes and use them in the adaptive immune response. There is no evidence for the presence of *TCR* genes in jawless vertebrates or in any invertebrates. The TCR-based immune response is therefore at least 450 my old. In bony fishes, amphibians and birds (reptiles have not been studied as yet), *TCR* genes are organized in a similar way to mammals. Each *TCR* locus contains many *V* segments, one or two *D* segments (if present), several *J* segments and one or two *C* segments. Families of *V* segments can be recognized in some of the vertebrate classes at least and some of the families may correspond to certain mammalian families, indicating that they may have diverged more than 350 my ago. In cartilaginous fishes, on the other hand, the organization is different: here one finds multiple clusters, each cluster containing a few *V* segments, possibly one *D* segment, a few *J* segments and one *C* segment (see Fig. 1.6a). In all these *TCR* gene systems, there is evidence for rearrangement preceding expression, even in cartilaginous fishes, in which it apparently occurs always within each of the clusters. These vertebrates all possess the *RAG1* and *RAG2* genes necessary for recombination of the segments. Moreover, there is some evidence that already in the sharks the rearranging segments can diversify further by N-nucleotide additions or deletions at the segmental junctions.

In contrast to the evolution of the α:β TCR, very little is known about the origin of γ:δ TCR. The latter is present in mammals and birds but has apparently assumed a more important function in some species than in others, as reflected in the different representations of γ:δ T cells and the size of the γ:δ TCR repertoire. Thus, in humans and mice, γ:δ T cells constitute only a minor fraction of T lymphocytes in most lymphoid organs, whereas in artiodactyls and in the fowl the α:β and γ:δ T cells are almost equally represented. Similarly, the repertoire of the human or mouse γ:δ T cells is much lower than that of the α:β T lymphocytes, but this may not be so in the sheep: in this species, a large number of *TCRG V* segments have been shown to rearrange with *DJ* segments. In both mammals and birds, however, the γ:δ TCR seems to specialize in the recognition of ligands frequent in certain epithelial tissues.

Pre-TCR

The mechanism of the rearrangement process apparently requires that first one and then the other of the two gene complexes specifying a given TCR heterodimer is recombined; simultaneous rearrangement of both genes could apparently lead to complications. In the case of the α:β TCR, the *TCRB* is rearranged first and only when this process has been successfully completed does the rearrangement of the *TCRA* complex follow. Whether a rearrangement has been successful (productive) can be tested only when the β chain encoded in the rearranged gene is expressed on the cell surface. This requirement, however, presents a problem because the β chain alone cannot reach the cell surface, at least not in a form in which it could undergo such a test. The immune system has solved this problem by the procurement of a surrogate α chain, the *pre-TCR α chain* (pTCRα). The gene specifying the surrogate α chain does not undergo rearrangement, but the chain does associate with the β polypeptide just like a true α polypeptide and assures β-chain delivery to the cell surface.

As expected, the *PTCRA* gene is expressed in precursor but not in mature T lymphocytes. Its absence, as in knockout mice, severely hampers α:β T-cell development, without affecting the generation of γ:δ lymphocytes. The gene consists of four exons, which encode the 5′UT region with the leader peptide (exon 1), single extracellular immunoglobulin-like domain (exon 2), connecting peptide (exon 3) and transmembrane region, cytoplasmic tail, as well as the 3′UT region (exon 4). The immunoglobulin-like domain contains two cysteine residues forming an intrachain disulphide bond in a manner characteristic of immunoglobulin-like proteins (Fig. 7.26), and sites for the addition of carbohydrate side-chains. (The molecule was originally described as a glycoprotein with relative molecular mass of 33 000 or *gp33*.) The connecting peptide is specified by 45 bp of sequence, exactly as in most of the TCR chains. It contains one cysteine residue capable of forming an interchain disulphide bond, again exactly in the same way as the bonds formed between α and β chains of the TCR. The transmembrane region, which is approximately 20 amino acid residues long, includes two positively charged residues (arginine and lysine) found in the same position also in the TCR α and δ chains (see Fig. 7.19) and believed to be involved in the interaction with the CD3 complex. The cytoplasmic tail differs from that of the TCR chain in its length of approximately 30 amino acid residues. It contains sites believed to be involved in signal transduction (two phosphorylation sites and an Src homology 3 or SH3-domain binding sequence; see Chapters 10 & 16). By its gene organization, as well as domain disposition and function, the *PTCRA* gene resembles the *TCRAC* gene segment, suggesting an origin of the two from a common ancestor. There is, however, no significant sequence similarity between the two genes. Also, the *PTCRA* gene has its own promoter region and a leader-encoding exon, which the gene encoding the constant region of the α chain lacks. The expression of the pre-TCR α:β heterodimer requires association with the CD3 complex. On the thymocyte surface, the pre-TCR is replaced by the mature TCR as soon as a functional α chain is produced by the cell.

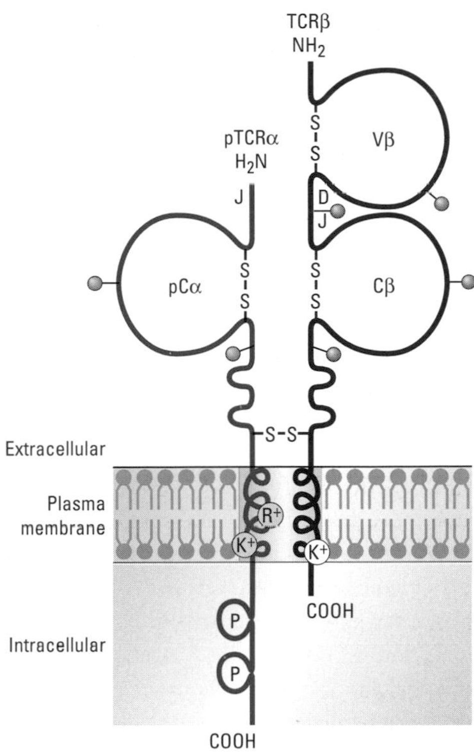

Figure 7.26 The pre-TCR: diagrammatic representation. S–S, disulphide bond; ●– and ●–, carbohydrate chains; R+ and K+, positively charged arginine and lysine residues, respectively; P, sites to which presumably phosphate groups are added by the enzyme protein tyrosine kinase.

Accessory TCR molecules and co-receptors

The function of the TCR is to receive a signal from another cell and pass it on to other molecules that ultimately activate the T lymphocyte. In this function it is assisted by *accessory molecules* (CD3 complex and the ζ and η proteins) and *co-receptors* (CD4 and CD8).

CD3 complex

The complex itself consists of three subunits, γ (gamma), δ

(delta) and ε (epsilon), but these are closely associated with two other proteins, ζ (zeta) and η (eta), and the five molecules are therefore usually considered together as if they were all part of one system (Fig. 7.27). The γ, δ and ε subunits are very similar to one another in structure (they all contain an immunoglobulin-like domain and resemble each other in sequence), whereas the ζ and η proteins are clearly unrelated to these three. The ζ chain-encoding gene, however, is related to the γ chain-encoding gene of the FcRγ (see Chapter 8). The genes encoding the human γ, δ and ε subunits all reside in a single, relatively short region of chromosome 11q23 and probably arose by tandem duplication from a single ancestral gene. The gene encoding the human ζ and η proteins is located on chromosome 1q22–q25 and is apparently of independent origin. The only thing all five chains have in common is the immune receptor tyrosine-based activation motif (ITAM) in their cytoplasmic regions (Fig. 7.28). This sequence interacts with the protein tyrosine kinase, which is known to be involved in signal transduction. The ζ and η proteins each contain three of these motifs, whereas the γ, δ and ε chains contain one each (see Fig. 7.27). The η protein is apparently specified by the same gene as the ζ protein, the difference between the two resulting from the way in which the transcript is processed: during the splicing some exons that are included in the mature mRNA of the η subunit are skipped in the production of the ζ mRNA (*differential splicing*). Consequently, the η polypeptide is longer than the ζ polypeptide (M_r of 22 000 and 16 000, respectively). The ζ protein, which is free of carbohydrates, has a very short extracellular domain (nine amino acid residues), a transmembrane region and a long cytoplasmic tail. One of the nine residues in the extracellular domain is cysteine, which is involved in the formation of an interchain disulphide bond in either ζ:ζ homodimers or ζ:η heterodimers. Each T lymphocyte appears to have both the homodimers and heterodimers at its surface at a ratio of 5 : 1 to 10 : 1. The transmembrane regions of the ζ and η chains contain one negatively charged residue each, which is believed to be involved in the formation of an ionic bond with the TCR β chain.

Of the three CD3 subunits, two (γ and δ) are glycosylated, each carrying two carbohydrate chains, whereas the third (ε) is not. The subunits assemble into two noncovalently associated heterodimers, γ:ε and δ:ε (see

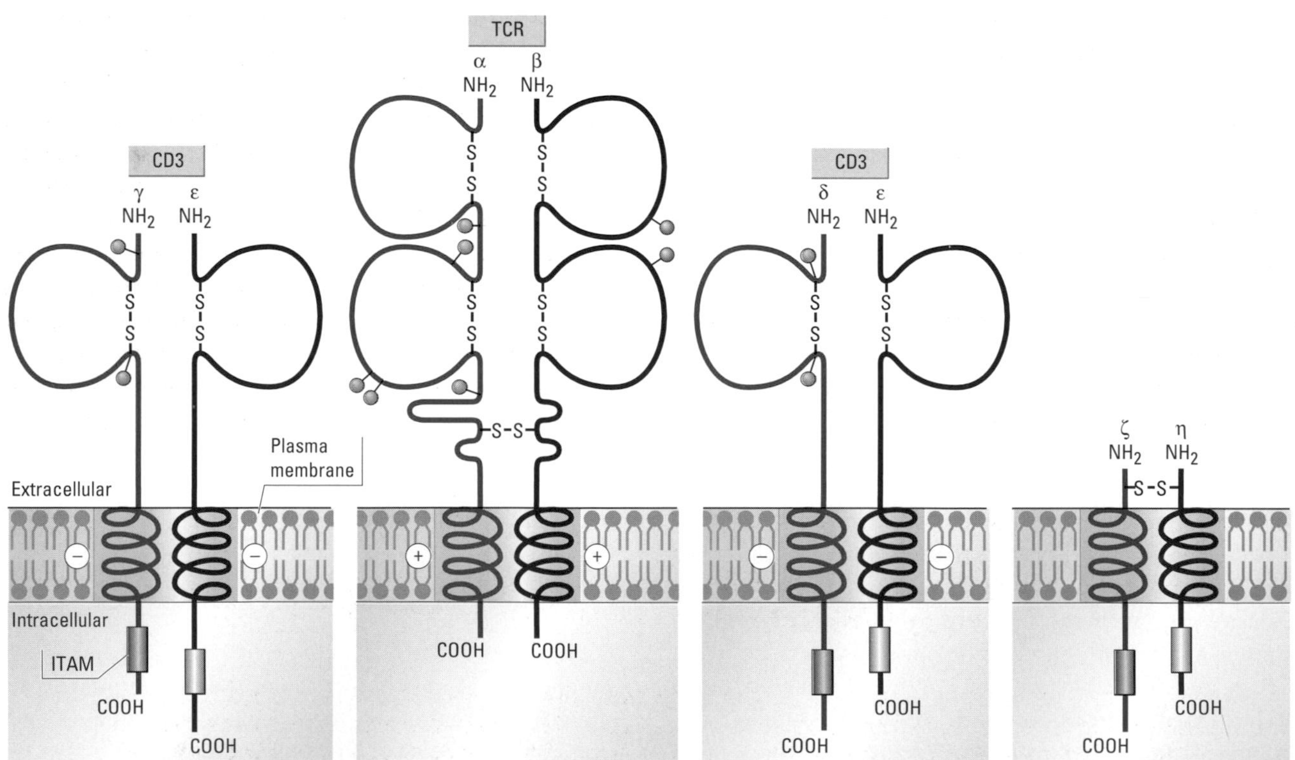

Figure 7.27 The TCR–CD3 complex. S–S, disulphide bond; and , carbohydrate chains; + and –, positively and negatively charged residues of transmembrane region; ITAM, immune receptor tyrosine-based activation motif; numbers indicate positions of marker residues (counting from the N- to the C-terminus). The transmembrane regions are exaggerated in this figure to show the interactions between the chains. The ζ and η chains in reality interact with the α and β TCR chains in the plasma membrane.

```
Human CD3γ        DKQTLLPNDQLYQPLKDREDDQYSHLQGNQLRRN
Human CD3δ        DTQALLRNDQVYQPLRDRDDAQYSHLGGNWARNK
Human CD3ε        KERPPPVPNPDYEPIRKGQRDLYSGL
Human ζ chain     PPAYQQGQNQLYNELNLGRREEYDVLDKRRGRDP
Mouse MB1         DMPDDYEDENLYEGLNLDDCSMYEDISRCLQGTY
Mouse B29         DGKAGMEEDHTYEGLNIDQTATYEDIVTLRTGEV
Rat Fcε γ chain   FERSKVPDDRLYEELHVYSPI-YSALEDTREASA
Rat Fcε β chain   DIASREKSDAVYTGLNTRNQETYETLKHEKPPQ
Human CD5         ENPTASHVDNEYSQPPRNSRLSYPALEGVLHRS
```

Figure 7.28 Partial amino acid sequence alignment of the cytoplasmic tails from the polypeptide chains constituting the CD3 complex, as well as a few other related molecules. The amino acid residues are given in the international single-letter code (see Appendix 1). Conserved residues shared by several sequences are highlighted. MB1 and B29 are molecules associated with the B-cell receptor (see Chapter 8); Fcε is a receptor for the Fc part of immunoglobulins (see Chapter 8) and CD5 is a scavenger receptor (see Chapter 21). (From Beyers, A.D. *et al.* (1992) *Trends in Cell Biology*, **2**, 253.)

Fig. 7.27). Each subunit consists of an extracellular domain, transmembrane region and a cytoplasmic tail. The extracellular domain has some sequence similarity with immunoglobulins, suggesting that it might form the immunoglobulin fold with disulphide bonds connecting two β-pleated sheets. This similarity in primary, and presumably also tertiary, structure places the γ, δ and ε chains into the immunoglobulin superfamily of proteins (see Chapter 8). The transmembrane regions of the three chains, like all the other chains of the TCR complex, contain a charged residue buried within a cluster of hydrophobic residues. The negatively charged residues of these three chains are believed to form salt bridges with the positively charged residues of the α and β chains (the interaction possibly occurs between the TCRβ and CD3γ chains on the one hand, as well as between the TCRα and CD3δ chains on the other). The cytoplasmic tail of the ε chain contains a large number of basic amino acids, followed by a stretch of prolines. The CD3 complex is assembled intracellularly before the *TCRA* and *TCRB* genes have completed their rearrangements, but it is not delivered to the cell surface without the TCR α and β chains.

CD4 and CD8 molecules

The CD4 and CD8 glycoproteins are expressed on a subset of thymocytes and mature T lymphocytes, CD4 primarily on T_H cells and CD8 on T_C cells. They are called 'co-receptors' because they bind the same MHC molecules as the TCR, the CD8 the class I and the CD4 the class II molecules. Upon interaction with MHC molecules, each TCR heterodimer associates with one molecule of either CD4 or CD8, each of which is associated, at its cytoplasmic tail, with molecules of a T-cell specific protein tyrosine kinase, Lck. The function of the CD4 and CD8 molecules is to stabilize the TCR–MHC–peptide interaction and to participate in signal transduction from TCR to intracellular proteins. Although they carry out similar functions, the two molecules and their encoding genes differ considerably in their organization. They both contain domains that resemble variable immunoglobulin domains in their primary (Fig. 7.29) and tertiary structures. The gene segments encoding these must have arisen by duplication from a common ancestral segment but the genes must have gone their separate ways for more than 400 my. This

```
IgVκ    DIQMTQSPSSLSASVGDRVTITCQASQD*IIKYLNWYQQTPG***KAPKLLIYE***A
CD8α     SQFRVSPLDRTWNLGETVELKCQVLLSNPTSGCSWLFQPRG*AAASPTFLLYLSQNK
CD8β       LQQTPAYIKYQTNKMVMLSCEAKISLSNMRIYWLRQRQAPSSDSHHEFLALWDSA
CD4             KKVVLGKKGDTVELTCTASQK*KSIQFHWKNS***N****QIKILGNQGSF
           |<--a-->|  |<--b-->|    |<--c-->|        |<--c'->|

IgVκ    SN*LQAGVP**SRFSGSGS***GTDYTFTISSLQPEDIATYYCQQYQSLPYTFGQGTKLQITR
CD8α    PK*AAEGLDT*QRFSGKRL***GDTFVLTLSDFRRENEGYYFCSALSNSIMYFSHFVPVFLPA
CD8β    KG*TIHGEEVEQEKIAVFR**DASRFILNLTSVKPEDSGIYFCMIVGSPELTFGKGTQLSVVD
CD4     LTKGPSKLN**DRADSRRSLWDQGNFPLIIKNLKIEDSDTYICE**VEDQKE***EVQLLVFG
        |<c''>|   |<--d-->|    |<-e->|      |<--f-->|   |<----g---->|
```

Figure 7.29 Amino acid sequence alignment of the immunoglobulin V and immunoglobulin-like domains from CD4 and CD8 polypeptide chains. Arrows indicate the positions of the β-strands (see Figs 7.31 & 7.34); asterisks show gaps introduced for optimal alignment. Amino acid residues are given in the international single-letter code (see Appendix 1).

conclusion is suggested by the observation that the immunoglobulin-like domain of CD8 is more closely related to immunoglobulins than any of the CD4 domains; if immunoglobulins emerged after the divergence of jawless and jawed vertebrates, CD8 must have diverged from CD4 before the emergence of jawed vertebrates. The ability to rearrange gene segments somatically before their expression apparently developed after the divergence of the *CD8* and immunoglobulin genes because only the latter can diversify by this mechanism.

The *CD4 glycoprotein* is a single-chain molecule with a rod-like extracellular part, a transmembrane region and a cytoplasmic tail (Fig. 7.30). The extracellular part consists of four immunoglobulin-like domains, D1–D4, two larger (D1 and D3) and two smaller (D2 and D4) ones. The tertiary structure of the D1 and D2 domains has been elucidated by X-ray diffraction analysis (Fig. 7.31). Each domain is organized into the sandwich of two β-pleated sheets like the immunoglobulin (and TCR) domains, but there are also important differences between the CD4 and immunoglobulin structures. First, there is no connecting 'hinge' between the two domains; instead, the last β-strand of D1 continues straight into the first strand of D2. Consequently, the two domains are closely packed against each other with a large hydrophobic interface between them. This arrangement contributes to the rod-like rigidity of the CD4 molecule. Second, the interconnecting loops, particularly of the D1 domain, are organized differently: some are shorter and others are longer than those of the immunoglobulins. The β-strands of the D2 domain are shorter than those of a typical immunoglobulin domain so that the domain's overall size is reduced (75 residues in D2 of CD4 as compared to about 100 residues in immunoglobulins). Third, the disulphide bond in the D2 domain does not connect the two β-pleated sheets; it is formed instead between the strands of the same sheet. And fourth, the D1 domain has an extra pair of β-strands that protrude on the surface that presumably interacts with the MHC class II molecule. The D1 domain resembles the V domain of an immunoglobulin light chain in sequence and the V domain of an immunoglobulin heavy chain in tertiary structure; the D2 domain resembles a modified C domain of an immunoglobulin molecule (see Chapter 8). The tertiary structure of the D3 and D4 domains is not known but is assumed, on the basis of sequence similarity, to be immunoglobulin-like as well. The entire extracellular part spans the distance from the plasma membrane of the T lymphocyte, along the entire extracellular length of the TCR, and then further along much of the extracellular part of the MHC class II molecule (see Fig. 7.30). In contrast to the transmembrane regions of the TCR and CD3 chains, the

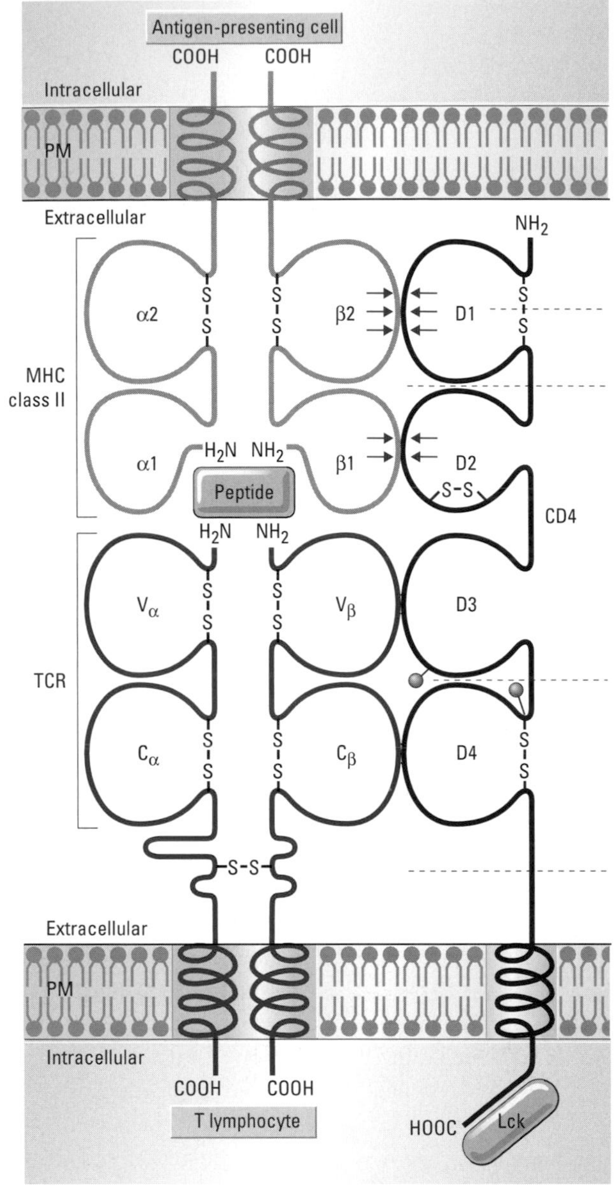

Figure 7.30 The co-receptor function of the CD4 molecule: the TCR of a T lymphocyte (the CD3 complex is omitted for simplicity) binds the peptide–MHC ligand of the antigen-presenting cell and the CD4 molecule interacts with the MHC class II molecule; whether it interacts also with the TCR remains an open question (arrows). The protein tyrosine kinase molecule (Lck) associated with the CD4 molecule is presumably involved in signal transduction. Broken lines indicate exon borders in the CD_4-encoding gene. S–S, disulphide bond; D1–D4, immunoglobulin-like domains of CD4; ⚬—, carbohydrate moieties (shown for the CD4 molecule only); lck, lymphoid T-cell protein tyrosine kinase.

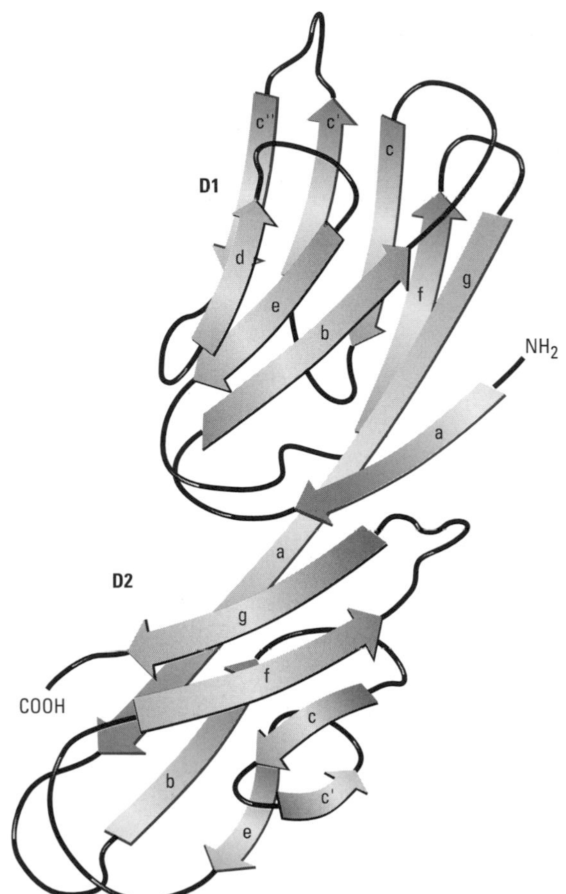

Figure 7.31 Tertiary structure of the CD4 D1 and D2 immunoglobulin-like domains: ribbon model. Lower-case letters indicate β-strands labelled in the order from the N- to the C-terminus, separately in each domain. Strands constituting the two β-pleated sheets in each domain are distinguished by shading. The D1 domain encompasses residues 1–98 and is composed of nine β-strands, three in one sheet and six in the other. The D2 domain encompasses residues 99–173 and is composed of seven strands, three arranged into one sheet and four into the other. (Modified from Ryu, S.-E. *et al.* (1990) *Nature*, **348**, 419.)

transmembrane region of CD4 (and CD8) does not contain any charged residues that could be involved in the formation of salt bridges. The CD4 (CD8) molecules apparently do not join the TCR–CD3 complex until both TCR and CD4 (CD8) have contacted the MHC molecule. When the CD4–MHC class II assemblage is established, the CD4 molecule may also interact (via its D3/D4 domains) with the V_β/C_β domains of the TCR (see Fig. 7.30), but direct evidence for these contacts is not available. The cytoplasmic tail of the CD4 polypeptide has a sequence recognized by the Lck protein tyrosine kinase, which transmits the signal resulting from CD4–MHC molecule interaction.

Several methods have been used to identify the CD4 residues involved in the interaction with the class II MHC molecule; the most sophisticated is *site-directed mutagenesis* (Fig. 7.32). The principle of this method is to create a *CD4* gene in which a single codon has been changed so that the product of the mutated gene differs from the standard (wild-type) gene in a single amino acid residue. The altered gene, together with sequences necessary for its expression, is introduced into a cell that does not express any *CD4* genes itself but does express *TCR* and *MHC* genes, and is allowed to integrate into the host cell chromosomes. The cell expressing the altered CD4 molecule is then tested for its ability to carry out functions which require the participation of this molecule. The experiments have demonstrated that CD4 binds to class II molecules via its D1 and D2 domains. Although changes in the D3 domain sometimes influence the binding, this effect is believed to be indirect by causing conformational alterations in the D1 and D2 domains. There is still, however, no agreement on the specific D1 and D2 residues involved in the binding; they may differ depending on the type of class II molecule with which the CD4 molecule interacts. The binding appears to involve a broad area of the CD4 molecule, the D1 domain interacting with the class II β2 domain and the D2 domain with the class II β1 domain (Fig. 7.30). In the D1 domain, a particularly strong involvement in the binding has been demonstrated for residues on the loops between the *c′* and *c″*, as well as between *c″* and *d* β-strands, and on the β-strand *a* (see Fig. 7.31). The CD4 molecule has acquired a certain notoriety since its recognition as the receptor via which the human immunodeficiency virus (HIV) gains entrance into the T_H lymphocytes. The interaction of the HIV gp120 surface component and the CD4 molecule occurs via a cluster of residues on the β-strand *c″* in the D1 domain of the latter (see Fig. 7.31).

In contrast to the CD4 molecule, the *CD8 molecule* is a dimer composed of either two identical α chains or one α and one β chain; a dimer of two β chains has not been observed. The two chains are encoded in at least three genes: one (*CD8A*) encoding the α chain and two (*CD8B1* and *CD8B2*) specifying two forms of the β chain. The *CD8A* and *CD8B1* genes are located on human chromosome 2p12 close to the *IGKV* gene, which codes for the variable region of one of two types of the immunoglobulin light chains (see Chapter 8). The *CD8B2* gene maps to 2q12, a position on the opposite side of the centromere from the *CD8B1* gene. (The human *CD4* gene resides on the short arm of chromosome 12.) The sequences of the CD8 α and β proteins are identical in 21% of residues only, but the exon–intron organization of the genes, as well as the domain organization of the proteins, is the same (the CD8 β1 and β2 proteins are identical in more than 98% of their

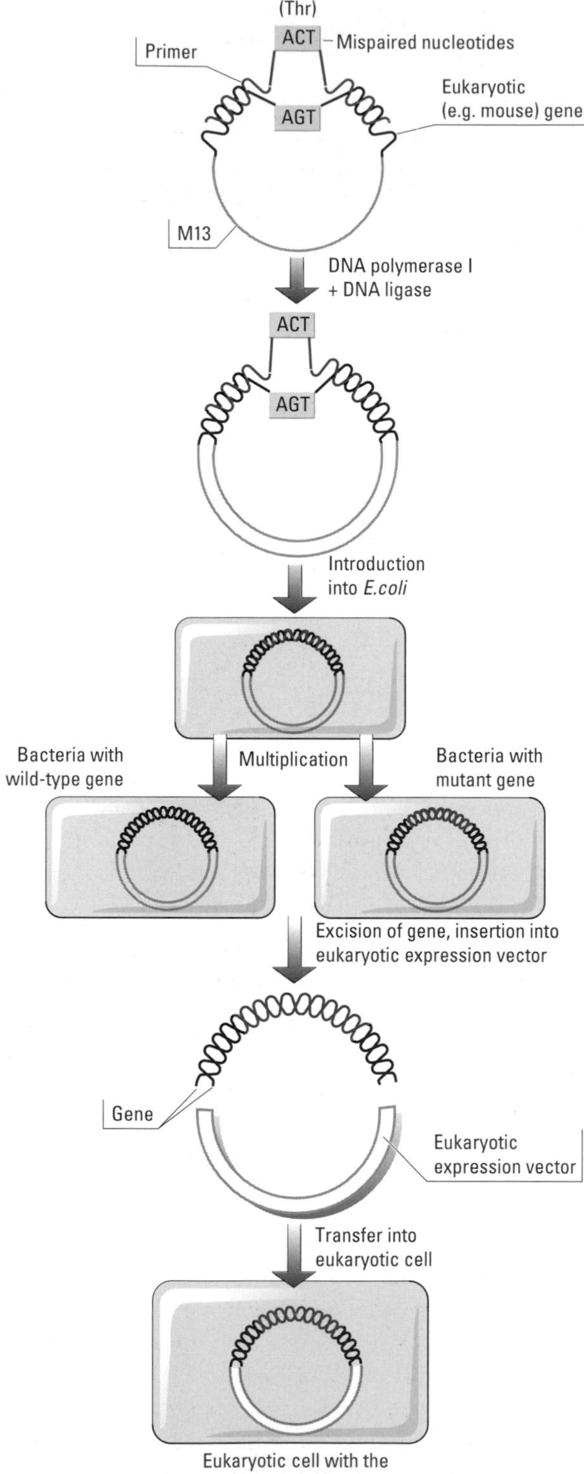

Figure 7.32 The principle of site-directed mutagenesis. To replace a specific amino acid residue in a particular protein, one of the two DNA strands of the gene encoding this protein is inserted into the circle of single-stranded bacteriophage DNA (the *M13 vector*). Simultaneously, a short stretch of nucleotides (*oligonucleotide*) is synthesized such that its sequence is complementary to the sequence of the gene in the region specifying the amino acid residue. The oligonucleotide matches the gene sequence exactly, except for one site. For example, if the aim is to replace serine encoded in the AGT triplet by threonine specified by the ACT codon, an oligonucleotide possessing the TGA triplet is used, which becomes ACT on the complementary strand. In the presence of DNA polymerase I, the oligonucleotide, which has annealed to the complementary region of the gene, serves as an initiator (*primer*) of DNA synthesis (the creation of the complementary strand of the entire circle). The double-stranded vector with the gene *insert* is then introduced into suitable bacteria and these are allowed to multiply. During multiplication, the vector with the insert (*plasmid*) replicates; some bacteria receive the plasmid with the unaltered gene and others the plasmid with the altered one. The latter are selected, their plasmids isolated and the inserts enzymatically excised from the vector. The inserts are then inserted into a new vector constructed in such a way that it allows expression of the insert in eukaryotic cells. This *eukaryotic expression vector* contains a promoter region of a gene expressed in a eukaryotic cell, the polyadenylation signal, an intron sequence and a sequence specifying a ribosome-binding site. The vector with the insert is introduced into a cultured eukaryotic cell, for example by exposing the cell suspension to a short electric pulse, which makes the plasma membrane transiently permeable to DNA molecules. The vector persists for a while in the cultured cells, providing an opportunity for transient expression of the inserted gene. More permanent expression requires integration of the gene into the host cell DNA. The *transformed cells* can be detected with the help of a suitable selection system and the expression of the gene can be demonstrated by an assay detecting the gene product.

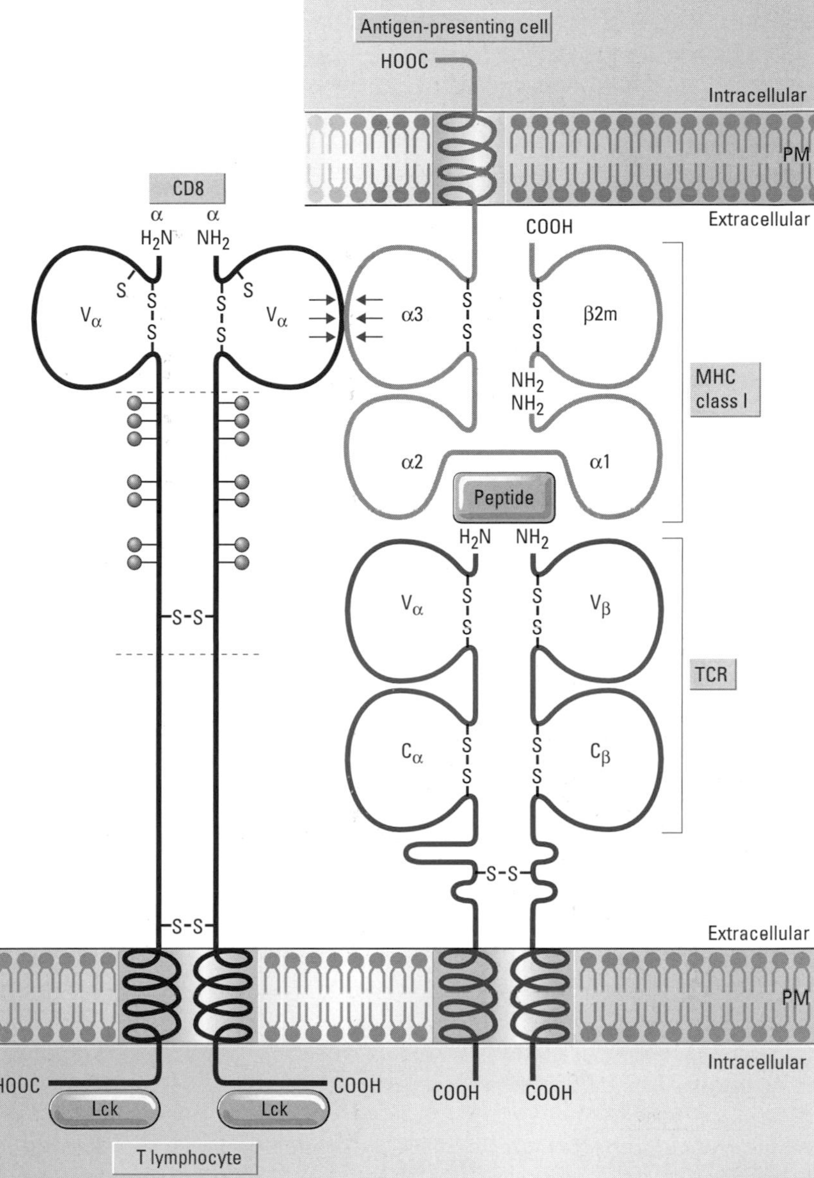

Figure 7.33 The co-receptor function of the CD8 molecule: the TCR of a T lymphocyte (the CD3 complex is omitted for simplicity) binds the peptide–MHC ligand of an antigen-presenting cell and the CD8 molecule interacts with the α3 domain of the MHC class I molecule (arrows). The protein tyrosine kinase molecule (Lck) associated with each of the two CD8 α chains (it does not associate with the CD8 β chains) are presumably involved in signal transduction. S–S, disulphide bonds; ●—, O-linked carbohydrate moieties (shown only for the CD8 homodimer); broken lines indicate exon borders in the CD8-encoding gene; lck, lymphoid T-cell protein tyrosine kinase.

residues.) Thus the *CD8A* and *CD8B* genes probably originated from the same ancestor, but diverged a long time ago.

Each CD8 chain consists of a single immunoglobulin-like domain, a long (48-residue) stalk region, a transmembrane region and a cytoplasmic tail (Fig. 7.33). The stalk region contains seven *O*-glycosylation sites, all of which are probably occupied by carbohydrate moieties with many negatively charged sialic acid residues. The residues may help to hold the stalk in an extended form and the negative charges may repel it from the plasma membrane. In the CD8 chain, as in the CD4 chain, charged residues are absent in the transmembrane region and the cytoplasmic tail contains a sequence motif for interaction with the Lck protein tyrosine kinase. The two chains of the dimer are held together by two disulphide bonds in the stalk region.

The tertiary structure of the immunoglobulin-like domain has been determined for the α_2 homodimers. The domain is shaped like a box with round edges and its organization closely resembles that of the V domain borne by the κ light chain type of immunoglobulin molecule (Fig. 7.34; for a description of the V_κ domain, see Chapter 8). The only major difference between the two domains is that in the CD8 V_α domain the loop corresponding to the CDR2 is extended by six residues (as in CD4) in comparison with the V_κ domain. The interface between the two V_α domains of the α_2 homodimer is formed by the *g* and *c′*

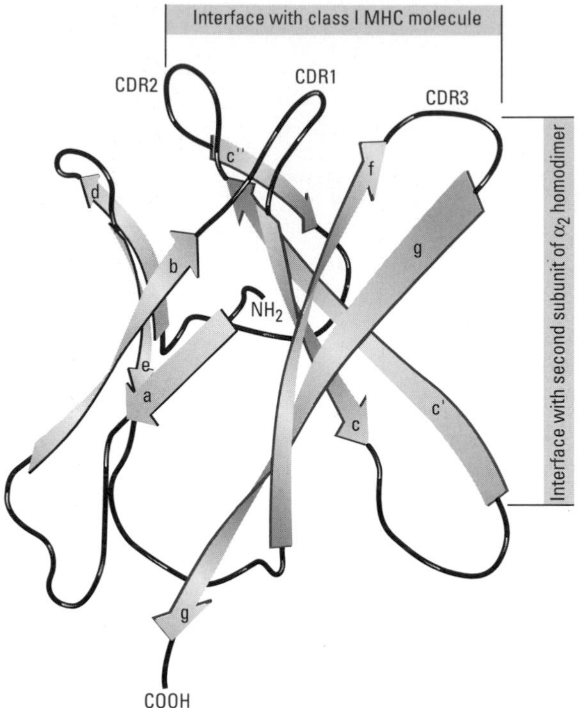

Figure 7.34 Tertiary structure of the CD8 immunoglobulin-like domain. Lower case letters indicate β-strands labelled in the order from N- to the C-terminus. CDR loops correspond to the complementarity-determining regions of the immunoglobulin light-chain variable domain. Strands constituting the two β-pleated sheets are distinguished by shading. The domain contains nine β-strands, four in one sheet and five in the other. (Based on Leahy, D.J. *et al.* (1992) *Cell*, **68**, 1145.)

strands of the different monomers (Fig. 7.34). The domain contains three cysteine residues, two of which are close together; it may exist in two versions depending on which of the cysteine residues are involved in disulphide bond formation.

Upon the engagement of the TCR with the class I MHC–peptide assemblage, the CD8 dimer binds to the α3 domain of the class I molecules (see Fig. 7.33). The identity of the interacting residues has been determined by site-directed mutagenesis. In the CD8 molecule, the participating residues reside in loops corresponding to the CDR of the immunoglobulin V domains, in particular in CDR1 and CDR2 (see Fig. 7.33). In the class I molecule, they reside for the most part in a seven-residue loop formed by predominantly negatively charged amino acid residues at positions 223–229. The latter are believed to interact electrostatically with the positively charged amino acids of the CD8 molecule. The interactions generate a signal that is transmitted to the cytoplasmic tail, picked up by the Lck molecule and then passed on to the cell's interior.

Natural killer cell receptors

Molecules on the surface of natural killer (NK) cells that are capable of binding ligands on other (target) cells and converting this interaction into an intracellular signal, either activatory or inhibitory, are referred to as *NK cell receptors* (NKCR). They are not members of the TCR family and differ from the TCR in many respects, one of which is their inability to rearrange their encoding gene segments. Instead, they achieve their diversity by providing a separate gene for each variant. The NKCR are not clonally distributed, as are TCR, but the expression of some of the *NKCR* genes at least is restricted to NK cell subsets, different genes being expressed in distinct subsets. (The members of each subset are apparently not identical and hence not clones.) The specificity of the NKCR is usually broader than that of the TCR. Finally, the NKCR-encoding genes have been recruited from different gene families and are therefore more heterogeneous than the *TCR* genes, which all constitute a single family.

Two structurally different families of NKCR have been identified: the lectin-type and the immunoglobulin-type families. The lectin-type NKCR are best known in the mouse but homologous genes and proteins have also been found in the rat and in humans. Some of them seem to recognize carbohydrate groups on thus far unidentified target cell glycoproteins or glycolipids; these function as *activating NKCR*. Others recognize certain MHC class I molecules (mainly H2D in the mouse) and act as *inhibitory NKCR*. It is not known what the lectin-type NKCR recognize on the MHC molecule: it is probably the protein part of the MHC molecule close to the peptide-binding site but the carbohydrates of the MHC glycoprotein may also contribute to the interaction. The NKCR of the immunoglobulin family, the *killer cell inhibitory receptors* (KIR), have been identified thus far only in humans and nearly all of them have been demonstrated to recognize certain allelic forms of either HLA-A, -B or -C molecules. Different subsets of NK cells express different members of the inhibitory receptor families (either of the lectin type in rodents or of the immunoglobulin type in humans) or their different combinations.

Lectin-type NKCR

The genes encoding this family of receptors appear to be clustered into a single chromosomal region, the *NK gene complex* (*NKC*). In the mouse, the *NKC* gene is located on chromosome 6; in humans, a homologous complex may be present on the short arm of chromosome 12 in the region 12p12.13–p13.2. Some of the receptors encoded by *NKC*

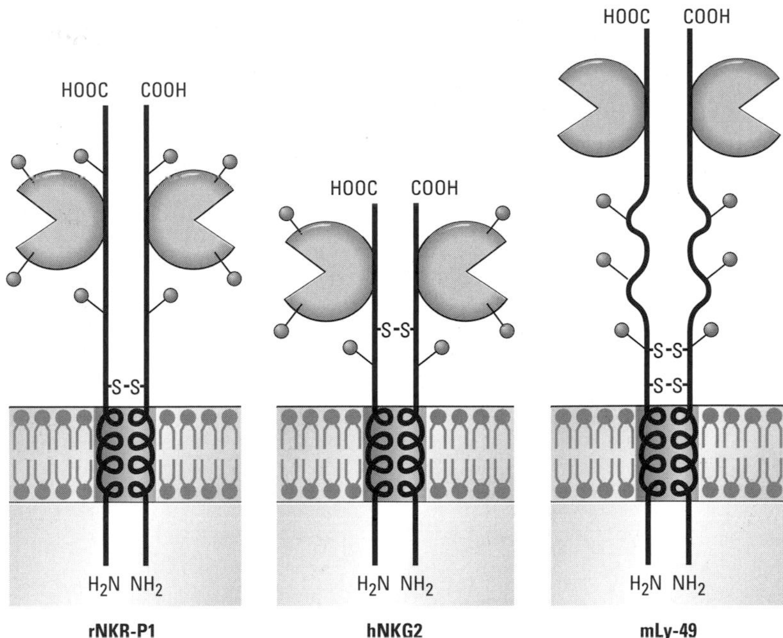

Figure 7.35 The lectin-type family of NK cell receptors. The lectin-binding domain is highlighted. ●–, carbohydrate moiety; S–S, disulphide bond; m, mouse; r, rat; h, human. (Based on Testin, R. *et al.* (1994) *Immunology Today*, 15, 479.)

genes are of the activatory, others of the inhibitory type. They include NKR-P1 of the rat, Ly49 of the mouse and CD94 and NKG2 of humans; another human receptor, CD69, whose expression is not restricted to NK cells, is also a member of this family. Their overall structure is very similar, each molecule being a disulphide-bonded homodimer or a CD94:NKG2 heterodimer and each monomer consisting of an extracellular part, transmembrane region and a cytoplasmic tail (Fig. 7.35). The extracellular part comprises a *carbohydrate-recognition domain* (CRD) found otherwise in the family of *calcium-dependent (C-type) lectins* (see Chapter 13) and a stalk region. The CRD is a stretch of about 120 amino acid residues that contains six conserved cysteine residues responsible for the overall folding of the domain. It binds carbohydrate in a Ca^{2+}-dependent manner; at least some of the domains, however, are also capable of binding non-carbohydrate moieties. Among the other members of the family are *selectins*, which play a crucial part in the recruitment of leucocytes into inflamed tissues (see Chapters 15 & 21), and CD23, which is a receptor for one class of immunoglobulin molecules (IgE; it is therefore also referred to as FcεRII; see Chapter 8). In contrast to most of the integral membrane proteins discussed so far, the C-type lectin family of proteins have their N-terminus in the cytoplasm and the C-terminus outside the cell. This orientation of integral membrane proteins (lectins) is referred to as *type II*.

NKR-P1 is a family of at least three glycoproteins designated A, B and C. The proteins are identical in 72–74% of

AsialoGM$_1$ (GA$_1$)	Galβ1→3GalNAcβ1→4Galβ1→4Glc
HNK-1	GlcAβ1→3Galβ1→4GlcNAcβ1→3Galβ1→4Glc ↓3 HSO_3
Sialyl Le^X	Galβ1→3GlcNAc ↓3 ↓1.4 HSO_3 Fucα

Figure 7.36 Three oligosaccharides bound by the lectin domain of the NKR-P1 molecule. Fuc, fucose; Gal, galactose; Glc, glucose; GlcA, glucuronic acid; HNK, human natural killer; Le, Lewis.

their amino acid residues and are presumably encoded in closely linked genes. They recognize asialo-GM, HNK-1 and sialyl-Le^x (Fig. 7.36) and other oligosaccharides that are constituents of gangliosides and glycosaminoglycans on tumour cells, for example. The mouse homologue of the rat NKR-P1 is termed NK1.1 and human NKR-P1 is also known. NKR-P1 is an activatory type of receptor.

Ly49 is another family of at least eight closely related glycoproteins (Ly49-A to Ly49-H), each apparently expressed on a different subset of NK cells. This differential expression has been referred to as 'allelic exclusion' but if some of the proteins are encoded in distinct loci, as seems very likely, this may be an inappropriate designation. Ly49 family members are an inhibitory type of receptor. Ly49-A recognizes H2D^d and H2D^k, Ly49^c H2 molecules probably encoded in the *D* or *L* genes of the *d*, *k*, *b* and *s* haplotypes, and Ly49-G H2D^d and H2D^k molecules.

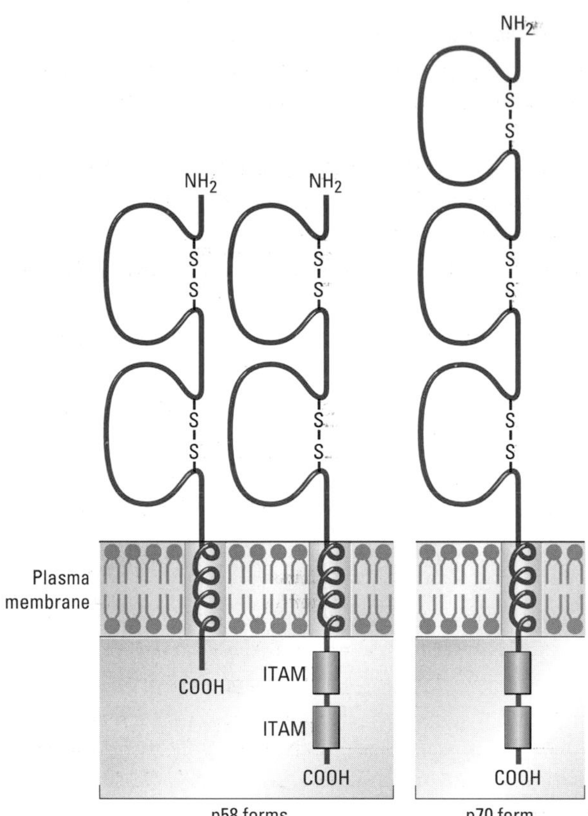

Figure 7.37 Representatives of the immunoglobulin-like family of NK cell receptors. Three different forms of the receptor are shown. S–S, disulphide bond; ITAM, immunoreceptor tyrosine-based activation motif.

NKG2 is a family of at least four human lectin-like NKCR, some of which are specified by distinct loci. All three families (NKR-P1, Ly49 and NKG2) are apparently distantly related to one another. One can therefore expect homologues of human NKG2 to exist also in the mouse (rat) and, conversely, homologues of mouse Ly49 can be expected to be present in humans.

Immunoglobulin-type NKCR (KIR)

Genes encoding at least 10 known members of this receptor family are clustered in a single region of human chromosome 19. These apparently monomeric receptors contain either two or three extracellular domains with a predicted tertiary structure similar to that of either the C or V domains present in immunoglobulin molecules (see Chapter 8) and are thus members of the immunoglobulin superfamily. The M_r of these receptors ranges from 58 000 (p58) to 70 000 (p70 or NKB1). Individual members of the KIR family differ profoundly in the structure of their intracellular domains. Most of them have long (approximately 80 amino acid residues) cytoplasmic domains containing a motif similar to the ITAM sequence found in CD3 chains, while others have only short cytoplasmic domains devoid of such sequences (Fig. 7.37). The p58 molecules seem to be associated with the ζ-chain dimers, which are also indispensable components of the signalling part of the TCR–CD3 complex. Mouse or rat homologues of human KIR have not been identified as yet. The KIR recognize and bind amino acid residues 74–83 of the class I α-helix in the carboxyl-terminal part of the α domain. Located near this segment is a highly conserved glycosylation site. The oligosaccharide chain attached to this site (Asn 86) is believed to direct the KIR of the NK cell to the protein segment.

NK cells possess another activating receptor belonging to the immunoglobulin superfamily, the FcγRIII (CD16), which binds the Fc region of immunoglobulin molecules; it will be described in Chapter 8.

Further reading (for additional references see Chapter 5)

Arden, B., Clark, S.P., Kabelitz, D. & Mak, T.W. (1995) Human T-cell receptor variable gene segment families. *Immunogenetics*, **42**, 455–500.

Arden, B., Clark, S.P., Kabelitz, D. & Mak, T.W. (1995) Mouse T-cell receptor variable gene segment families. *Immunogenetics*, **42**, 501–530.

Bentley, G.A., Boulot, G., Karjalainen, K. & Mariuzza, R.A. (1995) Crystal structure of the β chain of a T cell antigen receptor. *Science*, **267**, 1984–1987.

Boismenu, R. & Havran, W. (1995) T-cell lineage commitment revisited. *Current Biology*, **5**, 829–831.

Chien, Y.-H. & Jores, R. (1995) T cells with B-cell-like recognition properties. *Current Biology*, **5**, 1116–1118.

Clark, S.P., Arden, B., Kabelitz, D. & Mak, T.W. (1995) Comparison of human and murine T-cell receptor variable gene segment subfamilies. *Immunogenetics*, **42**, 531–540.

Cullity, B.D. (1978) *Elements of X-ray Diffraction*, 2nd edn. Addison-Wesley, Reading, MA.

Davis, M.M. (1990) T cell receptor gene diversity and selection. *Annual Review of Biochemistry*, **59**, 475–496.

Dudley, E.C., Girardi, M., Owen, M.J. & Hayday, A.C. (1995) αβ and γδ T cells can share a late common precursor. *Current Biology*, **5**, 659–669.

Fields, B.A., Ober, B., Malchiodi, E.L., *et al.* (1995) Crystal structure of the V_α domain of a T cell antigen receptor. *Science*, **270**, 1821–1824.

Godfrey, D.I. & Zlotnik, A. (1993) Control points in early T-cell development. *Immunology Today*, **14**, 547–553.

Groettrup, M. & von Boehmer, H. (1993) A role for a pre-T-cell receptor in T-cell development. *Immunology Today*, **14**, 610–614.

Gumperz, J.E. & Parham, P. (1995) The enigma of the natural killer cell. *Nature*, **378**, 245–248.

Haas, W. & Tonegawa, S. (1992) Development and selection of γδ T cells. *Current Opinion in Immunology*, **4**, 147–155.

Jameson, S.C., Hogquist, K.A. & Bevan, M.J. (1995) Positive selection of thymocytes. *Annual Review of Immunology*, **13**, 93–126.

Jorgensen, J.L., Reay, P.A., Ehrlich, E.W. & Davis, M.M. (1992) Molecular components of T-cell recognition. *Annual Review of Immunology*, **10**, 835–873.

Kearse, K.P., Roberts, J.P., Wiest, D.L. & Singer, A. (1995) Developmental regulation of αβ T cell antigen receptor assembly in immature CD4+CD8+ thymocytes. *BioEssays*, **17**, 1049–1054.

Kersh, G.J. & Allen, P.M. (1996) Essential flexibility in the T-cell recognition of antigen. *Nature*, **380**, 495–498.

Kruisbeek, A.M. (1993) Development of αβ T cells. *Current Opinion in Immunology*, **5**, 227–234.

Lanier, L.L. & Phillips, J.H. (1996) Inhibitory MHC class I receptors on NK cells and T cells. *Immunology Today*, **2**, 86–91.

Lefranc, M.-P. & Rabbits, T.H. (1989) The human T-cell receptor γ (TRG) genes. *Trends in Biochemical Sciences*, **14**, 214–218.

Leiden, J.M. (1993) Transcriptional regulation of T cell receptor genes. *Annual Review of Immunology*, **11**, 539–570.

Lieber, M. (1996) Immunoglobulin diversity: rearranging by cutting and repairing. *Current Biology*, **6**, 134–136.

Matis, L.A. (1990) The molecular basis of T-cell specificity. *Annual Review of Immunology*, **8**, 65–82.

Miceli, M.C. & Parnes, J.R. (1993) Role of CD4 and CD8 in T cell activation and differentiation. *Advances in Immunology*, **53**, 59–122.

Moss, P.A.H., Rosenberg, W.M.C. & Bell, J.I. (1992) The human T-cell receptor in health and disease. *Annual Review of Immunology*, **10**, 71–96.

Parham, P. (1994) Accentuating the positive. *Current Biology*, **4**, 444–447.

Raulet, D.H. (1994) How γδ T cells make a living. *Current Biology*, **4**, 246–248.

Rocha, B., Guy-Grand, D. & Vassalli, P. (1995) Extrathymic T cell differentiation. *Current Biology*, **7**, 235–242.

Spits, H., Lanier, L.L. & Phillips, J.H. (1995) Development of human T and natural killer cells. *Blood*, **85**, 2654–2670.

Sprent, J. & Webb, S.R. (1995) Intrathymic and extrathymic clonal deletion of T cells. *Current Biology*, **7**, 196–205.

Trinchieri, G. (1994) Recognition of major histocompatibility complex class I antigens by natural killer cells. *Journal of Experimental Medicine*, **180**, 417–421.

WHO–IUIS Nomenclature Subcommittee on TCR Designation (1993) Nomenclature for T-cell receptor (TCR) gene segments of the immune system. *Bulletin of the World Health Organization*, **71**, 113–115.

Yokoyama, W.M. (1995) Hybrid resistance and the Ly-49 family of natural killer cell receptors. *Journal of Experimental Medicine*, **182**, 273–277.

Yokoyama, W.M. & Seaman, W.E. (1993) The Ly-49 and NKR-P1 gene families encoding lectin-like receptors on natural killer cells: the *NK* gene complex. *Annual Review of Immunology*, **11**, 613–635.

chapter 8 B-cell receptors, immunoglobulins and Fc receptors

The *B-cell receptor* (BCR) is the third member of the molecular trio that carries the basic tune of adaptive immunity. To appreciate how the BCR fits into the orchestra to which the immune system is often compared, recall what happens when a parasite invades an organism. A set of specialized antigen-presenting cells processes some of the parasite's proteins and displays the peptides bound to major histocompatibility complex (MHC) molecules on their surfaces. T-cell receptors (TCRs) recognize these non-self peptide–self MHC ligands and are thereby activated. In the meantime, B lymphocytes, too, recognize the foreign molecules (antigens) via their antigen-specific receptors, the BCRs. Their activation, however, is dependent on a delivery of signals from the activated T lymphocytes. The signals come from soluble molecules, cytokines, for which the B lymphocyte also possesses specialized receptors, as well as from direct contact between the two cell types, contact mediated by cell-surface adhesion molecules and their ligands. These events, the recognition of the antigen by the BCR and the engagement of the cytokine receptors and of the adhesion molelcules, induce the mature B lymphocyte to differentiate into the plasma cell, which then produces a secretory version of the BCR, the *antibodies*. The BCR and the antibodies are jointly referred to as *immunoglobulins*.

In this chapter, we describe the common features of the membrane-bound and secreted immunoglobulins, their specific characteristics, the evolution of immunoglobulin molecules, and the superfamily to which they belong. The chapter ends with the description of receptors that specifically recognize immunoglobulin molecules.

How immunoglobulins came by their name

Chemists have known for some time that if a neutral salt such as ammonium sulphate is added in small doses to blood serum or plasma, at a certain salt concentration an insoluble material begins to separate (*precipitate*) from the solution. The reason for this 'salting out' is that the serum contains a large number of proteins which remain in solution because their molecules interact with molecules of water and so are kept apart. If salts are added to the serum, however, more and more water binds to the ammonium sulphate, until a point is reached at which not enough water is available to interact with the proteins. At this point, the protein molecules begin to interact with one another, forming large aggregates that fall out of the solution. Since different proteins have different affinities for neutral salts, they precipitate at different salt concentrations. The first protein fraction that precipitated out of the serum was called *globulin* because it was thought, erroneously as it turned out, to be related to haemoglobin, the red pigment of erythrocytes. The protein that precipitated at higher ammonium sulphate concentrations was termed *albumin* because, when heated, it coagulated into a substance resembling egg-white, *album ovi*.

Globulins and albumin can also be separated from each other by *electrophoresis*. In the original version of this method, *moving boundary electrophoresis*, the serum sample was placed in a U-shaped tube connected to a source of electric current, one arm to a positively charged anode and the other to a negatively charged cathode. Since the proteins in the serum carry electrical charges imparted to them by the amino acid side-chains, they migrate either to the anode or the cathode, depending on their net charge. Furthermore, since different proteins carry different charges determined by their amino acid composition, they migrate at different speeds, so that proteins carrying a greater charge migrate faster than proteins with a lesser charge. The individual proteins separate from one another, with sharp boundaries between them. Since the refraction index of the solution changes dramatically at these boundaries, it provides information about the direction of migration and the concentration of each protein (Fig. 8.1). The moving boundary of a protein mixture then appears as a series of peaks separated by valleys (Fig. 8.2a). Serum fractionation by moving boundary electrophoresis not only separated globulins from albumin, but also differentiated the former into three peaks, which were labelled α, β and γ, starting from the one closest to albumin. More sophisticated electrophoretic techniques can separate the three

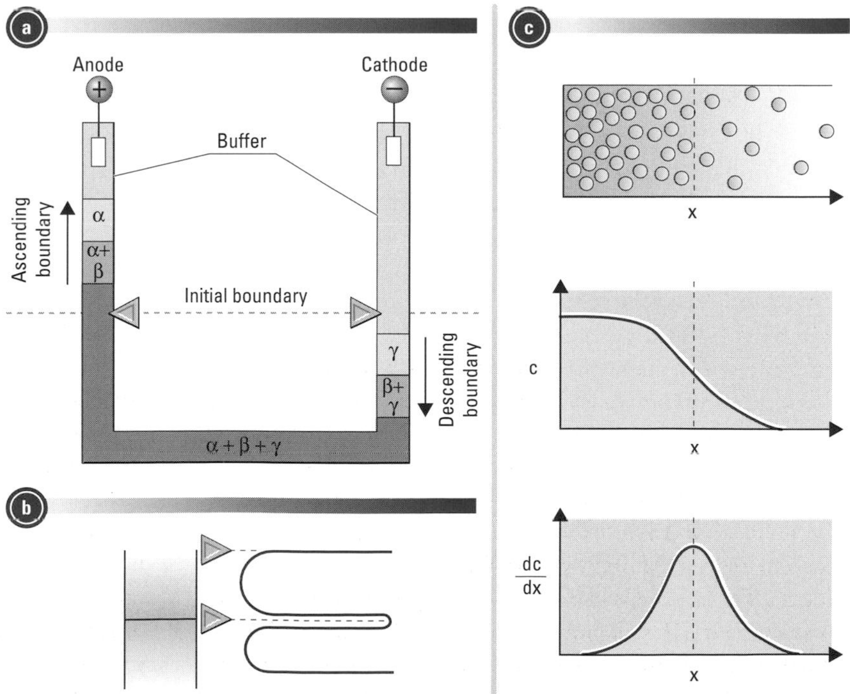

Figure 8.1 A bit of history: moving-boundary electrophoresis used in earlier times to separate serum into fractions α, β, and γ. (a) Schematic view of the apparatus and of the movement of negatively charged proteins (the 'boundary') towards the anode. (b) Optical record of moving boundaries (note the sharp change in refraction indices at the boundary; only one is shown here). (c) Transformation of concentration gradient curves.

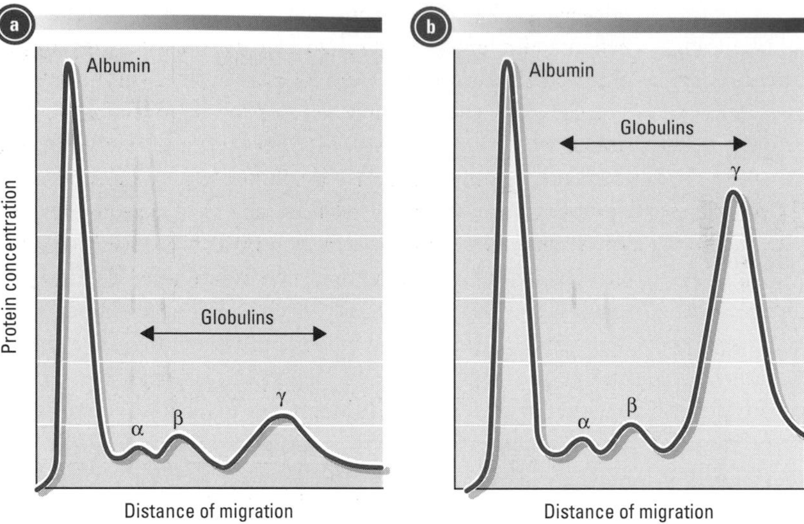

Figure 8.2 Serum fractionation by moving-boundary electrophoresis. (a) Normal serum. (b) Immune serum (antiserum). After absorption of the antiserum by the immunizing antigen, the electrophoretic pattern shown in (b) changes to that seen in (a). (Based on Tiselius, A. & Kabat, E.A. (1939) *Journal of Experimental Medicine*, **69**, 119.)

globulin peaks further into subfractions designated α1, α2, β1, β2 and so on.

In the late 1940s, researchers noticed that when they injected a foreign substance (*antigen*), for instance a suspension of bacteria, into an animal, the γ-globulin peak increased in height, often dramatically (Fig. 8.2b). They attributed this increase to the presence of *antibodies*, proteins produced by the animal in response to the inoculated antigen and capable of binding this antigen specifically. When they then added the antigen to the *antiserum* (i.e. serum known to contain antibodies specific for a tested antigen in contradistinction to a *normal serum*, which lacks these antibodies), a precipitate formed, and the protein profile of the serum in moving boundary electrophoresis returned to that of a normal serum. (The procedure by which antibodies are removed from an antiserum by the addition of an antigen is termed *absorption*.) Obviously, the antibodies were part of the γ-globulin fraction. Although some antibodies were also found later in the slowly migrating subfraction of β-globulins, the overwhelming majority proved to be associated with the γ-globulin peak. Not all γ-globulins are antibodies, however, and to distinguish the antibody-containing globulins from the rest the term *immune globulins* or *immunoglobulins* (abbreviated Ig) was introduced for the former.

Immunoglobulin genes

Human immunoglobulin molecules are encoded in three clusters of gene segments (*loci*) on three different chromosomes: the *IGH cluster* (H for 'heavy') on chromosome 14q32; the *IGK cluster* (K for 'kappa') on chromosome 2p12–p11; and the *IGL cluster* (L for 'lambda') on chromosome 22q11 (Fig. 8.3). The *IGH* cluster consists of four types of segments: *V* (for 'variable'), *D* (for 'diversity'), *J* (for 'joining') and *C* (for 'constant'). The *IGK* and *IGL* clusters each consist of three types of segments: *V*, *J* and *C*. The *IGH* cluster is thus located on the same chromosome as the *TCRA/D* cluster but this fact has probably no functional significance because the distance between the two regions is very large and because in other species *IGH* and *TCRA/D* are on different chromosomes. The *D* and *J* segments each consist of a single exon; the *V* and *C* segments consist of more than one exon.

The *IGH locus* stretches over a region encompassing some 1.1 million nucleotide pairs (1100 kb or 1.1 Mb). The entire region has been physically mapped. The major part of the *IGH* locus (about 900 kb) is taken up by the *V* segments (Fig. 8.4). There are approximately 95 *V* segments plus or minus a few representing insertion/deletion polymorphism in individual humans. However, only about 50 of the 95 *V* segments are believed to be functional; the remaining segments are pseudogenes. In addition to these, there are at least 24 orphons, *V* segments not part of the major cluster on chromosome 14. The orphons are clustered in two regions on chromosomes 15 and 16. Although not all of the orphons are pseudogenes rendered inactive by structural defects, it is unlikely that any of them are functional. Their expression would require interchromosomal (as opposed to intrachromosomal) recombination for the assembly of a functional unit and this has never been observed.

The 95 *IGHV* segments have been divided into three *subgroups* and these into seven *families* (Table 8.1). The subgroups were originally defined by amino acid sequence similarity of proteins; the definition of families is based largely on nucleotide sequence similarity using the same

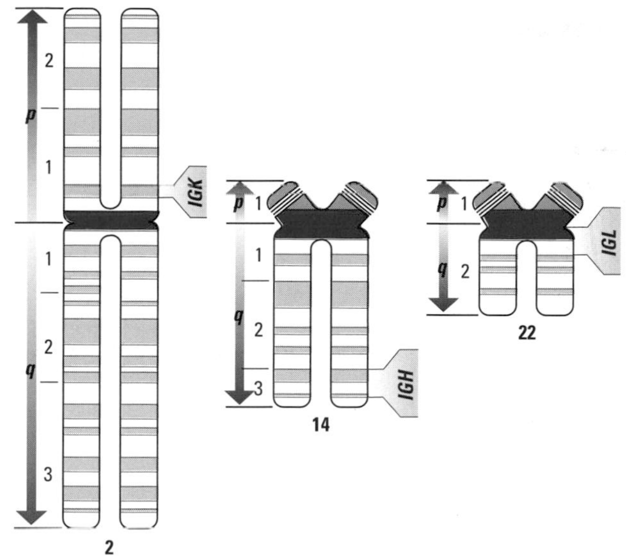

Figure 8.3 Location of functional immunoglobulin loci on human chromosomes.

criteria as for TCR segments. Most of the families are present also in the mouse, so the divergence of the duplicated segments from which the families evolved must have occurred before the separation of the primate and rodent lineages some 60–80 million years (my) ago. However, the mouse has some families, the homologues of which are apparently not represented in humans. (There are at least 15 *V*-segment families in the mouse, organized into the same three subgroups as in humans; in the rabbit, a repre-

Table 8.1 Number of gene segments in human and mouse immunoglobulin loci.

	Number of segments (human/mouse)			
Locus	*V*	*D*	*J*	*C*
IGH	95/110	23/12	9/4	11/8
IGK	90/100	0	5/4	1/1
IGL	60/2	0	7/4	7/4

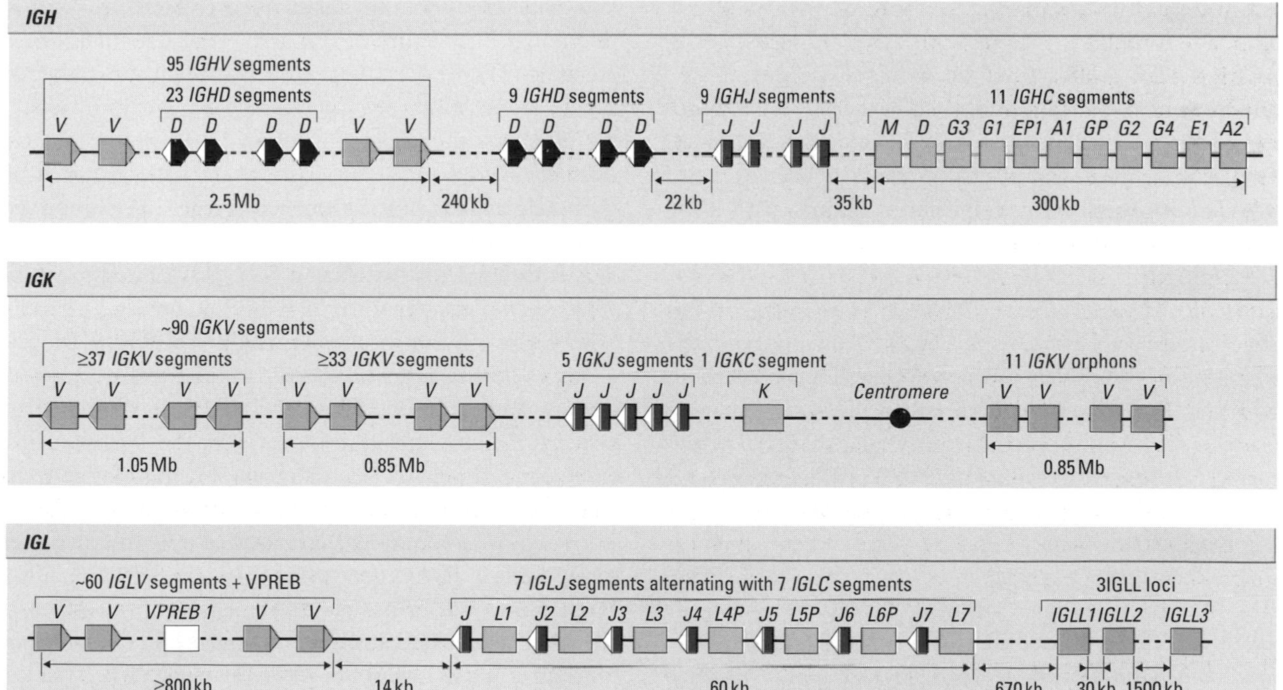

Figure 8.4 Organization of the human immunoglobulin loci. Rectangles represent individual gene segments, triangles recombination signal sequences (open triangles, 12-bp spacer signals; closed triangles, 23-bp spacer signals). Interconnecting lines indicate intervening sequences; dotted lines indicate segments not shown. Double-headed arrows give an estimate of distances in kilobase pairs (kb) or megabase pairs (Mb).

sentative of the Lagomorpha, all *V* segments seem to be members of one highly conserved family.) Another difference between the mouse and humans is that in the mouse, *V* segments belonging to the same family tend to cluster together in discrete regions of the chromosome, whereas in humans members of different families are intermingled physically. The *V* region of the *IGH* locus must therefore have undergone many rearrangements during primate evolution, mostly duplications, deletions and transposition. The fact that all the *IGHV* segments have the same transcriptional orientation indicates that no inversions occurred. The density of *V* segments at the human *IGH* locus is, on average, one segment per 10–17 kb.

The human *IGHD segments* are found at two positions in the *IGH* locus: one cluster is in the *V* region and another in the region between the *V* and *J* clusters (see Fig. 8.4). The former, the 'D5 cluster', consists of two subclusters that originated by an internal duplication. Each subcluster contains five *D* segments. The *V* segments located downstream from the *D5* cluster are physically barred from rearranging with any of these *D* segments. Originally, four *D* segments were identified in the second *D* cluster (*D1–D4*); later, more were added and currently 12 functional segments and one pseudogene are known, but there may be more.

The human *IGHJ region* contains six functional *J* segments and three pseudogenes, all clustered in a tract only about 3 kb long (see Fig. 8.4). Because segments corresponding to the pseudogenes are also pseudogenes in the mouse, the inactivation must have taken place > 60 my ago. Some 6 kb downstream from the *J* region is the *IGHC region*, which consists of nine functional *C* segments and two pseudogenes (see Fig. 8.4). The segments are (in the order in which they are arranged on the chromosome): *IGHM*, *IGHD*, *IGHG3*, *IGHG1*, *IGHEP1*, *IGHA1*, *IGHGP*, *IGHG2*, *IGHG4*, *IGHE1* and *IGHA2*. The *IGHEP1* and *IGHGP* are, as the letter 'P' signifies, pseudogenes. There is another 'processed' pseudogene (without introns), *IGHEP2*, on chromosome 9. This arrangement arose by a series of duplications, the most recent of which occurred before the divergence of Old World monkeys (represented, for example, by the macaque) and hominoids more than 20 my ago (Fig. 8.5). The recent duplication involved the segment *G–G–E–A* of the original *M–D–G–G–E–A* segment. It appears that the *E* gene segment is allowed to exist in only one functional copy per chromosome (for possible reasons, see Chapter 23) and so the second copy has been inactivated by various means (deletion, truncation) in different hominoid species.

The human *IGK locus* occupies a region on the short arm of chromosome 2 approximately 2 Mb in length (see Fig. 8.4). The locus consists of about 90 *V*, five *J* and one *C* segment. In addition to the main cluster of *V* segments, there are 12 *V* orphons on the long arm of chromosome 2, five on chromosome 22 and at least eight on chromosome 1, and perhaps on other chromsomes as well. The 20 orphons that have been sequenced are all pseudogenes. Of the 70 *V* segments in the *IGK* locus, some 43% are also pseudogenes. The *V* region takes up most of the *IGK* locus. It can be divided into two parts, one about 1 Mb long and containing at least 37 *V* segments, and the other 0.85 Mb long with at least 33 V segments. Because the *V* segments in the two parts are oriented transcriptionally in opposite directions and because they are closely related, it is believed that they arose by a large, relatively recent duplication. The human *V* sequences fall into 47 families, which are interspersed along the entire region. The mouse *V* segments comprise 16 families, of which at least seven pre-date the primate–rodent divergence.

The human *IGL locus* occupies a region on the long arm of chromosome 22 approximately 880 kb long (the *V* region alone takes up 850 kb) and contains approximately 60 *V*, seven *J* and seven *C* segments (see Fig. 8.4). A special feature of the locus is that *J* segments alternate with *C* segments so that *J* and *C* segments form seven pairs. Segments *IGLC1*, *2*, *3* and *7* are functional; segments *IGLC4*, *5* and *6* are pseudogenes. The *V* segments fall into three clusterers and nine families, the members of which are probably intermingled. Families 1, 2, 3 and 7 are particularly rich in members. Of the 60 *V* segments, 30 are known to be functional, seven might be functional, 20 are known to be pseudogenes and three are suspected to be pseudogenes. Additional, decaying pseudogenes may be scattered over the entire region. At least four haplotypes have been identified differing in the presence or absence of certain segments.

Associated with the human *IGL* locus on chromosome 22 are genes encoding the *pre-BCR* chains, V_{preB} and the homologue of the mouse λ5 chain (see Fig. 8.4). These genes, in contradistinction to the *IGL* genes, are expressed only in preB cells (see Chapter 5). The two known V_{preB} genes, *VPREB1* and *2*, are located in the *V* region of the *IGL* locus; the genes encoding the λ5 homologue termed *IGL*-like genes (*IGLL1*, *2* and *3*, of which only the first one is known to be functional) are located 670 kb downstream from the last *IGLC* gene (*IGLC7*). The *VPREB* and the *IGLL* genes are translated from separate transcripts (i.e. the genes do not undergo rearrangement). In the mouse, the *VPREB* and *IGLL* genes reside in the one region outside the *IGL locus* and are only 5 kb apart.

Like the *TCR* genes, the immunoglobulin genes rearrange before they are expressed on the cell surface. At the *IGH* locus, one of the *D* segments transposes to and joins with one of the *J* segments and the *D–J* segment is then joined by

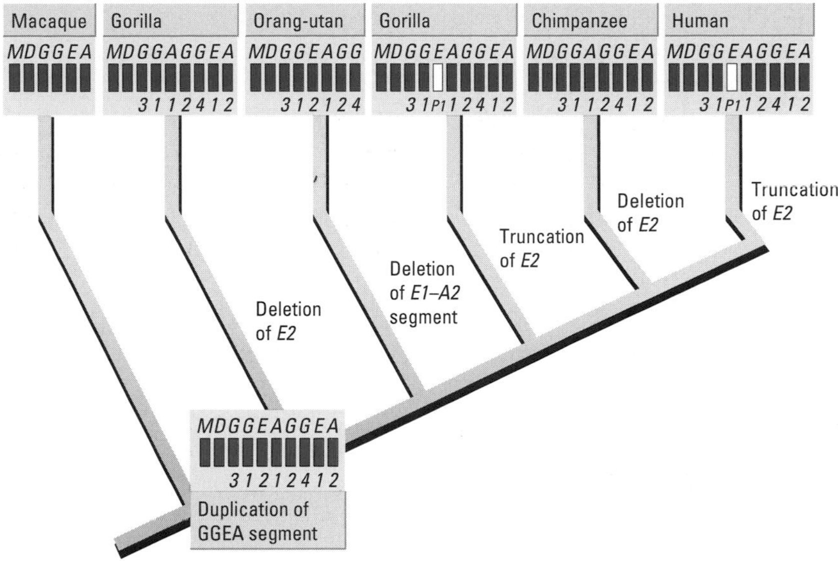

Figure 8.5 Evolution of primate *IGHC* segments. Closed rectangles indicate functional segments, open rectangles pseudogenes. Letters above and numbers beneath rectangles are the names of the segments. Truncation of *IGHC E1* in the lineages leading to the gorilla and humans consisted of two independent events that deleted different parts of the segment. The *IGHGP* segment has been omitted from this diagram because it is not known when it arose and when it became a pseudogene. The processed *IGHEP2* segment arose before the divergence of New World and Old World monkeys. (Based on data from Kawamura, S. & Ueda, S. (1992) *Genomics*, **13**, 194.)

one of the *V* segments. The productively rearranged *IGH* gene is transcribed and one of the nine C segments is chosen for expression. In this way, nine different types of heavy (H) chain can be produced (μ, δ, γ3, γ1, α1, γ2, γ4, ε1 or α2) depending on whether the *IGHCM, D, G3, G1, A1, G2, G4, E1* or *A2* segments are used. After *IGH*, either the *IGK* or *IGL* loci are rearranged. If the *IGK* recombination is productive, the cell produces an immunoglobulin molecule that consists of two identical H and two identical κ (kappa) chains. If not, and the *IGL* locus rearrangement succeeds, the cell synthesizes immunoglobulin molecules with two identical H chains and two identical λ (lambda) chains. In both instances, the cell will be making immunoglobulin molecules with two H chains (of one of nine possible types) and two light (L) chains (of one of two possible types). A more detailed description of these processes follows.

Gene activation, transcription and rearrangement

In the germ line and in most of the somatic cells, the human *IG* genes are arranged as shown in Fig. 8.4 and they are all silent (inactive). The parts of the chromatin fibres they occupy are wound around the histone octamers and the nucleosomes are tightly packed (see Fig. 7.4). In addition, the enhancers responsible for gene activation might be occupied by repressors, assuring the silence of the genes. It is only in the bone marrow that certain progenitor cells set on a course ultimately leading to the expression of *IG* genes and thus to the differentiation of the progenitors into B lymphocytes. What exactly happens in the progenitors committed to the B-lymphocytic lineage is not known, but from the limited data available and from analogy with other genes, a crude picture of *IG* gene activation can be sketched out.

At some point in its development, the progenitor begins to synthesize proteins that enter the nucleus and begin to assemble at the *IGH* locus of the chromatin, specifically in regions containing the *enhancer* sequences. There are three such regions at the *IGH* locus (at least in the mouse, in which most of the studies on *IG* gene activation have been performed): one (and the main) region in the intron between the most downstream J_H segment and the *IGHM* segment (ENH_{iH} region); another downstream of the *IGHA2* segment ($ENH_{3'H}$ region); and another still in the promoter region just upstream of every *IGHV* segment (Fig. 8.6, which also shows the position of the enhancer regions at the *IGK* and *IGL* loci; these are discussed later). The proteins are variously referred to as 'activators', 'transcription factors', or simply 'nuclear proteins'; they correspond to the *activators* in Fig. 7.14. Each of them contains a region via which it can recognize and bind to a short DNA sequence in the enhancer region of the *IGH* locus (this sequence is the 'enhancer element' or simply *enhancer*). There are nine such sequences in the ENH_{iH} (Fig. 8.7), and six in each of the *IGHV* promoter regions (Fig. 8.8). Each enhancer can bind several different activators (Fig. 8.7). At least 16 activators that bind to the enhancers in the ENH_{iH} region have already been identified by methods such as *electrophoretic mobility shift analysis* (Fig. 8.9), *DNA footprinting* (Fig. 8.10) and the *CAT assay* (Fig. 8.11). The proteins belong to several different families and bear a bewildering variety of names and synonyms whose origins are known only to a sect of experts and sometimes not even to them (see Fig. 8.4). Most of the proteins are synthesized not only by cells of the B lineage but by other cells as well; a few are, however, B-cell specific (Fig. 8.7). The presence of activators specific for *IG* enhancers in non-B cells in which *IG* genes are inactive is baffling. It is thought that in these cells the activators actually inactivate the *IG* genes by interacting with repressor proteins. At least one such repressor protein (ZEB) has been identified. The overall activity of the *IGH* enhancer may be the sum total of interactions among a wide array of proteins. Be that as it may, the production of certain B cell-specific activators by the progenitor apparently shifts the regulatory effects from negative to positive.

How the activators gain access to the enhancer sequences in the tightly packed chromatin is unclear. One possibility is that they compete with the histones for DNA binding in this region and gradually replace them. The transiently histone-free region becomes accessible to the enzyme DNase and DNase hypersensitive sites, a hallmark of gene activation, are thus generated. The local displacement of histones and the assembly of activators in the enhancer regions changes the structure of the chromatin from closed to open.

The congress of the activators into the *IGH* enhancer regions is the beginning of the assembly of the transcription apparatus. The activators are then presumably followed by co-activators and these by the basal factors (see Fig. 7.14). The basal factors bind to the promoter region of one of the *IGHV* segments, which may be a large distance from the enhancer, as measured in numbers of nucleotide pairs. The promoter and enhancer regions are, however, brought together by looping-out the intervening sequence, perhaps by the interaction of special DNA sequences (*matrix-associated regions*; MAR) with the proteins of the nuclear scaffolding. The MAR of the *IGH* locus flank the enhancer and promoter regions. The main component of the promoter region is the *TATA box*, the site of the *TATA-box binding protein* attachment (see Fig. 8.8). The region, however, contains several other sequence motifs ('boxes') that bind proteins involved in the regulation of transcription and hence can be classified as enhancers. The octamer motif is also present in the ENH_{iH} and $ENH_{3'H}$, where it binds the Oct-1 and Oct-2 activator proteins. To assess the activity of a promoter such as that of the *IGH* gene, molecular biologists use the CAT assay (see Fig. 8.11).

Once the transcription apparatus is assembled, transcription can begin. The first RNA molecules synthesized at the *IGH* locus after the opening of the chromatin are not translated into proteins and are therefore referred to as *sterile transcripts*. Their function is not known but they may be

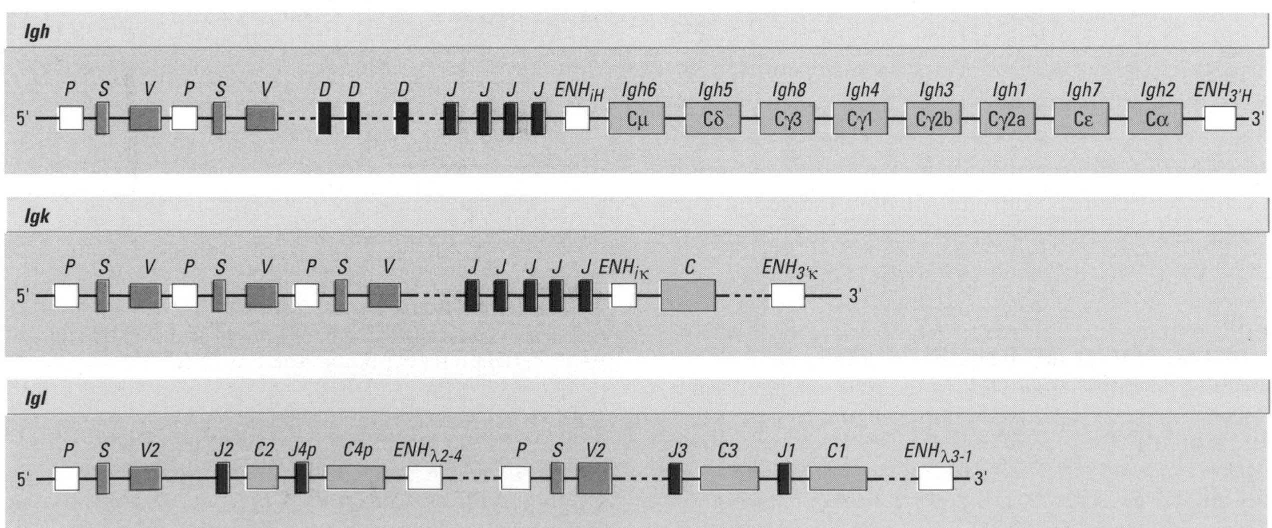

Figure 8.6 Location of the promoter (P) and enhancer (ENH) regions in the mouse immunoglobulin loci. S, exon encoding the signal peptide; dots indicate unspecified length of DNA; p, pseudogene; for heavy-chain-encoding loci the chain designations are given within the boxes.

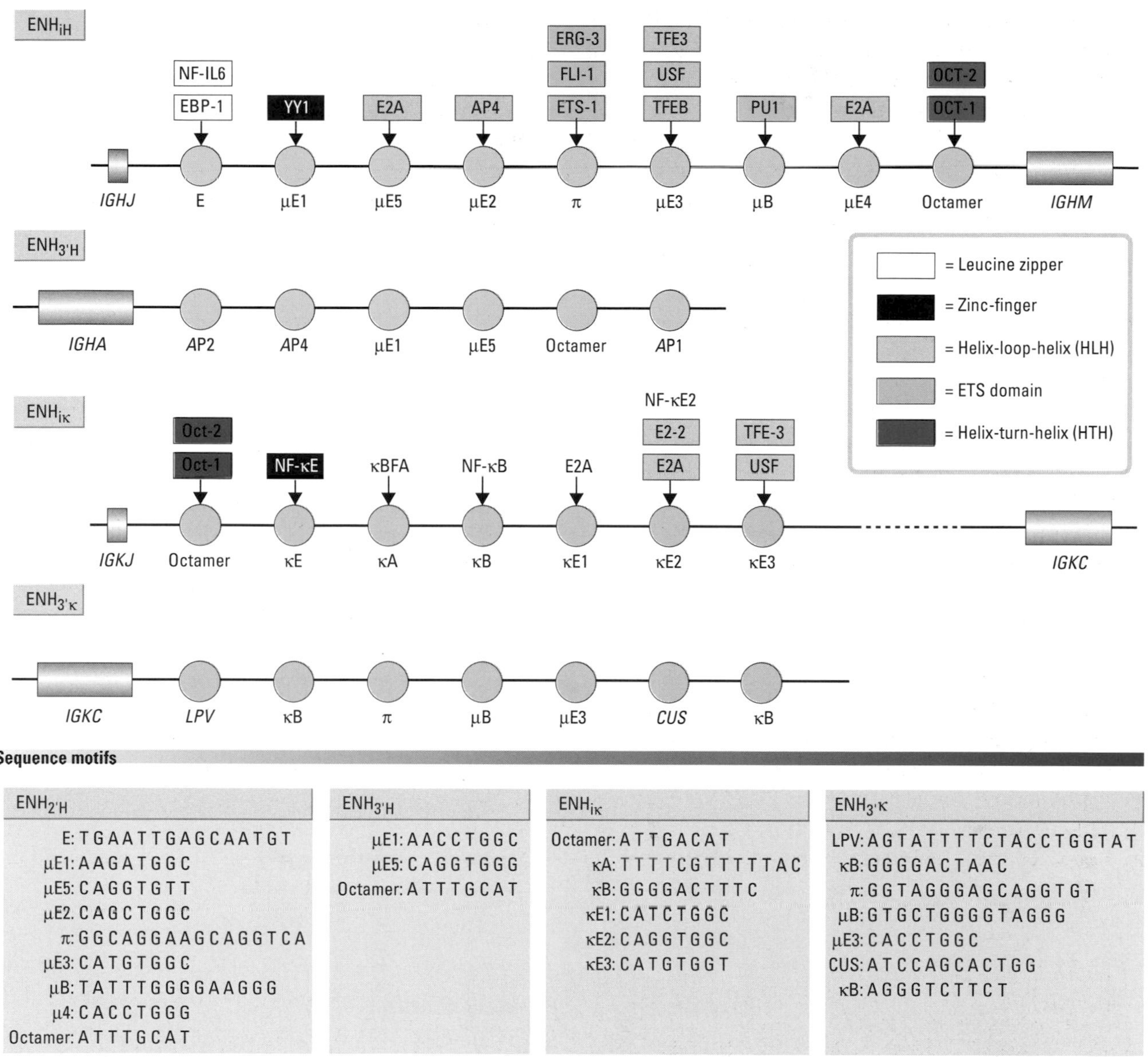

Figure 8.7 Protein-binding sites (small circles) in the enhancer regions of mouse immunoglobulin genes. The proteins known to bind to these sites are also shown (rectangles above arrows). For location of the enhancer regions in the different *IG* loci, see Fig. 8.6. The families of the proteins are indicated by the different coloured rectangles (see key). (For description of the families, see Fig. 7.12.) The E2A protein occurs in different forms (E12, E47, E2–5 or ITF1) that are the products of alternative splicing of a transcript derived from the same gene. Derivation of some of the designations: 3′, enhancer located in the 3′ region of the gene; *AP*, activator protein; *CUS*, conserved upstream sequence; *E* boxes, named after Anna Ephrussi, the first author of the publication in which this group of sequence motifs was reported; EBP, enhancer-binding protein; ENH, enhancer; ERG, *e*ts-*r*elated *g*ene; ETS, *E-twenty-s*ix (protooncogene homologous to an oncogene in retrovirus E26); FLI, Friend leukaemia integration (oncogene) homologue; H, heavy-chain gene; i, intron; κ, kappa chain encoded in the *IGK* segment; κBFA, factor binding to the κA box; *LPV*, region homologous to the enhancer of human lymphotrophic papovirus; μ, mu chain encoded in the *IGHM* segment; NF-κE, nuclear factor binding to the κE box; NF-IL6, nuclear factor induced by interleukin-6; Oct, octamer; π, preB-cell motif (confers strong enhancement in preB cells but not in mature B cells); PU, protooncogene product recognizing a purine-rich sequence; TFE, transcription factor binding to the E-box; USF, upstream stimulatory factor; YY, homologue of human GLI-Krüppel protein; no explanation for choice of letters given.

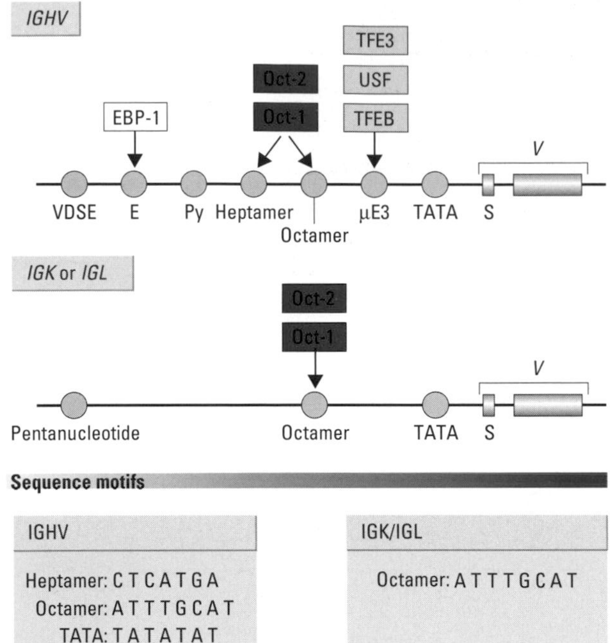

Figure 8.8 Promoter regions of immunoglobulin genes. Protein-binding sites located upstream of every *V* segment are indicated as circles. Proteins known to bind to these sites are indicated by the symbols above the arrows. The Oct-2 protein is B-cell lineage specific; the other proteins are also found in non-B cells. E, Ephrussi box; EBP, enhancer-binding protein; Oct, octamer; Py, pyrimidine-rich motif; TFE, transcription factor binding to E box; USF, upstream stimulating factor; VDSE, vitamin D sensitive element; S, exon encoding the signal peptide.

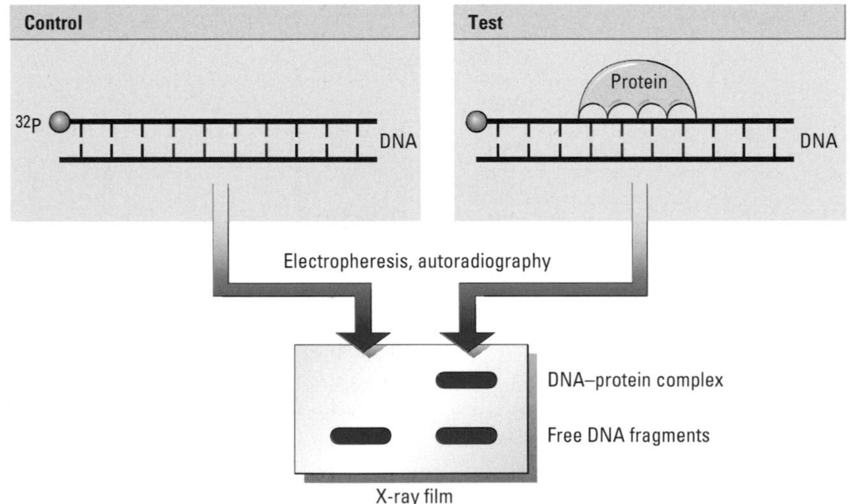

Figure 8.9 Electrophoretic mobility shift analysis, also referred to as gel retardation (retention, shift) assay. To determine whether a cellular extract contains a protein that binds to motif sequences in a given DNA fragment (e.g. an activator binding to an enhancer sequence), the extract is incubated with the DNA fragment, which has been labelled by the attachment of radioactive atoms (^{32}P) to one end of one of the two strands. After washing to remove unattached proteins, the DNA is subjected to gel electrophoresis. As a control, DNA that has not been exposed to the extract is electrophoresed in a lane next to the test lane. An X-ray film is then exposed to the gel. Attachment of the protein makes the DNA heavier and bulkier so that the complex migrates more slowly (it moves a shorter distance away from the 'origin', the slot into which the sample was loaded) than the uncomplexed DNA. An extra band of radioactive material is therefore seen on the X-ray film in the test lane in comparison with the control lane.

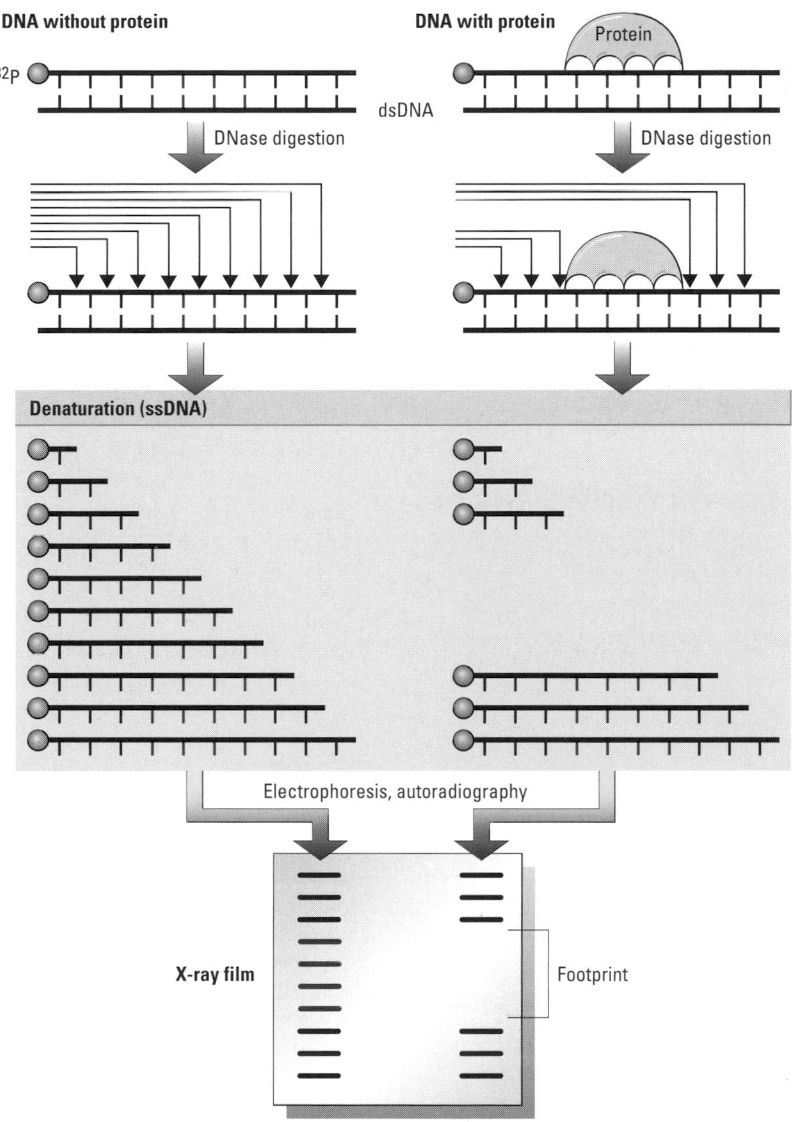

Figure 8.10 DNA footprinting. To identify the sequence motif that a DNA-binding protein recognizes, the DNA fragment is labelled by the attachment of radioactive ^{32}P atoms to one end of one of its two strands and incubated with the protein. After washing to remove the unattached protein, the DNA is digested with DNase. The conditions of the digestion (enzyme concentration, duration of treatment, etc.) are such that the DNase has time to nick (break one of the two strands indicated by arrows) each DNA molecule in the suspension only once. Because the selection of sites for nicking is entirely random, in the control DNA (which has not been incubated with the protein) every two neighbouring nucleotides in a DNA strand have the same probability of having the bond between them broken. At the end of the treatment, there will therefore be DNA molecules in the control suspension in which the nick occurred between the first two nucleotides, others which were nicked between the second and third nucleotide, and so on (indicated by horizontal lines connected to arrows). When the two strands are then separated (the DNA is denatured, for example by heating) and subjected to gel electrophoresis, a 'ladder' of bands containing strands of increasing length appears, the increment being one nucleotide. The ladder can then be visualized by the exposure of an X-ray film to the gel (*autoradiography*). The same thing happens in the DNA exposed to the protein, except that the sequence to which the protein is attached is inaccessible to the DNase and thus is protected from nicking. On the gel (film), the fragments that in the control result from nicking in this region are missing in the test lane. This blank region is a *footprint* of a protein that has attached to a specific region of the DNA molecule. If the sequence of the DNA fragment is known, the sequence of the binding motif (highlighted) can be read off from the footprint. There are several different versions of the DNA footprinting assay, not all of which use DNase to pinpoint the protected region. ds, double-stranded; ss, single-stranded.

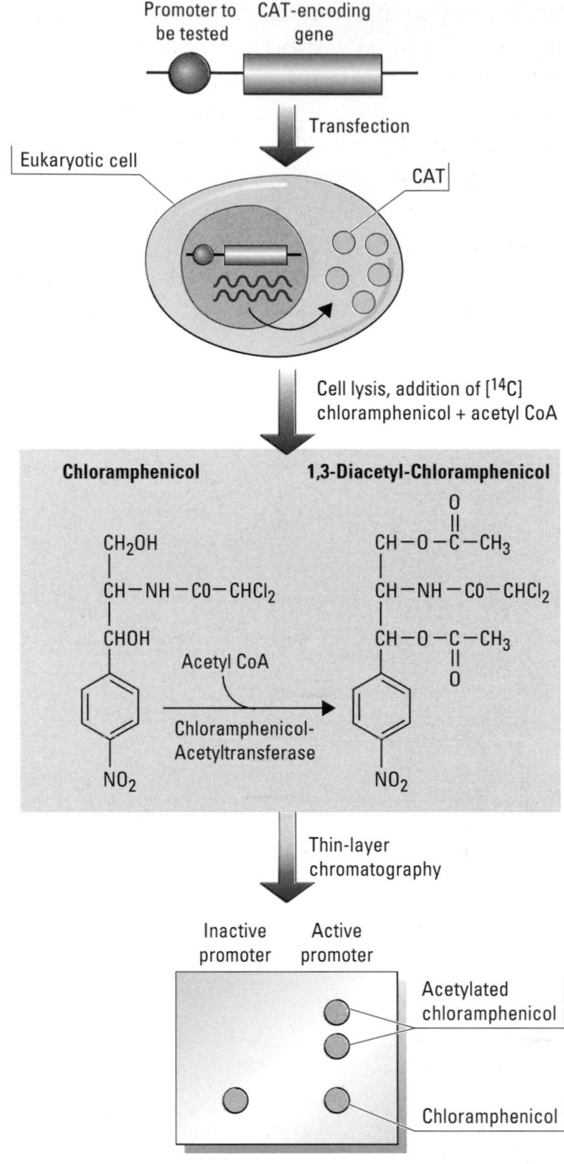

Figure 8.11 CAT assay. To measure the strength of a promoter (i.e. its efficiency in promoting the transcription of an adjacent gene), the promoter region is excised from its gene and placed next to a *reporter gene* whose activity can be quantitated easily. A commonly used reporter is the *chloramphenicol acetyltransferase* (*CAT*) gene, which codes for an enzyme that transfers acetyl groups (CH_3CO) to the antibiotic chloramphenicol. The construct containing the tested promoter and the reporter gene is transferred (*transfected*) into eukaryotic cells, where it produces the enzyme. The cells are then lysed, radioactively labelled, chloramphenicol and acetyl-CoA are added to the lysate and the quantity of produced acetylated chloramphenicol is determined by thin-layer chromatography. (In this technique, a drop of lysate is placed at one edge of a plate coated with a thin layer of a solid material such as an ion exchanger, gel filtration agent or physical adsorbent; see Figs 8.23 & 8.43. The plate is then lowered into a container with a mixture of organic solvents such as chloroform and alcohol. As the solvents move up through the coating by capillary action, they take some of the substances in the lysate with them and separate them according to their migration speeds.)

involved in the *VDJ* recombination process. Although rearranging loci are transcribed before or concomitantly with their recombination, a causal link between these two events has not been demonstrated formally. It has been speculated, however, that transcription makes the locus accessible to the recombination factors (RAG1, RAG2 and others).

Normally, *IGH* genes rearrange first, *IGK* genes next and *IGL* genes last. Occasionally, however, the L chain-encoding genes rearrange before the *IGH* genes. At the *IGH* locus, the temporal order is the $D \rightarrow J_H$ transposition first and $V_H \rightarrow DJ_H$ transposition next (Fig. 8.12). For unknown reasons, the transposition of a V_H segment to an unrearranged *D* segment does not occur. At the L chain-encoding loci, which do not have *D* segments, the *V* segments are transposed directly to the *J* segments. The transposition occurs with the help of recombination signals that consist, as in the case of the *TCR* loci, of heptamer–spacer–nonamer sequences, where the spacer can be either 12 bp or 23 bp long. And just as in the case of the *TCR* loci, the heptamers are variations on the theme CACAGTG and the nonamers deviate very little from the consensus sequence ACACAAACC. At the *IGL* locus, the signals are arranged as at the *TCR* loci: a signal with a 23-bp spacer flanks the 3′ end of each *IGLV* segment and a signal with a 12-bp spacer flanks the 5′ end of each *IGLJ* segment. At the *IGK* and *IGH* loci, the signals are arranged somewhat differently (Fig. 8.13). Each *IGKV* segment is flanked at its 3′ end by a signal with the 12-bp spacer and each *IGKJ* segment at the 5′ end by a signal with the 23-bp spacer. The distribution of the signals enables the *IGL* loci to obey the *12/23 joining rule*: two segments can be joined only when one of them is flanked by the 12-bp spacer signal and the other by the 23-bp spacer signal. Because of this rule, one *V* segment cannot be joined to another *V* segment, one *D* cannot join another *D*, and one *J* cannot join another *J*. Similarly, an *IGHV* segment cannot join an *IGHJ* segment directly without *IGHJ* first joining *IGHD*. The joining of *IGHV* to *IGHD* segments is permitted by the 12/23 rule but, as already mentioned, for some reason normally does not occur.

The mechanism of signal-mediated recombination is apparently the same for the *TCR* and *IG* loci and probably is mediated by the same set of proteins, including the RAG1 and RAG2 proteins. To recapitulate what was described at length in Chapter 7, the mechanism involves the following four steps (see Figs 7.7–7.9). First, proteins, at least some of which might be part of the transcription apparatus, assemble near two distant gene segments, and their

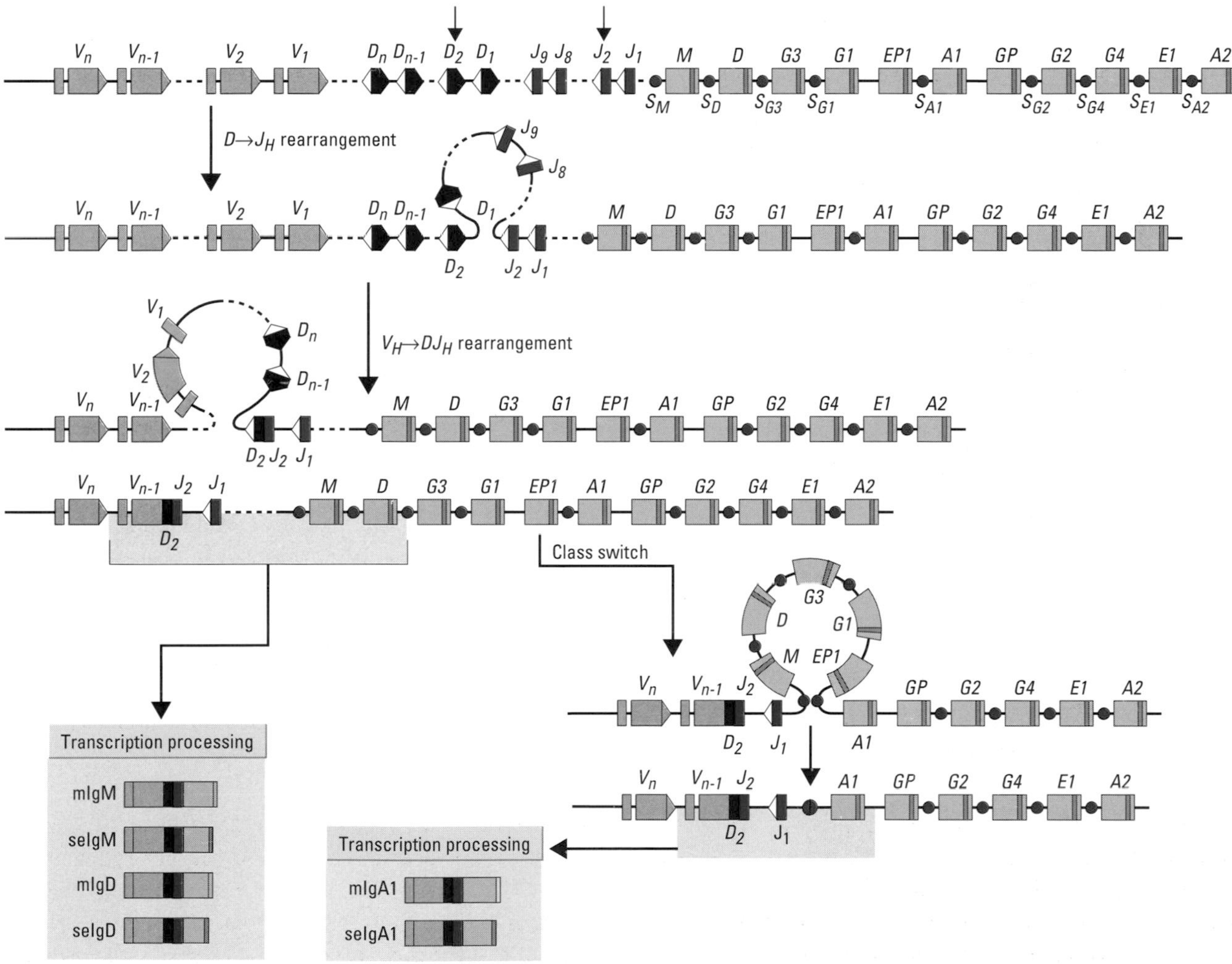

Figure 8.12 Rearrangements at the human *IGH* locus. Three types of recombination take place at the *IGH* loci. First, one of the *D* segments is joined with one of the J_H segments ($D \rightarrow J_H$ rearrangement). Second, one of the V_H segments is fused with the DJ_H joint ($V_H \rightarrow DJ_H$ rearrangement). And third, the V_HDJ_H joint is transposed to the vicinity of one of the C_H segments (class switch; described later in this chapter). In all three instances, recombination involves removal of the intervening, looped-out DNA sequence. Each recombination is preceded and followed by transcription (only the transcription preceding and following the class switch is shown here). The transcripts of the C_H segments can be spliced in alternative ways to produce either membrane-bound (*m*) or secreted (*se*) heavy immunoglobulin chains (this point, too, is discussed later). *V* and *D* segments are numbered arbitrarily (*n*, unspecified number). Short arrows mark segments chosen for joining. Rectangles indicate segments; triangles indicate recombination signal sequences; circles indicate class switch signals; dotted lines indicate unspecific intervening sequence. (Here, the '*C*' symbol in the C_H segment designations is omitted.)

interactions bring the two segments together by looping-out the intervening DNA sequence. The segments align with each other in such a way that their recombination signal sequences (one with the 12-bp and the other with the 23-bp spacer) become juxtaposed. If the recombination signals of the two segments were originally arranged head-to-head (see Fig. 7.9a), the intervening sequence forms a simple loop; if they were in a head-to-tail arrangement, it forms an inversion loop (see Fig. 7.9b). Second, double-stranded breaks occur between each of the two signal sequences and the coding sequences; the breaks are probably effected by a multiprotein enzyme ('recombinase'), one component of which might be the RAG proteins. Third, the free ends are ligated: signal to signal and coding sequence to coding sequence. In the case of a simple loop, this step results in the deletion of the signals and of the intervening sequence in the form of a non-replicating circle; in the case of an inversion loop, the intervening sequence, together with the signals, is inverted and remains part of the chromosome. Inversional rearrangements occur in one-half of the recombinations involving *IGKV* segments (those that have been duplicated and inverted); rearrangements by deletional mechanisms take place in the other half of the *IGKV* segments and in all rearrangements at the human *IGH* and *IGL* loci. Fourth, the ligation of the signals is usually not accompanied by any changes in the sequence, whereas the joining of the coding ends is. The latter undergo *junctional diversification* by the addition of P-nucleotides and addition and/or deletion of N-nucleotides. The P-nucleotides are templated by the overhanging single strands generated by the cleavage of the hairpin structure; the N-nucleotides result from the non-templated action of terminal deoxynucleotidyl transferase and of other enzymes (see Chapter 7 and discussion later in this chapter).

The rearrangements of the *IG* genes are, however, preceded by the expression of pre-BCRs, which consist of surrogate L chains combined with the H chains (see Fig. 8.53). The surrogate L chain is encoded in the *VPREB* and the *IGLL* ('λ5') genes.

The rearrangement of the *IGH* locus proceeds in two steps: in the first step, a randomly chosen *D* segment is moved to a randomly chosen *J* segment; in the second step, a randomly chosen V_H segment is moved to the DJ_H joint and the segment from the V_HDJ_H joint to, and including, the C_M segment is transcribed and translated into a full-length H (μ) chain. The product is then tested for its ability to associate with the surrogate L chain. The C_M segment contains one exon, which is required for membrane integration of the H chain. If this exon is missing or if its translation is garbled, the chain cannot be inserted into the membrane. In this case, or in any other situation in which the H chain proves to be non-functional, new rounds of rearrangements involving some of the remaining V_H, *D* and J_H segments (i.e. those that have not been deleted in previous rounds) are carried out until a functional H chain is produced. If they all fail and the supply of segments is exhausted, the cell dies by programmed cell death. If, on the other hand, a functional H chain is produced and a pre-BCR consisting of the H and surrogate L chains becomes integrated into the plasma membrane, further rearrangements stop and the cell begins to proliferate. The rearrangements resume only at the end of the proliferation phase, when the cells enter a resting stage and *RAG1/RAG2*, downregulated at the beginning of the phase, are upregulated again. However, the resumption concerns the L chain-encoding loci, *IGK* and *IGL*; the *IGH* can no longer recombine. The phases of recombination of the *IGH* and *IGK/IGL* loci are thus clearly separated from each other by

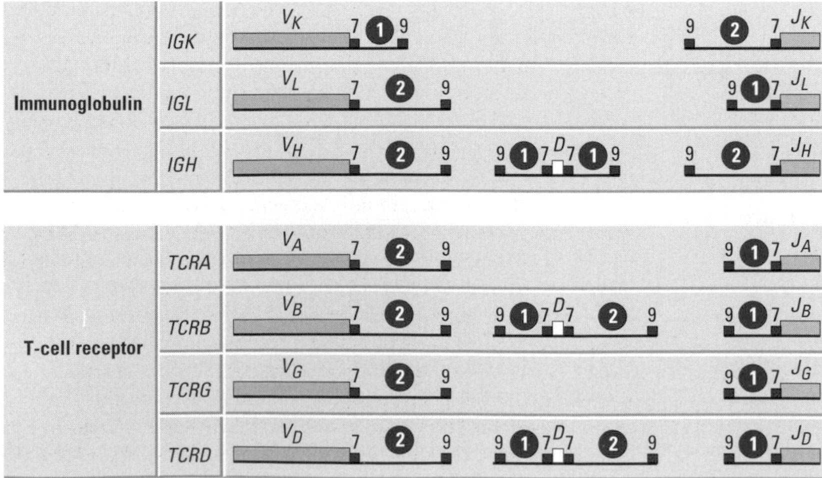

Figure 8.13 Comparison of recombination signal sequences flanking gene segments at immunoglobulin and T-cell receptor loci: 7, heptamer; 9, nonamer; 1, one-turn (12 ± 1 bp) spacer; 2, two-turn (23 ± 1 bp) spacer. (Modified from Kronenberg, M. *et al.* (1986) *Annual Review of Immunology*, 4, 529.)

a period of intense proliferation during which the recombination machinery is shut off. This situation closely parallels that described for the *TCRB* and *TCRA* loci in the preceding chapter.

During the second rearrangement phase it remains unresolved whether both L chain-encoding loci rearrange more or less simultaneously or whether the *IGK* locus recombines before the *IGL* locus; perhaps both situations occur. In either case, each rearranged version is tested for the ability of its product to associate with the H chain and to produce the BCR. If the rearrangement turns out to be non-functional (non-productive), new rounds of recombination follow until the cell exhausts its supply of *IGK/IGL V* and *J* segments. When that happens, the cell dies by apoptosis. However, even if one of the rearrangements turns out to be productive, the cell does not shut off the recombination machinery immediately. Instead it keeps it going for a while, in the event that ligand binding reveals the BCR to be unsuitable. In this case, the BCR L chain might be substituted by another one produced from subsequently rearranged genes (*editing*, in analogy to similar events taking place in the thymocytes). Only after final selection of the L chain has been made is the recombination machinery permanently shut off. The developing B cell thus passes through the same two checkpoints as the developing thymocyte: regulations at checkpoint 1 are effected by the pre-BCR and those at checkpoint 2 by the BCR (see Fig. 7.17).

Each preB cell has, of course, two versions of the chromosomes carrying the three *IGG* loci. The two chromosomes carrying the *IGH* locus rearrange their *IGH* genes simultaneously, but since there is only about 30% chance of any one rearrangement being productive, the probability of both chromosomes achieving productive rearrangements at the same time in both the $D \rightarrow J_H$ and $V_H \rightarrow DJ_H$ steps is low. And since further *IGH* rearrangements in a given preB cell are stopped once a productive rearrangement is achieved, only one of the two *IGH* alleles is normally expressed. The other allele is excluded from expression by the stochastic nature of the rearrangement process (*allelic exclusions*; Fig. 8.14). Similarly, since the chances that any two of the four chromosomes carrying the two L chain-encoding loci will accomplish productive rearrangement simultaneously are small, normally only one of the two *IGK* or *IGL* alleles becomes expressed. If a functional κ chain is produced, the BCR of the immature B cell becomes type $(\mu\kappa)_2$ and no further rearrangements occur. If a functional λ chain is produced before a κ chain, the BCR becomes type $(\mu\lambda)_2$. The signals that bring about the cessation of both activities remain unidentified.

The human *IGK* locus contains only one C_K segment (see Fig. 8.4) so that all the κ chains have the same constant region. The human *IGL* locus contains four functional C_L segments so that the λ chain can occur in four versions differing in their constant regions. The selection of the C_L segment for expression is tied together with the rearrangement. Because each C_L segment is associated with one J_L segment, rearrangement to a particular J_L segment leads to the use of the C_L segment associated with this J_L segment. The human *IGH* locus comprises nine functional C_H segments. The BCR of an immature B cell always uses the C_H segment closest to the J_H region for expression, which is the C_M, so that the receptor's H chain is always of the μ type (and the receptor is of the IgM class). When the cell matures, however, it switches to the use of other C_H segments and produces receptors containing other H chains. In these new versions, the cell retains the same H-chain variable region determined by the V_HDJ_H combination, but links it up with different constant regions. It thus keeps the same antigen-binding specificity (determined by the variable region) but combines it with different effector functions (determined, as described later, by the constant regions). The switch from expressing one C_H segment to the expression of another segment is achieved by another type of gene rearrangement, the *switch recombination*.

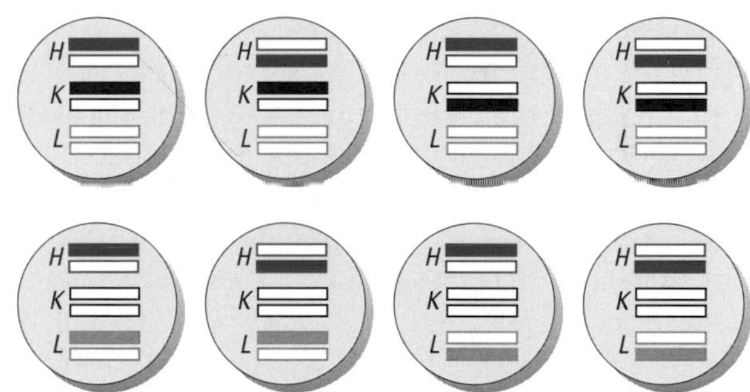

Figure 8.14 Principle of allelic and *IGK/IGL* locus exclusion. Of the two alleles at each locus (*H*, *K* or *L*), only one is expressed to produce functional immunoglobulin chains (closed rectangles) in a given B lymphocyte (circle); the other remains silent (open rectangles). Of the two light-chain-encoding loci (*K* and *L*), only one (either *K* or *L*) provides one functional allele in a given B lymphocyte; both alleles at the other locus remain silent. Consequently, immunoglobulin molecules have two identical heavy chains associated with two identical light chains, either κ or λ. Different cells express different combinations of alleles and light-chain-encoding loci. The diagram shows the eight combinations that would be theoretically possible if the choice of alleles and *L/K* loci for expression were random. Each cell will end up with only one of the eight combinations because once an *H* locus gene has been rearranged productively, further rearrangements of both alleles stop. Similarly, once a *K* gene is rearranged, rearrangement (and thus expression) of the *L* locus usually no longer take place.

Switch recombination

The first H chain expressed by the differentiating B cells is μ. As soon as a productive rearrangement of the D and V_H segments is achieved, transcription into RNA begins from the V_HDJ_H joint and continues downstream over the remaining J_H segments (if there are any left), across the long intervening sequence, and towards the first two C_H segments, C_M and C_D. Where it stops is not clear. It certainly includes the entire C_M segment with all its exons and introns, and it may also include the intervening sequence between C_M and C_D, as well as the entire C_D segment. A long transcript of more than 15 kb is thus produced which is then shortened by splicing out all the non-coding sequences (see Fig. 8.12). In the resulting mRNA therefore the coding sequences V_H, D, J_H and C_M become contiguous. The mRNA then leaves the nucleus and in the cytoplasm is translated into a protein, the μ chain. If the initial transcript encompassed the C_D segment, this is not included in the mRNA and hence not translated at this stage, so that the immature B cell synthesizes only the μH chains in the cytoplasm and expresses only IgM-type receptors on the cell surface (see Fig. 5.20).

In a later stage, the cell extends the transcription to include the C_D segment (if it has not done so earlier already) and splices the transcript in two ways: in one it cuts out the C_D segment and produces mRNA that is translated into the μ chain as before; in the other it excises the C_M segment and joins the V_HDJ_H sequence with the C_D segment (the mechanism responsible for this *alternative splicing* is explained later). The mRNA of the latter version is translated into the δ chain. Both H chains associate with the same L chains and the resulting IgM and IgD tetramers are delivered to the cell surface. The simultaneous expression of IgM and IgD receptors on the surface is the hallmark of the *mature B lymphocyte*. The two receptors have the same antigen-recognition sites (because they bear the same variable regions); they differ only in their constant regions.

Some evidence suggests that the cell may sometimes extend the region it transcribes even further downstream to include additional C_H segments and to produce monumentally long (180 kb or longer) transcripts. It may then join by alternative splicing one of these other C_H segments to the V_HDJ_H segment and produce other H-chain types. However, this evidence is controversial, and if this additional alternative splicing does occur it clearly is not the orthodox way of producing new H-chain types. The orthodox *class switch* (the change from the expression of one immunoglobulin class to another) is through additional DNA rearrangement (recombination). The rearrangement, however, does not occur unless the mature B lymphocyte is stimulated, by antigen, mitogen or some other means. If the lymphocyte does not encounter any of the activating agents, its algorithm takes it ultimately to apoptosis. Activation, on the other hand, initiates a chain of reactions, some of which presumably open the chromatin at one of the C_H segments downstream of the C_M and C_D segments. The choice of downstream segment is apparently determined by the nature of the activating stimulus and by the cytokine acting on the target cell during its stimulation. Thus, for example, it has been observed that bacterial lipopolysaccharide (LPS) in combination with interleukin-4 stimulates mouse cells to produce γ1 chains and, to a much lesser degree, ε chains; LPS in combination with interferon-γ leads to the production of γ2a chains; LPS combined with transforming growth factor β enhances a switch to α-chain production; and so on. Presumably different combinations of antigen and cytokine effect different class switches by stimulating the production of distinct nuclear proteins capable of binding to specific DNA sequences in the region upstream of the individual C_H segments. Several of these proteins have indeed been isolated and their specificity for sequence motifs in the C_H regions demonstrated.

Analysis of the sequences upstream of the individual C_H segments has led to the discovery of regions that contain several tandemly repeated motifs punctuated by unique or less repetitive sequences (Fig. 8.15). These *switch* (*S*) *regions*, which range in length from 1 to 10 kb, are found upstream of every C_H segment except C_D (which is joined to the V_HDJ_H segment not by recombination, but by alternative splicing). The individual switch regions are designated according to the segments with which they are associated: S_M, S_{G3}, S_{G1}, S_{A1}, etc., or less correctly (because they represent genetic rather than protein elements) S_μ, $S_\gamma3$, $S_\gamma1$, $S_\alpha1$, etc. The number of repeated motifs and their length varies from region to region, as does the sequence similarity of the motifs. All the *S* regions contain the pentamers GAGCT and GGGGT, repeated a different number of times in different regions. Three other pentamers (ACCAG, GCAGC and TGAGC), as well as one heptamer (YAGGTTG, where Y stands for 'pyrimidine') are also common. The overall sequence similarity of S_G regions to S_M regions is much lower than that of the S_E or S_A regions. The similarity of the mouse S_G to S_M regions decreases with the position along the chromosome ($S_{G3} > S_{G1} > S_{G2b} > S_{G2a}$).

The switch from one class to another is usually accompanied by the deletion of the intervening sequence. Thus, for example, human cells that have switched from μ-chain production to γ-chain production lack the entire piece of DNA from C_M to C_{G4} in one of their chromosomes. The rearranged chromosome contains a sequence from the

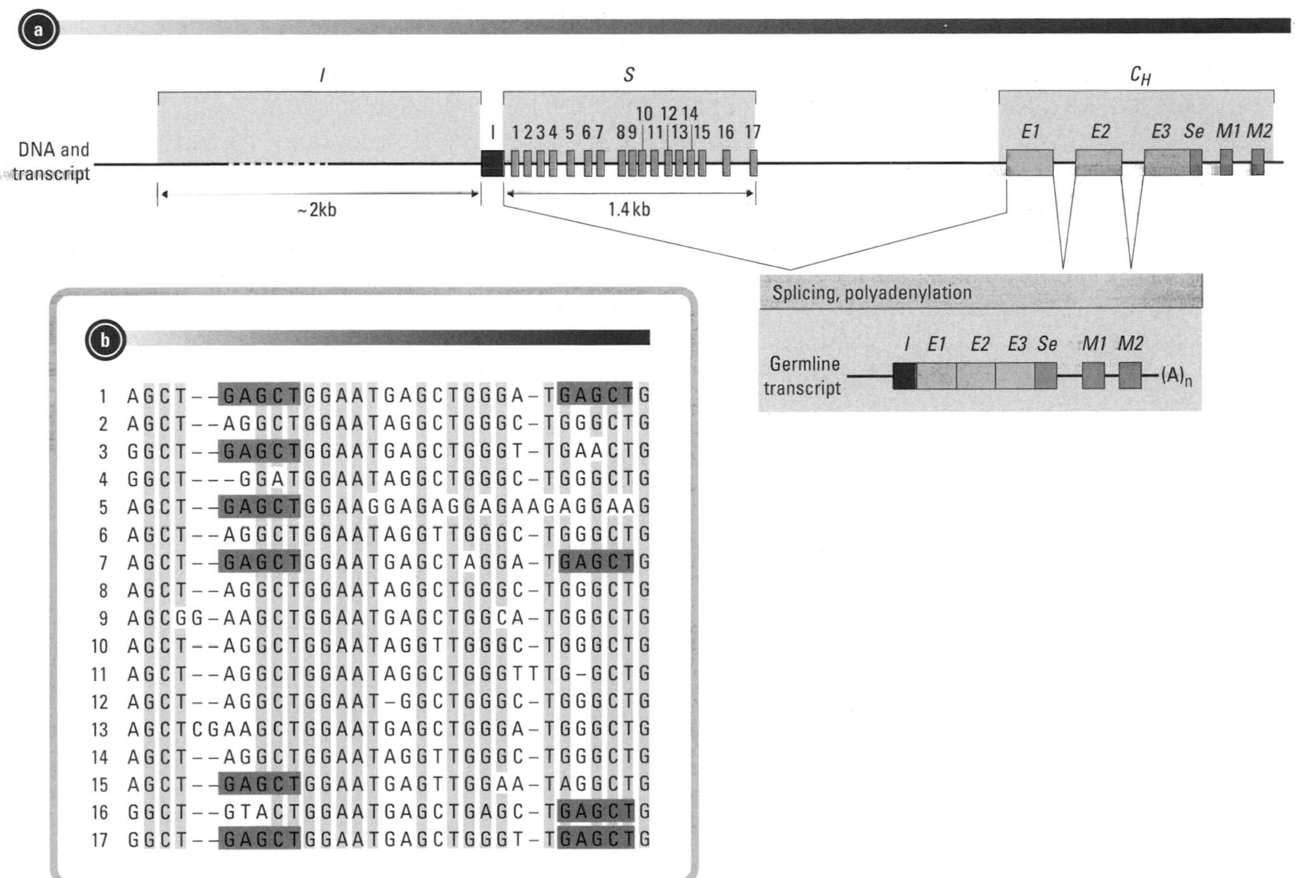

Figure 8.15 Organization of the chromosomal tract involved in the class switch and located upstream from the mouse C_A segment (a), and sequences of the repetitive elements found in this tract (b). The tract consists of two parts, the *I* region and the *S* region. The *I region* contains conserved sequences, some of which bind specific transcription factors and others which carry out promoter functions. Transcription can be initiated at different sites and part of the region then becomes the *I exon* of the *germ-line transcript* (discussed later). The *S region* contains a series (here 17, numbered 1–17) of repeats (pink rectangles) that show high sequence similarity to one another. The sequences listed in (a) are aligned in (b) according to corresponding numbers; shared nucleotides are highlighted. The repeats contain certain motifs that are shared by most of the *S* regions (here the GAGCT motif is enclosed in a rectangle). The V-shaped symbols indicate joining of exons by splicing the primary transcript to produce the germ-line transcript. The *E*, *Se* and *M* letters indicate exons of the C_H segment (see text); $(A)_n$ indicates a poly (A) tail.

upstream part of the S_M region joined directly to a sequence from the downstream part of the S_{G4} region. The breakpoint (joint) between these two parts occurs within one of the repetitive sequence motifs in the S_M region and one of the motifs in the S_{G4} region. Similar observations have been made for most of the switches: the breakpoint nearly always occurs within or near the repetitive sequences in the two regions involved in the switch. Moreover, in the cells that have undergone a class switch, the deleted DNA can often be found in an extrachromosomal circle, which the cell sooner or later degrades (sometimes, however, the circle integrates back into the chromosome in an inverted orientation). These observations have been interpreted in terms of a *deletional model* of switch recombination (Fig. 8.16a): in preparation for the switch one of the repetitive sequences in the S_M (donor) region is brought close to one of the repeats in the *S* (acceptor) region of a selected downstream C_H segment (the intervening sequence being looped out), double-stranded breaks are introduced by unidentified recombinases into the DNA of the two repeats, and the loose ends are then ligated in such a way that the intervening sequence is excised from the chromosome in the form of a circular DNA. Much less frequently, the switch may occur by *unequal sister chromatid exchange* (Fig. 8.16b). Chromatids, you will recall, are the two DNA molecules (with all the accessory material) held together by a centromere of a chromosome in early phases of cell division. Normally, crossing-over occurs between one chromatid of one chromosome and one chromatid of a homologous chromosome (i.e. between non-sister chromatids).

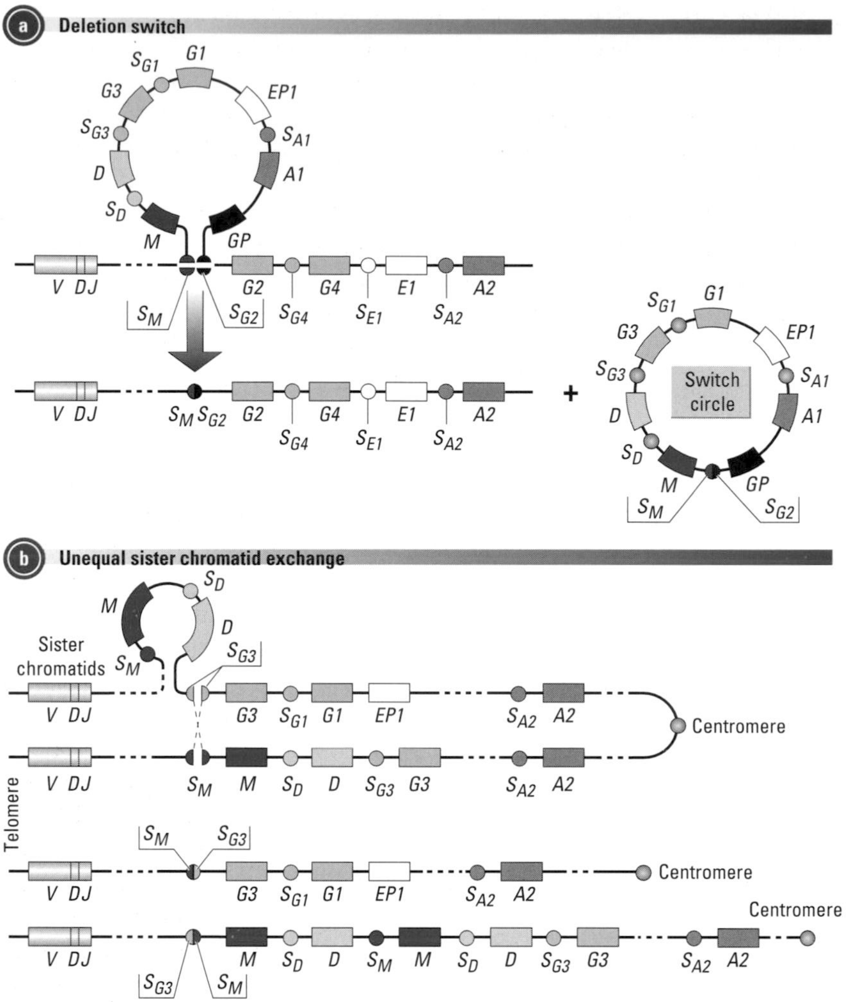

Figure 8.16 Two mechanisms of switch recombination. In the *deletion switch* mechanism (a) elements of two different switch regions (here S_M and S_{G2}) are brought together by looping out the intervening DNA, each suffers a double-stranded break, and the ends thus generated rejoin in a reciprocal manner (part of the S_M element with part of the S_{G2} element). A circular DNA (the *switch circle*) is thus formed by the material excised from the chromosome in which the S_{G2} segment now becomes closest to the V_HDJ_H segment. In the *unequal sister chromatid exchange mechanism* (b), two C_H segments (here C_M and S_{G3}) come together by a misalignment of chromatids in the same chromosome and their *S* regions suffer a break and reunion in a reciprocal fashion. One of the resulting chromosomes thus undergoes a loss of the C_M and C_D segments, while in the other chromosome these two segments are duplicated. (The 'C' symbol of the C-segment designations is omitted.)

Sometimes, however, chromatids of the same chromosome (i.e. sister chromatids) exchange genetic material. In the case of the class switch, the exchange would have to be unequal in the sense that an upstream region of one chromatid would align with a downstream region of the sister chromatid and following the exchange one chromatid would gain and the other lose genetic material.

The molecular mechanism of switch recombination remains elusive. Two, not necessarily mutually exclusive views have been expressed. According to one, the joining of the *S* regions is effected by region-specific recombinases, which enter the open chromatin, choose segments for the switch, bring them together, excise the intervening sequence and mend the ends. The expression of the specific recombinases is controlled by factors that regulate the class switch (cytokines, mitogens). According to another view, the *accessibility model*, the recombination is effected by an *S*-region complex (*S-recombinase*) that does not differentiate between the individual regions but acts on those that have become accessible by local opening of the chromatin. The accessibility of chromatin is controlled by the switch regulators. This hypothesis is consistent with most of the observations thus far. An important element of the mechanism appears to be the transcription of the C_H segment to which the cell will be switching. The transcripts are initiated at different sites within the *I-region*, a sequence approximately 2 kb long upstream from the *S* region. They then proceed through the *S* region and terminate downstream of the C_H segment. They are referred to as *sterile transcripts* (because they are not translated into proteins) or *germ-line transcripts* (because they are made before the region rearranges). The germ-line transcripts are processed to stable forms in which an exon derived from the *I*-region is spliced to the C_H segment. Nearly all of them contain a stop codon in the C_H segment so that translation into a long peptide is not possible. The transcripts seem to be somehow related to the process of switch recombination: they may participate in the opening of the chromatin or they may target *S* region for recombination.

Although the switch recombination resembles the *V*(*D*)*J* recombination superficially, the mechanisms of the two processes are probably different. The major difference between the two events is that the class switch is not restricted to a single site as it is in the case of *V*(*D*)*J* recombination: although the switch recombination is restricted to the *S* region, it can occur at many different sites within this region and involve different sequences.

Most of the class switches are from C_M to one of the downstream C_H segments. Switches between downstream segments, however, also occur. For example, in the mouse most of the B lymphocytes that express the ε chain first switch from C_M to C_{G1} and then from C_{G1} to C_ε.

Membrane-bound and secreted forms of H chains

After *VDJ* recombination and class switch, the *IGH* genes perform one other antic. Up until now the discussion has dealt exclusively with H chains that are inserted into the membrane and become part of the BCR. However, there are also H chains that, after they have combined with L chains, are discharged (*secreted*) by the cell in a soluble form as *antibodies*. These two forms, membrane-bound and secreted, are manufactured right from the beginning of immunoglobulin synthesis in preB cells, but their ratio changes during further differentiation. In preB, immature and mature B cells, almost all the H chains are integrated into the membranes and very few form soluble immunoglobulin molecules. After the stimulation of the B lymphocyte (and class switch), but in particular in the terminal stages of differentiation into plasma cells, the ratio shifts towards the other extreme: now most of the H chains of any class are manufactured for secretion as antibodies.

The membrane-bound and the secreted H chains are encoded in the same genes. Furthermore, there is also no difference between the primary transcripts ultimately translated in either of the two forms. It is only during RNA processing that the decision is made as to which form of the H chain will be produced. To understand *how* the choice between membrane-bound and secreted forms is made, we must have a look at the organization of the rearranged *IGH* gene.

After *VDJ* recombination, all that remains of the *IGH* locus are the unused and inactive V_H segments upstream of the one involved in the final productive rearrangement, the *VDJ* joint, possibly some remaining unused *J* segments downstream of the joint, an intervening sequence and finally the region occupied by the C_H segments (see Fig. 8.12). The *VDJ* joint itself consists of two exons, one specifying the bulk of the signal sequence and the other coding for the variable region of the H chain (Fig. 8.17). Each of the C_H segments consists of a variable number of exons and introns, depending on the particular segment. The C_M segment is composed of six exons, four of which (E_M1–E_M4) encode the four domains of the μ chain's extracellular part (discussed later). The 3′ end (the 'Se part') of exon E_M4 specifies also a short sequence of some 20, mostly hydrophobic, amino acid residues (Fig. 8.17). This sequence appears only in the secreted and not in the membrane-bound form of the μ chain. The sequence encoded in the last two exons, designated M_M1 and M_M2, on the other hand, appears in the membrane-bound μ chain (where it constitutes the peptide connecting the fourth domain to the membrane, the transmembrane region and the cytoplasmic tail), but not in the secreted form of the μ chain.

The rearranged *IGM* gene is normally transcribed all the way to a point downstream of the M_M2 exon so that the primary transcript contains the information for both the secreted and membrane-bound versions of the μ chain. However, the processing (splicing) of the primary transcript then occurs in two alternative ways, distinguished by the use of different polyadenylation sites. There are two such sites at the 3′ end of the *IGM* gene, one (site 1) downstream of the E_M4 exon and another (site 2) downstream of the M_M2 exon (Fig. 8.17). The use of site 1 results in the excision from the primary transcript of the entire sequence downstream of this site, including exons M_M1 and M_M2. Splicing of the remaining exons then produces mRNA that encodes the secreted μ chain. The use of site 2 leaves the M_M1 and M_M2 exons in the mRNA but removes the 3′ end (the Se part) of E_M4. The removal is possible because exon 4 has the sequence GGTAAA at the site where its Se part begins. This sequence codes for the residues glycine (GGT) and lysine (AAA), but it is also a variant of the splicing signal G/GTAAG at the donor splice site. If site 1 polyadenylation signal is used, the GGTAAA sequence is ignored by the splicing enzymes (which recognize it only if another splice signal lies downstream) and is translated into glycine and lysine (followed by the remaining 20 amino acid residues of the secreted form). If, on the other hand, signal 2 is used, the splicing enzymes recognize the G/GTAAA sequence, cleave it at the 'slash' site (between the two Gs) and join E_M4 at this site with M_M1. The decision as to which of the two polyadenylation sites will be used seems to be made by the proteins that regulate polyadenylation. The factors required for polyadenylation begin to assemble at the polyadenylation sequence as soon as it is transcribed

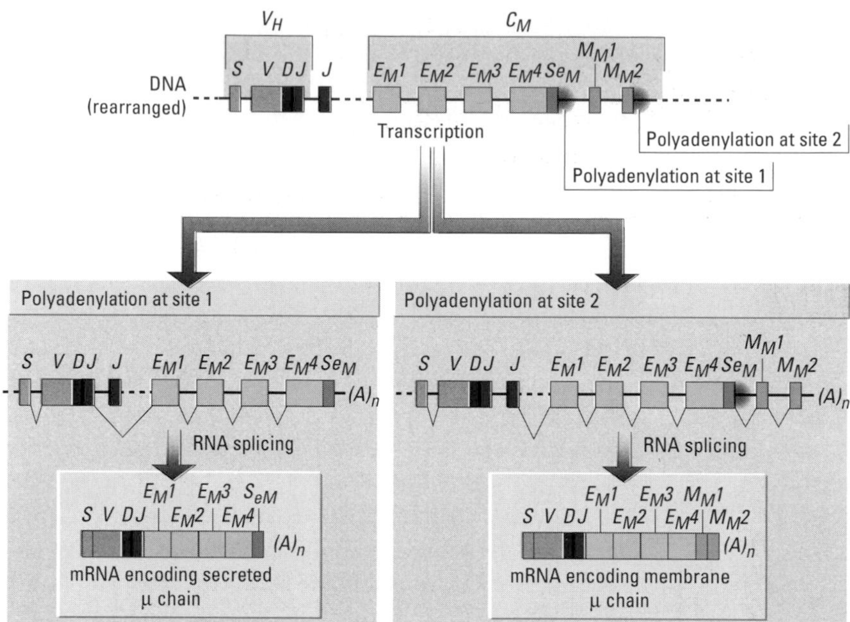

Figure 8.17 Alternative splicing of a primary transcript derived from the *IGH* locus interval extending from the V_HDJ_H segment to the 3′ end of the C_M segment. Polyadenylation of the transcript at site 2 leads to removal of the Se_μ portion of the transcript and produces mRNA that codes for the membrane (m) version of the μ chain. Polyadenylation at site 1 removes M_M1 and M_M2 exons and produces mRNA that is translated in the secreted form of the μ chain. $(A)_n$, poly (A) tail; *E*, exon; *M* and *Se*, exons coding for the part characteristic of membrane-bound and secreted heavy chains, respectively. The V-shaped lines mark spliced-out regions.

from the DNA. Hence, if there are two such sequences, the one in the upstream position is used preferentially because the polyadenylation apparatus is assembled here earlier than at the downstream site. At the *IGM* locus, however, the upstream site is apparently occupied by an inhibitor protein that destabilizes it and thus allows the downstream site to win the competition for the proteins of the apparatus. It is only at the B-cell terminal differentiation stage that synthesis of the inhibitor ceases and the upstream site begins to be used preferentially.

Similar differential use of polyadenylation sites may also explain how immature B cells may exclude the C_D segment from expression and how mature B cells manage to express both the μ and δ H chains. The C_D gene segment has also two polyadenylation sites (sites 3 and 4 in Fig. 8.18), one downstream of exon E_D3 and another downstream of exon E_D2. The regulated use of sites 1, 2, 3 or 4 of a transcript that initially includes the C_D segment can produce secreted μ, membrane-bound μ, secreted δ, or membrane-bound δ chains, respectively.

The organization of the other C_H gene segments is similar to that of the C_M and C_D segments. All the segments have *Se*, *M1* and *M2* exons, as well as two polyadenylation sites so that in each case the primary transcript can be alternatively spliced to produce either secreted or membrane-bound α, γ or ε chains. The primary transcripts are, however, produced selectively after the switch recombination involving a particular C_H segment. Thus, both the BCR and the antibodies can be of different isotypes (classes and subclasses).

Immunoglobulin (BCR) diversity and repertoire

Immunoglobulins in either membrane-bound or secreted form acquire their diversity by the same processes as TCRs, that is by combinatorial and junctional diversification. However, they also use a third mechanism that TCRs do not, somatic diversification. *Combinatorial diversification* exploits the diversity contained in the germ line in the form of different *V*, *D* and *J* segments. It creates one set of diverse combinations by picking one segment each from the *V*, *D*, *J* pools and amalgamating them in a chimeric segment that encodes the variable region of the H chain. It creates another set by picking one segment each from the two other *V* and *J* pools and fusing them into a joint that encodes the variable region of the L chain. The random combination of H and L chains in a complete immunoglobulin molecule then becomes yet another source of combinatorial diversification. Assuming that there are 50 V_H, 12 *D* and 6 J_H segments (counting only the functional ones) at the human *IGH* locus, their random associations would provide the potential for creating $50 \times 12 \times 6 = 3600$ different H chains. Similarly, random combinations of *V* and *J* segments could potentially generate $40 \times 5 = 200$ κ chains and $30 \times 5 = 150$ λ chains. The combinations of different H and L chains could then create $3600 \times (200 + 150) \approx 1.2 \times 10^6$ different immunoglobulin molecules. This would give the maximal size of the B-cell repertoire if it was generated exclusively from different combinations of gene segments present in the germ line. In reality, this number is probably lower than the

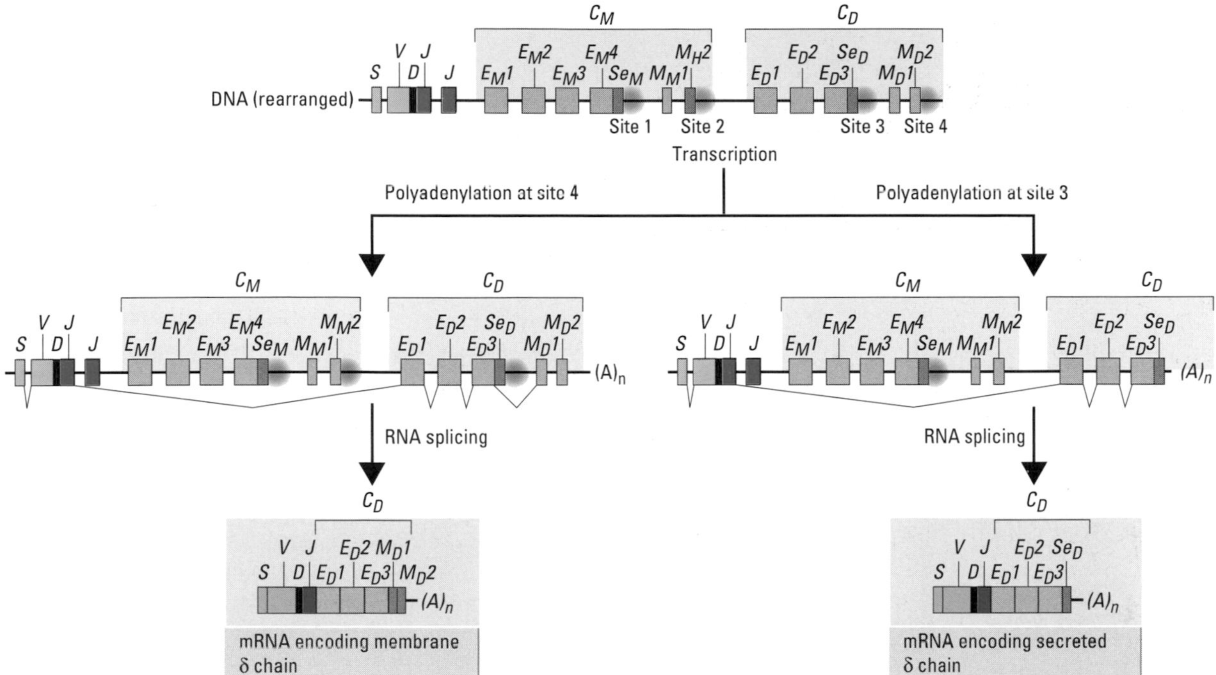

Figure 8.18 Alternative splicing of a primary transcript that encompasses the V_HDJ_H, C_M and C_D segments. Polyadenylation at site 4 leads to the removal of the *Se* part of exon 4 in the C_D segment and the production of the membrane-bound version of the δ chain from those transcripts from which the entire C_M segment has been spliced out. Polyadenylation at site 3 removes the M_D1 and M_D2 exons and leads to the production of the secreted form of the δ chain, if the C_M region has been spliced out from the transcript. The decision whether to remove the C_M segment from the transcript is controlled by unidentified factors. $(A)_n$, poly (A) tail; *E*, exon; *M* and *Se*, exons coding for the parts characteristic of membrane-bound and secreted heavy chains, respectively. The V-shaped lines mark spliced-out regions.

estimate because of non-randomness in segment selection and because of other limiting factors.

The combinatorial diversity is, however, augmented by *junctional diversification*, which occurs during the fusion of the recombining *V(D)J* segments. The genes diversify at the segmental junctions by two processes: the imprecise joining of the coding sequences (contrasting with the precise joining of the recombination signal sequences) and the addition/deletion of new nucleotides by terminal deoxynucleotidyl transferase, endonuclease and other enzymes. Both processes can create sequences in the rearranged genes that are absent in the germ line. Because of its unpredictability, the contribution of junctional diversification to the overall diversification of the B-cell repertoire is difficult to estimate. Much of the junctional diversification renders the *IGH* rearrangements non-productive by shifting the reading frame of the D_H segments; by contrast, the *D* segments of the TCR can be read in three different frames without loss of functionality. Almost all of the productive rearrangements represent new sequences in the junctional regions and thus increase the multifariousness of the repertoire. An increase by an order of magnitude is perhaps not an exaggerated estimate. (For a detailed description of junctional diversification, see Chapter 7.)

Additional augmentation of the B-cell repertoire is achieved by the process of *somatic hypermutation*. Once the DNA rearrangements are completed and the immunoglobulin molecules are expressed on the cell surface, the B lymphocyte is ready for an encounter with antigen. When that happens, the lymphocyte divides repeatedly, replicating its DNA before each division. During replication, errors occur in the form of a wrong nucleotide being incorporated here and there into the DNA. If the error is not corrected by a proof-reading mechanism, it is perpetuated through all the progeny of the particular cell, i.e. it becomes a *somatic mutation* limited to the particular individual (in contradistinction to a *germ-line mutation*, which can be passed on from one individual to another). Somatic mutations occur in all dividing cells, but their frequency is low. In B cells, however, they occur at a rate of 10^{-3} mutations per nucleotide pair per cell division, which is approximately 1 million times higher than in other cells. This high rate is restricted to the rearranged *IG* loci and in these to the variable regions (Fig. 8.19); other genes in the B cell and the

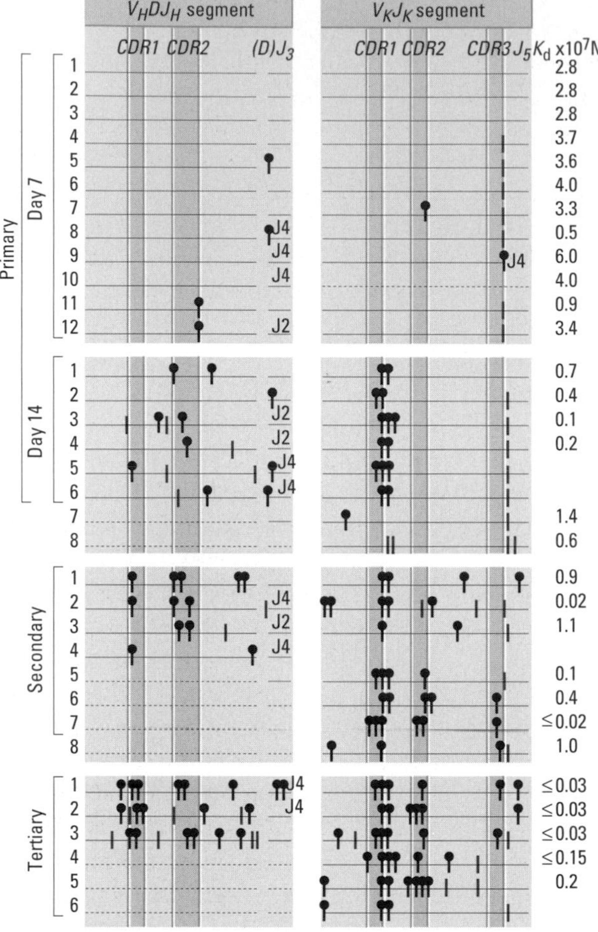

Figure 8.19 Experimental evidence for somatic hypermutation in *IGHV* and *IGKV* segments. Mice were divided into four groups and all were given a single injection of a chemically simple antigen (oxazolone). At 7 and 14 days after the injection, B lymphocytes were taken from the first and second group, respectively (primary response). The third and fourth groups were given one (secondary response) or two (tertiary response) additional injections, respectively, and their B cells, too, were taken out 7 days after the last injection. In all cases, the individual B cells were immortalized, their *IGH* and *IGK* genes isolated and the V_H and V_K segments sequenced. One characteristic of the response to oxazolone is that the majority of the antibodies produced use a single V_H and a single V_K segment. The diagram depicts how the sequence of the *IGHV* and *IGKV* segments changed progressively with time after the injections. The sequence found in unimmunized animals is symbolized by a simple horizontal line; differences from this sequence are symbolized by short, vertical lines at positions where mutations have been found. Vertical lines with circles indicate mutations that lead to amino acid replacements (non-synonymous substitutions); lines without circles indicate synonymous substitutions that do not change the amino acid sequence. The dotted lines indicate sequences derived from different *V* segments. The last column gives antibody affinities, a concept that is introduced in Chapter 14; see also Chapter 17. The increase in the number of mutated sites during the primary response and particularly after the secondary and tertiary responses is clearly evident. CDR, complementarity-determining regions. (Modified from Berek, C. & Milstein, C. (1987) *Immunological Reviews*, **96**, 23.)

constant regions of the *IG* loci mutate at the standard rate. Although both the productively and non-productively rearranged regions display the high mutation rate, the pattern of mutations in these two regions is different. In the productively rearranged regions, mutations leading to amino acid replacements in the encoded proteins (*non-synonymous mutations*) are found to be clustered in regions of the proteins that come in contact with the antigen (the complementarity-determining regions, CDR), whereas mutations that do not change the amino acid sequence (*synonymous mutations*) are scattered throughout the entire *V*(*D*)*J* segment. In the non-productively rearranged genes, both kinds of mutations are randomly scattered throughout the segment. This difference does not arise from the differential susceptibility of different *V*(*D*)*J* regions to the mutational process. Rather, initially both kinds of mutations occur randomly over the entire region, but the antigen then selects cells with altered CDRs preferentially for further proliferation. The affinity of the BCR for the immunizing antigen is indeed 100–1000 times higher after it has been diversified by hypermutation in comparison with its previous affinity. The hypermutation region is about 2 kb long; it begins rather distinctly in the promoter region upstream of the *V* segment and trails off into the intron downstream of the *J* segment. Most of the changes are point mutations (alteration of one nucleotide to another); deletions or additions of nucleotides are rare. When the *V* segment of an *IG* gene is replaced by a segment from an unrelated gene, and the construct is used to create a transgenic mouse, some of the replaced parts mutate at an increased rate but others do not. Hypermutation is restricted to B cells that after the first encounter with antigen migrate to germinal centres in lymphoid organs and become memory cells. (For discussion of the impact of somatic mutations on the B-cell's immune response, see Chapter 17.) The mechanism by which the mutation rate is increased has not been explained. It has, however, been demonstrated that somatic hypermutation is linked to the initiation of transcription. According to one hypothesis, mutating B cells contain a putative *mutator factor*, which binds to the transcription initiation complex assembled at the promoter region. The factor has two functions: it increases the inherent tendency of the RNA polymerase in the complex to pause; and it aids in the recruitment of transcription-coupled repair factors to the transcribed DNA strand. (Indeed, it has been demonstrated in other systems that cells contain a transcription repair coupling factor that overcomes the repair inhibitory effect of the stalled RNA polymerase and recruits repair enzymes to such sites.) The repair factors increase the probability of generating point mutations simply by the repair of those replication errors that have arisen. As the transcription machinery reaches the region beyond the *J* segments, the mutator factor dissociates from the complex and, subsequent to this event, repairs replication errors at a rate characteristic of most somatic cells.

Which of the theoretically possible BCR and immunoglobulin variants are actually expressed in an individual has been tested by the analysis of transcripts (cDNA) obtained from a pool of lymphocytes, by the analysis of individual immortalized B-cell clones and by polymerase chain reaction (PCR) analysis of individual B cells from the blood. The data obtained in these studies are, however, still incomplete and the conclusions drawn from them ambiguous. The studies show that the *BCR repertoire* is not random but rather that it reflects the number of members in each V_H family: the more numerous families are also more frequently represented in the repertoire, the order being $V_H3 > V_H4 > V_H1 > V_H5 > V_H2 > V_H6$ for the human genes. Furthermore, in at least some of the immune responses, a limited set of the available V_H family members is used, and often one particular V_H segment is highly preferred. The human V_H3 family contains some 46% of all the functional V_H segments but it is found to be used by some 56% of B lymphocytes. Thus, this family appears to be positively selected, probably at the molecular level, because a similar bias has been documented for both the productively and non-productively rearranged genes. Perhaps the members of this family are associated with particularly strong enhancers that favour their transcription and thus also their involvement in recombination. Some evidence for negative selection affecting the B-cell repertoire has also been reported, but remains controversial. Unsettled also is the issue as to whether the frequency of participation in *V(D)J* recombination depends on the position of the *V* segments on the chromosome. Preferential involvement of *V* segments proximal to the *D–J* segments has been reported by some investigators.

Synthesis and assembly of immunoglobulins

The primary transcripts of the rearranged *IGH*, *IGK* and *IGL* genes are processed in the nucleus and the resulting mRNA molecules are dispatched into the cytoplasm. There they become the focus for the assembly of ribosomes and all the other components of the translation apparatus. The ribosomes dock the complex on the outer surface of the rough endoplasmic reticulum (RER), where the translation of the mRNA into polypeptides takes place (Fig. 8.20). Since the H and L chains are encoded in separate mRNA molecules, they are also synthesized separately. The synthesis of an L chain takes about 1 min, that of an H chain about 2 min. The L chain-encoding mRNA accommodates four to eight ribosomes, the H-chain mRNA 11–20. The complexes of mRNA and multiple ribosomes are referred to as *polyribosomes*.

Translation begins from the 5′ end of the mRNA and synthesis of the protein from its N-terminus. The first 20 or so, mostly hydrophobic, amino acid residues of each protein (the *signal peptide*) guide the chain into the lumen of the RER, where they are cleaved off and degraded. As the chain comes off the polyribosome, it assumes its characteristic tertiary structure, which is secured with the formation of intrachain disulphide bonds. The pathway leading to the assumption of the quaternary structure depends on the class of participating H chain. In the case of IgM each H chain associates first with one L chain, and then the two half molecules combine into a tetramer (pathway: $H + L \rightarrow HL$; $HL + HL \rightarrow H_2L_2$). In the case of IgG and IgA, the predominant pathway of assembly is: $H + H \rightarrow H_2$; $H_2 + L \rightarrow H_2L$; $H_2L + L \rightarrow H_2L_2$. The assembly, interchain disulphide bond formation and partial glycosylation all take place on the luminal side of the RER. The partially glycosylated immunoglobulin tetramers are packaged into transport vesicles and delivered to the *cis* face of the Golgi complex.

Travelling through the Golgi apparatus, the immunoglobulin molecules complete their glycosylation and at the *trans* face of the apparatus are collected in exocytic vesicles that then deliver them to the cell surface. If the H chain contains the transmembrane region near its C-terminus, it remains anchored by this piece in the membrane throughout the entire journey, including the final stage when the exocytic vesicle fuses with the plasma membrane. If, on the other hand, it contains the hydrophobic sequence characteristic of secreted immunoglobulins, it remains a free molecule that is released into the extracellular space when the secretory vesicle opens up by fusing with the plasma membrane.

Structure of the immunoglobulin molecule

Science has created its own heraldry, a set of insignia that typifies achievements, fields, fashions and trends. In the biology of our time, the two most stylish emblems are the

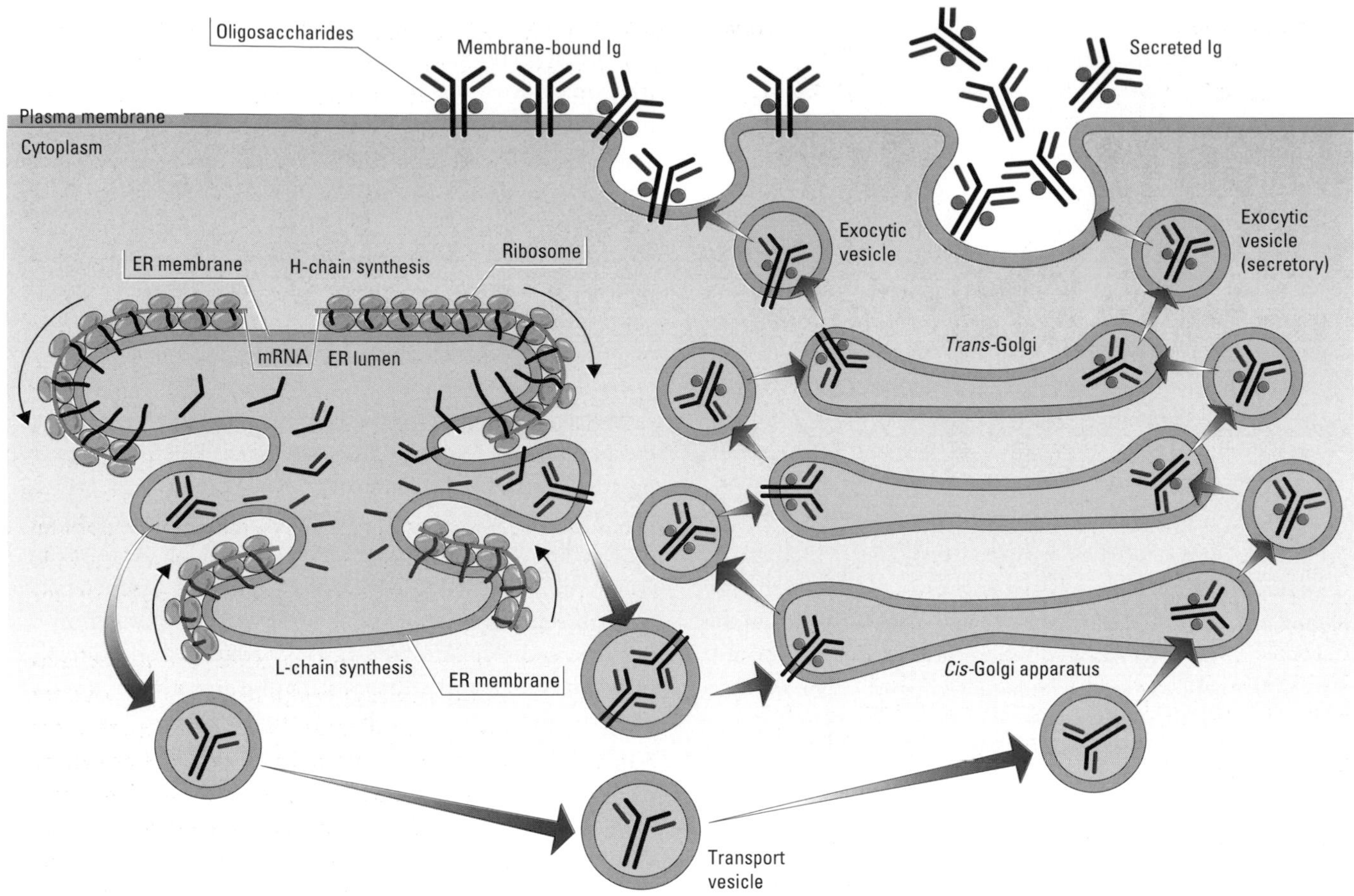

Figure 8.20 Intracellular pathways (arrows) in the synthesis and assembly of immunoglobulin molecules. Both the synthesis of membrane-bound and secreted immunoglobulin molecules are depicted. ER, rough endoplasmic reticulum.

DNA double helix and the Y-shape of the immunoglobulin molecule. Figure 8.21 shows one version of the Y-shape, a structure consisting of two H and two L chains. On the following pages, other figures will show other versions, emphasizing different aspects of the structure. The Y-shape is one of the best characterized molecules and books have been written about it. Here, we concentrate only on the principal features of the molecule: the chains, the fragments, the domains, the regions and the bonds. These features are described using the human IgG molecule as a model.

Chains

Each of the two identical H chains in the tetrameric immunoglobulin molecule has a relative molecular mass (M_r) of about 50 000 and each of the two identical L chains has an M_r of approximately 20 000; the basic immunoglobulin molecule has an M_r of 150 000. When spun in a high-speed centrifuge, the molecules move in the centrifugal field with a velocity seven times greater than that of the basic unit, the *sedimentation coefficient* (S). Biochemists therefore say that IgG is a 7S molecule.

There are nine kinds of H chains in human immunoglobulin molecules: μ, δ, γ1, γ2, γ3, γ4, α1, α2 and ε, each encoded in a separate C_H gene segment. They divide immunoglobulin molecules into classes and subclasses. The five classes are IgM, IgD, IgG, IgA and IgE, corresponding to the H chains μ, δ, γ, α and ε, respectively. The IgG class is divided further into four subclasses, IgG1, IgG2, IgG3 and IgG4, corresponding to the H chains γ1, γ2, γ3 and γ4, respectively. The difference between classes and subclasses is in the degree of kinship: subclasses of a given class are more similar to one another than they are to other classes. The subclasses and classes were originally defined by a combination of serological and physicochemical methods. Biochemists managed to separate some of the classes and subclasses of immunoglobulin molecules on the basis of their size, density and charge; immunologists succeeded in producing antibodies against the individual classes or sub-

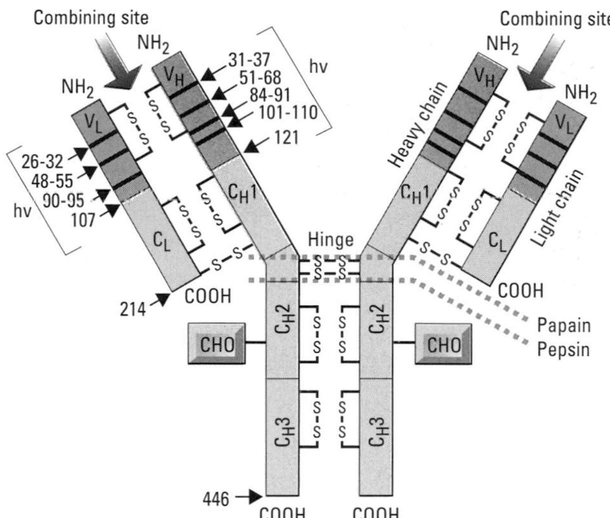

Figure 8.21 Diagram of the human IgG molecule. Shaded bars indicate polypeptide chains, S–S disulphide bonds, dotted lines places of enzymatic cleavage and numbers amino acid positions. C, constant region; CHO, carbohydrate; COOH, carboxyl end; H, heavy chain; L, light chain; hv, hypervariable region; NH_2, amino end; V, variable region. (Modified from Klein, J. (1982) *Immunology: The Science of Self–Nonself Discrimination*. John Wiley & Sons, New York.)

classes by cross-species immunization (e.g. rabbit antibodies against human immunoglobulin). Specific antibodies are still the fastest means of determining the class and subclass of a given antibody. The antibodies recognize amino acids that differentiate the donor from the recipient in their immunoglobulin molecules. The number of classes and subclasses may vary from species to species. As we learn later, the different immunoglobulin classes and subclasses tend to specialize in somewhat different functions and the variation in their numbers apparently reflects the species' response to variation in the functional requirements.

The L chains are of two kinds, κ or λ. Since there is only one human C_κ-encoding gene segment, there is only one type of κ chain. On the other hand, since there are four functional C_λ-encoding gene segments, there are four types of λ chain, λ1, λ2, λ3 and λ6. These do not define classes and subclasses (only H chains do so); they define isotypes (the different class- and subclass-defining H chains are also isotypes). The human λ1, λ2, λ3 and λ6 chains are also referred to as Mcg, Ke^-Oz^-, Ke^-Oz^+ and Ke^+Oz^-, respectively (Ke is sometimes written as KERN). These symbols are derived from the designations of myeloma proteins (described later). The $C_\lambda Oz^+$ chain differs from Oz^- in that the former has Lys and the latter Arg at position 188; Ke^+ and Ke^- chains have a Gly and Ser, respectively, at position 157. Since a given H chain can associate with different L chains, molecules of a particular class or subclass can be of the κ, λ1, λ2, λ3 or λ6 type; hybrid molecules of the type κλ or $\lambda_x\lambda_y$ do not occur. The ratio of κ : λ molecules varies from class to class, subclass to subclass and species to species. In mice, for example, most of the immunoglobulin (over 95%) is of the κ type, while the overall κ : λ ratio in humans is 6 : 4. In the horse, more than 95% of the immunoglobulin is of the λ type.

In an intact immunoglobulin molecule, the four chains are held together by covalent (disulphide) and non-covalent bonds. To break the disulphide bond and separate the chains from one another, biochemists expose the protein to a large excess of a reducing agent such as 2-mercaptoethanol (Fig. 8.22). To prevent spontaneous reformation of the broken bonds, the reduction must be followed immediately by alkylation, for example with iodoacetamide. However, the reduction of most of the immunoglobulin molecules under these conditions is only partial, and the chains remain held together by non-covalent bonds. To achieve complete chain dissociation, a denaturing agent such as urea or guanidine hydrochloride, must be added:

$$H_2N-\overset{\displaystyle O}{\overset{\|}{C}}-NH_2 \qquad\qquad H_2N-\overset{\displaystyle NH_2^+Cl^-}{\overset{\|}{C}}-NH_2$$

Urea — Guanidine hydrochloride

These agents, however, disrupt non-covalent bonds between as well as within the chains, with the result that the

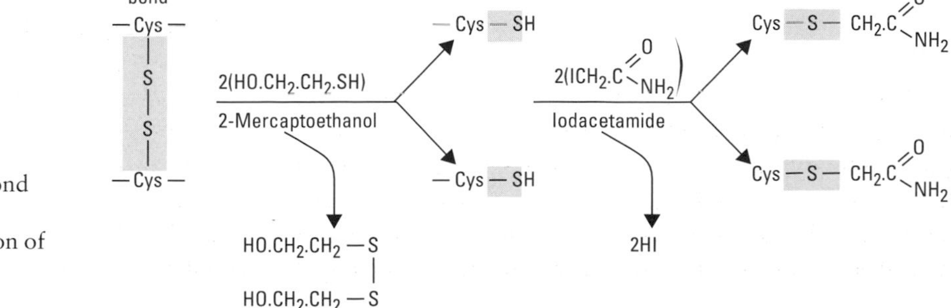

Figure 8.22 Breakage of the disulphide bond by exposure to the reducing agent 2-mercaptoethanol. Spontaneous reformation of the bond is prevented by alkylation with iodacetamide.

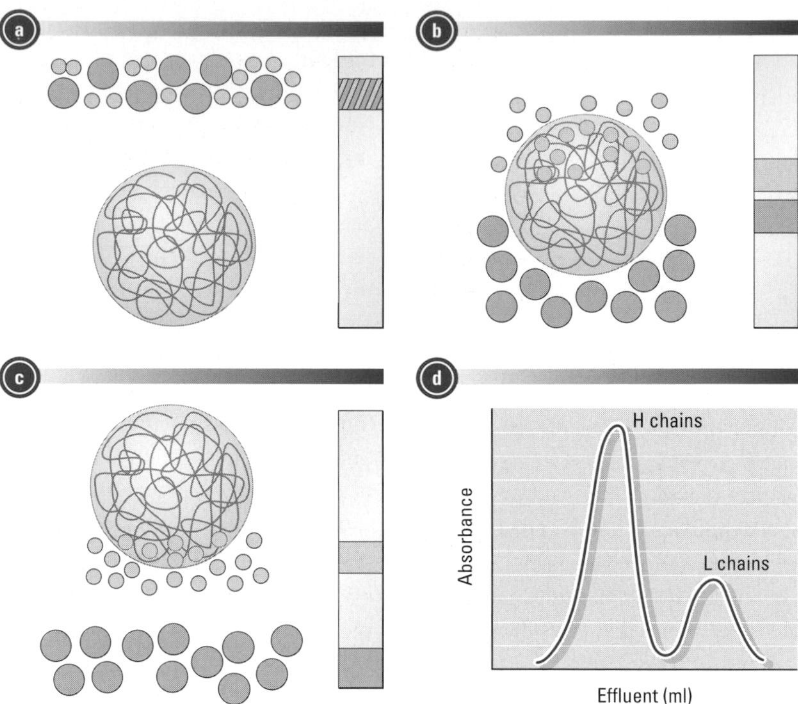

Figure 8.23 Principle of exclusion (gel-filtration) chromatography. The separation of chemical substances by differential movement through a column of some suitable adsorbent is termed *column chromatography*. More strongly adsorbed substances are retarded in their movement and emerge from the column later than less strongly adsorbed substances. In *exclusion (gel-filtration) chromatography*, the adsorbents are cross-linked carbohydrate polymers (such as Sephadex, a trade name for cross-linked polymeric dextran) made into beads. When allowed to swell in a buffer solution, they form a gel, which can be packed in a column. The sample is applied to the top of the column and the buffer solution is percolated through the gel at a constant rate. The swollen beads function as thousands of little filters because of the intertwined threads inside them. Large molecules in the sample cannot enter the beads because they are larger than the interstices formed by the filaments; they pass down the larger spaces between the beads relatively quickly and without much resistance and are eluted from the column. Since this group of molecules is excluded from entering the beads, it is referred to as the *excluded fraction*. Small molecules that enter the beads through the interstices are retarded in their movement, and are thus separated from the more rapidly moving larger molecules (they represent the *included fraction*.) The degree of retardation depends on how much time the molecules spend inside the beads; this time is determined by the size of the molecules and the diameter of the interstices. By using polymers cross-linked to various degrees (Sephadex G10–G200), one can manipulate the size of these openings and the resulting degree of separation of large from small molecules. The eluate is collected in small fractions and the amount of protein present in each fraction is determined optically by its capacity to absorb ultraviolet light. In a–c, the left-hand portions of the figure shows separation of molecules by a single bead; the right-hand side depicts a column loaded with the sample. (a–c) Different stages of separation; (d) absorbance peaks seen after the separation of immunoglobulin heavy and light chains.

chains lose their native conformation and acquire the configuration of a random coil. The free H and L chains can then be separated by gel filtration chromatography (for example on a Sephadex G-200 column; Fig. 8.23).

By mixing the separated H and L chains, partial reassociation occurs. The degree of reassociation depends largely on the harshness of the treatment used for dissociation. Completely denatured chains reassociate only via non-covalent interactions, whereas chains that have been dissociated gently can even reconstitute some of the disulphide bonds. Dissociation and reassociation of H and L chains have been used to study antigen binding. The surprising result of these studies is that even after a complete loss of ordered structure, the chains regain some antibody activity upon reassociation.

Fragments and regions

Another way of taking the IgG molecule apart is to attack it with enzymes and break it into pieces. Protein-specific enzymes break the covalent peptide bond between two amino acid residues in the polypeptide chain (they function as proteolytic enzymes or proteases), each enzyme having a special preference for a particular residue or residues. The two enzymes commonly used are *papain*, isolated from the latex of the papaya tree *Carica papaya*, and *pepsin*, isolated from stomach juice. Papain splits the immunoglobulin molecule into three pieces of equal size (M_r of approximately 45 000; Fig. 8.24). Two of these pieces are identical and are able to bind antigen; the third piece is different and is not capable of antigen binding. The former are the *Fab pieces* (Fab for 'fragment antigen binding') and the latter is the *Fc piece* (Fc for 'fragment crystalline' because it can be crystallized from a solution as a homogeneous substance; Fabs prepared from a pool of serum IgG molecules cannot be crystallized because they are such a heterogeneous bunch).

Pepsin breaks the Fc part of the IgG molecule into small pieces, while leaving a larger piece intact (Fig. 8.24). The latter is approximately twice the size of one Fab piece. Because it consists of two Fabs held together by a disulphide bond, it is referred to as the *F(ab′)*$_2$. The two enzymes thus act on approximately the same region of the IgG molecule, but papain splits the molecule on one side of the disulphide bond that holds the two Fabs together, whereas pepsin splits it on the other (Fig. 8.24).

2-Mercaptoethanol treatment of Fab yields two smaller fragments, one of which is the L chain while the other is slightly larger than the L chain. The latter is designated *Fd* because *d* follows *a*, *b* and *c* in the alphabet. Prolonged treatment of Fc with papain cleaves this fragment further to produce the *Fc′*. Other immunoglobulin classes and IgG molecules of other species behave differently when treated with proteolytic enzymes. By special chemical treatment it is also possible to produce *Fv* pieces (*v* for variable), which consist of the V_H and V_L domains held together by non-covalent bonds and which contain one antigen-combining site (are monovalent).

Domains

An important observation made on the basis of this enzymatic splintering of the IgG molecule is that the molecule breaks into modules or *domains*. The regions between the individual modules seem to be more vulnerable to an enzymatic attack because they are more accessible to the enzyme than the compact module itself.

The organization into domains correlates well with the exons of the individual *IG* genes in that there is roughly one exon for each domain (Fig. 8.25). Since, as we learn shortly, the major domains are all constructed on the same principle, it is likely that the corresponding exons evolved by multiple duplications from a single ancestral exon.

The human IgG molecule consists of six pairs of domains adding up to 12 domains altogether. An L chain consists of two domains, V_L and C_L, whereas an H chain consists of four domains, V_γ, $C_\gamma1$, $C_\gamma2$ and $C_\gamma3$. A pivotal element in the formation of each domain is the amino acid cysteine. Each of the domains contains two cysteine residues in

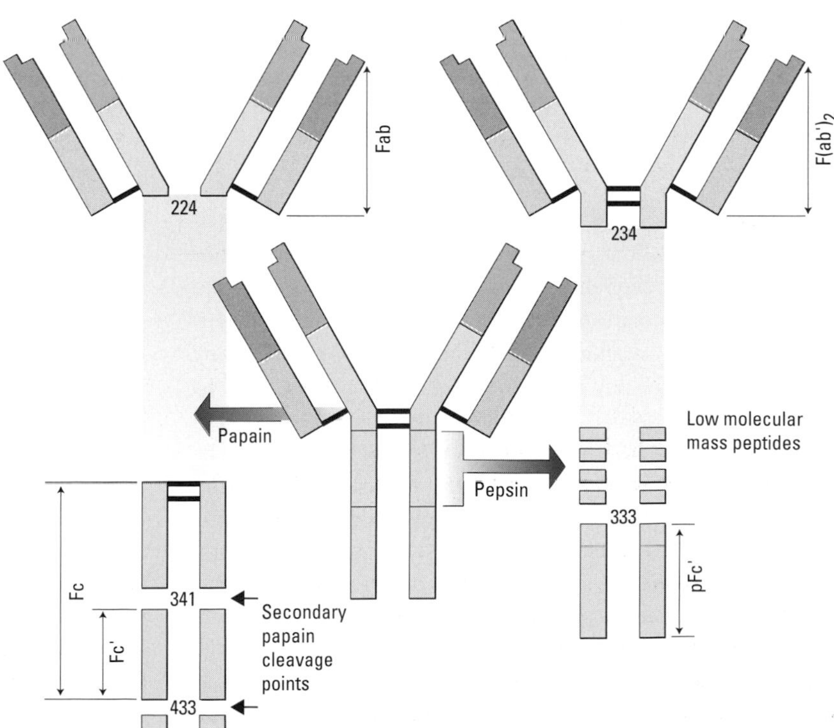

Figure 8.24 Fragmentation of the IgG molecule by the proteolytic enzymes papain and pepsin. The resulting fragments are designated Fab, Fc, Fc′, F(ab′)$_2$ and pFc′. The numbers indicate amino acid positions in the heavy (γ) chain.

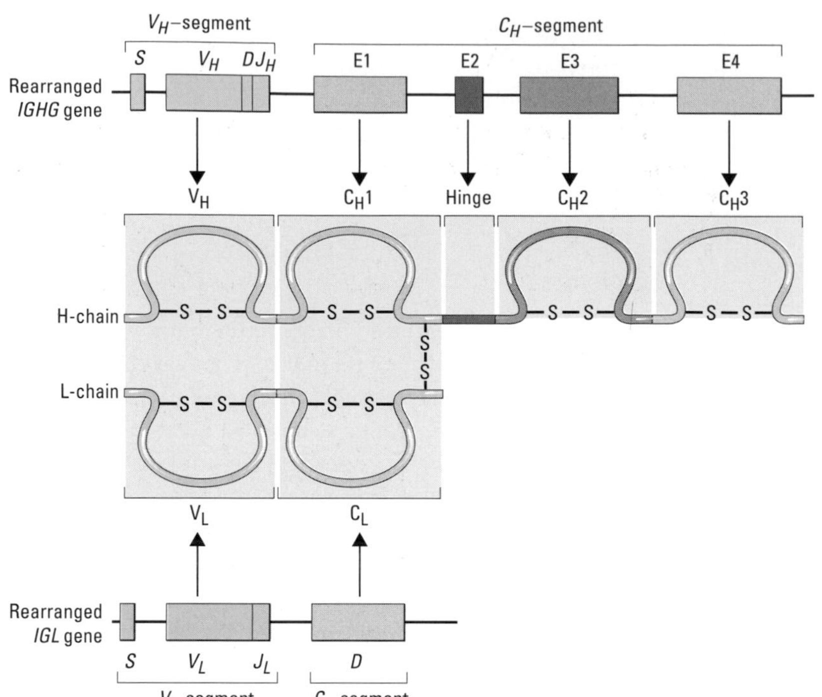

Figure 8.25 Correspondence between exons of the *IGHG* and *IGL* genes and domains of heavy (H) and light (L) chains in IgG half molecules.

approximately the same positions. The domain is about 110 amino acid residues long, and the two cysteine residues are separated by about 60 residues, leaving approximately 25 residues at each end of the polypeptide. The 60 residues loop out and the two cysteine residues are then brought together close enough for a disulphide bond to form between them (Fig. 8.26). The number of domains per chain and per molecule varies among the different immunoglobulin classes.

Regions

Figure 8.27 depicts the amino acid sequence of a group of human κ chains. It is apparent that in the left-hand portion of the figure the sequences vary considerably from chain to chain. Beyond position 108, however, the variability stops abruptly, and from there to position 214 there is hardly any variation at all. Each of the κ chains thus consists of two *regions*, an N-terminal *variable* (V) *region* and a C-terminal *constant* (C) *region*. The chains of other isotypes can also be divided into V and C regions. In the L chains, each V and each C region consists of one domain; in the H chains, the V region consists of one domain, whereas the C region consists of three or four domains, depending on the immunoglobulin class. Note, however, that the V and C regions of polypeptide chains do not correspond to the *V* and *C* segments of polynucleotide chains. The V region is encoded in the *V(D)J* segments joined together in the rearranged gene. The C_H region is encoded in the C_H segment but it lacks either the *Se-* or the *M*-encoded section, depending on whether it is part of the secreted or membrane-bound chain. The C_κ and C_λ regions do correspond to the C_K and C_L segments, respectively.

Examination of the sequences in Fig. 8.27 reveals that certain positions of the V region vary more than others. The Wu–Kabat plot reveals that the variability is highest at positions 31–35, 50–65 and 95–102 in the H chains and at positions 24–34, 50–56 and 89–97 in the L chains (Fig. 8.28). These positions represent the *hypervariable regions*, hv1–hv3, in both the H and L chains (Fig. 8.29). They are the *complementarity-determining regions*, CDR1, CDR2 and CDR3, the segments that contact the antigen.

The sequences of the V region not included in the hypervariable region constitute the *framework regions*. They comprise approximately 75% of the total V region and display an average variability of 5%. Their function is to place the hypervariable regions into the right position for contact with antigen and to bring stability to the three-dimensional structure of the V region.

Hinge region

The immunoglobulin molecule consists of the Fab and Fc parts; the point at which these join together in the H chain is the *hinge region*. Like a hinge that allows a door to open and close, the hinge region permits the outstretched Fab

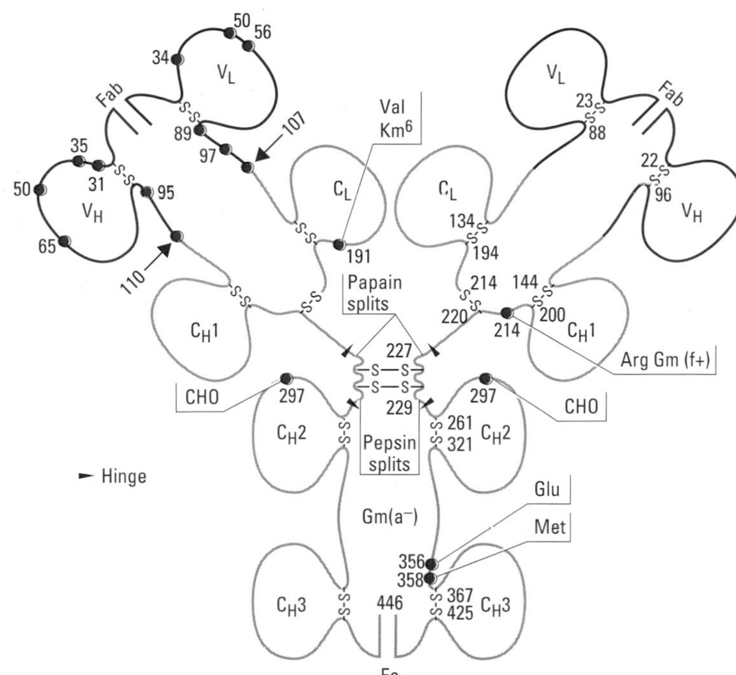

Figure 8.26 Diagram of the human IgG molecule showing the looping out of the polypeptide chains around the disulphide bonds (S—S). Numbers indicate amino acid positions; CHO, carbohydrate; arrows at residues 107 and 110 denote transition from variable (*V*) to constant (*C*) regions; Gm and Km, allotypic markers discussed later. (Modified from Kabat, E. A. (1978) *Advances in Protein Chemistry*, **32**, 1.)

arms of an IgG molecule to wave and rotate, the Fab elbow to bend and the Fc tail to wag (Fig. 8.30). The hinge region of the human IgG molecule consists of three parts: the upper, middle and lower hinge (Fig. 8.31). The upper and middle (core) hinge are encoded in a separate exon located between the C_G1 and C_G2 exons; the lower hinge is contributed by the 5′ end of the C_G2 exon. The two predominant amino acids in the hinge region are cysteine and proline. The cysteine residues form disulphide bonds that hold the two H chains together and prevent any significant degree of folding. It is this absence of folding that makes the region highly susceptible to enzymatic attack by papain or pepsin. The number of interchain disulphide bonds in the hinge region varies from 1 to 15, depending on the isotype and the species. The prolines form the rigid part of the hinge, around which the arms flap. The ring structure of this amino acid hinders rotation around the peptide bond that connects the proline residue with adjacent amino acids. Proline-rich polypeptides twist into *polyproline helices*, and two or three such segments can intertwine to form double or triple helices. Flexibility in the hinge region, on the other hand, is imparted by glycine, the simplest amino acid with very limited demands on positioning in space. Glycine residues are believed to function as the ‘elbows’ and ‘knees’ for the ‘arms’ and ‘legs’ of the H chain.

There is a considerable amount of variation in amino acid sequence, length and carbohydrate content among the hinge regions of the various H chains (Table 8.2) and of different species. Although there is at least a 20–25% similarity in the amino acid sequence of the chains in different classes in the rest of the molecule, in the hinge region there is no significant similarity at all. These properties have led to speculations that the region might represent the remnants of a collapsed ancient domain that could have been related to the C_H1 and C_H2 domains of the μ chain. The IgM (and also the IgE) molecule does, indeed, have an extra domain in the same position as the hinge region of the IgG (IgD and IgA) molecule. Although there are short, flexible sequences at each end of this extra domain, the IgM (IgE) molecule otherwise has no clearly defined hinge region.

The γ1 hinge region consists of a short flexible segment, forming one open turn of a helix easily accessible to solvents (*upper hinge*). The segment is followed by a rigid, cross-linked stretch of polyproline double helix (*middle hinge*) and then again by a flexible part (*lower hinge*). The human γ3 hinge region is approximately 70 amino acid residues long and contains 21 proline and 11 cysteine residues. Its basic polyproline unit is repeated four times (Table 8.2).

Carboxyl termini of membrane-bound and secreted immunoglobulins

The H chains of all isotypes can occur in two forms, membrane-bound and secreted, which differ at their carboxyl ends. Each of the membrane-bound H chains ends with

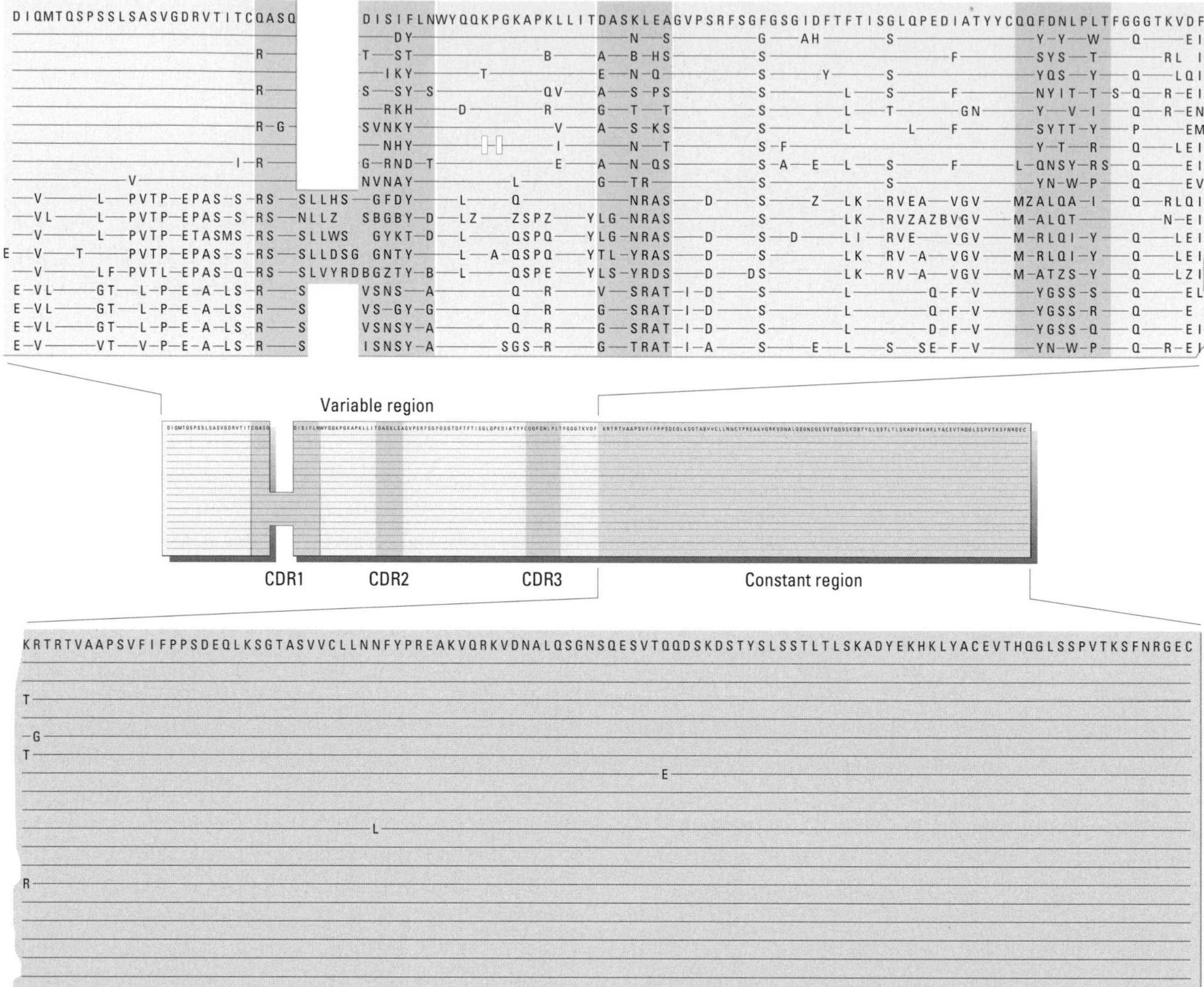

Figure 8.27 Amino acid sequences of 19 human immunoglobulin κ chains. The complete sequence is given for the first chain (ROY) only (the top line). For all other chains, amino acid residues are specified only if different from the one in the top line at the corresponding position; identity with top-line amino acids is indicated by horizontal lines. Hypervariable (complementarity-determining) regions (CDR1, CDR2, CDR3) within the variable region are highlighted. Amino acid residues are given in the international single-letter code (see Appendix 1).

some 40 amino acid residues encoded in the *M1* and *M2* exons. The residues can be divided into three parts: a short extracellular *connecting peptide* ('spacer'), a transmembrane region and a cytoplasmic tail (Fig. 8.32a). The largely hydrophilic *connecting peptide* links the membrane-proximal domain to the plasma membrane. The *transmembrane region* consists of 26 largely hydrophilic residues. The *cytoplasmic tail* varies in length among H-chain isotypes but is generally short. In the secreted forms of H chains, this 40-residue sequence at the C-terminus is replaced by about a 20-residue sequence encoded in the *Se* part of the last C_H exon (Fig. 8.32b).

Disulphide bonds

Bonds between cysteine residues link the two H chains together, link the L with the H chain and also bridge distant regions within a domain. The interchain bonds are somewhat weaker than the intrachain bonds and for this reason they can be reduced selectively without denaturing the chains. Most of the H chain–H chain disulphide bonds are located in the hinge region, but in some immunoglobulin classes (e.g. human IgM), they can also form at the carboxyl end of the H chain. The number of disulphide bonds in the hinge region varies from class to class and from subclass to

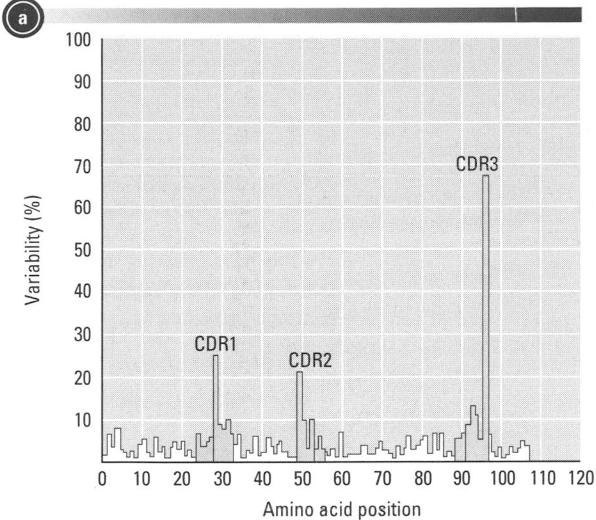

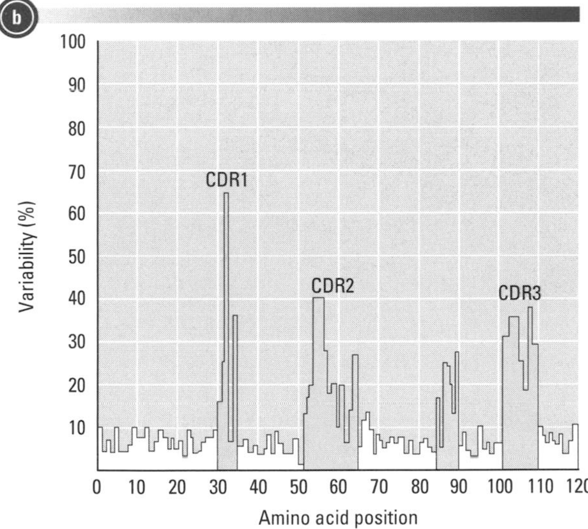

Figure 8.28 Variability (Wu–Kabat) plots for amino acids in the V region of immunoglobulin light (a) and heavy (b) chains. Hypervariable (complementarity-determining) regions (CDR) are highlighted. (Modified from Capra, J.D. & Edmundson, A.B. (1977) *Scientific American*, **236**, 50.)

subclass (Fig. 8.33). Human γ1 and γ2 chains, for example, are connected by two disulphide bonds, whereas γ3 chains are held together by 15 bonds.

In most immunoglobulin molecules, the L chain is attached to the H chain by one disulphide bond. One form of the human IgA2 molecule, however, contains no disulphide bonds between H and L chains. Where it is present, the disulphide bond forms between a cysteine residue in the H chain and either the C-terminal cysteine residue of the κ chain or the penultimate cysteine residue of the λ chain. The H-chain cysteine residue can be located close to the middle of the chain, as in the human IgG1 molecule, or nearer to the N-terminus, as in most other immunoglobulins. In pathological conditions, disulphide bonds can also form between two L chains.

Carbohydrates

All immunoglobulin molecules contain a small amount of carbohydrate and hence can be classified as glycoproteins. The sugars are arranged into short chains, *oligosaccharides* or *glycans*, which are attached at specific places to the polypeptide chains. Some immunoglobulins (human IgA1, human IgD and rabbit IgG) are among the few serum proteins known to contain both N- and O-linked oligosaccharides. Most other globulins have only N-linked oligosaccharides.

The O-linked oligosaccharides are heterogeneous in structure, but are all relatively small, with an M_r of approximately 750. They are attached at multiple, closely spaced sites to the hinge region of the human α1 and δ chains. The more common N-linked oligosaccharides are larger. They have an M_r of approximately 2500–3000 and usually consist of fewer than 15 monosaccharides.

More than 20 different oligosaccharide side-chains have been identified in various immunoglobulin molecules. Their number per molecule, their type and the site of their attachment are characteristic of each immunoglobulin class (Fig. 8.34). Regardless of subclass and species, IgG molecules always have only one N-linked oligosaccharide approximately at position 300 in the γ chain. Other H chains have two to five oligosaccharides per molecule. Normally, oligosaccharides are restricted to the C region of the H chains.

Immunoglobulins without L chains

The H_2L_2 tetrameric structure is so emblematic of the immunoglobulins that a dimeric antibody seems unimaginable. Yet, such antibodies do occur, under both pathological conditions, in cases of the so-called 'heavy chain disease' (discussed later), and physiological conditions in at least one group of vertebrates, the camelids, represented in the Old World by the camel and in the New World by the lama. Although camelid serum contains the standard tetrameric IgG1 molecules, it also contains considerable amounts of IgG2 and IgG3 molecules that lack L chains and the C_H1 domain of the H chain. In the dimers, the last framework (FR4) residues of the V_H region connect directly to the hinge region. The IgG3 dimers have a short hinge (Fig. 8.35a), whereas in the hinge of the IgG2 dimers the Pro-X motif (where X is Gln, Glu or Lys) is repeated 12

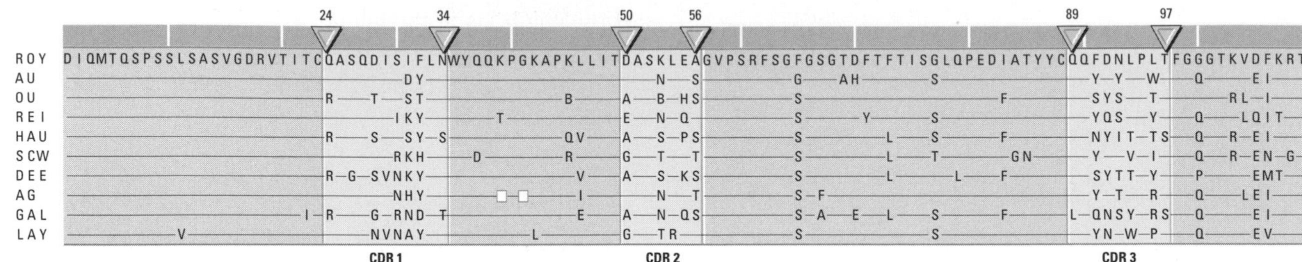

Figure 8.29 Amino acid sequence of the V region of 10 human immunoglobulin κ chains selected and enlarged from Fig. 8.27. The complementarity-determining regions (CDR1, CDR2 and CDR3) are highlighted. Identity with top-line sequence is indicated by horizontal lines. Numbers indicate amino acid positions. Abbreviations of amino acid residues are in the international single-letter code (see Appendix 1).

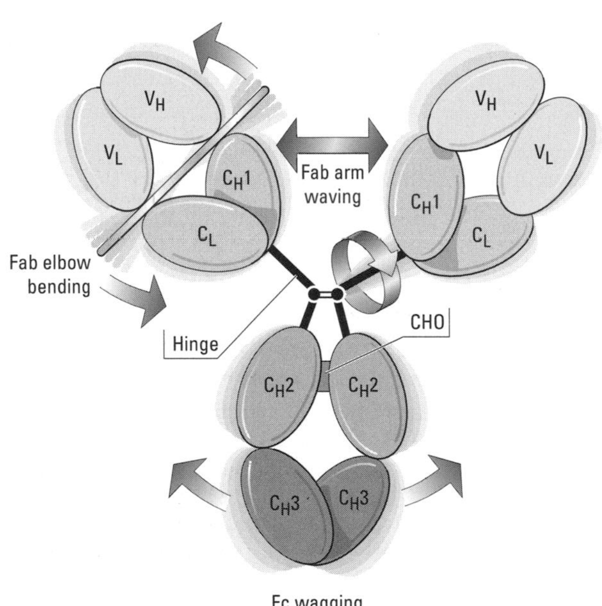

Figure 8.30 Movements of parts of the human IgG molecule (arrows) allowed by the flexibility of the hinge region. CHO, carbohydrate moiety. Disulphide bonds are indicated by lines connecting the hinge regions of the two heavy chains. (Modified from Brekke, O.H., Michaelsen, T.E. & Sandlie, I. (1995) *Immunology Today*, **16**, 85.)

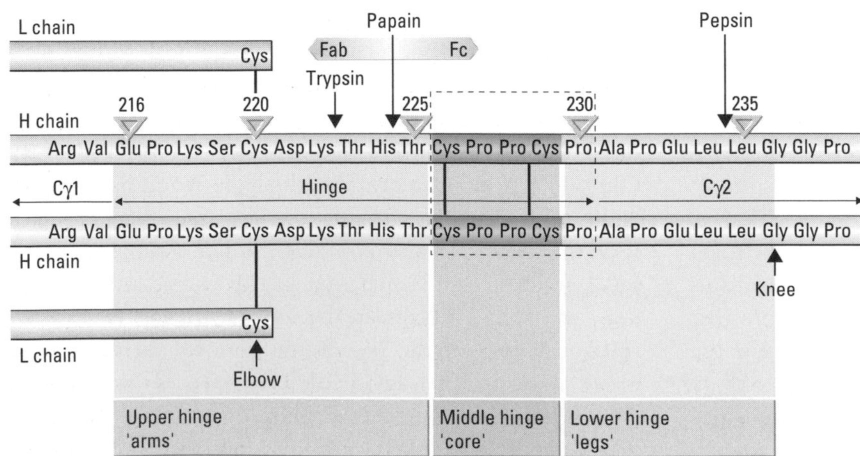

Figure 8.31 The hinge region of the human IgG1 molecule. The broken line rectangle delineates the core region, numbers indicate amino acid positions, vertical arrows sites of cleavage by the indicated enzymes and horizontal pink arrows the border between the Fab and Fc regions.

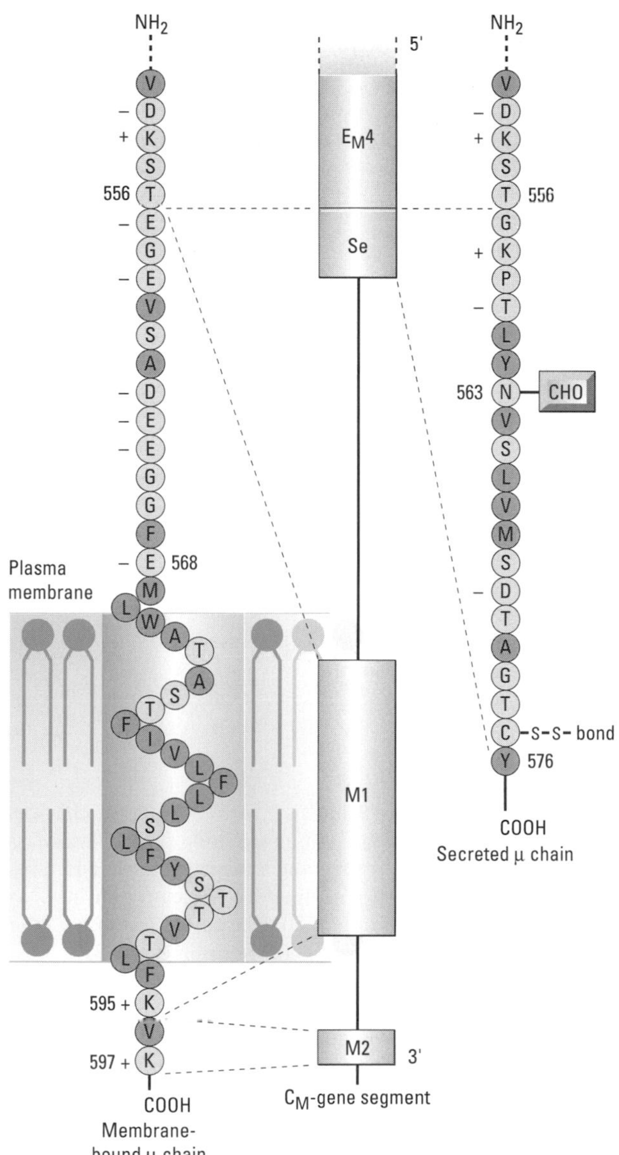

Figure 8.32 The C-terminus of the human immunoglobulin μ chain: comparison of the membrane-bound with the secreted form. The middle part of the figure shows the 3′ end of the C_M gene segment (3′ end of exon 4 with the *Se* part, as well as exons M1 and M2). Letters in circles indicate amino acid residues in the single-letter code (dark and light circles represent hydrophobic and hydrophilic uncharged residues, respectively; + and – signs indicate positively and negatively charged residues, respectively). Numbers indicate amino acid positions counted from the N-terminus. CHO, carbohydrate; S—S, disulphide bond.

times and forms a rigid rod that compensates for the absence of the C_H1 domain. In the dimers, the H chains apparently carry out the same functions that are normally effected by the combination of H and L chains.

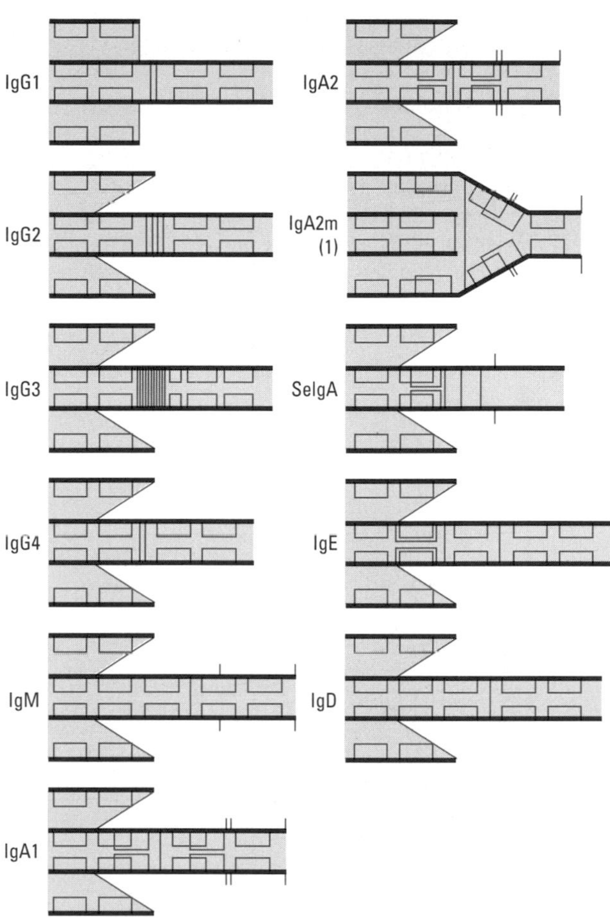

Figure 8.33 Distribution of disulphide bonds in human immunoglobulins of various classes and subclasses. Thick black lines denote heavy and light chains, thin red lines disulphide bonds. (Modified from Klein, J. (1982) *Immunology: The Science of Self–Nonself Discrimination*. John Wiley & Sons, New York.)

Tertiary structure of immunoglobulin molecules

Immunoglobulin molecules are composed of *domains*. As already mentioned, the human IgG molecule consists of 12 domains: two comprising each of the two L chains (V_L and C_L) and four comprising the extracellular part of each of the two H chains (V_H, C_H1, C_H2 and C_H3; see Fig. 8.26). H chains of other classes (e.g. IgM) have a fifth domain (C_H4). The Fab is composed of four domains (V_L, C_L, V_H, C_H1), the Fc of another four (two C_H2 and two C_H3) domains (see Fig. 8.24). The intact immunoglobulin molecule is difficult to crystallize because the hinge region of different molecules is in different conformational forms and this heterogeneity disturbs the crystallization process. Efforts have therefore concentrated on Fab or Fc, which are relatively easy to crystallize. Some IgG molecules, however, spontaneously lose the rigid part of their hinge regions and

Subclass	Upper hinge	Middle hinge	Lower hinge
IgG1	EPKSCDKTHT	CPPCP	APELLGGP
IgG2	ERK	CCVECPPCP	APPVAGP
IgG3	ELKTPLGDTTGT	$(CPRCP)_4(EPKSCDTPPPCPRCP)_3$	APELLGGP
IgG4	ESKYGPP	CPSCP	APEFLGGP

In the γ3 chain of the IgG3 molecule, the motif EPKSCDTPPPCPRCP is repeated three times and the motif CPRCP four times. The amino acids are given in the international single-letter code (see Appendix 1). The first residue in the γ1 sequence is at position 216, the last at position 238.

Table 8.2 Amino acid sequence of human IgG heavy chains in the hinge region.

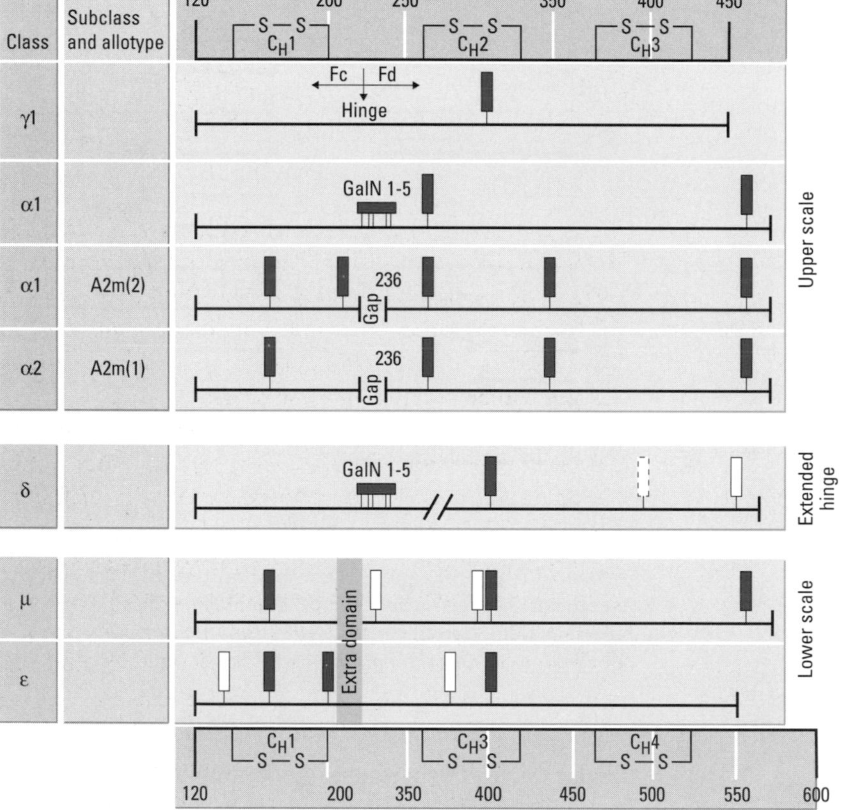

Figure 8.34 Distribution of oligosaccharides in human immunoglobulin heavy chains. Solid red rectangles denote mannose-rich type and open rectangles complex-type oligosaccharides. The dotted rectangle in the δ chain indicates the position of the oligosaccharide on only about half of the IgD molecules. Horizontal rectangles denote O-linked oligosaccharides. Numbers in the upper and lower scales indicate the residue positions in the chains (note that the extra domains have been omitted in the μ and ε chains). (Modified from Putnam, F.W. *et al.* (1982) *Annals of the New York Academy of Sciences*, 399, 41.)

these can then be used to obtain crystals of the entire IgG molecule.

X-ray diffraction analysis of the various crystals has revealed all the immunoglobulin domains to be organized on a similar principle, that of the *immunoglobulin fold*. In each domain, the polypeptide chain forms either seven (C domain) or nine (V domain) *β-strands* folded into two *β-sheets* in such a way that neighbouring strands run in opposite directions to each other (they are antiparallel; Figs 8.36 & 8.37). The β-strands are connected by *loops*, which vary in length and structure among the different domains of a given molecule and among molecules of different classes; some form tight turns, some are helical and others have an irregular structure. In each C domain, one β-sheet is composed of three and the other of four antiparallel β-strands; in each V domain, one sheet contains four and the other five antiparallel β-strands (Fig. 8.38). The strands are either numbered or designated by letters in the order in which they connect with each other (via the loops) starting from the N-terminus of the polypeptide chain. In the letter designations, sheet I of the C domain is composed of strands d–e–b–a; sheet II of strands g–f–c; sheet I of the V domain is composed of strands d–c–b–a and sheet II of strands g–f–c–c′–c″, where c′ and c″ are the two extra strands that the V domain possesses in comparison with the C domain. The two additional strands have been inserted into the loop

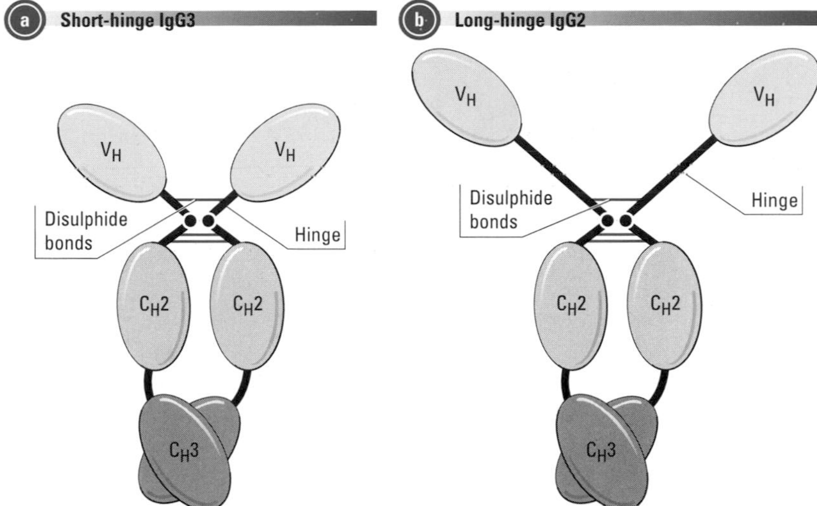

Figure 8.35 Immunoglobulins without light chains. Two versions of these dimeric immunoglobulin molecules have been found in camelid serum: IgG3 molecules with short hinge (a) and IgG3 molecules with long hinge (b). Note that the C_H1 domain is also missing. (From Hamers-Casterman, C. *et al.* (1993) *Nature*, 363, 446.)

that in the C domain connects the strands c and d. (The C_H2 and C_H3 domains contain a short, three residues long, β-strand that contributes to one of the two sheets so that each of them can be considered as having four strands.) In topological diagrams, the two β-sheets are depicted as being in one plane (Fig. 8.38). They then resemble an ornamental motif used by the ancient Greeks to decorate pottery, the *Greek key motif*. In reality, the two sheets are arranged into a sandwich that is twisted into a barrel, the *Greek key β-barrel* (Fig. 8.39). The dimensions of the barrel are 40×25×25 Å. In the *β-sandwich*, the side-chains of hydrophobic amino acid residues are located between the two sheets and form its 'butter', the hydrophobic core. The side-chains of the hydrophilic residues are on the surface of the barrel. The two β-sheets are connected by the *disulphide bond*, the toothpick holding the two slices of the sandwich together. The loops connecting β-strands b and c, c′ and c″, f and g protrude from the V_H and V_L barrels like the fingers of two grasping hands (Fig. 8.40). They are formed by the residues that constitute the hypervariable regions of the V domains, and are the 'fingers' by which the immunoglobulin molecules grasp the antigen, i.e. the *complementarity-determining regions*: CDR1 (loop b → c), CDR2 (loop c′ → c″) and CDR3 (loop f → g). Each of the two V domains (V_H and V_L) on each of the 'arms' of the IgG molecule provides three 'fingers', so that altogether there are six 'fingers' to grasp an antigen. The area in which the two V domains contact the antigen is termed the *combining site*. The loops can vary in amino acid composition, in length and in orientation, particularly CDR3, which encompasses the V(D)J junctions. It is this variability that imposes on each combining site the ability to interact with only a limited number of antigens, i.e. its *specificity*. Hence the specificity of antigen binding by antibodies is determined mostly, if not exclusively, by the CDRs of both the V_H and V_L regions; the framework regions act mainly as a scaffold that props the CDRs into the right position for interaction with antigen. The nature of the interaction between the antibody and the antigen will be discussed in Chapter 14.

The V_L and C_L, as well as the V_H and C_H1 domains, are connected by a short, flexible *switch peptide*, which allows the domains to arrange at different angles with each other, somewhat like an elbow allows the lower arm to move against the upper arm. This flexibility is important for correct positioning of the V domains when they react with the antigen. The C_H1 and C_H2 domains are connected via the hinge, another flexible region in the IgG molecule. The connection between the C_H2 and C_H3 domains, on the other hand, is somewhat rigid. The two C_H2 domains are separated from each other by the carbohydrate chain so that there is very little contact between them (see Fig. 8.30). All the other domain pairs contact each other over wide surface areas (Table 8.3) and interact via non-covalent bonds. The amino acid residues whose side-chains are involved in these interactions are mostly conserved among the different immunoglobulin classes.

Table 8.3 Contacts between immunoglobulin (IgG) domains.

Domain pair	Area of contact ($Å^2$)	No. of residues involved per domain	Contacting sheets
V_H–V_L	1800		5 stranded
C_H1–C_L	500	6 and 7	4 stranded
C_H3–C_H3	2200	20	
C_H2–C_H3	780	7	

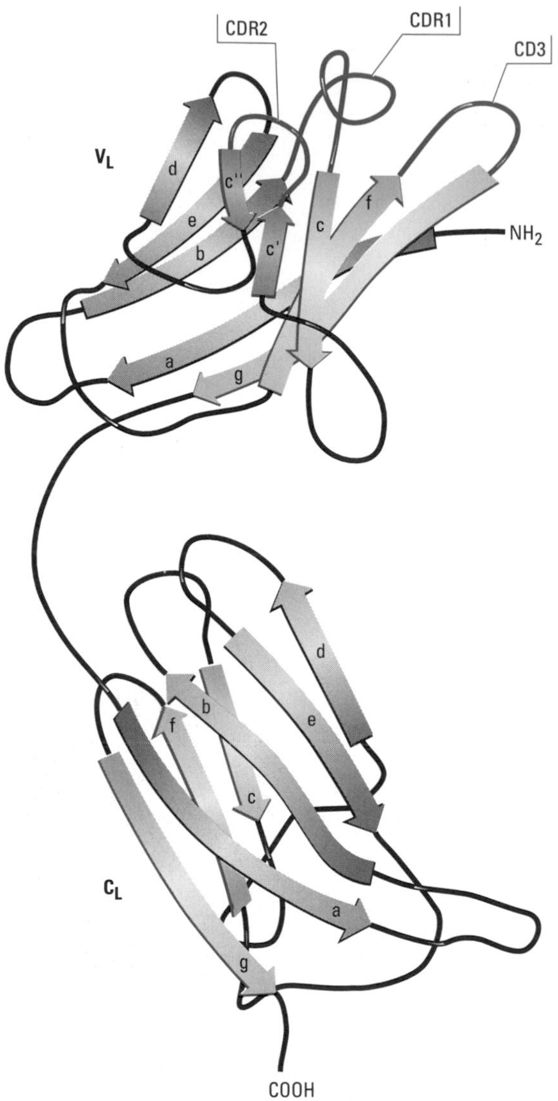

Figure 8.36 Tertiary structure (ribbon model) of immunoglobulin light chains. Small letters indicate individual β-strands, arrows their orientation. Shading distinguishes the two β-pleated sheets. (Modified from Branden, C. & Tooze, J. (1991) *Introduction to Protein Structure*. Garland Publishing, New York.)

The overall shape of the immunoglobulin molecule can be deduced from X-ray diffraction analysis. It can also be observed directly by electron microscopy. When electron microscopists examined immunoglobulin molecules alone, all they saw were irregular globular particles lacking any internal structure. To stretch them out, investigators combined them with antigens. Since bulky antigens, such as virus particles, obscured the antibody, investigators replaced them by *haptens*, small molecules that can bind antibodies but alone cannot induce their formation. In the *bifunctional hapten technique* (see Fig. 8.33), two haptens separated by a spacer of eight or more carbon atoms are used. An example of a bifunctional hapten is the polyethylenediamine chain with an immunologically active (functional) dinitrophenyl group attached at each end. The bifunctional hapten is so small that it cannot be seen in an electron micrograph and one has an unobscured view of the stretched-out immunoglobulin molecules. Since both the hapten and the immunoglobulin molecules have two binding sites, one bifunctional hapten can interact with two immunoglobulin molecules, and one immunoglobulin molecule can interact with two different haptens, so that dimers and rings of three, four, five or more immunoglobulin molecules can form (Fig. 8.41). The investigations have shown that in an antigen–antibody complex, the angle between the two arms of the IgG molecule varies from 90 to 180° and the configuration of the molecule from a Y to a T shape. After trypsin digestion, the molecules become V-shaped. The T-shaped or 'clicked open' form is frequently seen in crystals, in which the immunoglobulin molecules form a regular lattice.

Properties of immunoglobulin classes and subclasses

From the description of the basic IgG molecule we now turn to the properties that distinguish the individual immunoglobulin classes and subclasses. The general properties are summarized in Table 8.4; the structural features of the polypeptide chains composing the different immunoglobulin molecules are shown in Figs 8.33 and 8.42.

Immunoglobulin G (IgG)

The IgG molecule has the structure of the basic H_2L_2 tetramer. In normal serum of most animals, IgG is the major immunoglobulin class, constituting about 75% of the total immunoglobulin. Human IgG has an M_r of 146 000 and a sedimentation constant of 6.6S (or roughly 7S). At alkaline pH (8.6), IgG has the slowest electrophoretic mobility of all major plasma proteins except complement component C1q, a fact that facilitates its isolation by ion-exchange chromatography (Fig. 8.43).

Human IgG falls into four subclasses (IgG1, IgG2, IgG3 and IgG4) that constitute 70%, 20%, 8% and 2%, respectively, of the total IgG. However, the proportion of each subclass varies from individual to individual and may be controlled genetically. IgG1 differs from all other IgG molecules in the position of the half-cystine linking the L and H chains: in IgG1 the half-cystine is at position 220; in other IgG molecules it is at position 131. The different subclasses also differ in the number of disulphide bonds (see Fig. 8.33).

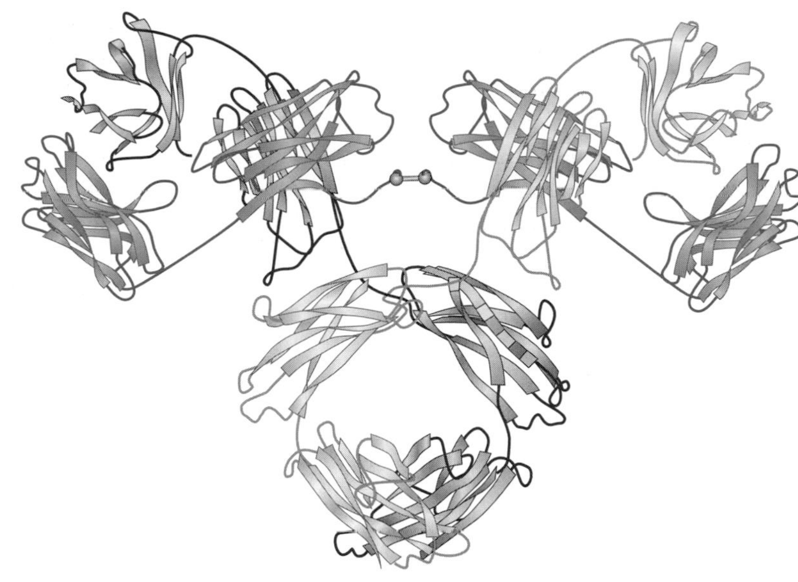

Figure 8.37 Tertiary structure (ribbon model) of IgG molecule. (From Guddat, L., Edmundson, A. and Andersen, K. *Immunology Today*, cover page, February issue, 1995).

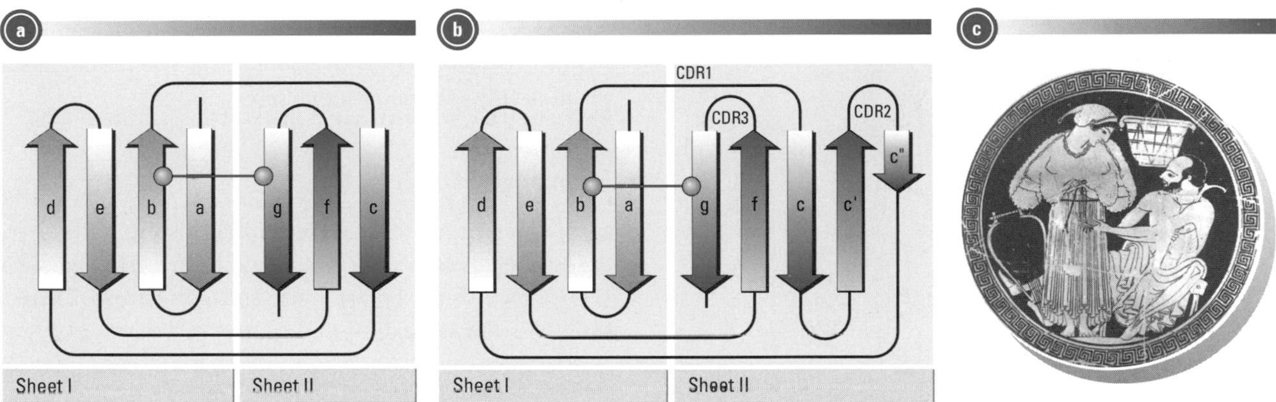

Figure 8.38 Topological diagrams of immunoglobulin constant (a) and variable (b) region structure. (c) Greek key motif on the inside of a cup from 500 BC found in an Etruscan necropolis (British Museum, London). Small letters indicate β-strands, closed circles cysteine residues connected by a disulphide bond. CDR, complementarity-determining regions.

The IgG3 molecule has 95 extra amino acid residues in the γ chain and is therefore heavier than the molecules of other IgG subclasses.

On average, subclasses are more than 95% similar to one another in their amino acid sequence. The greatest differences are found in the hinge region, both in terms of sequence and in the number of residues (IgG1, 15; IgG2, 12; IgG3, 62; IgG4, 12). In IgG1, the hinge is flexible enough to allow the Fab arms to flap about and spin around their axis. In IgG2, on the other hand, the double disulphide bond right at the base of the Fab arms and the loss of a glycine in the 'knee' together make the arms rather rigid. In IgG3, the long hinge keeps the Fab arms well clear of the Fc region and allows them free movement. The flexibility of IgG4 is somewhere between that of IgG1 and IgG2.

Four IgG subclasses are known in the mouse: IgG1, IgG2a, IgG2b and IgG3. The two IgG2 subclasses are structurally very similar and are therefore difficult to separate from one another. Of the total IgG, IgG2a represents the largest and IgG3 the smallest fraction.

Immunoglobulin M (IgM)

Human serum IgM has an M_r of 970 000 and a sedimentation coefficient of 19S. Each IgM molecule is a pentamer composed of five subunits (monomers), each with an M_r of about 180 000 and a sedimentation coefficient of 7.8S. The subunits are joined by disulphide bonds and by an extra piece, the *joining* or *J chain* (discussed later). (In the absence of the J chain the subunits assemble into functionally active

IgM hexamers.) The pentamer can be split into monomers by mild reduction, for example by using 0.01 M 2-mercaptoethanol at neutral pH. Each subunit has the same basic structure, which consists of two H (μ) and two L chains, so that the 'monomer' is in fact itself a tetramer. The H chains are each composed of five domains: one variable (V_H) and four constant ($C_\mu 1$–$C_\mu 4$). They have thus one domain more than the H chain of IgG, if the IgG hinge region is not counted as a separate domain. The $C_\mu 4$ domain contains 18 extra amino acid residues that form the 'tail' of the μ chain. The molecule is rich in carbohydrates, containing five oligosaccharide moieties per μ chain. There are two disulphide bonds connecting H chains of adjacent monomers (positions 414 in the $C_\mu 3$ domain and 575 in the tail of the $C_\mu 4$ domain) and one bond connecting the two H chains of each monomer (position 337 in the $C_\mu 2$ domain). (The μ chain consists of 576 amino acid residues, so the monomer-linking cystine is in the penultimate position.) The linkage of the J chain with the monomers is controversial. According to the *clasp model* (see Fig. 8.42h), the hairpin-shaped J chain functions as a clip that closes the circle of five monomers, linking only two of them.

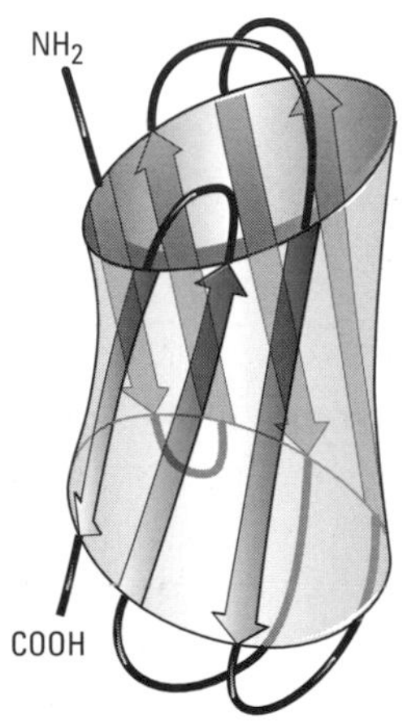

Figure 8.39 The β-barrel configuration of an immunoglobulin constant domain (From Branden, C. & Tooze, J. (1991) *Introduction to Protein Structure*. Garland Publishing, New York.)

Although the IgM molecule has 10 antigen-combining sites (two in each monomer), it often uses only five of these (for strong binding at least). One possible reason for this is the lack of flexibility of the $F(ab')_2$ arms, which limits the molecule's binding abilities. The characteristic *starfish-shaped* appearance of the free IgM molecule changes when it binds to an antigen with multiple sites, such as bacterial flagella. The arms are then dislocated below the plane of the Fc_5 disc formed by the Fc regions of the five monomers and the molecule assumes a *staple shape*.

Immunoglobulin A (IgA)

IgA is present not only in serum but also in various body fluids, such as saliva, intestinal and bronchial mucus, nasal secretions, sweat, breast milk and colostrum. There are thus two forms of IgA, serum and secretory. (All serum

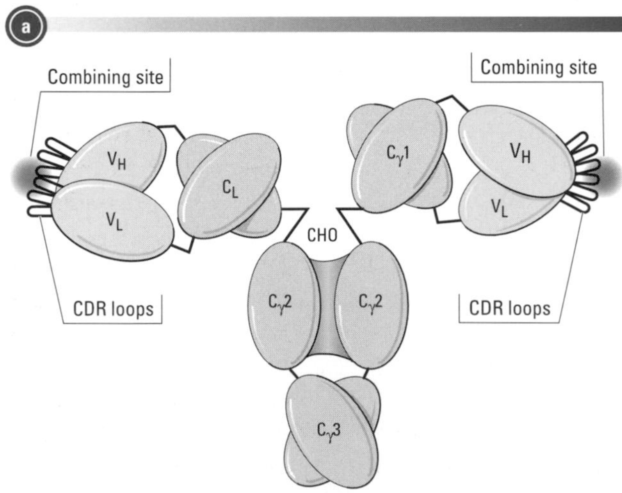

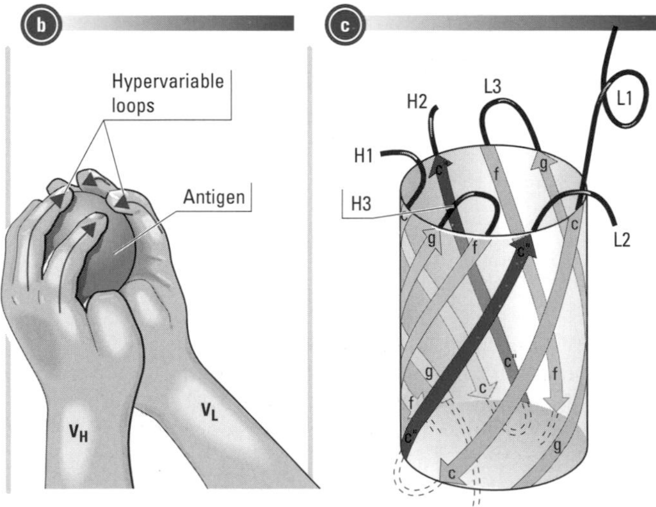

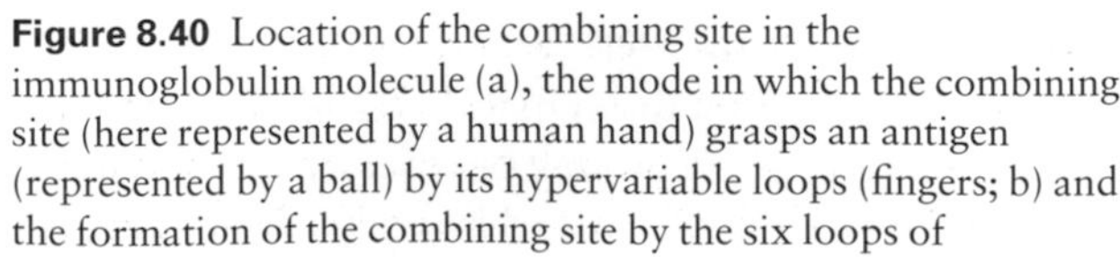

Figure 8.40 Location of the combining site in the immunoglobulin molecule (a), the mode in which the combining site (here represented by a human hand) grasps an antigen (represented by a ball) by its hypervariable loops (fingers; b) and the formation of the combining site by the six loops of complementarity-determining regions (CDR) contributed by the variable regions of the heavy (H) and light (L) chains (c). CHO, carbohydrate moiety. (a and b, Modified from Branden, C. & Tooze, J. (1991) *Introduction to Protein Structure*. Garland Publishing, New York.)

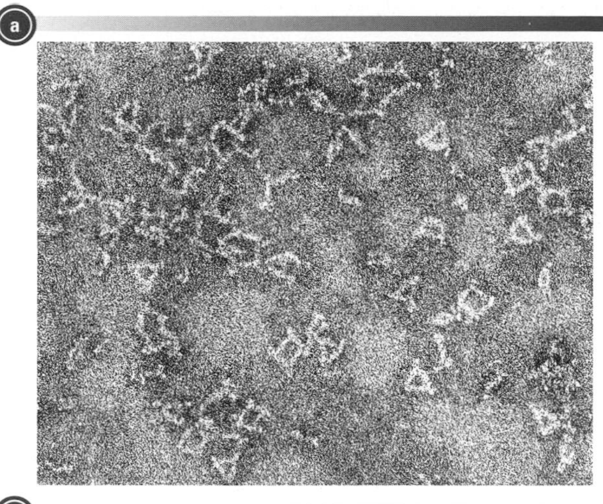

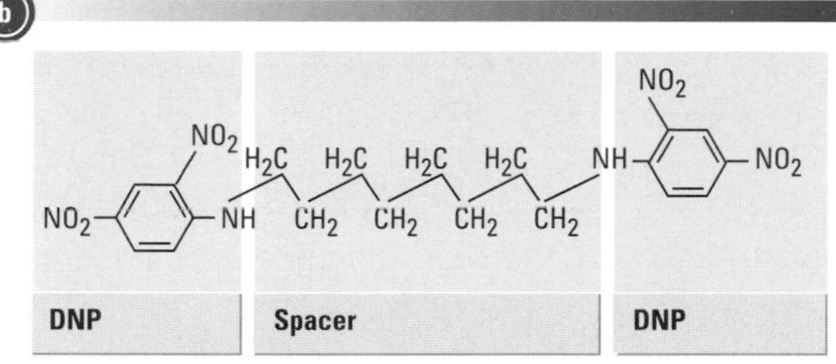

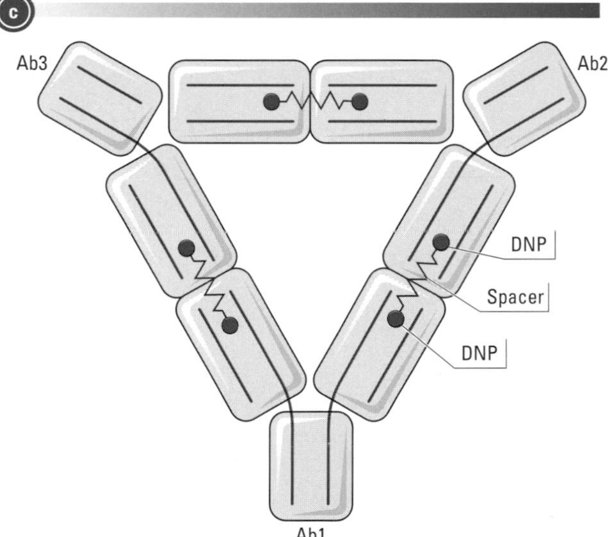

Figure 8.41 Bifunctional hapten technique for the visualization of immunoglobulin molecules in electron microscope. (a) Electron micrograph of IgG molecules joined into molecular complexes. Magnification 500 000×. (b) Structure of a bifunctional hapten with dinitrophenyl (DNP) at both ends. (c) Diagram of one of the complexes seen in (a). Ab, antibody. (a, courtesy of Dr N.M. Green.)

immunoglobulins are secreted forms, in contrast to membrane-bound forms, but IgA exists, in addition, in a 'secretory' form.) Human *serum IgA* constitutes 15–20% of the total immunoglobulin pool. More than 80% of it is in a monomeric form; the rest is polymeric. The monomers have the typical four-chain structure, an M_r of some 160 000 (the α chain, like the γ chain, consists of four domains), a sedimentation coefficient of 7S and a relatively high carbohydrate content (see Fig. 8.42g). The two α chains are joined by a single disulphide bond. Polymeric IgA occurs in the form of dimers, trimers, tetramers or pentamers, in which the two, three, four or five monomeric units are held together by disulphide bonds and by the J chain (always one J chain per molecule); the chain is identical to that found in pentameric IgM molecules.

Human serum IgA falls into two subclasses, IgA1 and IgA2, the former occurring at a higher concentration than the latter. The two subclasses differ in electrophoretic mobility (the α2 chains are more negatively charged than the α1 chains), in carbohydrate content (α1 chains have galactosamine-containing carbohydrates attached to them whereas α2 chains do not), in M_r (the α2 chain is slightly heavier than the α1 chain) and in amino acid sequence (12 amino acid residues present in the hinge region of α1 are deleted in α2, and the α1 hinge region contains a duplicated stretch of seven amino acid residues that is absent in the α2 chain hinge region). The IgA2 subclass occurs in two forms: in A2m(1), the two L chains are joined by disulphide bonds instead of being bonded to H chains; in A2m(2), normal H–L chain disulphide bonds occur. The Fab arms of the IgA1 molecule can flap; the IgA2 molecule, on the other hand, is more restricted in its flexibility.

The α1 chain contains 17 half-cystines (see Fig. 8.33), of which one forms a disulphide bond with the L chain, one with the H chain, one with the J chain and two with the so-called *secretory component* (see below); the remaining half-cystines participate in the formation of intra-H-chain disulphide bonds.

Most *secretory IgA molecules* consist of two IgA monomers (each having the basic four-chain immunoglobulin structure), one J chain and one secretory component (Fig. 8.44). The molecule has an M_r of 390 000 and a sedimentation coefficient of 11S. The two monomers can either be stacked on top of each other (less frequent YY form) or joined by their Fc ends (more prevalent >–< form). The J chain forms a disulphide bond with the penultimate half-cystine of the α chain, and the secretory component forms similar bonds with the half-cystines at positions 304 and 314. A small proportion (10–20%) of secretory IgA occurs in the form of higher polymers (tetramers and hexamers); another 10% is of the 7S type and is derived in part

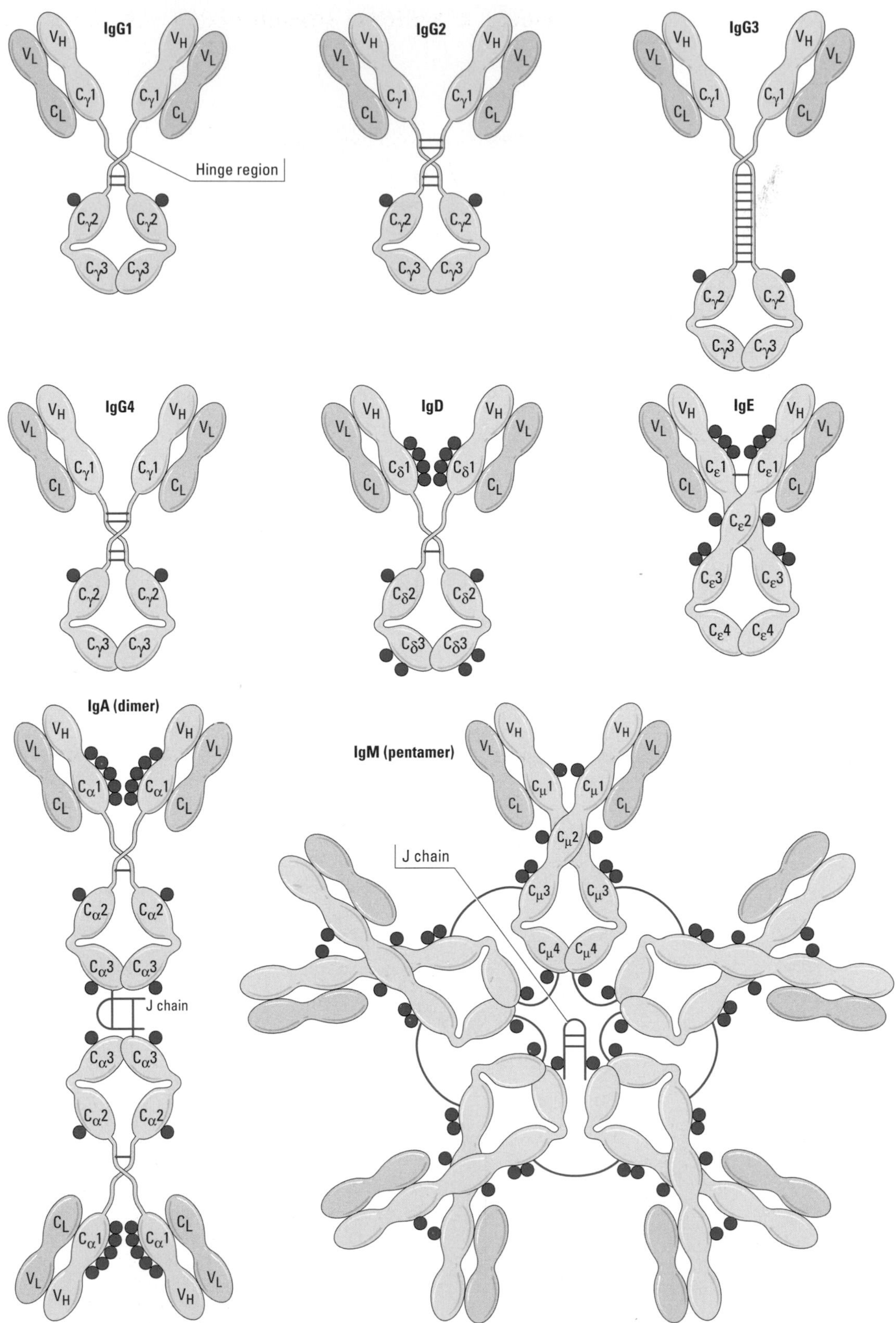

Figure 8.42 Quaternary structure of human immunoglobulin classes and subclasses found in the serum. Heavy and light chains are shaded grey and pink, respectively. Red circles represent carbohydrate moieties, connecting lines interchain disulphide bonds (only those between heavy chains or between heavy and J chains are shown). The secretory component in the IgA dimer is omitted.

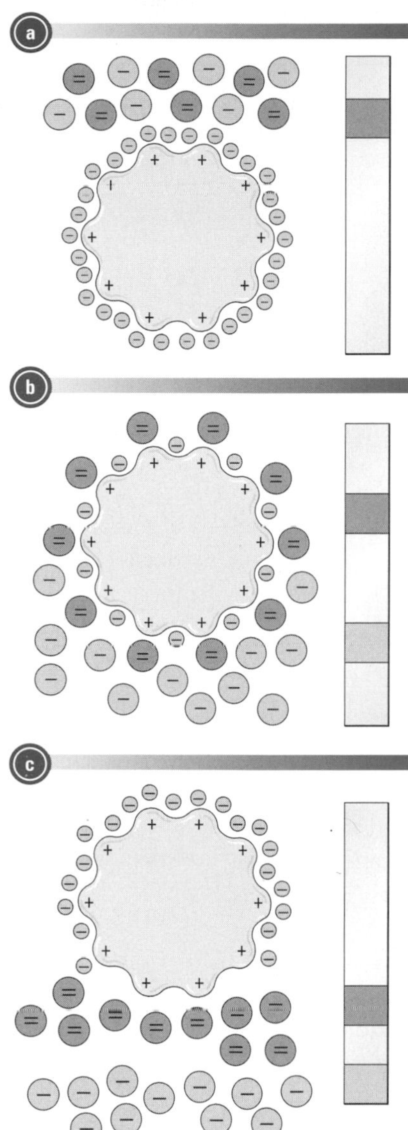

Figure 8.43 Principle of ion-exchange chromatography. The separation of molecules from a mixture occurs on an electrostatically charged adsorbent (ion exchanger), according to the molecule's net charge at a given ionic strength. The ion exchanger consists of an insoluble matrix (a synthetic resin, a polysaccharide or a protein) to which positive (in the case of an anion exchanger) or negative (in the case of a cation exchanger) functional groups are covalently bound. In the commonly used anionic exchanger diethyl aminoethyl (DEAE) cellulose, the insoluble matrix is cellulose and the charged functional groups are the DEAE ions. The DEAE-cellulose is allowed to swell in a medium that can provide suitable counterions, in this instance in a buffer containing NaCl. The chloride anions bind to the DEAE cations on the cellulose and establish an equilibrium:

$$\text{Cellulose-DEAE}^{+} + \text{Cl}^{-} \leftrightarrow \text{Cellulose-DEAE}^{+}\text{Cl}^{-}$$

The swollen cellulose is packed into a column and the protein sample, dissolved in a suitable buffer, is applied to the top and eluted with buffers of increasing or decreasing pH, or by keeping pH constant and varying ionic strength. Positively charged proteins and proteins bearing no net charge pass through the column unretarded. Negatively charged proteins compete with the Cl^- ions and displace them on the cellulose, the degree of displacement being dependent on the net protein charge and on the pH and salt concentration of the eluting buffer. By changing the pH of the buffer and thus affecting the net charge of the proteins or by increasing the molarity of the buffer and thus introducing more ions to compete with the proteins for the charged groups, one can ultimately release all the proteins from the exchanger. However, the interaction of proteins with the exchanger retards their movement down the column, and since some proteins are retarded more than others the individual protein species separate from one another. The left-hand part of the figure depicts the exchange of ions on a single bead; the right-hand part depicts a column with fractions of the sample in different stages of separation (a–c). (From Klein, J. (1982) *Immunology: The Science of Self–Nonself Discrimination*. John Wiley & Sons, New York.)

Table 8.4 Physicochemical and metabolic properties of human immunoglobulins.

Immunoglobulin	Heavy chain	Sedimentation coefficient	M_r (× 10^3)	Number of H-chain domains	Carbohydrate content (%)	Number of oligosaccharides per H chain	Average electrophoretic mobility (pH 8.6)	Serum level (mean, adult, mg/ml)	Half-life (days)	Catabolic rate	Synthetic rate (mg/kg daily)
IgG1	γ1	7S	146	4	2–3	1	γ	9	23	7	33
IgG2	γ2	7S	146	4	2–3	1	γ	3	23	7	33
IgG3	γ3	7S	170	4	2–3	1	γ	1	8	17	33
IgG4	γ4	7S	146	4	2–3	1	γ	0.5	21	7	33
IgM	μ	19S	970	5	12	5	Fast γ to β	0.5–2	5	8.8	3.3
IgA1	α1	7S	160	4	7–11	8	Fast γ to β	3.0	6	25	24
IgA2	α2	7S	160	4	7–11	8	Fast γ to β	0.5	6	25	24
sIgA	α1 or α2	11S	385	4	7–11	?	—	0.05	—	—	—
IgD	δ	7S	184	4	9–14	3	Fast γ	0.03	3	37	0.4
IgE	ε	8S	188	5	12	6	Fast γ	0.00005	2	71	0.002

from serum and possibly also from secreted and dissociated 11S IgA.

Secretory component and the receptor for polymeric immunoglobulins

IgA molecules are synthesized by plasma cells in the submucosa of the intestine or of an exocrine gland (Fig. 8.45). They then dimerize and cross through the epithelial cells of the mucosa into the lumen. While crossing the epithelial cells, the dimers acquire an extra glycoprotein chain, the *secretory component*, with which they remain associated as secretory IgA molecules. A similar secretory component participates in the transport of pentameric IgM molecules across epithelial cells. Like IgA, IgM exists in two forms, serum and secretory, although the concentration of IgM in secretions is much lower than that of IgA. And like IgA, IgM molecules acquire the secretory component during their journey across the epithelial cell. By wrapping around the Fc regions of IgA and IgM molecules, the secretory component masks sites susceptible to cleavage by proteolytic enzymes and thus protects molecules from the proteases that are abundant in the mucosal environment.

The secretory component is a remnant of the *receptor for polymeric immunoglobulin (poly-Ig)* (Fig. 8.46), which binds poly-Ig molecules at the submucosal surface of the epithelial cells. The receptor–ligand complex then undergoes endocytosis, is transported across the cell in vesicles, and exocytosed at the opposite cell surface. During this process of *transcytosis* the ligand-binding domain of the receptor is proteolytically cleaved off and discharged into external secretions in association with the poly-Ig. The cleaved-off part of the receptor then constitutes the secretory component (see Fig. 8.45).

The human poly-Ig receptor (i.e. the membrane-bound version of the secretory component) is encoded in a gene on chromosome 1q31–q42. It is 764 amino acid residues long of which 18 (the signal peptide) are cleaved off after its synthesis in the epithelial cells (see Figs 8.45 & 8.46). It consists of an extracellular part, a transmembrane region and a relatively long (103 residues) cytoplasmic tail. The extracellular part is believed to be organized into five domains (D1–D5), each domain being about 110 residues long and presumably arranged into the immunoglobulin fold. The molecule con-

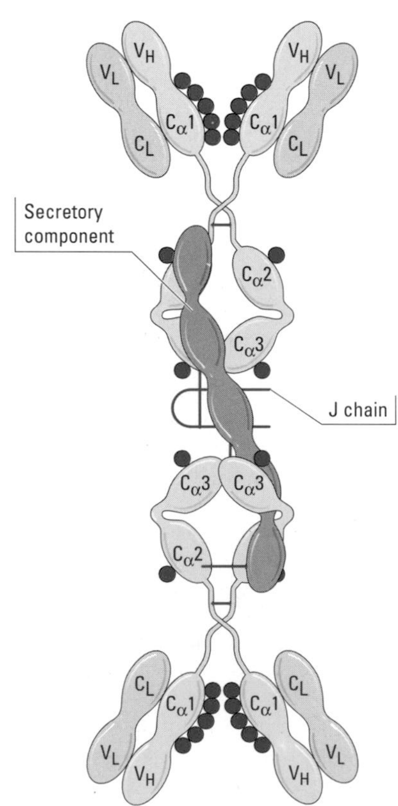

Figure 8.44 Structure of secretory IgA molecule (dimer). Closed circles represent carbohydrate moieties, interconnecting lines interchain disulphide bonds.

tains 20 cysteine residues, of which half are believed to be involved in intradomain folding (i.e. functioning as 'toothpicks' holding together the two 'slices of the sandwich'). The cleavage that produces the free secretory component after it binds to polymeric IgG or IgM molecules probably occurs near the membrane so that the free component contains most of the extracellular part, some 600 residues long. This part is glycosylated and may contain seven carbohydrate moieties. The component is believed to interact with the $C_\alpha2$ and $C_\alpha3$ domains of the IgA H chain, initially probably non-covalently and then via a disulphide exchange reaction between D5 of the component and $C_\alpha2$ of one IgA subunit.

J chain

The *joining (J) chain* is a 136 or 137 residue polypeptide (depending on the species) with one carbohydrate moiety (M_r 15 000). It is rich in acidic residues (aspartic and glutamic acids) and poor in glycine, serine and phenylalanine; it lacks tryptophan. It contains eight cysteine residues, six of which are involved in the formation of three intrachain disulphide bonds. The remaining two cysteine residues near the chain's N-terminus link up with the penultimate cysteine residues of the α or μ chains. The J chain is believed to fold into an eight-stranded antiparallel β-barrel comprising a single immunoglobulin-like domain.

The gene coding for the human J chain (*IGJ*) is on chromosome 4q21 and consists of four exons. Similar genes have been found in other vertebrates: cartilaginous and bony fish, amphibians, reptiles, birds and mammals. The genes of the different taxa are quite conserved in their sequences. The gene is expressed in B lymphocytes and in plasma cells, but not in epithelial cells. J chains are synthe-

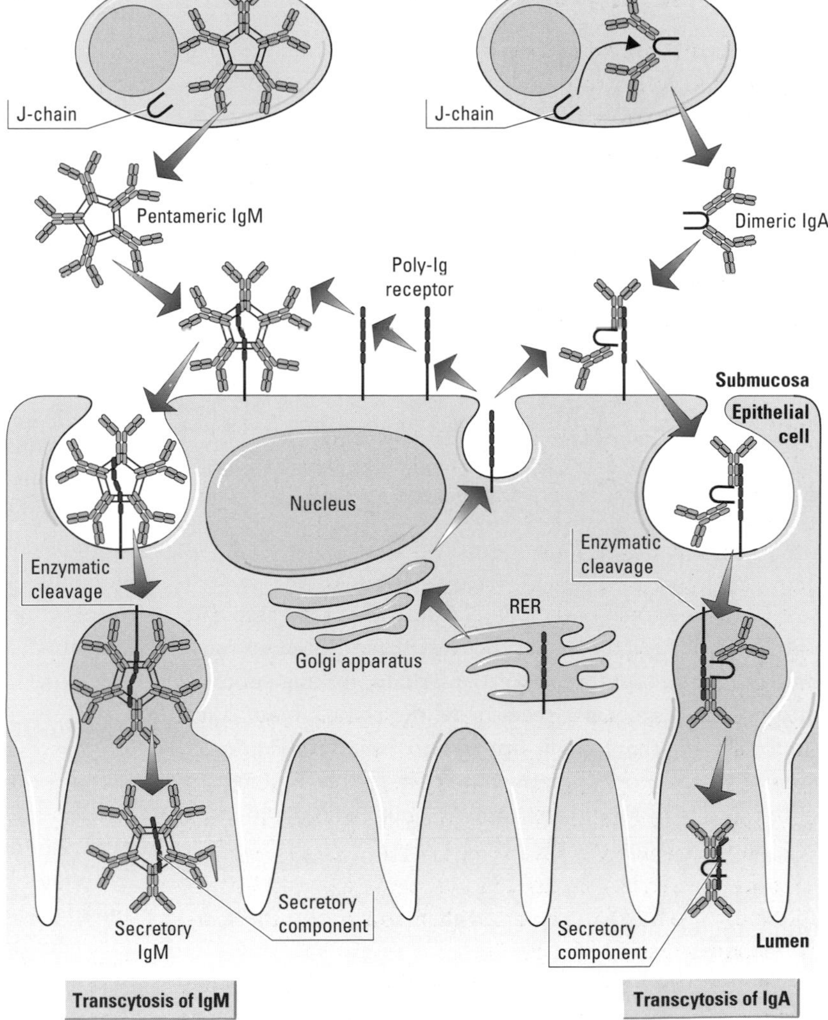

Figure 8.45 Transport of IgA and IgM molecules across epithelial cells of the mucous membrane. Both molecules and the J chain are synthesized by plasma cells in the submucosa. The tetrameric subunits polymerize, with the help of the J chain, into dimers (IgA) or pentamers (IgM) and these are secreted onto the mucosal surface. Simultaneously, the epithelial cells synthesize on their rough endoplasmic reticulum (RER), the receptor for polymeric immunoglobulin (poly-Ig) molecules. After glycosylation in the Golgi apparatus, the receptors are transported by exocytosis to the submucosal surface, where they associate with the polymeric IgA and IgM molecules. The complexes are endocytosed and the endocytic vesicles are transported to the luminal surface of the epithelial cells. The vesicles open up by exocytosis and the poly-Ig receptor is enzymatically cleaved so that only its immunoglobulin-like part (the *secretory component*) remains associated with the immunoglobulin molecules. The immunoglobulins are thus released as secretory IgA and IgM into the lumen.

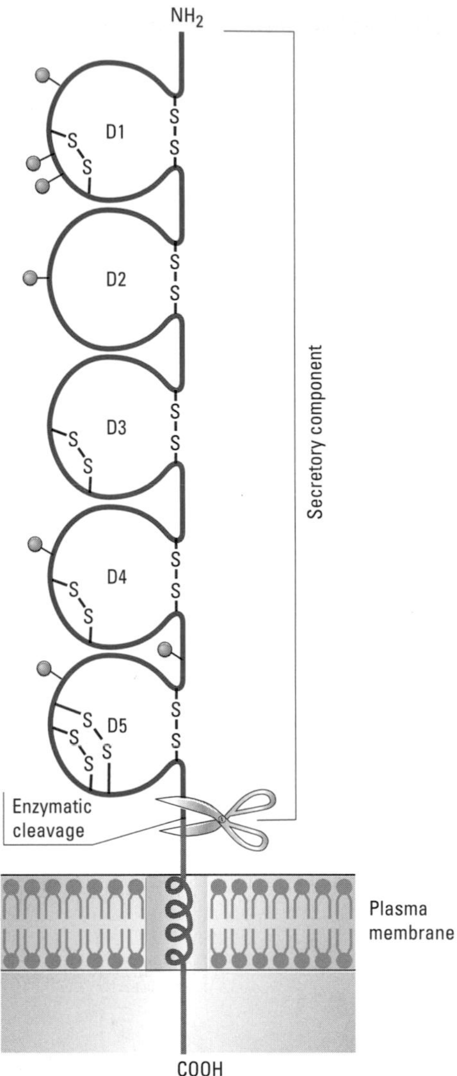

Figure 8.46 Structure of the receptor for polymeric immunoglobulins. D1–D5, immunoglobulin-like domains; S—S, disulphide bond; ●–, carbohydrate moiety.

sized in a free form in the cytoplasm, where they associate with IgA and IgM molecules. Because these molecules polymerize even in the absence of the J chain, linking subunits into polymers does not seem to be the chain's main function. Instead, the J chain appears to be essential for the binding of secretory component to poly-Ig. The binding site of the secretory component on poly-Ig includes, in addition to C_α and C_μ domains, the J chain.

Immunoglobulin D (IgD)

The concentration of IgD in serum is variable but generally low (μg/ml compared with mg/ml of IgG). As a result of this, and also because of its susceptibility to proteolysis by serum plasmin, IgD is difficult to isolate. On the membrane, IgD is co-expressed with IgM and its appearance heralds the transformation of an immature into a mature B cell. Like IgG, the IgD molecule is a four-chain ($L_2\delta_2$) 'monomer', with an M_r of 175 000–185 000 and a sedimentation coefficient of 7S. In comparison with IgG, the M_r of IgD is higher but the sedimentation coefficient is about the same, indicating that the IgD molecule must be less compact than the IgG molecule. The human δ chain consists of four domains (V_δ, $C_\delta1$, $C_\delta2$ and $C_\delta3$) and a hinge region located between $C_\delta1$ and $C_\delta2$ (see Fig. 8.42). The mouse δ chain consists of only three domains (V_δ, $C_\delta1$ and $C_\delta2$) and a hinge region. In both species, the two H chains are linked by a single disulphide bond. The molecule is rich in carbohydrates and, like IgA1, contains multiple O-linked oligosaccharides attached to serine and threonine in the hinge region, in addition to N-linked oligosaccharides at residues 354 in $C_\delta1$ as well as 445 and 496 in $C_\delta3$. Curiously, although present in serum, no antibody activity has as yet been associated with the IgD molecule.

Immunoglobulin E (IgE)

Of all the immunoglobulins, IgE occurs in serum at the lowest concentration. IgE molecules are monomers with an M_r of about 190 000, a sedimentation coefficient of 8S and the electrophoretic mobility of fast γ-globulins. As with other immunoglobulins, IgE monomers consist of two L chains and two H (ε) chains. Each ε chain consists of five domains (V_H and $C_\varepsilon1$–$C_\varepsilon4$) and contains 15 half-cystines (see Fig. 8.42), one participating in the disulphide bond with the L chain, two in H–H bonds and the rest in intrachain bonds. An unusual feature of the IgE molecule is the separation of the two inter-H-chain disulphide bonds by one complete domain (there is no hinge region in IgE and the molecule is among the least flexible of the immunoglobulins): one bond is located between $C_\varepsilon1$ and $C_\varepsilon2$ and the other between $C_\varepsilon2$ and $C_\varepsilon3$. There is also an extra intra-H-chain disulphide bond in the $C_\varepsilon1$ domain.

Antibodies as antigens

Like any other protein, immunoglobulins can, under certain circumstances, function as antigens and elicit the formation of antibodies. The antigenic determinants detected by these antibodies are of three principal types—isotypes, allotypes and idiotypes (Fig. 8.47)—depending on the genetic difference between the recipient and the donor.

Isotypes (Greek *isos*, the same) are antigenic sites that differentiate C regions encoded in *C*-gene segments. The term

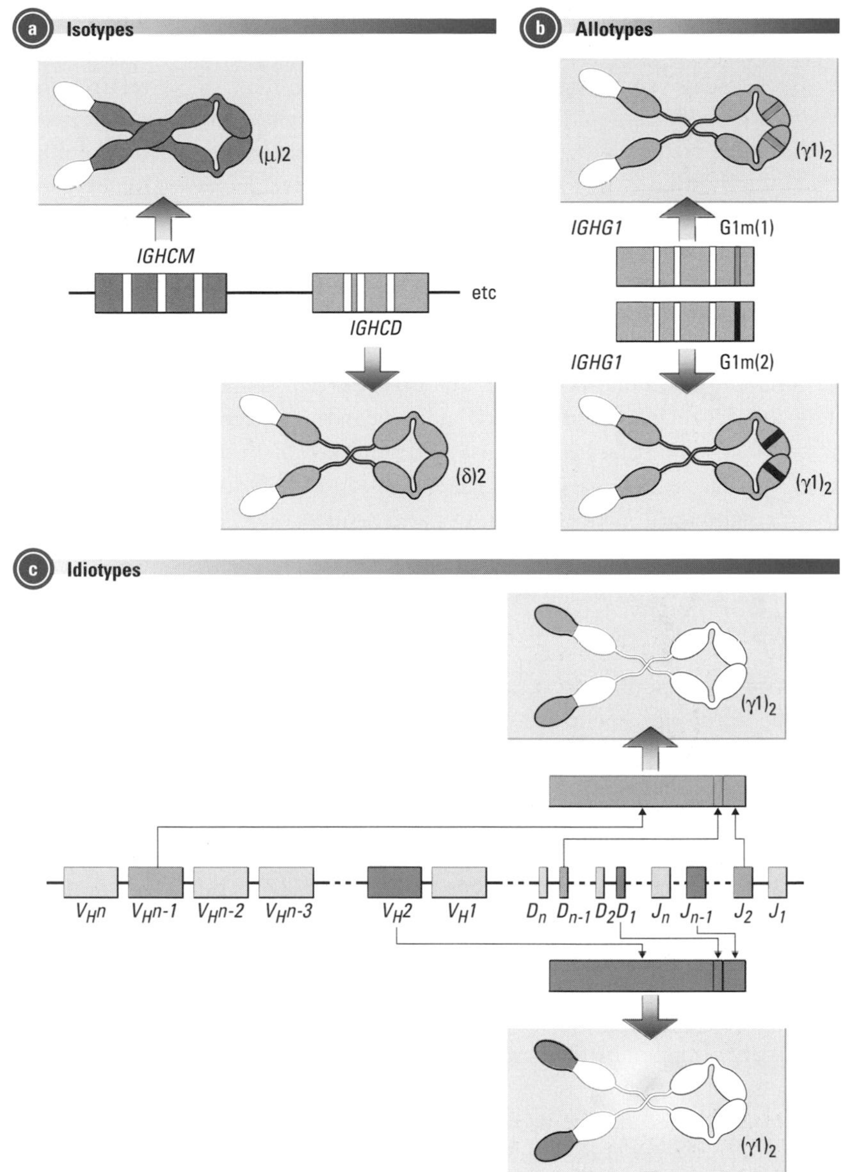

Figure 8.47 The difference between isotype (a), allotype (b) and idiotype (c). Each section shows the relevant genes and the proteins encoded in them. Light chains are omitted for simplicity.

is usually restricted to the products of the *C* segments at the *IGH* locus, i.e. to the constant regions of the H chains, and *isotypes* are then synonymous with immunoglobulin *(sub)classes*. However, it can be applied also to the constant regions of the L chains. The immune system of an animal into which human serum has been inoculated produces antibodies specifically reacting with the individual human immunoglobulin classes. The inoculation of whole serum, of course, results in a mixture of antibodies, some reacting with the IgM fraction, others with the IgG1 fraction, and so on. However, the polyspecific antiserum can be rendered monospecific (i.e. reactive with only IgM or only IgG1) by judicious absorption — removal of some of the antibodies after they have bound to their corresponding antigens. Isotype-specific antibodies have played an important part in the distinction and definition of individual isotypes.

Allotypes (Greek *allos*, other) are antigenic sites that differentiate individuals of the same species; the differences are encoded in alleles at the same locus or a gene segment. The term can be applied to any such differences, on immunoglobulins or any other proteins; it is, however, most commonly used in the context of immunoglobulins. Most of the immunoglobulin allotypes reflect amino acid differences between constant regions of a given isotype but some allotypic differences have also been described for the framework parts of the variable region. The constant region of a given isotype is not absolutely identical in all the individuals of a species. Small variation, usually limited to a single nucleotide pair (amino acid residue), does occur in most of the *C* segments (regions) and this, too, can be detected by the immune system. When blood is exchanged between two individuals differing in, say, their Cγ1 regions, the recipients produce antibodies that recognize specifically this single amino acid difference between the IgG1 proteins.

Idiotypes (Greek *idios*, one's own, personal) are antigenic sites that differentiate the V regions of immunoglobulins produced by one clone of B lymphocytes from V regions of immunoglobulins produced by other B-cell clones. The difference is always located at or near the antigen-combining site. It arises because different B-cell clones choose different *V(D)J* segments for expression and because the recombination process creates unique sequences at the *V(D)J* junction.

Allotypes

Intentional immunization is rarely used to obtain allotype-specific antibodies in humans. Instead, investigators take advantage of accidental immunizations such as those that occur as a consequence of multiple transfusions or multiple pregnancies (see Chapter 6). An additional source are patients with rheumatoid arthritis who produce antibodies against their own immunoglobulins (see Chapter 25). The antibodies can be detected using the *haemagglutination inhibition assay* in which the allotype-specific antibody competes with another antibody for binding (the assay is described in Chapter 14). In animals, allotype-specific antibodies are obtained by deliberate immunizations with purified immunoglobulins of a particular class, and their detection is based on the use of more direct assays. More and more, however, these conventional serological methods of allotype detection are being replaced by DNA-based techniques. In one of the latter, the DNA encompassing the site responsible for the allotypic difference is amplified by PCR and the amplification product blotted onto a filter, which is then hybridized with a labelled, allele specific oligonucleotide.

Individual human allotypes were originally designated by letters (or letters with numbers; the so-called *alfameric system*) but because such nomenclature is cumbersome, a committee of experts working under the auspices of the World Health Organization later introduced a *numerical system*. In both systems the symbol is prefixed by an abbreviation of the chain that controls the allotype (G1m, Mm, Km, etc. for allotypes borne by the γ1, μ, κ chains, respectively, where 'm' stands for 'marker'). Human immunoglobulin allotypes have been described for the H chains α2, γ1, γ2, γ3, γ4 and ε and for the κL chain (Table 8.5). Because the *C* segments encoding the H-chain allotypes all occupy a relatively short region of the chromosome in which crossing-over occurs infrequently, human populations differ in the combinations of allotype-specifying alleles (*haplotypes*) in the same way as they differ in *HLA* haplotypes (see Chapter 6). The allotypic haplotypes and their frequencies, as well as the frequencies of individual allotypes, are important population characteristics, which can be used, together with other markers, to inquire into the origin of human ethnic groups. Other applications of allotypes include paternity testing, forensic typing and monitoring of graft survival in bone marrow transplantation.

Idiotypes

The individual sites recognized by antibodies in or near the combining site of other antibodies are called *idiotypic determinants* or *idiotopes*. A collection of idiotopes of a given immunoglobulin molecule is an *idiotype*. The antigen-combining site of an antibody is the *paratope*. The antibody that binds to an idiotope is referred to as anti-idiotypic antibody; here it will be called idiotope-specific antibody.

An idiotope can reside either within a combining site or on the outside but in the vicinity of the site. In the former, but not the latter, the interaction between the idiotope and anti-idiotope is inhibited by the antigen that the combining site recognizes. Some idiotopes are formed by either H or L chains alone, but many require the contribution of both chains, i.e. they are *conformational determinants*. The amino acid residues that contribute to the formation of an idiotope map mostly to the loops that constitute the CDRs but framework residues also play their part. Although the presence or absence of an idiotope correlates with specific single amino acid replacements, several other residues shared by molecules that differ in an idiotope also participate in the formation of the determinant.

Idiotopes that result from a unique sequence created by *V(D)J* recombination are restricted to a single individual of a given species (*individual idiotopes*). They are restricted to antibodies produced by a single B-lymphocyte clone and are a somatic phenomenon: progeny of the individual with the idiotope lack the determinant on their immunoglobulins. Idiotopes encoded in a *V* segment of the germ line are expressed in several individuals of the same and sometimes also of different species (*cross-reactive idiotopes,* CRI or IdX). Their distribution reflects the repeated usage of the particular *V* segment by different individuals. They are inherited according to Mendel's laws and can thus serve as markers for the germ-line gene segments. Usually, antibodies bearing a particular cross-reactive idiotope bind the same antigen (they are of the same specificity). A given idiotope can be shared by antibodies belonging to different immunoglobulin classes because the same *V(D)J* segment can be expressed with different *C* segments as a result of class switch. Some idiotypes are found on the majority of antibodies reacting with a given antigen (*dominant idiotopes*), while others are present only on a small fraction of antibodies of a given specificity (*minor idiotopes*). Other idiotopes still are normally undetectable but can become dominant if the B-cell clone is activated by idiotope-specific antibodies or by a special immunization regimen (*silent idiotopes*).

The presence of certain idiotopes in the combining site

Table 8.5 Human immunoglobulin allotypes.

Chain	Gene	Allotype designation: Numeric	Alfameric	Location	Amino acid at position
γ1	*G1m*	1	a	$C_\gamma 3$	Asp 356 Leu 358
		−1	Non-a	$C_\gamma 3$	Glu 356 Met 358
		2	x	$C_\gamma 3$	
		4 (3)	f(b^w, b^2)	$C_\gamma 1$	Arg 214
		7	r	C_H	
		17	z	$C_\gamma 1$	Lys 214
		18	Rouen 2	C_H	
		20	San Francisco 2	C_H	
γ2	*G2m*	23	n	$C_\gamma 2$	
		−23	Non n	$C_\gamma 2$	
		5 (12)	b,b^1(b$^\gamma$)	$C_\gamma 2$	
γ3	*G3m*	−5	Non-b,b^1	$C_\gamma 2$	
		6	c(c^3)	$C_\gamma 3$	
		11	b$^\beta$(b^0)	$C_\gamma 3$	Phe 436
		−11	Non-b$^\beta$(non b^0)	$C_\gamma 3$	Tyr 436
		13 (10)	b^3(b$^\alpha$)	$C_\gamma 3$	
		14	b^4	$C_\gamma 3$	
		15	s	$C_\gamma 2$	
		16	t	$C_\gamma 2$	
		21	g	$C_\gamma 2$	Tyr 296
		−21	Non-g	$C_\gamma 2$	Phe 296
		24	c^5	C_H	
		25	Bet	C_H	
		26	u	C_H	
		27	v	C_H	
		28	g5	C_H	
γ4	*G4m*	1	4a	$C_\gamma 2$	Leu 309
		−1	4b	$C_\gamma 2$	Gap 309
Unclassified	*Gm*	7	γ	C_H	
		8	e	C_H	
		9	P	C_H	
		12	bγ	C_H	
		18	Ro^2	C_H	
		19	Ro^3	C_H	
		20	z (S.F.)	C_H	
α2	*A2m*	1	1	C_H	131 No bridge to L chain
		2	2	$C_\alpha 1$	131 Bridge to L chain
ε	*Em*	1		C_H	
κ	*Km*	1	1	C_κ	
		2	2	C_κ	
		3	3	C_κ	Ala 153 Val 191

has led to the prediction that the antibody specific to such idiotopes should mimic epitopes of the antigen structurally (it should be an *internal image* of the antigen). The concept of internal image has played an important part in speculations concerning the regulation of the immune response (see Chapter 19). However, X-ray diffraction analyses of idiotope–anti-idiotope complexes have thus far provided only limited support for epitope anti-idiotope mimicry.

Monoclonal antibodies

Immunoglobulins secreted by plasma cells accumulate in blood plasma and other body fluids. The plasma (normal serum) thus contains a heterogeneous immunoglobulin mixture that reflects the individual's previous encounters with a variety of antigens. Immunization, whether natural or deliberate, increases the concentration of antibodies specific for the immunizing antigen, but even this fraction is heterogeneous because it has been contributed to by many different B-cell clones stimulated by the antigen: the antiserum is said to be of polyclonal origin or simply *polyclonal*. There are many situations in immunology in which a *monoclonal antibody*, consisting of immunoglobulins produced by the stimulation of a single B-cell clone, is more desirable than a polyclonal antiserum. For one thing, the homogeneity of a monoclonal antibody removes some of the variables associated with the use of polyclonal antibodies and thus enhances reproducibility of an experiment or a clinical trial. For another, it offers a potential for producing stronger and more effective reagents than do the polyclonal antibodies. It has therefore been an immunologist's dream to replace polyclonal by monoclonal antibodies.

The first step towards fulfilment of the dream was the exploitation of normal B lymphocytes accidentally transformed into tumour cells. Such accidents occur, from time to time, in both humans and animals, and when they affect B cells in terminal stages of differentiation they result in the appearance of *plasma cell tumours* (*plasmacytomas*, *myelomas*), which secrete large quantities of immunoglobulins into blood plasma (see Chapter 26). The immunoglobulins, the *myeloma proteins*, appear as a distinct band on electrophoresis of the patient's serum and can therefore be isolated and purified easily. They can consist of complete immunoglobulin molecules, free L chains (*Bence-Jones proteins*, named after Henry Bence-Jones, 1814–1873, an English physician who first described them) or a mixture of both. Myeloma proteins are homogeneous, but an experimenter has no control over their specificity. It is, in fact, a laborious undertaking to determine which antigen a myeloma protein might be specific for. They were therefore helpful in efforts to elucidate immunoglobulin structure but were not of much use in situations in which they were needed to act as antibodies. Plasmacytomas, however, contributed to the realization of the dream of producing monoclonal antibodies with predetermined specificity by providing one of the essential components for the *B-cell hybridoma technique*.

The principle of the technique is to fuse two cells: one is programmed to secrete antibodies of a single specificity, but is mortal; the other does not secrete immunoglobulins, but allows the expression of immunoglobulin genes, and is immortal (Fig. 8.48). The product of the fusion, a hybrid cell or *hybridoma*, combines the properties of both input cells, i.e. it continues to produce antibodies of the desired specificity and it is immortal. By growing the hybridomas in culture or in suitable animals, a resource is available for producing virtually unlimited amounts of antibodies, all of which are identical. The two input cells are a *B lymphocyte* activated by a given antigen and a *plasmacytoma cell* engineered to facilitate the selection of antibody-secreting *B-cell hybridomas* after the fusion (Fig. 8.48). The activated B lymphocyte is obtained from the spleen of an animal (usually a mouse) immunized against the particular antigen.

The new system of monoclonal antibody production has been exploited quickly by experimentalists of different callings: cell biologists, geneticists, microbiologists, biochemists and, of course, immunologists. The application of the system to human clinical situations has been hampered, however, by difficulties in setting up human B-cell hybridoma systems. One can immunize a mouse against human antigens and produce mouse monoclonal antibodies specific for such antigens. However, when such antibodies are introduced into human blood, they are recognized as foreign by the human immune system and eliminated. The main problems in producing human monoclonal antibodies have been, first, that humans cannot be immunized deliberately and at will; second, that in immunized volunteers, spleen cannot be used as a source of activated B cells; and third, that the plasmacytoma fusion partner has proved difficult to engineer.

An alternative to the use of plasmacytomas is to transform activated human B lymphocytes with the *Epstein–Barr virus* (EBV) *in vitro*. EBV is a widespread human herpes virus that normally replicates in the epithelial cells of the nasopharynx and parotid gland, but infects also B lymphocytes. Its DNA does not integrate into the host chromosome but instead persists in EBV-infected cells in a free ring-like form (episomes). The infected B lymphocytes produce their own growth factors and thus continue to divide in tissue culture as *lymphoblastoid cell lines* (LCLs). Some of the LCLs secrete antibodies into the culture super-

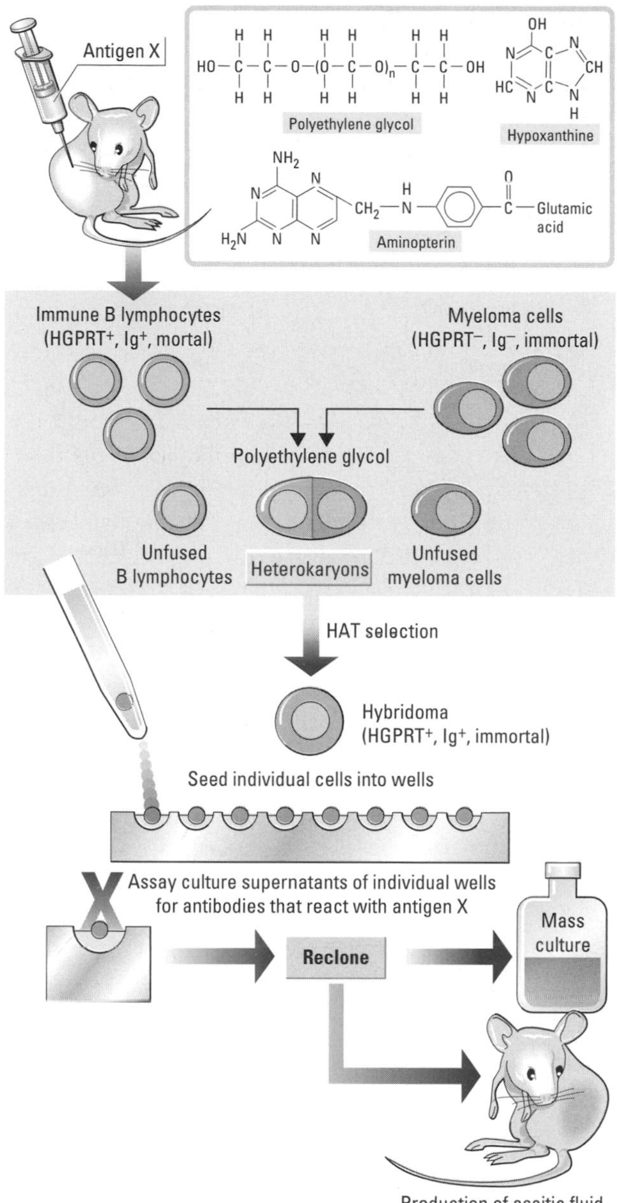

Figure 8.48 Production of a monoclonal antibody. An antigen inoculated into a mouse stimulates the recipient's B lymphocytes that express cell-surface receptors (immunoglobulins) specific for it. The lymphocytes are cultured with mouse myeloma cells in the presence of *polyethylene glycol* (PEG), an agent that promotes fusion of cells by bridging their membranes. With the help of PEG, some of the myeloma cells fuse with some of the B lymphocytes to form *heterokaryons*, cells with nuclei derived from different cells. Subsequently, the nuclei fuse as well and B-lymphocyte × myeloma cell hybrids or *B-cell hybridomas* arise. The culture then contains three types of cells: unfused B lymphocytes, unfused myeloma cells and hybridomas. Since the goal is to obtain cells that, like myelomas, are immortal but that produce antibodies as the B lymphocyte would if it were to differentiate further, the hybridomas must be selected out from the rest of the cells. To get rid of the unfused B cells is not a problem because they die in the culture unless they are restimulated by exposure to antigen. But to separate the hybridomas from the myeloma cells, a special trick has to be used. The myeloma cells have been mutated to render them incapable of producing the enzyme *hypoxanthine guanine phosphoribosyl transferase* (HGPRT), which is involved in one of two biochemical pathways the cell uses to synthesize nucleotides. In the *endogenous pathway*, the nitrogenous bases of the nucleotides are synthesized de novo from amino acids. This pathway can be blocked by *aminopterin*, a substance that structurally resembles a substrate on which at least two enzymes in this pathway act. The enzymes bind aminopterin but cannot convert it into the desired product and the endogenous pathway thus comes to a standstill. In the *salvage pathway*, in which nucleotides produced by degradation of nucleic acids are reused, HGPRT converts guanine and hypoxanthine into guanosine monophosphate (GMP) and inosine monophosphate (IMP), respectively. The special trick consists of culturing the cell mixture in a medium that contains hypoxanthine, aminopterin and thymidine (*HAT medium*). The HGPRT-defective myeloma cells synthesize nucleotides via the endogenous pathway and hence grow normally in an ordinary medium. But when placed in HAT medium, aminopterin blocks the endogenous pathway and, since the salvage pathway is blocked because of the defective HGPRT, the cells die for lack of nucleotides. In the hybridoma cells, on the other hand, the B cell-derived chromosomes provide an active HGPRT that enables the hybrid to use the hypoxanthine in the medium via the salvage pathway (the endogenous pathway is blocked by aminopterin in these cells, too). Thus only the hybridomas will grow in the culture. The thymidine in the medium is, in this case, not relevant to the selection. It becomes relevant in other systems, in which a gene coding for another enzyme of the salvage pathway, thymidine kinase (which converts thymidine into thymidine monophosphate) is inactivated. Of course, the culture may also contain hybrid cells that do not produce any antibodies or that produce antibodies of no interest to the experimenter. (The production of antibodies encoded in the myeloma cell chromosomes is precluded by another mutation.) The hybridomas must therefore be *cloned* (colonies established from individual cells in the wells of a plate designed for this purpose) and the presence of desired antibodies tested in the supernatant of individual clones. Clones producing the right *monoclonal antibodies* are then expanded and large amounts of the antibody are obtained either from a mass culture or by inoculating the hybridoma cells into the peritoneal cavity of genetically or immunologically compatible mice. The growth of the tumour cells stimulates the host to produce antibody-containing *ascitic fluid* (from Greek *ascités*, bag-like) that fills the cavity.

natant. The level of antibody production is generally low, however, and usually the production stops after a few months. Attempts to replace *in vivo* immunization by exposure to antigen in tissue culture have only been partially successful. Normally, such immunizations are difficult because the *in vitro* system lacks the microenvironment necessary for B-cell activation and the responses are limited to IgM antibodies which bind antigen poorly. However, an improvement has been achieved by mixing lymphocytes from two unrelated individuals. T lymphocytes in the mixture recognize, via their TCRs, the disparate MHC molecules of the partner and become activated to produce cytokines, which then help B cells to switch from IgM to IgG production and to produce antibodies that bind the antigen more strongly.

An alternative solution to the problem of producing human monoclonal antibodies takes advantage of the availability of *scid mice*. These animals have suffered a mutation in a gene required for the completion of *V(D)J* recombination in both *IG* and *TCR* genes. In mice carrying two defective copies of the gene, mature T and B cells fail to develop and the mice suffer from *severe combined immunodeficiency disease* (*scid*). Because the mouse hosts lack their own T lymphocytes, they do not reject transplants of human fetal liver cells (see Chapter 24) and the human stem cells differentiate in the thymus into T cells that recognize mouse molecules as self. This *scid–human mouse* can be immunized and the stimulated human B cells used to produce B-cell hybridomas that secrete human monoclonal antibodies.

Since its introduction in 1975, the B-cell hybridoma technique has been modified in numerous ways, in particular by combining it with various recombinant DNA methods. Thus, to render mouse antibodies (Fig. 8.49c) less antigenic for the human body, the antibody genes can be redesigned by replacing the mouse *C* segments of both H and L chain-encoding genes by human *C* segments (Fig. 8.49a,d). One can also perform more drastic molecular surgery and replace, in addition, the *V* segment except for the CDRs (Fig. 8.49b). The engineered gene can then be introduced into the genome of a myeloma cell that itself does not synthesize any immunoglobulins. The antibodies secreted by the transfected cells are then basically human (they have been *humanized*) except for the part that determines their specificity. And if the surgery in the *V* segment has adversely influenced the specificity of the antibody, one can attempt to restore or even improve antigen binding by substituting key amino acids in the V region using methods of site-directed mutagenesis. If an antibody of a particular class is sluggish in carrying out certain effector functions (e.g. binding to Fc receptors, of which more later), one can replace (at the gene level) the Fc with a corresponding part from another immunoglobulin class. One can also replace part of the *C* segment by a gene coding for an immunotoxin (Fig. 8.49e) and thus impose a function on an antibody that it normally does not have, i.e. direct killing of the cell to which it binds. Finally, antibodies can be engineered to contain one combining site that binds one antigen (e.g. the CD3–TCR complex) and another combining site that binds another antigen (e.g. a tumour-specific antigen; Fig. 8.49f). Such *bispecific* or *bifunctional antibodies* can bind with one arm to one cell (a T lymphocyte) and with the other arm to another (a tumour cell) and thus facilitate their interaction (e.g. killing of the tumour cell by the cytotoxic T lymphocyte). Hybrid antibodies, in which one half of the molecule binds one antigen and the other half another antigen, can also be obtained by the fusion of two hybridomas producing these

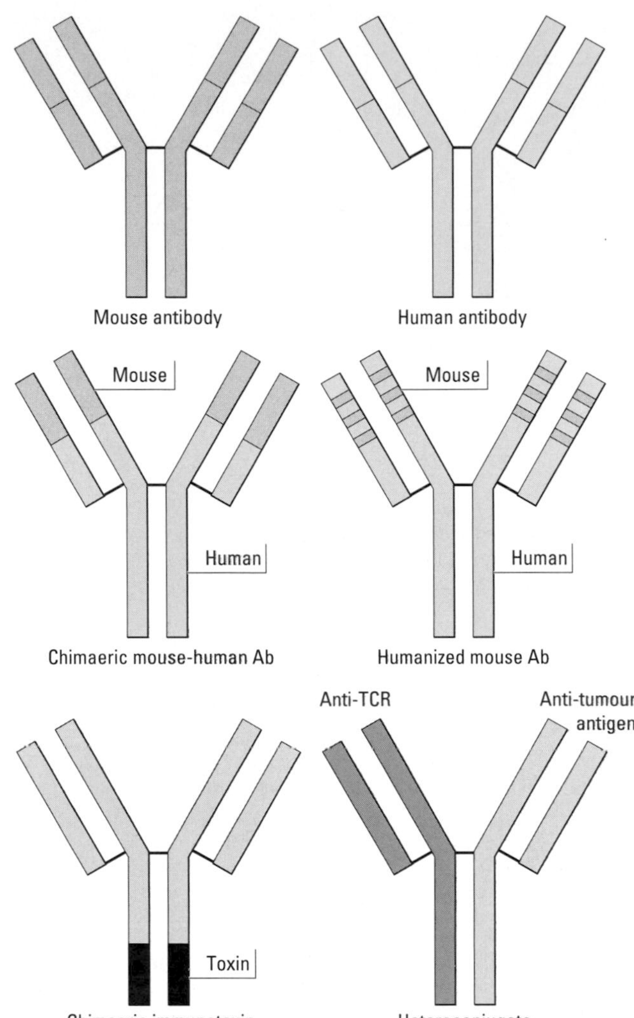

Figure 8.49 Antibodies (Ab) engineered by recombinant DNA techniques.

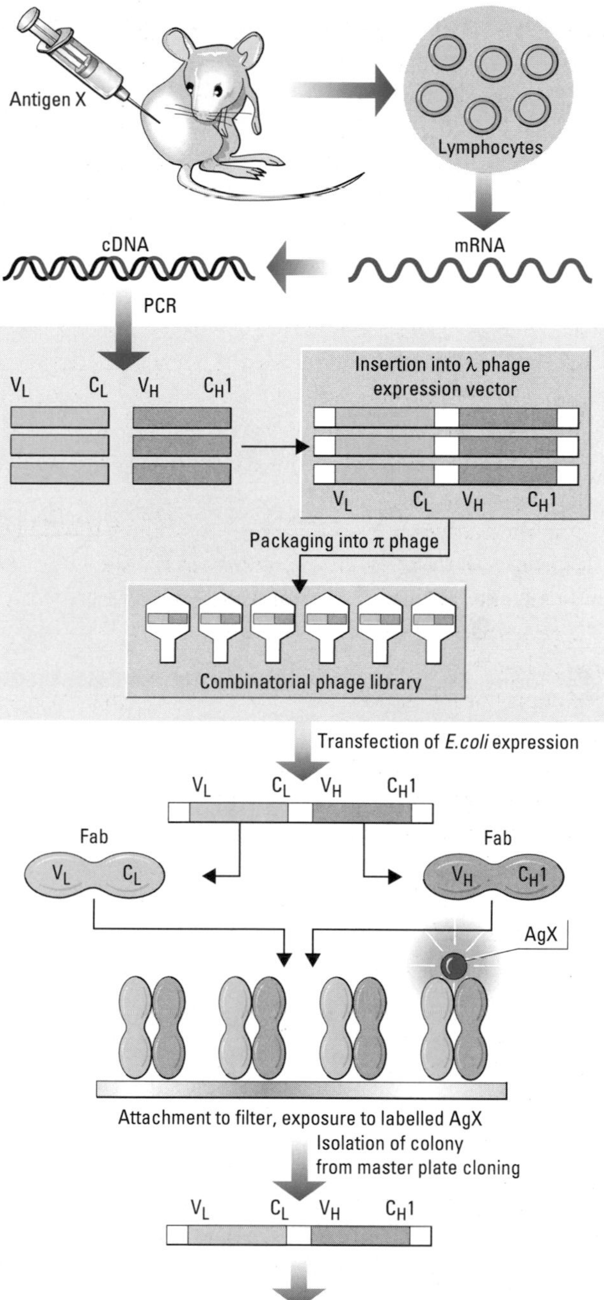

Figure 8.50 Procedure for the generation of combinatorial antibody libraries. Messenger RNA is isolated from spleen cells of a mouse immunized against an antigen X. The single-stranded mRNA is converted (with the help of reverse transcriptase) into double-stranded complementary DNA and the sequence coding for the immunoglobulin light chain (V_LC_L) and the Fab part of the heavy chain (V_HC_H1) are amplified by the polymerase chain reaction (PCR) using primers specific for the 5′ and 3′ ends of the corresponding DNA segments (including the promoter region). The amplified products are inserted into λ phage expression vectors, always one V_LC_L and one V_HC_H1 segment into one vector molecule. The vectors with the inserts are packaged into phages, the phages used to infect *Escherichia coli* bacteria and the bacteria grown into discrete colonies in a culture dish. The infected bacteria produce V_LC_L and V_HC_H1 proteins, which associate spontaneously into Fab molecules. A filter placed on top of the culture (*replica filter*) will capture some of the proteins produced by the bacteria at positions corresponding to the location of the individual colonies. Exposure of the filter to labelled antigen X will then identify the colony that produces Fab molecules with combining sites capable of binding this antigen. The DNA segments specifying these Fab molecules can be isolated and used to transfect bacteria or eukaryotic cells and thus to produce large quantities of the antibody fragments. In another version of the procedure, λ phage is replaced by the M13 phage, which displays the antibody fragments on its surface along with its own proteins. This variant allows large-scale screening for antibodies of the desired specificity in a solution rather than on a culture plate.

two types of antibodies. As such hybridomas are derived ultimately from four parental cells, they are called *quadromas*.

Attempts are also being made to replace altogether the hybridoma methods by recombinant DNA techniques. One such attempt (Fig. 8.50) focuses on the gene segments that specify the Fab of an immunoglobulin molecule, the V_HC_H1 and V_LC_L. These segments can be amplified by PCR from many different mRNA (cDNA) molecules expressed in a population of cells undergoing an immune response, the amplified segments cloned and paired randomly (always one V_HC_H1 with one V_LC_L, in a suitable vector) and the pairs translated into proteins (Fabs). Screening of this *combinatorial library of antibodies* with a labelled antigen then identifies those combinations that bind this antigen. The identified V_HC_H1–V_LC_L pairs are then placed into an expression vector, either bacterial or mammalian, and used to produce large quantities of anti-

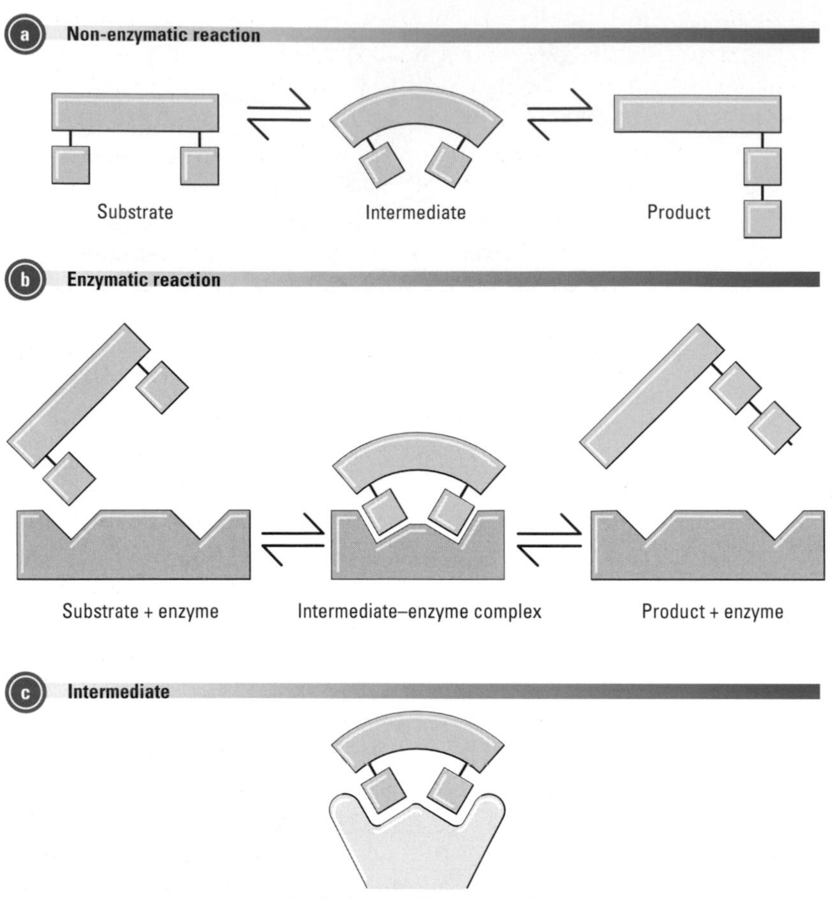

Figure 8.51 Principle of enzymatic reaction (a, b) and of substituting enzymes by catalytic antibodies (c). A chemical reaction constitutes transfer of an atom or an atomic group from one place in a molecule (substrate) to another to generate a different molecule (product). For this transfer to occur, the substrate must assume an unstable intermediate form. In an ordinary reaction (a), the probability of occurrence of the intermediate form is low and the reaction slow. In an enzymatic reaction (b), the intermediate enzyme complex is more stable than the substrate–enzyme complex and the reaction is accelerated dramatically. The combining site of catalytic antibody (c) mimics the active site of an enzyme and so it, too, accelerates the chemical reaction.

bodies with selected specificity. It is also possible to use engineered Fv instead of Fab. Although in some Fv the V_H and V_L domains remain stably associated via non-covalent bonds, in others the domains come apart easily. This problem has been circumvented by either site-directed mutagenesis, which is used to introduce cysteine residues into the domains so that they become linked together via disulphide bonds, or fusing the V_H and V_L segments at the DNA level via a stretch of nucleotides that encodes a polypeptide linker. At the protein level, the linker then joins the two domains into *single-chain Fv (scFv) protein*. However, methods of this type still suffer from certain technical problems and, until these are solved, hybridoma methods will remain in wide use. Monoclonal antibodies have found many applications for a variety of purposes: mapping of epitopes on antigenic molecules, purification and identification of proteins (e.g. those of the CD system), identification and isolation of lymphocyte subpopulations and clones, tumour detection and imaging, tumour killing (e.g. by immunotoxins), production of diagnostic reagents, to name just a few. A whole industry has grown up around the use of monoclonal antibodies.

A particularly innovative application of monoclonal antibodies is to employ them instead of enzymes to catalyse chemical reactions (Fig. 8.51). In an ordinary chemical reaction, a molecule ('substrate') must assume an unstable intermediate form ('transition state' structure) before it changes into another molecule ('product'). Because the intermediate represents a state of high energy content, the probability that the transition structure will form and last long enough for the change to occur is low and the reaction is slow. An enzyme binds the transition structure, stabilizes it and thus increases the rate at which a reaction approaches an equilibrium, i.e. it catalyses the reaction. The interaction between the enzyme and the intermediate is the function of the *active site*, a cleft or crevice on the surface of the enzyme molecule complementary to the critical part of the transition state structure. The active site and its manner of interaction with the intermediate closely resembles the combining site of an antibody and its interaction with the antigen. Hence, if antibodies could be found that bind to transition state structures, they would be expected to accelerate chemical reactions just like or even better than enzymes, i.e. they would act as *catalytic antibodies* or *abzymes*. The possibility of designing catalysts at will would find many applications in the chemical and pharmaceutical industries. Several groups of investigators are therefore trying to design small molecules (haptens) that mimic transition state structures and then find antibodies specifically reacting with these molecules that can accelerate chemical reactions. Screening for the suitable antibody is facilitated by the use of combinatorial libraries.

Function of antibodies

Free immunoglobulins protect a vertebrate body either directly or indirectly. *Direct protection* is effected via the ability of antibodies to interfere with the activities of the parasite and can assume a variety of forms, depending on the circumstances (see Chapter 21). Thus, many bacteria secrete molecules (*toxins*) that bind to host cells via specific receptors and disrupt the cell's function. Antibodies (*antitoxins*) may attach to the receptor-binding domain of the toxin and thus neutralize its effect (*neutralizing antibodies*). Many bacteria also need to attach themselves to host cells to survive in the body. The attachment relies on the interaction between specialized molecules on the bacteria surface (*adhesins*) and a ligand on the host cell. Antibodies against bacterial adhesins can block the attachment. Finally, viruses use specialized molecules to interact with the host cell's receptor and with their help to enter the cell. Antibodies against these molecules interfere with this interaction and thus contribute to the containment of the infection.

In *indirect protection*, the antibody focuses other molecules onto the parasite by binding to antigens on the parasite's surface; the actual attack is then mediated by these *effector molecules*. A prerequisite for this form of protection is that the effector molecules interact with the antibody only when the latter itself is bound to the antigen. If they were to interact with antibodies in the absence of antigen, their actions could, directly or indirectly, damage the body. An antibody interacts with an antigen via the combining site and with the effector molecule via its Fc portion. The two main types of effector molecules that interact with the Fc region of immunoglobulins are complement components and Fc receptors. *Complement* is a set of plasma proteins that act as a team to attack an extracellular parasite either by puncturing its cell membranes or by making the parasite more palatable to phagocytes. The complement system can act independently of immunoglobulins, but antibodies bound to a parasite make its actions more effective. The complement system is described in Chapter 12.

Fc receptors are a set of heterogeneous molecules whose common characteristic is that they all bind to specific sites on the Fc part of the immunoglobulin molecule. When this happens, the receptors generate a signal that activates the cell expressing them. Since different cells express a variety of Fc receptors that bind to different immunoglobulin classes, distinct responses can be generated depending on the circumstances. Activation of phagocytes leads to ingestion and intracellular killing of the parasite; activation of natural killer cells results in target cell lysis; and activation of mast cells triggers the release of toxic substances. Fc receptors are described in more detail in the final section of this chapter.

The Fc part of an immunoglobulin can also interact with molecules borne by parasites themselves, particularly by certain bacteria. The best known of these *bacterial Fc receptors* is *protein A*, a cell wall component of *Staphylococcus aureus*. The interaction of bacterial Fc receptors with antibodies leads to the activation of the complement system (see Chapter 12).

Because the Fc parts of the various immunoglobulin classes differ in their ability to interact with effector molecules, the classes participate in different effector functions. A brief description of the different functions follows (see also Table 8.6). *IgM antibodies* are good at binding complement after they have combined with an antigen. *IgG antibodies* excel in preparing cells or particles for ingestion by phagocytic cells, such as neutrophils and macrophages. The antibody binds by its $F(ab')_2$ region to antigens on the target cell surface and with its Fc region to Fc receptors on the surface of the phagocytic cell and thus assists in engulfing the coated particle. Of the four subclasses, IgG1 and IgG3 show the highest affinity for Fc receptors, IgG4 has intermediate affinity and IgG2 very low affinity. IgG molecules can, like IgM molecules, also bind the C1q component of the complement pathway. The binding affinity decreases among the IgG subclasses in the order: IgG3 > IgG1 > IgG2 > IgG4. Human IgG3 and IgG1 activate the complement cascade almost as efficiently as IgM, IgG2 activates it less efficiently and IgG4 does not activate it at all. However, the Fc part of IgG4, when used without the $F(ab')_2$ fragment, does activate the complement molecule, indicating that in this subclass the Clq binding site is normally obstructed by the Fab arms. IgG molecules also contain a binding site for protein A and can therefore bind directly to certain Gram-positive bacteria. In humans, all four IgG subclasses can bind protein A, although in IgG3 the binding depends on the presence of a particular allotype. Individuals with an allotype characterized by His at position 435 (virtually all Mongoloids) bind protein A, whereas individuals with Arg at this position (most Caucasoids) do not.

IgA antibodies function at body surfaces such as those of the digestive, respiratory and reproductive tracts. They are also the first antibodies the fetus and later the newborn

Table 8.6 Properties of human serum immunoglobulins relevant for their function.

Property	IgM	IgD	IgG1	IgG2	IgG3	IgG4	IgA1	IgA2	IgE
Presence on membranes of mature B cells	+	+	–	–	–	–	–	–	–
Activation of classical complement pathway	+++	–	+	+/–	++	–	–	–	–
Transplacental crossing	–	–	+	+/–	+	+	–	–	–
Binding to macrophage Fc receptors	+	–	++	+/–	++	+	–	–	–
Presence in secretions	+	–	–	–	–	–	++	++	–
Induction of mast cell degranulation	–	–	–	–	–	–	–	–	+
Reactivity with staphylococcal protein A	–	–	+	+	–	+	–	–	–

Activity levels: +++ and ++, high; +, moderate; +/–, minimal; –, absent.

receive passively from the mother. To reach the surfaces, the fetus and the mother's milk, IgA molecules must pass through tissues, cells and membranes. They have adapted to this passage by restructuring their Fc regions and by acquiring the J chain and the secretory component. Once at the surface, IgA molecules glue pathogens together and thus prevent their entry into the body (see Chapter 18). They also facilitate phagocytosis by binding, via their Fc parts, to Fc receptors on phagocytes.

IgE antibodies bind to Fc receptors on mast cells and basophils. When an antigen comes along, it cross-links the antibodies, clusters the receptors and triggers the cells to release substances that can cause muscles to contract and thus expel the parasites lodged in them. Unfortunately, in some individuals cross-linking of the bound antibodies can also occur via certain environmental antigens, such as pollen; the triggered release of substances from mast cells and basophils can then damage body tissues and lead to an allergic reaction (see Chapter 23).

The function of *IgD antibodies* is not known. Although they are well represented on the cell surface at a certain stage of B-lymphocyte development, they are only present in minute quantities in the serum. Various suggestions have been made as regards their function, both on the cell surface and in the serum, but so far none have been supported unambiguously by experimental evidence.

The B-cell receptor

The membrane-bound version of immunoglobulins is referred to as the *B-cell receptor*. It differs from secreted immunoglobulins in two ways: the secretory part of the H chain is replaced by the membrane-anchoring part, consisting of a short connecting peptide, transmembrane region and short cytoplasmic tail; and the H_2L_2 tetramer is associated non-covalently with additional polypeptide chains that function in the transmission of the signal from the cell surface to the cell's interior. The cytoplasmic tail is apparently too short (it is less than 10 amino acid residues long) for signal transmission and so this function has been taken over by the associated chains. The number of associated molecules is uncertain, as not all of them have been identified as yet. Two of the accessory molecules are co-expressed with the H_2L_2 tetramers on the cell surface; all the others are loosely associated with the tetramer in the cytoplasm beneath the surface. The two accessory molecules (each in itself being a dimer; see below), together with the H_2L_2 tetramer, are therefore regarded as constituting the *minimal BCR* (Fig. 8.52). The two molecules have been designated Igα and Igβ and their encoding genes *IGA* and *IGB*, respectively. The H chain of the minimal BCR can be of different isotype depending on the differentiation stage of the B cell: immature B cells bear μ chains on their surface, mature B cells μ and δ chains, and activated B cells α, γ (γ1, γ2, γ3, γ4) or ε chains. The Igα and Igβ chains are required for the expression of all these H chains so that the BCR of any class (IgM, IgD, IgA, IgG, IgE) always has the minimal structure of eight chains (two H, two L, two Igα and two Igβ).

The function of the BCR is to receive a signal via its combining site and transmit it to the cell's interior. The cell's response then depends on the nature of the signal and also on the nature of the signals perceived by other receptors on the B-lymphocyte surface. The B cell can be activated or inactivated, induced to proliferate or arrested in its growth, induced or inhibited to secrete antibodies. It can also take up a protein, process it and present the ensuing peptides to T lymphocytes and thus induce or enhance T-cell responses. All these and other options are discussed in Chapter 17. In the bone marrow, signalling via the BCR steers the devel-

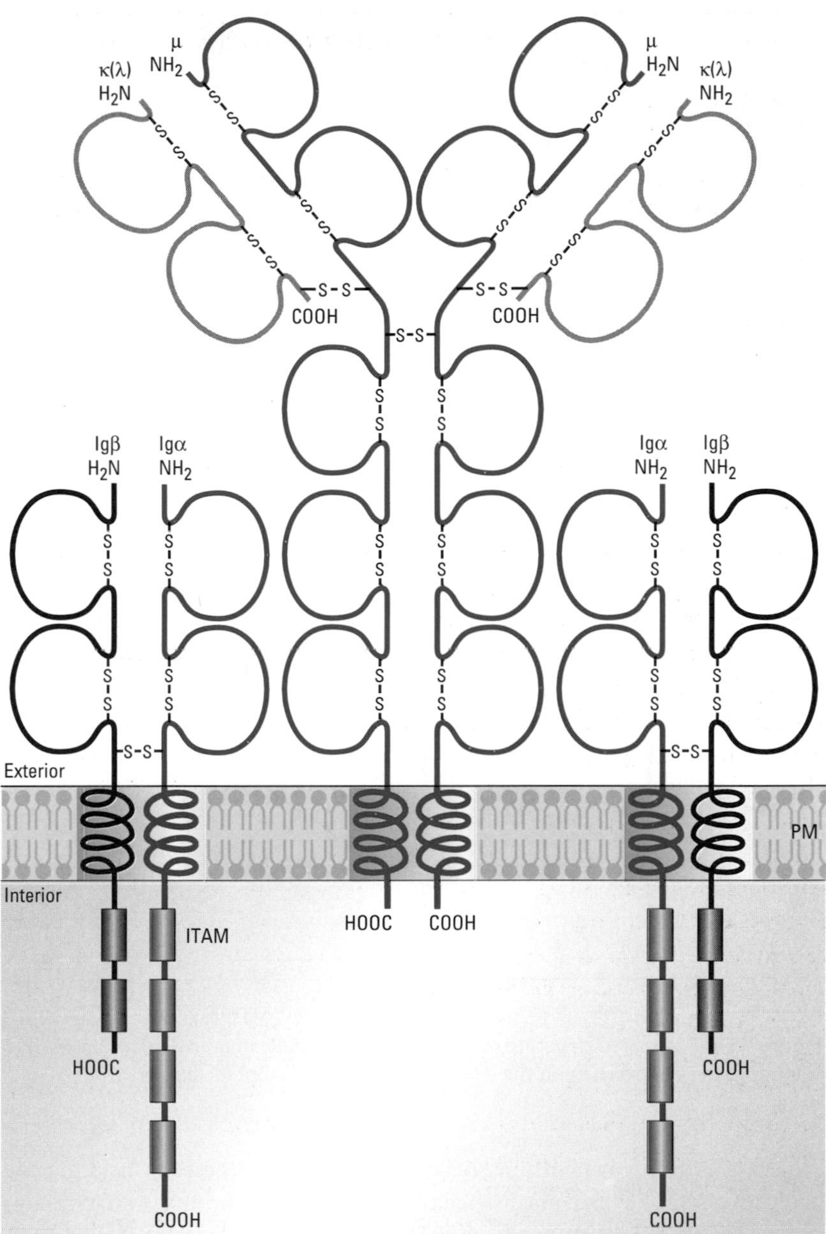

Figure 8.52 The B-cell receptor (IgM) with its accessory molecules (Igα and Igβ). The rectangles in the cytoplasmic tail indicate sequence motifs (ITAMs) recognized by protein tyrosine kinase. S—S, disulphide bond; ITAM, immune receptor tyrosine-based activation motif.

oping B cells through the differentiation stages or, when necessary, sets them on the course towards programmed cell death.

The expression of the BCR during B-cell differentiation is preceded by the cell-surface appearance of pre-BCR, in which the L chain is substituted by a surrogate chain. Description of the Igα and Igβ chains as well as of the surrogate chain follows; the BCR-associated intracellular molecules are dealt with in Chapter 17.

Accessory BCR molecules

There are certain parallels between the accessory molecules of the TCR (the CD3 complex) and BCR (the Igα:β complex): both types are involved in signal transduction; both are non-covalently associated with the receptor in the plasma membrane; both are necessary for the surface expression of the receptor (in the absence of Igα and Igβ molecules the immunoglobulin H chains are retained in the endoplasmic reticulum and are degraded); both are invariant; and both contain chains that are members of the immunoglobulin superfamily. These shared features of CD3 γ, δ and ε and Igα and Igβ chains may reflect an origin from a common ancestral protein.

The Igα and Igβ chains form heterodimers covalently linked by a single disulphide bond (see Fig. 8.52). Each BCR

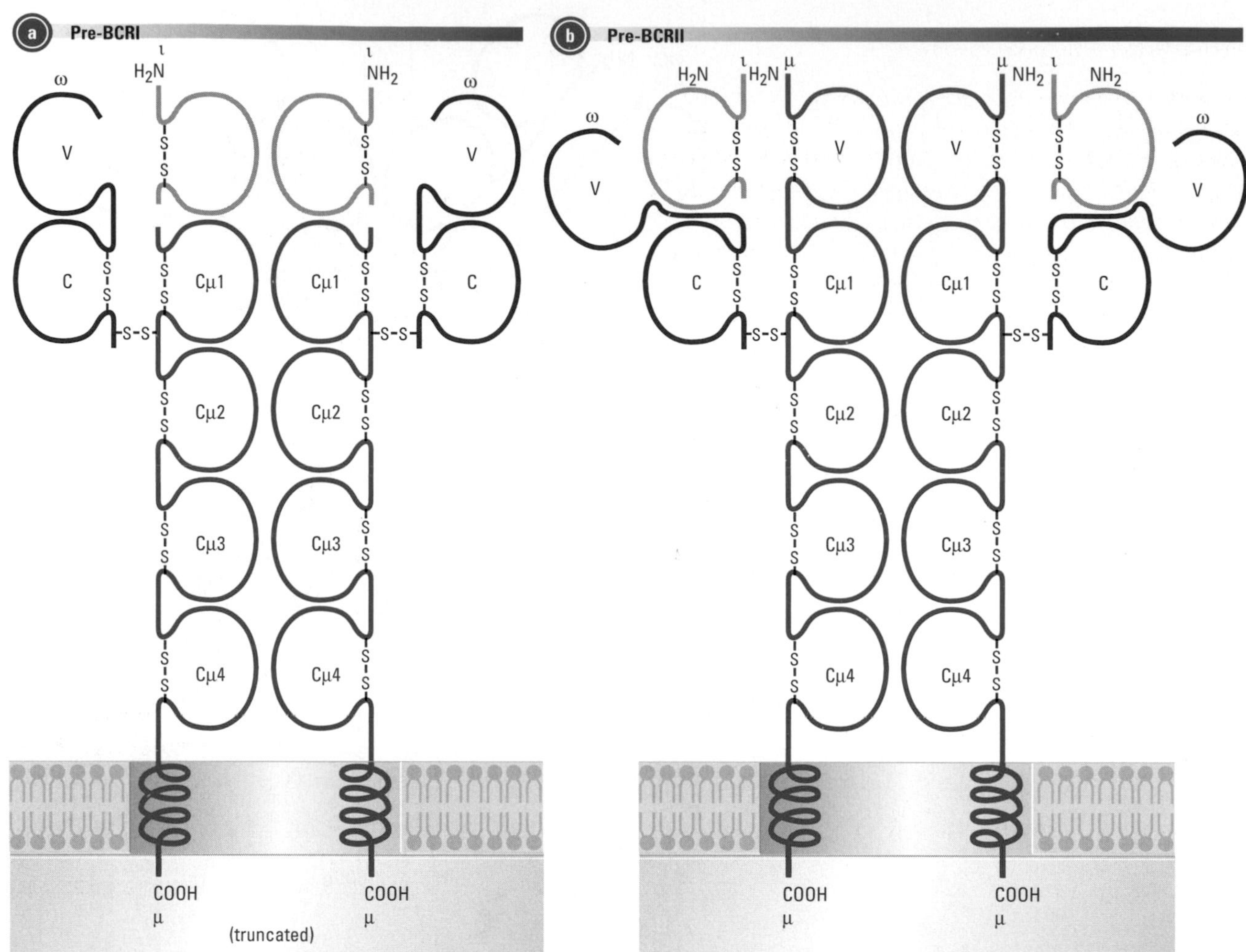

Figure 8.53 Postulated structure of B-cell receptors (BCR) in preB-I (a) and preB-II (b) cells. The ω (omega) chain is encoded in the *IGLL* (λ5) gene, the ι (iota) chain in the *VPREB* gene. S—S, disulphide bonds.

molecule is non-covalently associated with two of these heterodimers. They become associated with the receptor in the preB-cell stage at the time when the cells express the H chain-containing pre-BCR. The expression of Igβ chains then persists all the way to the terminally differentiated plasma cells; the expression of Igα chains is terminated before the onset of terminal differentiation.

Both the Igα and Igβ chains consist of two extracellular immunoglobulin-like domains (which are most similar to the V domain of κ chains), a connecting peptide (which contains the cysteine residue involved in the interchain disulphide bond formation), a transmembrane region and relatively long cytoplasmic tail. The tertiary structure of the immunoglobulin-like domain has not been determined but, based on comparisons of its primary structure with that of other immunoglobulin-like domains, it is believed to contain seven β-strands organized into two β-pleated sheets held together by a single disulphide bond. The cytoplasmic tail contains multiple immunoreceptor tyrosine-based activation motif (ITAM) sequences (see Chapter 10) with which protein tyrosine kinase molecules are believed to interact during signal transduction. The transmembrane and cytoplasmic regions of Igα and Igβ are also the most conserved parts of the molecules; the amino acid sequence similarity between the corresponding human and mouse chains is greater than 90%. The two chains are encoded in separate genes: the human *IGA* locus is on chromosome 19q13.2; the human *IGB* locus on chromosome 17q23. The Igβ chain may exist in several different forms, presumably produced by alternative splicing of the encoding mRNA. The M_r of the predominant β form is 37 000; the M_r of the α chain is 47 000 (both chains are glycosylated). The Igα and Igβ chains are also referred to as CD79a and CD79b, respectively.

Surrogate immunoglobulin chain

The surrogate component of the pre-BCR is composed of two chains: ι (iota) encoded in the *VPREB* gene; and ω (omega) encoded in the *IGLL* ('λ5') gene (Fig. 8.53). The ι *(V_{preB}) chain* consists of a single immunoglobulin-like domain believed to have the tertiary structure of a V_λ domain, except that the last β-strand (g) and part of the CDR3 loop are replaced by a sequence not related to any known immunoglobulin protein (Fig. 8.54b). The *ω (λ5) protein* consists of two immunoglobulin-like domains, one of which is postulated to contain four (d, e, f and g) of the seven β-strands of an immunoglobulin domain, and another which may have the tertiary structure resembling that of an L-chain constant domain (Fig. 8.54a). In the first of these two ω domains, the missing β-strands (the N-terminal part of the domain) are substituted by a sequence unrelated to any known immunoglobulin sequence. The ω chain is thought to be linked to the μ chain of the pre-BCR via a disulphide bond, whereas the ι chain is associated with the μ chain non-covalently (Fig. 8.54a).

The 'chimeric' nature of the ι and ω chains is a reflection of an abrupt change in sequence similarity in the encoding genes. In the mouse, in which the *VPREB1* and *IGLL* genes are close together (separated by only 10 kb of DNA), the former gene consists of two and the latter of three exons (Fig. 8.55). The nucleotide sequence of *VPREB1* exon 1, intron 1 and most of exon 2 is similar to that of an *IGVL* segment. The nucleotide sequence of *IGLL* exon 3, intron 2 and the 5′ part of exon 2 is related to that of *IGJL–IGCL* segments. But the sequence starting from the 3′ part of *VPREB1* exon 2 and extending to the 5′ part of *IGLL* exon 2 is dissimilar to any known sequence. It seems as if the *VPREB* and *IGLL* genes originated from a $V_LJ_LC_L$ gene by replacement of the 3′ part in the V_L and 5′ part in the J_L segment (and of the intervening region) with a sequence of unidentified origin. Separate duplications (and transpositions) of the newly created *VPREB* and *IGLL* genes then created the gene organizations now observed in mouse and humans (see Fig. 8.4).

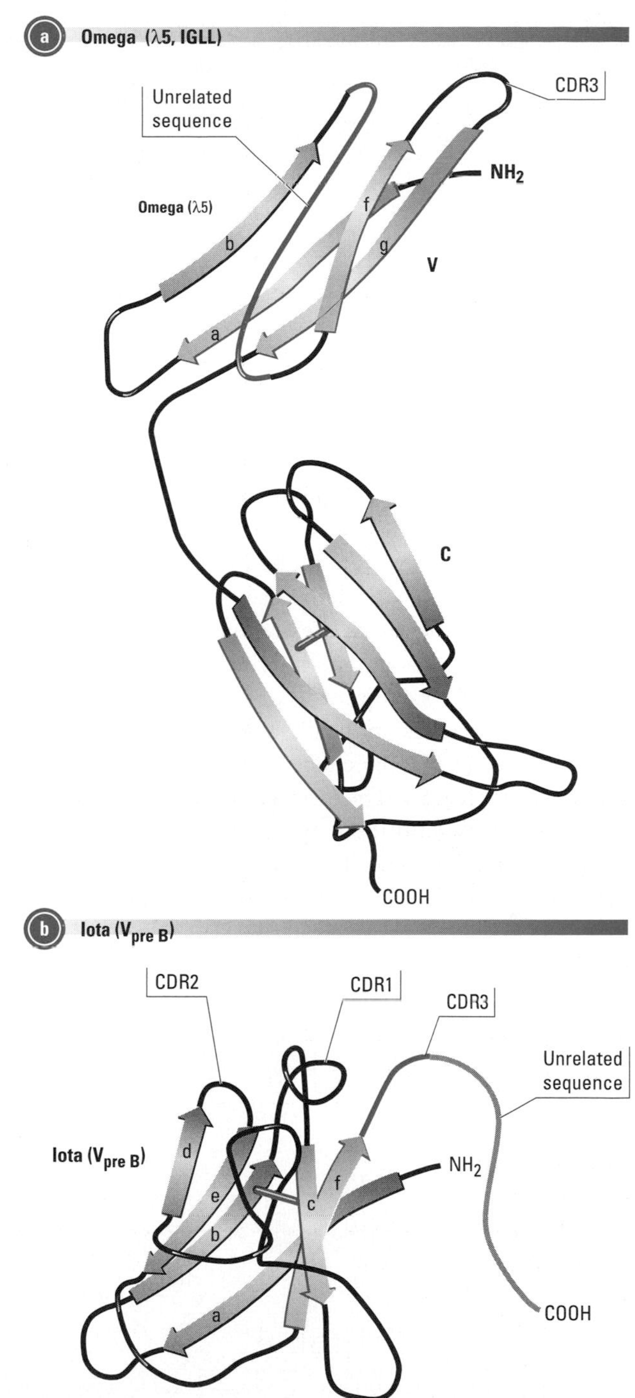

Figure 8.54 Predicted structure of the ω (omega) and ι (iota) chains encoded in the *IGLL* (λ5) and *VPREB* genes, respectively. CDR, complementarity-determining regions; red bars, disulphide bond connecting the two β-pleated sheets of the immunoglobulin fold. The light grey line represents a sequence with no similarity to any known sequence. (Modified from Melchers, F. *et al.* (1993) *Immunology Today*, **14**, 60.)

Evolution of immunoglobulins

Immunoglobulins have been found in all classes of jawed vertebrates; all efforts to find immunoglobulins in jawless vertebrates and invertebrates have failed. In the jawed vertebrates that have been studied, and these include cartilaginous fishes, bony fishes, dipnoans, crossopterygians, amphibians, reptiles, birds and mammals, immunoglobulins exist in both the membrane-bound and secreted forms and have the same tetrameric structure of two H and two L

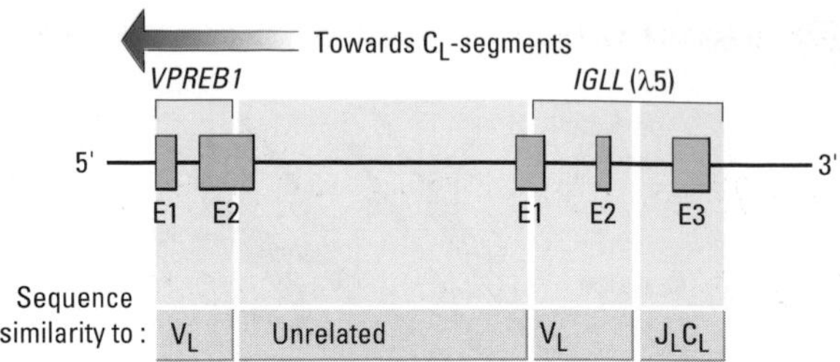

Figure 8.55 Sequence similarities of the mouse *VPREB1* and *IGLL* (λ*5*) genes. E, exon.

chains. The only known exceptions to the latter rule are the immunoglobulins of camelids (which, as stated earlier, lack L chains) and the immunoglobulin-like molecules of sharks. Designated tentatively as *new* or *nurse shark antigen receptor* (*NAR*), shark immunoglobulin-like molecules are dimers in which each chain consists of five domains, the N-terminal domain resembling the immunoglobulin V domain and the remaining four domains resembling those of the immunoglobulin constant region. There is an indication that *NAR* genes may somatically rearrange and that amino acid substitutions may be clustered in three regions corresponding to the CDRs. The NARs are thus far known only in a secreted form and there appears to be only one *NAR* gene in the shark genome. The phylogenetic position of the NAR is uncertain: it appears to lie between immunoglobulins and TCRs.

The organization of the bona fide immunoglobulins varies among the different classes of jawed vertebrates, being most extreme in cartilaginous fishes (sharks, skates and rays) (Fig. 8.56). *Cartilaginous fishes* (chondrichthyans) possess two types of H chain and one type of L chain. One of the H-chain isotypes is related to the mammalian μ chain, the other is unrelated to any other known isotype; the L chain is related to the mammalian κ chain. The two classes formed by these chain isotypes are referred to as IgM and IgX. The secreted IgM molecules occur either as pentamers or monomers of the basic four-chain subunits. The organization of the gene segments encoding chondrichthyan H and L chains differs from that of all other vertebrate classes. Instead of having a single H chain-encoding locus and one or two L chain-encoding loci, cartilaginous fishes have multiple loci on different chromosomes for both chains. Each locus, again in contrast to the *IG* loci of other vertebrates, consists of a single *V*, single *J* and single *C* segment; the H chain-encoding loci each have, in addition, two *D* segments located between *V* and *J* (Fig. 8.57). In some of the H and L chain-encoding loci, all the segments are separated by short (~ 400 bp) intervening sequences; in others, some of the intervening sequence has been removed and the segments joined, with the following combinations found: *(VD)–J–C*, *(VDJ)–C* and *(VD)–(DJ)–C* at the H-chain loci, and *(VJ)–C* at the L-chain loci (parentheses indicate joined segments, the dashes intervening sequences). The joining is apparently the result of *V(D)J*

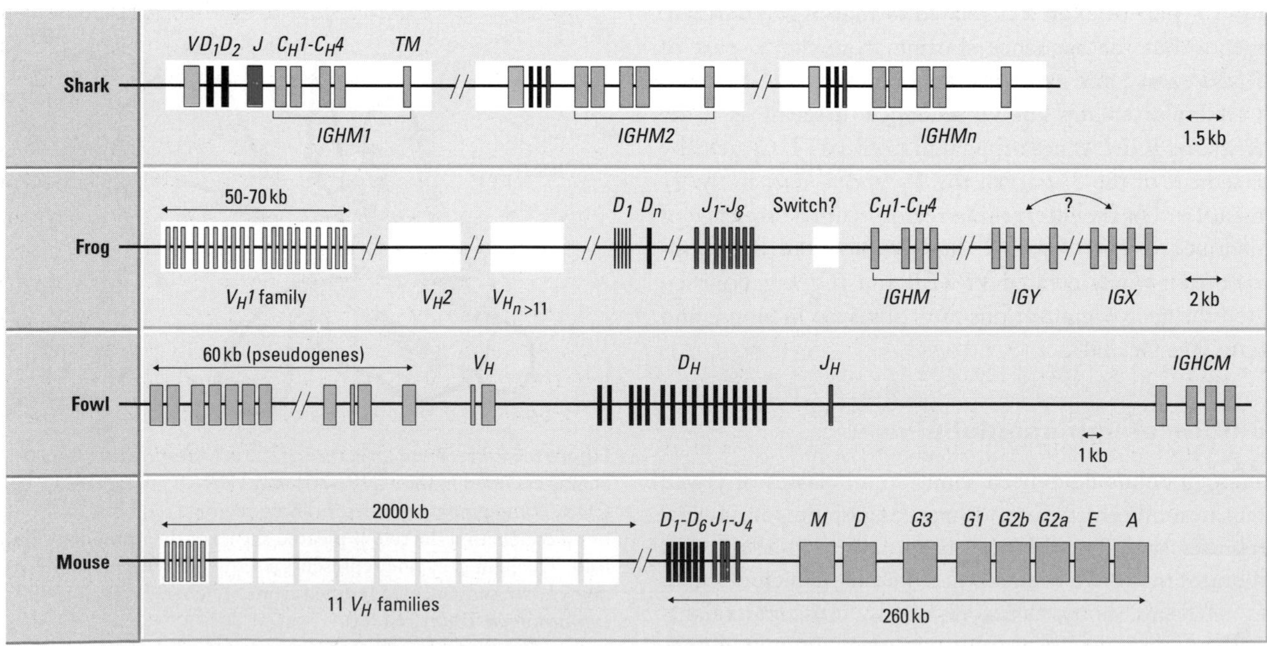

Figure 8.56 Organization of *IGH* loci in representatives of different vertebrate classes: cartilaginous fishes (shark), amphibians (frog), birds (domestic fowl) and mammals (mouse). (From Parham, P. (1995) *Current Biology*, 5, 696.)

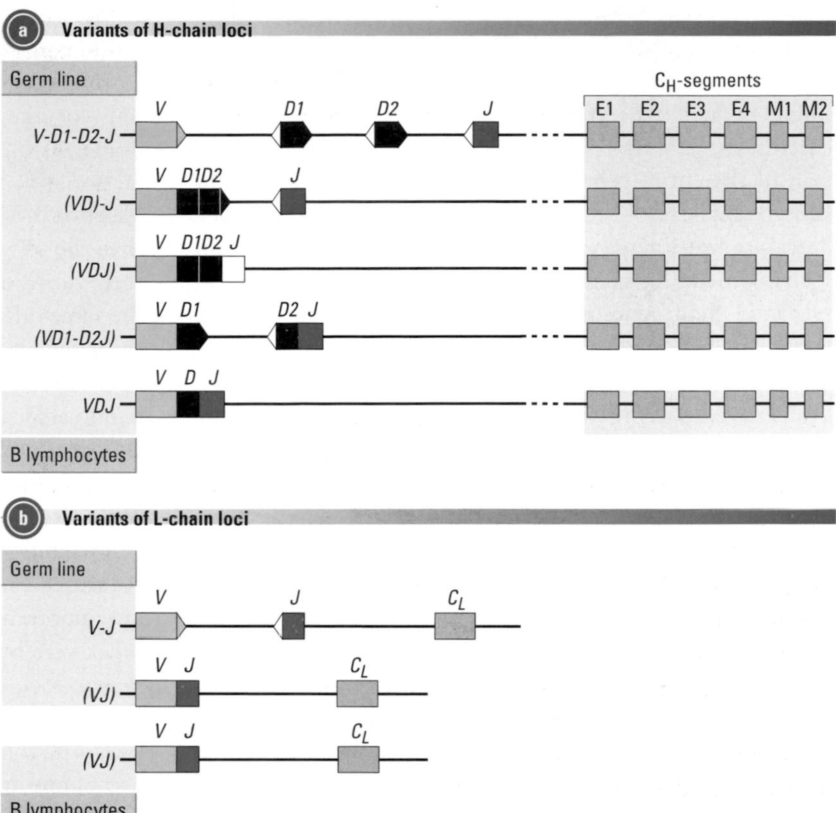

Figure 8.57 Organization of heavy (a) and light (b) chain-encoding loci in cartilaginous fishes. Only a few loci representing the different types of organization are shown; many such loci on different chromosomes exist in the fish genome. Rectangles represent exons or gene segments, triangles recombination signal sequences.

recombination, but it is not known when the rearrangement occurred (the joined segments are present in the germ line). The segments not joined in the germ line recombine somatically apparently by the same mechanism and using the same recombination signal sequences as their mammalian counterparts. Recombination occurs always within one locus (presumably one locus per B cell) and never between different loci. The arrangement of the recombination signal sequences is such that in one family of H chain-encoding loci either the *D1* or *D1* and *D2*, but not *D2* alone, participate in the rearrangement, and in the other family either *D2* or *D1* and *D2*, but not *D1* alone, participates. The two families also differ in the sequences of their segments with only about 60% nucleotide sequence similarity between them, which is approximately the same as that between chondrichthyan and mammalian gene segments. The families must therefore be quite ancient.

Three families of loci are known at the chondrichthyan L chain-encoding loci, one of which is related to the mammalian κ chain-encoding genes. The other two are equidistant from both the κ- and λ-encoding gene segments. The κ, λ and the three chondrichthyan L-chain gene families must have therefore diverged before the separation of cartilaginous and bony fishes more than 450 my ago.

The gene rearrangement in both the H and L chain-encoding segments is accompanied by both P- and N-type diversification and is followed by diversification through somatic hypermutations; however, this does not seem to be associated with antigen-driven selection (affinity maturation; see Chapter 17).

The *C* segment encoding the μ chain consists of four exons (E_M1–E_M4), followed by two exons (M1 and M2) necessary for the expression of the membrane-bound form; E_M4 contains the *Se* part necessary for the expression of the secreted form by alternative splicing. The *C* segment encoding the H chain of the IgX molecule consists of three exons with the *Se* part in the third exon (the *M* exons have as yet not been identified). IgM and IgX are expressed together in immature B cells; mature cells express either IgM or IgX, but no class switch signals have been identified.

All other jawed vertebrates (bony fishes, dipnoans, crossopterygians, amphibians, reptiles, birds and mammals) have a limited number of H and L chain-encoding loci, each locus consisting of multiple, tandemly arranged *V*, (*D*) and *J* segments, followed by *C* exons. But each vertebrate group has its own idiosyncracies in terms of *IG* locus organization and expression. Thus, some *bony fishes* (*teleosts*) have only one H chain-encoding locus, but others have two, both specifying a μ chain of the IgM class. (The secreted IgM is a tetramer rather than pentamer, as it is in other vertebrates.) The presence of the second locus might be a relic of an event postulated to have occurred early in the evolution of this vertebrate group: the duplication of the entire genome (*tetraploidization*), followed by subsequent loss of some of the duplicated chromosomes. Tetraploidization may also explain the presence of multiple L chain-encoding loci in bony fishes. A unique feature of the teleost H-chain genes is that exons encoding the membrane-anchoring region are spliced with the C_H3 rather than with the C_H4 exon.

The *crossopterygians*, represented by the coelacanth *Latimeria chalumnae*, have their H-chain genes arranged like the bony fishes, but many of the *V* segments are associated with their own *D* segments in a *V–D–V–D* . . . arrangement. Although this organization is somewhat reminiscent of that found in cartilaginous fishes, it probably arose independently either by duplication or *V–D* recombination. Crossopterygian L-chain genes have not been identified as yet.

The *dipnoans*, represented by the African lungfish, are still poorly characterized. It is known, however, that their H chains occur in at least two different isotypes, μ and ν (nu), and their immunoglobulins in two classes, IgM and IgY, respectively.

Amphibians, represented by the South African clawed toad *Xenopus laevis*, have three H-chain isotypes, μ, υ (upsilon) and χ (chi), and the corresponding classes IgM, IgY and IgX (note, however, that χ does not correspond linguistically to X). The last two of the three have no mammalian counterparts and the IgX of cartilaginous fishes and of amphibians are different. Amphibians also have two different L chains encoded in separate loci: σ (sigma), which associates preferentially with the μ chain; and ρ (rho), which combines with the υ chain. This kind of L-chain preference for certain H chains has thus far been documented only for amphibians.

Reptiles, like amphibians, have three H-chain isotypes, μ, υ and ν, and three corresponding classes IgM, IgY and IgN. The homology relationships of the ν chain are uncertain, although it is believed to be related to the lungfish ν chain; the υ chain corresponds to the amphibian υ chain. The L chains remain uncharacterized.

Birds, too, possess three different H chain isotypes, μ, α and υ, and the corresponding classes IgM, IgA and IgY; they have only one L-chain type (λ). The μ, α and λ chains are homologous to the corresponding mammalian chains; the υ chain is homologous to the amphibian and reptilian υ chain. The υ chain occurs in three forms: in addition to the standard membrane-bound and secreted forms, both of which contain one V_υ domain and four C-region extracellular domains ($C_\upsilon1$–$C_\upsilon4$), there is a third version that occurs in anserine birds, such as ducks and geese, which consists only of the V_υ domain combined with two C-region domains, $C_\upsilon1$ and $C_\upsilon2$. It is designated υ(ΔFc) because it lacks the Fc part of the υ chain (here, delta (Δ) stands for 'deletion'). The IgY molecule containing the υ(ΔFc) chain is thus the structural equivalent of mammalian $F(ab')_2$. The three forms of the υ chain arise by alternative splicing from the same mRNA (Fig. 8.58). To produce the υ(ΔFc) form, a short sequence (the so-called 'terminal exon') in the intron between the $C_\upsilon2$ and $C_\upsilon3$ exons is translated into two amino acid residues, glutamic acid and phenylalanine. The cleavage/polyadenylation signal in the 3′ untranslated region associated with the terminal exon ensures that none of the exons further downstream is translated.

Although both the H and L chain-encoding genes are organized similarly to their mammalian counterparts, there are important differences that set the birds apart from all other vertebrates. The bird H-chain locus, like the mammalian loci, contains multiple V_H segments, multiple (but nearly identical) *D* segments and a single *J* segment, followed by the *C* segments. However, all of the *V* segments except one are pseudogenes. The V_H region thus consists of a 60–80 kb cluster of multiple non-functional and single functional V_H segments (Fig. 8.59); the same is true for the V_L region. The pseudogenes lack recombination signal sequences, are truncated at their 5′ ends, lack the signal peptide sequence and vary in their transcriptional orientation. Some of the V_H segments appear to be fused to *D* segments and possibly also to parts of *J* segments. C_HDJ_H recombination always involves the one functional V_H segment, one of the *D* segments and the single J_H segment. This arrangement would normally mean that birds would be deprived of all the diversity provided in other vertebrates by the presence of multiple V_H and V_L segments. In fact, the birds have found a way to diversify their repertoire even when all but one of the *V* segments are non-functional. During or after *V(D)J* recombination (which occurs in the bursa of Fabricius and only during a short period of ontogenic development in contrast to mammals, in which the life-long process continues in the bone marrow), blocks of sequences are transferred from the pseudogenes to the functional *V* segment (Fig. 8.58). The transfer, referred to as *gene conversion*, takes place by means of an unknown mechanism and is not entirely random. Because the pseudogenes differ from one another in their sequences, diversification of the functional gene segment is accomplished by the transfer. A similar mechanism might also be operating in the rabbit, although on a more limited scale.

The distribution of immunoglobulin classes among verte-

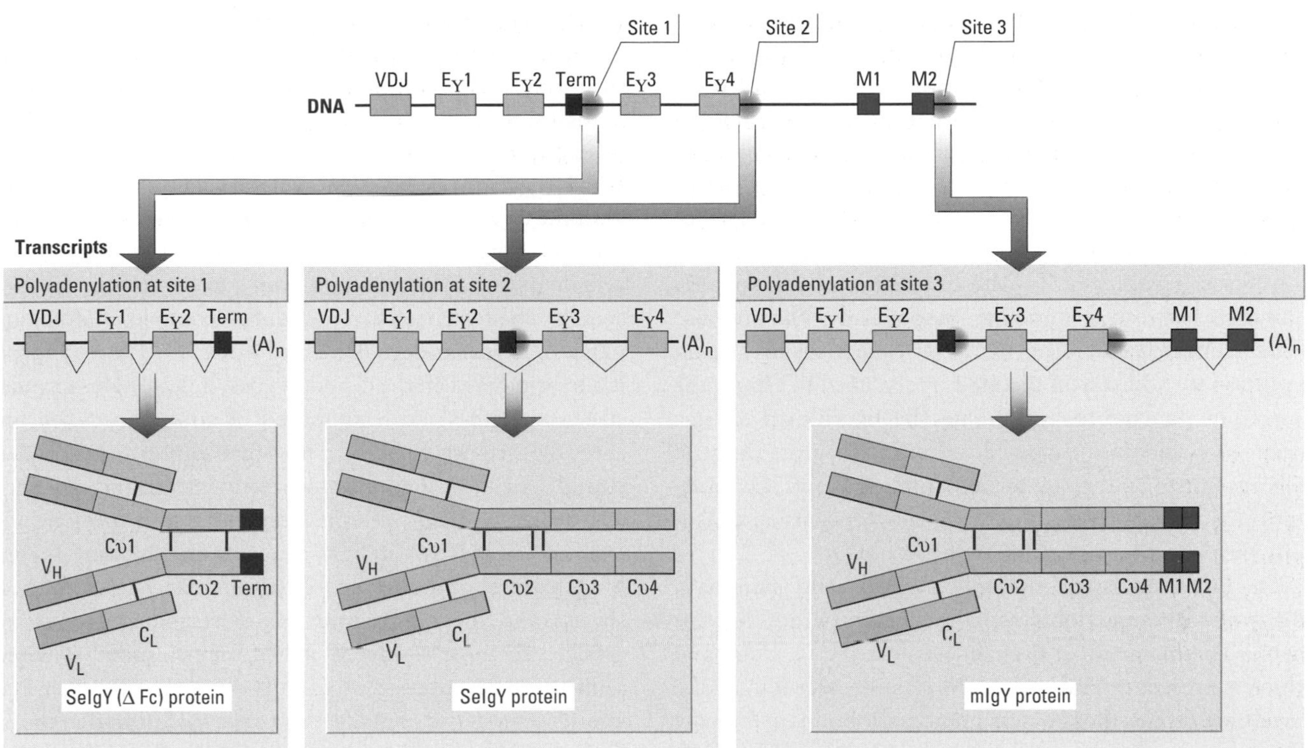

Figure 8.58 The rearranged immunoglobulin *Y* locus, its transcripts and different forms of heavy chains (υ) translated from them. The light chain is encoded in another locus which is not shown; 1–3 are cleavage/polyadenylation sites. The *term exon* encodes two C-terminal amino acid residues that occur only in the ΔFc form. Splicing is indicated by V-shaped lines. E, exon; M, exons encoding the membrane-anchoring part of the υ chain. Chain-connecting lines indicate interchain disulphide bonds.

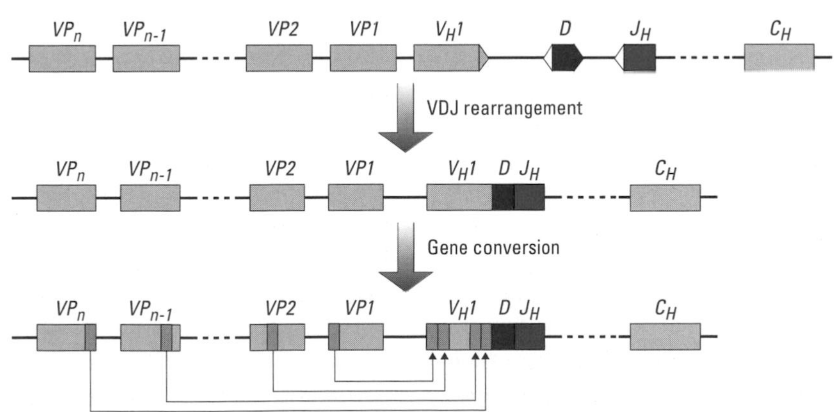

Figure 8.59 Organization of heavy-chain-encoding locus in birds. All *VPs* are non-functional pseudogenes; V_H1 is the only functional *V* segment with recombination signal sequences (triangles). *VDJ* recombination is followed by gene conversion that replaces parts of the V_H1 segment by sequences from the different *V* pseudogene segments. The light-chain-encoding locus of birds is organized in a similar fashion (but without *D* segments) and it, too, undergoes gene conversion after V_L1–*J* rearrangement.

brate taxa apparently reflects the evolution of the H chains. The IgG and IgE classes are restricted to mammals. They appear in evolution when the IgY class, which is present in dipnoans, amphibians, reptiles and birds, disappears. Sequence comparisons indicate that the $C_\gamma2$ and $C_\gamma3$ domains of IgG are most closely related to the $C_\upsilon3$ and $C_\upsilon4$ domains of IgY, respectively. However, IgY also resembles IgE, for example in the number of exons, exon lengths and the positions of disulphide bonds. Moreover, IgY resembles both IgG and IgE in the length and sequence of the exons that code for the membrane-anchoring regions. All these and several other features suggest that IgY is a forerunner of both IgG and IgE. IgG may have evolved from IgY by compaction of the $C_\upsilon 2$ exon into one that encodes the hinge region. Avian IgY appears to have a dual function: defence against infectious diseases and involvement in allergic reactions (see Chapter 23). These functions are split in mammals between IgG and IgE, respectively. The presence of the truncated IgY form (υΔFc) in some birds may be an evolutionary adjustment dictated by the need to reduce the danger of damage to host tissues by overblown allergic reactions (which are triggered when Fc receptors on mast cells recognize Fc regions of full-length IgY and IgE molecules). Mammals reduce this danger by decreasing drastically the concentration of IgE in the serum.

The IgA class is present only in birds and mammals. (Birds add immunoglobulins to their eggs before they lay them.) The mammalian α chain has lost the $C_\alpha 2$ domain, which is present in birds. The IgM class is present in all the vertebrate groups that possess immunoglobulins and μ may therefore represent one of the original H chains. How IgX, IgN and IgD fit into this scheme is uncertain. (IgD has thus far been found only in mammals.) The λ and κ L chains are at least as ancient as the μH chain.

Immunoglobulin superfamily

Immunoglobulins, TCRs and MHC molecules are all members of the *immunoglobulin superfamily*, a group of proteins related in structure and presumably origin as well. The structural feature uniting all these members into one superfamily is the *immunoglobulin fold*, a set of seven to nine β-strands arranged sandwich-like into two β-pleated sheets. Any molecule that has at least one domain tacked into the immunoglobulin fold qualifies for membership in the superfamily; most members have several such domains (Table 8.7). The fold occurs in at least six different variants among the various members and domains: c, v, s, h, i and a (Fig. 8.60). The epitome of the *c-type fold* (also referred to as *C1-fold*) is provided by the immunoglobulin constant domain with its seven β-strands arranged into one sheet (I) containing four antiparallel strands (*d–e–b–a*) and another (II) containing three antiparallel strands (*g–f–c*). The *v-type fold* is exemplified by the immunoglobulin variable domain, an eight- or nine-stranded structure in which one sheet is formed by four antiparallel β-strands (*d–e–b–a*) and the other by four or five (*g–f–c–c′–c″*) β-strands. The fold can occur in two subvariants, depending on the position of strand *a*, which can be part of either sheet I in antiparallel pairing with strand *b* so that each of the sheets has four strands, or sheet II in parallel pairing with strand *g* (the classical four plus five strand arrangement of sheets). In some domains, strand *c″* is reduced to a loop. The *s-type fold* (also referred to as *C2-fold*) is a seven-stranded structure in which the fourth strand has switched sheets in comparison with the c-type so that sheet I has three strands (*e–b–a*) and sheet II four strands (*g–f–c–c′*). The designation of the switched strand then changes from *d* to *c′* to reflect the sheet switch. The fold has been found, for example, in domain 2 of CD2, as well as domains 2 and 4 of CD4. The *h-type fold* is a hybrid between the c- and s-types. It is an eight-stranded structure with sheet I composed of strands *d–e–b–a* and sheet II of strands *g–f–c–c′*. This organization arises because strand *c′* of sheet II continues directly into strand *d* of sheet I. The *i-type fold* ('i' for intermediate) is present, for example, in the myosin light-chain kinase (telokin). It combines features of the v-type fold (the *a* strand shared by both sheets) and the c-type fold (no *c″* strand and *c′* strand reduced to three residues). It is a nine-stranded structure with sheet I composed of strands *d–e–b–a* and sheet II of strands *a′–g–f–c–c′*. Finally, the *a-type fold*, found in the V_α TCR domain, resembles the v-type fold but differs from it in that the *c″* strand is associated with the *d* strand of the adjacent sheet. The two sheets in these six variants are usually, but not always, held together by disulphide bonds. The position of the disulphide bonds, when they are present, can vary among the different domains.

The immunoglobulin superfamily now has more than 100 members but the number continues to grow. It has been estimated that some 40% of proteins on the surface of human leucocytes may contain immunoglobulin-like domains. But proteins with immunoglobulin-like domains are not restricted to leucocytes or to cell surfaces. Some are components of the intercellular matrix (e.g. tenascin, fibronectin) and others are located intracellularly (e.g. myosin light-chain kinase or telokin). Furthermore, they are not restricted to vertebrates but occur also in insects, molluscs, worms and other invertebrates, as well as in bacteria and even viruses. The origin of the immunoglobulin superfamily therefore apparently pre-dates the emergence of the MHC–TCR–immunoglobulin-based immune system. It is doubtful, however, whether it can be traced back all the way to prokaryotes. The possibility remains that the immunoglobulin-like organization arose independently several times by *convergent evolution* so that the superfamily now contains members with a similar tertiary domain structure but of different origin. It is difficult to distinguish which members derive from the same ancestor as the immunoglobulin molecules and which do not. Members sharing not only tertiary structure but also showing signifi-

Table 8.7 Members of the immunoglobulin family possessing V- and C-type domains. (Modified from Kuma, K. *et al.* (1991) *Current Opinion in Structural Biology*, 1, 384.)

Protein (species)	Number of domains	Protein (species)	Number of domains	Protein (species)	Number of domains
Proteins involved in the		CD32 (FcγRII) (H)	2	*Carcinoembryonic*	
immune system		CD33 (H)	2	*antigen (CEA)-related*	
Igκ (H)	2	CD47 (IAP) (H)	1	*proteins*	
FcεRI (H)	2	CD48 (H)	2	CEA (H)	7
Poly-IgR (Rb)	5	CD50 (ICAM-3) (H)	5	NCA (H)	3
V_{preB} (H)	1	CD54 (ICAM-1) (H)	5	CD66 (H)	4
TCRα (H)	2	CD56 (H)	5	PSβG (H)	5
TCRβ (H)	2	CD58 (LFA-3) (H)	2	Ecto-ATPase (R)	3
TCRγ (H)	2	CD64 (FcγRI) (H)	3	T1 (M)	2
TCRδ (H)	2	CD79a (mb-1, Igα) (H)	1		
MHC class I (H)	1	CD79b (B29, Igβ) (H)	1	*Protein tyrosine*	
MHC class II α (H)	1	CD80 (B7, BB1) (H)	2	*kinases*	
MHC class II β (H)	1	CD83 (H)	1	CSF1R (*c-fms*) (M)	5
β_2-microglobulin (H)	1	CD86 (B7.2) (H)	2	PDGFR-A (H)	5
2B4 (M)	2	CD89 (FcαR) (H)	2	*c-kit* (H)	5
DNAM-1 (H)	2	CD96 (H)	3	bFGFR (F)	3
G-CSFR (H)	1	CD100 (H)	1	FLT3 (H)	5
IL-1R (CD121a) (H)	3	CD101 (H)	7		
IL-6R (CD126) (H)	1	CD102 (ICAM-2) (H)	2	*Protein tyrosine*	
IL-6R (β chain; gp130;		CD106 (VCAM-1) (H)	7	*phosphatases*	
CD130)	1	CD147 (OX-47, M6) (H)	2	DLAR (D)	3
IL-11R (H)	1	CDw150 (SLAM)	2	DPTP (D)	2
LAG-3 (H)	4	CD152 (CTLA-4)	1		
Ly-9 (M)	4	CD166 (ALCAM)	5	*Intracellular proteins*	
MAdCAM-1 (H)	2			C-protein (F)	6
Sialoadhesin (M)	17	*Proteins involved in*		smMLCK (F)	3
CD1 (H)	1	*the neural system*		Twitchin (Ce)	26
CD2 (H)	2	NCAM (R)	5		
CD3γ (H)	1	Fasciclin II (G)	5	*Others*	
CD3δ (H)	1	Contactin (F)	6	BPG7 (M)	8
CD3ε (H)	1	F3 (M)	6	α1B (H)	5
CD4 (H)	4	TAG-1 (R)	6	Hemolin (SM)	4
CD7 (H)	1	L1 (M)	6	Poliovirus R (H)	3
CD8 (H)	1	Neuroglian (D)	6	gp42 (M)	2
CD16 (FcγRIII) (H)	2	MAG (R)	5	Cartilage link	
CD19 (H)	2	*amalgam* (D)	3	protein (F)	1
CD22 (H)	7	Thy (CD90) 1 (H)	1	Versican (H)	1
CD28 (H)	1	MRC OX-2 (R)	2		
CD31 (PECAM-1) (H)	6				

ALCAM, activated leucocyte cell adhesion molecule; BPG, biphosphoglycerate phosphatase; c-fms, cellular homologue of McDonough feline sarcoma virus oncogene; c-kit, cellular oncogene homologue of protein kinase (tyrosine); CD, cluster of differentiation; Ce, *Caenorhabditis elegans*; CEA, carcinoembryonic antigen; CSFR, colony stimulating factor receptor; CTLA, cytotoxic T lymphocyte antigen; D, *Drosophila*; DLAR, *Drosophila* leucocyte common antigen-related phosphatase; DNAM, DNAX accessory molecule; DPTP, *Drosophila* protein tyrosine phosphatase; F, domestic fowl (chicken); FcR, Fc receptor; FGFR, fibroblast growth factor receptor; G, grasshopper; gp, glycoprotein; H, human; IAP, integrin associated protein; ICAM, intercellular adhesion molecule; Ig, immunoglobulin; IL, interleukin; LAG, lymphocyte activation gene; M, mouse; MAdCAM, mucosal addressin cell adhesion molecule; MAG, myelin-associated glycoprotein; MLCK, myosin light chain kinase (skeletal muscle); MRC OX, Medical Research Council, Oxford; NCA, nonspecific crossreacting antigen (subgroup of CEA); NCAM, neural cell adhesion molecule; PDGFR, platelet-derived growth factor receptor; PECAM, platelet endothelial cell adhesion molecule; Poly-IgR, poly-immunoglobulin receptor; PSβG, P-selectin βG; R, rat; Rb, rabbit; SLAM, surface lymphocyte activation molecule; SM, silk moth; TAG, transiently expressed axonal surface glycoprotein (axonin); TCR, T-cell receptor; Thy, thymus; VCAM, vascular cell adhesion molecule.

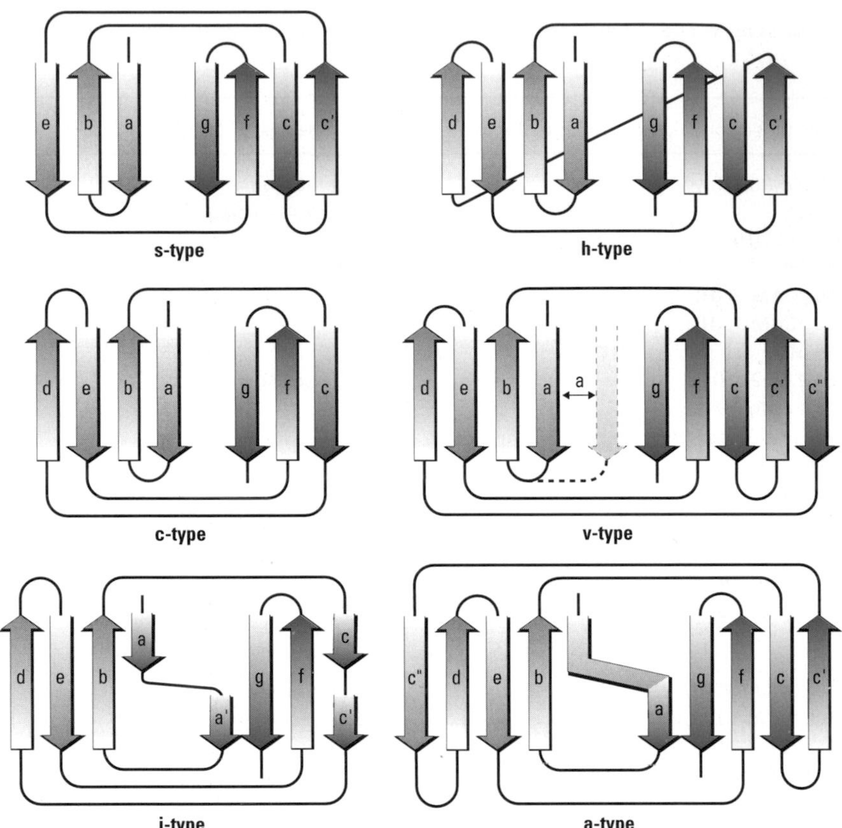

Figure 8.60 Six different topologies of the immunoglobulin fold. In the v-type, the *a*-strand can also move to the position indicated by the broken arrow and thus become part of the second β-pleated sheet. (Modified from Bork, P., Holm, L. & Sander, C. (1994) *Journal of Molecular Biology*, **242**, 309.)

cant sequence similarity are usually regarded as bona fide members, but this criterion is not fully reliable. It is known that during evolution sequence changes faster than tertiary structure and when sequence similarity drops below 25% it is no longer considered significant. On the other hand, it is conceivable that similarity not only in tertiary but also in primary structure can arise independently by convergent evolution.

Although members of the immunoglobulin superfamily cover a wide spectrum of diverse proteins involved in different functions, the immunoglobulin-like domains are all involved in binding. They bind short peptides, as in the case of the MHC, large proteins and carbohydrates, as in the case of immunoglobulins, or giant proteins such as the titin oligomers bound by actin and myosin. They bind antigens, hormones and various cell-surface molecules, including immunoglobulins themselves. In most instances, binding occurs via the β-pleated sheets but some domains have evolved special binding sites such as the CDR loops in TCR and immunoglobulin molecules. Apparently, any part of the surface can be adapted by the immunoglobulin-like domain for interaction with other molecules. Often different domains of the same protein have diverse binding functions. Ligand binding can serve different functions, but most of these are part of either the immune response or the intercellular communication system.

Fc receptors

Among the immunoglobulin-superfamily members involved in the immune response are the *Fc receptors* (FcR). These are cell-surface molecules that bind to specific sites in the Fc region of immunoglobulins. They are classified according to the immunoglobulin class (H-chain isotype) that they recognize (indicated by the Greek-letter designation of the isotype) and the strength of binding (affinity; indicated by Roman numerals). Some Fc receptors have also been identified by antibodies and given CD designations. Fc receptors have been described for all human immunoglobulin classes and subclasses. Of these, however, only receptors for the IgG, IgE and IgA classes are well characterized; receptors for the IgM and IgD classes have been defined functionally but not structurally. There are two high-affinity Fc receptors in humans (FcγRI and FcεRI) and several low-affinity receptors (FcγRII, FcγRIII, FcεRII, FcαR; see Table 8.8 & Fig. 8.61). Only high-affinity Fc receptors can bind 'monomeric' immunoglobulin molecules (i.e. molecules consisting of a single H_2L_2 tetramer). Both

Table 8.8 Designations and properties of human Fc receptors.

Receptor	CD designation	Gene	Chromosome	Alternative splicing forms	Chains	M_r ($\times 10^3$)	Amino acid residues (total)	Length of domains SP	EC	TM	CY	Affinity (K_d) (M^{-1})	Specificity	Expression	Function
FcγRIA	CD64	*FCG1A*	1q23			72	374	15	273	21	63	10^{-8}–10^{-9}	IgG3, IgG1	Mo, Ma, Ne	Cell activation, endocytosis
FcγRIIA	CD32	*FCG2A*	1q23	FcγIIa1		40	325	35	186	28	76	$<10^{-7}$	IgG1, IgG3	Ne, Mo, Pl, LC	Endocytosis, phagocytosis, cell activation
				FcγRIIa2		40	297	35	186	0	76	$<10^{-7}$	IgG1, IgG2, IgG3	—	
FcγRIIB		*FCG2B*	1q23	FcγIIb1		40	310	44	180	23	63	$<10^{-7}$	IgG1, IgG3	Ly, Ma	Negative reaction of BC
				FcγIIb2		40	291	44	180	23	49	$<10^{-7}$	IgG1, IgG3	Ly, Ma	
FcγRIIC		*FCG2C*	1q23			40	321	42	178	23	78	$<10^{-7}$		My	Endocytosis
FcγRIIIA	CD16a	*FCG3A*	1q23			50–70	254	17	191	21	25	$<10^{-7}$	IgG1, IgG3	NK, Mo, Ma	Cell activation, endocytosis
FcγRIIIB	CD16b	*FCG3B*	1q23			50–70	233	17	191	21	4	$<10^{-7}$	IgG1, IgG3	Ne	
FcεRI		*FCE1A*	1q23		α	45–65	260	28	181	21	31	$<10^{-10}$	IgE	Mc, Ba, LC	Mast cell activation
		FCE1B	11q13		β	32									
		FCE1G	1q23		γ	9									
FcεRIIa	CD23	*FCE2A*	19p13.3	FcεRIIa		43	321		277	21	23	$<10^{-7}$	IgE, CD21	BC	Endocytosis
		FCE2B		FcεRIIb		43	320		277	21	22	$<10^{-8}$	IgE, CD21	Mo, Ly, Pl, Eo, LC	Phagocytosis, cell activation
FcαR		*FCA*	10q13.4			60	287	21	206	19	41	5×10^{-7}	IgA	Mo, Ne	Phagocytosis, cell activation
PolyIgR		*PIGR*	1q31–41			82	733	18	629	19	103	5×10^{-7}	IgA, IgM	Ec	Transcytosis

Ba, basophils; BC, B cells; CY, cytoplasmic tail; Ec, epithelial cells; EC, extracellular domain; Eo, eosinophils; K_d, equilibrium dissociation constant; LC, Langerhans' cells; Ly, lymphocytes; Ma, macrophages; Mc, mast cells; Mo, monocytes; M_r, relative molecular mass; My, myeloid cells; Ne, neutrophils; NK, natural killer cells; Pl, platelets; SP, signal peptide; TM, transmembrane region. For information on MHC-like Fc receptor, see Chapter 6.

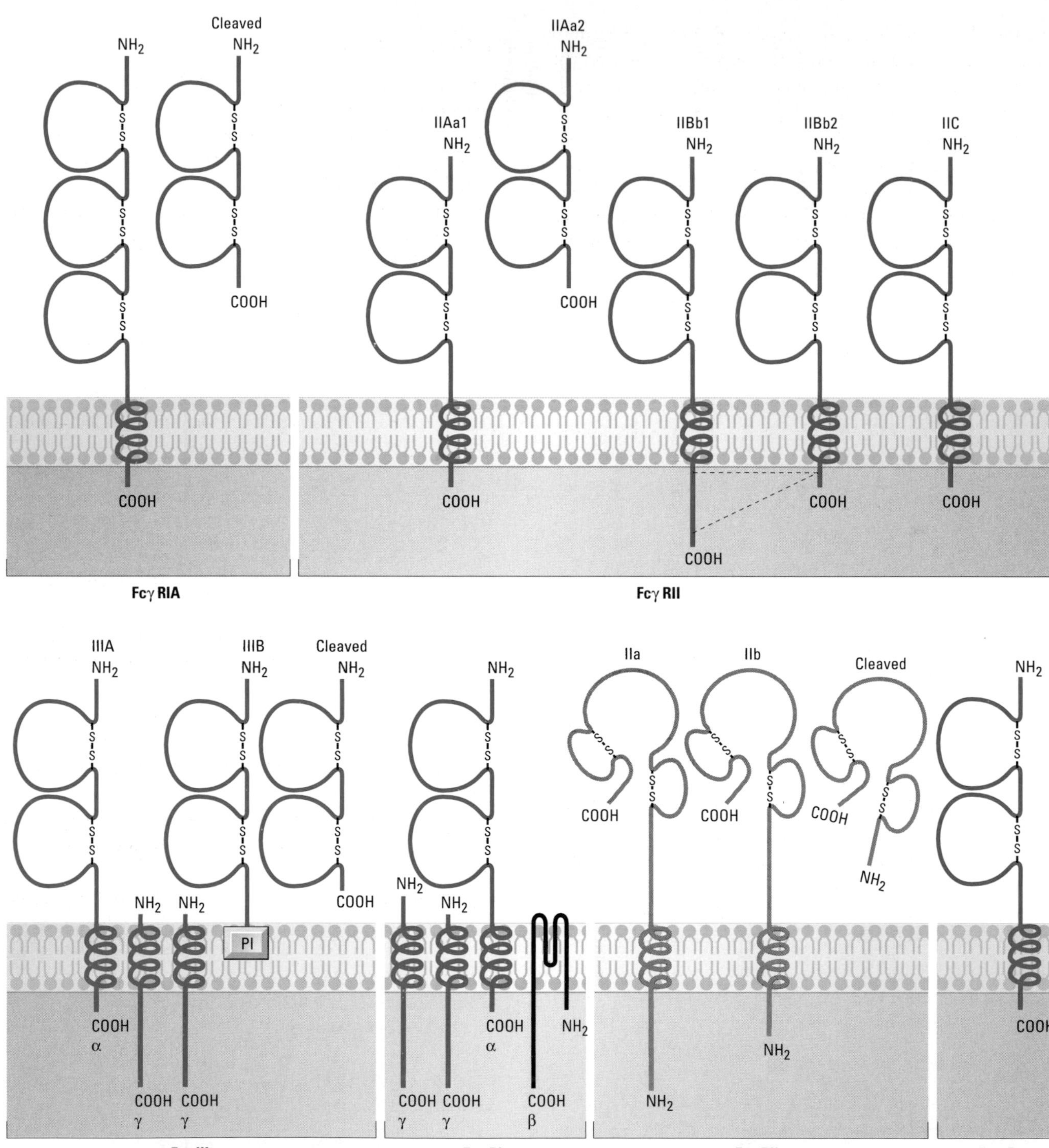

Figure 8.61 Human Fc receptors. PI, phosphatidylinositol anchor; S—S, disulphide bond.

classes of receptor trigger a response only when cross-linked by immunoglobulin molecules. This happens when either immunoglobulins are clustered into aggregates or many immunoglobulin molecules are bound via their combining site to a parasite or an effector cell. The signals generated by such multiple interactions can lead, depending on the cell type and the immunoglobulin class involved, to phagocytosis, killing of the immunoglobulin-coated pathogen, tumour cell or virus-infected cell, release of mediators of an inflammatory reaction (see Chapter 21) or a reaction that regulates the immune response. They may, under certain circumstances, also trigger an attack on the host's own tissues (autoimmunity; see Chapter 25) or allergic reactions (see Chapter 23). These responses will be described later in this book.

All Fc receptors are membrane-bound molecules, at least in their original form (Fig. 8.61). Most of them are single-chain structures consisting of an extracellular part, a transmembrane region and a cytoplasmic tail. The extracellular part is composed of one to three immunoglobulin-like domains. Alternative splicing of the same mRNA, however, produces in some cases (FcγRII) forms without the transmembrane region. Free FcR fragments are also produced by enzymatic cleavage of the membrane-bound forms (FcγRIII, FcεRII). Some of the chains devoid of the transmembrane regions are attached to the membrane via the phosphatidylinositol (PI) anchor (FcγRIII); see Fig. 12.35. Further diversity has been achieved by the duplication and divergence of some of the receptor genes (FcγRIIA, B and C; FcγRIIIA and B).

The FcγRIII and FcεRI molecules each consist of three types of chains, α, β and γ, of which only the α chain contains immunoglobulin-like domains and is involved in interactions with immunoglobulins. The β and γ chains, which are shared by these two receptors, are probably involved in signal transmission. All three chains are encoded in separate genes. Each of the FcγRIII and FcεRI molecules has one β and two disulphide-linked γ chains associated non-covalently with the α chain. The β chain, which crosses the membrane four times, is related to CD20, both being encoded by closely linked genes on human chromosome 19. (CD20 is a molecule expressed on B lymphocytes and possibly involved in B-cell activation.) The γ chains dimerize through their N-terminal cysteine residues located on the outside of the cell close to the plasma membrane. They resemble the ζ chain associated with the TCR. The γ- and ζ-encoding genes belong to the same family; their encoding genes are closely linked to each other on human chromosome 1. The third member of this family, the η chain, is also associated with the TCR (see Chapter 7). The cytoplasmic tails of these chains contain characteristic sequence motifs (ITAMs) involved in interaction with protein tyrosine kinases. The Fc receptor for poly-Ig molecules, which is expressed on epithelial cells of the mucosa, was described earlier in this chapter. The Fc receptor for IgG molecules, which is expressed on the epithelial cells of the small intestine in newborn mammals, was described in Chapter 6.

Further reading

Alt, F.W., Oltz, E.M., Young, F. *et al.* (1992) VDJ recombination. *Immunology Today*, **13**, 306–314.

Banchereau, J. & Rousset, F. (1992) Human B lymphocytes: phenotype, proliferation, and differentiation. *Advances in Immunology*, **52**, 125–262.

Bork, P., Holm, L. & Sander, C. (1994) The immunoglobulin fold. Stuctural classification, sequence patterns and common core. *Journal of Molecular Biology*, **242**, 309–320.

Burton, D.R. & Woof, J.M. (1992) Human antibody effector function. *Advances in Immunology*, **51**, 1–84.

Calabe, F. & Neuberger, M.S. (eds) (1987) *Molecular Genetics of Immunoglobulins*. Elsevier, Amsterdam.

Chen, J. & Alt, F.W. (1993) Gene rearrangement and B-cell development. *Current Opinion in Immunology*, **5**, 194–200.

Cook, G.P. & Tomlinson, I.M. (1995) The human immunoglobulin V_H repertoire. *Immunology Today*, **16**, 237–313.

Cook, G.P., Tomlinson, I.M., Walter, G. *et al.* (1994) A map of the human immunoglobulin V_H locus completed by analysis of the telomeric region of chromosome 14q. *Nature Genetics*, **7**, 162–168.

Harriman, W., Völk, H., Defranoux, N. & Wabl, M. (1993) Immunoglobulin class switch recombination. *Annual Review of Immunology*, **11**, 361–402.

Honjo, T., Alt, F.W. & Rabbits, T.H. (eds) (1989) *Immunoglobulin Genes*. Academic Press, New York.

Kindt, T.J. & Capra, J.D. (1984) *The Antibody Enigma*. Plenum Press, New York.

Kinet, J.-P. (1992) The γ–ζ dimers of Fc receptors as connectors to signal transduction. *Current Opinion in Immunology*, **4**, 43–48.

Koop, v.F., Richards, J.E., Durfee, T.D. *et al.* (1996) Analysis and comparison of the mouse and human immunoglobulin heavy chain J_H–C_μ–C_δ locus. *Molecular Phylogenetics and Evolution*, **5**, 33–49.

Lai, E., Wilson, R.K. & Hood, L.E. (1989) Physical maps of the mouse and human immunoglobulin-like loci. *Advances in Immunology*, **46**, 1–59.

Lewis, S.M. (1994) The mechanism of V(D)J joining: lessons from molecular, immunological, and comparative analyses. *Advances in Immunology*, **56**, 27–151.

Lieber, M. (1996) Immunoglobulin diversity: rearranging by cutting and repairing. *Current Biology*, **6**, 134–136.

Lin, W.-C. & Desiderio, S. (1995) V(D)J recombination and the cell cycle. *Immunology Today*, **16**, 279–289.

Maizels, N. (1995) Somatic hypermutation: how many mechanisms diversify V region sequences? *Cell*, **83**, 9–12.

Melchers, F., Rolink, A., Grawunder, U. *et al.* (1995) Positive and negative selection events during B lymphopoiesis. *Current Opinion in Immunology*, **7**, 214–227.

Melchers, F., Karasuyama, H., Haasner, D. *et al.* (1993) The surrogate light chain in B-cell development. *Immunology Today*, **14**, 60–68.

Neuberger, M.S. & Milstein, C. (1995) Somatic hypermutation. *Current Opinion in Immunology*, 7, 248–254.

Oettinger, M.A. (1992) Activation of V(D)J recombination by RAG1 and RAG2. *Trends in Genetics*, **8**, 413–415.

Pan, Y., Yuhasz, C. & Amzel, L.M. (1995) Anti-idiotypic antibodies: biological function and structural studies. *FASEB Journal*, **9**, 43–49.

Parham, P. (1995) A boost to immunity from nurse sharks. *Current Biology*, **5**, 696–699

Pascual, V. & Capra, J.D. (1991) Human immunoglobulin heavy-chain variable region genes: organization, polymorphism, and expression. *Advances in Immunology*, **49**, 1–74.

Reth, M. (1992) Antigen receptors on B lymphocytes. *Annual Review of Immunology*, **10**, 97–121.

Reth, M. (1995) The B-cell antigen receptor complex and co-receptors. *Immunology Today*, **16**, 310–313.

Rolink, A. & Melchers, F. (1993) B lymphopoiesis in the mouse. *Advances in Immunology*, **53**, 123–156.

Rolink, A., Andersson, J., Ghia, P. *et al.* (1995) B-cell development in mouse and man. *Immunologist*, **3/4**, 125–128.

Roth, D.B., Lindahl, T. & Gellert, M. (1995) How to make ends meet. *Current Biology*, **5**, 496–499.

Schatz, D.G., Oettinger, M.A. & Schlissel, M.S. (1992) V(D)J recombination: molecular biology and regulation. *Annual Review of Immunology*, **10**, 359–383.

Sakaguchi, N., Matuso, T., Nomura, J., Kuwahara, K., Igarashi, H. & Inui, S. (1993) Immunoglobulin receptor-associated molecules. *Advances in Immunology*, **54**, 337–392.

Staudt, L.M. & Lenardo, M.J. (1991) Immunoglobulin gene transcription. *Annual Review of Immunology*, **9**, 373–398.

Warr, G.W., Magor, K.E. & Higgins, D.A. (1995) IgY: clues to the origin of modern antibodies. *Immunology Today*, **16**, 392–398.

Weaver, D. T. (1995) V(D)J recombination and double-strand break repair. *Advances in Immunology*, **58**, 29–85.

Winter, D.B. & Gearhart, P.J. (1995) Another piece in the hypermutation puzzle. *Current Biology*, **5**, 1345–1346.

chapter 9

Cell adhesion molecules

Major histocompatibility complex (MHC) components, T-cell receptors (TCRs) and immunoglobulins are the three principal molecules that initiate and execute adaptive immune responses. In addition to these three, the immune system employs numerous other molecules, most of which participate in both adaptive and non-adaptive responses. They include molecules that mediate contact between cells, transmit messages between them and carry out attacks on non-self elements. These will be the subject of the next four chapters. Here the focus is on molecules that make cells adhere to each other. Adhesions of leucocytes to other cell types and adhesions between different types of leucocytes are involved in nearly all immune responses: leucocytes have to attach to stromal cells in the bone marrow and in the thymus to receive proper differentiation signals; later they must attach to endothelial cells as they leave the blood circulation and enter tissues; and in the tissues they adhere to macromolecules of the extracellular matrix. T cells have to contact antigen-presenting cells (APCs) to become activated (see Chapter 16); mature effector T_H1 and T_H2 (helper T) cells must bind to macrophages and to B cells, respectively, to stimulate them; effector cytotoxic T (T_C) cells and natural killer (NK) cells have to fasten firmly to their targets to kill them; and memory B lymphocytes must hitch to follicular dendritic cells to receive stimulatory signals triggering the secondary antibody response (see Chapter 17). All these adhesive intercellular interactions are mediated by various pairs of adhesion molecules. These act not just as a passive molecular 'glue' but in most cases also as elicitors of signals that change the behaviour of the interacting cells. The signals can be stimulatory and lead, for example, to cell proliferation, execution of an effector function or oriented migration; in other cases, the signals may be negative and suppress these activities or even induce cell death. In a sense, molecules such as the TCR and its co-receptors CD4 and CD8 or the MHC molecules discussed in previous chapters could also be considered as adhesion molecules because they contribute to specific contact between T cells and APCs.

Adhesion molecules in leucocyte–endothelial cell interactions

The main players in the immune response, both adaptive and non-adaptive, are the white blood cells or *leucocytes*. They are mobile cells that originate in the bone marrow, enter the bloodstream, are carried with the blood to different organs and selectively enter various tissues of the body. Some of the cells (specifically lymphocytes) can re-enter the bloodstream via lymphatics and repeat this circuit (blood → tissues → lymph → blood) many times over, i.e. they *recirculate*. Others (granulocytes and monocytes) stay in the tissues; once they have *emigrated* from the blood they cannot re-enter it. Even recirculating lymphocytes show a predilection to exit the bloodstream at specific sites, usually those at which they encountered antigen for the first time; they are said to *home* for these sites. The stream of leucocytes is directed and regulated by a set of *cell adhesion molecules* (CAMs) which act as traffic lights, instructing the moving cells where they should slow down, stop and enter the exit ramp. CAMs are not restricted to the cells of the immune system; they regulate many other processes, particularly embryogenesis and interaction between cells of the nervous system. Before turning to the CAMs that regulate leucocyte traffic, we must familiarize ourselves with the main routes frequented by leucocytes, lymphocytes in particular.

Lymphocyte circulation

Lymphocytes are like migratory birds: they settle down only temporarily before moving on further, but keep coming back to the same place. Let us now follow their migratory routes, starting from their birthplace (Fig. 9.1). Human B lymphocytes are born in the bone marrow, which they leave as immature cells, entering the blood circulation and maturing on the way. They take up short residence in the B-cell areas of the spleen, lymph nodes, Peyer's patches or other regions of the mucosa-associated lymphoid tissue (MALT). If they do not encounter antigen, they die; if they do, they become activated and either differentiate into plasma cells

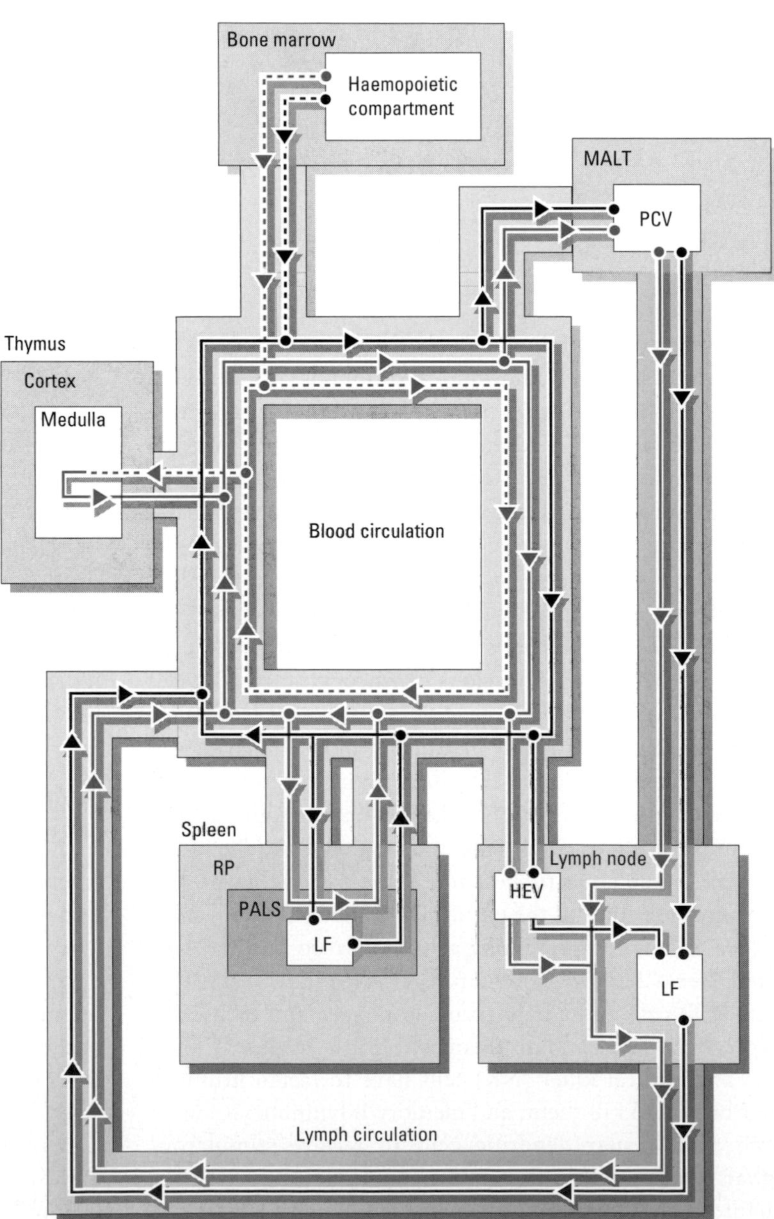

Figure 9.1 Lymphocyte circulation. Only the main pathways are shown. Broken lines indicate pathways of lymphocyte precursors, solid lines pathways of mature cells. Red lines indicate pathways of T lymphocytes, black lines those of B lymphocytes. HEV, high endothelial venule; LF, lymphoid follicle; MALT, mucosa-associated lymphoid tissue; PALS, periarteriolar lymphoid sheath; PCV, postcapillary venule; RP, red pulp.

or turn into memory cells. Depending on the site of residence of the original mature cells, the differentiating plasma cells move into the medulla of a lymph node, red pulp of the spleen or the submucosa and lamina propria of the gastrointestinal and respiratory tracts. At these sites, the plasma cells secrete antibodies for a while and then die. The memory cells accumulate in the central portion of the lymphoid follicle, form the germinal centre and thus transform the follicle into a secondary one. After their short residence in the germinal centre, the memory cells leave the lymph node (spleen or the MALT) through the mantle of the secondary follicle. Cells leaving the lymph node or the lymphoid tissues of the MALT are picked up by the lymph and carried by the efferent lymphatics into the thoracic duct (or the right lymphatic duct) and from there into the bloodstream. Memory B cells leaving the spleen join the blood directly. All memory B cells may circulate for a while and then leave the blood either in the lymph nodes, Peyer's patches or elsewhere in the MALT. They then head for the B-lymphocyte zones in these individual organs and tissues, passing through fields of APCs. If they encounter the right antigen, they are restimulated and the whole cycle is repeated. If they fail to make contact with the antigen, they rest for a while in that organ and then move on to make additional rounds in the lymph and bloodstream.

Human T lymphocytes are also conceived in the bone marrow, which they leave, however, very early, not as adolescents, like the B cells, but as 'embryos' (Fig. 9.1). The progenitors are selectively extracted by chemotaxis from the blood by the thymus, where they differentiate. Most of the progeny die but a small percentage becomes properly indoctrinated and educated and these cells leave the thymus as mature or almost mature T lymphocytes. They enter the thymic venules and join the blood circulation. As the blood brings them into lymphoid organs and tissues, they leave the high endothelial venules and head through the field of APCs, into the T-cell zones. If they fail to encounter antigen on the way, they die; cells stimulated by the proper antigen turn into either effector or memory cells. After a short pause, both cell types then re-enter the blood circulation: cells from the spleen directly, cells from other organs and tissues via the lymphatic system. Effector cells may respond to chemical signals and leave the blood at different sites in non-lymphoid or lymphoid tissues where an infection has taken hold, and then die in these tissues after carrying out their function. Memory cells leave the blood via the high endothelial venules, enter the lymphoid organs and tissues and recirculate on and on, until they again encounter antigen.

Both B and T lymphocytes leave the blood and cross over into the lymphoid tissues at special ferrying points, the *high endothelial venules* (HEV). These are very thin blood vessels inserted between capillaries and veins, i.e. they are *postcapillary venules*. Whereas other venules are lined with flat, thin endothelium, the endothelial cells of the HEV are high (hence the name), large and columnar (see Fig. 3.15). HEV occur constitutively in the lymph node, Peyer's patches and probably in other tissues of the MALT; they fail to develop, however, if the lymphoid organs are deprived of lymphocytes and appear only after lymphocytes begin to circulate through the organs. The rate of lymphocyte emigration through the 'flat' endothelium of blood vessels is very low except in those tissues that become inflamed (see Chapter 21). Mature circulating lymphocytes possess special *homing receptors* for molecules expressed by the endothelial cells of the different types of HEV and for endothelia of blood vessels in inflamed tissues. As the lymphocytes pass through the HEV, they collide randomly with its walls and their homing receptors grasp corresponding ligands of the lining endothelial cells. If a few receptors on each cell manage to grasp the ligands, the cell comes to a halt and begins immediately to burrow into the wall and to cross it. Originally, it was thought that lymphocytes crossed directly through the endothelial cells (*transcellular crossing*) but later, evidence was obtained for lymphocyte passage between the cells (*intercellular crossing*). However, transcellular crossing may occur in some instances. After passing though the endothelial cell layer, the lymphocytes cross the basement membrane and enter the surrounding tissue.

Different lymphocytes have different homing receptors that allow them to home for a particular lymphoid organ or inflamed tissue. Thus, some B lymphocytes have receptors for ligands expressed by the HEV of Peyer's patches, whereas others have different receptors for ligands on the HEV of peripheral lymph nodes. The receptors are expressed on the microvilli of mature, migrating lymphocytes and not on immature cells. The binding between the receptor and its corresponding ligand leads to the apposition of the microvilli to shallow pits on the luminal surface of the HEV in a process requiring energy and calcium, and involving the lymphocyte cytoskeleton.

Emigration of granulocytes

Monocytes and granulocytes leave the bloodstream in response to stimuli from the surrounding tissue that are released when the tissue is damaged by infection, injury or both. An infected or injured vascularized tissue responds to the insult in a characteristic way referred to as *inflammation* (Latin *inflammare*, to set on fire). The cardinal signs of inflammation are redness, swelling, localized heat (hence the name), pain, fever and often impairment of function (see Chapter 21). Inflammation is a complex set of events accompanied by the release of many different soluble substances that diffuse away from the site of their production. Some of the substances induce the expression of CAMs on the endothelium. Others cause movement of cells in the direction of the molecules' increasing concentration (*chemotaxis*); they act as *chemoattractants*. Leucocytes are known to respond to a number of chemoattractants and to sense concentration differences of 1% across their diameter. The leucocyte-affecting chemoattractants can be divided broadly into two categories: the *classical chemoattractants*, which have been known for some time, and the more recently described *chemoattractive cytokines* or *chemokines* (Table 9.1). The latter are polypeptides, 70–80 amino acid residues long, with specificity for leucocyte subsets. They belong to two different families defined by sequence similarity in the region of cysteine (C) residues. The C-X-C or *α chemokines* (where 'X' stands for any amino acid residue) tend to attract neutrophils, whereas the C-C or *β chemokines* attract monocytes and, to a lesser degree, eosinophils and certain lymphocytes. Non-covalent interactions of chemoattractants with certain proteoglycan molecules of the blood vessel wall ensure that blood flow does not sweep them away.

The changes effected by the soluble substances influence leucocyte traffic in the local blood vessels. Granulocytes and monocytes, presumably guided by the chemoattractants, begin to move towards the periphery (margins) of the bloodstream (*margination*; Fig. 9.2), where they come in contact with endothelial cells of blood vessel walls. The interaction between the CAMs of the endothelial cells and their corresponding ligands on the leucocytes provides a kind of tether, like the rope fastened to a donkey to keep it within bounds. But it is a weak tether; the force of the bloodstream breaks it easily, only for it to form again downstream, where the leucocyte's ligands create new bonds with the CAMs of the endothelial cells. This on–off formation of bonds (*tethering*) causes the leucocyte to tumble end over end along the endothelium (*rolling*; see Fig. 9.2). The marginated, rolling leucocytes are now exposed to a relatively high concentration of chemoattractants, some of which induce the expression of a new set of CAMs. The interaction between the new CAMs of the leucocytes and the CAMs of the endothelial cells leads to a firm attachment (*adhesion*) of the leucocytes to the endothelium (see Fig. 9.2). The leucocytes then pass between the endothelial

Table 9.1 Leucocyte chemoattractants. (From Springer, T.A. (1994) *Cell*, 76, 301.)

Chemoattractant	Origin	Responding cells
Classical chemoattractants		
N-formyl peptides	Bacterial protein processing	Monocyte, neutrophil, eosinophil, basophil
C5a	Complement activation	Monocyte, neutrophil, eosinophil, basophil
Leukotriene B_4	Arachidonate metabolism	Monocyte, neutrophil
Platelet-activating factor	Phosphatidylcholine metabolism	Monocyte, neutrophil, eosinophil
C-X-C chemokines		
IL-8/NAP-1	T lymphocyte, monocyte, endothelial cell, fibroblast, keratinocyte, chondrocyte, mesothelial cell	Neutrophil, basophil
CTAP-III/β-thromboglobulin/NAP2	Successive N-terminal cleavage of platelet basic protein released from α granules	Neutrophil, basophil, fibroblast
gro/MGSA	Fibroblast, melanomas, endothelial cell, monocyte	Neutrophil, melanomas, fibroblast
ENA-78	Epithelium	Neutrophil
C-C chemokines		
MCP-1	T lymphocyte, monocyte, fibroblast, endothelial cell, smooth muscle	Monocyte, basophil
MIP-1α,β	Monocyte, T lymphocyte, basophil	Monocyte, neutrophil, T-lymphocyte subpopulation, basophil, eosinophil
RANTES	T lymphocyte, platelets	Moncyte, T-lymphocyte subpopulation, eosinophil
I-309	T lymphocyte, mast cell	Monocyte

C5a, complement component (fragment) 5a; CTAP, *c*onnective *t*issue *a*ctivating *p*eptide; ENA, *e*pithelial cell line-derived *n*eutrophil *a*ctivating (peptide); gro, *gro*wth regulatory; I, integrin (family protein); IL, interleukin; MCP, *m*onocyte *c*hemoattractant *p*rotein; MGSA, *m*elanoma *g*rowth *s*timulating *a*ctivity; MIP, *m*acrophage *i*nflammatory *p*rotein; NAP, *n*eutrophil *a*ctivating *p*eptide; RANTES, *r*egulated upon *a*ctivation, *n*ormal *T*-*e*xpressed and presumably *s*ecreted.

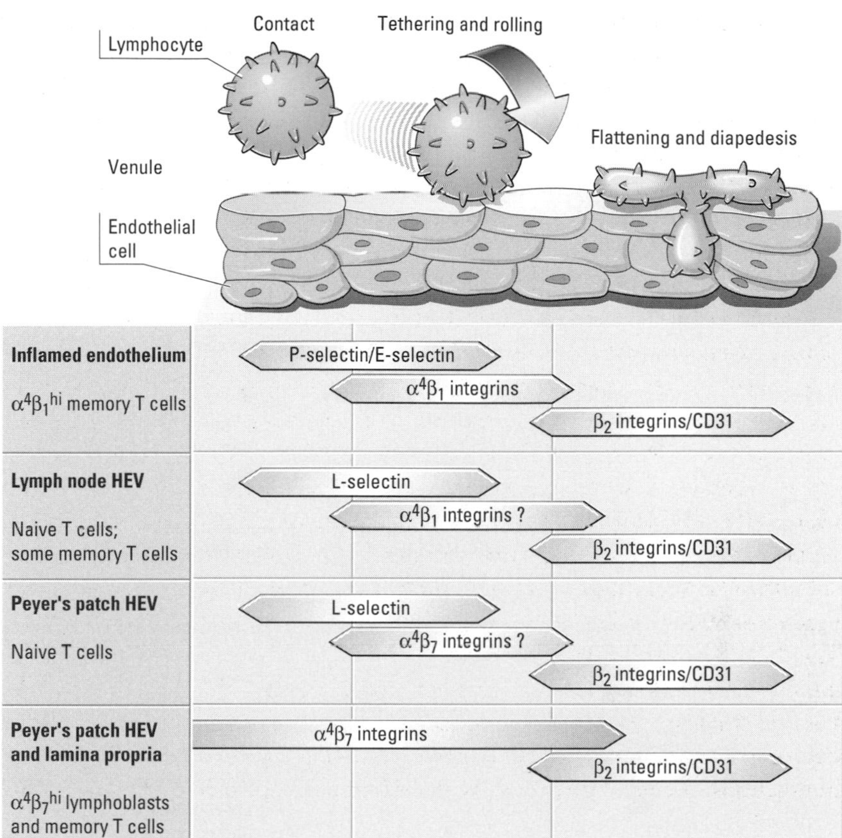

Figure 9.2 Lymphocyte tethering, rolling and diapedesis and the involvement of selectins/integrins in these processes in different vascular endothelia. (From Mackay, C. (1995) *Current Biology*, 5, 733.)

cells and enter the inflamed tissue (*extravasation* or 'leakage of blood from a vessel'; Latin *vas*, vessel). The interaction between leucocytes and endothelial cells may also involve *haptotaxis* (Greek *haptein*, to cling to; *taxis*, an ordering, arranging), in which cells migrate to the region of highest adhesion (highest density of ligands on the endothelium).

Families of adhesion molecules

Several structurally distinct families of CAMs are known to be involved in leucocyte interaction with endothelial cells: selectins, mucins (the ligands of selectins), integrins, members of the immunoglobulin superfamily, the glycoprotein CD44 and several other molecules (Table 9.2). The concept of a receptor and its ligand is not very useful as far as CAMs are concerned, because in most instances it is arbitrary to refer to one partner as a receptor and the other as its ligand. For this reason, the terms *receptor* and *counter-receptor* are sometimes used instead. Selectins and mucins (but also some integrins and their ligands) are involved in the initial phases of leucocyte emigration (tethering and rolling); the other CAMs in the final phases (adhesion and extravasation; Fig. 9.3). The description of the individual families follows and includes some members involved in adhesions other than those between leucocytes and endothelia.

Selectins

Selectins are a group of at least three glycoproteins, each with a distinct function and characteristic distribution (Table 9.2): *L-selectin*, expressed on all leucocytes except for subpopulations of memory lymphocytes; *P-selectin*, stored in the α-granules of platelets and the so-called Weibel–Palade bodies of endothelial cells; and *E-selectin*, induced on endothelial cells by cytokines such as interleukin-1, as well as by the bacterial lipopolysaccharides and tumour necrosis factor. L-selectin mediates binding of granulocytes, lymphocytes and monocytes to the endothelium at inflammatory sites; E-selectin is involved in the initial binding of neutrophils, monocytes and $CD4^+$ memory T lymphocytes to the vascular endothelium; and P-selectin mediates adhesion of neutrophils and monocytes to activated platelets and endothelial cells.

The three selectins have a similar structure, each consisting of a single, glycosylated, membrane-bound polypeptide chain (Fig. 9.4). The relative molecular mass (M_r) of each selectin ranges from 74 000 to 140 000. Each mature

Table 9.2 Leucocyte surface adhesion molecules and their ligands*.

Name	Other names	Cellular distribution	Structural characteristics	Ligands	Polypeptide size (amino acid residues)	M_r (×10³) (SDS-PAGE)
Selectins						
E-selectin	CD62E, ELAM-1	Activated endothelium	One C-type lectin, one EGF-like, six CRP domains	sLeˣ oligosaccharides on leucocyte PSGL-1 and ESL-1	589	115
L-selectin	CD62L, LAM-1	Leucocytes	One C-type lectin, one EGF-like, two CRP domains	sLeˣ oligosaccharides on endothelial mucins, GlyCAM-1, CD34 and MAdCAM-1	334	75
P-selectin	CD62P, PADGEM	Activated endothelium, platelets	One C-type lectin, one EGF-like, nine CRP domains	sLeˣ oligosaccharides on leucocyte PSGL-1	759	150
Mucins						
GlyCAM-1		High endothelium	Secreted mucin	L-selectin	132	50
CD34		Endothelium, haematopoietic precursors	Membrane-anchored mucin	L-selectin	354	105–120
PSGL-1		Leucocytes	Covalent dimer of a membrane-anchored mucin	P-selectin E-selectin	384	120 (monomer)
MAdCAM-1		Endothelia of mucosal lymphoid tissue venules	Three Ig domains, one mucin domain	L-selectin, VLA-4 (α4β1 integrin)	384	58–66
CD43	Leukosialin, sialophorin	Leucocytes	Membrane-anchored mucin; variably glycosylated in different cells	ICAM-1; probably also others	385	95–135
β1 integrins						
VLA-1	α1β1; CD49a/CD29	Activated T cells, monocytes	Integrin family; I-domain in α1 chain	Collagen, laminin	1153 (α1); 778 (β1)	210 + 130
VLA-2	α2β1; CD49b/CD29	B cells, monocytes, thrombocytes	Integrin family; I-domain in α2 chain	Collagen, laminin	1150 (α2); 778 (β1)	170 + 130
VLA-3	α3β1; CD49c/CD29	B cells	Integrin family	Fibrinogen, laminin, collagen	1119 (α3); 778 (β1)	(1125 + 30)† + 130
VLA-4	α4β1; CD49d/CD29	Leucocytes	Integrin family	Fibronectin, VCAM-1	999 (α4); 778 (β1)	150 + 130
VLA-5	α5β1; CD49e/CD29	Memory T cells, monocytes, platelets	Integrin family	Fibronectin	1008 (α5); 778 (β1)	(135 + 25)† + 130
VLA-6	α6β1; CD49f/CD29	Memory T cells, platelets	Integrin family	Laminin	1050 (α6); 778 (β1)	(120 + 30)† + 130
β2 integrins						
LFA-1	α1β2; CD11a/CD18	Leucocytes	Integrin family; I-domain in αL chain	ICAM-1, -2, -3	1145 (αL); 747 (β2)	180 + 95
Mac-1	αMβ2; CD11b/CD18; CR3	Myeloid cells, natural killer cells	Integrin family; I-domain in αM chain	ICAM-1, -2, -3, iC3b, fibrinogen, factor X, LPS, β-glucans, CD23	1137 (αM); 747 (β2)	170 + 95
p150,95	αXβ2; CD11c/CD18; CR4	Myeloid cells, dendritic cells	Integrin family; I-domain in αX chain	ICAM-1, C3b, fibrinogen	1124 (αX); 747 (β2)	150 + 95
αDβ2	αD/CD18	Myeloid cells	Integrin family; I-domain in αD chain	ICAM-3, ICAM-1	1145 (αD); 747 (β2)	170 + 95
β3 integrins						
gpIIb/IIIa	αIIβ3; CD41/CD61	Platelets	Integrin family	Fibrinogen, fibronectin, von Willebrand factor, thrombospondin	1008 (αIIb); 762 (β3)	(120 + 22)† + 110

(*Continued on p. 277.*)

Table 9.2 (*Continued.*)

Name	Other names	Cellular distribution	Structural characteristics	Ligands	Polypeptide size (amino acid residues)	M_r (×10³) (SDS-PAGE)
β3 integrins (*Continued.*)						
Vitronectin receptor	αVβ3; CD51/CD61	Endothelia, platelets, fibroblasts	Integrin family	Vitronectin, fibronectin, fibrinogen, thrombospondin, CD31	1018 (αV); 762 (β3)	(125 + 25)† + 110
β7 integrins						
LPAM-1	α4β7	Lymphocyte subpopulations	Integrin family	VCAM-1, MAdCAM-1	999 (α4); 770 (β7)	150 + 120
HML-1	αEβ7	Intestinal epithelial lymphocytes	Integrin family; I-domain in αE chain	E-cadherin	1160 (αE); 779 (β7)	(150 + 25)† + 120
Ig superfamily proteins						
CD2	LFA-2	T cells, natural killer cells	Two Ig domains	LFA-3, CD48, CD59	327	45–55
ICAM-1	CD54	Leucocytes, activated endothelium	Five Ig domains	LFA-1, Mac-1, p150,95, CD43	507	90
ICAM-2	CD102	Endothelium, monocytes, subset of lymphocytes	Two Ig domains	LFA-1, Mac-1	254	55–65
ICAM-3	CD50	Leucocytes	Five Ig domains	LFA-1	518	130
LW blood group protein	ICAM-4	Erythrocytes, leucocytes	Two Ig domains	LFA-1, Mac-1	241	60
LFA-3	CD58	Many cell types	Two Ig domains; a fraction GPI-anchored	CD2	222 (TM-form)	40–65
CD48	Blast-1	Leucocytes	Two Ig domains; GPI-anchored	CD2	217	45–50
CD31	PECAM-1	Endothelia, platelets, myeloid cells, lymphocyte subsets	Six Ig domains	Glycosaminoglycans, αVβ3 integrin, CD31 (homotypic)	711	130
VCAM-1	CD106	Endothelia	Six or seven Ig domains (variant forms)	VLA-4, LPAM-1	623 (6-domain form) 715 (7-domain form)	95 110
MAdCAM-1 (see Mucins)						
CD22	BLCAM	B cells	Five (α-form) or seven (β-form) Ig domains	Sialylated glycoproteins (e.g. CD45)	628 (α-form) 828 (β-form)	130 140
CD28		T cells	One Ig domain; covalent dimer	CD80, CD86	202	44 (monomer)
CTLA-4		Activated T cells	One Ig domain; covalent dimer	CD80, CD86	186	43 (monomer)
CD80	B7/BB1	Activated B and T cells, monocytes, dendritic cells	Two Ig domains	CD28, CTLA-4	262	60
CD86	B7.2	Dendritic cells, monocytes, activated B cells	Two Ig domains	CD28, CTLA-4	306	80
ALCAM		Activated leucocytes, thymic epithelium	Five Ig domains	CD6	556	100
Other adhesion molecules						
CD44	Pgp-1	Leucocytes, erythrocytes	Heavily glycosylated protein (mucin-like)	Hyaluronate	274 or 341 (alternative forms)	80–95
VAP-1		Endothelia		Unknown		180
L-VAP-2	CD73	Endothelia, activated lymphocytes	5′-Nucleotidase; GPI-anchored	Unknown	548	70
ESL-1	CFR	Myeloid cells		E-selectin	1148	150
CD5	T1	T cells, B1 cells	Three scavenger receptor domains	CD72	471	67
CD6	T12	T cells, B-cell subset	Three scavenger receptor domains	ALCAM	444	110

(*Continued on p. 278.*)

Table 9.2 (*Continued.*)

Name	Other names	Cellular distribution	Structural characteristics	Ligands	Polypeptide size (amino acid residues)	M_r (×10³) (SDS-PAGE)
CD72		B cells	C-type lectin (covalent dimer)	CD5	359	42 (monomer)
CD21	CR2	B cells, follicular dendritic cells	15 or 16 CRP domains	CD23, C3d, C3dg	1067	140
CD23	FcεRII; Blast 2	B-cell subset, activated macrophages, follicular dendritic cells	C-type lectin	CD21, IgE	321	45

* A number of other leucocyte adhesion molecules whose functions are less clearly defined, such as CD26, CD33, CD36, CD56, the CD66 group, CDw90, CD99, CD105 (see Appendix 3) are not included.
† The α-chains are post-translationally cleaved into two fragments held together by a disulphide bond.
ALCAM, activated leucocyte cell adhesion molecule; BLCAM, B lymphocyte cell adhesion molecule; CFR, cysteine-rich fibroblast growth factor receptor; CR, complement receptor; CRP, complement regulatory protein; CTLA, cytotoxic T lymphocyte antigen; EGF, epidermal growth factor; ELAM, endothelial cell adhesion molecule; ESL, E-selectin ligand; GlyCAM, glycosylation-dependent cell adhesion molecule; gp, glycoprotein, GPI, glycosyl phosphatidylinositol; HML, human mucosal lymphocyte; ICAM, intercellular adhesion molecule; Ig, immunoglobulin; LAM, leucocyte adhesion molecule; LFA, leucocyte function associated; LPAM, lymphocyte Peyer's patch adhesion molecule; LPS, lipopolysaccharide; L-VAP, leucocyte–vascular adhesion protein; Mac, macrophage (antigen); MAdCAM, mucosal addressin (adherence) cell adhesion molecule; M_r, relative molecular mass; PADGEM, platelet activation-dependent granule external membrane; PECAM, platelet–endothelial cell adhesion molecule; Pgp, phagocytic glycoprotein; PSGL, P-selectin glycoprotein; SDS-PAGE, sodium dodecyl sulphate polyacrylamide gel electrophoresis; sLe^x, sialyl Lewis x; TM, transmembrane; VAP, vascular adhesion protein; VCAM, vascular cell adhesion molecule; VLA, very late activation antigen.

polypeptide chain consists of a single N-terminal C-type *lectin-like domain* (a structure found otherwise in proteins that bind carbohydrates in a calcium-dependent manner); a single *EGF-like domain* (a structure first described in the epidermal cell growth factor); a varying number of *CCP repeats* (structures present in complement regulatory proteins; E-, L- and S-selectins contain six, two and nine CCP repeats, respectively); a single *transmembrane region*; and a short *cytoplasmic tail*. The number of CCP repeats largely determines the variation in the length of the polypeptide chain (610, 372 and 795 residues for E-, L- and P-selectins, respectively). It is also responsible for the variation in molecular mass; additional variation is imposed by the different numbers of carbohydrate moieties attached to the polypeptide chain. The lectin, EGF, CCP repeat, transmembrane and cytoplasmic domains are 17–19, 32–38, 58–62, 21–23 and 16–35 residues long, respectively. Each domain is encoded in a separate exon of genes that in humans reside in a single region of chromosome 1; the three genes probably arose by duplication from a single ancestral gene.

The ligands of the selectins are certain mucins, which are described below. The interaction between selectins and mucins involves the lectin domains of the former and the sialylated carbohydrate moiety of the latter. The EGF domain of the selectins may contribute to the binding by interacting with the protein part of the mucin. The CCP repeats are believed to provide the flexibility and extension of the selectin molecule necessary to span the space between the interacting cells. The interaction between the receptors and counter-receptors is very rapid (within milliseconds) and is characterized by high association and dissociation constants (hence the tethering and rolling of the marginated leucocyte that is characteristic of the initial phase of emigration). At least some selectins are not only adhesion but also signalling molecules.

Mucin-like carriers of selectin ligands

Mucoproteins or *mucins* are somewhat obsolete terms for glycoproteins whose solution is highly viscous; the preferred term is *proteoglycans*. They differ from other glycoproteins in that they contain numerous carbohydrate moieties and each moiety is a polysaccharide rather than oligosaccharide (see Chapter 11). Each proteoglycan molecule consists of a serine- and threonine-rich, membrane-bound polypeptide (*core protein*) from which several long, serine- or threonine-linked *carbohydrate side-chains* emanate (Fig. 9.5). Many of the proteoglycans are sulphated (i.e. sulphate groups are attached to their glycans). Sulphation is critical for the high affinity and selectivity of selectin-binding reactions.

L-selectin has been shown to bind to carbohydrates of three different mucin-like molecules (see Table 9.2): GlyCAM, CD34 and MAdCAM-1 (Fig. 9.5). ***Glycosylation-dependent cell adhesion molecule-1*** or *GlyCAM-1* is expressed exclusively on cells of the HEV in

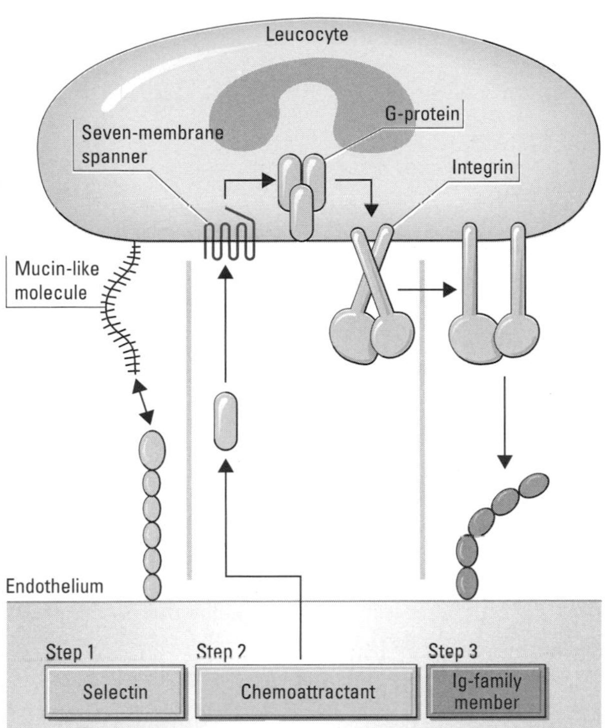

Figure 9.3 The three main pairs of molecules involved in the three steps of leucocyte adhesion to vascular endothelium. In the first step (tethering and rolling), selectins bind transiently to carbohydrates borne by mucin-like proteoglycan molecules. In the second step, chemoattractants released by cells in the tissues surrounding the blood vessel diffuse into the vessel and form a concentration gradient near the surface of the endothelial cells. Tethering and rolling leucocytes bind the chemoattractants via specialized receptors, which are molecules that cross the plasma membrane seven times. The binding generates a signal that is transmitted via specialized G-proteins to the integrins and effects the activation of the latter. In the third step, activated integrins bind to proteins of the immunoglobulin superfamily, establishing a firm link between the leucocytes and the endothelial cells. (Slightly modified from Springer, T.A. (1994) *Cell*, **76**, 301.)

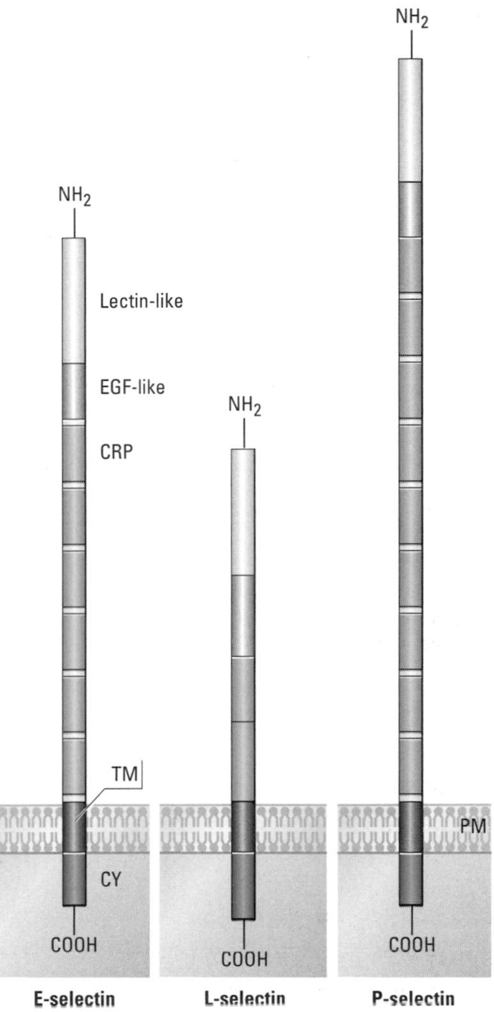

Figure 9.4 Domain organization of three selectin polypeptides. CRP, complement regulatory protein (domain); CY, cytoplasmic domain; EGF, epidermal growth factor (domain); TM, transmembrane region; PM, plasma membrane. Domains are distinguished by shading. (Based on Piggott, R. & Power, C. (1993) *The Adhesion Molecule Facts Book*. Academic Press, London.)

lymph nodes. It is a secreted, rather than membrane-anchored, molecule and its actual role in L-selectin-mediated adhesion is not clear; it may either support the adhesion, if it adheres to some structures on the endothelial cells, or inhibit adhesion by blocking the binding sites of L-selectin molecules. *CD34* is expressed on endothelial cells, including those of the HEV; it contains a globular domain that may have an immunoglobulin-like structure. The ***mucosal addressin cell adhesion molecule-1*** or *MAdCAM-1* is found on venules of lymphoid tissues in the mucosa; it is a hybrid between a mucin and an immunoglobulin-superfamily membrane protein (Fig. 9.5). The three molecules guide the entry of lymphocytes into lymphoid tissues (homing); in the case of MAdCAM-1 this occurs specifically into the lymphoid tissue of the mucosa (e.g. that of the gut).

P-selectin binds to the *P-selectin glycoprotein-1* or *PSGL-1*, which is a dimer of two disulphide-bonded subunits (Fig. 9.5), each with an M_r of 120 000. The carbohydrates that interact with the three selectins have been identified as *sialyl Lewis*^{x} and *sialyl Lewis*^{a}, which are fucosylated *N*-acetyl-lactosamines (see Fig. 7.38). They are borne by several different leucocyte glycolipids and glycoproteins and are variants of the Lewis blood group antigens originally described by antibodies found in the serum of a patient called Mrs Lewis.

A major leucocyte surface ligand of E-selectin is the *E-selectin ligand* or *ESL-1*, which is structurally distinct from mucins and is similar to the cysteine-rich fibroblast growth

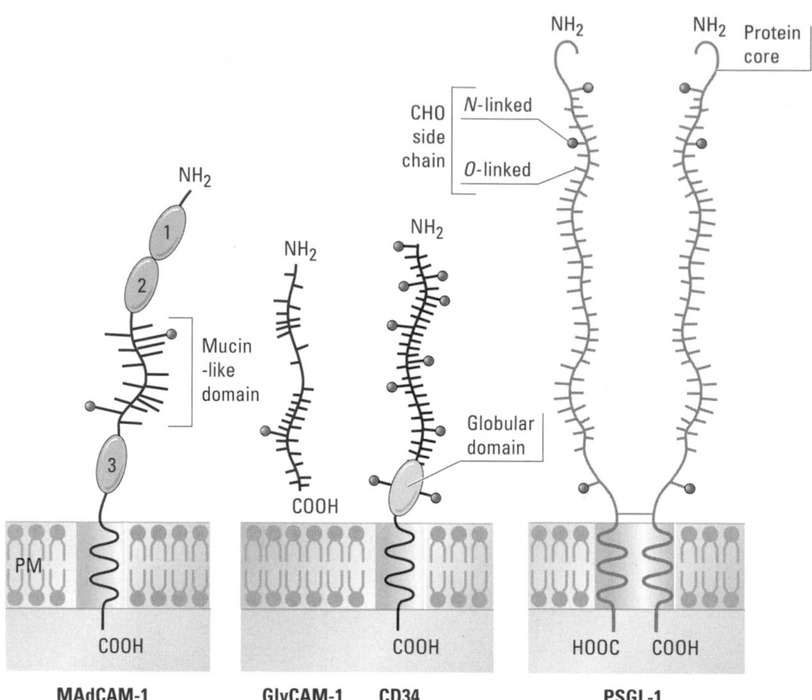

Figure 9.5 Examples of mucin-like molecules bearing carbohydrates bound by selectins of the vascular endothelium. CHO, carbohydrate; GlyCAM, glycosylation-dependent cell adhesion molecule (soluble form); MAdCAM-1, mucosal addressin cell adhesion molecule-1; PM, plasma membrane of leucocyte; PSGL-1, P-selectin glycoprotein-1. (Modified from Springer, T.A. (1994) *Cell*, 76, 301.)

factor receptor (see Table 9.2). The interaction with E-selectin involves the oligosaccharide chains of the ESL-1.

Integrins

Integrins are heterodimers of two non-covalently associated subunits, α and β (Fig. 9.6). Most of them participate in adhesive interactions between cells of the immune system as well as those involving other cell types. They are key elements in maintaining the integrity of the developing embryo and of some parts of the mature organism (hence the name). At least eight different β subunits and 15 α subunits have been identified (Fig. 9.6). Each subunit is a glycoprotein in which the polypeptide chain has an extracellular part, a transmembrane region and a cytoplasmic tail some 40–50 amino acid residues long. The extracellular part of each α subunit consists of seven repeating domains, each of which is 24–45 residues long; the domains are spaced 20–35 residues apart. Some α subunits contain an insert (the *I-domain*) of some 200 extra residues. The N-terminal domain contains three to four binding sites for divalent cations such as Mg^{2+}. The extracellular part of the β subunit contains four repeating subunits and altogether 56 conserved cysteine residues. Integrins are classified into families based on the type of their β subunits (β1–β8 integrins). In most of these families, a single β subunit can be paired with several different α subunits (Fig. 9.7). Some of the α subunits, too, are 'promiscuous' and can bind to more than one β subunit (Fig. 9.7). As a result, at least 22 different dimers are known of which 13 can be found on various types of leucocytes. Only β2 and β7 families are expressed exclusively on leucocytes.

Integrins bind two main types of ligands: proteins of the extracellular matrix (fibrinogen, fibronectin, laminin, collagen, thrombospondin, vitronectin, von Willebrand factor and others); and proteins of the immunoglobulin superfamily (ICAMs and VCAMs, which will be described shortly; Fig. 9.8). Most integrins bind more than one ligand and have different specificities depending on the type of cell that expresses them. Many recognize the RGD sequence (the tripeptide Arg-Gly-Asp) on the extracellular matrix proteins. Ligand binding requires the participation of divalent cations. The cytoplasmic tail of the α and β subunits appears to bind to the components of the cytoskeleton and thus participates in the transduction of signals. Phosphorylation of the cytoplasmic tail may regulate signal transduction.

Integrins function in platelet aggregation, inflammation (see Chapter 21), wound healing, tumour metastasis, cell migration during embryogenesis and immune response. Many integrins exist in two conformational states differing in the affinity of their interaction with their counter-receptors. The structural basis of the difference between these two states is not known but it seems likely that the high-affinity state may result from clustering of the integrin molecules. The conversion from the low-affinity to the

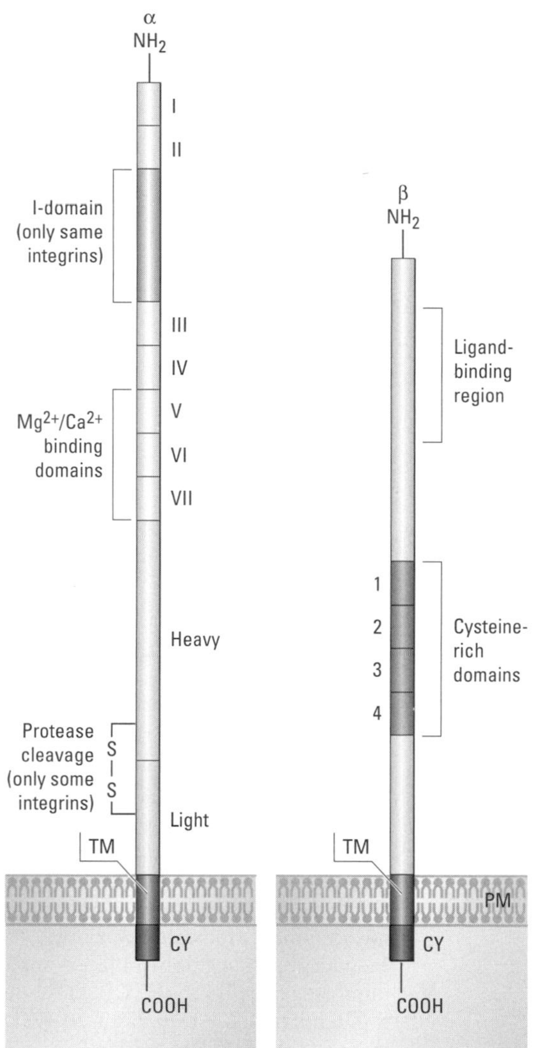

Figure 9.6 General structure of an integrin α:β heterodimer. Some integrin α chains contain a site at which they can be cleaved by proteases. When this happens, the single chain splits into heavy and light chains held together by a disulphide bond (S–S). I–VII are seven repeated domains; repeats II and III are separated by an inserted (I) region in some α chains. CY, cytoplasmic domain; PM, plasma membrane; TM, transmembrane region.

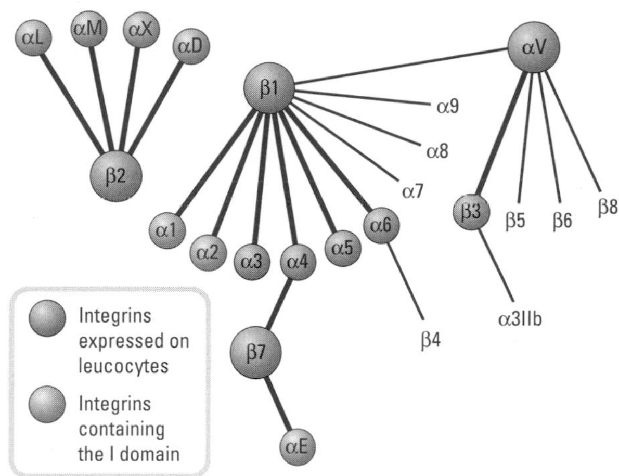

Figure 9.7 Dimer formation (connecting lines) between different integrin α and β chains. Thick lines denote α:β pairing on leucocytes. (From Stewart, M. *et al.* (1995) *Current Opinion in Cell Biology*, 7, 690.)

high-affinity state is induced by signals provided to the cell through various receptors. For example, one of the consequences of TCR ligation is the conversion of the major leucocyte integrin LFA-1 into the high-affinity state. Similarly, activation of neutrophils by IL-8 or other chemotactic substances also leads to the conversion of LFA-1 to the high-affinity state. Because the consequences of intracellular signalling reactions are manifested at the cell surface, this phenomenon is referred to as *inside-out signalling*. Since most integrins can bind more than one adhesion counter-receptor and vice versa, the integrin-based adhesive system shows remarkable plasticity and versatility. In addition to functioning as adhesion molecules, some integrins also have other functions based on their binding of different ligands. Thus, two β2 integrins (Mac-1 or CD11b/CD18 and p150,95 or CD11c/CD18) bind the complement fragment iC3b and therefore act as complement type 3 and 4 receptors (CR3 and CR4), respectively (see Chapter 12). As such, they are involved in phagocytosis of complement-opsonized particles (see Chapter 15). Moreover, Mac-1 binds certain carbohydrate structures and is identical to the β-glucan receptor of phagocytes, which is involved in the recognition of some microbial surface polysaccharides by these cells.

In addition to their adhesive function, integrins also contribute to signal transduction inside the cells. These signalling functions are poorly understood but probably involve association with intracellular enzymes, *protein kinases* (see Chapter 10) and intimate collaboration with other surface receptors, such as Fc receptors on phagocytic cells (see Chapter 15).

Integrins can be divided into several groups based on their β subunits. The properties of some of these molecules relevant for the immune system and especially for leucocyte–endothelial cell interactions are briefly described below and summarized in Table 9.2.

β1 Integrins are also called VLA molecules (*v*ery *l*ate *a*ctivation antigens in reference to their appearance up to 2 weeks after T-cell activation *in vitro*). At least nine members of this group are known, each being a non-covalently linked heterodimer of the β1 subunit (CD29; M_r 130 000) and one of the α1–α9 subunits (the α1–α6 subunits are also called CD49a–CD49f; see Table 9.2). Most of these molecules are expressed on cells that do not belong to

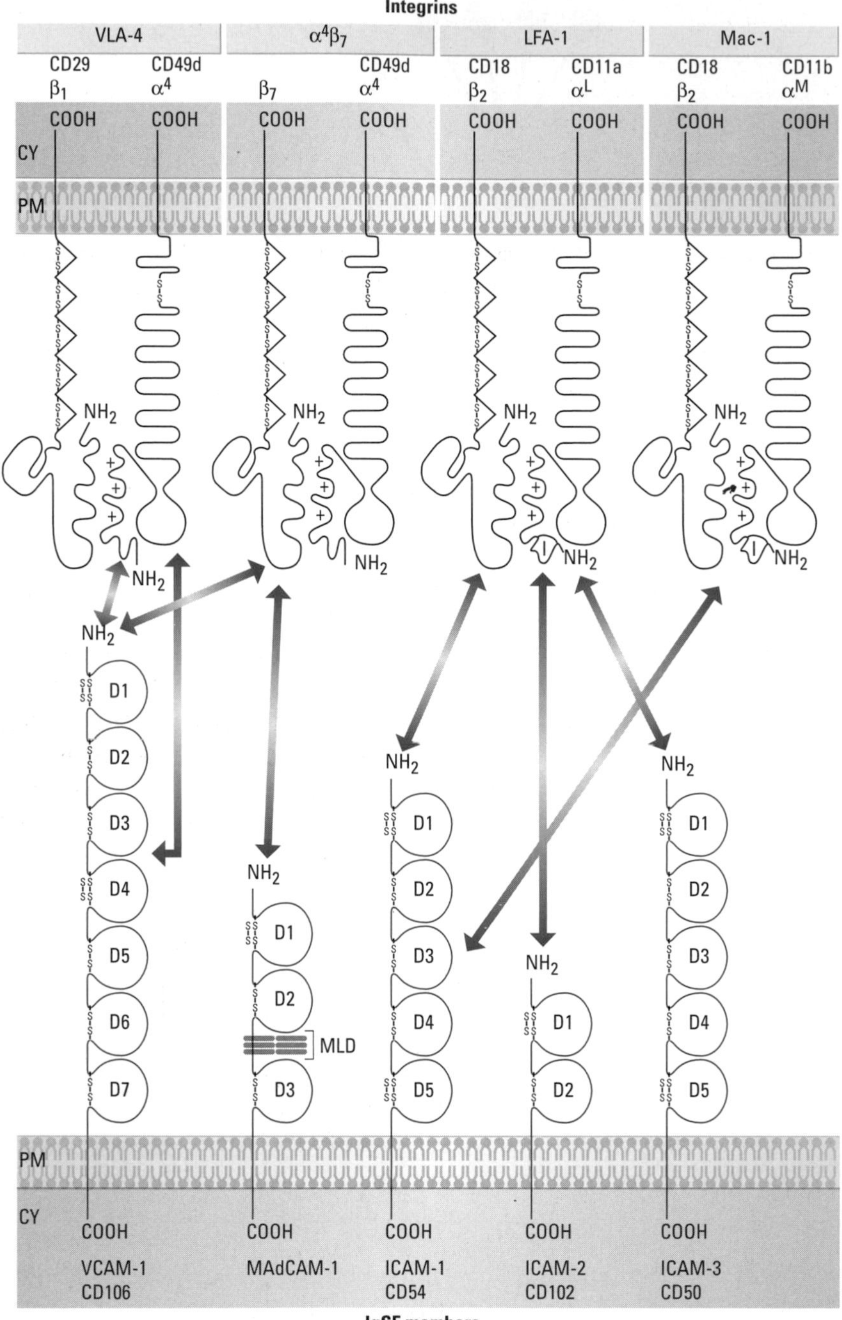

Figure 9.8 Immunologically important cell adhesion molecules of the immunoglobulin superfamily. The integrin counter-receptors of the individual immunoglobulin-superfamily (IgSF) molecules are shown at the top and interactions are indicated by arrows. Individual immunoglobulin-like domains are numbered from D1 to D7. CD, cluster of differentiation; CY, cytoplasmic domain; I, inserted region; ICAM, intercellular adhesion molecule; LFA, lymphocyte function associated; Mac-1, macrophage adhesion molecule; MAdCAM, mucosal addressin cell adhesion molecule; MLD, mucin-like domain; PM, plasma membrane; S–S, disulphide bond; VCAM, vascular cell adhesion molecule; VLA, very late antigen. Mg^{2+}/Ca^{2+}-binding domains are indicated by +. (From de Fougerolles, A. & Springer, T.A. (1995) *Chemistry and Biology*, **2**, 639.)

the immune system, such as fibroblasts, and only some of them play a part in leucocyte adhesion. For example, integrins are involved in the adhesion of activated and memory T cells to several proteins of the extracellular matrix (see Table 9.2). These interactions help to guide activated effector T cells as they move through tissues and the signals provided via the adhesion receptors synergize with the signals emanating from the TCR. The β1 integrins are associated with another membrane protein, CD9 (M_r 24 000), which belongs to the *tetraspan* or *four-transmembrane (4TM) superfamily*, characterized by a polypeptide chain crossing the plasma membrane four times. This protein seems to be involved in linking the integrin molecules to the cytoskeleton and to intracellular signalling molecules. One of the β1 integrins, VLA-4 (α4β1; CD49d/CD29) is involved in interactions of lymphocytes, monocytes and eosinophils with endothelial cells. It binds to VCAM-1 (vascular cell adhesion molecule; CD106), an integral membrane glycoprotein of the immunoglobulin superfamily (see Table 9.2 & Fig. 9.8). VLA-4 participates in the early stage of the leucocyte–endothelial cell interaction (tethering and rolling), as well as in later phases (firm adhesion and extravasation). Binding of T cells to VCAM-1 generates activating signals synergizing with those provided via the TCR. The α4 subunit also pairs with another integrin chain, β7, producing a dimer involved in lymphocyte adhesion to specialized endothelia, as described below.

β2 Integrins are often called *leucocyte integrins*. Four members of this group are known, each being a non-covalent heterodimer of the β2 subunit (CD18; M_r 95 000) and one of the α subunits called αL (CD11a), αM (CD11b), αX (CD11c) and αD. The αLβ2 integrin, commonly known as *LFA-1 (leucocyte function-associated antigen-1)*, recognizes at least three counter-receptors (intercellular adhesion molecules, ICAM-1, -2 and -3) of the immunoglobulin superfamily (see Fig. 9.8). The αMβ2 (also called Mac-1) and αXβ2 (p150,95) molecules serve similar adhesion functions as LFA-1 mainly on myeloid cells and function also as complement type 3 and 4 receptors (CR3, CR4), respectively. The Mac-1 molecule has a remarkably broad repertoire of binding sites. In addition to ICAM-1, it binds the iC3b fragment of complement, components of the blood clotting system (fibrinogen and factor X), bacterial lipopolysaccharides and β-glucans. The β2 integrins are, in their high-affinity conformation, key adhesion receptors mediating firm attachment of leucocytes to endothelia following initial tethering and rolling mediated by selectins (and to some extent by VLA-4); they are also involved in leucocyte adhesion to other cells.

A defect in β2 integrins is responsible for *leucocyte adhesion deficiency* (LAD). It results from an abnormal splicing of RNA or a missense mutation in the gene coding for the β2 (CD18) subunit. The absence of functional β2 integrins impairs leucocyte function, especially migration of neutrophils to inflammatory sites, and phagocytosis of complement-opsonized bacteria. As a result, the affected person suffers from recurrent bacterial infections, some of which may be fatal (see Chapter 26).

β3 Integrins include two molecules, αIIbβ3 and αVβ3, both sharing the β3 chain (CD61; M_r 105 000) and distinguished by the α chains. The αIIbβ3 heterodimer (CD41/CD61; gpIIb/IIIa) is the major platelet receptor mediating platelet attachment to several proteins of the extracellular matrix (see Chapter 21). The αVβ3 (CD51/CD61) heterodimer is the major receptor of many cell types for the extracellular matrix protein vitronectin; it also binds the CD31 (to be described later) on endothelial cells. Several additional forms of vitronectin receptors exist, in which the αV subunit is paired with β1, β5, β6 or β8 subunits. The β3 integrins are associated with a structurally unusual molecule, the integrin-associated protein, IAP (CD47; M_r 50 000). The extracellular, N-terminal part of this molecule contains an immunoglobulin-like domain, while its C-terminal half crosses the membrane five times (Fig. 9.9). IAP contributes through its extracellular domain to binding of extracellular matrix proteins; its multiple membrane-spanning domains and intracellular loops probably participate in interactions of the β3 integrin complex with cytoskeletal and signalling molecules. Vitronectin receptor and its associated IAP are involved in trans-endothelial migration of granulocytes and in the activation of phagocytes at the site of inflammation.

Two *β7 integrins* control the adhesion of specific lymphocyte subsets to mucosal HEV. They are expressed exclusively on leucocytes and consist of the shared β7 chains and either the α4 (CD49d) chain (also used in the VLA-4 integrin) or the αE chain (CD103). The *α4β7 integrin* or the *lymphocyte Peyer's patch adhesion molecule-1* (LPAM-1) is expressed on subsets of lymphocytes homing to mucosal lymphoid tissues. It binds to two mucosal endothelial surface counter-receptors, VCAM-1 and MAdCAM-1, both members of the immunoglobulin superfamily (see Fig. 9.8). The αEβ7 integrin, the human mucosal lymphocyte-1 (HML-1) binds to E-cadherin, an epithelial

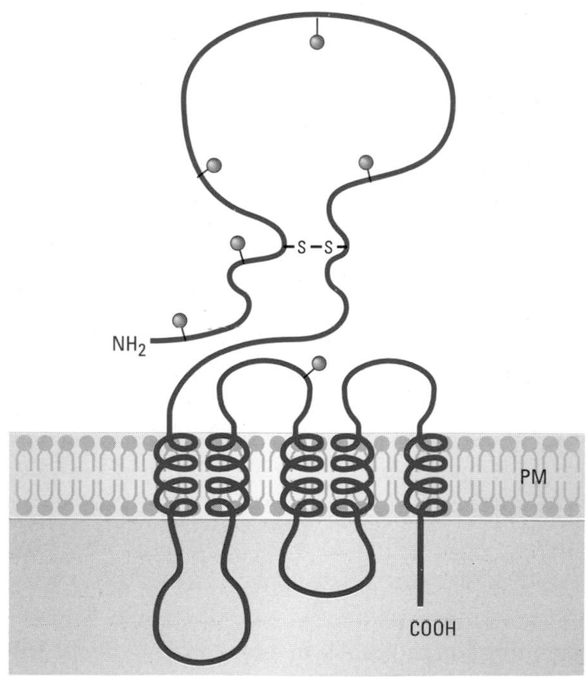

Figure 9.9 Structure of the integrin-associated protein (IAP). PM, plasma membrane; ●—, oligosaccharide chains; S–S, disulphide bond. (Based on Lindberg, F. P. *et al.* (1993) *Journal of Cell Biology*, **123**, 485.)

cell adhesion molecule, and is therefore responsible for specific intraepithelial retention of some T cells (see Chapters 16 & 18).

Molecules of the immunoglobulin superfamily

The immunoglobulin superfamily encompasses all molecules with at least one domain organized in the immunoglobulin-fold form (see Chapter 8 & Table 9.2). Among the more than 100 known members of the immunoglobulin superfamily are some that function as cell adhesion molecules in embryonic development and immunity. Some of the immunoglobulin-superfamily CAMs specialize in adhesion, others function in adhesion as well as signal transduction and others still specialize exclusively in signal transduction. As pointed out in Chapter 8, all the immunoglobulin-superfamily domains seem to be derived from a single common ancestor. The function of the ancestral immunoglobulin-superfamily molecules might have been the mediation of cell–cell contact by the apposition of identical immunoglobulin-like domains between molecules of two cells. Such *homophilic* or *homotypic interactions* are still common among members of the immunoglobulin superfamily. Subsequent diversification of the domains led to interactions between non-identical members of the immunoglobulin superfamily (*heterophilic* or *heterotypic interactions*) and to the generation of molecules with multiple immunoglobulin-like domains.

Several members of this superfamily have been mentioned already as counter-receptors of certain integrins. To reiterate, three ICAMs (ICAM-1, -2, -3) serve as ligands of β2 integrins; of these, *ICAM-2* and *ICAM-1* participate in leucocyte–endothelial interaction. *VCAM-1* and *MAdCAM-1* are the ligands of VLA-4 and α4β7 integrins (see Fig. 9.8). The platelet endothelial cell adhesion molecule-1, *PECAM-1* (CD31; Fig. 9.10), is expressed on endothelial cells, monocytes, granulocytes, platelets and subpopulations of lymphocytes. The extracellular part of this receptor consists of six immunoglobulin-like domains and binds several ligands, such as glycosaminoglycans (heparin, chondroitin sulphate) of the connective tissue and αVβ3 integrin; it also interacts in a homotypic fashion with other CD31 molecules. Other adhesion molecules of the immunoglobulin superfamily will be discussed later.

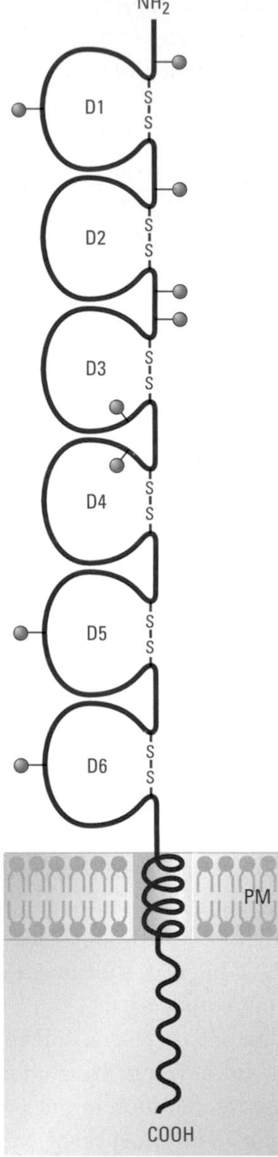

Figure 9.10 Structure of the platelet endothelial cell adhesion molecule-1 (PECAM-1; CD31). D1–D6, immunoglobulin-like domains 1–6; PM, plasma membrane; ●–, oligosaccharide chains; S–S, disulphide bond.

Other adhesion molecules involved in leucocyte–endothelial cell interactions

The *phagocytic glycoprotein-1* (Pgp-1; CD44) is expressed on leucocytes and other cell types. It is a heavily glycosylated integral membrane protein in which over 50% of the total mass is contributed by N-linked, O-linked and chondroitin sulphate carbohydrate chains. It is the receptor for hyaluronate, a glycosaminoglycan present on endothelial cell surfaces; it contributes to the firm adherence of leucocytes to endothelia. Larger forms of CD44 produced by alternative splicing of mRNA are expressed by epithelial cells; one of them appears to confer metastatic potential to some carcinomas.

Other endothelial surface molecules participating in interaction with leucocytes are *endoglin* (CD105), a strongly glycosylated homodimer of M_r 95 000 subunits;

VAP-1 (*vascular adhesion protein*-1; M_r 180 000) of so far unknown primary structure; and *L-VAP-2* (*lymphocyte-vascular adhesion protein*-2; CD73; M_r 70 000). Counter-receptors of these molecules on leucocytes are not known.

Area code model of leucocyte emigration

Cell adhesion molecules appear to act in sequence rather than in parallel. At least three, partially overlapping steps have been distinguished and each has been shown to involve different sets of CAMs (see Fig. 9.3). The first step, which may actually represent a combination of two distinct steps (tethering and rolling), involves the interaction between selectins and their carbohydrate ligands on mucin-like (proteoglycan) molecules. The second step involves activation of the cellular mechanisms that lead to the third step, adhesion and extravasation. These mechanisms are triggered by the interaction between chemoattractants and their receptors. The latter are molecules that span the leucocyte membrane seven times and are coupled with specialized signal transduction molecules, the *G-proteins*. The signals generated by the interaction of chemoattractants with their specific receptors activate integrins, which in the third step bind molecules of the immunoglobulin superfamily and thus mediate the firm attachment of leucocytes to endothelial cells.

At each of these three steps, the interacting cells have a choice of multiple receptors or ligands differentially expressed on the various leucocyte types and endothelial cells. This differential expression regulates the traffic of leucocytes by channelling different leucocyte types into distinct tissues. The multiplicity of CAMs and their ligands (counter-receptors) allows for great combinatorial diversity of possible interactions and thus for selectivity in leucocyte localization into different organs. The principle of leucocyte localization can be compared to that of the area code system in telecommunications. In the USA, an area code consists of three digits, where the hundreds, tens and ones specify progressively smaller areas in the country (they localize the call into that area). The CAMs and their ligands may function in much the same way, with the three steps of leucocyte–endothelium interactions corresponding to the three digits of the area code (Fig. 9.11). In the first step (corresponding to the hundreds in the area code), the particular combination of interacting selectins and mucin-like molecules specifies the destination of the 'call' very roughly by slowing down the movement of leucocytes in the particular part of the body. In the second step (the tens in the area code), the presence of particular chemoattractants in a specific tissue and the expression of certain receptors on the leucocyte directs leucocytes to a more circumscribed area in the body. Finally, in the third step, the expression of specific integrins and molecules of the immunoglobulin superfamily (the single numbers, 'ones', of the area code) localizes leucocytes very precisely to a specific vascular endothelium. Inflammation alters the expression and localization of signals in the endothelium via the production of distinct sets of chemoattractants. The changed signals in turn alter the traffic of leucocytes in the bloodstream and draw certain leucocytes directly to the inflamed site.

Area code model of lymphocyte homing

The three-step area code model can be extended to include the targeted return of circulating lymphocytes to specific organs and tissues. Most lymphocytes cruise through the body in search of intruders. The moment they encounter one in the form of a foreign antigen, they change both their behaviour and their route. This is brought about by the expression of sets of surface molecules that differ according to the tissue in which the encounter took place. As a result, naive lymphocytes (those that have not yet encountered antigen) and memory cells (those generated after the encounter with antigen) follow somewhat different recirculation pathways (Fig. 9.12). Moreover, memory cells generated in a particular tissue tend to home preferentially for that tissue, so that there are separate streams of lymphocytes circulating through the skin, the gut and the lungs, which drain into the lymphoid tissues associated with these organs and tissues (Fig. 9.12). Naive lymphocytes enter the lymph nodes via the HEV and drain via the efferent lymphatics. Memory cells, by contrast, emigrate via the 'flat' endothelium in the tissues and drain via the afferent lymphatics. Emigration into the spleen involves the endothelium of the sinuses. The HEV specialize in facilitating the emigration of lymphocytes into the peripheral lymph nodes that drain the skin and the lymphoid tissues of the mucosa (Peyer's patches, tonsils, appendix). The HEV develop in response to intense antigenic stimulation and the composition of the molecules they express is developmentally regulated.

The signals that guide lymphocytes to specific tissues are the same as those used for other leucocytes; only the combinations (the area codes) are different (Fig. 9.13). The process of lymphocyte emigration, like that of other leucocytes, is believed to occur in three or four steps, the first step involving selectin–mucin-like molecule interactions, the second chemoattractant–receptor interactions and the third integrin–immunoglobulin-superfamily molecule interactions. Each tissue, the peripheral lymph node HEV, Peyer's patch HEV, skin and gut, expresses a unique combination of CAMs and chemoattractants that interact with unique

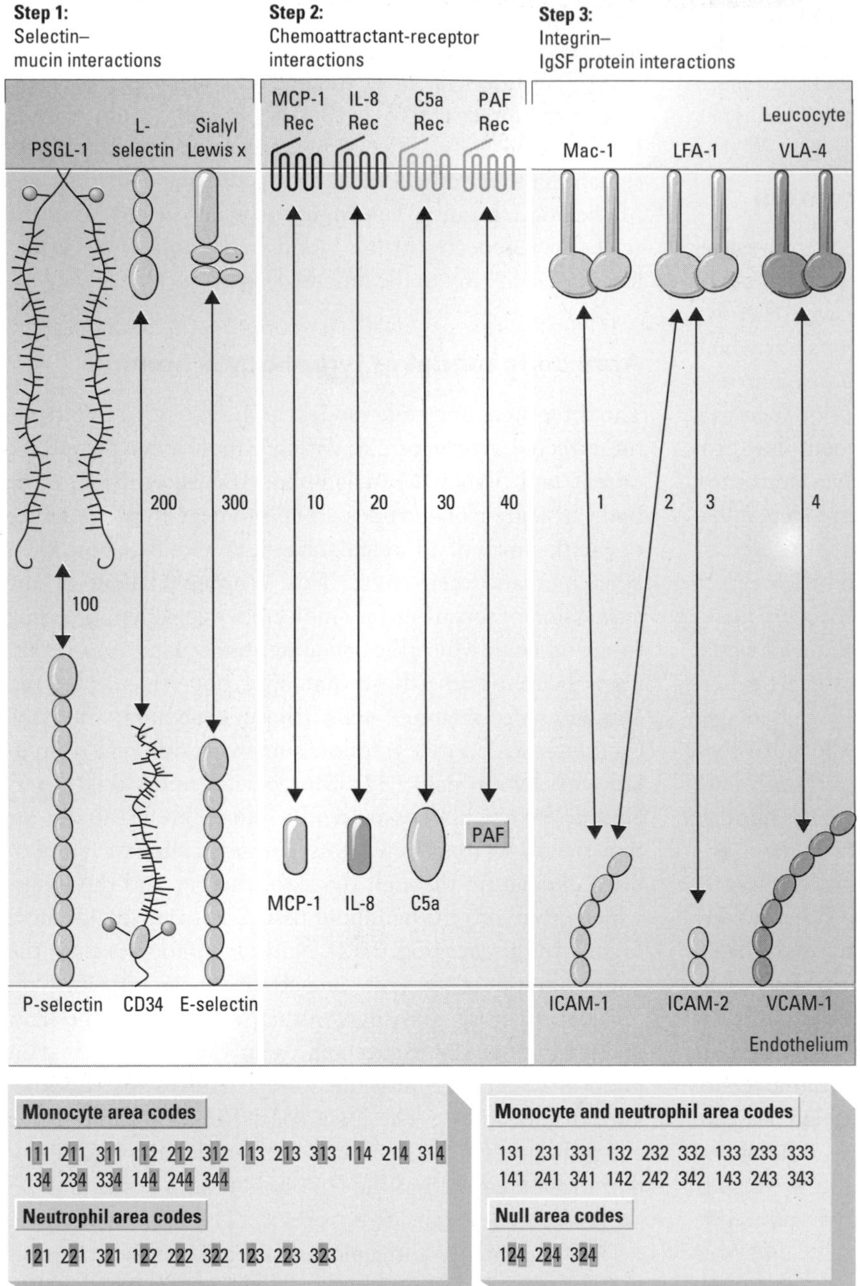

Figure 9.11 The area code model of monocyte/neutrophil interaction with vascular endothelium. The use of different combinations of receptors and counter-receptors (ligands) at each of the three successive stages of leucocyte emigration directs the cell into different tissues. The combinations thus function as area codes localizing the 'call' into a progressively more circumscribed region. Here, hundreds represent selectin–mucin interactions; tens, chemoattractant–receptor interactions; and ones, integrin–immunoglobulin-superfamily protein interactions. C5a, complement component 5 fragment a; ICAM, intercellular adhesion molecule; IgSF, immunoglobulin superfamily; IL, interleukin; LFA, leucocyte function associated; Mac, macrophage adhesion molecule; MCP, monocyte chemoattractant protein; PAF, platelet activating factor; PSGL, P-selectin glycoprotein; VCAM, vascular cell adhesion molecule; VLA, very late antigen; ⚬–, N-linked carbohydrate moiety; ═══, O-linked carbohydrate moiety. (Slightly modified from Springer, T.A. (1994) *Cell*, 76, 301.)

combinations of receptors, counter-receptors and ligands distinguishing individual lymphocyte sets and subsets (Fig. 9.13). These distinctive combinations serve as area codes for the circulating lymphocytes guiding their different sets and subsets to specific organs and tissues.

Molecules involved in leucocyte–leucocyte and leucocyte–other cell adhesion

As pointed out earlier, adhesion between various types of leucocytes and between leucocytes and the cells targeted by them is indispensable in nearly all functions of the immune system. These adhesion interactions are nearly always linked to signal transduction into one or both cells in contact. Some of the adhesion/signalling molecules are, in fact, more properly classified as membrane cytokines and their receptors, and so they are described in Chapter 10.

Among the adhesion molecules participating in the *T cell–APC interaction* are leucocyte integrin LFA-1, scavenger receptor family proteins CD5 and CD6, immunoglobulin-superfamily receptors CD2, CD28 and CTLA-4, and ligands (counter-receptors) of these receptors.

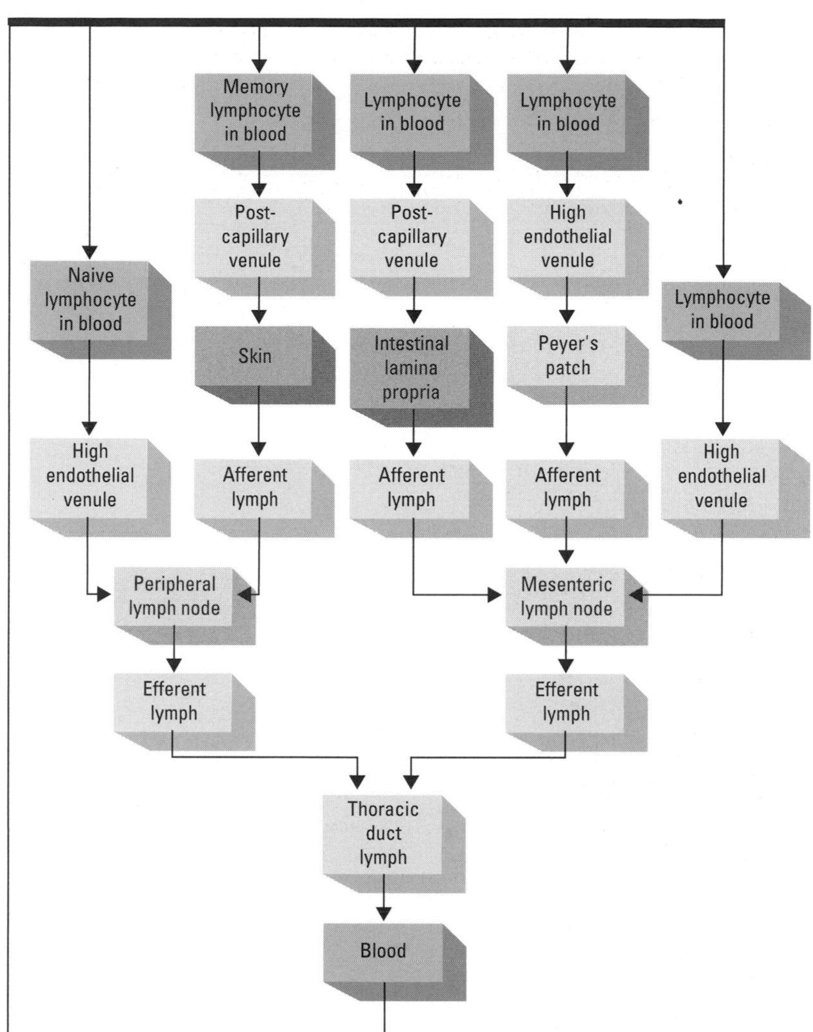

Figure 9.12 Lymphocyte recirculation routes. (Slightly modified from Springer, T. A. (1994) *Cell*, 76, 301.)

The β2 integrin LFA-1 may contribute to T cell–APC interaction from both sides. It binds to ICAM-1 and ICAM-3 (see Fig. 9.8) and less commonly to ICAM-2, which is expressed mainly on endothelial cells.

The *CD2 glycoprotein* expressed on the surface of T cells and NK cells is structurally similar to its broadly expressed ligand, the *LFA-3 (CD58) molecule*. It contains two immunoglobulin-like domains in its extracellular part (Fig. 9.14), a transmembrane region and a 25-residue long cytoplasmic tail. In addition to CD58, human CD2 binds (with lower affinity) to the *CD48* and *CD59 molecules*. The former is structurally similar to CD2 and CD58 in its extracellular part but has no transmembrane and cytoplasmic parts. Instead, it is anchored in the membrane via a lipid, glycosyl phosphatidylinositol (GPI, see Fig. 12.35), attached covalently to the C-terminal amino acid residue of CD58. The CD59 protein, which is structurally different from CD2/CD58, is one of the major complement-regulatory proteins (see Chapter 12); it, too, is a GPI-anchored protein. The only known ligand of CD2 in the mouse and rat is the CD48 glycoprotein. Binding of CD2 to its ligands elicits regulatory signals in the T cell that synergize with those provided by the TCR.

The *CD5 receptor* (M_r 67 000) has an extracellular part consisting of three scavenger receptor type domains (Fig. 9.15). It is expressed on T cells and B1 cells. It binds the B-cell surface molecule, *CD72*, a member of the C-type lectin family. The signals delivered to the T cell via CD5 are inhibitory and help to dampen the ongoing response. The structure of the T-cell surface *CD6 molecule* (M_r 100 000–130 000) is similar to that of CD5 (Fig. 9.15). The molecule binds to the activated leucocyte cell adhesion molecule (ALCAM), expressed on thymic epithelium and activated leucocytes. The extracellular part of ALCAM consists of five immunoglobulin-like domains. The CD6-mediated signals appear to contribute to T-cell activation.

The *CD28 glycoprotein* is a covalent dimer of an M_r 44 000 membrane glycoprotein, the extracellular part

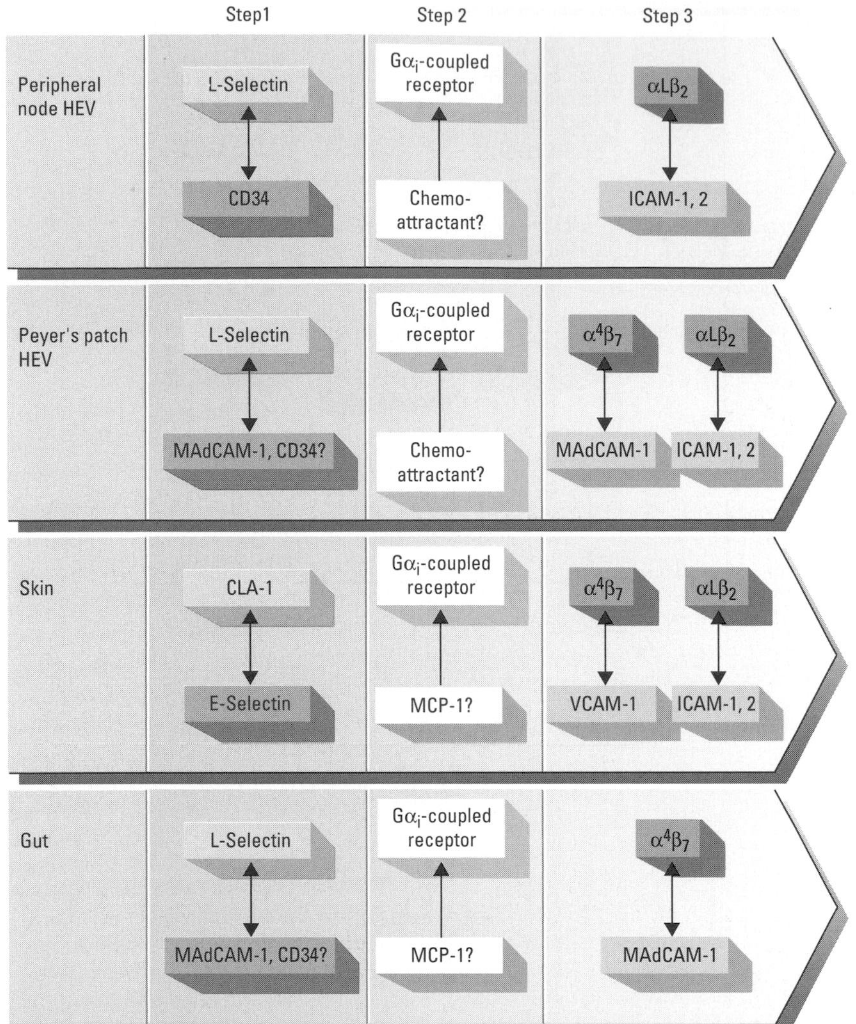

Figure 9.13 The three-step model of lymphocyte homing. Molecular interactions in each step in different organs are shown. α and β, integrins; CLA, CD36 and LIMPII (lysosomal integral membrane protein II) analogous; HEV, high endothelial venule; ICAM, intercellular adhesion molecule; MAdCAM, mucosal addressin cell adhesion molecule; MCP, monocyte chemoattractant protein; VCAM, vascular cell adhesion molecule. (From Springer, T. A. (1994) *Cell*, **76**, 301.)

of which contains one immunoglobulin-like domain (Fig. 9.16). It is constitutively expressed on T cells and binds at least two ligands on APCs, CD80 (B7/BB1; M_r 60 000; Fig. 9.16) and CD86 (B7.2; M_r 80 000), both of which are members of the immunoglobulin superfamily. Ligation of the CD28 receptor with CD80 or CD86 provides co-stimulatory signals to T cells that received the first signals via the TCR. In the presence of CD28-mediated signals the T cell becomes fully activated, divides and differentiates into mature effector cells; in the absence of CD28-based signals the T cell becomes anergic or may even die by apoptosis (see Chapter 16). A receptor structurally closely related to CD28 and called *cytotoxic T lymphocyte antigen-4* (CTLA-4; Fig. 9.16) is expressed on activated T cells. Like CD28, it interacts with the CD80 and CD86 counter-receptors, but the affinities of these interactions are up to 100-fold higher than in the case of CD28. The signals provided to the activated T cell via the CTLA-4 receptor inhibit further activation and proliferation. Thus, CTLA-4 appears to be a negative regulator or 'brake' of the T-cell activation process. It is a matter of semantics whether one calls CD28 and CTLA-4 adhesion/signalling receptors or cytokine receptors, and CD80 and CD86 adhesion/signalling ligands or membrane-bound cytokines (see Chapter 10).

Several adhesion molecules are involved in interactions of B lymphocytes with other cells, such as stromal cells of bone marrow, follicular dendritic cells and T_H cells (see Chapter 17). Some pairs of these adhesion molecules have already been discussed (e.g. CD2–CD58; LFA-1–ICAM-1; CD28–CD80/CD86; CD5–CD72). An additional B-cell surface adhesion receptor is the immunoglobulin-superfamily protein *CD22*, which acts as a sialic acid-specific lectin. It recognizes sialic acid, which is often present as a terminal monosaccharide residue on various oligosaccharide chains decorating cell-surface glycolipids and glycoproteins. CD22

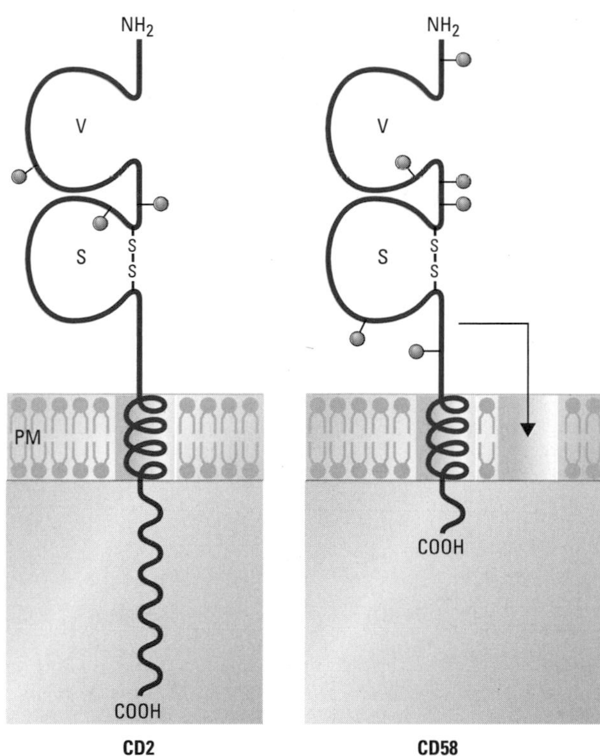

Figure 9.14 Structure of CD2 and CD58 molecules. There are two alternative forms of CD58 molecules produced by alternative splicing: a transmembrane form (shown), and a glycosylphosphatidylinositol-anchored form (indicated by arrows). PM, plasma membrane; S—S, disulphide bonds; S, s(C2)-type fold of immunoglobulin-like domain; V, v-type fold of immunoglobulin-like domain; ⚬–, oligosaccharide chain. (Based on Barclay, A.N. *et al.* (1993) *The Leucocyte Antigen Facts Book*. Academic Press, London.)

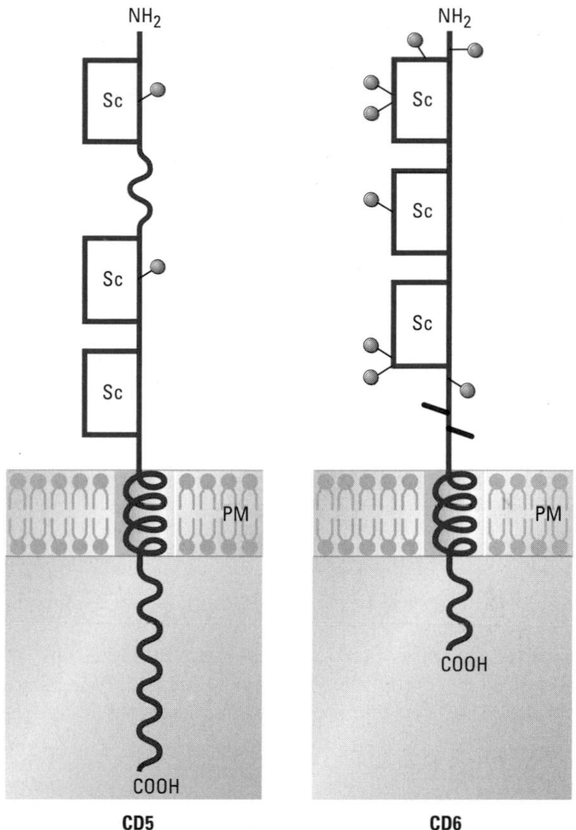

Figure 9.15 Structure of CD5 and CD6 molecules. PM, plasma membrane; Sc, scavenger receptor molecule (domain). ⚬– and ═══, oligosaccharide chains, *N*- and *O*-linked, respectively. (Based on Barclay, A. N. *et al.* (1993) *The Leucocyte Antigen Facts Book*. Academic Press, London.)

seems to contribute to the adhesion of B cells to various cell types involved in different phases of B-cell maturation and differentiation.

Interactions between B lymphocytes and T_H cells and between B lymphocytes and follicular dendritic cells are also dependent, in part, on adhesions mediated by a pair of molecules that have other functions, *CD21* and *CD23*. The former is the complement type-2 receptor (CR2) of B cells (see Chapter 12); the latter is a low-affinity IgE receptor expressed on B cells, activated T lymphocytes, follicular dendritic cells, activated macrophages and thrombocytes (see Chapter 8). The CD23 receptor is a member of the C-type lectin family; its carbohydrate-binding site recognizes oligosaccharide chains on the CD21 (CR2) molecule.

Soluble forms of adhesion molecules

Several adhesion molecules described in this chapter are released from the cell surface by specific proteases, a process referred to as *shedding*. By this process, which often accompanies cell activation, cells may dispose of adhesion receptors that are no longer useful or that are even undesired. If their local concentration is high enough, some of the soluble forms may inhibit cell adhesion by competing with counter-receptors. Certain tumour cells seem to shed some of their adhesion molecules in order to 'blind' the corresponding counter-receptors on leucocytes and thus avoid an attack by the immune system (see Chapter 22). Increased concentrations of adhesion molecules (e.g. ICAM-1, -2 and -3, VCAM-1, CD44 or LFA-3) in body fluids of patients with chronic inflammatory diseases, autoimmune diseases and some tumours are the basis of certain diagnostic tests.

Some of the soluble forms have their own specific functions, apparently unrelated to the adhesion functions of their membrane-associated forms. Thus, the soluble forms of CD23 are regulators of B-cell activation (see Chapter 17), and soluble forms of E-selectin and VCAM-1 are potent inducers of angiogenesis (formation of new blood

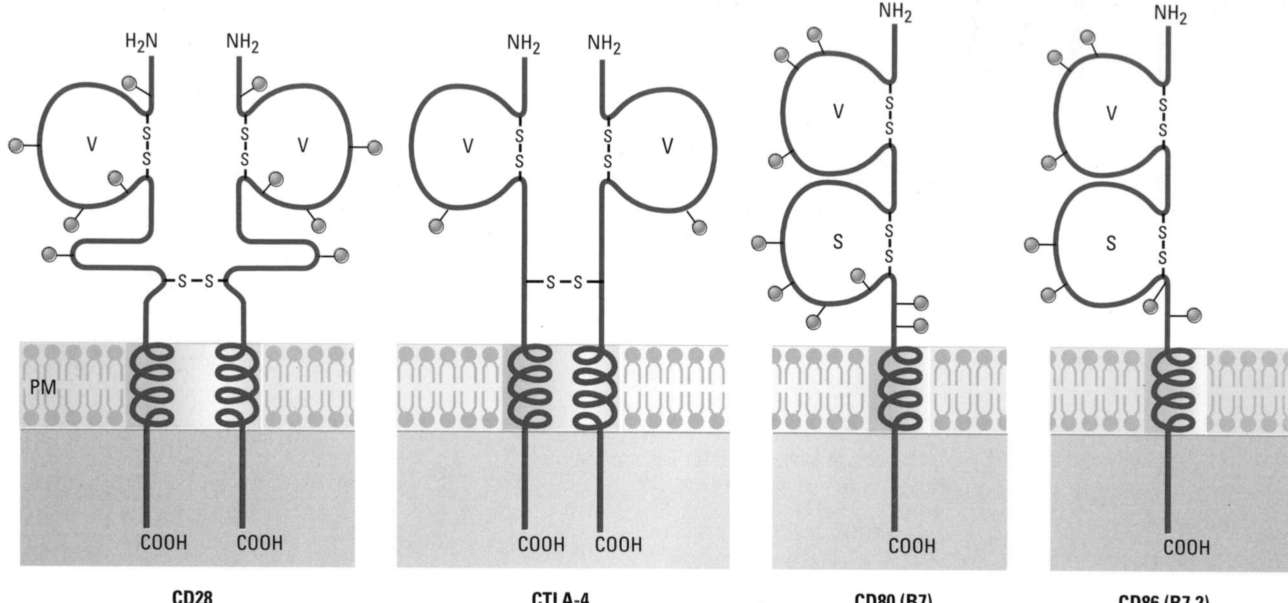

Figure 9.16 Structure of CD28, CTLA-4, CD80 and CD86 molecules. CTLA, cytotoxic T lymphocyte antigen; PM, plasma membrane; V and S, v- and s(C2)-type immunoglobulin fold; S–S, disulphide bond. ●—, oligosaccharide chains. (Based on Barclay, A.N. *et al.* (1993) *The Leucocyte Antigen Facts Book*. Academic Press, London.)

vessels in wound repair, tumour growth and in inflamed tissues). In this respect, soluble molecules act as cytokines.

Further reading

Bertozzi, C.B. (1995) Cracking the carbohydrate code for selectin recognition. *Chemistry and Biology*, **2**, 703–708.

Bevilacqua, M.P. (1993) Endothelial–leucocyte adhesion molecules. *Annual Review of Immunology*, **11**, 767–804.

Fougerolles, A. de & Springer, T.A. (1995) Ideas crystallized on immunoglobulin superfamily—integrin interactions. *Chemistry and Biology*, **2**, 639–643.

Lasky, L.A. (1992) Selectins: interpreters of cell-specific carbohydrate information during inflammation. *Science*, **258**, 964–969.

Lasky, L.A. (1995) Selectin–carbohydrate interactions and the initiation of the inflammatory response. *Annual Review of Biochemistry*, **64**, 113–139.

Mackay, C.R. (1992) Migration pathways and immunologic memory among T lymphocytes. *Seminars in Immunology*, **4**, 51–58.

Mackay, C. (1995) A new spin on lymphocyte homing. *Current Biology*, **5**, 733–736.

McEver, R.P., Moore, K.L. & Cummings, R.D. (1995) Leukocyte trafficking mediated by selectin–carbohydrate interactions. *Journal of Biological Chemistry*, **270**, 11025–11028.

Miller, M.D. & Krangel, M.S. (1992) Biology and biochemistry of the chemokines: a family of chemotactic and inflammatory cytokines. *CRC Critical Reviews in Immunology*, **12**, 17–46.

Pigott, R. & Power, C. (1993) *The Adhesion Molecule Facts Book*. Academic Press, London.

Picker, L.J. & Butcher, E.C. (1992) Physiological and molecular mechanisms of lymphocyte homing. *Annual Review of Immunology*, **10**, 561–591.

Rosen, S.D. & Bertozzi, C.R. (1994) The selectins and their ligands. *Current Opinion in Cell Biology*, **6**, 663–673.

Rosen, S.D. & Bertozzi, C.R. (1996) Leukocyte adhesion: two selectins converge on sulphate. *Current Biology*, **6**, 261–264.

Springer, T.A. (1994) Traffic signals for lymphocyte recirculation and leucocyte emigration: the multistep paradigm. *Cell*, **76**, 301–314.

Stewart, M., Thiel, M. & Hogg, N. (1995) Leukocyte integrins. *Current Opinion in Cell Biology*, **7**, 690–696.

Tedder, T.F., Steeber, D.A., Chen, A. & Engel, P. (1995) The selectins: vascular adhesion molecules. *FASEB Journal*, **9**, 866–873.

Varki, A. (1994) Selectin ligands. *Proceedings of the National Academy of Sciences USA*, **91**, 7390–7397.

chapter 10 Cytokines and their receptors

Cells can intercommunicate in one of two ways. One cell can either contact another and send a signal via cell-surface adhesion receptors or entrust the message to a water-soluble molecule and dispatch the messenger to seek out the target. Immune system cells use both forms of information transfer. Having covered the first option in the previous chapter, let us now turn to communication via soluble molecules.

Definition

The messengers running errands between immune system cells were originally called *interleukins* (literally, molecules that move between leucocytes) and were differentiated into *lymphokines*, produced by lymphocytes, and *monokines*, produced by monocytes. When it was later discovered that similar messengers run errands not only for leucocytes but also for other cells such as fibroblasts, endothelial cells and keratinocytes, the term was broadened and became *cytokines*, to include communication molecules carrying messages between *any* kind of cell. Cytokines, then, are soluble proteins or glycoproteins made by cells to affect the behaviour of other cells. Here, we consider only cytokines produced by the cells of the immune system (leucocytes, inflammatory cells and haemopoietic cells), which are also among the best characterized.

Cytokines should be distinguished from other biologically active water-soluble molecules — hormones, growth factors and chemokines. *Hormones* are produced by specialized glands and are carried by the blood throughout the entire body to act at sites removed from the locus of their production; they tend to act on one or only very few cell types. Cytokines, by contrast, are produced by scattered cells and act over short distances but on a variety of cell types. *Growth factors* stimulate the growth of other cells and tend to be produced constitutively, whereas cytokines have a variety of effects on their target cells and are usually produced only after stimulation of a cell. *Chemokines* are molecules involved in the migration of cells. However, the demarcation lines between these categories are indistinct because some cytokines can travel long distances, like hormones, stimulate cell growth, like growth factors, and influence cell migration, like chemokines. In fact, some growth factors and certain chemokines are often included among the cytokines. The difficulties regarding cytokine classification stem from the artificiality of the category: structurally, cytokines are a very heterogeneous group of unrelated molecules unified by one rather superficial functional characteristic, their influence on the behaviour of other cells.

Properties

Most cytokines are glycosylated proteins with relative molecular mass (M_r) of between 10 000 and 25 000; chemokines are even smaller, with M_r of between 8000 and 10 000. They are highly potent molecules that mediate biological effects at picomolar concentrations and act via cell-surface receptors with which they combine with high affinity; the dissociation constant (K_d) of the interaction (see Chapter 14) ranges from 10^{-10} to 10^{-12} M. Most cytokines are secreted, but a few are expressed on the plasma membrane or are held in reservoirs in the extracellular matrix. The bulk are manufactured on stimulation of the producing cell; only a few are synthesized constitutively. After stimulation, production lasts only a few days. Cytokines introduced artificially into the circulation have a very short half-life.

All cytokines act via specific target cell *receptors*. The distribution of receptors among the different cell types determines the cytokine's range of influence. The receptors are coupled to intracellular signal transduction machineries activated by the receptor–ligand interaction. The intracellular signal thus generated then influences the cell's physiology, in part by activating some genes in the nucleus and silencing others. Following stimulation, the cell may begin to grow and divide; it may differentiate into another cell type; or it may begin to produce and secrete other cytokines. Other effects may be rapid and more direct, not requiring changes in gene transcription, such as changes in the cell's shape, adhesiveness, movement in a specific direction or exocytosis of cytoplasmic granules. The actions of the target cell may have a domino effect upon the behaviour of other cells until the initially local event ultimately translates, via a chain of reactions, into a systemic effect such as fever, change in blood pressure or blood clotting.

Most cytokines are *paracrines*, i.e. they act on target cells that happen to be present in the neighbourhood of the producing cell and that express the appropriate receptor. Some cytokines are *autocrines*, i.e. they act on the same cell that produced them. A few are *endocrines*, i.e. they act on target cells at a distance from the producing cell. Cytokine actions are characterized by pleiotropy, redundancy, synergy and antagonism. Very often a single cytokine acts on several different types of target cell and stimulates different responses (*pleiotropy*). Frequently, however, two different cytokines can also induce a similar response (*redundancy*). The combined effect of some cytokines is sometimes greater than might be expected on the basis of the cumulative effects of the individual cytokines (*synergy*). And there are also cytokines that offset the effects of other cytokines (*antagonism*). Antagonistic interactions are among the mechanisms by which the actions of cytokines are regulated. The need for control is obvious: overproduction of cytokines could easily turn beneficial effects into harmful ones.

Methods of detection

In the laboratory, cytokines can be monitored by one of several techniques that can be classified into three categories according to their underlying principles. The first category encompasses techniques based on the use of monoclonal or polyclonal antibodies specific for individual cytokines (*immunoassays*). The principle of immunoassays, such as the enzyme-linked immunosorbent assay (ELISA) and the immunoradiometric assay (IRMA), is described in Chapter 14. In essence, a cytokine-specific antibody is first attached to a solid substrate such as a plastic plate or beads, the cytokine is then allowed to bind to it and the bound cytokine is detected by another specific antibody tagged with a visible label.

The second category includes techniques that measure the effect of a cytokine on appropriate target cells in culture (*bioassays*). The detection system consists of at least two cell types: the cytokine-producing cells activated by a suitable stimulus and the target cell (a cell line whenever possible) capable of responding to the cytokine. The method of measuring cytokine production varies depending on the activity of the product. The presence of a cytokine that promotes cell proliferation can be revealed by the incorporation of tritiated thymidine into the DNA of the dividing target cells (see Chapter 24). The production of cytokines that stimulate antibody secretion by B-cell hybridomas can be ascertained by assaying for the particular immunoglobulins in the culture supernatant. The effects of cytokines that promote differentiation of progenitors into certain types of colonies of haemopoietic cells can be assayed microscopically by counting such colonies.

In the third category of assays, the presence of cytokines with effector functions can be revealed by assaying target-cell viability, by the inhibition of virus replication (prevention of viral damage to the cultured cell) or some other such detection system. Cytokines can also be assayed by determining their ability to compete with the binding of a labelled cytokine to its receptor.

Structure: cytokine families

In spite of their heterogeneity, cytokines can be divided into several families, where members of the same family have a similar tertiary (and usually also primary) structure and act on a group of structurally related receptors. The main cytokine families are the haemopoietin, interferon, epidermal growth factor, interleukin-1, tumour necrosis factor, transforming growth factor and chemokine families; a few cytokines remain unassigned (Table 10.1). The various cytokines bear a bewildering variety of names and acronyms. In particular, the reader should be aware that cytokines bearing similar designations are not necessarily related. In the interleukin series, for instance, more than a dozen cytokines bear the designation IL-1 through IL-17, although their actions are not restricted to leucocytes and many of them are unrelated to one another, both structurally and functionally. The characteristics of the immunologically most important cytokines are given in Table 10.2. A brief description of the structural features characterizing the cytokine families follows.

Haemopoietins

This family includes several cytokines involved in the growth and differentiation of haemopoietic cells (see Chapter 4). Representative members of the family are interleukin (IL)-4, IL-2 and IL-3. *IL-4* is a glycoprotein with an M_r of 15 000–19 000 and a mature polypeptide chain consisting of 129 amino acid residues. It was first described as the *B-cell stimulating factor-1* (*BSF-1*) because of its ability to induce the secretion of antibodies by B cells. Later, however, it was recognized as one of the pleiotropic cytokines that acts not only on B lymphocytes but also on T lymphocytes and many non-lymphoid cells, including monocytes, endothelial cells and fibroblasts. IL-4 causes B cells to switch to IgE production and is therefore one of the key factors in allergic responses (see Chapter 23). In addition, it is an essential regulator of helper T-cell responses that selectively stimulates T_H2 cell differentiation and suppresses T_H1 cell development (see Chapters 16 and 21). Most IL-4 activities are shared also by IL-13. IL-4 is produced by T_H2 and T_H0 lymphocytes, mast cells and bone marrow stromal cells. The polypeptide chain of the IL-4 molecule is folded into a compact globule with a hydrophobic core (Fig. 10.1). The four α-helices (A–D), which range in length from 15 to 25 residues and are connected by three loops (AB, BC and CD), are a dominant feature of the structure. Residues 27–31 and 105–108 within the two longer loops form short β-strands arranged into a small antiparallel β-sheet. The four α-helices are packed against each other to form a left-handed antiparallel *four-helix bundle* with an up–up–down–down topology (Fig. 10.1). Together they donate 18 hydrophobic residues to the interior of the bundle to form the hydrophobic core. The structure is held together by three disulphide bonds and by hydrogen bonds; one of the disulphide bonds connects the N and C termini of the molecule. Human IL-4 contains two potential N-linked glycosylation sites.

IL-2 is secreted by activated T_H1 cells. It was originally believed to be a specific *T-cell growth factor* but now is known to stimulate growth and differentiation not only of

Table 10.1 Families of immunologically relevant cytokines.

Family (structural motif)	Members	Receptor type
Haemopoietins (four-helix bundle)	IL-2, IL-3, IL-4, IL-5, IL-6, IL-7, IL-9, IL-11, IL-12 (p35), IL-15, G-CSF, GM-CSF, OSM, LIF	Cytokine receptor type I
	M-CSF	Ig/tyrosine kinase
Interferons (four-helix bundle)	IFN-α, IFN-β, IFN-γ, IL-10	Cytokine receptor type II
Interleukin-1 (β-trefoil)	IL-1α, IL-1β, IL-1Rα	Ig
TNF (jelly-roll motif)	TNF-α, TNF-β, LT-β, CD30L, CD40L, FasL, CD70, OX-40L, 4-1BBL	TNFR
TGF-β (cysteine knot)	TGF-β	Ser/Thr kinase
Chemokines (Greek key)	IL-8, MIP-1α, MIP-1β, MIP-2, PF-4, PBP, I-309/TCA-3, MCP-1, MCP-2, MCP-3, γIP-10, RANTES	Seven membrane-spanning
Other	IL-12 (p40), IL-14, IL-17, MIF	
	SCF	Ig/tyrosine kinase
	IL-16	Ig

Abbreviations are explained in Table 10.2 on page 294.

Table 10.2 Characteristics of immunologically relevant cytokines*.

Abbreviation	Name	Synonyms	M_r (× 10^3) mature	Form	No. of amino acid residues precursor/ mature	CHO	S—S bonds	Chromosome	Producing cell	Main target cell (tissue)	Main biological effects
Haemopoietins											
IL-2	Interleukin-2	T-cell growth factor (TCGF)	15–20	M	153/133	0	1	4q26–27	T_H1 lymphocytes	Activated T_H and T_C cells	Proliferation
IL-3	Interleukin-3	Mast cell growth factor (MCGF), multicolony-stimulating factor (multi-CSF), eosinophil-CSF (E-CSF) and others	14–30	M	152/133	2	1	5q23–31	Activated T cells, mast cells, eosinophils	Haemopoietic cells	Growth and differentiation
IL-4	Interleukin-4	B-cell stimulating factor-1 (BSF-1)	15–19	M	153/129	2	3	5q31	T_H2 lymphocytes	Antigen-primed B cells, activated B cells	B-cell activation, IgG1 and IgE switch
IL-5	Interleukin-5	B-cell growth factor II (BCGFII), eosinophil differentiation factor (EDF), E-CSF and others	45	$(M)_2$	134/115	2	2	5q23–31	T_H2 cells, mast cells, eosinophils	Activated B cells, eosinophils	Proliferation and differentiation
IL-6	Interleukin-6	Interferon-β2 (IFN-β2), B-cell stimulatory factor-2 (BSF-2), B-cell differentiation factor (BCDF) and others	26	M	212/183	2	2	7q21p14	Monocytes, macrophages, T_H2 cells, bone marrow stromal cells	Proliferating B cells, plasma cells, myeloid stem cells, hepatocytes	T and B cell growth and differentiation, acute phase reaction
IL-7	Interleukin-7	Lymphopoietin-1 (LP-1), preB-cell growth factor	20–28	M	177/152	3	3	8q12–13	Bone marrow, thymic cells, spleen cells	Lymphoid stem cells, resting T cells	Growth of preB and preT cells
IL-9	Interleukin-9	p40	32–39	M	144/126	4	5	5q31.1	T_H2 cells	T cells	Proliferation
IL-11	Interleukin-11	Adipogenesis inhibitory factor	23	M	199/179	0	0	19q13.3–13.4	Bone marrow stromal cells	Progenitor B cells, megakaryocytes	Differentiation, acute phase reaction
IL-12	Interleukin-12	Natural killer stimulatory factor (NKSF)		HeDi							
		Cytotoxic lymphocyte maturation factor (CLAF)							B cells, macrophages	T cells, natural killer cells	Proliferation, activation
		p35 subunit	35		253/196	3	3	3p12–q13.2			
		p40 subunit	40		328/306	4	5	4c31			
IL-13	Interleukin-13		9/17	M	132/112	4	2	5c31	T_H cells	Macrophages	Inhibition of activation of T_H1 cells and cytokine release
IL-15	Interleukin-15	TCGF	14–15	M	162/114	2	2		Epithelial cells, monocytes	T cells	Proliferation
G-CSF	Granulocyte colony-stimulating factor	Colony-stimulating factor β (CSFβ), pluripoietin β	21	M	207/177 (174)	0	2	17q21–22	Macrophages, fibroblasts, endothelial cells, bone marrow stromal cells	Neutrophil precursors	Growth and differentiation, activation

GM-CSF	Granulocyte–monocyte colony-stimulating factor	Colony-stimulating factor α (CSFα), pluripoietin α	22	M	144/127	2	2	5q21–32	Macrophages, T cells, fibroblasts, endothelial cells	Haemopoietic progenitor cells	Growth and differentiation, activation
OSM	Oncostatin M		32, 36	M	252/227 (196)	2	2	22q12	Activated T cells, monocytes	Fibroblasts, smooth muscle cells	Growth and proliferation
LIF	Leukaemia inhibitory factor	Human interleukin for DA (HILDA)	45	M	202/180	6	3	22q14	Bone marrow stroma, fibroblasts, T cells	Haemopoietic stem cells	Proliferation and differentiation
M-CSF	Macrophage colony-stimulating factor	Colony stimulating factor-1 (CSF-1)	45–50	$(M)_2$	554/522 (406,224)	3	7–9	5q33.1	Lymphocytes, monocytes, fibroblasts, endothelial cells	Macrophages and their progenitors	Growth and differentiation, activation
Interferons											
IFN-α	Interferon-α	Type I interferon, leucocyte interferon	16–27	M	188(189)/165(166)	0	2	9p22	Lymphocytes, monocytes, macrophages	Uninfected cells	Inhibition of viral replication; see Table 10.3
INF-β	Interferon-β	Type I interferon, fibroblast interferon	20	M	187/166	1	1	9p22	Fibroblasts, some epithelial cells	Uninfected cells	Inhibition of viral replication
IFN-γ	Interferon-γ	Immune interferon, type II interferon	40–70	$(M)_2$	166/143	2	0	12q24.1	T_H1 cells, natural killer cells	Uninfected cells	See Table 10.3
IL-10	Interleukin-10	Cytokine synthesis inhibitory factor (CSIF)	35–40	$(M)_2$	178/160	1	2	1	T_H2 cells, monocytes, macrophages	Macrophages, T_H1 cells	Suppression of macrophage and T_H1 cell function
Interleukin-1 family											
IL-1α	Interleukin-1α	Lymphocyte-activating factor (LAF), endogenous pyrogen (EP), leucocyte endogenous mediator (LEM), mononuclear cell factor (MCF), catabolin	17.5 (?)	M	271/159	2	0	2q12–21	Macrophages, epithelial cells	See Fig. 10.7	
IL-1β	Interleukin-1β	LAF, EP, LEM, MCF, catabolin	17.3 (?)	M	269/153	1	0	2q13–21	Macrophages, epithelial cells	See Fig. 10.7	
Tumour necrosis factor family											
TNF	Tumour necrosis factor	Cachectin, macrophage cytotoxin, necrosin, TNF-α	52	$(M)_3$	233/157	0	1	6p21.3	Macrophages, monocytes, natural killer cells T cells, B cells	See Fig. 10.9	Local inflammation, endothelial cell activation
LT-α	Lymphotoxin-α	Tumour necrosis factor-β		$(M)_3$	205/71	1	0	6p21.3		Tumour cells	Killing, endothelial cell activation
LT-β	Lymphotoxin-β		33	$(M)_3$	244/244 (240)	1	0	6p21.3	Activated T and B cells	?	?
CD30L	CD30 ligand (membrane-bound)		40	$(M)_2$	234/234	5	3?	9q33	Activated T cells, monocytes	Activated lymphocytes	Activation, apoptosis, induction?
CD40L	CD40 ligand (membrane-bound)	gp39	40	?	261/261	1	1	Xq26.3	Activated T cells, thymus stroma	B cells, monocytes, thymocytes	Activation, induction of somatic mutations, switching and memory in B cells

(Continued on p. 296.)

Table 10.2 (*Continued.*)

Abbreviation	Name	Synonyms	M_r (× 10^3) mature	Form	No. of amino acid residues precursor/ mature	CHO	S—S bonds	Chromosome	Producing cell	Main target cell (tissue)	Main biological effects
FasL	Fas ligand (membrane-bound)	CD95L	40	?	281/281	3	1	1q23	T_C and some other cells	Many cell types	Apoptosis or activation
CD70		CD27L	50	$(M)_n$	193/193	2	2(?)	19p13	Activated lymphocytes	T cells	Activation?
OX-40L	OX-40 ligand (membrane-bound)	gp34	34	?	183/183	4	1	1q25	Some transformed lymphoid cell lines	T cells?	Activation
4-1BBL	4-1BB ligand		50	$(M)_2$	254/254	0	1	19p13.3	Various cell types	T cells	Activation
Transforming growth factor family											
TGF-β	Transforming growth factor-β	Glioblastoma-derived T-cell suppressor factor	25	$(M)_2$	414/112	0	1	19q13.1	Platelets, macrophages, T cells	Monocytes, macrophages, B cells	Inhibition of cell growth, anti-inflammatory effect, switch to IgA
Others											
IL-14	Interleukin-14	High molecular weight B-cell growth factor (HMW-BCGF)	60	M	498/483	3	?	?	T cells	B cells	Proliferation, inhibition of Ig secretion
IL-16	Interleukin-16	Lymphocyte chemoattractant protein (LCP)	14	$(M)_n$	130/130	1	0	2q31	$CD8^+$ T cells	$CD4^+$ T cells	Chemotaxis
L-17	Interleukin-17		17.5	$(M)_2$	155/136	1	3	?	$CD4^+$ T cells	Fibroblasts, other cells?	IL-6 and IL-8 production, upregulation of ICAM-1
MIF	Migration inhibition factor		12.5	$(M)_n$	115/?	2	1	19	T cells	Macrophages	Activation, inhibition of migration
SCF	Stem cell factor	Mast cell growth factor (MGF), *kit* ligand (KL), *steel* factor (SLF)	28–35	$(M)_2$	273/248	5	2	12q22–24	Bone marrow stromal cells, brain, liver, kidney and others	Haemopoietic progenitor cells	Differentiation

*All data refer to human cytokines.

M, monomer; $(M)_2$, homodimer; $(M)_3$, homotrimer; $(M)_n$, undefined oligomer; HeDi, heterodimer; CHO, number of potential *N*-linked glycosylation (carbohydrate) sites; S–S bonds, number of disulphide bonds.

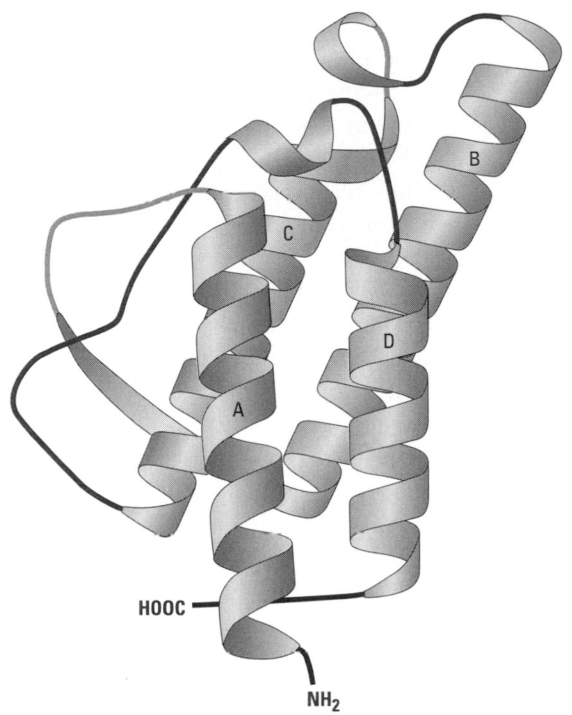

Figure 10.1 Tertiary structure of the human interleukin-4 (IL-4) molecule: a ribbon model. The structure consists of a four-helix bundle (A–D), one β-strand (arrow) and connecting loops. (From the Protein Data Bank Swiss 3-D; based on data from Powers, R. *et al.* (1992) *Science*, **256**, 1673.)

T cells, natural killer (NK) cells and B cells, but also some myeloid cells. Its activities are similar to those of *IL-15*.

IL-3, originally called *multi-colony stimulating factor* (*multi-CSF*), is produced by activated T cells, eosinophils and mast cells. It is a haemopoietic growth factor with a broad range of action. It participates, together with lineage-specific haemopoietins, in committing progenitor cells to distinct differentiation pathways. IL-3 has been used clinically to stimulate haemopoietic progenitor cells after bone marrow transplantation.

IL-5 is secreted mainly by activated T_H2 cells as a cysteine-linked homodimer. It is involved in eosinophil differentiation but also stimulates B-cell growth and differentiation in certain species (mouse) although not in others (humans).

IL-6 is a multifunctional cytokine produced by several cell types. It is a mediator of acute phase reaction (see Chapter 21), co-stimulator of haemopoiesis and an essential factor in plasma cell development. IL-6 is also an indispensable component of culture media supporting the growth of B-cell hybridomas secreting monoclonal antibodies. The activities of IL-6 are partially overlapped by those of *IL-11*, *oncostatin M* (*OSM*) and *leukaemia inhibitory factor* (*LIF*).

IL-7 is produced mainly by bone marrow and thymic stromal cells. It is an essential growth and differentiation factor of preB cells and early thymocytes but it also contributes to activation of mature T cells.

Granulocyte colony-stimulating factor (G-CSF) is produced by bone marrow stromal cells, macrophages, fibroblasts and endothelial cells. It stimulates development of neutrophil granulocytes from their myeloid precursors and contributes to mature granulocyte activation; it also stimulates proliferation of endothelial cells.

Granulocyte–monocyte colony-stimulating factor (GM-CSF), produced by T cells, macrophages, fibroblasts and endothelial cells, stimulates survival and growth of haemopoietic stem cells from their myeloid precursors and activation of a variety of other cells. Systemic administration of this cytokine causes mobilization of haemopoietic stem cells from bone marrow to blood circulation; such blood can then be used (after partial purification of the stem cells) for transplantation instead of bone marrow. GM-CSF, in conjunction with IL-4, efficiently stimulates *in vitro* development of dendritic cells, presumably from monocytes.

Monocyte colony-stimulating factor (M-CSF, CSF-1) is produced by many cell types as a transmembrane precursor. The soluble cytokine is released by proteolytic cleavage and is active as a disulphide-bonded homodimer. M-CSF is a growth and differentiation factor of monocytes, macrophages and their myeloid progenitors. It also acts as an activator of these cells.

Interferon family

Virologists have long known that individuals suffering from one viral disease rarely contract another one simultaneously. Similar *viral interference* can also be demonstrated *in vitro*: cells in cultures infected with one virus usually cannot be superinfected with another. One of the mediators of such interference is a family of soluble factors produced by virally infected cells, the *interferons* (IFNs).

The secretion of IFNs can be induced not only by viruses but also by other stimuli, some of which act both *in vivo* and *in vitro* (e.g. certain synthetic or natural polyribonucleotides), while others act only *in vivo*, presumably because they stimulate cells that are either absent or poorly represented in culture. The latter category of stimuli includes certain bacteria and bacterial products (e.g. endotoxin), rickettsiae, protozoa, organic compounds (e.g. pyran copolymers, polyacrylic acid copolymers, vinyl copolymers and polyvinylsulphate), antibiotics, polysaccharides, mitogens and antigens. There may be two mechanisms involved in IFN induction: a specific one mediated primarily by viruses and a more general one mediated by stimuli that alter cell metabolism.

The three main cell types capable of producing IFNs are fibroblasts, T lymphocytes and macrophages (monocytes). The ability to produce IFN is probably present in all vertebrates; production by invertebrate cells has not been demonstrated. Prokaryotes definitely do not produce IFNs, and although plants produce a substance that resembles it functionally the similarity may be superficial.

With few exceptions, IFN are species specific. Thus, human IFN functions in humans but not in most other vertebrate species and mouse IFNs work in the mouse but are otherwise ineffective, even in the rat. The reason for the species specificity could be species-specific differences in the receptors via which IFNs act. IFNs and their receptors have co-evolved in each species and so can interact within species limits but usually not beyond them. On the other hand, IFNs are not virus specific: IFNs induced by one virus can render cells resistant to other viruses. All viruses are probably sensitive to IFNs, though not all to the same degree. The variation in sensitivity is not dependent on the inducing virus; a virus may be relatively resistant to the IFN that it has induced, but this very same IFN may act as a strong inhibitor of a different virus.

There are three IFN types, designated by the Greek letters α, β and γ. *IFN-α* was originally discovered as a product of leucocytes and is therefore referred to as *leucocyte interferon (LeIF)*. *IFN-β* was discovered as a product of virus-infected fibroblasts and so is also referred to as *fibroblast interferon (FIF)*. IFN-α and IFN-β are sometimes grouped together into a single category of *type I interferons*. (IFN-β was originally split into two subtypes, IFN-β1 and IFN-β2. Later, however, IFN-β2 was shown to be identical to IL-6.) *IFN-γ*, the *immune* or *type II interferon*, is produced by mitogen- or antigen-stimulated T lymphocytes. It differs from IFN-α and IFN-β in that it is labile at pH 2 and has more pronounced anticellular than antiviral activity. The IFN types can be distinguished by specific antibodies: certain antibodies react only with α but not with β or γ IFNs; others react with β but not with α or γ; others still react only with IFN-γ.

The genes coding for IFN-α and IFN-β are similar in about 30% of their sequence; they may have diverged 250 million years ago, after the divergence of birds and mammals. The IFN-γ-encoding gene shows no significant sequence similarity to IFN-α- and IFN-β-encoding genes but it codes for a similarly sized protein in which certain single amino acid residues occupy the same position as in IFN-α and IFN-β. Therefore, the IFN-γ-encoding gene presumably diverged from a common ancestor even earlier than IFN-α- and IFN-β-encoding genes.

In the human genome there are more than 24 IFN-α-encoding genes and pseudogenes and at least one IFN-β- and one IFN-γ-encoding gene. All the functional IFN-α-encoding genes are in a single cluster on human chromosome 9; the IFN-β- and IFN-γ-encoding genes are on chromosomes 9 and 12, respectively. The individual genes in the IFN-α-encoding cluster are similar in 80–90% of their sequence; they probably diverged from a common ancestor not more than 25 million years ago, long after the emergence of primates in mammalian evolution. The IFN-α- and IFN-β-encoding genes are functional even though they lack introns; the IFN-γ-encoding genes have introns. Of the IFN-α-encoding genes 18 specify proteins that are each 166 residues long; the remaining six genes specify proteins containing 172 residues each. The IFN-γ protein is 146 residues long. IFN-α is an unglycosylated protein, whereas IFN-β and IFN-γ are glycoproteins but the oligosaccharide moieties are not essential for their biological activity. All mammals studied have been shown to contain several IFN-α-encoding genes but only one or two IFN-β-encoding genes, with the exception of bovids which possess multiple IFN-β-encoding genes, probably as a result of recent duplications. Other vertebrates contain IFN-β- but no IFN-α-encoding genes.

The tertiary structure of IFN-α has not yet been resolved but considerations of primary structure suggest that it is similar to that of IFN-β, which has been elucidated. The folding topology of IFN-β, in turn, resembles that of IL-4 from the haemopoietin family. Whether this resemblance means that the haemopoietins and IFNs are derived from a common ancestor remains an open question. The single polypeptide chain of IFN-β is folded into five (rather than four as in IL-4) α-helices (A–E), which are further clustered into a bundle held together by two disulphide bonds (Fig. 10.2). The five helices are interconnected by four loops (AB, BC, CD, DE) of which the AB loop is the longest. The A and B helices run parallel to each other; the three remaining helices are arranged in an antiparallel fashion. Four of the helices (A, E, B and C) correspond to the IL-4 bundle; the fifth helix (D) is appended to this structure. Loop AB, helix D and part of the DE loop form a contiguous site by which the molecule binds to its receptor.

In the tertiary structure of IFN-γ, the four-helix bundle motif is no longer recognizable, although 62% of the molecule is composed of α-helical regions. The IFN-γ molecule is a homodimer, each of the two identical subunits consisting of six α-helices ranging in length from 9 to 21 residues (Fig. 10.3). All helices of one subunit run parallel to each other but antiparallel to those of the second subunit. The helices are connected by short, non-helical segments and the whole structure is held together by extensive interhelical

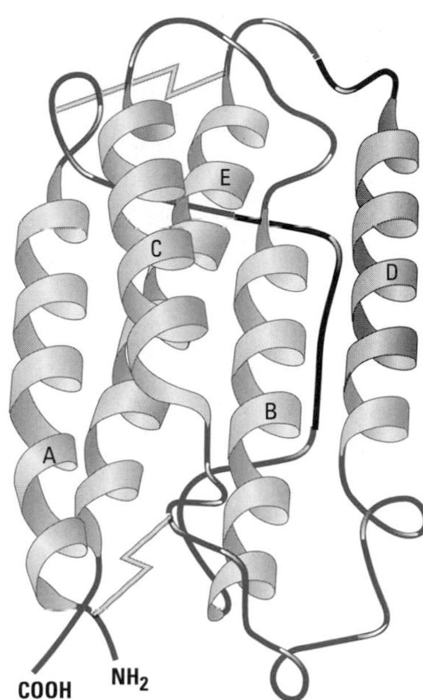

Figure 10.2 Tertiary structure of interferon-β (IFN-β): a ribbon model. The four helices of the bundle are labelled A, B, C, E; D is the extra α-helix outside the bundle. The two disulphide bonds are indicated by ⚡. The area interacting with the IFN-β receptor is highlighted. (From Senda, T. *et al.* (1992) *EMBO Journal*, **11**, 3193.)

contacts but there are no disulphide bonds in the molecule. Each subunit has a flattened, elliptical shape but the overall structure of the dimer is that of a compact globule.

All IFNs have both antiviral and anticellular activities, i.e. they interfere with the multiplication of viruses and regulate a variety of cellular functions (Table 10.3). Various IFNs are equally effective in inducing the antiviral state. The regulatory activity of IFN-γ, however, is much more potent than that of IFN-α and IFN-β.

The mechanism of antiviral activity is still not fully understood. Two enzymes have been implicated thus far, but other mechanisms probably contribute to the induction of the antiviral state. An infecting virus adsorbs to the host cell, penetrates the plasma membrane, releases its genetic material and replicates in the cell (Fig. 10.4). The new viruses leave the cell, enter the surrounding fluid and penetrate other cells. During the early stages of infection, the virus causes a series of changes in the metabolism of the host cell, some of which lead to activation of the IFN genes in the host's genome. The activated genes produce mRNA, which then leaves the nucleus for the cytoplasm where it is translated into IFN protein by ribosomes. The cytokine is secreted by the infected cell; it binds to IFN receptors on the cell that produced it, then to other nearby infected as well as uninfected cells. Signals triggered via the receptor then stimulate the synthesis of several enzymes, two of which seem to be especially important: protein kinase and 2-5A synthetase (Fig. 10.5). The first of these, *IF-2 protein kinase* (also called *PKR*, for protein kinase RNA-dependent because it is activated by double-stranded RNA), transfers a phosphate group to an initiation factor, IF-2, which is involved, along with other factors, in protein synthesis. IF-2 normally holds together the initiation complex of protein synthesis, which consists of the strand of mRNA to be

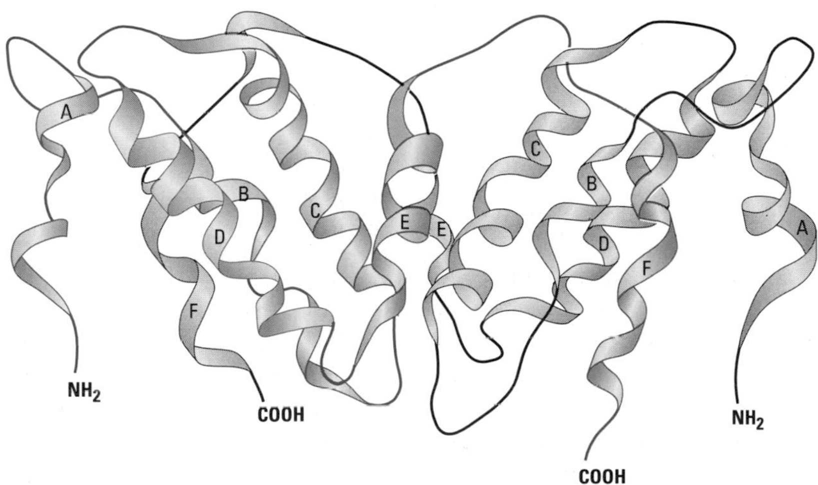

Figure 10.3 Tertiary structure of an interferon-γ (IFN-γ) dimer: a ribbon model. The two subunits are distinguished by colour shading. The α-helices in one subunit are labelled A–F. N and C are the two termini of each of the two polypeptide chains. (From the Protein Data Bank, Swiss 3-D; based on data from Ealick, S.E. *et al.* (1991) *Science*, **252**, 698.)

Table 10.3 Selected biological effects of interferons.

Effect	IFN-α/β	IFN-γ
Induction of antiviral state	++	++
Expression:		
2′,5′-oligoadenylate synthase	++	++
HLA class I	++	+
HLA class II	–	++
β_2-microglobulin	++	+
Complement factor B	+	+
ds RNA-dependent protein kinase	++	++
Fc-receptor	+	++
Activation of:		
cytotoxic T lymphocytes	++	–
granulocytes	–	++
macrophages	+	++
natural killer cells	+	++
Modulation of B-lymphocyte activity	+	+
Inhibition of cell growth	+	+

–, no effect; +, weak effect; ++, strong effect; ds, double-stranded; HLA, human leucocyte antigen; IFN, interferon.

translated, the smaller of the two ribosomal subunits and the initiator tRNA. The phosphorylated form of IF-2 can no longer assist in the formation of the initiation complex and when the cell is infected by the virus the viral mRNA remains untranslated; it is then attacked by ribonucleases and degraded. The protein kinase requires double-stranded RNA for its action and this is supplied by the viral mRNA. The latter, although single-stranded, loops back on itself to form double-stranded regions. The host's mRNA molecules lack such regions and are therefore protected from the action of the protein kinase.

The second enzyme, *2′,5′-oligoadenylate synthetase* (*2-5A synthetase*), catalyses the polymerization of adenine nucleotides into a long chain of adenine units, the 2,5-oligoadenylic acid. The oligonucleotide activates ribonucleases normally present in the cell in an inactive form, which then degrade viral mRNA. The presence of these enzymes makes uninfected cells resistant to virus attack (the cells are said to have acquired an *antiviral state*). In the infected cells these enzymes may help to suppress viral replication. IFN-γ also inhibits viral infection by another mechanism: in mouse macrophages infected by viruses such as ectromelia, vaccinia and herpes simplex-1, it induces the enzyme *nitric oxide synthase*, which produces nitric oxide (NO) and efficiently blocks viral replication (see Chapter 15).

Shortly after the first IFN is produced, yet another gene is activated and a regulatory protein is produced that eventually inactivates the IFN gene and thus halts IFN production. Hence, IFN serves as an intercellular messenger that brings the news of foreign invasion to other cells and mobilizes defence forces. It is an extremely effective messenger: only

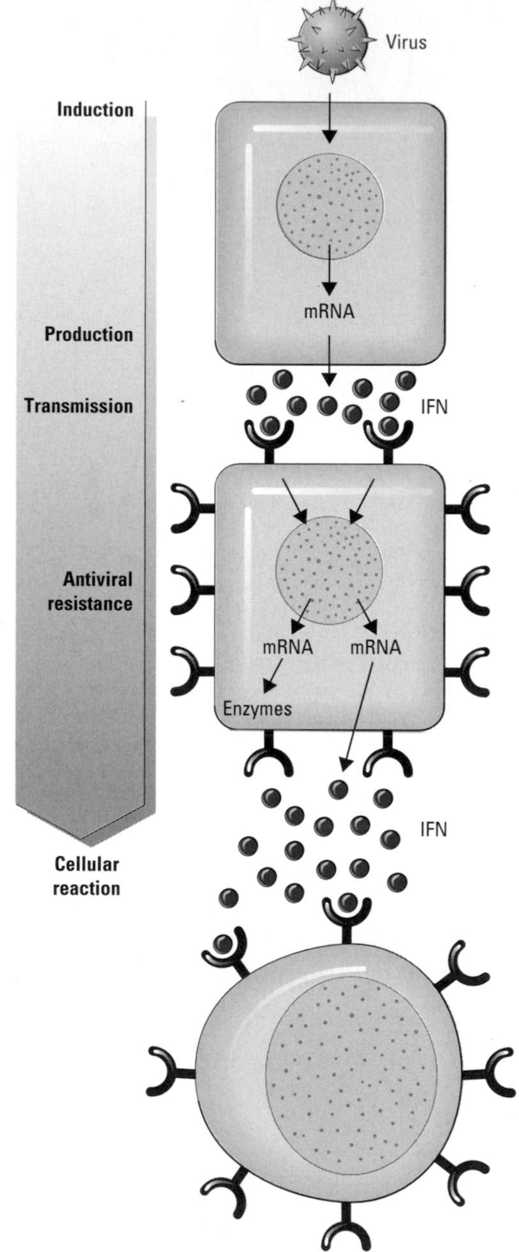

Figure 10.4 Interferon (IFN) induction, production, transmission and action. IFN inducers (viral nucleic acids) derepress *IFN* genes of the target cell and the activated genes produce mRNA that is subsequently translated into protein. The secreted IFN interacts with membrane-bound IFN receptors; the interaction activates the cell and derepresses genes coding for antiviral effector molecules. The diffusing IFN binds to receptors on neighbouring cells and induces antiviral resistance in them also.

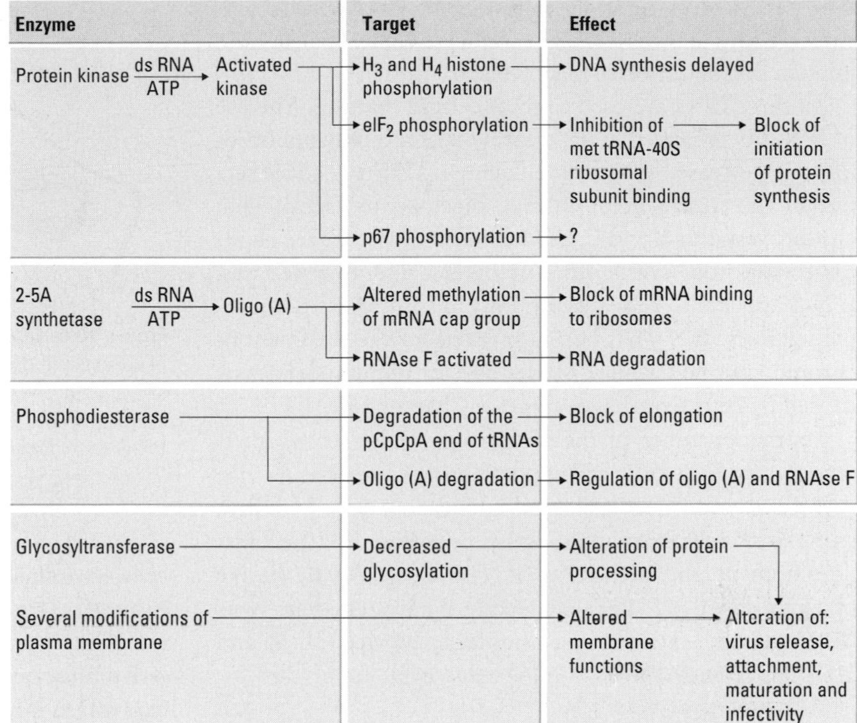

Enzyme
Target
Effect
Protein kinase
ds RNA
ATP
Activated kinase
H3 and H4 histone phosphorylation
DNA synthesis delayed
eIF2 phosphorylation
Inhibition of met tRNA-40S ribosomal subunit binding
Block of initiation of protein synthesis
p67 phosphorylation
?
2-5A synthetase
ds RNA
ATP
Oligo (A)
Altered methylation of mRNA cap group
Block of mRNA binding to ribosomes
RNAse F activated
RNA degradation
Phosphodiesterase
Degradation of the pCpCpA end of tRNAs
Block of elongation
Oligo (A) degradation
Regulation of oligo (A) and RNAse F
Glycosyltransferase
Decreased glycosylation
Alteration of protein processing
Several modifications of plasma membrane
Altered membrane functions
Alteration of: virus release, attachment, maturation and infectivity

Figure 10.5 Enzymes believed to be involved in the induction of antiviral resistance by interferon. ATP, adenosine triphosphate; ds, double-stranded; eIF_2, eukaryotic initiation factor 2. (Modified from Dianzani, F. (1985) *EOS: Rivista di Immunologia ed Immunofarmacologia*, 5, 59.)

1–10 IFN molecules are required to protect a cell against an IFN-sensitive virus.

The mechanism by which interferon *inhibits cell growth* is not known. One possibility is that inhibition occurs via the 2-5A system: the 2-5A synthetase is capable of adding adenosine monophosphate (AMP) to a variety of important metabolites, such as nicotinamide adenine dinucleotide (NAD) or adenosine diphosphate (ADP), and the dephosphorylated core of 2-5A inhibits DNA synthesis. Thus, via the 2-5A system, IFN has access to mechanisms that regulate normal cell growth.

The highly pleiotropic *anticellular activities* of IFNs are summarized in Table 10.3. Some of these activities are mediated by all three IFN types, but IFN-γ is effective at doses several orders of magnitude lower than those required for IFN-α or IFN-β action. Other activities are mediated only by IFN-γ and not by the two other IFNs. Some of the effects are inhibitory, others stimulatory. One of the first anticellular effects attributed to IFNs was their *ability to inhibit growth of neoplastic and normal cells*. The effects of IFN-γ are particularly striking in this regard, although IFN may not be the actual agent that arrests or kills the cells. IFN-γ has a strong synergistic effect with lymphotoxin (described later), which then acts directly on the cells.

Of all the *stimulatory effects* of IFN-γ, the most extensively studied is *induction of gene expression*. Cells exposed to IFN, particularly IFN-γ, begin to express previously silent genes. Among them are several that code for cell-surface markers and receptors, in particular the class II major histocompatibility complex (MHC) molecules. Although all three IFN types induce the appearance of class II molecules, IFN-γ does so more efficiently than the other two. It induces the expression of class II molecules in a wide variety of cells, including myelomonocytic cells, T lymphocytes, mast cells, fibroblasts, neurons, melanocytes and a number of tumour-derived cell lines. Since the appearance of class II molecules enables many of these cells to present foreign antigens to T lymphocytes, IFN-γ is thought to function as one of the regulators of immune response.

One further possible immunoregulatory function of IFN-γ involves high-affinity *Fc receptors* for monomeric IgG. IFN either induces the expression of Fc receptors on cells that previously lacked them or enhances the expression of already active genes. Strong effects are observed on immature myeloid cells at various stages of differentiation, from myeloblasts to mature granulocytes. The effect has been documented for both normal and neoplastic myeloid cells.

IFN-γ also *acts on different cells of the immune system*, influencing their growth and/or differentiation. It participates in the activation of cytotoxic T lymphocytes, causes an increase in NK cell activity and has a potentiating effect on immunoglobulin secretion by B cells in the late phase of immune response *in vitro*. Together with other cytokines,

IFN-γ induces maturation of resting B lymphocytes, activates mature neutrophils and monocytes/macrophages and inhibits the migration of macrophages.

All three IFNs are used to treat certain diseases. The use of IFN-α is preferred in the treatment of a rare lymphoproliferative disease, hairy cell leukaemia. IFN-α is also effective in the treatment of chronic myelogenous leukaemia, chronic hepatitis B and C, genital warts caused by the papilloma virus and several other malignant and viral diseases. IFN-β appears to relieve symptoms in some cases of multiple sclerosis. IFN-γ has been approved for the treatment of chronic granulomatous diseases and an immunodeficiency caused by defective phagocytes (see Chapter 15).

Another member of the IFN family is *IL-10*, which is secreted by T_H2 cells. It supports proliferation of B cells, thymocytes and mast cells and cooperates with TGF-β to stimulate B cells to switch to IgA production. IL-10 inhibits development and activation of T_H1 cells. An IL-10-like cytokine called *vIL-10* is encoded in the Epstein–Barr virus (EBV) genome. The sequence similarity between IL-10 and vIL-10 is about 70%.

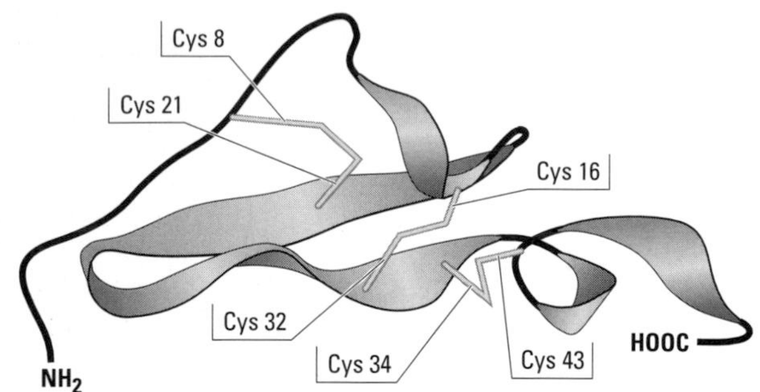

Figure 10.6 Tertiary structure of transforming growth factor-α (TGF-α): ribbon model. The broad segments represent β-strands arranged in two antiparallel β-sheets connected by disulphide bonds (══). (Based on data from Campbell, I.D. *et al.* (1989) *Progress in Growth Factors Research*, **1**, 13.)

Epidermal growth factor family

Epidermal growth factor (EGF) and *transforming growth factor α* (TGF-α), the two members of this family, are only peripherally involved in immunity. They are mitogenic molecules that play an important part in the control of normal cell growth; hence they are also involved in wound healing and in the inflammatory response. The TGF-α precursor is produced by monocytes, keratinocytes and many other cell types. The 160-residue precursor polypeptide is proteolytically cleaved into a 50-residue soluble molecule. Approximately 22% of the structure consists of β-strands, the rest comprises loops and regions with no clearly recognizable structural motifs; there are no α-helical regions in the molecule (Fig. 10.6). The four β-strands are organized into two antiparallel β-sheets, one major (four to five residues long) and one minor (two residues long). The structure is held together by three disulphide bonds. EGF and TGF-α act via the same receptor.

Interleukin-1 family

IL-1 is produced by a wide variety of cells including monocytes, tissue macrophages, Langerhans' cells, dendritic cells, T and B lymphocytes, NK cells, vascular endothelium, smooth muscle cells, fibroblasts, thymic epithelial cells, cells of the nervous system, keratinocytes and chondrocytes. Its range of action is equally extensive; it includes T and B lymphocytes, monocytes, macrophages, neutrophils, epidermal cells, endothelial cells, osteoblasts and hepatocytes among its targets (Fig. 10.7). It participates in the activation of T_H lymphocytes, promotes maturation and clonal expansion of B lymphocytes, enhances NK-cell activity, increases the expression of intercellular adhesion molecules (ICAMs) on vascular endothelial cells, chemotactically attracts macrophages and neutrophils to sites of inflammatory response, induces the synthesis of acute-phase proteins by hepatocytes (see Chapter 21), enhances collagen synthesis by epidermal cells, induces osteoblast proliferation, promotes bone resorption by osteoblasts, stimulates collagenase release from chondrocytes, induces prostaglandin production by muscle cells, influences the thermoregulatory centres in the hypothalamus and thus acts as a fever-inducing substance (pyrogen), and affects cells of the central nervous system causing somnolence (drowsiness, sleepiness) and anorexia (lack or loss of appetite).

IL-1 occurs in two different forms, IL-1α and IL-1β, encoded in different genes. Although both forms show only 20% sequence similarity, they bind to the same receptor and have similar, if not identical, biological properties. The mature human IL-1β chain folds into a tetrahedron with each triangular face formed by three antiparallel β-strands and each edge formed by two antiparallel β-strands, one on each adjoining side (so that altogether there are 12 β-strands connected by loops; see Fig. 10.8). The interior of the tetrahedron is filled with hydrophobic side-chains. The structure of the IL-1α molecule is similar to that of IL-1β despite containing 14 β-strands and one short helical region. IL-1α is mostly cell-associated while IL-1β is mainly released from cells.

Another member of this cytokine family is the *IL-1 receptor antagonist* (*IL-1Ra*) which is structurally related to IL-1β. This protein is produced by the same cells that produce

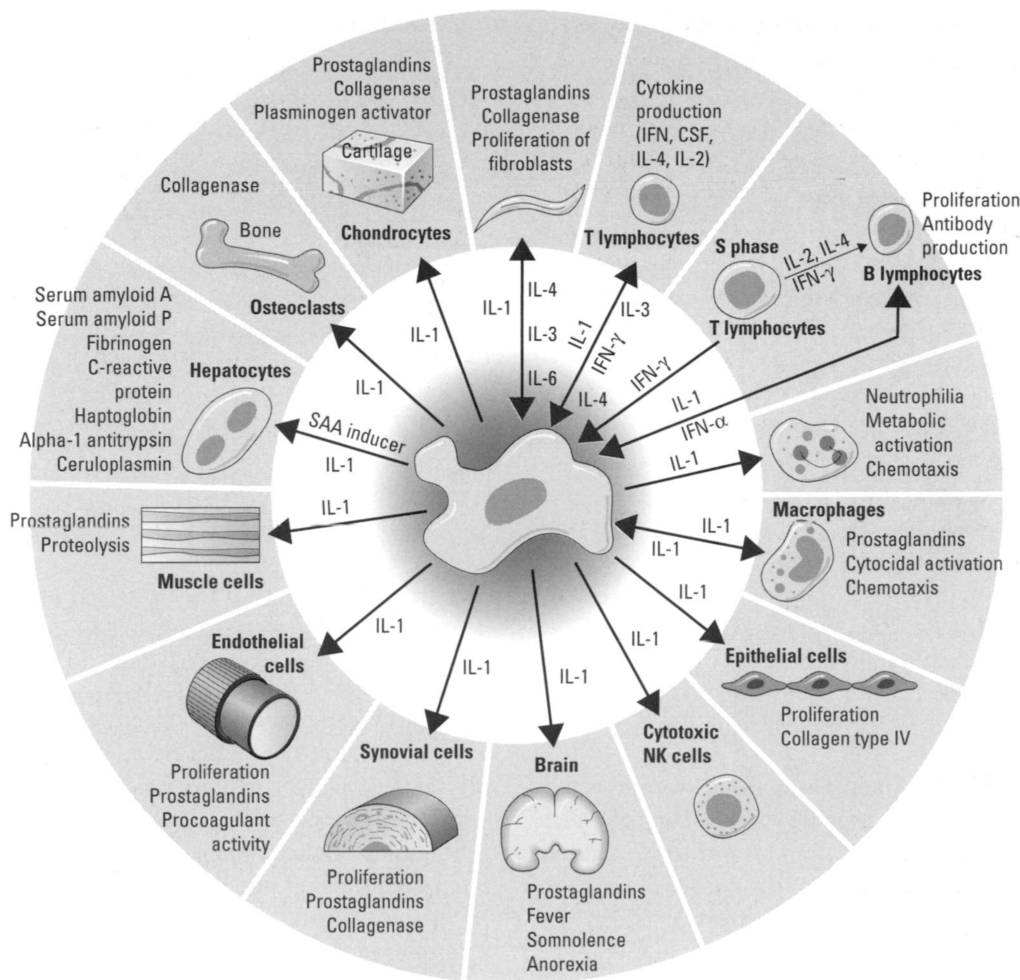

Figure 10.7 Biological effects of interleukin-1 (IL-1) on target cells and tissues. Several of the effects now known to be mediated by IL-1 were previously ascribed to other factors bearing different names. Some of the interactions between the IL-1 producing and the target cells are unidirectional (single arrows), others bidirectional (double arrows). CSF, colony-stimulating factor; IFN, interferon; IL, interleukin; SAA, serum amyloid A. (Modified from Oppenheim, J.J. *et al.* (1986) *Immunology Today*, 7, 45.)

IL-1 and binds to the IL-1 receptor, but this event does not lead to signalling. The competition between IL-1 and IL-1Ra dampens the activities of IL-1.

Tumour necrosis factor family

The three members of this family are tumour necrosis factor (TNF, also known as tumour necrosis factor-α or TNF-α), lymphotoxin-α (LT-α, also referred to as tumour necrosis factor-β or TNF-β) and lymphotoxin-β (LT-β). They are encoded in three closely linked genes within the MHC. The order of these genes, in the direction from centromere to telomere, is *LTB* . . . *TNF* . . . *LTA*. The three genes and the proteins they encode are related to each other in their sequence. LT-β is an integral membrane glycoprotein, LT-α is a secreted glycoprotein and TNF-α is a protein that can remain attached to the membrane by its long signal sequence until it is processed by a matrix metalloproteinase. The length of the human proteins LT-β, LT-α and TNF is 244 (240), 171 and 152 amino acid residues, respectively. LT-β forms complexes with LT-α on the cell surface but their function is unknown. LT-α and TNF are very similar in their biological activities. They owe their different names to the assays by which they were discovered. The inoculation of the bacillus Calmette–Guérin (BCG) into mice or rabbits, followed by an injection of endotoxin, elicits the appearance of a factor which, when inoculated into mice, causes the complete regression of transplantable tumours. Examination of the regressing tumours reveals extensive bleeding (haemorrhage) and tissue death (necrosis). The

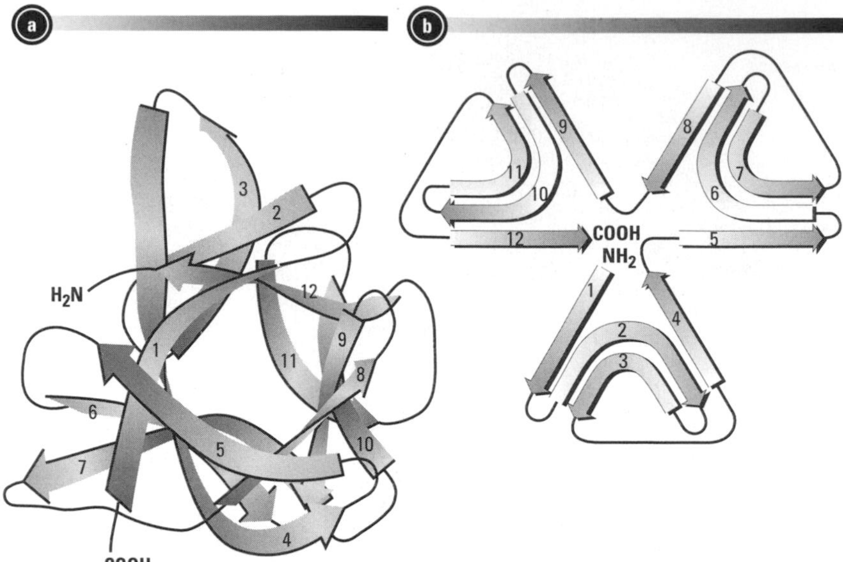

Figure 10.8 Tertiary structure of interleukin-1β (IL-1β). (a) Ribbon model of the tetrahedron molecule. (b) Diagram of the folding pattern showing the faces of the tetrahedron. β-strands are numbered from 1 to 12 (flat arrows). N and C are the termini of the single polypeptide chain. (From Priestle, J.P. *et al.* (1988) *EMBO Journal*, 7, 339.)

cytokine responsible for this effect was therefore named *tumour necrosis factor*. TNF-like activity can also be demonstrated in the media of monocyte cultures stimulated with BCG and endotoxin.

The activation of T lymphocytes by antigen or mitogen *in vitro* leads to the release of several cytokines, one of which was shown to kill certain tumour and transformed cells, as well as bystander normal cells, in particular fibroblasts and some lymphocytes. Because of its cytotoxic effect, the cytokine was designated *lymphotoxin*.

TNF is produced by monocytes and macrophages, as well as by many other cells including T and B lymphocytes and fibroblasts. LT-α is produced mainly by activated T and B lymphocytes. A potent stimulator of TNF production is the lipopolysaccharide (LPS), the cell-wall constituent of Gram-negative bacteria. In fact, effects such as fever, shock and activation of neutrophils, which accompany infections with Gram-negative bacteria, are probably directly or indirectly caused by TNF. The LPS of the bacteria stimulates macrophages to produce TNF which subsequently stimulates the production of IL-1, probably in addition to having a direct effect on tissues (Fig. 10.9). Activated macrophages have long been known to inhibit the growth of tumour cells. It now appears that most, if not all, of this inhibition is mediated by the TNF that the macrophages produce. The basis for haemorrhagic necrosis of tumours by TNF is the direct effect of TNF on endothelial cells. TNF alters the growth and morphology of endothelial cells that line the blood vessels supplying the tumour, increases the synthesis of factors favouring blood clotting and enhances endothelial cell adhesiveness for inflammatory cells (see Chapter 21). However, TNF also has cytotoxic or cytostatic effects on tumour cells, probably mediated by prostaglandins, proteases, free radicals and lysosomal enzymes, whose synthesis or release it stimulates.

TNF is identical with *cachectin*, a factor largely responsible for *cachexia* or physical wasting, usually associated with chronic or neoplastic diseases. Cachectin, produced by LPS-stimulated macrophages, was demonstrated to inhibit lipoprotein lipase, an enzyme involved in lipid storage in fat tissues. Furthermore, TNF is also identical with a macrophage-derived factor that activates eosinophils to kill parasites, such as schistosomes, in the presence of antibodies. Elevated TNF levels have been demonstrated in the blood of patients with visceral leishmaniasis and malaria. Finally, TNF may also have antiviral effects, although it is possible that these are actually mediated by IL-6, whose production it stimulates. Indeed, the versatility of TNF's effects stems mainly from the fact that it is part of a network of interactive signals operating in inflammatory or immune responses (see Chapter 21). The biological effects of LT are very similar to those of TNF-α, which is not surprising since both cytokines act via the same receptor.

TNF and LT are also similar in their tertiary structure. TNF forms homotrimers, with each subunit composed of a 157-residue polypeptide (Fig. 10.10). The wedge-shaped subunits are tightly packed into a conical-shaped trimer, the edge of one wedge interacting with the face of the neighbouring wedge. In each subunit, the polypeptide is folded into a structure referred to as the *jelly roll (Swiss roll) motif*, which was originally discovered in the coat proteins of certain spherical plant and animal viruses. The motif also occurs in the lectin concanavalin A and in the haemagglutinin protein of the influenza virus. A Swiss roll is a thin

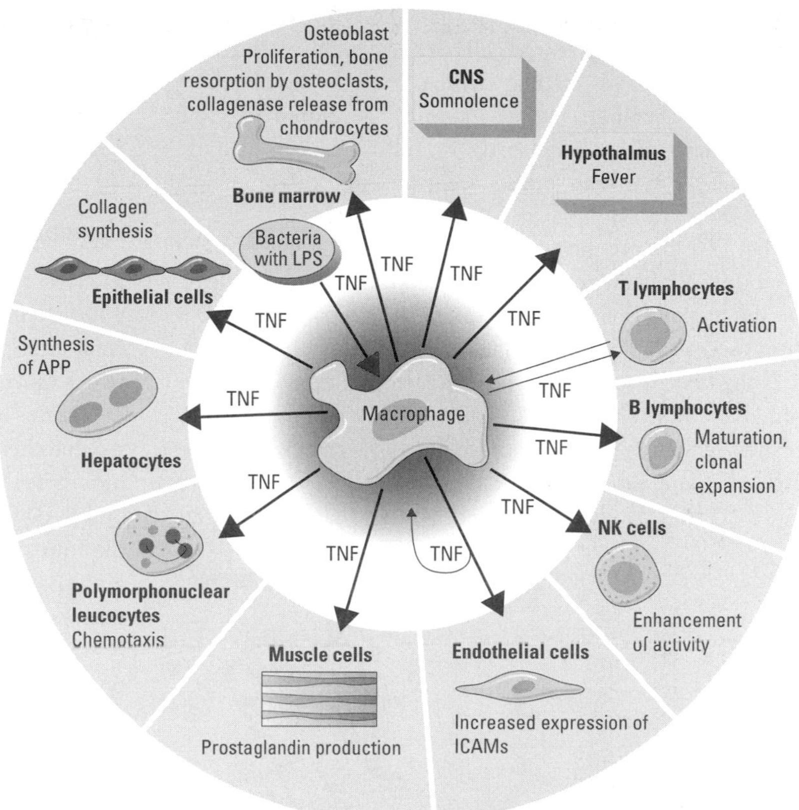

Figure 10.9 Biological effects of tumour necrosis factor-α (TNF-α) on target cells. APP, acute phase proteins (see Chapter 21); CNS, central nervous system; ICAM, intercellular adhesion molecules; NK, natural killer.

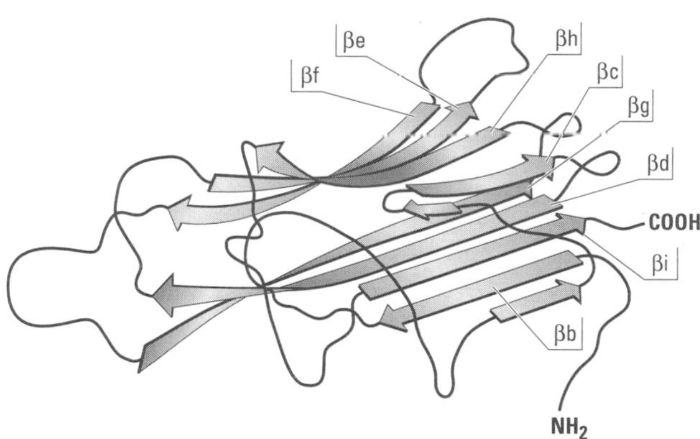

Figure 10.10 Tertiary structure of tumour necrosis factor-α (TNF-α). Ribbon model of one subunit. β-Strands are shown as flat arrows and are designated by letters corresponding to those used for homologous viral protein structures. (From Jones, E.Y., Stuart, D.I. & Walker, N.P.C. (1989) *Nature*, **338**, 225.)

layer of sponge cake spread with jelly and rolled up to form several round layers. You would need a strong imagination, however, to discern a jelly roll in the structure depicted in Fig. 10.10. It looks more like a sandwich formed by two antiparallel β-pleated sheets. The upper sheet contains three long and two short β-strands; the lower sheet is formed by five β-strands of gradually decreasing length.

Other TNF family members are the transmembrane proteins FasL (ligand of the 'death receptor' Fas or CD95), CD70 (ligand of the lymphocyte receptor CD27), CD30L (ligand of the receptor CD30), CD40L (gp39; ligand of the B-cell surface receptor CD40), 4-1BBL (ligand of the lymphocyte receptor 4-1BB), OX-40L (ligand of the receptor OX-40) and TRAIL (*T*NF-*r*elated *a*poptosis-*i*nducing *l*igand). The interactions of these mostly membrane-bound proteins with their receptors (which all belong to the TNF receptor family) have characteristic cytokine-like activatory or inhibitory effects on the target cells.

Transforming growth factor β family

The name *transforming growth factor* (*TGF*) has been given to two different kinds of molecules, now differentiated by the designations α and β. The TGF-α molecule is a member of the EGF family with which it shares biological and structural properties. The TGF-β molecules form a family of their own. Human TGF-β molecules occur in five different but related (66–80% sequence identity) forms designated TGF-β1 through TGF-β5, all encoded in different genes on distinct chromosomes. The TGF-β cytokines are produced by most nucleated cells and are highly pleiotropic in their biological effects, which include involvement in wound healing, tissue repair, development and haemopoiesis. They act mostly by inhibiting cell growth. The TGF-β2 cytokine is also a class switch factor in IgA synthesis.

The TGF-βs are secreted as inactive, disulphide-linked homodimers. They are then activated by proteolytic cleavage but remain in a dimeric form in which each subunit is composed of 112 amino acid residues and has a characteristic elongated structure that has been compared to a slightly folded left hand (Fig. 10.11). The structure contains nine β-strands, which form the four fingers (β1 and β2 the first finger, β3 and β4 the second finger, β5 and β6 the third finger, β7 and β8 the fourth fingers, these last two fingers being crossed), and three α-helices, of which α1 forms the thumb and α3 the heel of the hand. Each subunit contains nine disulphide-bonded cysteine residues in the palm of the hand. In the dimer, the α3 helix (the heel of the hand) of one subunit lies against the curved β-sheet of the other subunit.

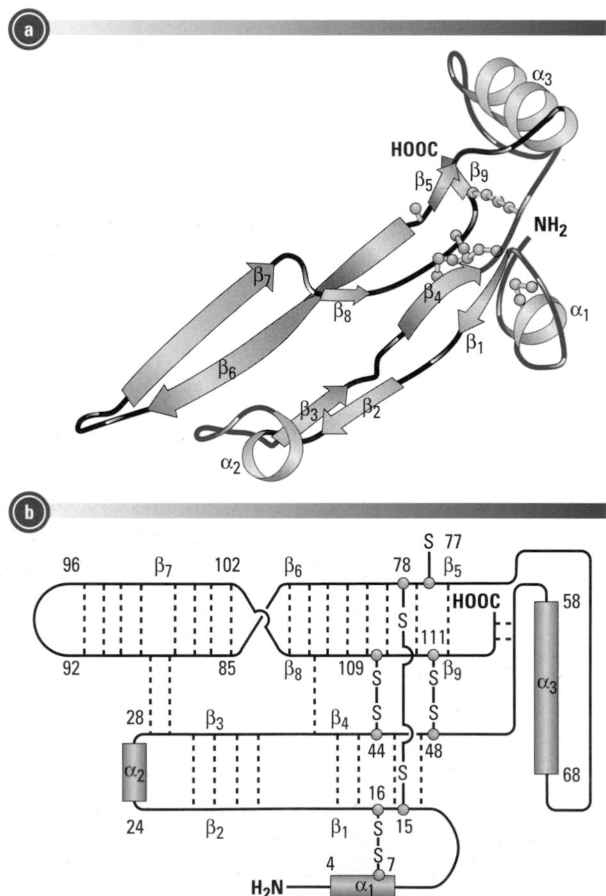

Figure 10.11 Tertiary structure of the transforming growth factor-β2 (TGF-β2) subunit. (a) Ribbon model. Cysteine residues are indicated by full circles, β-strands by numbered flat arrows; α-helices are numbered α1–α3. (b) Diagram of the strand topology showing disposition of disulphide bonds (S—S) and hydrogen bonds (dotted lines). Important residues are highlighted by numbers. Other symbols are as in (a). (From Daopin, S. *et al.* (1992) *Science*, 257, 369.)

Chemokine family

Members of this family are small molecules (M_r 8000–10 000) which, when bound to their receptors on vascular endothelial cells, form a concentration gradient down which leucocytes can migrate (see Chapter 21). The immobilization brought about by the receptors prevents the soluble chemokines from being washed away rapidly by the bloodstream. The family is divided into two subfamilies, α and β, distinguished by the organization of the first two of the four cysteine residues. In the α subfamily, the cysteines are separated by another residue X (C-X-C organization), whereas in the β subfamily, the two cysteines are adjacent (C-C organization). Both subfamilies are encoded in genes on distinct chromosomes: the α subfamily (which includes chemokines IL-8, GRO/MGSA, PF4, NAP-II, ENA-78) on human chromosome 4q12–21; and the β subfamily (with members MIP-1α, MIP-1β, MCAF/MCP-1, RANTES, I-309; see Table 9.1 for full designations) on chromosome 17q11–32. Both subfamilies differ also in their biological activities: α-subfamily members are potent chemoattractants and activators of neutrophils but not monocytes, whereas β-subfamily members are chemoattractants for monocytes and lymphocytes but not neutrophils. Some β-subfamily members also activate T cells. Individual members within each subfamily are 25–75% similar in their amino acid sequence; the sequence similarity between members of different subfamilies ranges from 20 to 40%. Each chemokine is either a dimer or tetramer (dimer of dimers) of identical subunits. The tertiary structure of the subunits in the subfamilies is very similar, whereas the organization of the subunits (the quaternary structure of the molecule) differs between the α and β subfamilies. Each subunit consists of a β-sheet formed by three antiparallel β-strands arranged into a Greek key motif, a long C-terminal α-helix positioned on top of the β-sheet and a series of irregular strands, turns and loops (Fig. 10.12). Dimers of the α subfamily assume a globular configuration that resembles the peptide-binding module of the MHC molecule (see Fig. 6.38): the three β-strands of each of the two subunits form a six-stranded β-sheet platform from which the two α-helices rise (Fig. 10.12). Dimers of the β subfamily form an elongated and cylindrical structure that has a different axis of symmetry from that of the α-subfamily globule and a different disposition of the α-helices

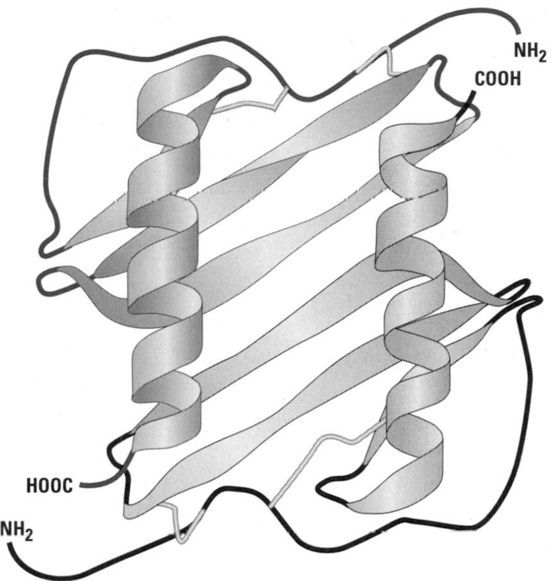

Figure 10.12 Tertiary structure of the interleukin-8 (IL-8) dimer: a ribbon model. The two subunits are differentiated by colour shading. Disulphide bonds are indicated by ═══ . Coils represent α-helices, flat ribbons β-strands. (From the Protein Data Bank Swiss 3-D; based on data from Baldwin, E.T. *et al.* (1991) *Proceedings of the National Academy of Sciences USA*, 88, 502.)

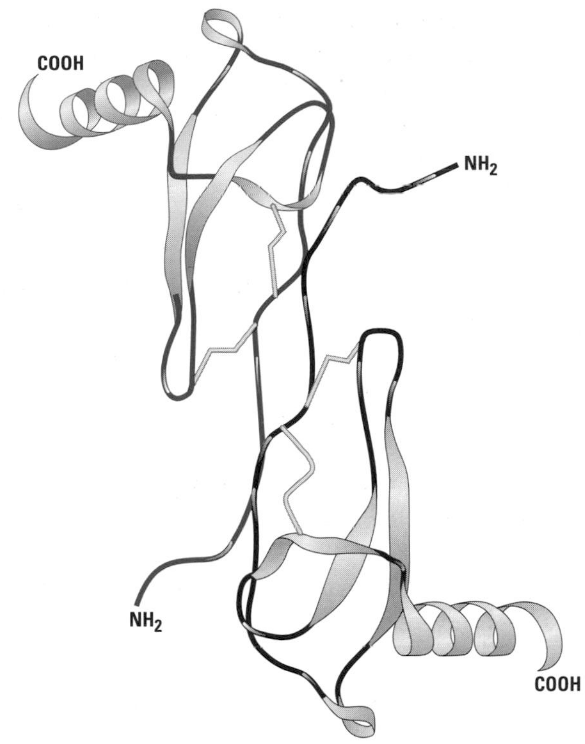

Figure 10.13 Tertiary structure of the macrophage inflammatory protein-1β (MIP-1β) dimer. The two subunits are distinguished by colour shading; disulphide bonds are indicated by ═══ . The coils represent α-helices, flat ribbons β-strands. (From the Protein Data Bank Swiss 3-D.)

(Fig. 10.13). The differences in quaternary structure between the α and β subfamilies explain why these subfamily members interact with different receptors and have different biological activities.

Other cytokines

IL-12 is a structurally unique cytokine made up of two disulphide-linked chains (p35 and p40); it is produced by monocytes, macrophages and B cells. It stimulates the development of NK and T_H1 cells and thus participates in the regulation of the immune response. The p35 chain is structurally related to the haemopoietin family, while p40 bears sequence similarity to the extracellular immunoglobulin-like and haemopoietin domains of the IL-6 receptor.

IL-14 is produced by T cells and some B-cell tumours and contributes to the activation of B cells. It is unrelated to other cytokines but shares significant similarity to the complement fragment Bb; IL-14 receptors also bind Bb.

IL-16 is produced by CD8+ T cells stimulated by histamine; it acts as a chemoattractant of CD4+ T cells. Preformed IL-16 is stored in cytoplasmic granules and is released rapidly upon stimulation. The biologically active form of this cytokine is an oligomeric aggregate that uses the CD4 molecule as its receptor. IL-16 appears to induce a state of resistance to HIV infection, possibly in part because of competition with the virus for the receptor.

IL-17, produced by activated CD4+ T cells, stimulates fibroblasts to secrete IL-6 and IL-8 and to express increased levels of the adhesion molecule ICAM-1. A molecule similar to IL-17 is encoded in the genome of *Herpes virus saimiri*.

Stem cell factor (SCF) is produced by many cell types, including bone marrow stromal cells, fibroblasts, hepatocytes, oocytes and others. It guides the development of haemopoietic, gonadal and pigment cell lineages. In haemopoiesis, it acts synergistically with IL-7 or GM-CSF. It is primarily produced in the form of two alternative transmembrane proteins but a secreted form also exists.

Migration inhibitory factor (MIF) is produced by activated T cells and possibly also other cells. Its name is derived from its ability to inhibit macrophage mobility. This property, however, is not unique to this cytokine; it is also exhibited by IL-4 and IFN-γ.

Certain other molecules, such as CD80 and CD86 (the ligands of CD28, the positive co-stimulatory receptor of T cells, and of CTLA-4, the negative regulatory receptor, respectively, see Chapter 16) can be regarded either as membrane-bound cytokines or as adhesion molecules (see Chapter 9).

Regulation

Several regulatory mechanisms have evolved to keep cytokines under tight control and to prevent beneficial effects from becoming harmful. Some mechanisms operate at the gene level, others at the level of product processing and others still at the level of mature products. As mentioned earlier, most cytokines are secreted after activation of the producing cells by appropriate stimuli: infectious agents, mechanical injury, toxic substances, antigens, bacterial products such as endotoxins, mediators of inflammation (see Chapter 11), complement components and cytokines themselves. By interacting with the producing cell, each of the stimuli initiates a complex set of reactions that ultimately lead (presumably via specialized transcription factors) to activation of the cytokine-encoding genes followed by secretion of the newly synthesized cytokine within hours after stimulation. The activated genes are then switched off again by another set of stimuli, which include glucocorticoid hormones and antagonistic cytokines. Much more rapid secretion is achieved by exocytosis of cytokines stored in cytoplasmic granules of various cell types.

At the level of product processing, regulation is achieved via the production of agents, mostly enzymes, that are responsible for conversion of the precursor form into a mature cytokine. Some cytokines (e.g. IL-1α, IL-1β, TNF-α, M-CSF and SCF) are initially inserted in the plasma membrane and are subsequently cleaved proteolytically and released as soluble molecules. In some cases, both the membrane-bound and soluble forms have biological activities, while in others only the soluble forms do. Other cytokines (e.g. TGF-β) are secreted in a biologically inactive form and are then activated enzymatically. The enzymes responsible for the processing remain unidentified (with the exception of a cysteine protease, the *IL-1 converting enzyme*, *ICE*, involved in IL-1β processing); they presumably become available during the immune and inflammatory responses.

Finally, at the level of mature cytokines, a number of molecules have been shown to exert a regulatory effect by binding to the cytokine. In addition to antagonistic cytokines, there are molecules in the blood and tissue fluids that either enhance or inhibit cytokine activities. Some of these molecules (e.g. the serum α_2-macroglobulin) act relatively non-specifically by binding to several cytokines, while others are highly specific. The latter include secreted forms of cytokine receptors such as TNF-R, IL-1R, IL-2R and IL-6R. The enhancing regulators achieve their effect, for example, by promoting cytokine secretion or by extending the half-life of the cytokine. The inhibitory regulators presumably block the active sites and thus prevent the cytokines from acting systemically; such is the case with IL-1Rα. Some cytokines (e.g. LIF and IL-1) are deposited on the extracellular matrix of the connective tissue, skin and bone; they can be released rapidly when the matrix breaks down during injury and tissue repair. Others (e.g. GM-CSF, SCF and IL-3) are bound to the stromal cells of the bone marrow and interact only with those haemopoietic cells with which they come directly into contact. Others still (e.g. MIP-1β and IL-8) are bound to the proteoglycans of the endothelial cells at inflammatory sites, where they promote leucocyte extravasation.

Cytokine activities are also regulated via cytokine receptors. The latter can be upregulated or downregulated by changing the expression of the encoding genes; they can be blocked by receptor antagonists that bind but do not initiate signal transduction; and their numbers can be reduced by internalization and shedding. Many cytokine receptors are reversible complexes of two or more subunits, one of which is often shared by several cytokines. Competition of cytokine receptors for the limited amount of the shared subunit (dependent on concentrations of the respective cytokines) also contributes to the regulation.

Some pathogens have learned how to subvert the regulatory mechanisms and alter them to their own advantage. Cowpox and vaccinia viruses, for example, produce a protein that binds to and inactivates IL-1β; the Shope fibroma virus secretes a protein that binds and inactivates TNF; and the myxoma virus produces a protein that resembles the IFN-γ receptor. EBV and cytomegalovirus contain genes homologous to the IL-10 and MIP-1α receptor genes, respectively, and presumably use them to upset the regulatory network and thus escape, or at least blunt, an immunological attack.

Function: the cytokine network

The function of cytokines is, in general, to coordinate the action of many different cell types participating in the immune and inflammatory responses. More specifically, their functions include the control of proliferation and differentiation of haemopoietic cells, recruitment of leucocytes to the site of infection and the activation of leucocytes and their effector mechanisms. Some cytokines also act directly as effector molecules: they arrest the growth of cells, contribute to target cell killing and have antiviral or antibacterial effects.

The release of cytokines follows the activation of the producing cell. The released cytokines induce a high level of receptor expression on the target cell and activate other producing cells. The latter produce different cytokines that again act on producing and target cells, and so the process continues until a large number of different cells have very rapidly become involved in the response. The cells and the cytokines act upon each other in a complex manner forming a *network* of interactions. The complexity of the network is a result of the production of multiple cytokines by the same cell; single cytokines acting on many different target cells; cytokines produced by one cell that stimulate the production of different cytokines from other cells; and cytokines interacting between themselves, some synergistically, others antagonistically.

The complexity of the cytokine network can be illustrated by focusing on two cell types that play a key part in the adaptive immune response: the macrophages and the T_H cells (Fig. 10.14). The encounter between macrophage and antigen in the presence of cytokines produced by stimulated T_H lymphocytes activates the cell. One consequence of activation is the secretion of more than a dozen different cytokines by the macrophage. These cytokines then act on a variety of cells: they assist T_H lymphocytes in their stimulation; they direct the differentiation of haemopoietic stem and progenitor cells; they act on neutrophils to effect their chemotaxis, adherence to vascular endothelium and extravasation; they promote the involvement of vascular endothelial cells and fibroblasts of the connective tissue in the inflammatory response; and they stimulate the hypothalamus to trigger systemic effects (see Chapter 21).

Activated T_H cells, too, secrete more than a dozen different cytokines, some of which are the same as those produced by macrophages (see Fig. 10.7). The various cytokines act on a number of different cells: other activated T_H cells, to boost their clonal expansion; cytotoxic T-cell precursors, to advance their differentiation into effector cells; NK cells, to promote their activation; haemopoietic stem and progenitor cells, to promote haemopoiesis; resting B lymphocytes, to effect, together with antigen, their activation; activated B cells, to assist in their differentiation into plasma cells; plasma cells, to help in immunoglobulin secretion; and eosinophils, to foster their growth and mediator release. The two types of T_H lymphocytes (T_H1 and T_H2) produce different cytokines that participate in distinct responses. The IL-2, IFN-γ and other cytokines produced by activated T_H1 cells participate primarily in cell-mediated and inflammatory responses and to a lesser degree in humoral responses. The IL-4, IL-5, IL-6, IL-10, IL-13 and other cytokines secreted by activated T_H2 cells mainly promote B-lymphocyte functions, favouring IgA and IgE responses against parasites and in allergic conditions. There is an antagonistic relationship between some of the cytokines produced by the two types of T_H lymphocytes.

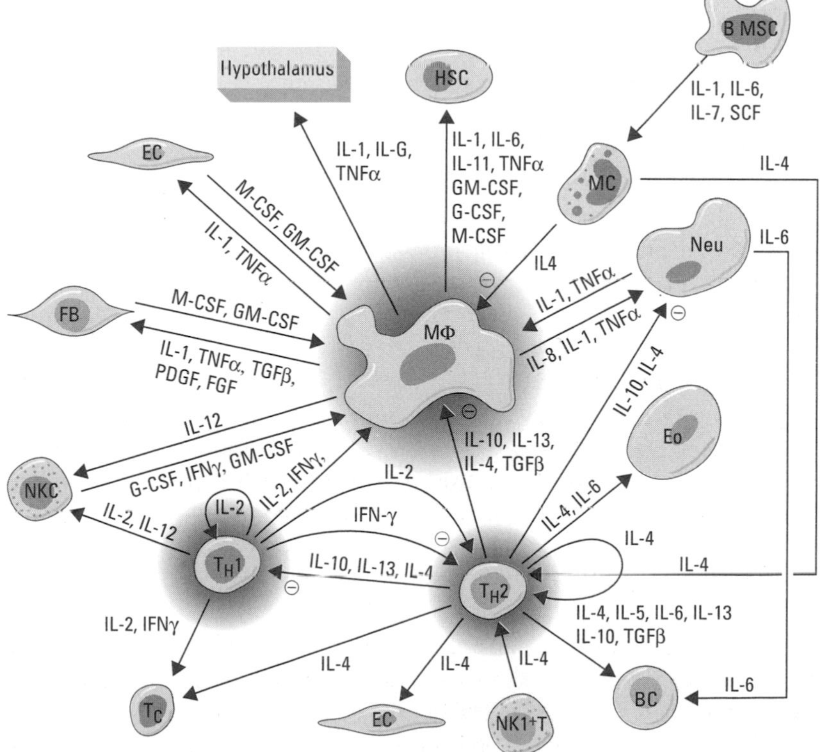

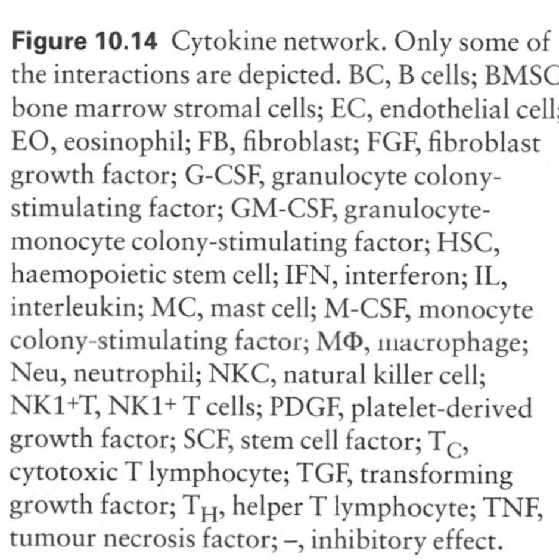

Figure 10.14 Cytokine network. Only some of the interactions are depicted. BC, B cells; BMSC, bone marrow stromal cells; EC, endothelial cell; EO, eosinophil; FB, fibroblast; FGF, fibroblast growth factor; G-CSF, granulocyte colony-stimulating factor; GM-CSF, granulocyte-monocyte colony-stimulating factor; HSC, haemopoietic stem cell; IFN, interferon; IL, interleukin; MC, mast cell; M-CSF, monocyte colony-stimulating factor; MΦ, macrophage; Neu, neutrophil; NKC, natural killer cell; NK1+T, NK1+ T cells; PDGF, platelet-derived growth factor; SCF, stem cell factor; T_C, cytotoxic T lymphocyte; TGF, transforming growth factor; T_H, helper T lymphocyte; TNF, tumour necrosis factor; –, inhibitory effect.

IFN-γ secreted by T_H1 cells, for example, inhibits cytokine production by T_H2 cells, whereas IL-4, IL-10 and IL-13 secreted by T_H2 cells inhibit cytokine production by T_H1 cells, probably via effects on antigen-presenting cells.

Cytokine receptors

Cytokines act via receptors on the surface of target cells. The distribution of the receptors among the various cell types fixes the range of the cytokine's action and determines the cytokine's biological effects. All receptor molecules consist of an extracellular, transmembrane and cytoplasmic part. The extracellular part of most receptors is composed of several domains or repeated units characterized by distinctive sequence motifs. Many receptors have a combination of different domains or repeats. Some receptors are single-polypeptide chain molecules, others consist of two or more chains differentiated by the Greek letters α, β and γ. Often one of the chains specializes in cytokine binding while the other functions in signal transduction, usually via its cytoplasmic domain. In several instances different α (ligand-binding) chains share the same β (signal-transduction) chain, a condition potentiating redundancy and antagonism in the cytokine's action.

Like cytokines, cytokine receptors, too, are classified into several families encompassing members with amino acid sequence similarity ranging from 15 to more than 50%. The classification is based on the type of extracellular domains, and since one receptor may have more than one domain type it can be a member of several families simultaneously. The main receptor families are the cytokine receptor family, interferon receptor family, immunoglobulin family, protein tyrosine kinase receptor family, tumour necrosis factor receptor family and seven transmembrane-spanning receptor family. A brief description of the individual families follows; the properties of the immunologically relevant receptors are summarized in Table 10.4.

Cytokine receptor family (CKR-F)

Also referred to as *cytokine receptor family type (class) I* or *haemopoietic receptor family*, this group includes receptors for IL-2, IL-3, IL-4, IL-5, IL-6, IL-7, IL-9, IL-12, IL-15, G-CSF, GM-CSF, LIF and several cytokine receptors not involved in immunity (Epo, CNTF, GH) among its members and represents the largest known collection of cytokine receptors (Fig. 10.15). The extracellular part of each of these receptors consists of two or three different types of domains: the *cytokine (CK) domain* characterized by the presence of the Cys-X-Trp motif and three additional conserved cysteine residues; the *fibronectin type III (FNIII) domain*, which contains a Trp-Ser-X-Trp-Ser or WSXWS motif essential for ligand binding and signal transduction; and (in some receptors) the s(*C2)-type immunoglobulin-like domain*. (Here, X stands for unspecified amino acid residue.) Each of these three domains is approximately 100 residues long and consists of two antiparallel β-pleated sheets of four and three β-strands. The tertiary structure of the immunoglobulin-like domain is described in Chapter 8; the CK and FNIII domains resemble the immunoglobulin-like domain but differ from it in the detailed arrangements of the β-strands (Fig. 10.16). The receptor molecules each consist of one to three glycosylated polypeptide chains. If more than one chain is present, one chain alone binds the ligand with low strength (affinity) and the second chain serves as an *affinity converter* that greatly increases the affinity of the receptor and effects signal transduction.

Some converter chains associate with different α (low-affinity) chains. Thus, IL-3R, IL-5R and GM-CSFR each have a distinctive α chain with a short cytoplasmic domain but all three associate with the same β chain (KH97). Similarly, IL-6R, IL-11R, LIFR, OSMR and CNTFR share a common signalling β subunit (gp130) that has structural similarity to G-CSFR. The IL-6–IL-6R complex binds two gp130 subunits which become disulphide linked; the dimerization leads to tyrosine phosphorylation necessary for signal transduction. IL-2R is a complex of three chains. The IL-2R α chain is not a member of the CKR-F; instead it has two complement control protein (CCP) domains. It binds IL-2 with low affinity but is unable to transmit the signal to other molecules. IL-2R β and γ chains are members of the CKR-F. The IL-2R β chain binds IL-2 with intermediate affinity, whereas the IL-2R γ chain does not bind IL-2 at all. The β and γ chains are involved in signalling. Mutations in the human γ chain-encoding gene cause X-linked severe combined immunodeficiency (X-SCID), a lethal condition characterized by the absence or greatly reduced number of T lymphocytes, and by severely depressed cellular and humoral immunity. The same γ chain is also part of IL-4R, IL-7R, IL-9R and IL-15R.

IFN receptor (cytokine receptor type II) family (IFNR-F)

The superfamily contains three IFN receptors (IFN-αBR, IFN-α/βR and IFN-γR) and the IL-10R. All four receptors are molecules with an extracellular part consisting of two to four FNIII domains (Fig. 10.17). The N-terminal FNIII domain of the receptors contains two conserved tryptophan and a pair of conserved cysteine residues. The second FNIII domain has a unique disulphide loop formed by another pair of conserved cysteine residues. This two-domain unit has apparently been duplicated in IFN-αBR to form a

Table 10.4 Characteristics of cytokine receptors*.

Name	M_r (× 10^3) mature	No. of amino acid residues precursor/mature	CHO	Chromosome	Affinity: K_d (M)
Type I cytokine receptor family (CKR-F)					
IL-2R					
α-chain (CD25)	55	272/251	2	10p15–14	10^{-8}
β-chain (CD122)	70–75	551/525	4	22q11.2–12	10^{-7}
γ-chain (CD132)	64	369/347	6	Xq13	None
IL-3R					
α-chain (CD123)	70	378/360	6	Xp22.3/Yp13.3	10^{-7}
β-chain (KH97) (CDw131)	120	897/881	3	22q12.2–13.1	None
IL-4R					
α-chain (CD124)	140	825/800	6	16p12.1–11.2	10^{-10}
IL-2R γ-chain (CD132)					
IL-5R					
α-chain (CDw125)	60	420/400	6	3p26	5×10^{-9}
β-chain (see IL-3Rβ)					
IL-6R					
α-chain (CD126)	80	468/449	5	1q21	10^{-9}
β-chain (gp130; CD130)	130	918/896	10	5q11	None
IL-7R					
α-chain (CD127)	68	459/439	5	5p13	High (2×10^{-10}), low (10^{-8})
IL-2R γ-chain (CD132)					
IL-9R					
α-chain	>57	522/482	2	Xq28/Yq12	1.9×10^{-10} (mouse)
IL-2R γ-chain (CD132)					
IL-11R					
α-chain (mouse)		432/409	2	9p13	10^{-8}
IL-6R β-chain (CD130)					
IL-12R					
α-chain					
β-chain	100	662/638	6	?	$2–5 \times 10^{-9}$
IL-13R					
IL-4R α-chain (CD124)					
IL-13Rβ-chain	65	427/406	11	X	10^{-8}
IL-15R					
α-chain (CD25-like)	60	268/231	1	10p15–14	10^{-11}
IL-2R β-chain (CD122)					None
IL-2R γ-chain (CD132)					None
G-CSFR (CD114)	150	836 (783)/812 (759)	9	1p35–34.3	1×10^{-10} to 5×10^{-10}
GM-CSFR					
α-chain (CD116)	80	400/378	11	Xp22.3/Yp13.3	3.2×10^{-9}
IL-3R β-chain (CDw131)					
LIFR					
α-chain	190	1097/1053	19	5p13–p12	High (0.15×10^{-10}), low (10^{-9})
IL-6R β-chain (CD130)					
Immunoglobulin family (IG-F) and protein tyrosine kinase receptor family (PTKR-F)					
IL-1R					
Type I (CD121a)	80	569/552	6	2q12	~10^{-9}
Type II (CD121b)	60–68	398/385	6	2q12–22	~10^{-9}
M-CSFR (Fms; CD115)	150	972/953	11	5q33–35	0.4×10^{-10}
SCFR (*Kit*; CD117)	145	976/954	10	4q12	?
IL-16R (CD4)	55	458/433	2	12pter–p12	
Tumour necrosis factor receptor family (TNFR-F)					
TNFR-I (p55) (CD120a)	55	455/426	3	12p13	5×10^{-10}
TNFR-II (p75) (CD120b)	75–80	461/439	2	1p36–32	10^{-10}

(*Continued on p. 312*)

Table 10.4 (*Continued.*)

Name	M_r (× 10^3) mature	No. of amino acid residues precursor/mature	CHO	Chromosome	Affinity: K_d (M)
CD27	50–55	260/240	1	12p12	
CD30	105–120	595/577	2	1p36	
CD40	50	265/245	2	20q12–13.2	
CD95 (Fas, APO-1)	43	335/319	2	10q24.1	
OX-40 (CD134)	48	277/249	2	1p36	
4-1BB (CDw137)	30	255/232	2	?	
Seven transmembrane-spanning receptor family (STSR-F)					
IL-8R					
High affinity	58–67	350/?	4	2q35	3.6×10^{-9}
Low affinity	>32	355/?	3	2q35	20× lower than that of high-affinity receptor
MIP-1αR	52	355/?	1	3p21	5×10^{-9}
Interferon receptor family (IFNR-F)					
IFN-αBR	95–110	557/530	11	21q22.1	10^{-9}–10^{-11}
IFN-α/βR (CD118)	102	331/305 (239)	5	21q22.1	?
IFN-γR					
α-chain (CDw119)	90	489/472	5	6q12–22	10^{-9}–10^{-10}
β-chain	>35	337/310	6	21q22	?
IL-10R	90–110	578/557	6	11q23.3	2×10^{-10}
Transforming growth factor β receptor family (TGFβ-F)					
TGF-βRI	53	503/479	1	9q33–34	5×10^{-12} to 30×10^{-12}
TGF-βRII	65	565/542	3	3p22	
TGF-βRIII (rat)	250–350	853/829	7	1p33–32	3×10^{-12} to 30×10^{-12}

* All data except those indicated refer to human receptors.
CD, cluster differentiation; CHO, number of potential *N*-glycosylation sites; CSF, colony stimulating factor; G-CSF, granulocyte colony-stimulating factor; GM, granulocyte-monocyte colony-stimulating factor; IFN, interferon; IL, interleukin; K_d, dissociation constant (see Chapter 14); *kit*-protein kinase (tyrosine); LIF, leukaemia inhibitory factor; M-CSF, monocyte colony-stimulating factor; MIP, macrophage inflammatory protein; R, receptor; TGF, transforming growth factor; TNF, tumour necrosis factor.

four-domain chain. (Note that the Greek letters in these designations refer to the ligand and not to the polypeptide chains comprising the receptor.) IFN-αBR binds one form of IFN-α encoded in one of the 24 IFN-α genes (IFN-α8). The IFN-α/βR binds IFN-α and IFN-β. Both receptors probably consist of more than one polypeptide chain; the human IFN-α/βR contains a disulphide-bonded homodimer. Biologically active IFN-γR is composed of at least two polypeptide chains, α and β, each containing two FNIII domains (Fig. 10.17). High-affinity interaction between IFN-γ and the IFN involves a single homodimer of the former and two molecules of the latter (the two α chains of the receptor do not interact with each other). How the β chain of the receptor fits into this complex is not known.

Immunoglobulin family (IG-F)

The extracellular parts of the receptors belonging to this family consist of either exclusively immunoglobulin-like domains (Fig. 10.18) or a combination of immunoglobulin-like and other domains (see Fig. 10.15). Members of the former category include IL-1R, M-CSFR, SCFR and CD4, the receptor for IL-16, as well as receptors for several cytokines acting on non-immune cells (PDGF, VEGF, FGF; abbreviations are explained in Fig. 10.18). Members of the latter category include IL-6R α and β chains, LIFR α and β (gp130) chains and possibly also IL-3Rα, IL-5Rα, IL-7Rα and GM-CSFRα (abbreviations are explained in Fig. 10.5). Each of these chains has one immunoglobulin-like domain in addition to CK and FNIII domains. The

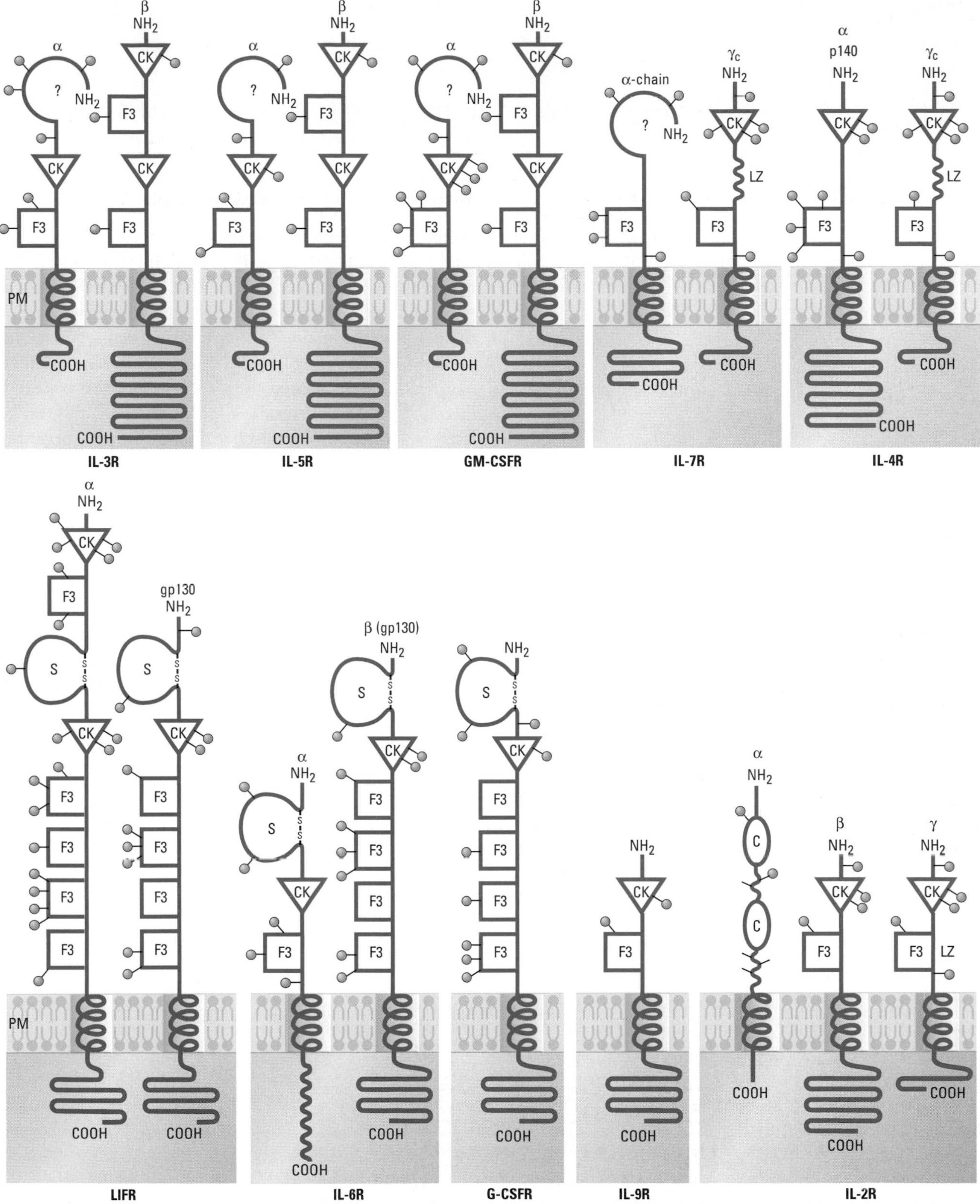

Figure 10.15 Cytokine receptor superfamily (CKR-F) type I. ⊸ and —, oligosaccharide chains, respectively. Domain designations: C, complement control protein; CK, cytokine domain; F3, fibronectin type III domain. Proteins: G-CSFR, granulocyte colony-stimulating factor receptor; GM-CSFR, granulocyte–monocyte colony-stimulating factor receptor; gp130, glycoprotein, M_r 130 000; IL, interleukin; LIFR, leukaemia inhibitory factor receptor; S, s(C2)-type immunoglobulin-like domain; LZ, leucine zipper; PM, plasma membrane. (Based on Callard, R. & Gearing, A. (1994) *The Cytokine Facts Book*. Academic Press, London.)

tertiary structure of the immunoglobulin-like domain is described in Chapter 8.

Protein tyrosine kinase receptor family (PTKR-F)

The characteristic feature of this family is the presence of the protein tyrosine kinase domain in the cytoplasmic region. Several receptors classified by their extracellular parts as belonging to the IG-F (M-CSFR, SCFR, VEGF, FGFR and EGFR) can also be classified by their cytoplasmic parts as belonging to PTKR-SF (Fig. 10.18).

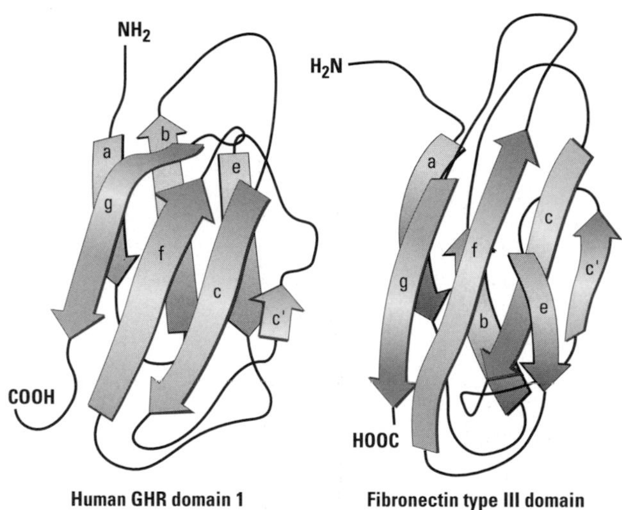

Figure 10.16 Tertiary structures of human growth hormone receptor (GHR) domain 1 (the cytokine or CK domains have a similar topology) and the fibronectin type III domain. β-Strands are designated by lower case letters. (Modified from Callard, R. & Gearing, A. (1994) *The Cytokine Facts Book*. Academic Press, London.)

Tumour necrosis factor receptor family (TNFR-F)

Prototype members of this family are the TNF receptors type I (TNFR-I) and type II (TNFR-II) (Fig. 10.19). The former is also known as p55 or CD120a and the latter as p75 or CD120b. Both are single-chain receptors with extracellular parts consisting of four cysteine-rich repeats, each some 40 residues long. TNFR-II has, in addition, a hinge-like region characterized by a high proportion of serine, threonine and proline residues, which are probably glycosylated by O-linked oligosaccharides. The repeat organization does not correspond to the exon organization of the encoding genes and the primordial gene encoding the four repeats is therefore thought to have arisen by unequal crossing-over. Sequence similarity between the two receptors is less than 25%, but both bind TNF and lymphotoxin. TNFR-I is found on most cell types, whereas TNFR-II is restricted to haemopoietic cells. Intracellular domains of the two TNF receptors are dissimilar, indicating that they use different signalling mechanisms. High-affinity interaction between the trimeric TNF and monomeric TNFR-I molecules occurs via clustering of three receptor molecules, each binding to one TNF monomer.

Among the other members of this receptor family are the leucocyte membrane molecules CD27, CD30, CD40, CD95 (Fas), OX-40 and 4-1BB. One of these receptors, CD40, is essential for the physiology of B cells (see Chapter 17). Another, CD95, is the major transducer of apoptotic signals in cytotoxic T (T_C) and NK cells (see Chapter 16); it is also

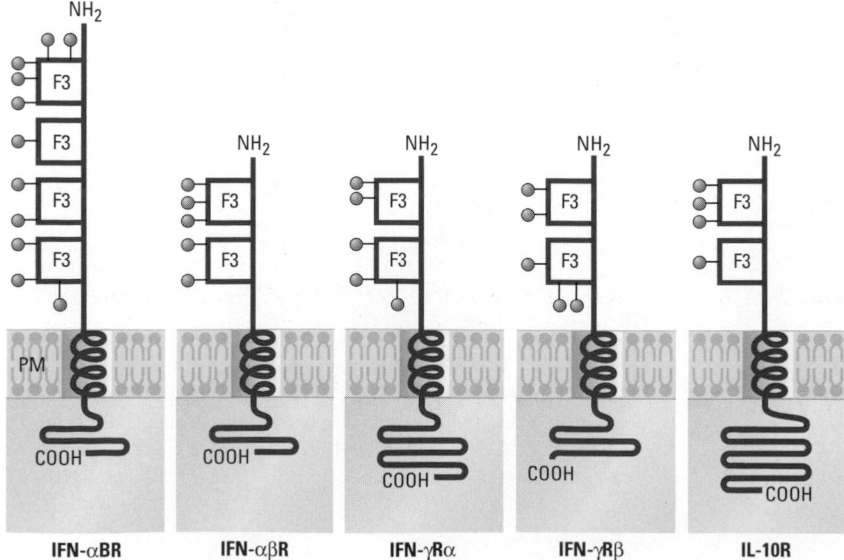

Figure 10.17 Interferon receptor family (IFNR-F). Only one chain of each receptor is shown. In reality, most of the receptors are homodimers or more complex structures. F3, fibronectin type III domain; ●–, oligosaccharide chains; IL, interleukin; PM, plasma membrane. (Based on Callard, R. & Gearing, A. (1994) *The Cytokine Facts Book*. Academic Press, London.)

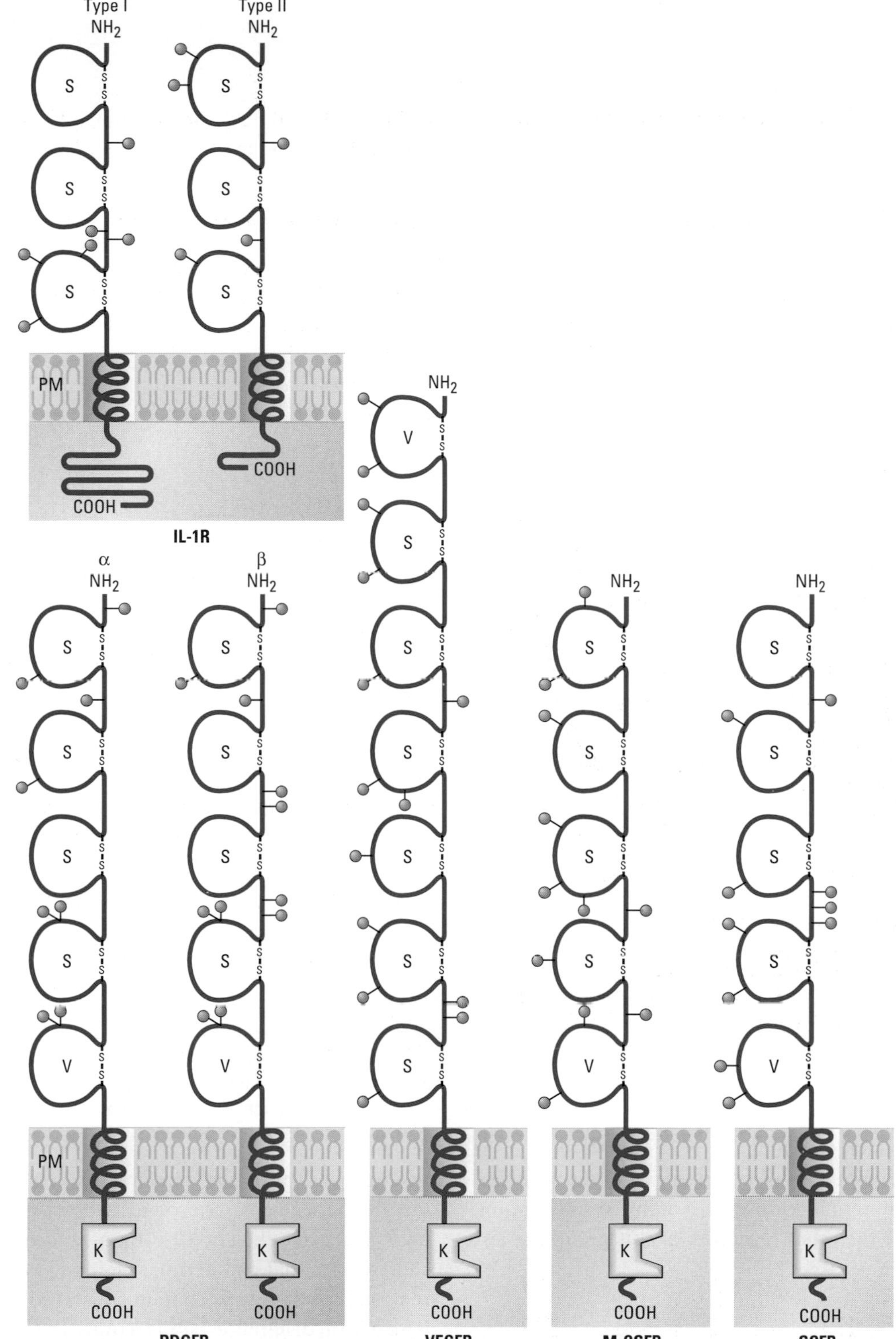

Figure 10.18 Immunoglobulin receptor family (IGR-F). V, v-type immunoglobulin-like domain; K, protein tyrosine kinase domain; ●—, oligosaccharide chain; IL-1R, interleukin-1 receptor; PDGFR, platelet-derived growth factor receptor; S, s(C2)-type immunoglobulin-like domain; VEGFR, vascular endothelial growth factor receptor; M-CSFR, monocyte colony-stimulating factor receptor; PM, plasma membrane; SCFR, stem cell factor receptor. (Based on Callard, R. & Gearing, A. (1994) *The Cytokine Facts Book*. Academic Press, London.)

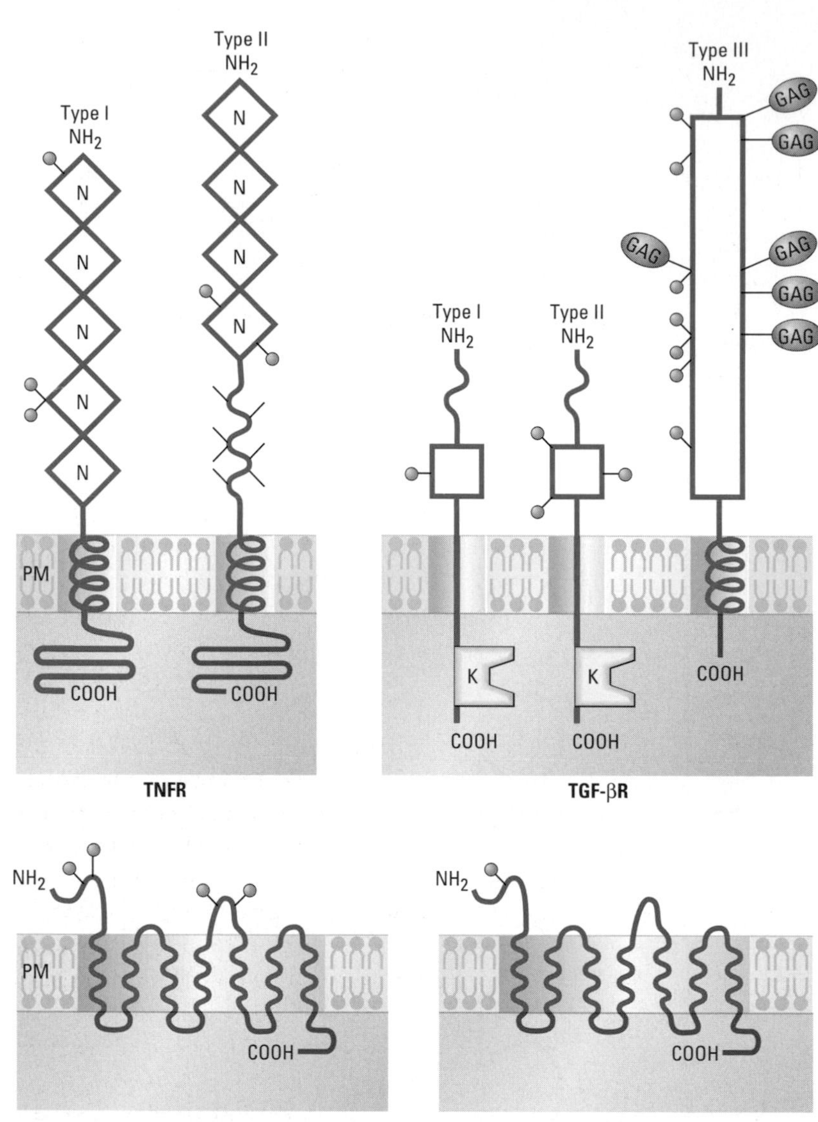

Figure 10.19 Tumour necrosis factor receptor family (TNFR-F), transforming growth factor-β receptor (TGF-βR) and seven membrane-spanning receptor superfamily (STSR-SF, here represented by IL-8R and MIP-1αR). GAG, glycosaminoglycan; K, tyrosine kinase domain; N, nerve growth factor receptor domain; IL, interleukin; MIP-1αR, macrophage inflammatory protein-1α receptor; PM, plasma membranes; ●–, *N*- and –, *O*-linked oligosaccharide chains, respectively. (Based on Callard, R. & Gearing, A. (1994) *The Cytokine Facts Book*. Academic Press, London.)

involved in the elimination of potentially autoreactive lymphocytes and the termination of T-lymphocyte activation. The functions of the other receptors of this group are less well understood.

Seven transmembrane-spanning receptor family (STSR-F)

This very large family comprises receptors that are only marginally involved in immunity. It does, however, contain receptors for chemokines such as IL-8 and macrophage inflammatory protein-1α (MIP-1α; see Fig. 10.9), the receptor for bacterial chemotactic peptides (fMLP; see Chapter 21) and the receptor for platelet-activating factor (PAF). The receptors are single-chain molecules with a short extracellular N-terminal region and a long transmembrane region that crosses the membrane seven times. The transmembrane segments are connected by three short extracellular and three intracellular loops and are followed by a short C-terminal cytoplasmic region. The N-terminus and the extracellular loops contain conserved cysteine residues, which form disulphide bonds required for ligand binding. It is believed that contact points between the ligand and the receptor include the transmembrane and intracellular regions of the latter. In the membrane, the receptors are associated with heterotrimeric GTP-binding proteins initiating signal transduction. The Duffy blood group antigen is also a member of this family; it binds IL-8 and related chemokines. Several chemokine receptors serve as co-receptors for the human immunodeficiency virus (see Chapter 26).

Other cytokine receptors

The receptor for *TGF-β (TGF-βR)*, which is peripherally involved in immunity, does not belong to the families described above. It occurs in three forms: high-affinity type I (M_r 55 000) and type II (M_r 80 000) and low-affinity type III (M_r 250 000–350 000) (see Fig. 10.19). The intracellular domains of the type I and II receptors possess serine/threonine kinase activity. Upon binding of TGF-β, the type I and II receptors associate with each other and jointly mediate signal transduction. The type III receptors do not transduce signals but concentrate TGF-β molecules on the cell surface and present them to the high-affinity receptors. The type III receptors include β-glycan, an integral membrane protein carrying glycosaminoglycan chains, and endoglin (CD105), a homodimer of two M_r 95 000 disulphide-linked subunits.

Intracellular signalling

The interaction of a cytokine with its receptor triggers a cascade of intracellular reactions that change the activities of the cell. In this regard, the cytokine–receptor system resembles many other ligand–receptor systems that convert an extracellular signal into a series of internal events leading ultimately to a cellular response, either positive or negative. There is a bewildering variety of signalling pathways which differ in the type of molecules they involve, the cellular compartments they traverse, the specifics of the interactions and the type of response they ultimately elicit. At the same time, however, they have certain features in common and their principal modes of operation are surprisingly few and simple. Since intracellular signalling has been referred to several times and occurs frequently in the following chapters, we use the cytokine–receptor system to explain the principles of intracellular signalling before proceeding to the specifics of cytokine-induced signalling.

General principles of signalling

Two reactions shared by diverse signalling pathways are phosphorylation and dephosphorylation. *Phosphorylation* is the substitution of a hydrogen atom by a phosphate group (PO_4^{3-}) in a particular molecule, in this context, a protein (Fig. 10.20); *dephosphorylation* is the removal of a phosphate group from a molecule (protein). The donor of the phosphate group is the *adenosine triphosphate (ATP)* molecule (Fig. 10.21a), which functions as an energy source. The recipients of the phosphate groups are the various proteins of the signalling pathway, different ones in distinct pathways. In a protein phosphorylation reaction, the hydrogen atom to be replaced is part of the hydroxyl

$$\text{ATP} + \boxed{\text{Protein}}-\text{OH} \xrightarrow{\text{Protein kinase}} \text{ADP} + \boxed{\text{Protein}}-\text{O}-\overset{\overset{\text{O}}{\|}}{\underset{\underset{\text{O}^-}{|}}{\text{P}}}-\text{O}^-$$

$$\text{H}_2\text{O} + \boxed{\text{Protein}}-\text{O}-\overset{\overset{\text{O}}{\|}}{\underset{\underset{\text{O}^-}{|}}{\text{P}}}-\text{O}^- \xrightarrow[\text{H}_2\text{O}]{\text{Protein phosphatase}} \boxed{\text{Protein}}-\text{OH} + \text{HO}-\overset{\overset{\text{O}}{\|}}{\underset{\underset{\text{O}^-}{|}}{\text{P}}}-\text{O}^-$$

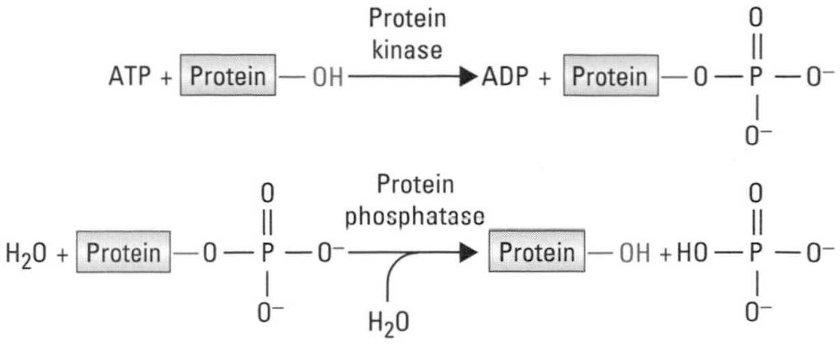

Figure 10.20 Phosphorylation and dephosphorylation of proteins. ADP, adenosine diphosphate; ATP, adenosine triphosphate.

(OH) group in an amino acid residue (Fig. 10.20). Proteins contain three amino acid residues with a free hydroxyl group: serine (Ser), threonine (Thr) and tyrosine (Tyr). All three residues can be phosphorylated, provided they are flanked by certain other residues. Why phosphorylation is so important in intracellular signalling is not entirely clear, but seems to have to do with the physicochemical properties of the phosphate group. The phosphate carries a strong negative charge and as such can interact with positively charged amino acid residues (e.g. lysine and arginine) in the protein and repel negatively charged groups (such as those of other phosphates and of aspartic and glutamic acid residues). These interactions may change the conformation of the protein and thus unmask previously concealed catalytic sites, alter the protein's ability to bind ions and create or abolish binding sites for other proteins. All these alterations influence the functional state of a protein.

Phosphorylation of a protein is an enzymatic reaction catalysed by *protein kinases* (PK). Similarly, dephosphorylation is catalysed by *protein phosphatases* (PP). The catalytic site of protein kinases recognizes the ATP molecule and a feature of the substrate — the phosphorylation motif of the protein. The enzymes can be classified into two broad categories according to the type of OH-bearing residue in the motif: the serine/threonine kinases and the tyrosine kinases.

In addition to protein kinases and phosphatases, the second principal components of signalling are the *guanosine triphosphate (GTP)-binding proteins (G-proteins)*. It is therefore possible to distinguish two types of signalling: one in which the receptor is coupled with G-proteins and another in which it is associated with protein kinases.

Signalling via G-protein-associated receptors

The receptors in this group belong to the STSR-F (also called *rhodopsin superfamily*, rhodopsin being the photon

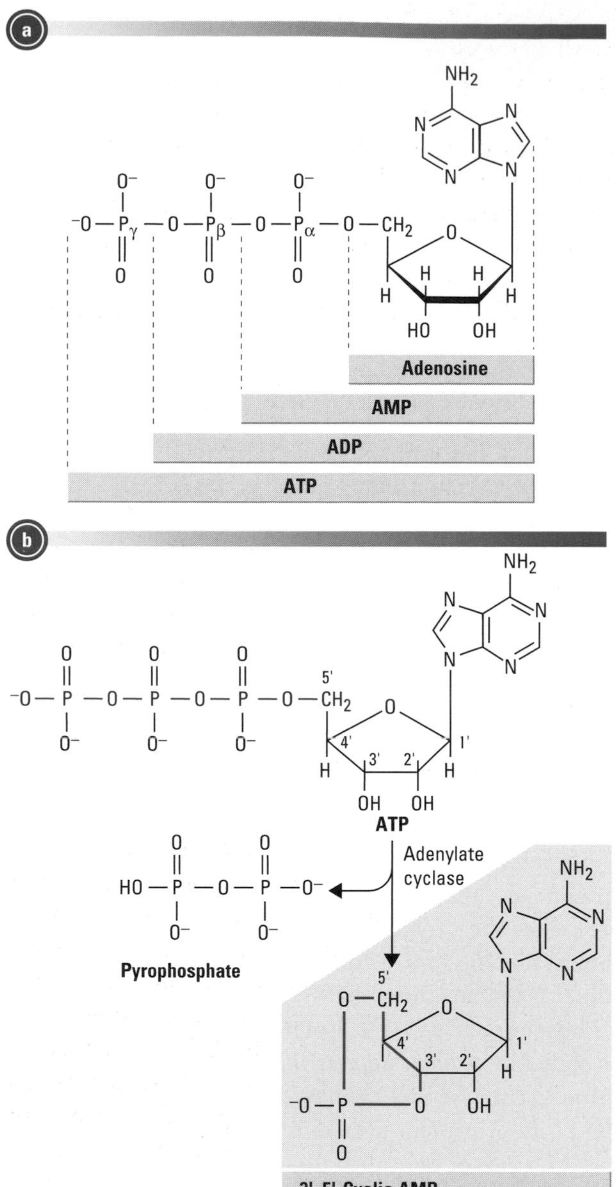

Figure 10.21 (a) Structure of adenosine triphosphate (ATP) and the relationship of ATP to adenosine diphosphate and monophosphate (ADP and AMP, respectively). (b) Synthesis of cyclic AMP from ATP. The cyclic structure is highlighted.

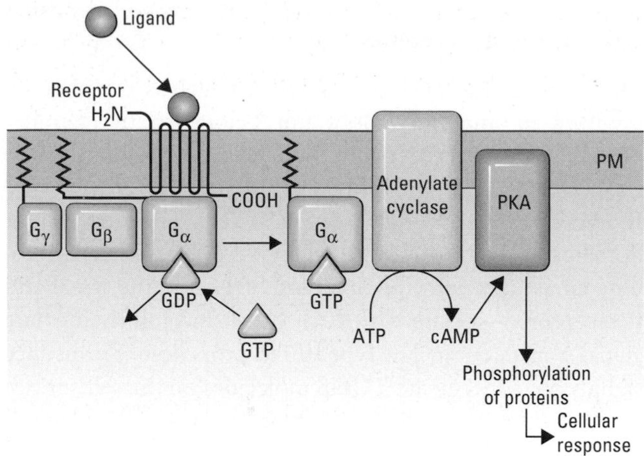

Figure 10.22 Signalling via adenylate cyclase (second messenger) and protein kinase A (PKA). Explanation in the text. G_α, G_β and G_γ are the subunits of the trimeric G-protein (note that the G_α and G_γ subunits are anchored in the plasma membrane (PM) by fatty acids: myristic and palmitic acids in the case of G_α and farnesyl acid in the case of G_γ). ATP, adenosine triphosphate; cAMP, cyclic adenosine monophosphate; GDP and GTP, guanosine diphosphate and triphosphate, respectively.

receptor in the retina). They include not only neurotransmitters, taste and olfactory receptors, but also chemokine receptors, receptors for chemotactic bacterial peptides and for complement fragment C5a, as well as the receptor for PAF. All these receptors are associated with the *trimeric G-proteins*, which each consist of three subunits: α (M_r 40 000–45 000), β (M_r 36 000) and γ (M_r 7000–8000) (see Fig. 10.22). The α and γ subunits anchor the trimer in the inner leaflet of the plasma membrane. The α subunit has a binding site for *guanosine diphosphate* and *triphosphate* (*GDP* and *GTP*, respectively). The G-protein cycles between two states, resting and active. In the resting state its α subunit is associated with GDP; in the active state GDP is replaced by GTP.

The sequence of events in signalling via this type of receptors is as follows (Fig. 10.22).

- Ligand binds to its receptor and the interaction induces a conformational change in the intracellular part of the receptor.
- The change detaches the α subunit from the βγ dimer of the trimeric G-protein associated with the receptor on the cytosolic face of the plasma membrane.
- The freed G_α subunit rapidly exchanges the bound GDP for GTP and the G_α–GTP complex binds to an effector molecule, i.e. an enzyme or membrane ion channel (see below), and activates it. The $G_{\beta\gamma}$ dimers may associate with other effector molecules and modify their activities.
- Eventually, the G_α subunit hydrolyses, via its own intrinsic GTPase activity, the GTP to GDP, the G_α–GDP complex dissociates from the effector molecule and joins the $G_{\beta\gamma}$ dimer, and the trimer returns to the resting state until another signalling event activates it again.
- The activated effector molecule then sets the signalling cascade into motion.

Among the enzymes regulated in this manner by G-proteins, most important are adenylate cyclase and some members of the phospholipase C family. *Adenylate cyclase* is an enzyme that converts ATP into cyclic adenosine monophosphate (cAMP) (Fig. 10.21b). This conversion leads to the release of two phosphate groups from ATP and cyclization (joining into a ring) of the third phosphate. cAMP generated by adenylate cyclase, which has been activated by the attachment of GTP–G_α (specifically, the G_α subunit of the $G_{\alpha s}$ subfamily), activates *protein kinase A (PKA)*. cAMP thus functions as a *second messenger* (the first messenger being the ligand) in the signal transduction pathway. Activated PKA phosphorylates various members of the cascade, i.e. intracellular proteins possessing a specific Ser/Thr-containing motif.

Phospholipase C (PLC) splits the bond between glycerol and phosphate and thus catalyses the removal of the head group from a phospholipid. (Phospholipases, which are components of the plasma membrane, are classified into types A1, A2 and C according to the bond they attack; the combined activity of A1 and A2 was originally referred to as phospholipase B; see Chapter 11.) There are several PLC groups distinguished by their structure and activities. Of these, PLCβ is activated by the G-protein; other PLCs (PLCγ) can be activated directly by certain types of receptors (see below). The target of PLCβ is *phosphatidylinositol 4,5-bisphosphate* (PIP_2, a minor component of the plasma membrane's inner leaflet), which is hydrolysed to *1,2-diacylglycerol* (DAG) and *inositol 1,4,5-trisphosphate* (IP_3) (Fig. 10.23). DAG and IP_3 are second messengers; the former is a membrane-bound molecule, the latter a soluble substance.

IP_3 diffuses into the cytosol, binds to a special receptor localized on the membranes of the endoplasmic reticulum (ER) and through it induces the release of calcium ions (Ca^{2+}) from intracellular stores (Fig. 10.23). Calcium is an abundant cation in the extracellular fluid and it also occurs at high concentrations in certain cellular organelles, particularly in elements of the smooth ER. Its cytosolic level, however, is kept extremely low because many cellular processes are dramatically affected by this ion. Because of its charge, the flexibility with which it establishes bonds with other substances and its high dehydration rate, calcium interacts readily with proteins and thus often effects a change in their conformation. Cellular functions can therefore be regulated by controlling cytosolic Ca^{2+} concentration. The controls operate via a variety of *calcium channels* (structures composed of integral membrane proteins responsible for the transport of substances across membranes; their opening and closing can be ligand operated), pumps (transmembrane proteins that use ATP or another nucleotide triphosphate as a source of energy to transport an ion against its gradient across the membrane) and other transporting systems. Upon interaction with its ER receptors, IP_3 effects the opening of the Ca^{2+} channels and thus the release of Ca^{2+} ions into the cytosol. The ions interact with *protein kinase C (PKC)*, another key signalling enzyme. In its inactive form, PKC is a soluble, cytosolic protein. Upon interaction with Ca^{2+} ions it binds to the cytoplasmic leaflet of the plasma membrane, where it can be activated by DAG. PKC activated by Ca^{2+} and DAG then phosphorylates several proteins possessing the Ser/Thr phosphorylation motif and the phosphorylated proteins alter the cell's activities. Ca^{2+} ions exiting through the open channels from the lumen of the ER into the cytosol bind also to a number of other proteins, thus changing their activities and affecting the cellular response. The effect of Ca^{2+} ions is mediated by *calmodulin*, a specialized Ca^{2+}-binding protein containing four helix–loop–helix Ca^{2+}-binding domains.

The pathway is regulated at several levels: by GTPase activating proteins acting on the $G_{\alpha q}$ protein; rapid hydrolysis of IP_3 to the inactive inositol 1,4-bisphosphate (IP_2); phosphorylation and then inactivation of the IP_3 receptor; and others.

Signalling via receptors linked to protein tyrosine kinases

Protein tyrosine kinases (PTKs) phosphorylate proteins at a tyrosine residue embedded in a specific sequence motif. They can be divided into two large groups: receptor-type and cytoplasmic PTKs. *Receptor-type PTKs* are integral membrane proteins whose extracellular part functions as a ligand-binding receptor, whereas the cytoplasmic part is a phosphorylating kinase. *Cytoplasmic PTKs* do not have a receptor function and are therefore able to process only signals received by the receptor-type PTKs or by other receptors. Although their entire molecules are located in the cytoplasm, some of them undergo post-translational modification and acquire fatty acid tails by which they anchor themselves in the inner leaflet of the plasma membrane.

Comparisons of sequences have revealed the existence of three highly conserved regions in the PTK proteins. Because the conservation was first noticed in comparisons with the Src (pronounced 'sarc') protein, the sequences are referred to as *Src homology regions 1–3* (SH1, SH2, SH3). (The Src protein is the product of the c-*src* proto-oncogene whose viral counterpart causes neoplastic transformation of chicken cells and the production of 'fleshy' appearing sarcomas.) Of the three Src homology regions, SH1 proved to be part of the catalytic domain by which the PTKs exert their enzymatic activity. The SH2 and SH3 regions contain sequences involved in protein–protein interactions. While the SH1 region occurs only in PTKs, the SH2 and SH3

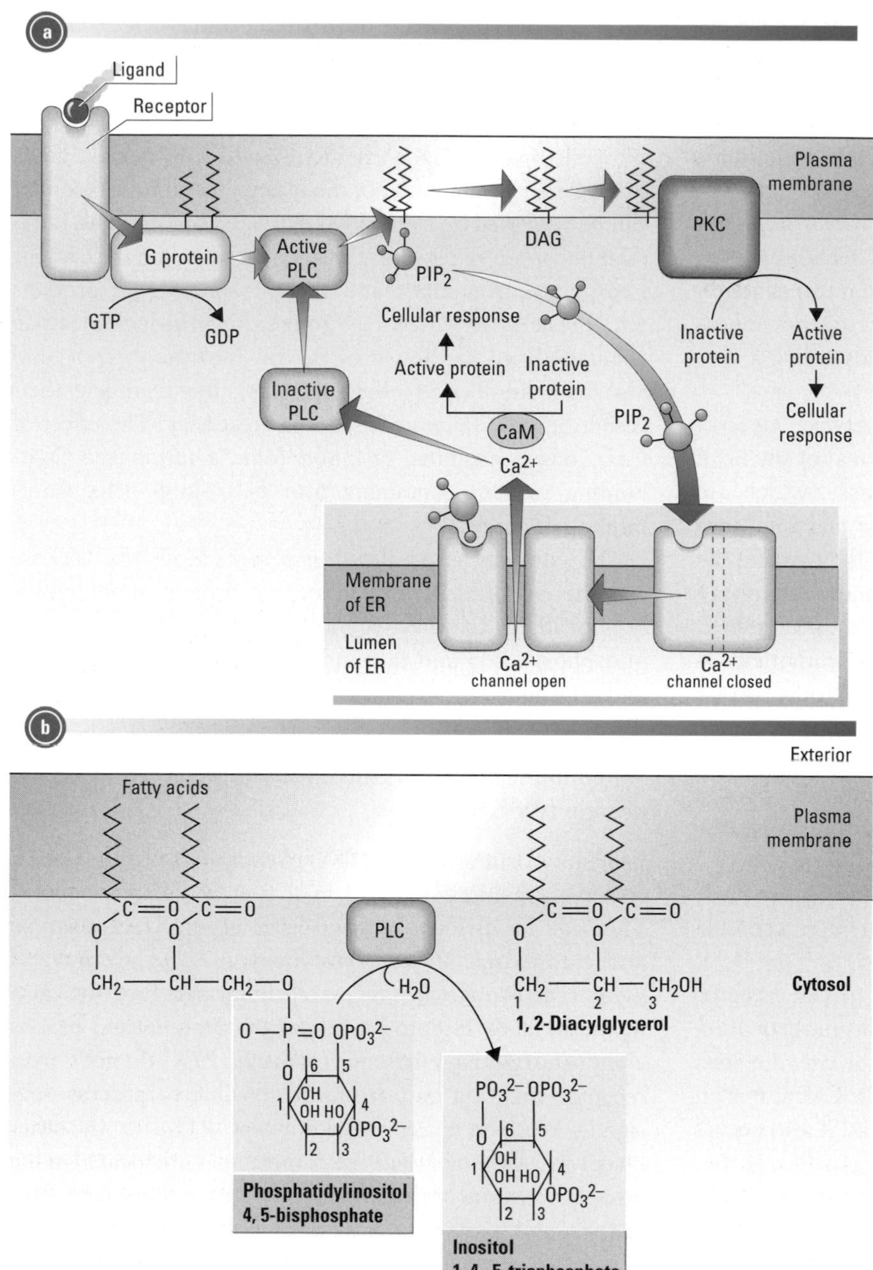

Figure 10.23 (a) Signalling via phospholipase C (PLC), 1,2-diacylglycerol (DAG), inositol 1,4,5-trisphosphate (IP_3) and protein kinase C (PKC). Explanation in the text. (b) Hydrolysis of plasma membrane phosphatidylinositol 4,5-bisphosphate (PIP_2) by phospholipase C (PLC). GDP and GTP, guanosine diphosphate and triphosphate, respectively. The G-protein consists in reality of three subunits (see Fig. 10.22). CaM, calmodulin; ER, enodoplasmic reticulum.

regions have been identified also in other enzymes (e.g. PLCγ, phosphatidylinositol 3-kinase (PI3K) and the protein tyrosine phosphatases, of which more later) and also in proteins that do not have any enzymatic activity but participate in signal transduction (some of these, too, are discussed later). In some proteins the SH2 and SH3 regions occur together, usually adjacent to each other; in others they exist separately. In addition to the SH2 and SH3 regions, at least two other protein interaction segments have been identified: the phosphotyrosine binding (PTB) and the pleckstrin homology (PH) domains (the 'pleckstrin' acronym derives from the term '*p*latelet and *le*u*k*ocyte *s*ubstrate'). However, these are not well characterized; the PTB domain appears to be a variant of the SH2 region.

The *SH2 domain* is approximately 100 amino acid residues long and is organized into one major antiparallel β-sheet flanked by two α-helices and one minor β-sheet formed by two β-strands. The structure binds to protein sequences containing phosphorylated tyrosine flanked by certain other amino acid residues. The binding is mediated by the main β-sheet, the intervening loops and one of the α-helices. The specific recognition of the phosphorylated tyrosine involves interactions between the side-chains of lysine and arginine and the ring system of tyrosine, as well as hydrogen-bonding interactions with the phosphate. (The SH2 domain recognizes the tyrosine only when the latter has been phosphorylated.) The interaction between the SH2 domain of one protein and the phosphorylated tyrosine-containing region of another protein is specific, so that a given protein binds only certain other proteins. The specificity of the binding is determined by the sequence of the SH2 domain and in the bound protein by the sequence flanking the phosphorylated tyrosine residue. Because of this specificity certain proteins can interact only with certain other proteins of the signalling cascade.

The *SH3 domain*, which is frequently located next to the SH2 domain, is approximately 50 amino acid residues long. It recognizes proline-rich sequences in various intracellular proteins. Like SH2, the SH3 domain mediates protein–protein interactions between intracellular signalling molecules. In both the SH2 and SH3 domain-mediated interactions, the binding leads to a conformational change of the SH domain-bearing protein and thus to a change of the protein's functional state.

The initiation of the signalling pathways occurs differently in cascades involving the receptor-type PTKs and those involving the cytoplasmic PTKs. The binding of a ligand to a *receptor-type PTK* leads to clustering of the receptors on the cell's surface, with the result that the receptors' cytoplasmic regions come close enough together to be able to interact with each other. The interaction leads to the activation of the catalytic region and mutual phosphorylation of multiple tyrosine residues in the cytoplasmic domains. The phosphorylated tyrosine residues and the flanking sequences are then recognized by different protein molecules located on the inner surface of the plasma membrane such as PLCγ, Ras-GAP and PI3K (Fig. 10.24). The recognition occurs via the SH2 regions of these proteins. Different receptors thus become associated with various combinations of intracellular proteins, depending on the sequences flanking their phosphorylated tyrosine residues. The proteins docked on the receptor's phosphotyrosine residues are subsequently phosphorylated by the PTKs, the phosphorylation activates the recruited proteins and initiates at least one of the three branches of the signalling cascade.

PLCγ, in contrast to PLCβ, does not require G-proteins to mediate its action. The phosphorylation-activated enzyme acts directly on PIP_2 in the inner leaflet of the plasma membrane, splitting it into DAG and IP_3. DAG then activates PKC and the rest of the pathway proceeds as described above.

The *Ras protein* was originally discovered as the product

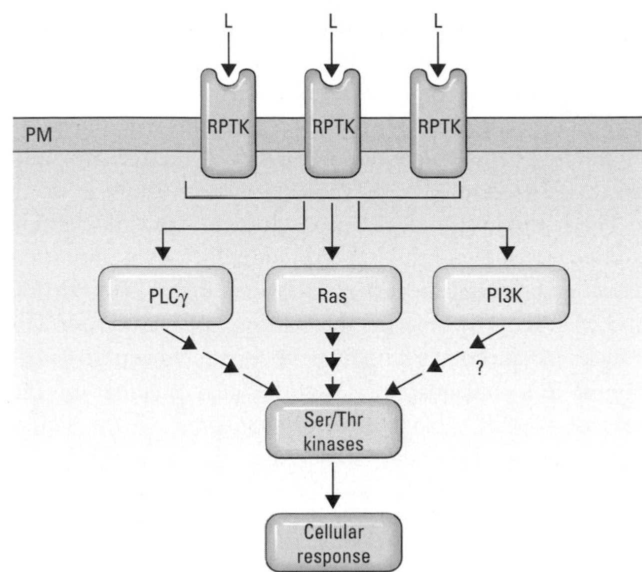

Figure 10.24 Generalized and greatly simplified scheme of the signalling pathway initiated by receptor-type protein tyrosine kinases (RPTK). L, ligand; PI3K, phosphatidylinositol 3-kinase; PLC, phospholipase C; PM, plasma membrane; Ras, rat sarcoma (oncogene homologue); Ser, serine; Thr, threonine.

of the viral oncogene responsible for the induction of *ra*t *s*arcomas. The protein, also referred to as $p21^{ras}$ because of its M_r of 21 000, is a member of the family of *small G-proteins*. In contrast to the trimeric G-proteins, the small G-proteins consist of a single polypeptide that corresponds to the G_α subunit of the trimeric G-proteins. Like G_α, Ras is a guanine nucleotide-binding protein. It cycles between an active growth-promoting state in which it is associated with GTP and an inactive state in which GTP has been replaced by GDP. This cycling is regulated by a number of proteins, some of which enhance the Ras activity while others mitigate it. The best characterized of these is the *GTPase-activating protein (GAP)*. This protein promotes the hydrolysis of Ras-bound GTP and hence speeds up Ras inactivation. The action of this negative regulator is counterbalanced by *guanine nucleotide exchange proteins*, which promote the loss of bound GDP and uptake of fresh GTP from cytosol and hence the reactivation of the Ras protein. Among these exchange-promoting proteins the best characterized is the *Sos* protein. Sos is a homologue of a protein originally identified in *Drosophila melanogaster* and designated *son of sevenless* because it was shown to be associated with the *sevenless* protein, a receptor-type PTK that in a mutated form leads to a characteristic defect in the development of the eye (the mutant lacks R7, one of the eight photoreceptor cells). Sos is associated with another molecule, the ***growth factor receptor-bound protein (Grb)***. Upon phosphorylation of the receptor PTK, the Sos/Grb, and at least one other ***SH2 domain-containing adaptor protein (Shc)***, interact via their SH2 domains with the phosphorylated tyrosine-containing motifs of the receptor and are thereby recruited to the membrane.

The complexes of adaptor proteins and nucleotide exchangers activate the Ras protein, which then initiates a cascade of three consecutively activated kinases (Raf, MEK and MAPK). The first member of this cascade, the Ser/Thr kinase *Raf*, becomes activated upon attachment to GTP-bound Ras. It phosphorylates the next member of the cascade, MEK (from ***m**itogen-activated, **e**xtracellular signal-regulated **k**inase*; sometimes also referred to as MAPKK). Phosphorylation-activated MEK has an unusual specificity — it phosphorylates a threonine and a tyrosine residue in the MAPK (***m**itogen-**a**ctivated **p**rotein **k**inase*, so named because it was originally discovered in mitogen-activated cells; it is also called *Erk* for *e*xtracellular signal *r*egulated *k*inase). MAPK ultimately phosphorylates several substrates, among them other protein kinases and transcription factors regulating the expression of specific genes (Fig. 10.25).

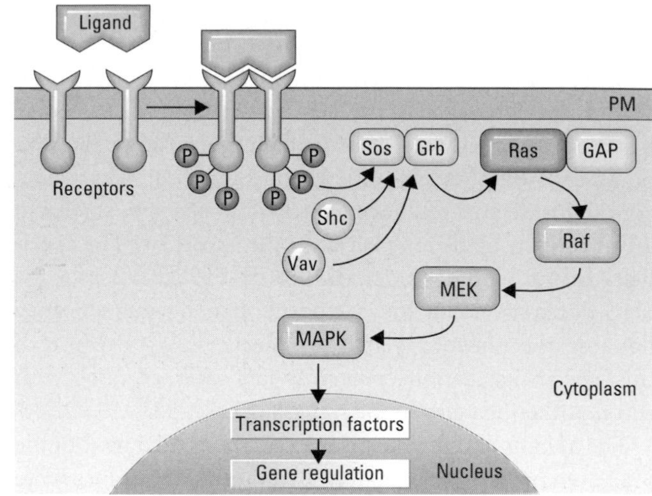

Figure 10.25 Signalling initiated by receptor-type protein tyrosine kinases and mediated by small G-proteins, here exemplified by the Ras protein (dark grey). Proteins regulating the G-protein (adaptor proteins) are indicated in light pink, serine/threonine protein kinases in light grey. GAP, GTPase-activating protein; Grb, growth factor receptor-bound (protein); MAPK, mitogen-activated protein kinase; MEK, mitogen-activated, extracellular signal-regulated kinase; P, phosphorylated tyrosine in the cytoplasmic domain of the receptor; PM, plasma membrane; Raf, rat fibrosarcoma protooncogene protein; Ras, rat sarcoma (protooncogene protein); Shc, SH2 domain-containing (adaptor protein); Sos, son of sevenless; Vav, sixth letter in Hebrew alphabet.

The third branch of receptor-type PTK-initiated signalling is mediated by the enzyme *PI3K*. PI3K is a complex of two proteins: p85, which is a regulatory subunit; and p110, which constitutes the catalytic subunit. The p85 subunit contains two SH2 domains, one SH3 domain and one *bcr* domain capable of interacting with small G-proteins (*bcr* stands for *b*reakpoint *c*luster *r*egion, a gene involved in the induction of chromosome translocations associated with chronic myelogenous leukaemia). It also contains tyrosine residues that can be phosphorylated by certain PTKs. PI3K is associated with a wide range of receptors and activated PTKs but its exact function in the signalling cascades is not known. It mediates transfer of the phosphate group from ATP to position 3 of the inositol ring in phosphoinositide lipids. The transfer can result in three products: phosphatidylinositol 3-phosphate [PtdIns (3)P]; phosphatidylinositol 3,4-bisphosphate [PtdIns $(3,4)P_2$]; and phosphatidylinositol 3,4,5-trisphosphate [PtdIns $(3,4,5)P_3$]. The last of these three compounds is believed to be an activator (second messenger) of certain types of PKC. In addition to its lipid-kinase activity, PI3K is also capable of phosphorylating certain proteins on Ser/Thr residues.

The *cytoplasmic PTKs*, which do not have a direct link to the extracellular environment and hence cannot receive primary signals from the outside, function by hitching up with transmembrane proteins, either the receptors themselves or, if these lack appropriately structured cytoplasmic tails, the chains associated with the receptors. The cytoplasmic tails of the receptors or their accompanying chains possess specific sequences that are recognized by the SH domains of PTKs and which mediate the binding. Each receptor is thus surrounded at its cytoplasmic part by a different entourage of cytoplasmic PTKs. The numerous cytoplasmic PTKs can be divided into eight subfamilies, which differ in the organization of their SH and catalytic domains, length, sequence homologies and function (Fig. 10.26). Cross-linking of the receptors by a ligand activates the receptor complex-associated cytoplasmic PTKs in a manner that is not entirely elucidated, but involves, in some cases at least, additional enzymes (e.g. certain phosphatases that are thought to remove inhibitory phosphate from the kinase). The activated PTKs then initiate one or several of the signalling cascades described on the preceding pages. In principle, the pathways may be initiated via phospholipases and the second messengers DAG, IP_3 and Ca^{2+} or via the Ras protein and the system of serine/threonine protein kinases.

The ultimate outcome of the signalling, the *cellular response*, depends on the ligand, the receptor and the signalling pathway chosen. The responses include: production

Family	M_r ($\times 10^{-3}$)	Members
Abl	150	Abl, Arg
Jak	120-130	Jak1, Jak2 Jak3, Tyk2
Fak	125	Fak
Fes	92-98	Fes/Fps, Fer
Syk	70-72	Syk, ZAP-70
Itk	62-77	Itk, Tec Btk (Atk)
Src	53-64	Src, Yes, Fyn, Lyn Lck, Blk, Hck, Fgr, Yrk
Csk	50	Csk, Lsk, Ntk

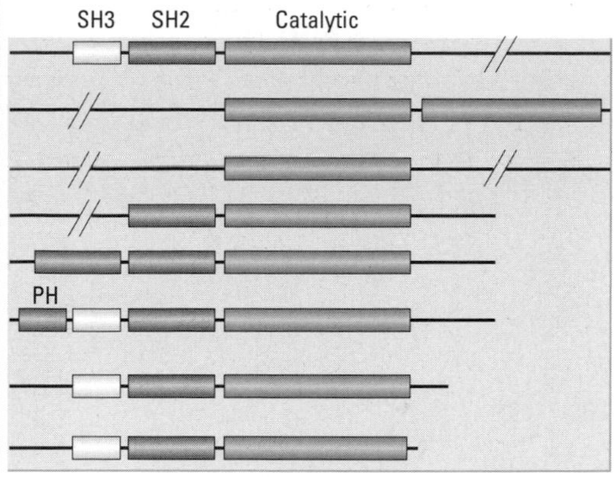

Figure 10.26 Subfamilies of cytoplasmic protein tyrosine kinases. Abl, Abelson leukaemia (protooncogene); Arg, Ab1-related gene; Atk, agammaglobulinaemia tyrosine kinase; Blk, B-lymphocyte specific protein kinase; Btk, Bruton's tyrosine kinase; Csk, C-terminal Src kinase; Fak, focal adhesion kinase; Fer, Fes/Fsp-related; Fes, feline sarcoma; Fgr, feline Gardner–Rasheed (sarcoma virus oncogene); Fps, Fujinami–PRCII sarcoma protooncogene protein; Fyn, protein related to Fgr and Yes; Fgr, Gardner–Rasheed sarcoma protooncogene protein; Hck, haematopoietic cell protein tyrosine kinase; Itk, interleukin-2 inducible kinase; Jak, Janus tyrosine kinase; Lck, lymphoid cell protein tyrosine kinase; Lsk, leucocyte C-terminal src kinase related gene; Lyn, Lck and Yes-related novel gene; Ntk, nervous tissue and lymphocyte kinase; PH, pleckstrin homology (domain); SH, src-homology (domain); Src, sarcoma (protooncogene); Syk, spleen tyrosine kinase; Tec, tyrosine kinase expressed in hepatocellular carcinoma; Tyk, tyrosine kinase; Yes, originally designated Yas, Yamaguchi sarcoma protooncogene protein; Yrk, Yes-related kinase; ZAP, zeta-associated protein. (Based on Bolen, J.B. (1993) *Oncogene*, 8, 2025.)

of transcription factors regulating gene expression; cell differentiation along a specific lineage; cell division (proliferation); induction of synthesis and secretion of molecules; expression of new cell-surface molecules; activation of cytoskeletal proteins leading to changes in cell shape and motility; and induction of programmed cell death.

The protein kinase activities are often counteracted by *protein phosphatases*. These, too, fall into two main groups: protein Ser/Thr phosphatases and protein tyrosine phosphatase. The latter, like protein kinases, can be either of the receptor or cytoplasmic type. Protein phosphatases exert their effect by removing inhibitory phosphates, dephosphorylating transcription factors and inhibiting protein kinases.

Signalling via cytokine receptors

A few cytokine receptors (e.g. M-CSFR and SCFR) possess PTK catalytic domains in their cytoplasmic parts. These then function as receptor-type PTKs and activate multiple signal-transduction pathways (Fig. 10.27). The pathways can be mediated by the Ras protein, PLCγ or PI3K. The ultimate outcome of signalling is gene regulation via transcription factors.

Most cytokine receptors lack intracellular PTK activity and function via cytoplasmic PTKs associated with their cytoplasmic tails. Cytokine receptors of the CKR-SF and IFNR-SF are associated with PTKs of the *Janus kinase* (*Jak*) family (Jak1, Jak2, Jak3 and Tyk2; Fig. 10.28; Table 10.5), each receptor subunit being associated with a specific Jak protein. Cytokine-induced receptor aggregation brings the Jak proteins in contact with one another and enables them to phosphorylate and thus activate each other. The activated Jak proteins then initiate multiple signal-transduction pathways. The shortest and possibly most important pathway begins with the phosphorylation of the cytoplasmic *Stat protein (signal transducer, activator of transcription)*, with M_r of between 84 000 and 113 000. The six known Stat proteins (Stat 1–Stat 6) are specific targets of various Jak family kinases. Upon tyrosine phosphorylation, the Stat proteins form homodimers, Stat-heterodimers or complexes with another cytoplasmic protein, p48. The dimers are translocated to the nucleus where they bind to regulatory sequences of various genes and act as transcription factors.

Jak family kinases also phosphorylate several tyrosine residues in the C-terminal parts of the cytokine receptor chains, and these serve as binding sites for several SH2 domain-containing proteins, such as Shc, PLCγ, PI3K, as well as tyrosine phosphatases PTP-1D and PTP-1C. The proteins are then phosphorylated and activated to initiate Ras–MAPK, PLCγ–PKC or PI3K pathways. Some of the cytokine receptors (e.g. IL-2R) are also associated, in addition to Jak, with Src and Syk family kinases and these, too,

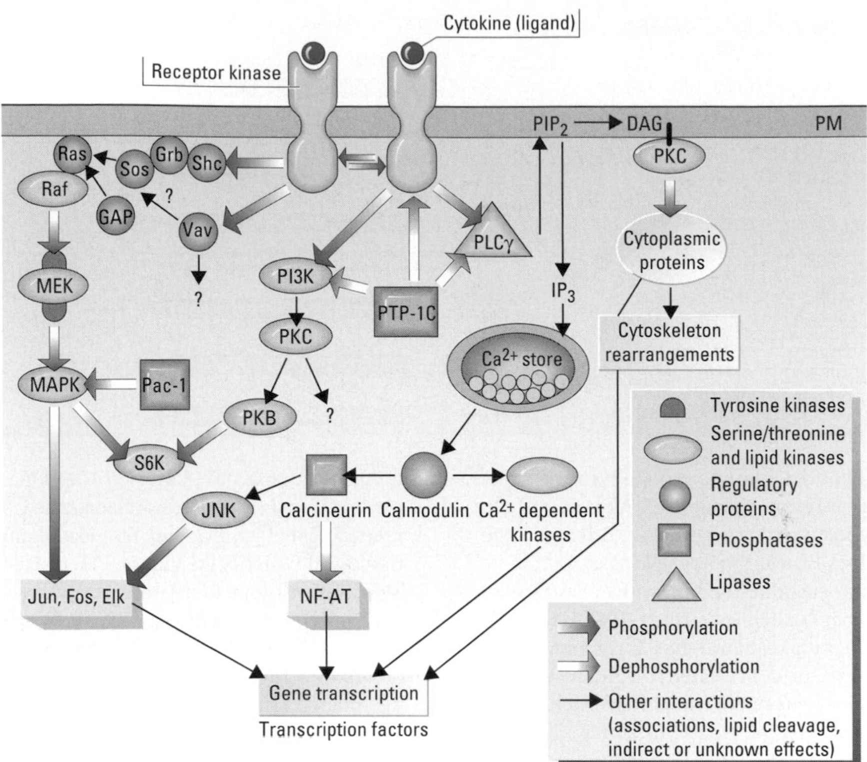

Figure 10.27 Signalling pathway triggered by the activation of cytokine receptors possessing protein tyrosine kinase catalytic domains in their cytoplasmic parts. DAG, 1,2-diacylglycerol; Elk, Eph-like kinase; Eph, kinase detected in 'erythropoietin-producing hepatoma'; Fos, FJB osteosarcoma (virus) protooncogene; GAP, GTPase-activating protein; Grb, growth factor receptor-bound (protein); JNK, Jun N-terminal kinase; Jun, *ju-nana*, Japanese '17'; MAPK, mitogen-activated protein kinase; MEK, mitogen-activated, extracellular signal-regulated kinase; NF-AT, nuclear factor of activated T cells; Pac-1, phosphatase of activated cells; PI3K, phosphatidylinositol 3-kinase; PKB, protein kinase B; PKC, protein kinase C; PIP_2, phosphatidylinositol 4,5-bisphosphate; PLCγ, phospholipase Cγ; PM, plasma membrane; PTP-1C, protein tyrosine phosphatase 1C; Raf, rat fibrosarcoma protooncogene protein; Ras, rat sarcoma (protooncogene protein); Shc, SH2 domain-containing (adaptor protein); Sos, son of sevenless (protein); S6K, S6 kinase; Vav, sixth letter of Hebrew alphabet.

contribute to the initiation of multiple signalling pathways. The Src and Syk family kinases are associated with the T-cell receptor, B-cell receptor and FcR complexes and mediate the initial steps in signalling through these receptors (see Chapters 7, 8, 15, 16 & 17). The activity of Src family kinases is regulated via phosphorylation and dephosphorylation of two critical tyrosine residues (Fig. 10.29). IL-4R, and probably also IL-9R, is unusual in that it uses as an early component of its signalling cascade a protein called *IRS-1 (insulin receptor substrate-1)*. The protein is associated with the IL-4R α chain and is phosphorylated by Jak 1 or Jak 3 at 21 tyrosine residues following receptor activation. The phosphorylated tyrosines serve as docking sites for several proteins with SH2 domains, including Grb2, PI3K and Syp. The accumulation of these proteins at the receptor-associated protein kinases facilitates their rapid phosphorylation and activation.

Negative regulation of all types of PTK-associated receptors is achieved by cytoplasmic phosphotyrosine phosphatases, such as PTP-1C. Several cytoplasmic phosphatases, such as Pac-1, dephosphorylate and thereby return to the resting, low-activity state the various intracellular proteins phosphorylated on serine and threonine residues during the course of the signalling cascade. However, not all phosphatases are necessarily negative regulators. Thus, for example, Src-family kinases are activated through dephosphorylation of phosphotyrosines at the C-termini by membrane-bound (CD45) or cytoplasmic (PTP-1C or PTP-1D) phosphatases.

Receptors of the TNFR-F contain a characteristic sequence of approximately 80 amino acid residues called the *death domain*, which is indispensable for apoptotic signalling. The domain is probably involved in association of two or more receptor molecules and in association with other cytoplasmic proteins carrying the death domains: *TRADD (TNFR associated death domain)* proteins,

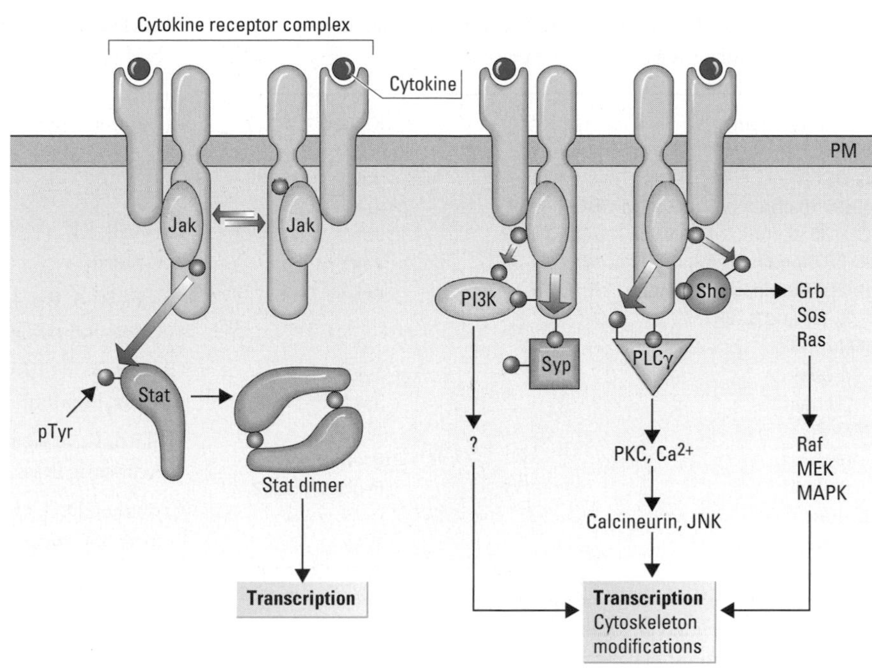

Figure 10.28 Signalling pathways triggered via cytokine receptors lacking protein tyrosine kinase catalytic domains but associated with cytoplasmic protein tyrosine kinases. Grb, growth factor receptor-bound protein; Jak, Janus tyrosine kinase; JNK, Jun N-terminal kinase; MAPK, mitogen-activated protein kinase; MEK, mitogen-activated, extracellular signal-regulated kinase; PI3K, phosphatidylinositol 3-kinase; PKC, protein kinase C; PLCγ, phospholipase Cγ; PM, plasma membrane; pTyr, phosphorylated tyrosine residue; Raf, rat fibrosarcoma protooncogene protein; Ras, rat sarcoma (protein); Shc, SH2 domain-containing (adaptor protein); Sos, son of sevenless (protooncogene protein); Stat, signal transducer, activator of transcription; Syp, SH2-containing phosphotyrosine phosphatase.

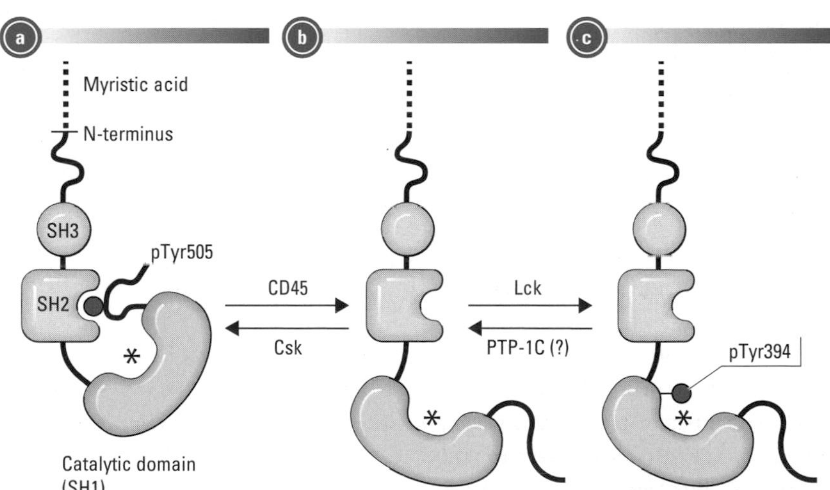

Figure 10.29 Regulation of the activities of Src-family kinases (here represented by Lck). In the inactive (resting) state (a), the tyrosine residue near the C-terminus (here number 505) is in a phosphorylated form, the phosphotyrosine residue is bound to the SH2 domain of the same molecule and the enzyme's catalytic site (asterisk) in the SH1 domain is blocked. Dephosphorylation of this negative regulatory tyrosine by the transmembrane tyrosine phosphatase CD45 relaxes the molecule and exposes the catalytic site (b). Such a partially active kinase can phosphorylate a positive regulatory tyrosine residue (here number 394) of another Lck molecule in its vicinity. The phosphorylation fully activates the second Lck molecule (c), which can then phosphorylate other molecules, for example proteins bearing the immunoreceptor tyrosine-based activation motif (ITAM). Phosphorylation of the negative (C-terminal) regulatory tyrosine is catalysed by the C-terminal Src kinase (Csk); dephosphorylation of the positive regulatory phosphotyrosine is probably catalysed by the cytoplasmic protein tyrosine phosphatase 1C (PTP-1C). CD, cluster of differentiation; LCK, lymphoid cell protein tyrosine kinase; SH, sarcoma (src) homology (region). (Adapted from Mustelin, J. & Burn, P. (1993) *Trends in Biochemical Sciences*, **18**, 215.)

Table 10.5 Janus kinase (Jak) family kinases associated with immunologically relevant cytokine receptors.

Receptor chain	Kinase
G-CSFR	Jak2
KH97 (β-chain of IL-3R, GM-CSFR, IL-5R)	Jak2
CD130 (β-chain of IL-6R, IL-11R and LIFR)	Jak1, Jak2, Tyk2
IL-2R β-chain, IL-4R, IL-7R, IL-9R	Jak1
IL-2Rγ (common chain of IL-2R, IL-4R, IL-7R, IL-9R and IL-5R)	Jak3
IFN-α/βR	
α-chain	Tyk2
β-chain	Jak1
IFN-γR	
α-chain	Probably Tyk2
β-chain	Probably Jak2
IL-10R	
α-chain	Tyk2
β-chain	Jak1

Jak1 is also associated with the immunoglobulin family protein kinase receptor members: monocyte-colony-stimulating factor receptor (M-CSFR), platelet-derived growth factor receptor (PD GFR) and epidermal growth factor receptor (EGFR).
CD, cluster of differentiation; G-CSFR, granulocyte colony-stimulating factor; GM-CSFR, granulocyte-monocyte colony-stimulating factor; IFN, interferon; IL, interleukin; KH97, laboratory clone designation; LIFR, leukaemia inhibitory factor; Tyk, tyrosine kinase.

FADD/MORT-1 (Fas associated death domain) protein and *RIP (receptor interaction protein)*. The manner by which these proteins propagate the signals is not known.

An early event triggered by TNFR is the activation of the *neutral sphingomyelinase*, an enzyme cleaving membrane lipid sphingomyelin into ceramide and phosphocholine. Ceramide activates a serine/threonine protein kinase (probably a type of PKC) and also a protein phosphatase. The ceramide-dependent protein kinase seems to activate the Raf–MEK–MAPK pathway and thus lead to the activation of the transcription factor NF-κB, phospholipase A_2 (the enzyme initiating prostaglandin synthesis; see Chapter 11) and numerous other effects. Ceramide is also critically involved in apoptotic signalling.

Chemokine receptors are coupled to trimeric G-proteins.

Further reading

Aggarwal, B.B. & Gutterman, J.U. (1992) *Human Cytokines: Handbook for Basic and Clinical Research*. Blackwell Scientific Publications, Oxford.

Aggarwal, B.B. & Vilcek, J. (1991) *Tumour Necrosis Factors: Structure, Function and Mechanism of Action*. Dekker, New York.

Akira, S., Taga, T. & Kishimoto, T. (1993) Interleukin-6 in biology and medicine. *Advances in Immunology*, **54**, 1–78.

Arend, W.P. (1993) Interleukin-1 receptor antagonist. *Advances in Immunology*, **54**, 167–228.

Baggiolini, M. & Sorg, C. (1991) *Neutrophil-activating Peptides and Other Chemotactic Cytokines*. Karger, Basel.

Balkwill, F.R. (1991) *Cytokines: A Practical Approach*. IRL Press, Oxford.

Baxter, A. & Ross, R. (1991) *Cytokine Interactions and their Control*. John Wiley & Sons, New York.

Callard, R.E. (1990) *Cytokines and B-lymphocytes*. Academic Press, London.

Callard, R. & Gearing, A. (1994) *The Cytokine Facts Book*. Academic Press, London.

Crowther, D.G. (1991) *Inteferons: Mechanisms of Action and Role in Cancer Therapy*. Springer-Verlag, Berlin.

Crumpton, M.J. & Dexter, M.T. (1990) *Growth Factors in Differentiation and Development*. Royal Society, London.

Dawson, M.M. (1991) *Lymphokines and Interleukins*. Open University Press, Milton Keynes.

Farrar, M.A. & Schreiber, R.D. (1993) The molecular cell biology of interferon-γ and its receptor. *Annual Review of Immunology*, **11**, 571–611.

Gold, M.R. & Matsuuchi, L. (1995) Signal transduction by the antigen receptors of B and T lymphocytes. *International Review of Cytology*, **157**, 181–276.

Hamblin, A.S. (1988) *Lymphokines*. IRL Press, Oxford.

Hamblin, A.S. (1994) *Cytokines and Cytokine Receptors: In Focus*. IRL Press, Oxford.

Kunkel, S.L. & Remmick, D.G. (1992) *Cytokines in Health and Disease*. Dekker, New York.

McKay, I.A. & Leigh, I. (1993) *Growth Factors: A Practical Approach*. IRL Press, Oxford.

Meager, A. (1990) *Cytokines*. Open University Press, Milton Keynes.

Minami, Y., Kono, T., Miyazaki, T. & Taniguchi, T. (1993) The IL-2 receptor complex: its structure, function, and target genes. *Annual Review of Immunology*, **11**, 245–267.

Moore, K.W., O'Garra, A., de Waal Malefyt, R., Vieira, P. & Mosmann, T.R. (1993) Interleukin-10. *Annual Review of Immunology*, **11**, 165–190.

Oppenheim, J.J., Rossio, J.L. & Gearing, A.J.H. (1993) *Clinical Applications of Cytokines: Role in Diagnosis, Pathogenesis and Therapy*. Oxford University Press, New York.

Renauld, J.-C., Houssiau, F., Louahed, J., Vink, A., van Snick, J. & Uyttenhove, C. (1993) Interleukin-9. *Advances in Immunology*, **54**, 79–98.

Sugamura, K., Asao, H., Kondo, M. *et al.* (1995) The common γ-chain for multiple cytokine receptors. *Advances in Immunology*, **59**, 225–277.

Taniguchi, T. (1995) Cytokine signaling through nonreceptor protein kinases. *Science*, **268**, 251–255.

Thomson, A.W. (1991) *Cytokine Handbook*. Academic Press, London.

Westwick, J. (1991) *Chemotactic Cytokines: Biology of the Inflammatory Peptide Supergene Family—International Symposium Proceedings*. Plenum Press, New York.

chapter 11 Mediators and messengers

Mediator is a rather ill-defined term for a biologically active compound participating in defence reactions. The expression 'biologically (pharmacologically) active' generally means that the particular compound elicits, often at very low concentrations, a marked response in living tissues and organs. The two biological activities usually associated with mediators are *contraction or relaxation of smooth muscles* and *increase or decrease in blood vessel wall (vascular) permeability*. The visible consequences of these activities may range from a rather inconspicuous change of skin colour at the site of injury to the spectacular shortening of a gut segment from a dissected guinea-pig. Sometimes a third activity is also attributed to mediators: the ability to attract cells to a particular spot in the tissue. The movement of cells towards the source of the mediator is referred to as *chemotaxis*. Some physiologists extend the term 'mediator' even further to include certain compounds with enzymatic or other activities.

The two broad categories of biological processes in which mediators are usually involved are inflammation and allergic reactions. *Inflammation* is a local reaction to tissue injury; *allergy* is, very roughly speaking, an altered reactivity (often an increased sensitivity or *hypersensitivity*) to a normally innocuous substance (see Chapter 23). These definitions are so vague that plenty of room is left for debate on what constitutes an inflammatory or allergic reaction and what does not. Inflammation is generally a beneficial defence reaction, whereas allergy is a pathological, harmful response, although the roles that these two phenomena play may sometimes be reversed.

Chemically, mediators are a mixed bag of compounds that can be divided into three broad categories: peptide mediators (kinins, anaphylatoxins); other low-molecular-mass mediators (products of arachidonic acid metabolism, biologically active amines and other miscellaneous compounds); and protein mediators (enzymes and other biologically active proteins). Cytokines should, technically, be included in this third category, but in this book they are treated as an independent group.

Mediators are released from cells upon *stimulation* either from specialized cellular compartments (usually *granules*), in which they are stored preformed, or after *de novo* synthesis. The release from granules is achieved by *exocytosis*, a process in which the granules migrate to the plasma membrane, fuse with it and open up to discharge their contents to the outside of the cell (*degranulation*). Many of the mediators are produced continuously as part of normal cell functions and are maintained at a regulated level; any excess is stored in the granules. The stimulus provided by the defence or allergic reactions leads to an excessive production of mediators and thus to the manifestation of their characteristic biological activities. The action of the mediator can be either short or long term. In the short-term action, the mediator is released at the time of the stimulation, acts for a relatively short period of time (often less than 1 hour) and then disappears rapidly. In the long-term action, effected by a strong or prolonged stimulation, the mediator-induced response may last for many hours.

The two main cell types that either release or synthesize mediators upon stimulation are *mast cells* and *basophils*.

The broadly defined mediators, however, can also be produced by eosinophils, neutrophils and platelets. Mast cells and basophils have a particularly efficient system of plasma-membrane receptors which, when occupied, initiate a chain reaction leading to mediator synthesis or release. Most important among these receptors are those that have high affinity for the Fc portion of IgE molecules. Individuals who, for unknown reasons, produce relatively high levels of IgE antibodies in response to particular stimuli are therefore prone to an excessive production of mediators and thus to allergic reactions. A description of some of the most important mediators follows.

Arachidonate metabolites

Phospholipids, the main constituents of the plasma membrane, consist of a polar head and two fatty acid tails. *Fatty acids* are long hydrocarbon chains with a carboxyl group (COOH) at one end and, in a free form, a CH_3 group at the other (Fig. 11.1). They differ in the length of the carbon atom chain and the number, position and orientation of the double (unsaturated) bonds (C=C). One of the fatty acids is *arachidonic acid*, so named because it was originally isolated from the peanut plant, *Arachis hypogaea*. Its chain is 20 carbons long and contains four double bonds at positions 5–6, 8–9, 11–12 and 14–15. Arachidonic acid is an integral part of phospholipids, triglycerol and cholesterol esters. Only when a cell is injured or stimulated is arachidonic acid cleaved off from these compounds and released (Fig. 11.2). The release mechanism is exquisitely sensitive; even a very mild, non-specific perturbation of the plasma membrane can lead to the partial release of the acid. This release, however, is relatively minor compared to the liberation triggered when a cell interacts with specific chemicals. There are thus two pathways of arachidonic acid release: a non-specific one liberating small amounts of the acid upon cell injury, and a specific one liberating large amounts upon cell stimulation. The non-specific disturbance of the plasma membrane may range from simple stretching to a frank rupture. Centrifugation, gel filtration or merely stirring with glass beads leads to the release of arachidonic acid from platelet phospholipids. Burns, ischaemia, electroconvulsive shocks, membrane-active venoms such as mellitin,

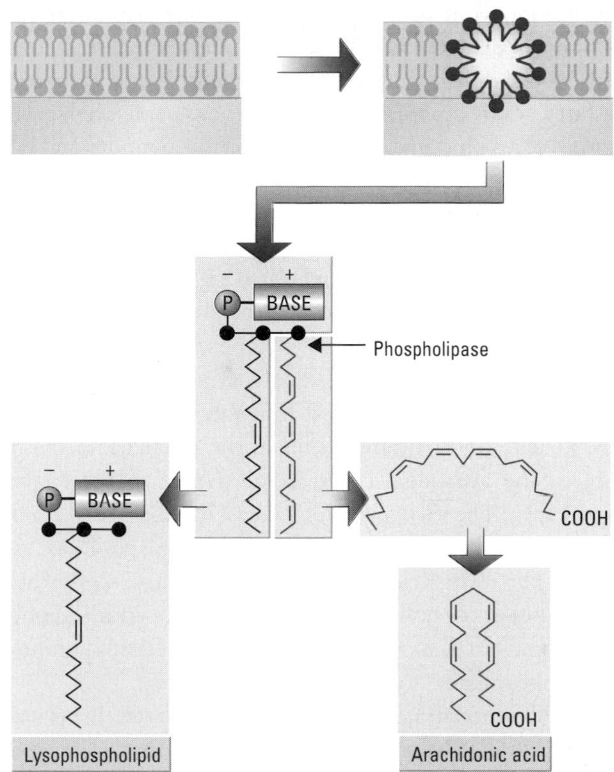

Figure 11.2 Release of arachidonic acid from plasma-membrane phospholipid. A local disturbance in the bilayer makes arachidonic acid-carrying phospholipids susceptible to attack by the enzyme phospholipase. The arachidonic acid is freed from the membrane and folds into the characteristic hairpin structure. The remainder of the molecule is referred to as lysophospholipid. P, phosphate.

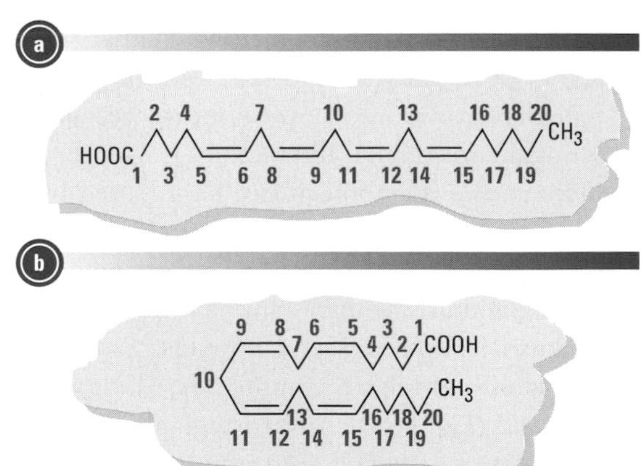

Figure 11.1 Structural formula of arachidonic acid. (a) Extended form. (b) Hairpin form. The molecule is an acid because it contains the COOH group, and since it has 20 carbon atoms it is an eicosa fatty acid (Greek *eikos*, twenty). The carbons are numbered consecutively starting from the COOH group. Because of the presence of four double bonds (C=C) and since the designation *enoyl* is used for unsaturation (i.e. for the presence of double bonds), the compound is tetraenoic acid. The double bonds emanate from carbon atoms 5, 8, 11 and 14, so that the full chemical name of the compound is 5-*cis*, 8-*cis*, 11-*cis*, 14-*cis*-eicosatetraenoic acid, the *cis* designation indicating a particular spatial arrangement of atoms.

Ca^{2+} ionophores such as A23187, tumour promoters such as phorbol esters or mechanical trauma may all lead to the turnover and degradation of phospholipids and the release of fatty acids, among them arachidonic acid. The specific stimuli of arachidonic acid release include peptides and hormones such as angiotensin II, bradykinin and adrenaline; proteases such as thrombin; and certain antigen–antibody complexes. Each of the cells responding to these stimuli has a specific set of receptors whose occupation initiates the response. The mechanism of non-specific release is unclear; specific release involves the enzyme *phospholipase*. The four types of phospholipase involved in the release of fatty acids from phospholipids are designated A_1, A_2, C and D. They each attack different sites in the polar head; the nature of the fatty acid chain is indifferent to the enzyme (Fig. 11.3). The two principal ways of liberating arachidonic acid from a phospholipid involve phospholipases A_2 and C. The former cleaves the polar heads at C-2; the latter hydrolyses phospholipids to produce diglycerides and phosphorylated bases such as inositol, choline, ethanolamine or serine phosphate.

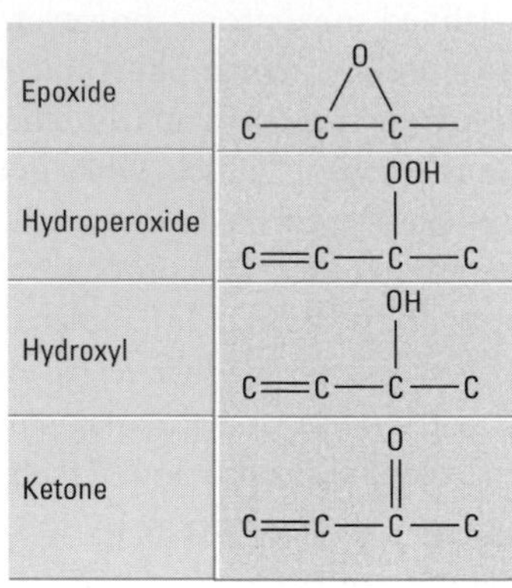

Figure 11.4 Highly active functional groups in unsaturated fatty acids such as arachidonic acid generated by the addition of oxygen atoms to various positions in the chain. The addition is catalysed by iron-containing enzymes. The positively charged Fe^{2+} associates with the negatively charged oxygen, which then associates with the double bond.

The liberated arachidonic acid is short-lived. It becomes the substrate of haem-containing enzymes that add oxygen atoms at various positions in the chain and thus create a variety of highly active functional groups such as epoxide, hydroperoxide, hydroxyl and ketone (Fig. 11.4). The reason why arachidonic acid oxidizes so easily is the presence of the double bonds in its chain. Oxygen bound to a metal ion, such as Fe^{2+}, in an enzyme tends to associate with a double bond. The oxygen atoms added to arachidonic acid vastly improve its ability to attach to metals or proteins and thus to modulate cellular functions. They also transform the highly lipophilic (membrane-soluble) arachidonic acid into compounds of intermediate lipid–water solubility and thus allow improved diffusion through water phases and better access to cytoplasmic constituents. One of the consequences of the oxidation is the formation of a five- or six-carbon ring in the middle of the chain, which makes part of the molecule considerably more rigid in comparison to the linear fatty acid. Rigidity is important for fitting the arachidonic acid derivatives into corresponding receptors and thus, once again, for cellular interactions.

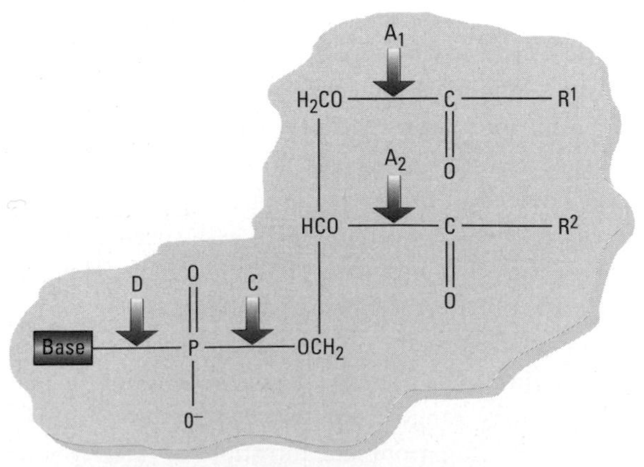

Figure 11.3 Sites of action (arrows) of phospholipases A_1, A_2, C and D on a typical phospholipid (phosphatidylcholine). R^1 and R^2 are the remains of the fatty acid chains.

Arachidonic acid metabolism can be initiated by either *cyclooxygenase (prostaglandin endoperoxide synthase)* or *lipoxygenase* (Figs 11.5 & 11.6). The former pathway generates prostaglandins, thromboxanes and prostacyclin; the latter produces leukotrienes and lipoxins. *Prostaglandins* are a large family of related compounds, all derived from *prostanoic acid* (Fig. 11.7). All prostaglandins possess 20 carbon atoms, five of which are arranged into a ring, the *cyclopentane*, and the rest into two fatty-acid (*aliphatic*) chains. Furthermore, they each have a double bond between C-13 and C-14, a hydroxyl group at C-15 in one of the side-chains and a terminal carboxyl group. Individual prostaglandins are designated by the symbol PG, followed by a third letter (A, B, C, D, E or F) to indicate the nature of the cyclopentane unit: whether it bears a hydroxyl at C-11 or a ketone group at C-9, and whether it is unsaturated or saturated. The three letters are followed by a numerical subscript to indicate the number of double bonds in the aliphatic chains emanating from the cyclopentane unit, and

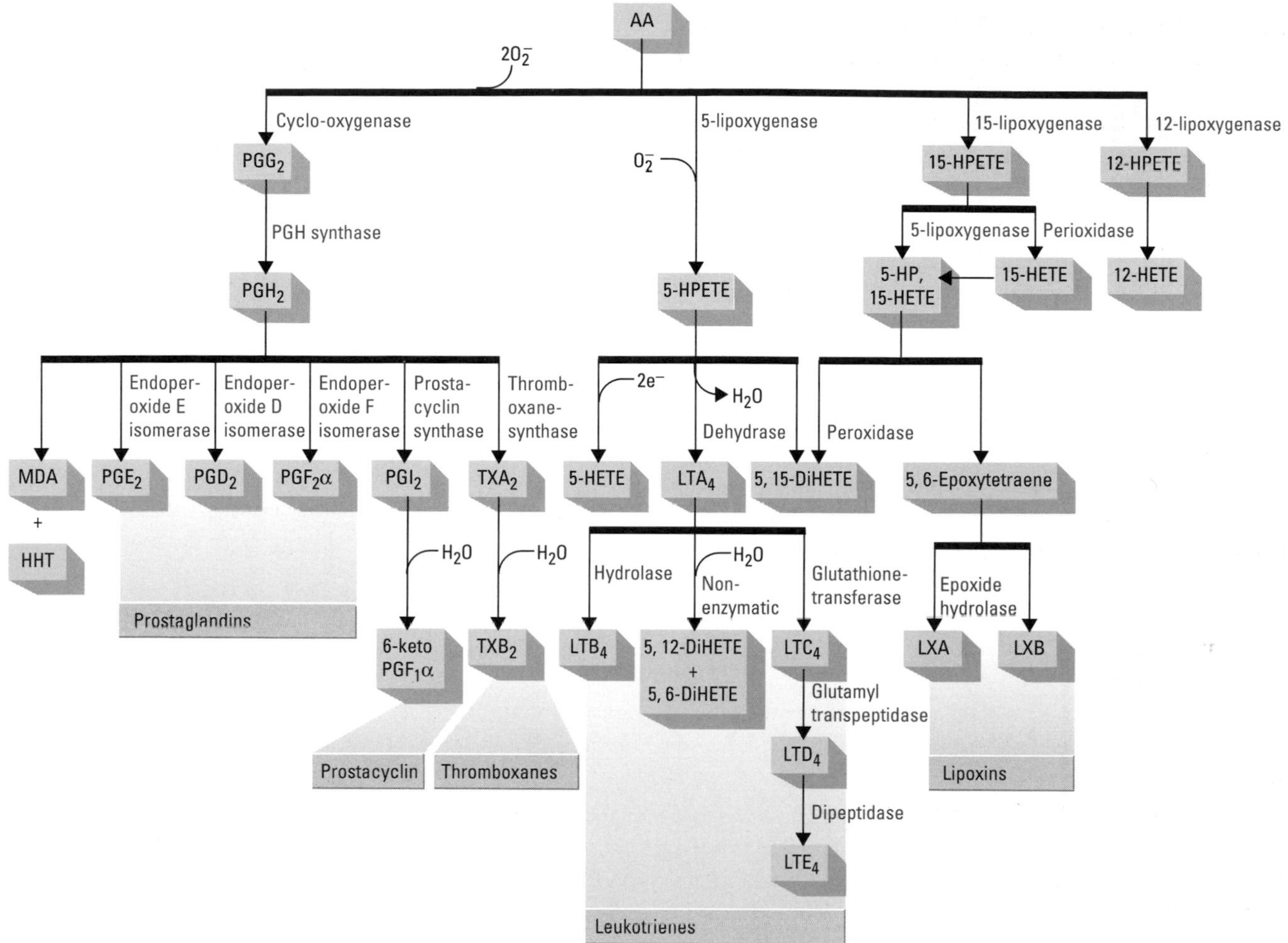

Figure 11.5 Arachidonic acid cascade: the verbal version. AA, arachidonic acid; DiHETE, dihydroxyeicosatetraenoic acid; HETE, hydroxyeicosatetraenoic acid; HHT, 12-hydroxy-5,8,10-heptadecatrienoic acid; HPETE, hydroperoxyeicosatetraenoic acid; LT, leukotriene; LX, lipoxin; MDA, malondialdehyde; PG, prostaglandin; TX, thromboxane. Participating enzymes are indicated in red.

in some symbols also by the Greek letter α, which indicates that the hydroxyl group at C-9 lies on the same side of the ring's plane as the carboxyl side-chain. The most prevalent prostaglandins are those possessing two double bonds (e.g. PGE_2 and $PGF_{2\alpha}$). Only some prostaglandins are derived from arachidonic acid. Another series of prostaglandins (e.g. PGE_1 and $PGF_{1\alpha}$) are derived from *8,11,14-eicosatrienoic acid* (dihomo-γ-linolenic acid) with three double bonds; a third series (e.g. PGE_3, $PGF_{3\alpha}$, PGI_3) is derived from *eicosapentaenoic acid* with five double bonds (Fig. 11.8; *eicosa*, the Greek word for 20 in the names of these acids, indicates that they each contain 20 carbon atoms). However, arachidonic acid, with its two double bonds, is the major source of physiologically important prostaglandins. Prostaglandins were originally identified as components of the seminal fluid capable of lowering blood pressure and stimulating contractions of uterine and intestinal smooth muscles. They derive their name from the false belief that they are produced in the prostate gland and stored in the seminal vesicle.

Prostacyclin (PGI_2) is in fact one of the prostaglandins; it received a separate name because it is functionally connected with thromboxane, which is not derived from prostanoic acid. *Thromboxanes* are derived from *thrombanoic acid*, which contains a six-carbon ring in place of the cyclopentane in prostaglandins (Fig. 11.9; the name refers to the fact that the substances are present predominantly in platelets or thrombocytes). The ring contains an oxygen bridge between the C-11 and C-12 atoms. Thromboxanes are designated by the symbol TX, followed by letters and

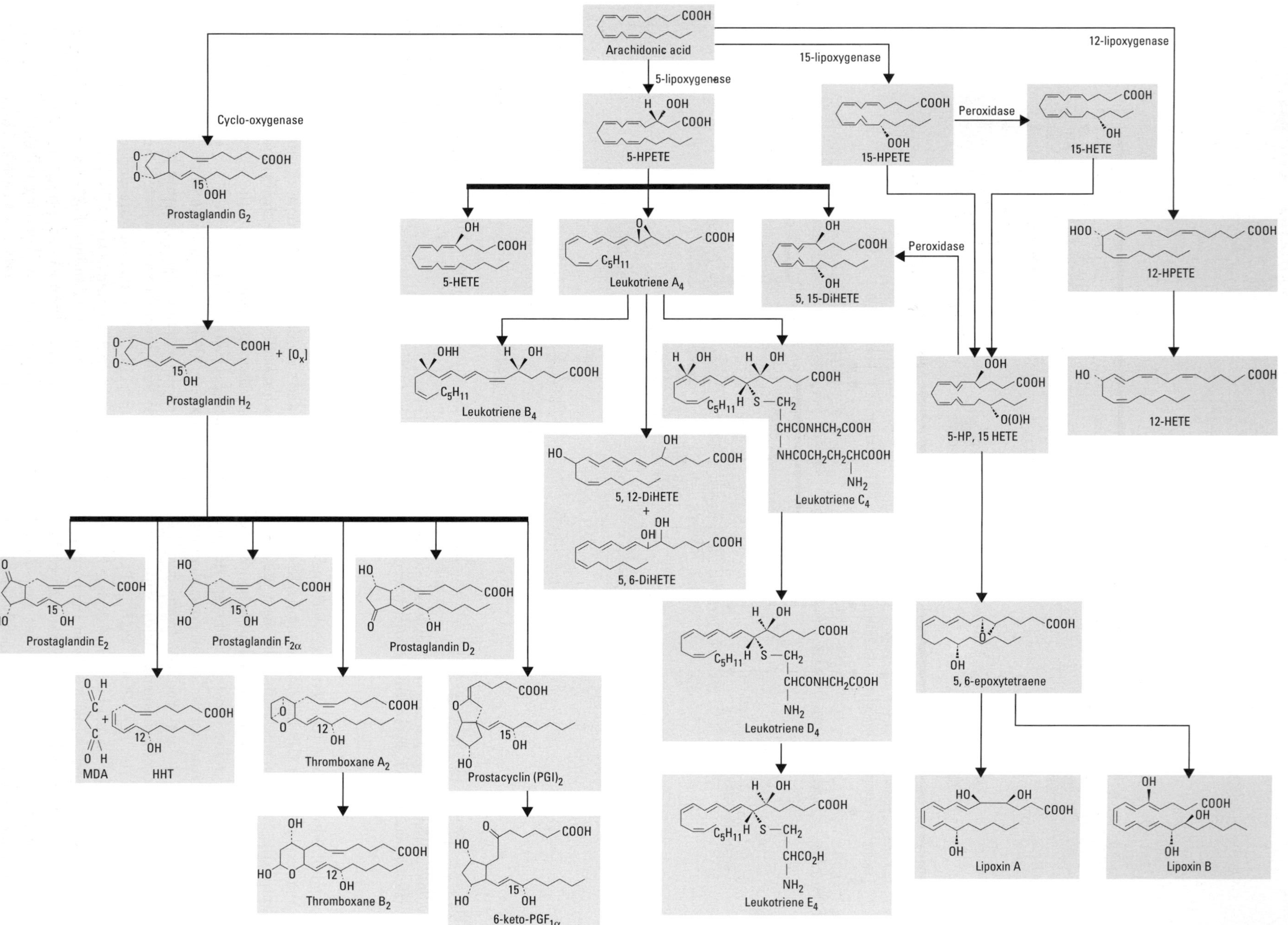

Figure 11.6 Arachidonic cascade: the chemical-formula version. DiHETE, dihydroxyeicosatetraenoic acid; HETE, hydroxyeicosatetraenoic acid; HHT, 12-hydroxy-5,8,10-heptadecatrienoic acid; HP, hydroperoxy; HPETE, hydroperoxyeicosatetraenoic acid; MDA, malondialdehyde.

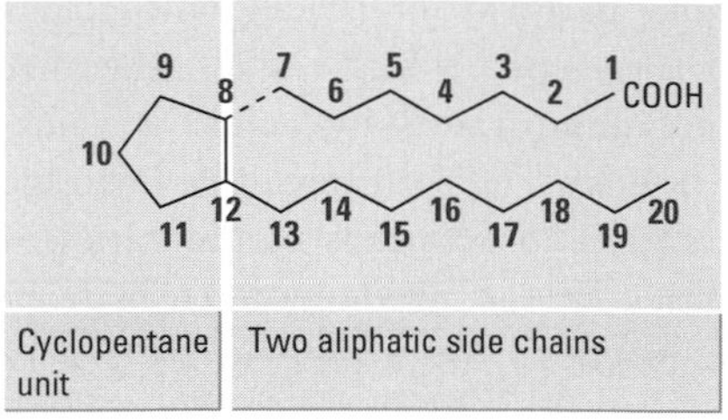

Figure 11.7 Prostanoic acid. Numbering of carbon atoms is indicated in red. Broken line indicates that the attached chain is below the plane of the carbons in the cyclopentane ring.

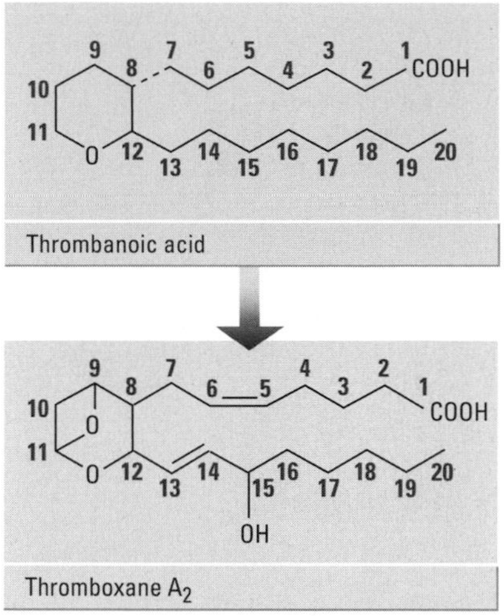

Figure 11.9 Derivation of thromboxane A_2 from thrombanoic acid. The numbering of carbon atoms is indicated in red. Broken line indicates that the chain is below the plane of the ring.

numbers similar to those used for prostaglandins. TXA_2, and its derivative TXB_2, are the only thromboxanes found in appreciable quantities in nature.

The first two steps in the *cyclooxygenase pathway* are the conversion of arachidonic acid to PGG_2, followed by the conversion of PGG_2 to PGH_2 (see Fig. 11.6). The first step is the *bisdioxygenase reaction*, in which two oxygen molecules are inserted into arachidonic acid to yield the endoperoxide PGG_2 (*cyclooxygenase activity*; endoperoxide is a compound with an internally located peroxide group, O—O). The second event is a two-electron reduction of the 15-hydroperoxide group of PGG_2 to yield PGH_2 (*hydroperoxidase activity*). Both the cyclooxygenase and hydroperoxidase activities are catalysed by the same haem-containing enzyme, the *cyclooxygenase (PG endoperoxidase synthase, PGH_2 synthase)*. The cyclooxygenase activity of the enzyme is inhibited by non-steroidal anti-inflammatory drugs such as aspirin and indomethacin. The drugs compete with arachidonic acid for the cyclooxygenase activity site. In addition, aspirin (acetylsalicylic acid) selectively acetylates a serine residue in or near the cyclooxygenase activity site and thus prevents the initial oxygen-insertion reaction (Fig. 11.10). The net result is inhibition of prostaglandin synthesis.

The PGH_2 generated in the first two steps of the cyclooxygenase pathway is then converted into biologically active prostaglandins, PGI_2 and thromboxanes, each reaction being catalysed by a specific enzyme (see Figs 11.5 & 11.6). The $PGH_2 \rightarrow PGD_2$ and $PGH_2 \rightarrow PGE_2$ conversions

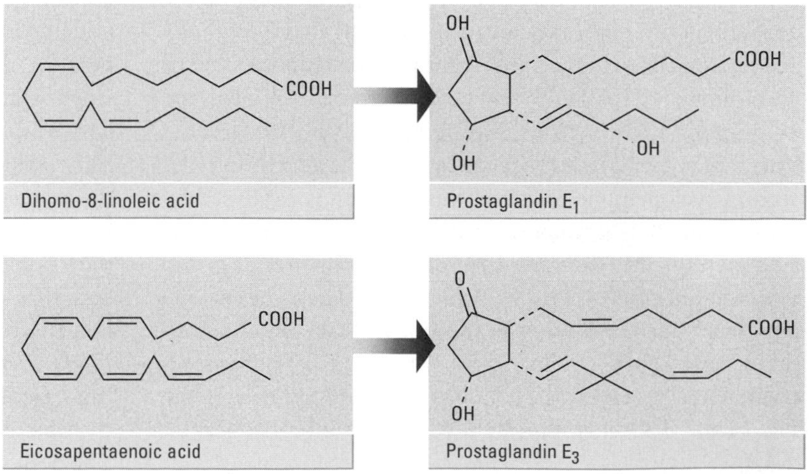

Figure 11.8 Alternative sources of prostaglandins. In addition to arachidonic acid, dihomo-8-linoleic acid (8,11,14-eicosatrienoic acid) and 5,8,11,14,17-eicosapentaenoic acid can also give rise to certain prostaglandins. Broken lines indicate that the chains are below the plane of the ring.

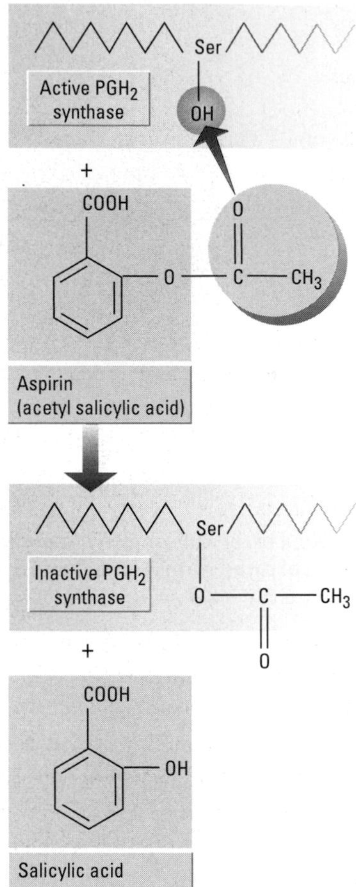

Figure 11.10 Inactivation of PGH_2 synthase (cyclooxygenase) by aspirin. The inactivation blocks prostaglandin synthesis and is one of the reasons for aspirin's anti-inflammatory effect.

involve rearrangements of atoms and atomic groups in a reaction that does not change the overall composition of the compounds. Such a reaction is called isomerization, the conversion of one isomer into another. The $PGH_2 \rightarrow PGE_2$ conversion requires the participation of the reduced form of glutathione (GSH). $PGH_2 \rightarrow PGF_{2\alpha}$ conversion involves the addition of two electrons, a process catalysed by a reductase. $PGH_2 \rightarrow PGI_2$ conversion involves the generation of a second cyclopentane ring and this reaction is catalysed by the enzyme PGI_2 synthase. Finally, $PGH_2 \rightarrow TXA_2$ conversion involves the rearrangement of the endoperoxide group in a reaction catalysed by TXA_2 synthase. The same enzyme apparently also catalyses the splitting of PGH_2 into malondialdehyde (MDA) and 12-hydroxy-5,8,10-heptadecatrienoic acid (HHT; it contains 17 carbon atoms; see Fig. 11.6). TXA_2 is rapidly hydrolysed into hemiacetal TXB_2.

The second pathway of arachidonic acid metabolism involves *lipoxygenases*, which catalyse the introduction of oxygen to polyunsaturated fatty acids (i.e. acids with multiple double bonds). The oxygen can be introduced into the C-5, C-12 and C-15 positions of the various eicosaenoic acids, resulting in the production of hydroperoxy fatty acids. The reactions are catalysed by 5-, 12- and 15-lipoxygenases, respectively, which are differentially expressed in cells and species. For example, pig polymorphonuclear leucocytes (PMN) display 5-, 12- and 15-lipoxygenase activity; human PMN possess 5- and 15-lipoxygenase activity; and human platelets display 12-lipoxygenase activity. The products formed by the action of the different lipoxygenases differ in their structure (see Fig. 11.6), although the principle of fatty acid oxygenation is the same. In the following account, we consider for simplicity only the reactions catalysed by 5- and 15-lipoxygenases.

5-Lipoxygenase is present in an inactive form in the cytosol. Cell activation via a receptor-mediated event leads to an increase of intracellular Ca^{2+} level and thus to activation of the enzyme. The activated enzyme then moves from the cytosol to the plasma membrane, where it interacts with *f*ive-*l*ipoxygenase-*a*ctivating *p*rotein (FLAP). With the help of FLAP, 5-lipoxygenase converts arachidonic acid to 5-hydroperoxy-6,8,11,14-eicosatetraenoic acid (5-HPETE), which can subsequently undergo one of three different transformations (see Fig. 11.6). Two-electron reduction of the hydroxyl group to an alcohol yields a 5-hydroxyeicosatetraenoic acid (5-HETE). Dehydration of 5-HETE produces an epoxy fatty acid called *leukotriene (LT)*A_4. Lipoxygenation at another position in the aliphatic chain yields, after reduction of two hydroperoxy groups, *5,15-dihydroxyeicosatetraenoic acid (5,15-diHETE)*. LTA_4 can undergo three further transformations (see Fig. 11.6). It can be hydrolysed non-enzymatically into various isomers of diHETEs, hydrolysed enzymatically to LTB_4 or it can undergo ring-opening in the presence of GSH to yield peptide derivatives in which GSH is attached via a sulphoether linkage to the fatty acid. The various peptide derivatives of LTA_4 are termed LTC_4, LTD_4, LTE_4 and LTF_4, depending on the nature of the peptide (Fig. 11.11; the numerical subscripts again indicate the total number of double bonds). The term 'leukotriene' reflects the fact that the compounds were originally isolated from leucocytes and that they contain at least three alternating double bonds (in fact, most leukotrienes have four double bonds). *Leukotrienes* are thus a family of acyclic (containing no ring) eicosanoid compounds derived from epoxyeicosatetraenoic acid and thus ultimately from arachidonic acid. The designation does not apply to diHETEs formed by two

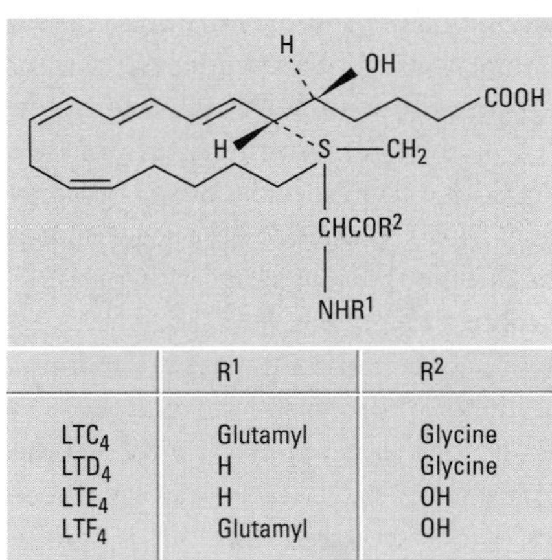

	R^1	R^2
LTC_4	Glutamyl	Glycine
LTD_4	H	Glycine
LTE_4	H	OH
LTF_4	Glutamyl	OH

Figure 11.11 Structure of leukotrienes LTC_4, LTD_4, LTE_4 and LTF_4 (the indices refer to the number of double bonds). R, radical.

consecutive lipoxygenase reactions, although some of these compounds do contain a triene unit. The combined action of 15- and 5-lipoxygenases on arachidonic acid produces 5-hydroperoxy-15-hydroxy-6,13-*trans*-8,11-*cis*-eicosatetraenoic acid (5-HP, 15-HETE), which is then converted into 5,6-epoxytetraene (see Fig. 11.6). This last compound is transformed into *lipoxins*, either lipoxin A (by the action of epoxide hydrolase) or lipoxin B (by attack on the C-14 position and generation of an 8-*cis* double bond). Lipoxin A is 5,6,15-trihydroxy-7,9,13-*trans*-11-*cis*-eicosatetraenoic acid, whereas lipoxin B is 5,14,15-trihydroxy-6,10,12-*trans*-8-*cis*-eicosatetraenoic acid. Lipoxins, like leukotrienes, are derived mostly from leucocytes.

Prostaglandins, PGI_2, thromboxanes, leukotrienes and lipoxins are formed in bursts in response to non-specific or specific stimuli. Normally, very little of these substances is present in an unstimulated cell. Upon stimulation, prostaglandins can be detected within 10–30 s, and their synthesis proceeds for 1–5 min and then stops. The synthesized substances are rapidly degraded, allowing them only a short period in which they can act and their action is restricted to the area around the site of synthesis, either the cell of origin or neighbouring cells. While virtually all animal organs produce prostaglandins, usually only certain cell types within each organ synthesize them. Each cell type is only able to form some of the various prostaglandins or thromboxanes. For example, platelets form TXA_2 almost exclusively; smooth muscle and arterial endothelial cells mainly form PGI_2; and renal tubule cells usually form PGE_2. The synthesis of HPETE and HETE, and hence of leukotrienes and lipoxins, is associated primarily with neutrophils, eosinophils, monocytes, mast cells and macrophages. Prostaglandins and thromboxanes are generated on the cytosolic side of various cell membranes: the endoplasmic reticulum, the nuclear membrane, the plasma membrane and possibly also the mitochondrial membrane. (Phospholipase C is a soluble protein but acts on the cytosolic surface of the membranes; phospholipase A_2, as well as most, if not all, of the enzymes involved in prostaglandin–thromboxane metabolism, are integral membrane proteins.)

Prostaglandins display a wide range of biological effects on the female reproductive system (steroidogenesis, ovulation, regression of corpus luteum, menstruation, parturition), gastric secretions, blood pressure and inflammatory processes. In inflamed tissues, they dilate blood vessels, increase vascular permeability and act on pain receptors and on the thermoregulatory centre in the hypothalamus causing fever. *Thromboxanes* and *prostacyclin* participate in blood clotting via their involvement in platelet activation (see Chapter 21). *LTC_4*, *LTD_4* and *LTE_4* effect smooth muscle contractions, particularly in the skin and lung microvasculature (they have been implicated as one component of an asthmatic reaction; see Chapter 23). The active principle responsible for contractions, released by lung tissues in response to an immunological challenge, was originally named the *slow-reacting substance of anaphylaxis* (*SRS-A*); it consists of a mixture of LTC_4, LTD_4 and LTE_4. The three leukotrienes are only marginally involved in inflammation because of their ability to increase blood vessel permeability in the skin and their influence on certain regulatory functions. LTB_4, on the other hand, plays an important part in inflammation by acting as a highly potent chemotactic factor for neutrophils. *Lipoxins* cause contraction of smooth muscles, dilation of microvasculature, chemotaxis, hypertension and hyperfiltration; they also inhibit natural killer cell activity.

Platelet-activating factor

When leucocytes from immunized rabbits are cultured with the antigen *in vitro* they produce soluble factors, some of which activate platelets, causing them to aggregate. The *platelet-activating factors* (*PAF*) are compounds derived from glycerol in a manner shown in Fig. 11.12. To each of the three principal carbon atoms of glycerol (*sn*1–*sn*3) a different radical is added: a remnant of fatty acid (an alkyl) is attached to *sn*1 via an ether linkage; an acetyl is linked to *sn*2; and a phosphocholine is joined to *sn*3. The resulting compound is therefore a 1-O-alkyl-2-acetyl-*sn*-glycero-3-phosphocholine or an *a*cetyl *a*lkyl *g*lycerol *e*ther analogue of *p*hosphatidyl*c*holine (*AGEPC*). A number of PAF variants have been identified that differ in both the length and

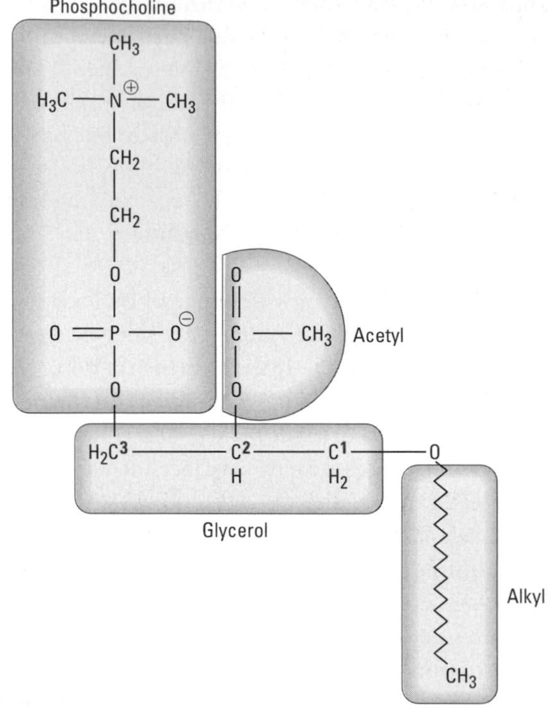

Figure 11.12 Structural formula of platelet-activating factor (PAF). The mode of PAF derivation from glycerol by substitutions at the three carbon atoms is shown in red.

number of double bonds in the fatty acid; the substituent at the *sn* position (instead of an acetyl, the various molecular species may have different acyls such as propionyl, butyryl, hexanoyl or palmitoyl); and the nature of the polar head group (the choline can be replaced by other groups). The two principal forms of interest here are the alkylacetylglycerophosphocholine (the original PAF) and the alkylacylglycerophosphocholine.

Alkylacyl-GPC is normally present in the membranes of unstimulated cells such as platelets, neutrophils, eosinophils, basophils, monocytes, mast cells and endothelial cells. *Alkylacetyl-GPC* (PAF) is normally absent in the membranes of unstimulated cells but is synthesized upon stimulation of the cells listed above. Alkylacyl-GPC is the precursor of PAF and the synthesis occurs via an intermediate, *alkyllyso-GPC* (lyso-PAF; Fig. 11.13). The conversion of alkylacyl-GPC to alkyllyso-GPC is catalysed by the enzyme phospholipase A_2 and the conversion of alkyllyso-GPC to PAF by the enzyme acetyltransferase. Both reactions are reversible: PAF can be converted back to alkyllyso-GPC in a reaction catalysed by an acetylhydrolase and alkyllyso-GPC can be converted back to alkylacyl-GPC in a reaction catalysed by an acyltransferase (Fig. 11.13). All four enzymes are widely distributed among the various tissues of the body, but acetyltransferase is normally present in an inactive form. To become active, it must be phosphorylated in a reaction catalysed by a protein kinase. This

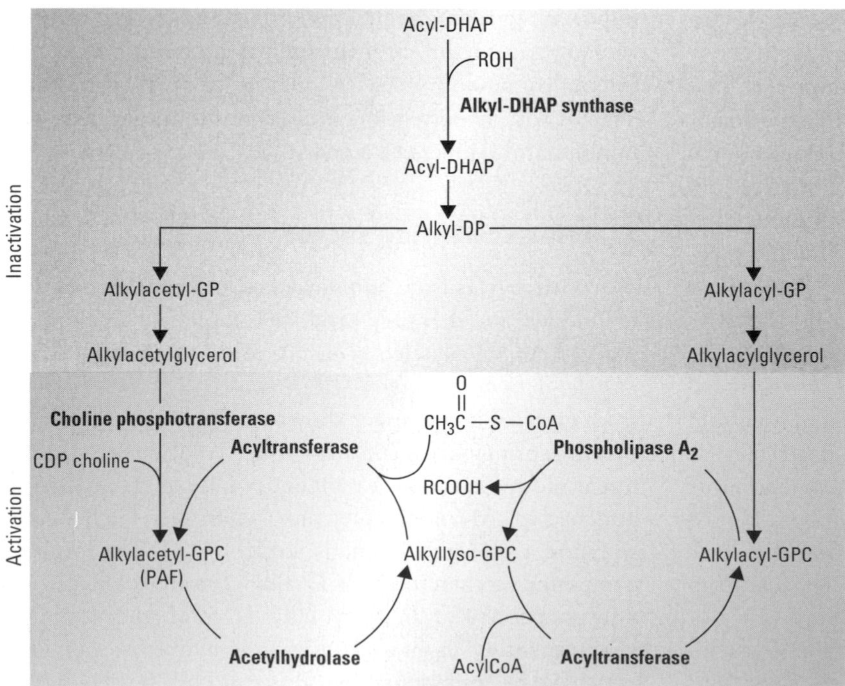

Figure 11.13 Biosynthesis and degradation of platelet-activating factor (PAF). CDP, cytosine diphosphate; CoA, coenzyme A; DHAP, dihydroxyacetone phosphate; DP, dihydroxyphosphate; GP, glycerophosphate; GPC, glycerophosphocholine; R, radical. Some of the participating enzymes are shown in red.

enzyme must be activated in turn by reactions initiated by the cell-activating stimulus. The phosphorylated acetyltransferase itself becomes a substrate for another enzyme, phosphohydrolase, which removes the added phosphate group and thus inactivates the acetyltransferase. In this manner, the production of PAF is tightly regulated. The stimulation of a cell with a high content of alkylacyl-GPC (e.g. a neutrophil) leads to the activation of a specific protein kinase, which in turn activates the specific acetyltransferase to produce PAF from lyso-PAF. Simultaneously, however, the activated acetyltransferase becomes the target of a specific phosphohydrolase that inactivates it again, and the production of PAF trails off. The produced PAF itself may become the substrate for acetylhydrolase and thus be converted back to lyso-PAF and subsequently to alkylacyl-GPC. However, if large quantities of PAF are produced as a result of cell stimulation, some of it is released from the membranes into the surrounding fluid (plasma in particular), where it becomes part of the mediator pool. The *de novo* generation of PAF is quite rapid: within 30 s after stimulation, PAF is demonstrable in the cell and within a few minutes it appears in the surrounding fluid. Since the acetylhydrolase is present not only in the cells but also in the plasma, the released PAF is inactivated rapidly, being converted by this enzyme to lyso-PAF. The plasma enzyme has a higher relative moleculer mass (M_r) than its corresponding cytosolic form, presumably because of added sugar residues that make it resistant to inactivation by proteases.

In addition to the pathway of PAF synthesis just described, there is also a *second pathway* which begins with alkylacetylglycerol phosphate (see Fig. 11.13). This compound is converted to alkylacetylglycerol, which in turn is converted to PAF in a reaction catalysed by the enzyme *choline phosphotransferase*. Both the acetyltransferase and the choline phosphotransferase are present at relatively high levels in most cells but only the former seems to be activated by the stimuli known to trigger the release of PAF. Different cell types may actually use different pathways of PAF synthesis and the selection of pathways could depend on the physiological state of the particular cell. Both pathways converge in a single compound, *alkyldihydroxyphosphate*, which itself is ultimately synthesized from acyldihydroxyacetone phosphate (acyl-DHAP; see Fig. 11.13).

Upon stimulation, PAF is released from platelets, granulocytes, monocytes, macrophages, mast cells, lymphocytes, endothelial cells and even bacteria (Fig. 11.14). It is an extremely potent mediator, being biologically active at

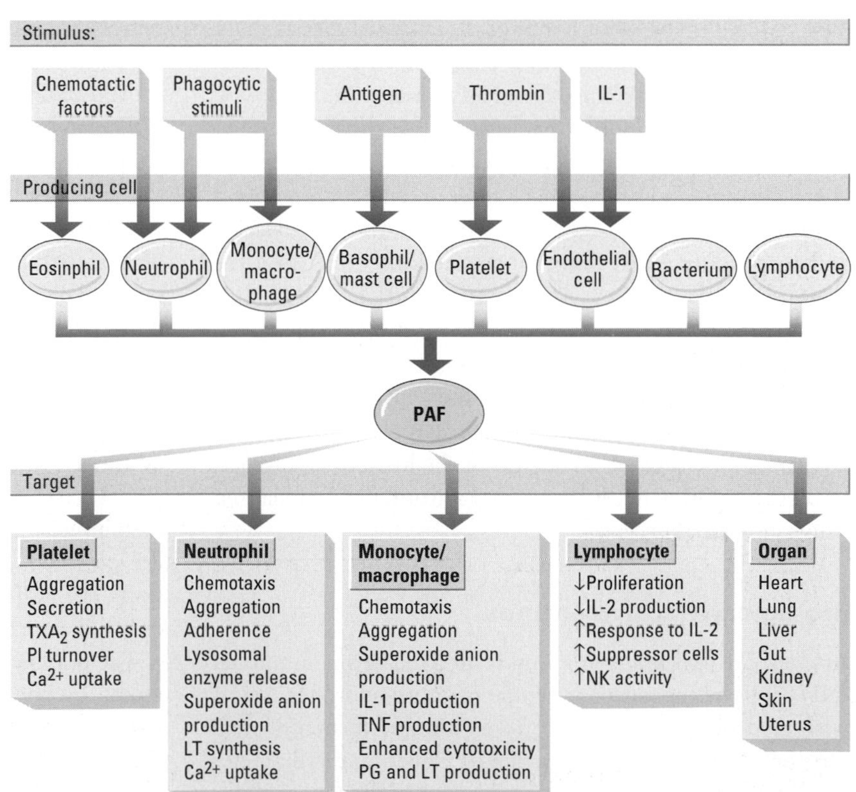

Figure 11.14 Stimuli and cells producing platelet-activating factor (PAF), as well as target cells or organs of PAF. IL, interleukin; LT, leukotriene; NK, natural killer; PG, prostaglandin; PI, phosphatidylinositol; TNF, tumour necrosis factor; TXA_2, thromboxane A_2; ↑, increase; ↓, decrease. (Modified from Braquet, P. & Rola-Pleszczynski, M. (1987) *Immunology Today*, **8**, 345.)

concentrations as low as 3×10^{-11} M. Its activity depends on all three of the groups attached to the glycerol backbone. The replacement of the acetyl group by propionyl, butyryl, hexanoyl or palmitoyl groups progressively decreases the activity of the compound in this order; the removal of the acetyl group renders the compound inactive. Similarly, the removal or replacement of the alkyl or phosphocholine groups results in a drastic decrease in activity or complete inactivation of the compound. The stimuli that lead to the generation of PAF can be immunological (e.g. antigen, interleukin (IL)-1 or IgE antibodies) as well as non-immunological (e.g. ionophore A23187, chemotactic factors, thrombin; see Fig. 11.14) in nature. The effects of PAF can be either direct or indirect. Directly, PAF binds to a cell-surface receptor, activates the cell and the activation can then be measured in terms of platelet aggregation, for example. Indirectly, PAF activates the cell, causing it to release another mediator whose effect is then measured (PAF can stimulate mast cells, for example, to release histamine, which then causes contraction of smooth muscles). The effects of PAF are manifold (see Fig. 11.14). In platelets, PAF causes activation, aggregation and degranulation leading to the release of substances such as serotonin and TXA_2. In neutrophils, it causes aggregation, degranulation, chemotaxis, increased cell adherence, enhanced respiratory burst, superoxide production (see Chapter 15) and the production of arachidonic acid metabolites via the lipoxygenase pathway. The main lymphocyte target of PAF is the T cell. (Normally, lymphocytes are unable to produce PAF, although they can produce lyso-PAF when stimulated with the A23187 ionophore; the reason for their failure to produce PAF may be the lack of acetyltransferase. This lack is not absolute, however, since under special circumstances lymphocytes can be forced to synthesize acetyltransferase and to produce PAF.) Some of the actions of PAF on the various T-cell subsets are summarized in Fig. 11.15. Directly or indirectly, PAF increases vascular permeability, induces constriction of smooth muscles in the gut and the lungs (smooth muscles seem to have PAF-specific receptors so part of this action at least can be considered as direct), stimulates glycogenolysis in the liver, causes hypertension, produces neutropenia and thrombocytopenia and causes intestinal necrosis.

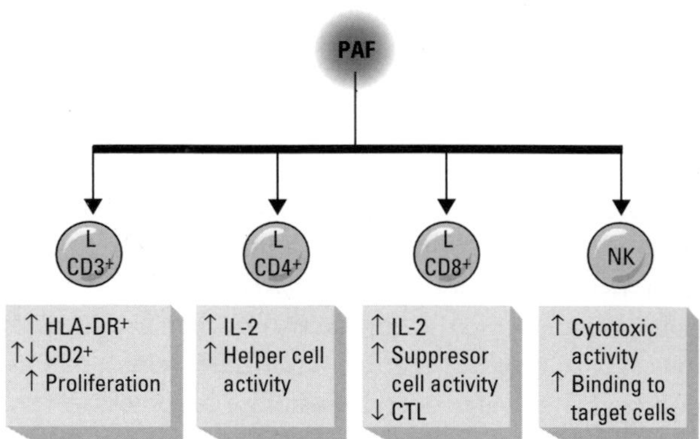

Figure 11.15 Effects of platelet-activating factor (PAF) on lymphocytes (L) and natural killer (NK) cells. CD, cluster of differentiation (antigen); CTL, cytotoxic T lymphocyte; IL-2, interleukin-2; ↑, increase; ↓, decrease. (Modified from Braquet, P. & Rola-Pleszczynski, M. (1987) *Immunology Today*, 8, 345.)

Biologically active amines

Amines are organic compounds derived from ammonia (NH_4) by the replacement of one or more hydrogen atoms with hydrocarbon radicals. Two amines, histamine and serotonin, are biologically active by affecting the diameter of blood vessels and the permeability of blood vessel walls. They are both synthesized from amino acids, histamine from histidine and serotonin from tryptophan.

Histamine (β-imidazolylethylamine)

The production of histamine from histidine involves the removal of CO_2 (decarboxylation), a reaction catalysed by the enzyme histidine decarboxylase (Fig. 11.16). Histamine is produced in tissue mast cells and circulating basophils, as well as in other cells of most body tissues (hence the name, from Greek *histos*, tissue). Mast cells and basophils store the produced histamine in metachromatic granules, in which it is associated, via ionic bonds, with carboxyl groups of proteoglycans and proteins in the granular matrix; it is released on degranulation. Histamine is degraded along one of two pathways: one, the predominant one in human tissues, initiated by the enzyme histamine-*N*-methyltransferase; and the other by the enzyme diamine oxidase (histaminase). The former pathway produces methylimidazole acetic acid and the latter riboside-*N*-3-imidazole acetic acid (Fig. 11.16), both of which are excreted in urine as inactive metabolites. The enzymes involved in these two pathways are prevalent throughout body tissues and in the circulation. The half-life of histamine produced in these tissues is only a few minutes.

The presence of histamine in a tissue extract can be determined by one of three methods. The oldest, and now outdated, method is to add the extract to part of the guinea-pig intestine (ileum) and to observe the shortening caused by contraction of smooth muscles in the intestine wall.

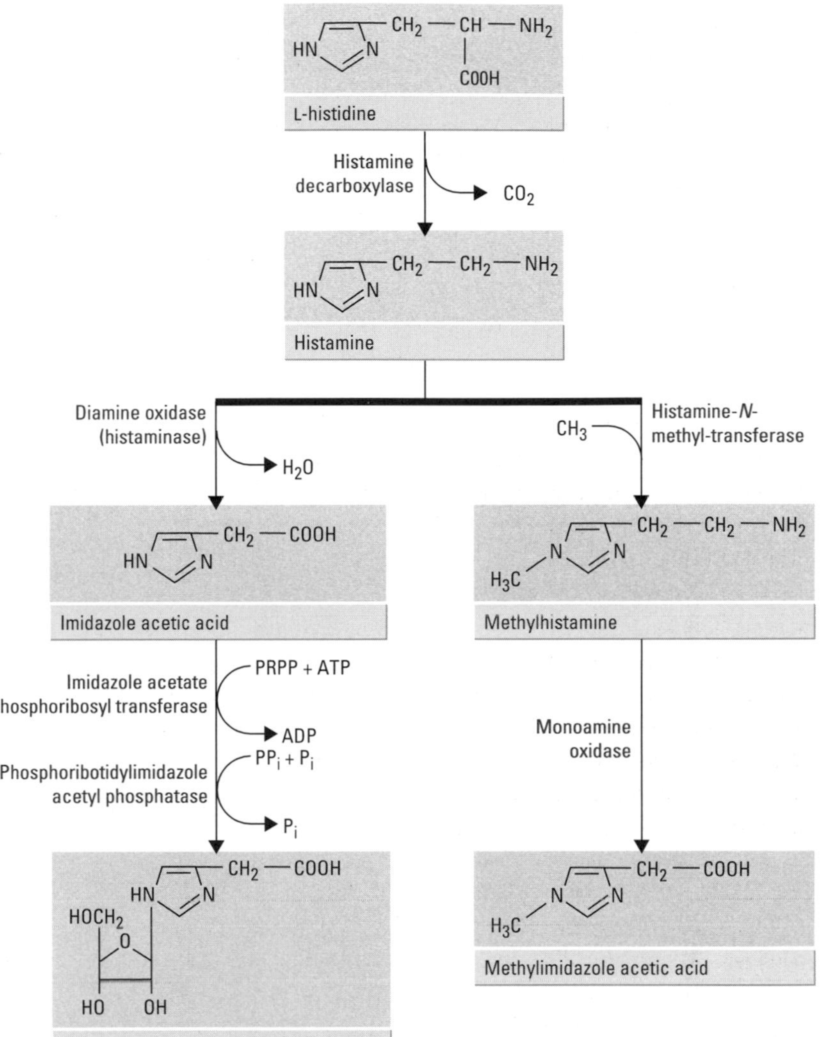

Figure 11.16 Histamine biosynthesis from histidine and its degradation to riboside-*N*-3 imidazole acetic acid and methylimidazole acetic acid. Participating enzymes are indicated in red. ADP, adenosine diphosphate; ATP, adenosine triphosphate; P_i, orthophosphate ion; PP_i, phyrophosphate ion; PRPP, 5-phosphoribosyl-α-pyrophosphate.

(Guinea-pigs are particularly sensitive to histamine action and are therefore the obvious choice in studying allergies.) In the second method, histamine is converted to a fluorescent product by the reaction with orthophthalic dialdehyde and the fluorescence of this product is then quantitated. In the third and most sensitive method, a radiolabelled methyl group is enzymatically transferred from 5-adenosyl methionine to histamine (a reaction catalysed by histamine methyltransferase) and the radioactivity of the resulting product is measured.

Histamine released by degranulation of mast cells and basophils exerts its biological effects via specific receptors on the surface of target cells. The binding of histamine to these receptors can be competitively inhibited by substances collectively known as *antihistamines*. There are now over 100 commercially available preparations with an antihistamine effect, most of which can be taken orally. The systemic effects of antihistamines become apparent 15–30 min after oral administration, peak at 1–2 hours and last for 3–12 hours, depending on the preparation. Antihistamines react with three kinds of histamine receptor, H_1, H_2 and H_3. Signals initiated by occupation of the H_1 receptor are transmitted via intracellular Ca^{2+} ions and the receptor can be blocked by the so-called *classical antihistamines* (the first group discovered), which all share the common structure of a substituted ethylamine (Fig. 11.17). The *H_2 receptor* acts via cyclic AMP and it can be blocked by a newer group of antihistamines, which are mostly polar or hydrophobic molecules (Fig. 11.17).

The histamine receptors determine the biological effects

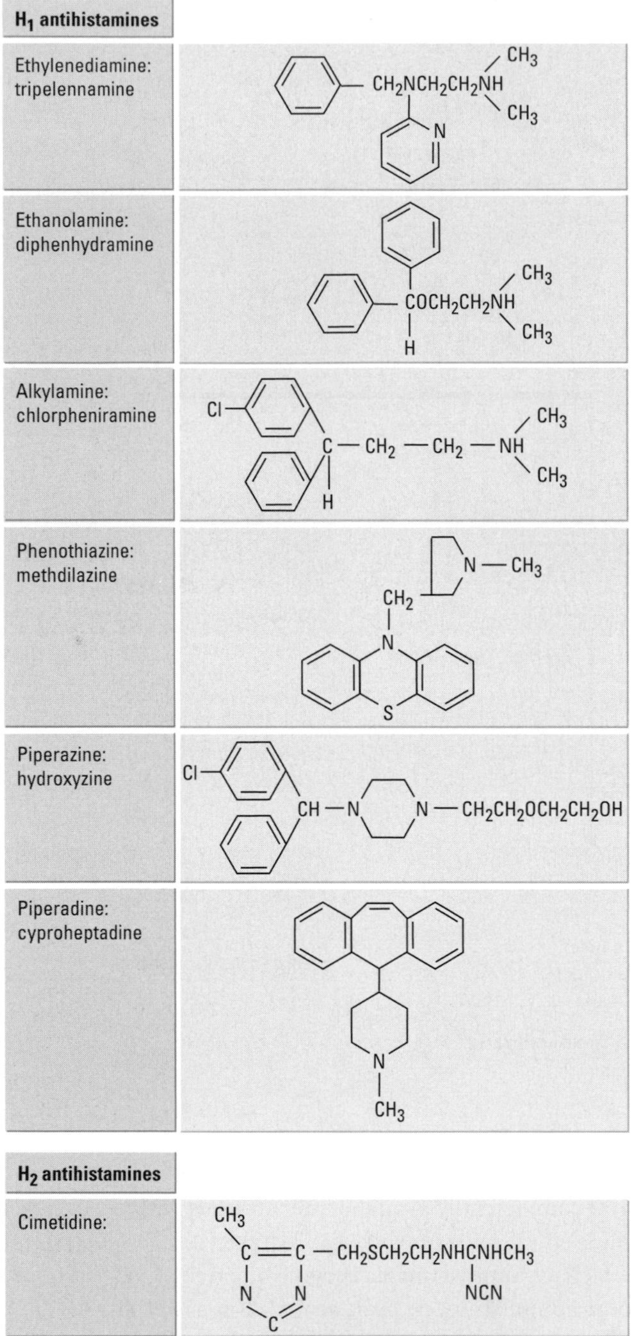

Figure 11.17 Structural formulas of H_1 and H_2 antihistamines.

of histamine (Fig. 11.18). The binding of histamine to H_1 receptors leads to the contraction of smooth muscles in the bronchi of the lungs and in the gastrointestinal tract. Histamine binding to H_2 receptors primarily stimulates the secretion of gastric acid by parietal cells, but it also has a variety of effects on the immune system. It suppresses or inhibits T cell-mediated cytotoxicity, cytokine (IL-1, IL-2, IL-6, TNF-α) production, granulocyte chemotaxis, release of lysosomal enzymes from neutrophils, lymphocyte proliferation and IgE-mediated release of histamine itself. One of the reasons for the diverse effects mediated by H_1 and H_2 receptors is the different tissue and cell distribution of these receptors (endothelial cells and smooth muscle cells express H_1 receptors, while other tissues, such as stomach glands, express H_2 receptors). The two receptors also mediate opposing effects of histamine on inflammation: the binding of histamine via H_1 receptors enhances inflammation, whereas binding via H_2 receptors inhibits it. The three main targets of histamine are blood vessels, smooth muscles and exocrine glands. The effect on the vascular system varies, depending on the size of the vessel and on the animal species. In general, large blood vessels and arterioles are constricted by histamine, whereas minute vessels, capillaries and venules are dilated. Histamine-induced arteriolar constriction is strong in rodents and slight in cats; in dogs, monkeys and humans, histamine causes arteriolar dilation. Fine-vessel dilation is brought about by the direct action of histamine on the musculature of the vessels, independent of innervation. Vasodilation is accompanied by an increase in permeability, leading to the seepage of plasma proteins and fluids into the extracellular spaces, and so to the formation of a swelling (oedema). In larger vessels, histamine increases permeability by causing the cells of the endothelial lining to separate, thereby generating intercellular spaces through which plasma can escape. When injected intravenously, histamine affects almost all capillaries in the body, but the response in humans is most conspicuous in the skin of the face and upper part of the body, the *blushing areas*, which become hot and red. The dilation of arterioles and capillaries results in a fall of blood pressure. Particularly sensitive to histamine are the muscles of the uterus and bronchioli. In most species, these muscles contract upon exposure to histamine; however in some species (e.g. the rat), histamine produces the opposite effect, i.e. muscle relaxation. Of the exocrine glands, the most strongly affected are those of the stomach. Histamine probably acts directly on the gland cells, inducing them to intensify their secretion.

Serotonin (5-hydroxytryptamine, 5-HT)

Serotonin is derived from tryptophan in two steps. First, tryptophan is converted to 5-hydroxytryptophan by the addition of one hydroxyl group to position 5, a reaction catalysed by the enzyme tryptophan-5-hydroxylase. In the second step, 5-hydroxytryptophan is converted to 5-hydroxytryptamine by the removal of CO_2 in a reaction catalysed by aromatic L-amino acid decarboxylase (Fig. 11.19). In tissues, serotonin is rapidly degraded, first

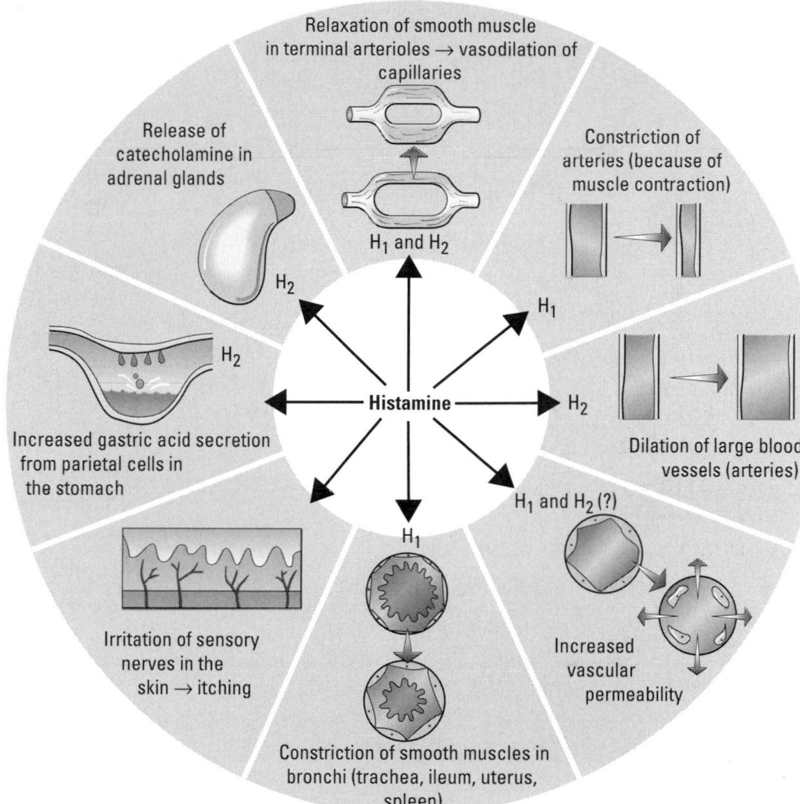

Figure 11.18 Some of the effects of histamine in humans.

to 5-hydroxyindole acetaldehyde in a reaction catalysed by monoamine oxidase and then to an inert metabolite, 5-hydroxyindole acetic acid, in a reaction catalysed by aldehyde dehydrogenase.

Diverse mammalian species contain serotonin in varying amounts in different cells. All species have serotonin in their central nervous system, where it functions as one of the neurotransmitters that carry messages across the gap between the dendrites of two neurons. Most mammals also have serotonin in platelet granules, from which it is released during blood clotting (it derives its name from the fact that it remains in the serum after the blood has been allowed to clot). In humans, serotonin is also found in the enterochromaffin cells of the gastrointestinal tract mucosa, but it is absent in mast cells. On the other hand, serotonin is present in rodents, bound to protein matrix, in the granules of some mast cells. Serotonin in tissues can be detected by one of three methods similar to those used for the detection of histamine (in the biological assay, one measures the contraction of the uterus dissected from rats in oestrus).

Serotonin effects a wide range of responses that vary not only between species but also between individuals of the same species. It acts in particular on smooth muscle cells and nerves, affecting primarily the cardiovascular, respiratory and digestive systems. Its effect on smooth muscles can be either direct or indirect via nerves. In the vascular system, serotonin causes leakage of venules by partially disjoining endothelial cells.

Granular proteoglycans

Like glycoproteins, proteoglycans (formerly *mucoproteins*) consist of proteins and carbohydrates; the differences between these two classes of organic compounds is in the protein-to-carbohydrate ratio. *Glycoproteins* usually contain 1–60% carbohydrate by weight in the form of short (generally less than 15 sugar residues) branched oligosaccharide chains of variable composition. *Proteoglycans*, on the other hand, usually contain 90–95% carbohydrate by weight in the form of many long, unbranched chains. A typical *proteoglycan aggregate* consists of a hyaluronic acid core from which many side-chains radiate like the bristles of a bottle-brush. Each 'bristle' consists of a single, serine-rich, 1900 amino acid residue *core protein* and more than 100

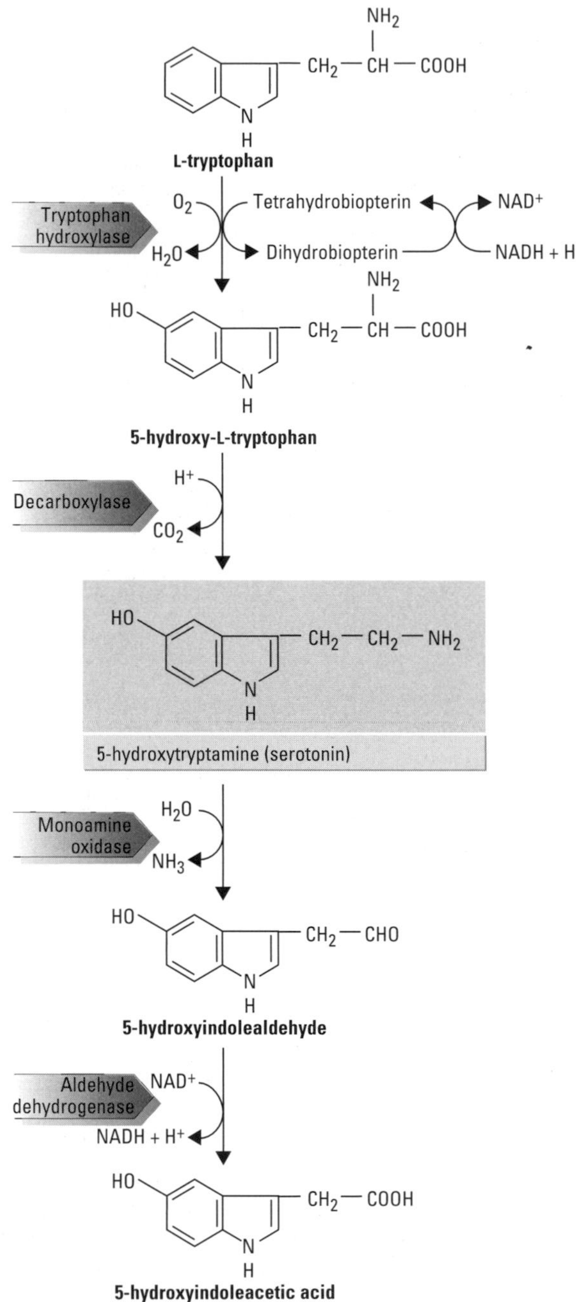

Figure 11.19 Biosynthesis of serotonin from tryptophan and its degradation to 5-hydroxyindole acetic acid. Participating enzymes are indicated by red arrows.

carbohydrate side-chains (Fig. 11.20), allowing approximately one carbohydrate side-chain for every 12 amino acid residues. Each carbohydrate chain consists of repeating disaccharide units, in which one of the two residues is always an amino sugar (*N*-acetylglucosamine or *N*-acetylgalactosamine) so that the chain represents a *glycosaminoglycan* (formerly *mucopolysaccharide*). The second sugar in the unit varies from one glycosaminoglycan to another. Each glycosaminoglycan chain is attached to the serine of the core protein via a *link trisaccharide* consisting of the sequence xylose-galactose-galactose. Before they are exported from the cell, some glycosaminoglycans are modified in the Golgi apparatus by the addition of sulphate groups (SO^-_3) to the amino sugar. The sulphate groups, together with the repeating carboxyl groups (COO^-) impart a high negative charge on the glycosaminoglycans. Proteoglycans are mainly present in the extracellular matrix, being part of connective tissue in a variety of organs. Some proteoglycans, however, form the matrix of intracellular granules. The matrix of mast cell granules is made of heparin, whereas the matrix of basophil granules is more complex, consisting of chondroitin sulphate, heparan sulphate and dermatan sulphate, with very little or no heparin, depending on the animal species.

Heparin

This proteoglycan derives its name from the fact that it was first isolated from the liver (Greek *hépar*). Nowadays, however, commercial preparations of heparin are produced from the intestinal mucosa and lungs. The source of heparin in all these tissues is mast cells, the only cells known to produce this mediator. The repeating disaccharide unit of heparin consists of *N*-acetyl-D-glucosamine and D-glucuronic or α-L-iduronic acid (these compounds are epimers: they differ only in the spatial arrangement of their carboxyl groups; Fig. 11.21). The chains are highly sulphated, so that the number of sulphate ions per disaccharide unit averages two to three. The length of each chain ranges from 4000 to 40 000 monosaccharide residues. (Further heterogeneity of heparin molecules is achieved by the proportion of the iduronic acid-containing disaccharides and the number of sulphate groups.) Heparin released by degranulation of mast cells is neutralized by protamines, myelin basic proteins and other positively charged protein molecules; it is degraded by the enzyme heparinase. The main function of heparin is the prevention of blood clotting. One of the key clotting factors is *thrombin*, a serine protease responsible for the conversion of fibrinogen to fibrin (see Chapter 21). The action of thrombin is opposed by *antithrombin III*, a protein whose arginyl residue is esterified by the serine in the thrombin active site. This process inactivates thrombin irreversibly in the thrombin–antithrombin complex. The reaction is slow but is greatly accelerated when antithrombin combines with heparin via a specific lysine residue (Fig. 11.22). The

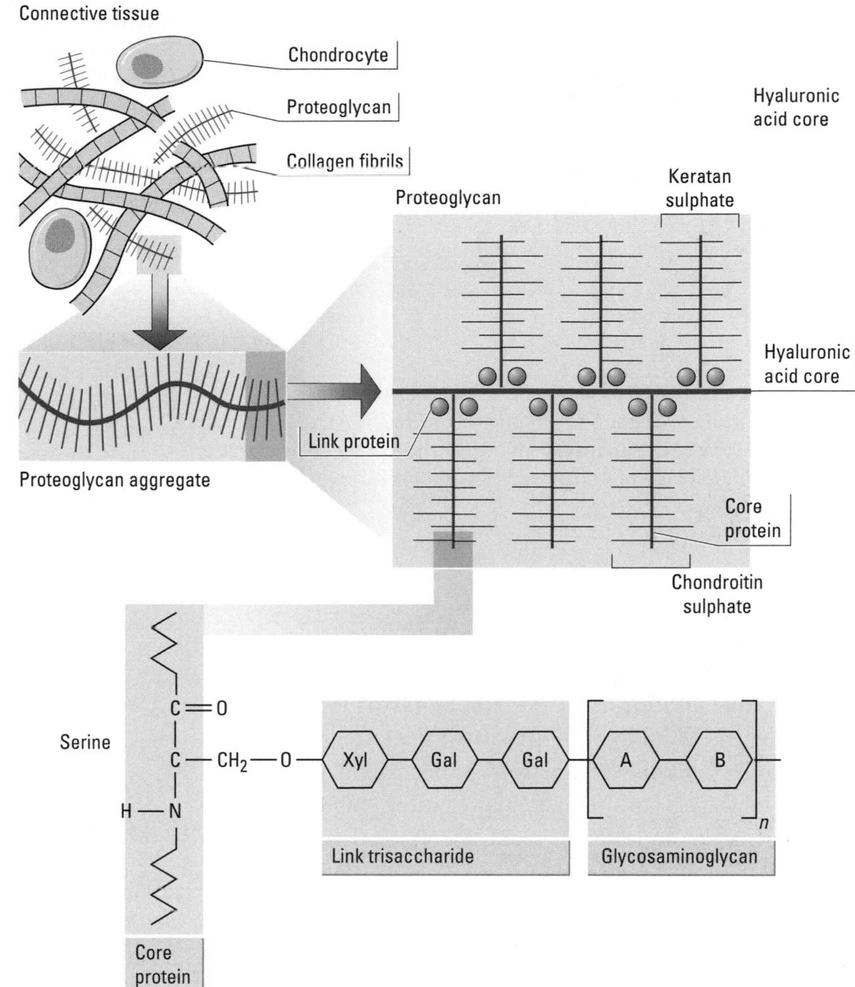

Figure 11.20 Schematic representation of a proteoglycan aggregate. A and B, two different monosaccharides; Gal, galactose; *n*, number of disaccharide units; Xyl, xylose.

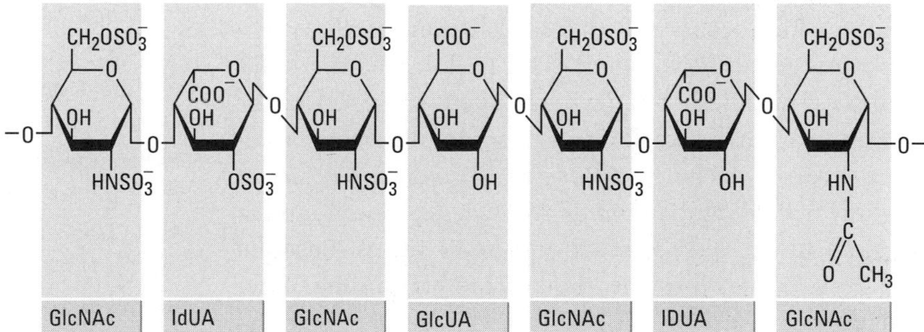

Figure 11.21 Fragment of the heparin chain. GlcNAc, *N*-acetylglucosamine; GlcUA, glucuronic acid; IdUA, iduronic acid.

binding of heparin is believed to induce a conformational change in the antithrombin III molecule and thus facilitate the interaction of the latter with thrombin. The heparin molecule then dissociates from the complex and can be reutilized by another antithrombin III molecule. Antithrombin III also binds to and activates other serine proteases involved in blood clotting: factors IXa, Xa, XIa and XIIa. The mechanism of inactivation is similar to that operating in the inactivation of thrombin. At high concentrations, however, heparin and heparin-like compounds can

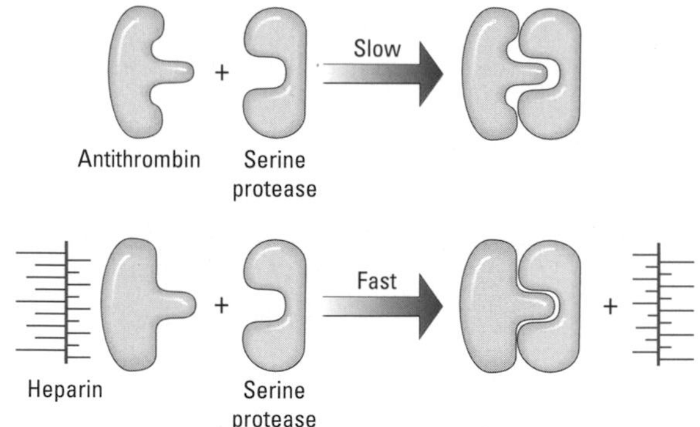

Figure 11.22 Postulated mechanism of heparin's participation in the blood clotting process. The binding of antithrombin to heparin induces a conformational change in the former and thus accelerates complexing of antithrombin with thrombin.

also prevent blood clotting by a different mechanism involving another anticoagulation molecule, *heparin co-factor II*. Like antithrombin, heparin co-factor II combines with thrombin to inhibit the activity of the latter, a process facilitated by heparin. Other effects of heparin include non-specific inhibition of platelet aggregation, inhibition of complement action, enhancement of elastase action and stimulation of phagocytosis.

Basophil sulphates

Basophil granules contain chondroitin sulphate, heparan sulphate and dermatan sulphate, which differ from heparin and from each other mainly in the composition of their disaccharide repeating units (Fig. 11.23). In contrast to heparin, which occurs only in mast cell granules, these proteoglycans are also found in the extracellular matrix of different tissues. Thus *chondroitin sulphate* is present in the cartilage, cornea, bone, skin and arterial walls; *heparan sulphate* occurs in the lungs, arteries and also on the surface of a variety of cells; and *dermatan sulphate* has been found in the skin, blood vessels, heart and heart valves. Basophil granule sulphates provide the matrix for storing other mediators.

Kinins

Kinins are small basic peptides so named because they have an effect on the contraction of smooth muscle (Greek *kinésis*, motion). They are produced from kininogens, large proteins present in the plasma, by the action of specialized arginine esterases known as *kallikreins* because they were originally isolated from the pancreas (Greek *kallikreas*, literally meaning 'a beautiful piece of meat'; see Chapter 21). Kininogens are single-chain glycoproteins with M_r ranging from 50 000 to 120 000, depending on the type and species of origin. Limited proteolysis by kallikreins at two sites within the molecule releases a short peptide, the *kinin*, and splits the single chain into two, heavy and light chains, held together by a disulphide bond. Kininogens are synthesized by hepatocytes and are then released into the plasma. In addition to releasing kinins, they function as co-factors in the contact phase of blood clotting, as potent inhibitors of cysteine proteases and as participants in the acute phase of the inflammatory response.

Three types of kininogens have been identified in mammalian plasma: high-molecular-mass kininogen (usually abbreviated to HMWK because of the original term 'weight' for 'mass'), low-molecular-mass kininogen

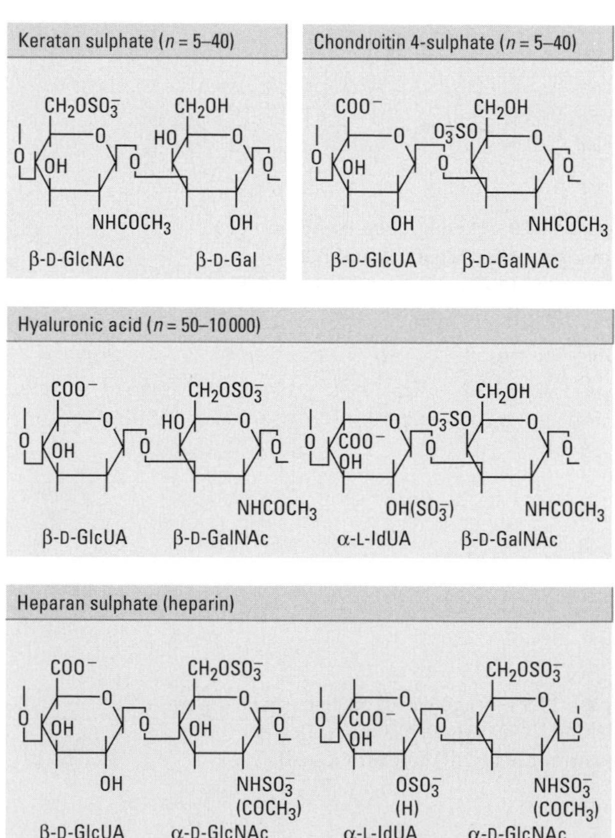

Figure 11.23 Composition of disaccharide repeating units in some of the mast cell and basophil glycosaminoglycans. Gal, galactose; GalNAc, *N*-acetylgalactosamine; GlcNAc, *N*-acetylglucosamine; GlcUA, glucuronic acid; IdUA, iduronic acid; *n*, number of disaccharide units.

(LMWK) and T-kininogen. HMWK and LMWK share their heavy chains, the kinin segment and a stretch of 12 amino acid residues distal from the kinin part; the C-termini of their light chains are completely different. T-kininogen is similar to LMWK throughout the molecule (Fig. 11.24). HMWK and LMWK are produced by alternative splicing from the same kininogen gene; T-kininogen is produced from a different gene. HMWK has a special histidine-rich region in its light chain that enables it to participate in the initiation phase of blood clotting. LMWK plays no part in blood clotting. T-kininogen is identical to the α_1 *major acute phase protein* (α_1-MAM) and the α_1 *acute phase globulin* (α_1-APG) of the rat.

Four types of kinin have been identified in the tissues, presumably released from kininogens by different kallikreins (Fig. 11.25). All four share a carboxylnonapeptide but differ in their N-termini. The best known of these four is *bradykinin*, so named because it causes slow contraction of the gut muscle (Greek *brady*, slow). *Kallidin* is released from kininogens by the action of kallikreins produced by endocrine or exocrine glands. The release of *T-kinin* correlates closely with inflammation, which leads to a dramatic increase of T-kininogen plasma concentrations. T-kininogen then sustains the inflammatory process by releasing T-kinin and, at the same time, inhibits inflammation by inhibiting cysteine proteases released from disintegrating cells. Kinins are rapidly degraded (they have a half-life of less than 30 s) by carboxypeptidases present in the plasma. The degradation of bradykinin involves the removal of arginine by *kinase I* (*carboxypeptidase N*) or of phenylalanine–arginine by *kinase II* (*angiotensin-converting enzyme, ACE*) from the C-terminus of the molecule. The seven-residue peptide produced by the action of kinase II is then

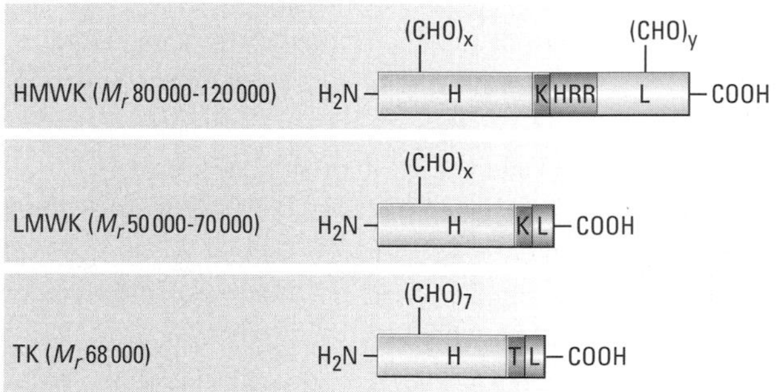

Figure 11.24 Comparison of the structure of high-molecular-mass kininogen (HMWK), low-molecular-mass kininogen (LMWK) and T-kininogen (TK). CHO, carbohydrate; H, heavy chain; HRR, histidine-rich region; K, kinin; L, light chain; T, portion of the chain corresponding to the kinin; x and y, unspecified numbers.

Bradykinin	H_2N– R P P G F S P F R –COOH
Kallidin	H_2N – K R P P G F S P F R –COOH
Met-Lys-bradykinin	H_2N–MK R P P G F S P F R –COOH
T-kinin (Ile-Ser-bradykinin)	H_2N– I S R P P G F S P F R –COOH

Figure 11.25 Amino acid sequence (expressed in one-letter code) of four kinins. Shared residues are highlighted.

reduced further to a pentapeptide. The des-Arg bradykinin is usually less active than bradykinin, whereas the des-Phe-Arg bradykinin and the pentapeptide are completely inactive.

Kinins cause smooth muscle contraction (which is slower than that induced by histamine and is unaffected by antihistamines), increased vascular permeability and vasodilation. They also induce pain when applied to the base of a blister, stimulate cellular glucose uptake and may cause hypotension as a consequence of arteriolar dilation. Bradykinin is able to activate phospholipase A_2 and so initiate arachidonic acid metabolism. Kinins act via receptors. A special category of *leukokinins* (peptides containing 20–25 amino acid residues) is released from plasma *leukokininogens* by the action of enzymes secreted by leucocytes (neutrophils, monocytes, lymphocytes and basophils).

Anaphylatoxins

These are described in Chapter 12.

Eosinophil chemotactic factors

Mast cell granules contain a number of peptides and polypeptides that, when released upon degranulation, cause granulocytes to migrate along the concentration gradient, i.e. they have chemotactic activity. Some of the factors react preferentially on certain types of granulocytes. The best characterized of these are two closely related tetrapeptides Val-Gly-Ser-Glu and Ala-Gly-Ser-Glu, which are particularly active on eosinophils and are therefore referred to as *eosinophil chemotactic factor-A* (*ECF-A*). The specificity of action of ECF-A is determined by the expression of eosinophil receptors. The peptide appears to attach itself to the receptor at two points: one involves the N-terminal amino acid, which binds to the receptor by hydrophobic interactions; the other involves the C-terminal amino acid, which binds to the receptor by ionic interactions between the carboxyl group and the receptor. If both sites are occupied, the receptor-bearing cell is stimulated; if only the C-terminus binds to the receptor, the cell is inhibited.

Table 11.1 Mediators produced by eosinophils not discussed in the text.

Name	Abbreviation	Intracellular location	Properties	Actions
Major basic protein	MBP	Core crystal of secondary granules; accounts for 55% of granule protein	pI 11.6; single polypeptide chain, 117 amino acid residues, 16% Arg; M_r 14 000	Toxic to parasites, tumour cells and many mammalian cells; causes histamine release from basophils and mast cells; neutralizes heparin
Eosinophilic cationic protein	ECP	Matrix of secondary granules	Basic; M_r 21 000; member of the RNase gene family	Shortens clotting time and alters fibrinolysis; kills certain parasites; potent neurotoxin; causes histamine release from mast cells; has weak RNase activity; inhibits culture of PBL
Eosinophil-derived neurotoxin (eosinophil protein X)	EDN (EPX)	Matrix of secondary granules	Basic; M_r 18 000–19 000; member of RNase gene family; high amino acid sequence similarity to ECP	Potent neurotoxin; kills parasites; inhibits cultures of PBL; has RNase activity

PBL, peripheral blood lymphocytes; pI, isolectric point.

Other biologically active peptides are listed in Table 11.1. The release of some of the mediators requires activation of the producing cells. Alternatively, some of the mediators function by activating or by contributing to the activation of their target cell.

Activation of cells

The cells of the immune system, as well as various other cells (e.g. platelets), can exist in one of two states, resting (quiescent, unstimulated) and activated (stimulated), the latter usually being of shorter duration than the former. The transition from resting to activated state is initiated by the binding of a ligand to a cell-surface receptor and everything that follows is a consequence of this process. The ligand can be a mediator, but also an antigen, and sometimes even an antibody, a hormone or one of several other categories of compounds. Mediators are excellent cell activators. The response of the activated cell depends on the genetic programme it has acquired during its differentiation — the type of organelles it has developed, the chemicals it has stored and the enzymes it is capable of producing. Activation is a way of manifesting this programme. A B lymphocyte activated by an antigen or a mitogen begins to secrete antibodies; a mast cell activated by histamine degranulates; a platelet activated by adenosine diphosphate begins to socialize with other platelets to form a plug that helps stop bleeding; and a neutrophil activated by an antibody engulfs the particle to which the antibody is attached. The remarkable fact, however, is that regardless of how variable the response to a stimulus may be, the initial phase of the activation process is very similar in different cells, both immune and non-immune.

Further reading

Bach, M.K. (1982) Mediators of anaphylaxis and inflammation. *Annual Review of Microbiology*, **36**, 371–413.

Beer, D.J. & Rocklin, R.E. (1987) Histamine modulation of lymphocyte biology: membrane receptors, signal transmission, and functions. *CRC Critical Reviews in Immunology*, **7**, 55–91.

Braquet, P. & Rola-Pleszczynski, M. (1987) Platelet-activating factor and cellular immune responses. *Immunology Today*, **8**, 345–352.

Gleich, G.J. (1988) Current understanding of eosinophil function. *Hospital Practice*, **23**, 137–160.

Hanahan, D.J. (1986) Platelet activating factor: a biologically active phosphoglyceride. *Annual Review of Biochemistry*, **55**, 483–509.

Kappler, D. (1992) Leukotrienes: biosynthesis, transport, inactivation and analysis. *Reviews of Physiology, Biochemistry and Pharmacology*, **121**, 1–30.

Larsen, G.L. & Henson, P.M. (1983) Mediators of inflammation. *Annual Review of Immunology*, **1**, 335–359.

Lee, T.H. & Austen, K.I. (1986) Arachidonic acid metabolism by the 5-lipoxygenase pathway and the effects of alternative dietary fatty acids. *Advances in Immunology*, **39**, 145–175.

Mangold, H.K. & Paultaut, F. (eds) (1983) *Ether Lipids. Biochemical and Biomedical Aspects*. Academic Press, New York.

Parker, C.W. (1987) Lipid mediators produced through the lipoxygenase pathway. *Annual Review of Immunology*, **5**, 65–84.

Poste, G. & Crooke, S.T. (eds) (1988) *Cellular and Molecular Aspects of Inflammation*. Plenum Press, New York.

Rola-Pleszczynski, M. (1985) Immunoregulation by leukotrienes and other lipoxygenase metabolites. *Immunology Today*, **6**, 302–307.

Samuelsson, B. (1983) Leukotrienes: mediators of immediate hypersensitivity reactions and inflammation. *Science*, **220**, 568–575.

Samuelsson, B., Dahlén, S.-E., Lindgren, J.A., Rouzler, C.A. & Serhan, C.N. (1987) Leukotrienes and lipoxins: structures, biosynthesis, and biological effects. *Science*, **237**, 1171–1175.

chapter 12 Complement and complement receptors

Towards the end of the nineteenth century, microbiologists learned that two substances in the antiserum were required to kill bacteria. One was heat stable and appeared only after exposure to bacteria, whereas the other was heat labile and was also present in the sera of non-immunized individuals. The heat-stable substance turned out to be antibody and the heat-labile substance was termed *complement* because it complemented the action of antibody on bacteria. Complement is not a single substance but a set of some 30 proteins, the *complement components*, coordinated in their functions like members of a relay-race team (Table 12.1). Normally, most of the proteins are in an inactive form, but a specific signal can activate the first protein of the team to leave its starting block and begin the race. By passing the baton, it activates the second protein, which then activates the third protein and this continues until the last member of the squad finishes the race by puncturing the membrane of a bacterium. Shown graphically, the activation sequence looks like a series of small waterfalls or a cascade, and this is why it is sometimes called the *complement cascade*.

For a long time, complement has been studied using a *model system* in which bacteria are replaced by sheep erythrocytes. The two other components of the system are heat-inactivated rabbit antiserum specific for sheep erythrocytes as the source of antibodies and normal guinea-pig serum as the source of complement. In this system, complement causes the lysis of antibody-coated erythrocytes or *haemolysis*, hence the term *haemolytic complement* used by earlier investigators. However, complement not only *lyses* cells; it also contributes to the destruction of foreign organisms in another way. Some of its components bind to the surface of foreign particles, thus making the coated particles more palatable for macrophages, i.e. they *opsonize* the particles and prepare them for efficient phagocytosis.

At first, researchers believed that complement could only be activated by antibodies, but evidence later accumulated suggesting that substances other than immunoglobulins could also serve as the starting signal in the complement relay race. The protein teams involved in the races initiated by antibodies and by non-immunoglobulin substances are different, with the result that there are two *complement pathways*. The pathway known for some time is called *classical* and the one discovered later *alternative*. The tracks of the classical and alternative complement pathways converge on the common track of the *lytic pathway* (Fig. 12.1). Since several of the complement components are enzymes with potential, when activated, to cause damage to the body, a system of *regulatory proteins* has evolved to keep the racers from running amok.

The complement components of the classical and effector

Table 12.1 Components of the complement pathway.

Symbol	Name	Function	Serum concentration (mg/ml)	M_r (× 10³)	M_r of polypeptide chains (× 10³)	Characteristics	Chromosome position of encoding gene
Classical pathway							
MBP	Mannose-binding protein	Binds to bacterial polysaccharides, activates MASP	143			Collagen-like structural protein	10q11.2–21
MASP	MBP-associated protein	Activates C4 and C2				Serine protease	
C1q	C1q	Binds to Ig in antibody–antigen complexes, activates C1r	80	410	6 × 24 6 × 23 6 × 22	Collagen-like structural protein	1p*
C1r	C1r	Activates C1s	50	90	2 × 85	Serine protease	12p13
C1s	C1s	Removes C4a fragment and thus activates C4; removes C2a and thus activates C2	50	85	85	Serine protease	12p13
C4	C4	Combines with C2	600	200	α95 β75 γ35	Thioester-containing structural protein	6p21
C2	C2	Cleaves C3 and C5	20	100	15	Serine protease	6p21
C3	C3	Combines with C5	1300	185	α100 β85	Thioester-containing structural protein	19p13.2–13.3
Alternative pathway							
Bf	Factor B	Combines with C3(H_2O); cleaves C3 and C5	210	92	92	Serine protease	6p21
D	Factor D	Activates factor B when B is in complex with C3b or C3(H_2O)	1	23	24	Serine protease	
Regulatory proteins in plasma							
H	Factor H	Inactivates the C3/C5 convertase by dissociating its subunits; also a co-factor for factor I	480	150	150	Structural protein	1q32
I	Factor I	Inactivates C3b with the aid of factor H and CR1	35	50 + 38 50 × 38	35 + 27	Serine protease	4q24–25
P	Properdin	Stabilizes the C3/C5 convertase by complexing with it	20	220	2–4 × 56	Structural protein	Xp11.23–p21.1
C1-INH	C1-inhibitor	Inactivation of C1r	200	104	53	Structural protein?	11p11.2–q13
C4bBP	C4b-binding protein	Masking of C2-binding site on C4	250	570	7 × 70	Structural protein?	1q3.2
DAF(CD55)	Decay-accelerating factor	Dissociation of C2 from C4	Cell bound	70	35	Membrane protein	1q3.2
MCP(CD46)	Membrane co-factor protein	Inactivation of C3b and C4b	Cell bound	51–68	34–40	Membrane protein	1q3.2
CR1(CD35)	Complement receptor 1	Inactivation of C3b and C4b, clearance of immune complexes, phagocytosis	Cell bound	190–280	220	Membrane protein	1q3.2

(Continued on p. 350.)

Table 12.1 *(Continued).*

Symbol	Name	Function	Serum concentration (mg/ml)	M_r (× 10^3)	M_r of polypeptide chains (× 10^3)	Characteristics	Chromosome position of encoding gene
CD59		Blocking of MAC assembly	Cell bound	19	12	Membrane protein	11p13
S	S protein	Forms soluble SC5b6789 complexes	0.25–0.45	83	83	Structural protein	17q11
	Clusterin	Forms soluble SC5b6787 complexes	0.35–1.05	80	35–40	Structural protein	8p21
Lytic pathway							
C5	C5	Anchoring molecule for C6	70	190	α124 β76	Structural protein, member of the thioester family but lacking the thioester	9q32–34
C6	C6	Anchoring molecule for C7	64	105–128	120	Structural protein	5p13
C7	C7	Anchoring molecule for C8	56	92–121	110	Structural protein	5p13
C8	C8	Anchoring molecule for C9	55	150	α77 β63 γ13	Structural protein	1p32*
C9	C9	Forms pores in the membrane	59	71	71	Structural protein	5p13

* Only the α- and β-chain genes; the γ-chain gene is located on a different chromosome.
CR, complement receptor; Ig, immunoglobulin; MAC, membrane attack complex.

pathways are designated C1 to C9. The numbering reflects the order of participation of the individual components in the cascade with the exception of C4, which was named before its position in the sequence was established (Fig. 12.1). All the components, with the exception of C1, are single proteins; the C1 component consists of three proteins designated C1q, C1r and C1s. Other components are designated by letters (e.g. B, D, H) or names (e.g. properdin, C1-inhibitor, C4b-binding protein). Several of the components are present in the serum in inactive forms. Activation usually takes place after the components have been split into fragments designated by the suffixes *a* (a smaller fragment released into body fluids) and *b* (a larger, membrane-bound fragment). For example, the C3 component splits into C3a and C3b fragments upon activation. The C3a and C3b fragments are further degraded into *c* (which is released into body fluids) and *d* (which remains membrane bound).

Activating substances

A race can be started with a pistol shot, a clap of hands or a verbal command. The complement cascade can be activated via an immunoglobulin, protein A, C-reactive protein, polyanions, certain bacteria and certain viruses. The classical pathway is activated by *immunoglobulins*, either attached to a surface (most commonly cell surface) or complexed with cell-free antigens (*immune complexes*). Free immunoglobulins alone do not activate complement and it would be a disaster if they did.

Protein A is a cell-wall protein found in many strains of *Staphylococcus aureus*; it consists of a single polypeptide chain that can be divided into two structural and functional parts (Fig. 12.2a). The N-terminal part contains four homologous regions, each of which binds one human IgG molecule. The C-terminal part anchors the protein in the cell wall. Because of its affinity for the Fc portion of certain immunoglobulins (human IgG1, IgG2, IgG4 and mouse IgG2a, IgG2b, IgG3), protein A has been used extensively in immunochemical studies. A single protein A molecule can bind two IgG molecules simultaneously and thus form complexes resembling antigen–antibody complexes. Like immune complexes, the protein A–immunoglobulin complexes activate the classical complement cascade.

C-reactive protein (Fig. 12.2b,c) is a β-globulin present in the sera of healthy individuals in trace amounts but at increased levels during infection and in the sera of patients suffering from certain inflammatory diseases such as

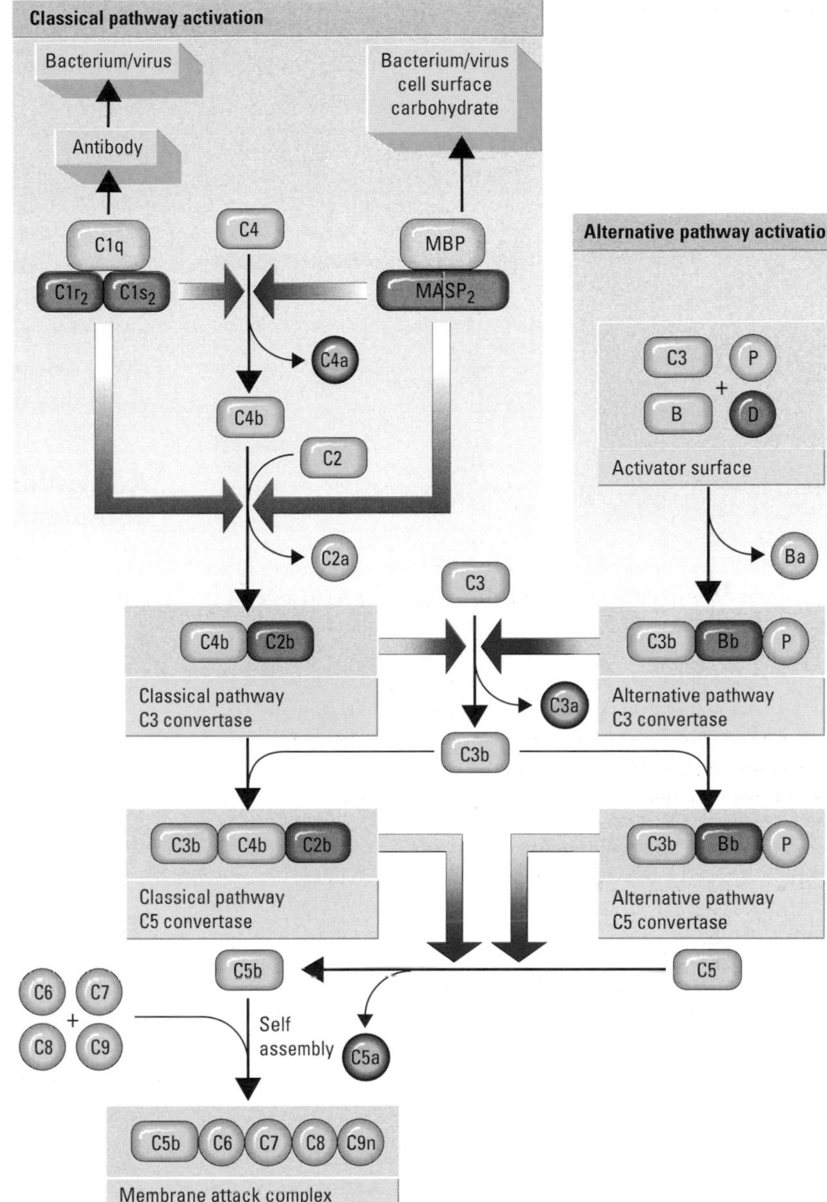

Figure 12.1 The complement cascade: an overview. Description in the text. Enzymatic reactions and enzymatically active components are indicated in red. Anaphylatoxins are indicated in dark grey circles, recognition proteins initiating the cascade in pink. MASP, MBP-associated serine protease; MBP, mannose-binding protein. The depiction should not give the impression that the MBP/MASP activation mode is equivalent, in terms of significance, to the C1 mode. Not enough is known about the biology of the MBP/MASP activation to draw such a conclusion. (From Reid, K. B. M. (1996) *Immunologist*, 3, 206.)

rheumatic fever. It characteristically binds (in the presence of calcium ions) to one of the polysaccharides (C) present in the cell wall of pneumococci. C-reactive protein consists of five identical, non-covalently associated subunits that show considerable amino acid sequence similarity among various mammalian species. Its synthesis by hepatocytes in the liver is accelerated 1000-fold by inflammatory stimuli. C-reactive protein activates the classical pathway by binding the C1 component directly. The same effect is achieved also by the *serum amyloid P* component (see Chapter 21).

The alternative pathway proceeds at a slow rate spontaneously but is accelerated dramatically by *activators*, in the absence of antibodies. Examples of activators are polyanions, as well as certain bacterial and viral substances. *Polyanions* are negatively charged compounds consisting of repeated subunits; they include deoxyribonucleic acid, polyinosinic acid, dextran sulphate, polyvinylsulphate, polyethanol sulphate, carrageenin and cellulose sulphate.

A prominent constituent of the outer membrane of Gram-negative bacteria is *lipopolysaccharide* (LPS). The

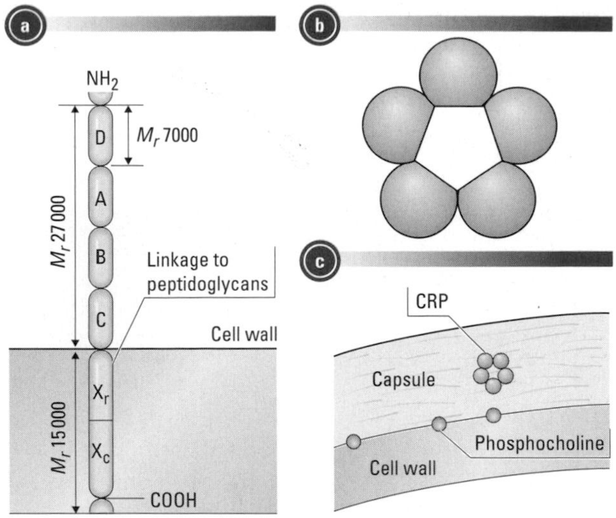

Figure 12.2 Examples of complement-activating substances other than immunoglobulins. (a) Protein A of *Staphylococcus aureus*. The protein consists of two regions, the N-terminal immunoglobulin-binding region (M_r 27 000) and the C-terminal region X_1 (M_r 15 000), which is covalently linked to the cell wall. The N-terminal region consists of four domains, D, A, B and C, each approximately 58 amino acid residues long. The domains are structurally very similar to one another. Each contains three parallel helical structures that interact hydrophobically with C_H2 and C_H3 domains of immunoglobulin; other regions of the domain interact electrostatically with the C_H3 domain. The X region is divided into two subregions, X_r and X_c. The X_r subregion consists of a unique sequence of 81 amino acid residues (for further details, see Uhlén, M. *et al.* (1984) *Immunology Today*, 5, 244). (b) Structure of C-reactive protein (CRP). (c) Location of CRP on the cell surface of *Streptococcus pneumoniae*. The CRP molecule is composed of five identical, non-covalently bound subunits, each with an M_r of 21 500 (the pentamer has an M_r of 110 000). Each subunit is 187 amino acid residues long. The CRP molecule attaches to phosphocholine in the cell wall of pneumococci via a specific binding site. Binding requires the participation of Ca^{2+} ions. (Modified from Gewurz, H. (1983), in *The Biology of Immunologic Disease* (Eds F.J. Dixon & D. W. Fisher), p. 139. Sinauer, Sunderland, MA.)

basic structural unit of the LPS molecule consists of three regions, the O side-chain, R core and lipid A (see also Chapters 13 & 21). The first two regions consist of sugars, the third of sugars and lipids. The lipid moiety of LPS binds the C1 component and thus directly activates the classical pathway. The polysaccharide constituent of LPS, on the other hand, activates the alternative pathway. *Gram-positive bacteria* do not contain LPS. Instead, the major constituents of their cell walls are peptidoglycans and teichoic acid. All Gram-positive cell walls activate the alternative pathway but opinions differ as to whether the peptidoglycan or the teichoic acid is responsible for activation.

A number of *viruses* activate either the classical or the alternative complement pathway, or both pathways in the absence of antibody. Good activators of the classical pathway are retroviruses, Sindbis virus and Newcastle disease virus. Among the activators of the alternative pathway are simian, Sindbis and vesicular stomatitis viruses. However, recent work has cast some doubt on whether viruses really do activate complement in the absence of antibody. There is, in some cases, good evidence, and in other cases, the suspicion that low-affinity carbohydrate-specific antibodies are involved in these activations.

Activation of the classical complement pathway

The classical complement pathway can be activated in two principal ways: indirectly by antibodies complexed with

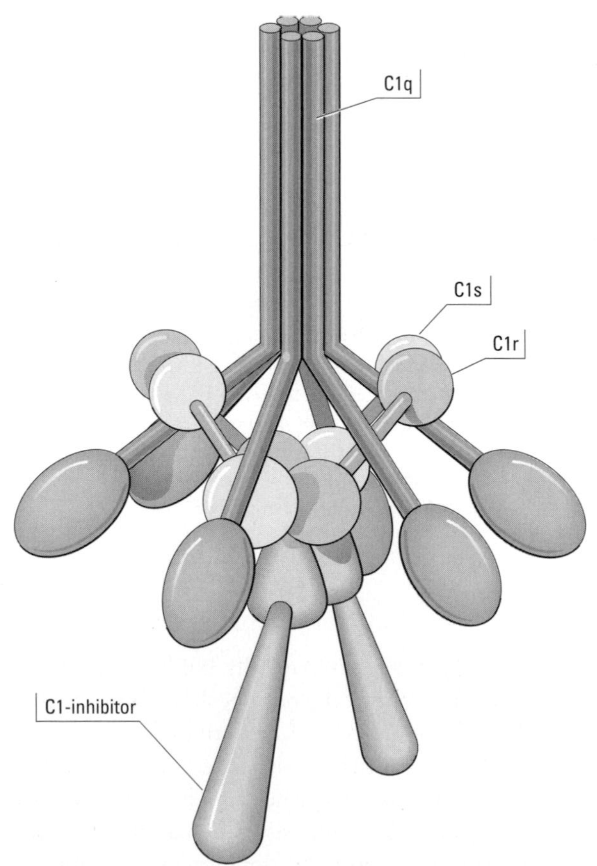

Figure 12.3 Model of the C1 component complexed with the C1-inhibitor. The C1 complex consists of one C1q molecule and a tetramer, $C1r_2C1s_2$, attached non-covalently to C1q.

an antigen, or directly by carbohydrates on the surface of bacteria and viruses (see Fig. 12.1). Antibody-mediated activation involves a complex of three proteins, the C1 component, consisting of the C1q, C1r and C1s proteins. Direct activation involves a complex of at least two proteins: the mannose-binding protein (MBP), which is homologous to C1q; and the MBP-associated serine protease (MASP), which is homologous to C1r (C1s). The MBP–MASP activation system may be the older of the two, but it has been discovered only recently and so much less is known about it than about the C1 activation system. We therefore begin the description of complement activation with the latter systems.

C1 component

To initiate the classical pathway, the antibody bound to an antigen on the cell surface or in an immune complex must interact with the first component of the classical pathway, C1 (Fig. 12.3). The C1 component consists of two structural and functional entities, the C1q protein and the $C1r_2C1s_2$ tetramer. The C1q protein is the recognition subunit that interacts with the immunoglobulin molecule; the $C1r_2C1s_2$ tetramer is the catalytic subunit that acquires enzymatic activity upon activation.

C1q is a most bizarre molecule (Fig. 12.4). It consists of 18 polypeptide chains of three kinds, A, B and C, each chain being about 200 amino acid residues long (Fig. 12.4). The first 90 residues represent repetition of the triplet Gly-X-Y, where X is often proline and Y is usually hydroxyproline or hydroxylysine. A similar sequence also occurs in the various collagens of connective tissue. Starting at position 90 and continuing towards the C-terminus, the regularity of the sequence is lost. This region contains one intrachain disulphide bond in each of the three polypeptide chains. Interchain disulphide bonds form at the N-terminus between the A and B chains and between the C chains. There is a high degree of sequence similarity between the three chains along their entire length, suggesting a common evolutionary origin. The 18 chains are arranged into six

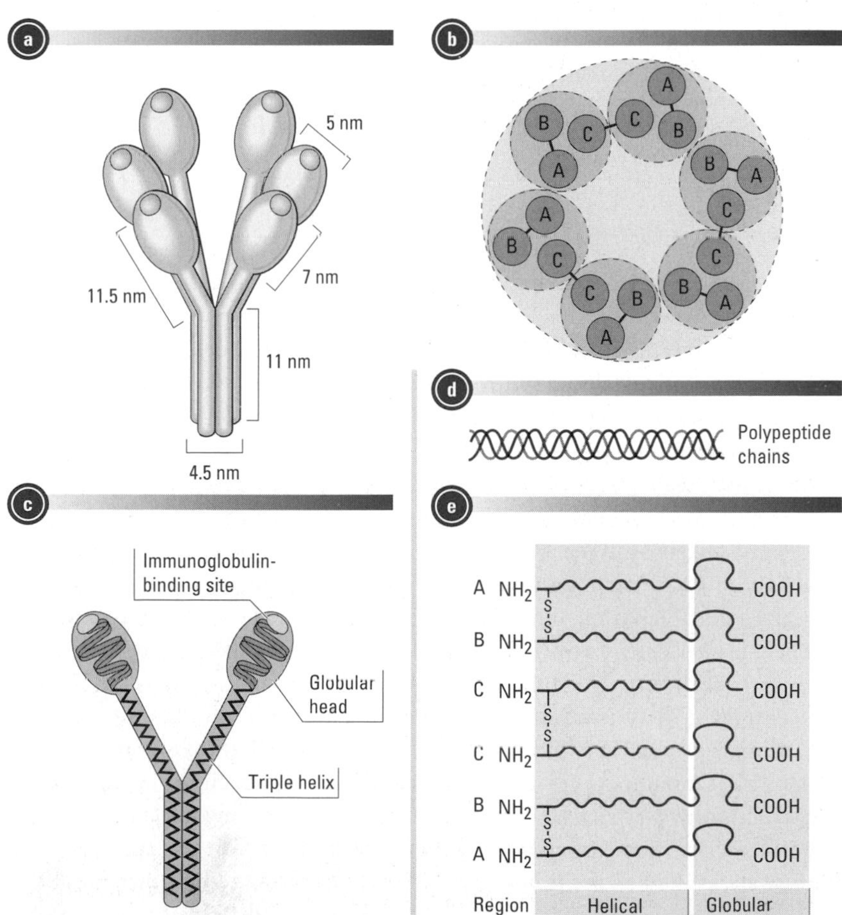

Figure 12.4 Structure of the C1q molecule. (a) A bouquet of tulips, each bloom formed by three polypeptide chains, A, B and C. (b) Cross-section through the 'stalks' of the bouquet. Each solid circle represents one polypeptide chain, the broken circles indicate chain grouping and the connecting lines indicate disulphide bonds. (c) Doublet of chains. (d) Triple helix in the collagen-like region of the molecule. (e) Interchain and intrachain disulphide bonds.

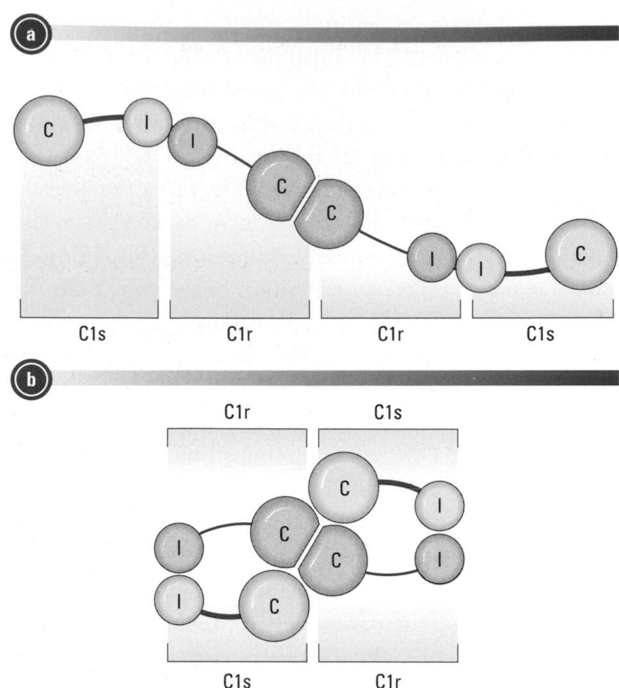

Figure 12.5 Two configurations of the $C1r_2C1s_2$ tetramer: (a) free, S-shaped form; (b) C1q-bound, 8-shaped form. Each C1s or C1r monomer consists of two compact globules, the larger catalytic (C) globule formed by the serine protease domain and the smaller interaction (I) globule formed by the CEC cassette (see text). The globules are connected by a rod formed by complement control protein repeats (CCPRs). (Based on Arland, G.J. *et al.* (1986) *Immunology Today*, 8, 106.)

triplets, each triplet consisting of one A, one B and one C chain. The triplets are then joined into pairs by the disulphide bond between their C chains. In each triplet, the three chains form a triple helix in the N-terminal region, whereas the rest of the molecule is globular so that the entire molecule resembles a bouquet of six tulips. The 'stalks', however, bend in the area in which the sequence regularity is interrupted and the flexibility in this region enables the triplets to assume angles between 40 and 160°, the most favoured angle being 100°. Each globular head has one binding site for the Fc portion of the immunoglobulin molecule.

The tetramer consists of two C1r and two C1s molecules arranged in tandem, where the C1r monomers are found in the centre and the C1s monomers at the ends; the order of the subunits is thus C1s–C1r–C1r–C1s (Fig. 12.5). Both the C1r and C1s monomers are single polypeptide chains which are structurally very similar, suggesting that their encoding genes arose by duplication from a common ancestor. The mature molecule has six domains of four kinds, arranged in the order C1r/s-1 . . . EGF . . . C1r/s-2 . . . CCP-1 . . . CCP-2 . . . serine protease (Fig. 12.6). The N-terminal *C1r/s-1 domain* (repeat) was originally believed to be restricted to the C1r and C1s molecules (hence the name) but was later shown to be present in a number of other proteins. Because it is involved in the interaction with the C1s molecule it is also known as the *IA domain*. It is followed in the chain by a segment homologous to the *epidermal growth factor* (*EGF*), which is also present in numerous other proteins beside EGF. It contains an asparagine residue which is post-translationally hydroxylated (converted into erythro-β-hydroxyasparagine) and which is characteristic of proteins capable of binding calcium ions. Next in row is a second C1r/s domain, *C1r/s-2*, and the combination of an EGF domain sandwiched between two C1r/s domains is referred to as the *CEC cassette* (for C1r/s . . . *EGF* . . . C1r/s). The cassette has also been found in proteins of different species ranging from the fruitfly to humans. The repeat that follows the C1r/s-2 domain has several aliases: *CCP (complement regulatory protein)*, SCR (short consensus repeat or short complement repeat) and B-type module (first described in factor B). The C-terminal domain is a *serine protease* (or proteinase), an enzyme with a serine residue in its catalytic site and the ability to cleave the peptide bond of proteins. It is similar in sequence to other serine proteases such as trypsin, chymotrypsin and elastase, as well as complement components C2 and factor B.

The C1r monomer is a dumbbell-shaped molecule in which the serine protease domain forms a large globule at one end and the CEC cassette a smaller globule at the other end. The two globules are connected by a rod formed by the two CCP repeats (see Fig. 12.5). Two C1r monomers associate non-covalently by their protease domains to form a $C1r_2$ dimer and the C1r/s domains of the dimers associate non-covalently with corresponding C1r/s domains of two C1s monomers to form a $C1r_2C1s_2$ tetramer (see Fig. 12.3). The two C1r/s domains also mediate binding of C1r (and of C1s) to the C1q molecule.

The structure of C1s is similar to that of C1r. The $C1r_2C1s_2$ tetramer can exist in a free S-shaped form when in solution or an 8-shaped form when attached to the C1q molecule (see Fig. 12.5). The transformation of the S- into an 8-shaped form apparently occurs via the catalytic domain of C1s in such a way that all four catalytic domains converge in a single cluster. The tetramer wraps itself around the arms of the C1q molecule so that the interaction domains of C1r and C1s lie outside the arms and the catalytic domains inside the cone formed by the C1q arms (see Fig. 12.3).

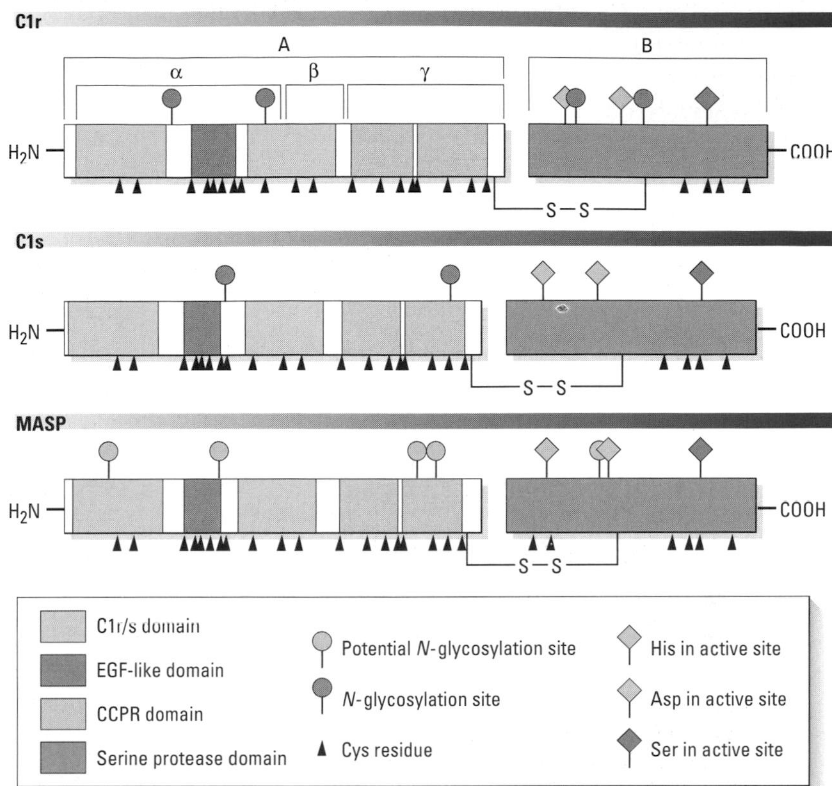

Figure 12.6 Organization of C1r, C1s and MBP-associated serine protease (MASP) subunits. CCPR, complement control protein repeat; EGF, epidermal growth factor; S—S, disulphide bond. (Slightly modified from Takayama, Y. *et al.* (1994) *Journal of Immunology*, **152**, 2308.)

Activation of the C1 component

The free S-shaped form of the $C1r_2C1s_2$ tetramer is inactive, perhaps because of the spatial arrangement of the catalytic units. The complex of the 8-shaped tetramer with the C1q molecule is also inactive because it is associated with another protein, the *C1-inhibitor*. The human C1-inhibitor is a single-chain, heavily glycosylated polypeptide (it contains about 35% carbohydrate, both N- and O-linked, which is more than most other plasma proteins). The C1-inhibitor molecule consists of a globular terminal part ('head') and a rod-like, N-terminal part ('tail'), kept rigid by many carbohydrate moieties attached to six or seven repeats of the tetrapeptide Glu (Gln)-Pro-Thr-Thr (see Fig. 12.3). The C-terminal domain contains the *reactive centre loop*, which is very sensitive to the action of proteolytic enzymes. Protease-mediated cleavage of a peptide bond within the loop alters many physical properties of the molecule and inactivates the inhibitor. A similar reactive centre loop is also present in other proteins that inhibit the activity of serine proteases and are therefore termed *serpins* (for *ser*ine *p*roteinase *in*hibitors). They are widely distributed among viruses, plants and animals. The C1-inhibitor has affinity for the catalytic domain of the C1r component; it binds non-covalently to the active site of this pro-enzyme via its globular region, two molecules of the inhibitor to one C1r dimer (see Fig. 12.3). The presence of the C1-inhibitor in the active site prevents activation of the C1 component. Furthermore, the rod-like domain of the inhibitor protrudes far beyond the base of the cone formed by the C1q arms and heads and thus sterically prevents interactions that may lead to C1 activation. The C1-inhibitor can be compared to a peg driven into a lobster's claws by fishermen: as long as the peg is in position, the shellfish is harmless, but remove the peg and you had better watch your fingers!

There is a dynamic equilibrium in the interaction between C1 and C1-inhibitor: the two components are continuously associating and dissociating. Normally, most of the C1 in the serum is associated with the C1-inhibitor and only a small proportion, perhaps less than 1%, of C1 is free. However, if immune complexes appear in the serum, the C1 molecules momentarily dissociated from the C1-inhibitor may bind tightly to the immunoglobulin in the complexes and thus be prevented from reassociating with the inhibitor.

As more and more C1 molecules bind to the antibodies and more C1-inhibitors are displaced, the equilibrium shifts towards activatable C1.

Antibodies interact via their Fc regions with binding sites on the globular heads of the C1q component (Fig. 12.7). The binding involves ionic interactions between amino acid residues Lys 90 Arg 101 of C1q and Glu 318 Lys 32 . . . Lys 322 Glu 333 of the IgG C_H2 domain. Weak binding between a single C1q and a single Fc site probably even occurs with free immunoglobulin molecules, but as it does not change the conformation of the C1 component it does not result in activation. For activation to occur, the shape of the C1q molecule must be distorted in a certain way, a process that depends on the attachment of the C1q heads to at least two Fc sites. Although IgG molecules do have two C1q-binding sites (one on each of the two heavy chains), the C1q molecule is not flexible enough to bind to both simultaneously. Bivalent binding can therefore only be achieved when C1q spans two IgG molecules. Furthermore, because the maximal armspan of C1q is 40 nm, the two IgG molecules must come very close together for a single C1q molecule to bridge them. On a cell coated with antibodies, the distances between neighbouring IgG molecules will depend on the density of the bound immunoglobulins. On an erythrocyte with 1000 molecules of bound IgG, only 1% of the molecules will be close enough to be spanned by C1q; with 20 000 molecules, 20% of the molecules can be spanned, and so on. The situation is somewhat different for IgM molecules. A pentameric IgM molecule has at least three binding sites for C1q and their spatial distribution allows a single C1q molecule to bind to a single IgM molecule firmly enough to be activated. Alas, in the free, star-shaped IgM molecule the binding sites are normally hidden. They become exposed only when the IgM molecule binds to antigen and assumes the staple-shaped configuration. (IgA, IgE and IgD molecules lack C1q-binding sites in their Fc regions; of the various human IgG subclasses, IgG3 and IgG1 bind and activate C1 readily, whereas IgG2 does so poorly and IgG4 hardly at all.)

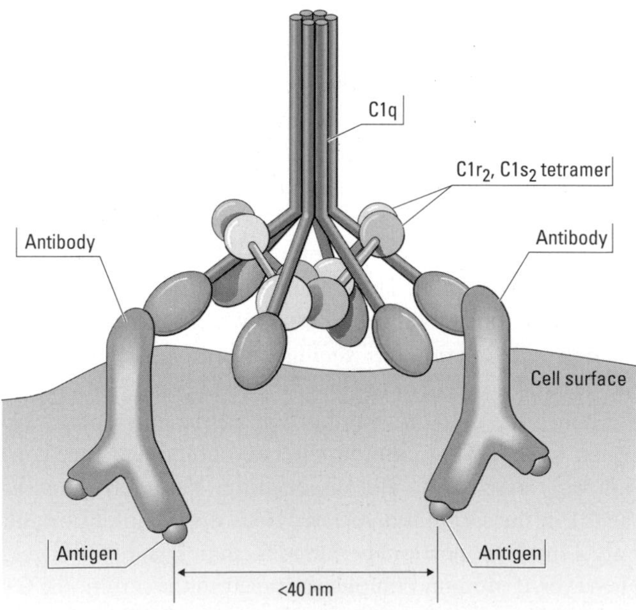

Figure 12.7 Bridging of two membrane-bound IgG molecules by the C1 component. Binding presumably distorts the C1 molecule and triggers its activation.

The multivalent binding of C1q to a cluster of Fc regions apparently results in the distortion of the symmetrical cone formed by the C1q arms and this distortion is then transmitted to the region occupied by the $C1r_2C1s_2$ tetramer. A change in the configuration of the tetramer favours spontaneous activation of one of the C1r molecules, presumably by exposing the active site. The activated C1r pro-enzyme then breaks a single Arg–Ile bond in its partner C1r polypeptide, but because the cleavage occurs in a region spanned by a disulphide bond the two fragments, A and B, remain disulphide linked. The breakage exposes the catalytic site and the cleaved C1r molecule then cleaves the first C1r molecule, following the principle 'You scratch my back, I'll scratch yours'. The two enzymatically active C1r molecules then cleave the two C1s molecules, again splitting each of them into two disulphide-linked chains (Fig. 12.8) and activating them (*autocatalytic activation*). Additional cleavages may follow at two other sites in the C1r chain breaking the A fragment into α, β and γ fragments (see Fig. 12.6). The cleavages leave the non-covalent bonds between the monomers intact so that fragments of the type $(\gamma\text{-B})_2$ appear, the so-called *C1rII fragments*.

Following the activation of C1s, the bonds between the tetramer and the cone break and the catalytic domains of C1s are exposed and ready to act on the next components of the cascade, C4 and C2. At the same time, however, the freed C1s domains are once again available for interaction with C1-inhibitor. This time, C1-inhibitor binds *covalently* to the catalytic sites of the C1r and C1s molecules (one of the C1-inhibitor's amino acid residues mimics the substrate of these two proteases) and the C1sC1r $(\text{C1-inhibitor})_2$ complex dissociates from the C1q molecule and is subsequently degraded. The activated C1 molecule thus has only a very short time to carry out its function (the activation of the C4 molecule) before it is inactivated again. Had it been otherwise, the protease could have caused considerable

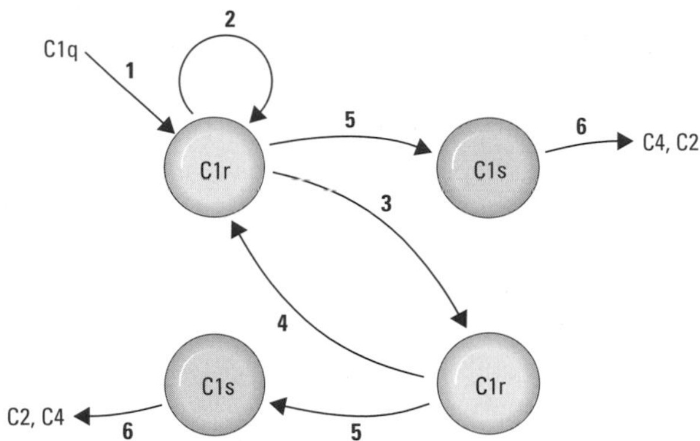

Figure 12.8 Activation of the C1 component of complement: postulated sequence of events. (1) Distortion of C1q caused by its bridging of Fc-binding sites is transmitted to one of the C1r monomers. (2) The distortion favours spontaneous activation of C1r. (3) The self-activated C1r enzymatically cleaves a peptide bond in the second C1r monomer. (4) The cleaved C1r molecule in turn cleaves the first C1r monomer. (5) The two cleaved C1r monomers cleave the two C1s monomers, thereby activating them. (6) The activated C1s molecules cleave first C4 and then C2 molecules.

damage to the body by cleaving other proteins. Understandably enough, the body does not like butchers with long knives running around and carving off its juiciest parts.

MBP–MASP complex

The serum of many vertebrate species has been shown to contain a complex of proteins that recognizes the Ra and R2 polysaccharides on the surfaces of many strains of Gram-negative bacteria such as *Salmonella typhimurium* and *Escherichia coli*. Upon recognition, the complex could be demonstrated to acquire serine protease activity that initiates reactions culminating in the killing of the bacteria. Because of its specificity, the complex has been designated *Ra-reactive factor* (*RaRF*).

Independently of these observations, in other studies it has been shown that an acute bacterial infection is often accompanied by an increased production of certain proteins in the liver and their release into the serum. One of these *acute phase proteins* (see Chapter 21) has been demonstrated to bind the sugar mannose, frequently found on the surface of bacteria but not on human cells. Ultimately, immunologists proved this ***mannose-binding protein*** (*MBP*) to be identical with the carbohydrate-binding component of RaRF. The enzymatically active component of RaRF has been designated ***MBP-associated serine protease*** (*MASP*). Elucidation of the structures of these two proteins has revealed MBP to be homologous to C1q and MASP to C1r (C1s). The homology pertains to both primary and tertiary structure.

The *MBP molecule* consists of trimers (Fig. 12.9) or tetramers of subunits that resemble the single 'tulip' of the C1q bouquet (the latter, however, contains six rather than three 'tulips'). In the MBP molecule, as in the C1q molecule, each subunit consists of an N-terminal collagen-like triple helix and a C-terminal globular recognition domain. Furthermore, C1q and MBP are members of a family of *collectins*, which resemble one another in structure. The *MASP molecule* resembles C1r and C1s molecules with which it shares 40% of its amino acid residues (see Fig. 12.6). MASP molecules, like C1r or C1s, are known to dimerize; whether they also form $C1r_2C1s_2$-like tetramers is not known.

Binding of MBP, via its globular part, to mannose and *N*-acetylglucosamine residues of bacterial polysaccharides activates the associated MASP in a manner that has not been elucidated. In particular, it is not known whether there are two types of MASP, one that autoactivates like C1r and a second which, upon activation, acts on C4 and C2 in the same manner as C1s. After MASP activation, however, the reaction proceeds in the same way as antibody-initiated C1 activation.

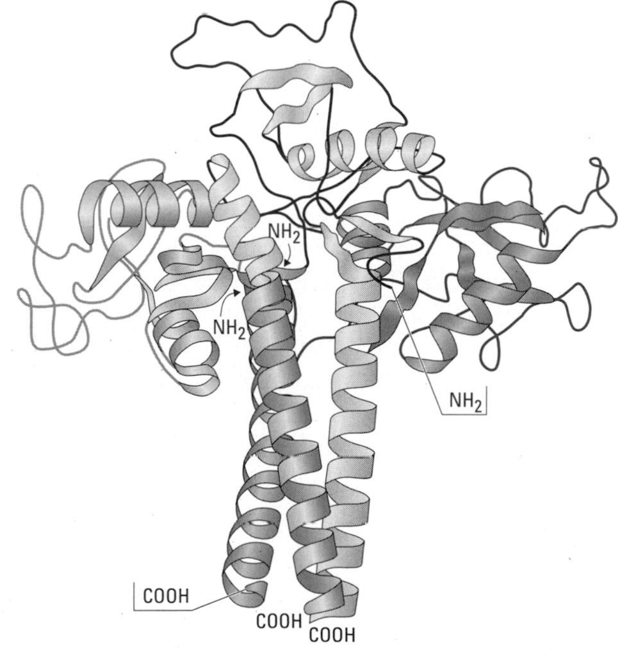

Figure 12.9 Structure of the mannose-binding protein (MBP). (Based on Protein Data Bank Swiss 3-D.)

Activation of the C4 component

The C4 component is synthesized as a single polypeptide chain that is then cleaved enzymatically into three chains, α, β and γ, held together by disulphide bonds (Fig. 12.10). When the activated C1s component encounters the mature C4 molecule, it recognizes the residues Arg 76 and Ala 77 in the α chain and breaks the peptide bond between them (Fig. 12.11). This cleavage releases a short *C4a fragment* from the N-terminus of the α chain, which then diffuses into the fluid phase to become active elsewhere. In the remainder of the molecule, now referred to as the *C4b fragment*, the removal of the C4a fragment unmasks a reactive site located on the α chain and characterized by the presence of a *thioester bond*. (A *thiol* is a monovalent radical containing sulphur attached to a carbon atom, and an *ester* is a compound formed by the elimination of H_2O during the interaction between the OH of an acid group, COOH, and the OH of an alcohol group.) In the C4 molecule, the thioester bond forms between the Cys and Gln residues in the sequence Cys-Gly-Glu-Gln (Fig. 12.11). The exposure of the previously hidden and protected thioester upon C4 activation has far-reaching consequences. The acyl (C=O) group of the thioester is highly electrophilic: it readily accepts electrons from nucleophilic (electron-donating) groups such as hydroxyl (OH) or amino (NH_2) groups. As long as it was hidden and buffered inside the molecule, the high reactivity of the thioester could not express itself. But now, when it is in the open, the thioester will interact with any component (protein, water or whatever else happens to be in its vicinity) carrying such groups. The bond between the sulphur atom of the Cys and the C=O group of the Gln breaks and the acyl instead links up with the electron donor via an ester bond (if the electron donor is an OH group) or an amide bond (if the donor is an NH_2 group) (Fig. 12.12). The transfer of the acyl group, however, is influenced by another amino acid residue residing at position 1106 in the human C4 molecule. There are two types of human C4, A and B, depending on the residue present at this position. C4A (and also α_2-macroglobulin, of which more later) has Asp and C4B (as well as C3, also discussed later) has His at this position. In the C4A molecule, transfer of the acyl group takes place directly, without the involvement of Asp 1106 (see Fig. 12.11). In C4B, on the other hand, the thioester is first attacked by the His 1106 group and an intermediate forms in which the acyl group is bound to the His side-chain. The released thiol (C–S) of the Cys residue then acts as a base to catalyse the transfer of the acyl group to an OH-carrying acceptor molecule or to water (see Fig. 12.11). Because of this effect of residue 1106, C4A binds predominantly to NH_2 groups, the reaction is relatively slow and the half-life of the activated thioester is in the order of 10 s. By contrast, C4B (and C3) binds mainly to OH groups or water molecules, the reaction is fast and the half-life of the thioester is very short (< 1 s). Furthermore, because the most likely molecule to be encountered first by the thioester of C4B and C3 is water, in more than 90% of cases the water molecules will neutralize the reactive group before it has a chance to establish a covalent bond with a protein. In some 10% of cases, however, the reactive thioesters of the C4B and C3 molecules manage to contact NH_2 or OH groups of carbohydrates or proteins on the surface of the cell on which the antigen–antibody–C1–C4 complex is assembling. On these relatively rare occasions, therefore, the C4b fragment becomes covalently bound to a cell-surface protein in the vicinity of the antigen. The chances of it attaching to proteins further away are even slimmer because it has only a fraction of a second to make contact with the membrane. If it does not manage to find a suitable acceptor in that short time, it is inactivated by the interaction with water molecules. Therefore, C4 activation and attachment is a rather inefficient process: it has been calculated that during the 60 μs of its lifetime, the activated molecule can only diffuse a distance of about 40 nm. Confinement of the reaction to a small circumscribed area is one further safeguard against the uncontrollable spreading of the attack.

The complement system compensates for the inefficiency by an *amplification process*: a single C1 molecule can activate and deposit approximately 30 C4 molecules. All these molecules settle down in a circular area with a radius of 40 nm and with the C1 molecule in the centre. As all other steps in the complement cascade depend on random diffusion of products, the clustering of activated fragments increases the probability that at least one of the deposited molecules will, in the end, deliver a lethal hit to the cell.

Activation of the C2 component

Activated C4 has an affinity for the C2 component, which in its pro-enzyme form is a single polypeptide chain with a relative molecular mass (M_r) of approximately 100 000. The polypeptide consists of three globular domains, each with unique functional properties (Fig. 12.13). The N-terminal *complement control protein repeat* (*CCPR*) *domain* contains three repeated regions, each approximately 60 residues long and has sites via which C2 interacts with C4b. The middle *von Willebrand type-A domain* is structurally homologous to a domain present in the von Willebrand factor, one of the plasma proteins involved in blood clotting (adhesion of platelets to surfaces and protection of one of the blood clotting factors); the domain is also

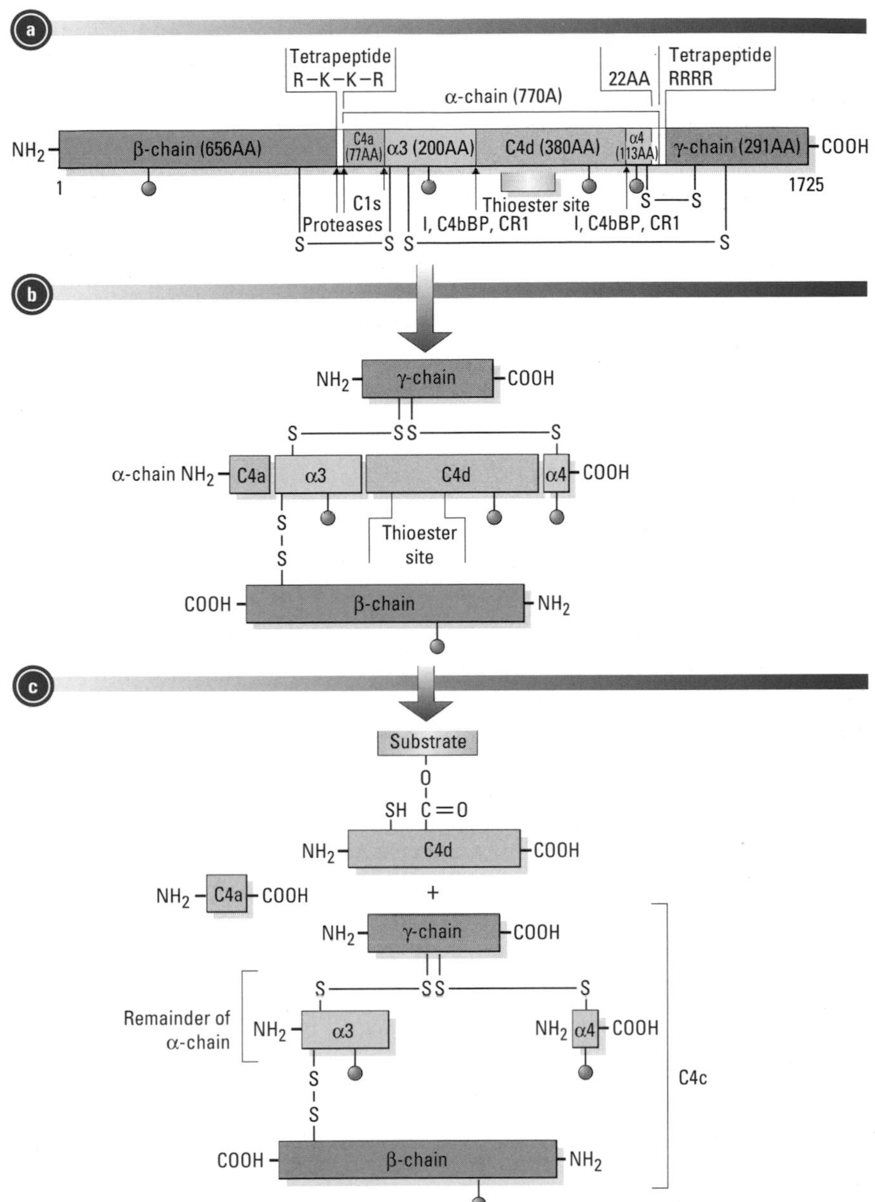

Figure 12.10 The C4 component. (a) The human *C4* gene specifies a protein (pre-pro-C4) that is 1744 amino acid (AA) residues long. The 19 N-terminal residues of this product constitute the signal peptide (not shown). After their removal, the 1725-residue pro-C4 is processed further. (b) Proteases cleave the pro-C4 chains at five sites and produce six fragments: the N-terminal β chain, followed by the tetrapeptide R-K-K-R, the α chain, the 22-residue peptide, the R-R-R-R tetrapeptide and finally the C-terminal γ chain. Both tetrapeptides and the 22-residue fragment drift off from the molecule, whereas the α, β and γ chains remain associated by disulphide bonds (the 22-residue peptide is sometimes considered to be part of the α-chain; without it, the chain is 765 residues long). (c) The three-chain structure attaches to a substrate via the thioester site in the α chain and C1s clips off a 77-residue fragment (C4a) from this chain, which drifts off, leaving behind the metastable C4b fragment. Factor I with cofactor C4b-binding protein (C4bBP) or complement receptor 1 (CR1) cleaves the α chain at two sites, releasing the C4c molecule into the fluid phase, while the remaining C4d fragment of 380 residues remains attached to the substrate by a covalent ester or amide bond. The thioester bond connects Lys 991 and Glu 994; ●–, potential *N*-glycosylation sites. Of the disulphide bonds (S—S) only those connecting the different fragments are shown. Several other disulphide bonds apparently exist in the C4 molecule but their distribution has not been determined. (Based on data from Yu, C.Y. (1991) *Journal of Immunology*, **146**, 1057.)

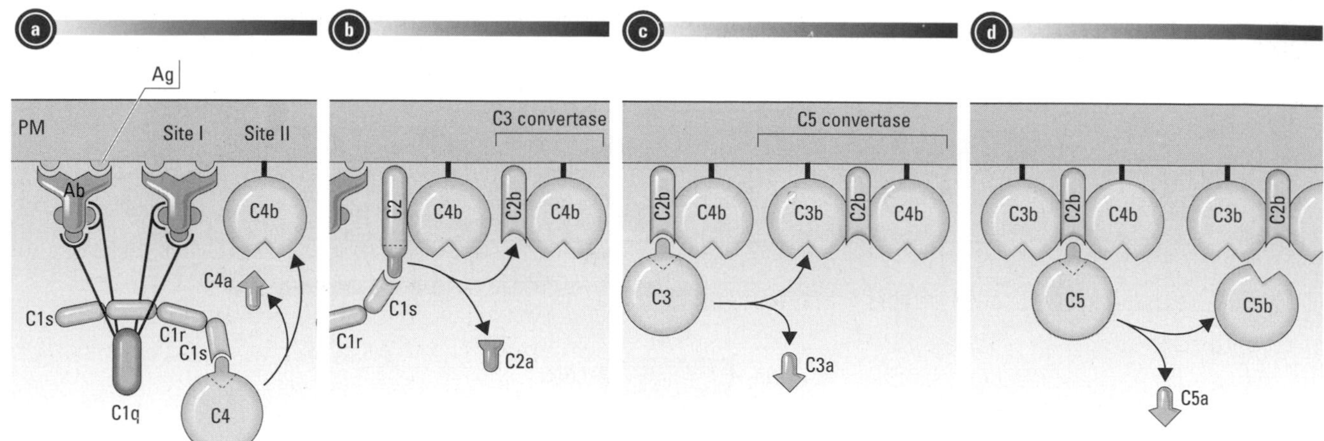

Figure 12.11 Stages in the activation of the classical complement pathway. (a) The C1 component, activated by the interaction with an antigen–antibody complex, cleaves the C4 component, splitting it into C4a, which drifts off, and C4b, which attaches to the plasma membrane (PM). (b) The C2 component attaches to the C4b molecule and is cleaved by the C1s component into C2a, which drifts off, and C2b, in which an enzymatically active site has been exposed by the cleavage. (c) The C3 component attaches to the C4bC2b complex and is cleaved by C2b into C3a, which drifts off, and C3b, which attaches itself to the membrane. (d) The C5 component binds to the C4bC2bC3b complex and is cleaved by C2b into C5a, which drifts off, and C5b, which remains attached to C3b on the membrane. There are three sites of complement interaction with the membrane: site I, at which C1 binds via the antibodies; site II, at which C4b (site IIA) and later C3b (site IIb) attaches; and site III (not shown), at which C5b, after it has attached to C6 and C7, later binds to the membrane via C7.

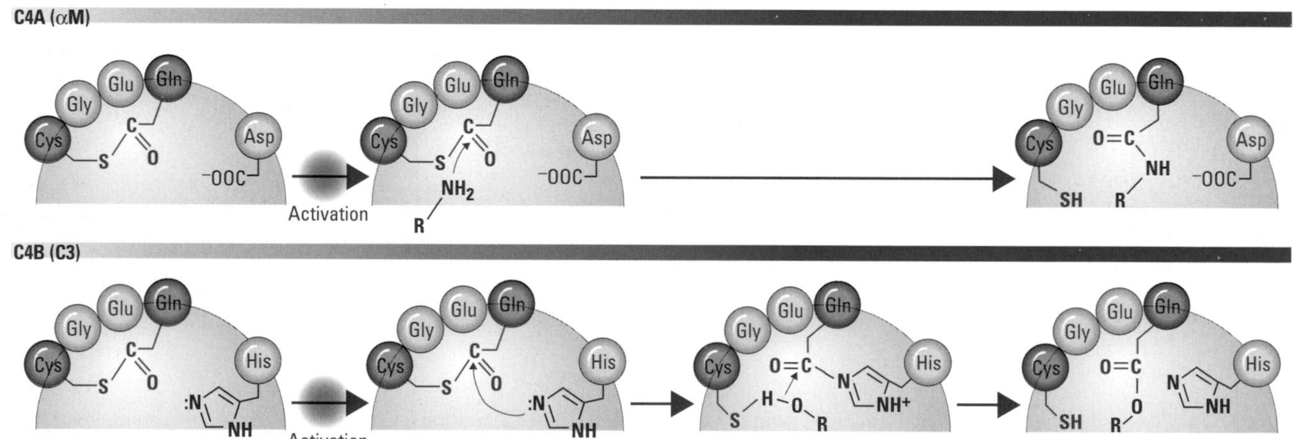

Figure 12.12 Binding of human C4A, C4B, α_2-macroglobulin (α_2M) and C3 molecules to water or proteins via the thioester site (positions 991–994). The residue at position 1106 that influences the binding is also shown. R denotes the rest of the molecule on the target cell or in the fluid phase. (Slightly modified from Law, S. K.A. & Dodds, A.W. (1996) *Immunology Today*, **17**, 105.)

found in several integrins and extracellular matrix proteins. It contains additional sites for binding of C2 and C2b to C4b. The C-terminal *serine protease domain* contains the catalytic site of the enzyme and is structurally homologous to members of the serine protease superfamily.

When a free C2 molecule accidentally hits the C4b fragment on the membrane, it binds to it with the aid of magnesium cations (Mg^{2+}) (see Fig. 12.11). Once a complex with C4b is formed, the C2 molecule is recognized by the catalytic site of the C1s protease and is cleaved into two fragments, the smaller C2a and the larger C2b fragment; the latter is thereby transformed into an active enzyme (Fig. 12.13). (Originally, the designations of C2 fragments were reversed in comparison with the

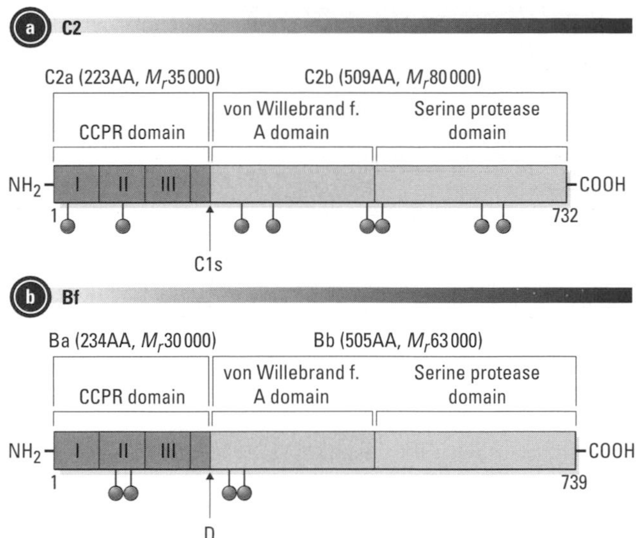

Figure 12.13 Complement component 2 (C2) and factor B (Bf). (a) The human C2 molecule consists of a single polypeptide chain that contains eight potential *N*-glycosylation sites (●–). C1s cleaves a single peptide bond between Arg 223 and Lys 224 producing two fragments, the N-terminal C2a and the C-terminal C2b. The two fragments are held together by non-covalent bonds only; there are no inter-fragment disulphide bonds. The C2a fragment consists of three repeats that are homologous to complement control protein repeats (CCPRs). The N-terminal part of the C2b fragment is homologous to the A domain of von Willebrand factor; the C-terminal part contains an enzymatically active site involving residues His 485, Asp 541 and Ser 659. This part is homologous to that of other serine proteases containing a similar catalytic site. (b) The human factor B molecule, like the C2 component, is a single-chain glycosylated protein (discussed later in the chapter). The two molecules resemble each other closely and are 39% identical in their sequence. The genes coding for the two proteins are closely linked. The native human factor B polypeptide is a 739-residue zymogen. It is converted into an active enzyme (serine protease) by the action of factor D, which breaks a single peptide bond between Arg 234 and Lys 235 and thus splits factor B into two fragments, the lighter Ba and the heavier Bb. The Ba fragment, like the C2a fragment, consists of three CCPRs; Bb, like C2b, consists of von Willebrand factor and serine protease domains. The catalytic site in the Bb fragment involves residues His 501, Asp 551 and Ser 674 (the numbers refer to the intact Bf chain).

designations of other complement component fragments; these older designations are still used by some researchers. The correct designations are, however, those used here.)

The fully extended $C1r_2C1s_2$ tetramer hangs from the C1q molecule like a snake from a tree, with the active C1s site (the snake's mouth) at the free end. The maximum distance it can extend is 60 nm; only C2 molecules found within this perimeter can therefore be activated. The C2 molecules bound to C4b but beyond the reach of C1q-bound C1 remain inactive. Free C2, not bound to C4, cannot be activated by C1. To be involved in the cascade, C2 must attach to C4b before it is cleaved by C1s. This prerequisite puts constraints on the number of C4bC2b complexes that can be formed. In fact, there may not be more than six such complexes around each C1 molecule. The complex composed of one molecule of both C4b and C2b held together by Mg^{2+} ions is termed the *C3 convertase*, for reasons that will become apparent shortly.

Both the activated C4 and the C3 convertase are unstable and short-lived. If it does not form a complex with C2, activated C4 becomes a target of the enzyme *factor I* (for 'inactivator'). Factor I is synthesized as a single polypeptide chain but is later split into two disulphide-bonded chains by the proteolytic removal of a tetrapeptide. The heavier of the two chains is a composite of several domains, at least some of which are also present in other proteins (Fig. 12.14). The light chain contains a catalytic site shared by the various serine proteases. In contrast to other members of the serine protease superfamily, however, factor I is not present in the plasma in an inactive zymogen form convertible into an active form by structural alterations. Rather, factor I circulates as an active protease. Because of its strict specificity for a small number of peptide bonds and the fact that it can act only in the presence of another factor (H or CR1, of which more later), circulating factor I normally does not cause any damage.

Factor I cleaves the bound C4b molecule at two sites in the α chain, leaving the C4d fragment attached to the substrate, while the remainder of the molecule (C4c) drifts off with the blood or lymph to perform other tasks (see Fig. 12.10c). C3 convertase decays rapidly, at a rate of 3% per second. The decay is, once again, a safeguard against a misguided attack on the body's own tissues. The convertase is inactivated in two stages. In the first stage, the C2b component dissociates itself from the C4b molecule and loses its enzymatic activity as well as its capacity to recombine with C4b. The dissociation occurs either spontaneously or by the action of three dissociation-promoting factors: C4b-binding protein, decay-accelerating factor and membrane co-factor protein. *C4b-binding protein (C4bBP)* is a complex molecule shaped like a shuttlecock (Fig. 12.15). It consists of one disc-shaped polypeptide (the 'cork' of the shuttlecock) from which seven extended polypeptides emanate (the 'feathers'). Each of the latter consists of eight repeats homologous to the CCPR domains of other molecules. Each C4bBP molecule can combine with up to six C4b molecules. Since it forms a complex with C4b at a site

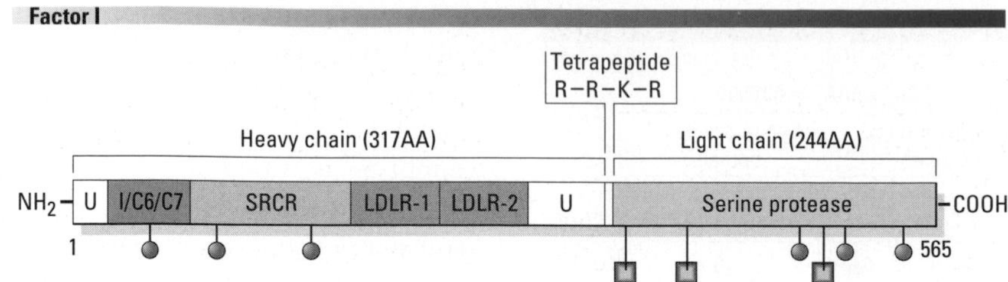

Figure 12.14 Complement factor I. The human factor I gene codes for a protein that, together with its leader sequence, is 583 amino acid residues long. The removal of the 18-residue leader leaves a single polypeptide chain composed of 565 residues. Proteolytic enzymes then cleave two peptide bonds, remove the tetrapeptide R-R-K-R and split the polypeptide into one heavy and one light chain held together by a disulphide bond. The heavy chain is composed of several domains (modules), some of which have also been found in other proteins: the I/C6/C7 domain in the C6 and C7 complement components; the scavenger receptor cysteine-rich (SRCR) domain in macrophage scavenger receptor (MSR) type I, CD5, CD6 and several other proteins; and the low-density lipoprotein receptor (LDLR) in proteins capable of binding lipoproteins with a relatively high content of cholesterol. The identity and origin of two other segments in the heavy chain (U, unknown) have still to be established. The heavy chain contains the catalytic site (residues His 362, Asp 411 and Ser 507, indicated by) characteristic of serine proteases. , potential *N*-glycosylation sites.

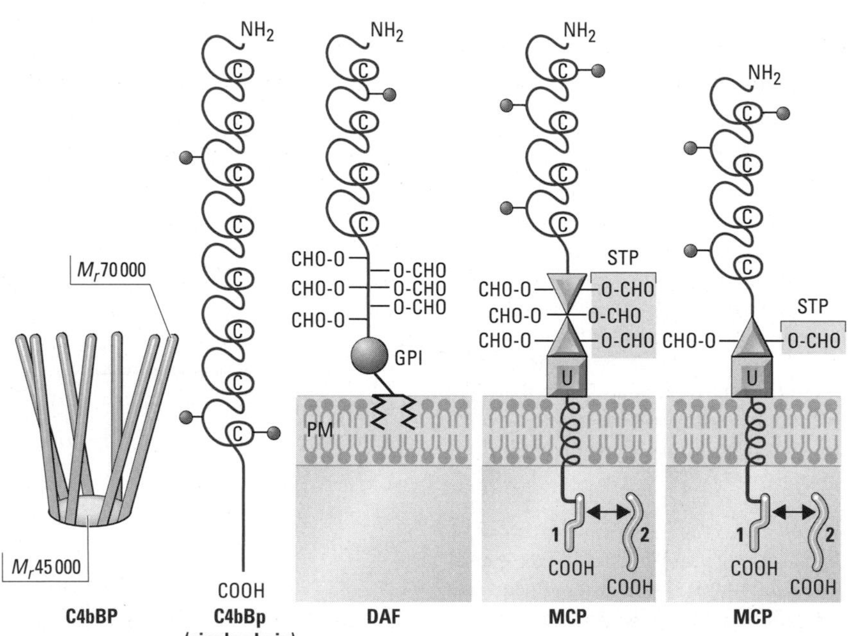

Figure 12.15 Three regulatory proteins of the complement cascade: C4b-binding protein (C4bBP), decay accelerating factor (DAF) and membrane co-factor protein (MCP). Shown from left to right: complete C4bBP molecule; single extended C4bBP chain; DAF molecule; and two forms of MCP produced by alternative splicing. Alternative splicing changes the length of the STP and the cytoplasmic regions of the MCP molecules, producing four different proteins from the same gene. The STP region of one version is 15 residues longer than the other and the cytoplasmic region of either of these two versions can be 16 or 23 residues long. C, complement control protein repeat domain; GPI, glycosylphosphatidylinositol; PM, plasma membrane; STP, serine, threonine, proline-rich domain; U, region of unknown function (12 residues long); , *N*-glycosylation sites. (Based in part on Liszewski, M.K. *et al.* (1996) *Advances in Immunology*, **61**, 201.)

close to that involved in the interaction with C2b, it interferes with C2b binding to C4b.

Decay accelerating factor (*DAF* or *CD55*; Fig. 12.15) is synthesized in the form of a transmembrane protein but without a cytoplasmic tail. In most molecules, the 28 C-terminal amino acid residues corresponding to the transmembrane region are removed post-translationally in the endoplasmic reticulum and are replaced by a preformed glycosylphosphatidylinositol (GPI) element consisting of ethanolamine, glucosamine, mannose, inositol and fatty acids (see Fig. 12.35). The insertion of the fatty acids into the outer leaflet of the membrane bilayer anchors the DAF molecule in the endoplasmic reticulum and the plasma membrane. The GPI is covalently linked to serine at position 319. The extracellular part of the protein consists of four CCPR domains followed by a stretch of 67 amino acid residues, 43% of which are either serine or threonine residues; the latter region is heavily O-glycosylated. DAF is expressed on all haemopoietic cells, endothelial cells, epithelial tissues, the central nervous system and the extracellular matrix. It is also present in a soluble form in the plasma and body fluids and in the placenta at the fetal–maternal interface. Its function is to accelerate the decay of C3 convertase. It leads to a rapid release of C2b from its binding site on C4b and thus to dissociation of the convertase. In contrast to C4bBP, however, it has no co-factor activity for factor I-mediated C4b and C3b degradation.

Membrane co-factor protein (*MCP* or *CD46*; Fig. 12.15) is structurally similar to DAF in that it consists of an extra cellular part composed of four CCPR domains followed by a highly O-glycosylated serine/threonine/proline (STP) region. The STP region occurs in two versions produced by alternative splicing: the removal of one exon (B) shortens the encoded protein by 15 amino acid residues. In contrast to DAF, however, the MCP molecule is normally anchored in the plasma membrane by a transmembrane region followed by a cytoplasmic tail, which can again occur in two versions produced by alternative splicing: in one version the tail is 16 and in the other 23 residues long. MCP molecules bind, via their CCPR domains, C4b and C3b components, especially if these occur in complexes constituting the convertases. MCP functions as a co-factor in factor-I mediated C4b and C3b degradation. It is widely distributed in the tissues, including (like DAF) the placenta. MCP is also the receptor for measles virus and is involved in the adherence to epithelial cells of group A *Streptococcus pyogenes*.

Cleavage of the C3 component

The target of C3 convertase is the complement component C3. The C4 and C3 components are related structurally and functionally and are encoded in genes that arose by duplication from a common ancestral element. The C3 molecule is synthesized as a single polypeptide chain that is later split into a larger α chain and a smaller β chain, the two chains being held together by disulphide bonds (Fig. 12.16).

When a C3 molecule in solution accidentally bumps into the C4bC2b complex on the membrane, it binds transiently to the complex and is cleaved by the catalytic site of the C2b fragment (see Fig. 12.11). The cleavage removes a 77-amino-acid peptide from the N-terminus of the α chain. The peptide, called the *C3a fragment* or *anaphylatoxin C3a*, diffuses away while the rest of the molecule, the *C3b fragment*, undergoes a conformational change to expose a labile *thioester bond*. The structure of the thioester site is similar to that found in the C4b molecule. The exposed bond breaks and the acyl group binds to either water molecules or the nearest protein via an ester or amide linkage (see Fig. 12.11). Membrane proteins within a radius of about 40 nm are most likely to become the anchoring sites for the C3b fragment. If the fragment diffuses further away, it interacts with water, loses its ability to attach to proteins and is eventually degraded. The anchoring process, like that of C4b, is very inefficient in that only some 20% of the cleaved C3 actually binds to cells. However, here again an amplification process compensates somewhat for the inefficiency: a single C4bC2b complex can cleave some 200 C3 molecules, which descend like a small shower on the membrane, clustering around the complex. Under optimal conditions of complement activation, more than 100 000 C3 molecules may be deposited on a sheep erythrocyte within 1 min.

The deposited C3b has two functions. First, it combines with C3 receptors on phagocytes and thus facilitates phagocytosis. The C3b molecule has two sites that allow it to interact with the C3 receptors, but phagocytosis will not take place until some 2000–4000 molecules cover the engulfed particle. Second, some of the C3b molecules bind to the C3 convertase to form a trimolecular complex C4bC2bC3b (also written as C4b2b3b), the *C5 convertase*. The C3b component of the C5 convertase binds the next component in the pathway, C5, and changes its conformation so that the C2b component can cleave it into C5a and C5b.

Membrane-bound C3b has a short lifespan. If it does not find its target within a minute or so, it is cleaved by factor I and inactivated so that it can no longer bind C5. The initial cleavage of C3b by factor I can only occur in the presence of a co-factor, either factor H or CR1. Factor I splits the α chain of C3b in two places, releasing a small intervening polypeptide, C3f. The rest of the now inactive C3b molecule is referred to as iC3b. Further cleavage by factor I in the presence of CR1 as a co-factor releases the bulk of the molecule from the cell surface as C3c, while a small fragment, C3dg, remains attached to the cell surface by the covalent bond of the binding site (see Fig. 12.16).

Cleavage of the C5 component

The C5 component, which is structurally related to the C4 and C3 components, is synthesized as a single polypeptide but is post-translationally cleaved into two chains, α and β, connected by disulphide bonds (Fig. 12.17). When a C5

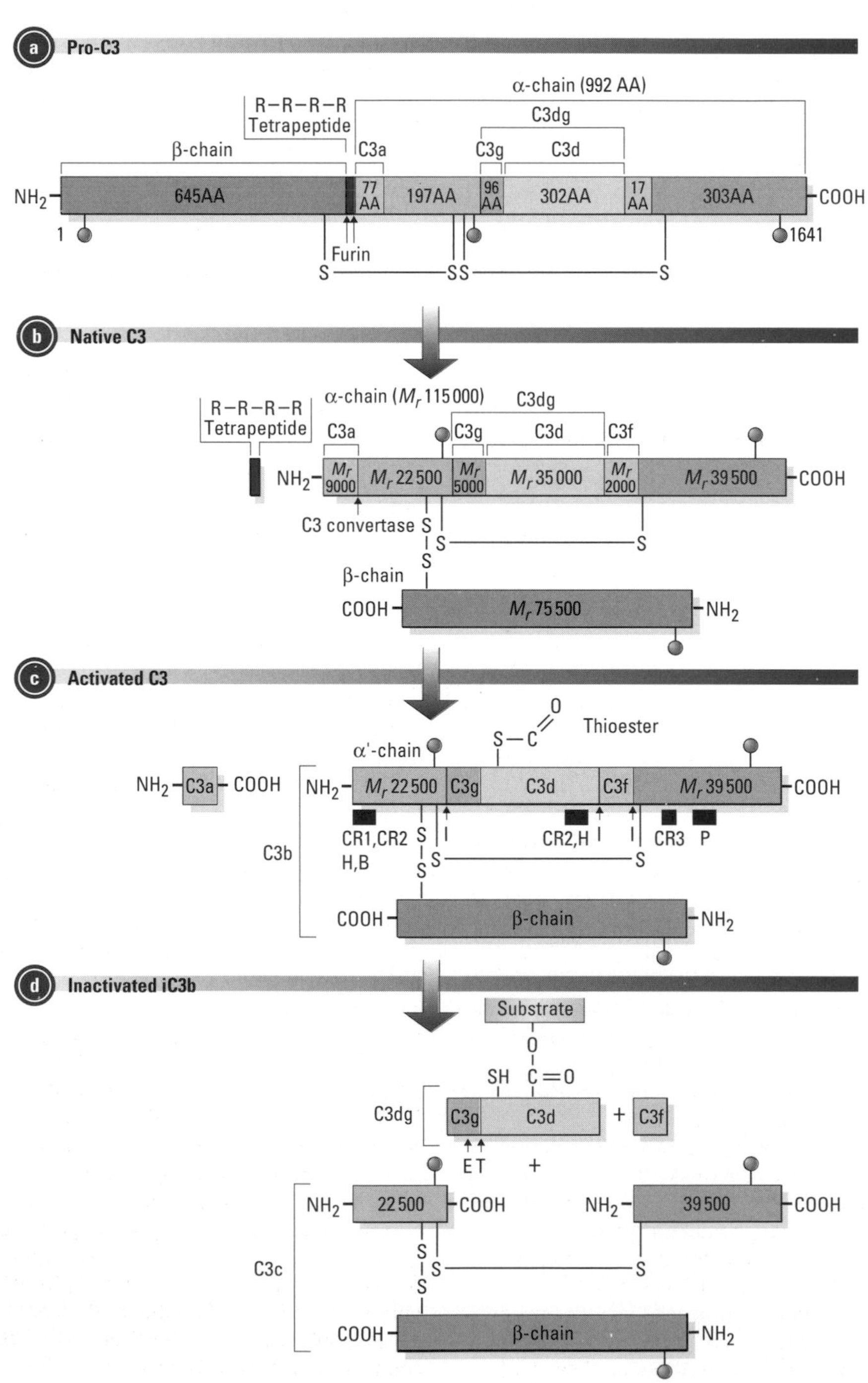

molecule in solution accidentally hits the C3b molecule on the cell surface, a transient bond is established between the two (see Fig. 12.11). While attached to C3b of the C5 convertase, the C5 molecule becomes the target for the C2b molecule. The catalytic site of the C2b molecule cleaves a single peptide bond in the α chain of the C5 molecule, releasing a fragment 74 amino acids long, the *anaphylatoxin C5a*, from the N-terminus. The rest of the molecule, the C5b fragment, then leaves the C5 convertase and initiates the assembly of the C5–C9 complex.

The activated C5 molecule is unstable. It undergoes inactivation while still bound to the membrane, its half-life being about 2 min at 37°C. It is stabilized, however, by the interaction with C6. It is a highly efficient molecule: only three to ten molecules attached to an erythrocyte are required to pierce a hole in the plasma membrane. The cleavage of the C5 component is the last enzymatic reaction in the cascade; none of the remaining steps require enzymatic activity. The enzymes of the classical pathway are the activated forms of C1r, C1s, MASP and C2; the C1q, MBP, C4 and C3 components have no enzymatic activity — they are structural proteins. The main steps in the classical pathway are summarized in Figs 12.1 and 12.11.

Alternative pathway

Initiation

One of the main differences between the classical and alternative pathways is that the initiation of the former requires the participation of activating substances (antibodies, MBP). The alternative pathway, by contrast, runs continuously and spontaneously at a low level in the absence of any activators; the latter merely amplify it by subverting the control mechanism. According to the *ticking-over hypothesis*, the alternative pathway is initiated by the spontaneous activation of the C3 component. In the plasma, the α chain of the C3 molecule spontaneously incorporates one molecule of water, with the result that the thioester bond is hydrolysed and a C3(H_2O) complex is formed (Fig. 12.18). The complex, which functionally behaves like C3b although it is not produced by the release of the C3a fragment, forms continuously at the very slow rate of 0.005% per minute. The C3(H_2O) molecule associates reversibly with *factor B* in the presence of physiological concentrations of Mg^{2+} ions. Factor B is a single-chain protein (Fig. 12.13), whose role in the alternative pathway is analogous to that of C2 in the classical pathway. The B and C2

Figure 12.16 (*Opposite.*) Complement component 3 (C3). (a) Human C3 is synthesized as a single-chain 1663-residue polypeptide. This *pre-pro-C3* molecule is post-translationally processed by the removal of 22 residues from the N-terminus (the signal peptide) and formation of the thioester bond in the sequence Cys 998-Gly-Glu-Gln 991 (numbers refer to the sequence of the mature protein). The thioester bond is the product of intramolecular transacetylation between the thiol group of Cys 998 and the γ-amide group of Gln 991. The processing steps also include removal of the tetrapeptide R-R-R-R from the *pro-C3 molecule*. The removal occurs by the breakage of two peptide bonds and is catalysed by a furin-like enzyme. It results in a two-chain molecule (*native C3*) in which the α and β peptides are held together by disulphide bonds. (b) In the native C3 molecule the labile thioester group is protected within a hydrophobic pocket, but cleavage of the α chain by C3 convertase exposes the highly reactive group. C3 convertase breaks a single peptide bond between Arg 726 and Ser 727 and thus releases a 77-residue peptide termed *C3a* from the N-terminus of the α chain; the remainder of the α chain is now referred to as *α′ chain* and the β–α′ molecule as *C3b*. (c) In contrast to native C3, the C3b molecule expresses multiple binding sites for other complement components, including C5, properdin, factors H, B and I, C4b-binding protein, C3b receptor and membrane co-factor protein (MCP). Binding of factor B (and of properdin in the presence of factor D) leads to amplification of C3 convertase; binding of C5 initiates the assembly of the membrane-attack complex; and binding of factor I inactivates C3b. Which of these events occurs depends on the surface that the exposed thioester group encounters. The group can react with nucleophilic groups present on the cell surface, on complex carbohydrates or on antigen–antibody (immune) complexes. The transacetylation reaction breaks the thioester bond and forms a new covalent bond with the substrate. (d) C3b components that fail to find a suitable substrate or which have accomplished their mission are inactivated in three steps by factor I with the participation of several co-factors. In the first two steps, factor I cleaves the α chain at two places, first between Arg 1281 and Ser 1282, and then between Arg 1298 and Ser 1299, releasing a short (17-residue) peptide termed *C3f*; the remainder of the molecule is now referred to as inactive C3b or *iC3b*. In the third step, factor I, in the presence of co-factors CR1 or H, breaks a single peptide bond between Arg 932 and Glu 933 of the α′ chain. This step generates a *C3dg* fragment from the α′ chain, which separates from the rest of the molecule now termed *C3c*. If iC3b was attached to the surface, the C3dg fragment remains fixed, whereas C3c is released back into the fluid phase. Further degradation of the C3dg fragment is accomplished by serum proteases such as trypsin (T) and elastase (E), which generate two fragments, C3d and C3g, from the original single one. ●–, *N*-glycosylation sites; AA, number of amino acid residues; S–S, disulphide bond; ■, binding site; ↑, cleavage site; P, properdin; B, factor B; CR, complement receptor; H, factor H.

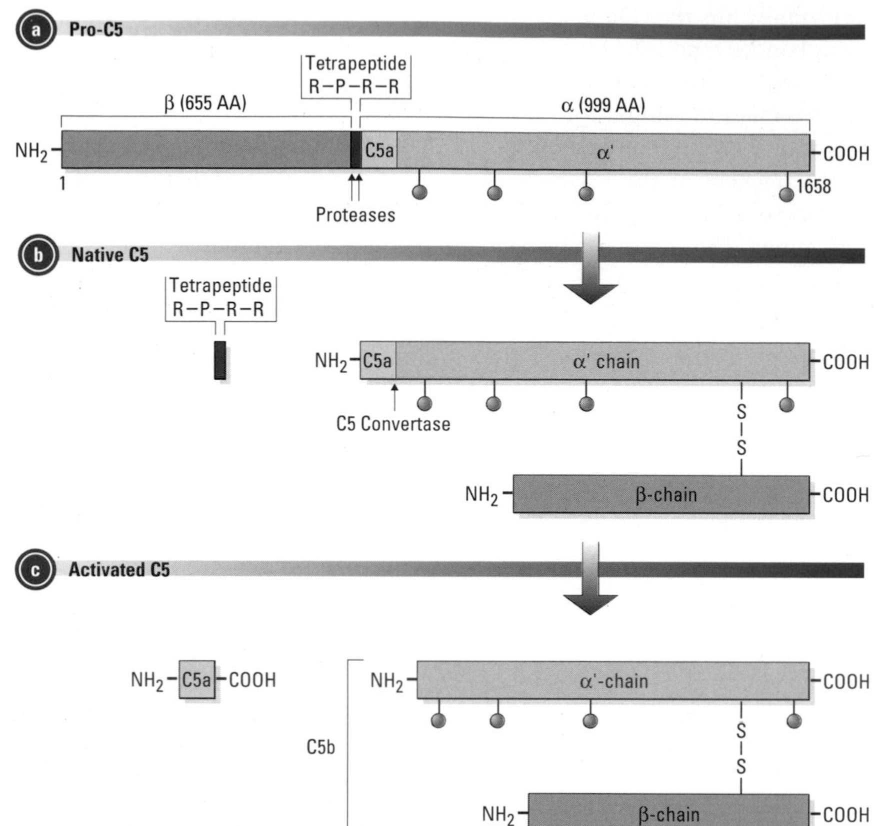

Figure 12.17 Complement component 5 (C5). Human *pre-pro-C5* is synthesized as a single-chain 1676-residue polypeptide. (a) After the removal of the 18-residue signal peptide, the 1658-residue *pro-C5* is cleaved by intracellular proteases into two chains: the N-terminal part becomes a 655-residue β chain and the C-terminal part a 999-residue α chain. (b) The chains remain connected by a single disulphide (S—S) bond. The cleavage breaks two peptide bonds and releases the R-P-R-R tetrapeptide from the β–α junction. The α chain contains four potential *N*-glycosylation sites (●–). The total carbohydrate content of the molecule is about 3%. The C5 polypeptide is similar in sequence and overall organization to the C4 and C3 polypeptides but in contrast to them it does not contain the thioester group. In human C5 there are serine and alanine residues at the positions corresponding to the cysteine and glutamine residues that form the thioester in C3 and C4. (c) *Native C5* is activated by the action of C5 convertase, which clips off a 74-residue fragment (C5a) from the N-terminus of the α chain by breaking a single peptide bond. The remaining part of the chain is denoted α′, and the entire molecule minus the C5a fragment C5b. AA, amino acid residue.

components are related both genetically and functionally. Like C2, factor B is a serine protease that occurs in the plasma in an inactive pro-enzyme form. Once associated with the C3(H_2O) molecule, factor B is attacked by factor D and activated. *Factor D* is also a serine protease that circulates in the blood in an active form (Fig. 12.19). It normally does no damage to the body because its concentration in the plasma is very low and it is highly specific for the Arg–Lys bond in factor B. It attacks factor B only when the latter is in a complex with the C3 molecule. The action of factor D on the C3(H_2O)B complex results in the cleavage of factor B into two fragments, Ba and Bb, followed by the release of the smaller Ba fragment from the complement cascade. The C3(H_2O)Bb complex, the *initiating (fluid-phase) C3 convertase*, then cleaves intact C3 molecules into C3a and C3b, just as the C3/C5 convertase does in the classical pathway. (The C3/C5 convertase, however, is composed of C4b and C2b fragments, whereas the fluid-phase C3 convertase consists of C3(H_2O) and Ba. In the alternative pathway, therefore, an enzyme containing C3 acts on C3.) Up to this point, all these events have been taking place in the fluid phase (again differing from the classical pathway) but now the metastable C3b fragment diffuses a distance of some 30 nm and if it encounters a suitable particle on the way it attaches itself to it via covalent ester or amide bonds.

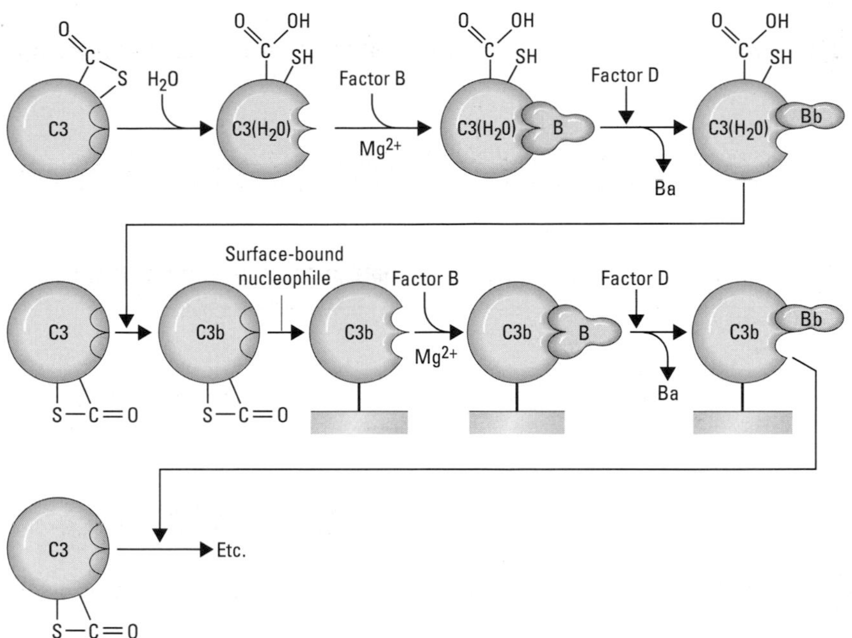

Figure 12.18 Initiation of the alternative complement activation pathway: the ticking-over model. A C3 molecule binds a molecule of water, its thioester bond breaks and a binding site for factor B is exposed. The bound factor B is attacked by factor D, which cleaves it into Ba and Bb fragments. The Ba fragment drifts off, while the Bb fragment remains non-covalently associated with $C3(H_2O)$, forming an initial C3 convertase $[C3(H_2O)Bb]$. The convertase attacks another native C3 molecule, releasing the C3a fragment from the latter. The exposed thioester of the remaining C3b molecule breaks, the molecule attaches to a surface provided by an activating agent and binds factor B in the presence of magnesium cations. The bound factor B is cleaved by factor D and the surface-bound C3 convertase (C3bBb) then attacks another native C3 molecule and so on. The activating agent thus accelerates (ticks over) a reaction that in its absence occurs at a slow rate. Factor B has three globular domains, one corresponding to the Ba and two to the Bb fragment. It binds to C3b via two contact sites, one in the Ba and another in the Bb fragment. The cleavage of factor B by factor D reduces the affinity of Ba interaction with C3b and the fragment leaves the complex; the exposed serine protease site of the Bb fragment is then ready to attack another C3 molecule. (Slightly modified from Halkier, T. (1991) *Mechanisms of Blood Coagulation, Fibrinolysis and the Complement System*. Cambridge University Press, Cambridge.)

The particles to which the activated C3b molecules become attached can be invading microorganisms but they may also be the body's own cells, because up to this stage the pathway does not discriminate between self and non-self. Discrimination is only possible from this point onwards: fluid-phase C3b and C3b bound to self particles are rapidly inactivated by factors H and I, whereas C3b deposited on foreign particles is relatively well protected from degradation by fluid-phase regulatory proteins. For reasons that are not entirely clear, factor H has a reduced affinity for C3b bound to many bacteria, fungi, certain viruses, virus-infected cells, certain tumour cells and eukaryotic parasites such as trypanosomes. The only two features these entities have in common are, first, the presence of carbohydrate and the absence of surface sialic acid and, second, the absence of regulatory proteins CR1, MCP and DAF. Regardless of the mechanism, a crude form of self–non-self discrimination does occur at this stage and the slow, random deposit of the first C3b is followed by a relatively rapid amplification of the reaction, but only on the surfaces that protect C3b from inactivation; these surfaces thus function as *activators* of the alternative pathway.

Amplification of C3b

The C3b fragment generated by the fluid-phase C3 convertase and bound covalently to the surface of the activating substance is joined by factor B, the latter is cleaved by factor D into Ba and Bb fragments, the Ba fragment diffuses away and the Bb fragment remains associated with the C3b fragment. The C3bBb complex, which is held together by Mg^{2+} ions, constitutes the *amplification C3 convertase*. It acts on other free C3 molecules, which in turn form further C3 convertases, which again act on C3 molecules, thus amplifying the initial event tremendously (see Fig. 12.18). The C3b molecules 'rain' on foreign particles, covering them quickly:

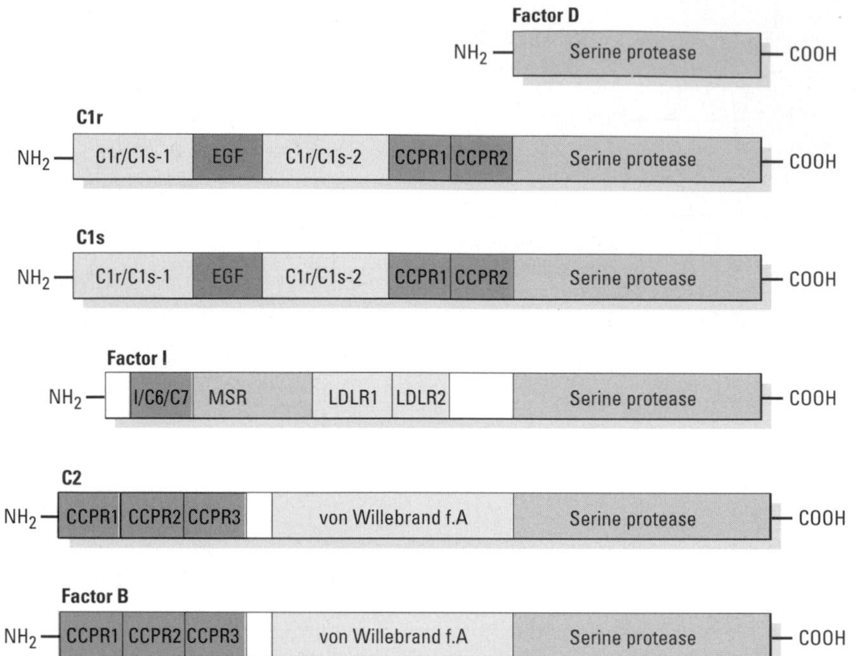

Figure 12.19 The family of serine proteases involved in the complement cascade. All except factor D were described earlier; they are depicted again here for comparison. Factor D differs from the other serine proteases in that it apparently does not contain additional domains with secondary functions. It is therefore correspondingly shorter than the other proteases. CCPR, complement control protein repeat; EGF, epidermal growth factor; LDLR, low-density lipoprotein receptor; MSR, macrophage scavenging receptor. Open rectangles represent regions without significant similarity to other proteins.

within 5 min after contact with serum, foreign erythrocytes become coated with 2×10^6 C3b molecules per cell.

The C3bBb complex is relatively labile. The subunits dissociate spontaneously and the freed (as well as the C3b-bound) Bb molecules lose their enzymatic activity irreversibly; the half-life of the fluid-phase and particle-bound C3bBb(Mg^{2+}) is about 90 s. The complexes are stabilized, however, by the interaction with *properdin (factor P)*. Native properdin is an oligomer composed of non-covalently bound subunits with an M_r of 56 000 (Fig. 12.20). It is present in the plasma as a mixture of dimers, trimers and tetramers associated head to tail in cyclic structures. Each monomer is composed of six *thrombospondin repeat (TSR) modules*, originally described in the cell adhesion protein thrombospondin. The binding of properdin to the C3 convertase stabilizes the latter by slowing down dissociation of the C3bBb(Mg^{2+}) complexes fivefold to tenfold. Properdin also protects the C3 convertase against degradation by factor I. It thus acts as a positive regulator of the complement cascade in contrast to other regulatory proteins that inhibit or degrade complement components and hence regulate the cascade negatively. The C3b convertase (C3bBb), stabilized by properdin, attacks additional C3 molecules, binds the resulting C3b fragments covalently via the α′ chain and thus forms $(C3b)_2Bb$ or $(C3b)_nBb$ complexes. During this process, the convertase loses its affinity for additional C3b molecules and acquires affinity for the C5 component. In other words, the C3 convertase becomes a *C5 convertase*. In the $(C3b)_2Bb$ complex, the extra C3b molecule binds the C5 component and the Bb component bound to the original C3b molecule then attacks the C5 molecule cleaving it into C5a and C5b fragments (Fig. 12.21). The C5a fragment dissociates from the convertase and drifts off; C5b becomes involved in the lytic pathway but ultimately (when C5b6 combines with C7; see below) dissociates from the convertase as well. C3b of the convertase becomes the target of an attack by factor I in the presence of factor H (patients suffering from factor H-deficiency undergo uncontrolled fluid-phase C3 activation). C3b is degraded into C3f and iC3b and subsequently degraded further in the manner described for the classical pathway. The alternative pathway is summarized in Fig. 12.22.

A particularly strong but artificial stabilization of C3

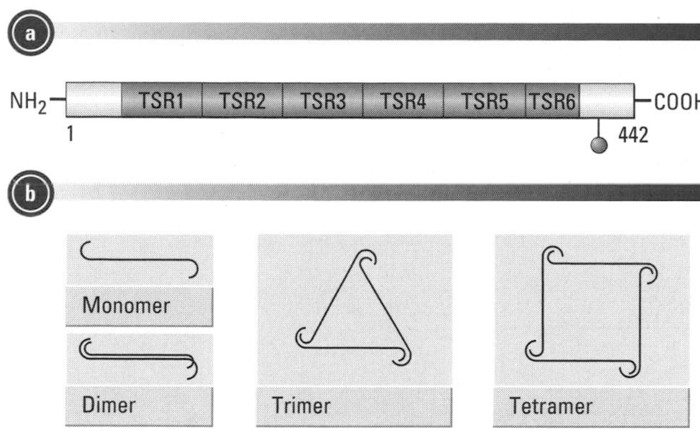

Figure 12.20 Properdin (factor P). (a) The monomer. More than 80% of the mature protein's sequence is organized into six modules (domains), each module being approximately 60 residues long and containing six conserved cysteine and three conserved tryptophan residues. Similar domains were originally found in the cell-adhesion protein thrombospondin and are therefore referred to as thrombospondin repeats (TSRs). They are also present in complement components C6, C7, C8α, C8β and C9 (see Fig. 12.24), as well as in *Eimeria tenella* (a fowl parasite) and certain malaria parasite proteins. All these proteins are involved in interactions with cell surfaces. The cell binding involves the sequence motif VTCG recognized in the cell surface CD36 receptor. Each of the six TSRs apparently represents an independent folding unit; the sixth TSR, however, is incomplete over its C-terminal part. The polypeptide contains a single *N*-glycosylation site ( ). (b) The oligomers. Properdin is present in plasma in the form of dimers (P_2), trimers (P_3) and tetramers (P_4) of the monomeric polypeptide; they occur in a ratio of 26 : 54 : 20, respectively. The oligomers form by strong, non-covalent head-to-tail interactions between the N- and C-termini of the monomers. The figure depicts a model of the possible interactions. (a, based on data from Nolan, F.K. *et al.* (1992) *Biochemistry Journal*, **287**, 291; b, based on data from Smith, S.A. *et al.* (1984) *Journal of Biological Chemistry*, **259**, 4582.)

convertase occurs after the addition of cobra venom to the serum. The venom contains a fragment of the snake C3 molecule, the *cobra venom factor* (CVF). The CVF–Bb complex has a half-life of 7 hours and is not affected by the regulatory proteins in the human plasma; it fails to bind mammalian factor H. Cobra venom therefore floods the system with excess C3b, which escapes the normal control mechanisms, amplifies the cascade and depletes the serum of C3 as well as of all components that follow C3 in the complement pathway.

Lytic pathway

The final outcome of both the classical and alternative pathways is the cleavage of the C5 components into C5a (which leaves the cascade) and C5b fragments. The removal of C5a from C5 leads to the transient expression of a binding site for *complement component 6* (C6) on the C5b fragment. C6 is one of four components involved in the assembly of the *membrane-attack complex* (MAC) in the lytic pathway. The other components are C7, C8 and C9 (Fig. 12.23). The C8 component is a three-chain molecule with α, β and γ chains, the first two of which are encoded in closely linked genes. C6, C7 and C9 are single-chain molecules. All four are *modular proteins*, which means that their polypeptide chains consist of modules (domains) found also in other proteins (Fig. 12.24). The modules include the TSR, the I/C6/C7 repeat, the CCPR, the EGF-like domain, the low-density lipoprotein receptor (LDLR) domain and the perforin domain. The *pore-forming protein* or *perforin* is a molecule stored in cytoplasmic granules of cytotoxic T lymphocytes and used by these cells to form cylindrical pores in the plasma membrane of the target cell with which they have made contact. Perforin thus carries out a function similar to that of the C9 molecule in the complement cascade (see below). The C6, C7, C8 and C9 molecules are all related to one another by their sequence and by the organization of their modules (Fig. 12.24). Upon binding to the C5b fragment, the C6 molecule undergoes a conformational change and thus acquires the ability to bind C7 (Fig. 12.25). If no C7 molecule is available, the C5b6 complex is released from the activating surface into the fluid phase, where it remains stable and active. (Note that in the symbol for the complex, the letter C is omitted from the C6, C7, C8 and C9 components.) If the released C5b6 complex

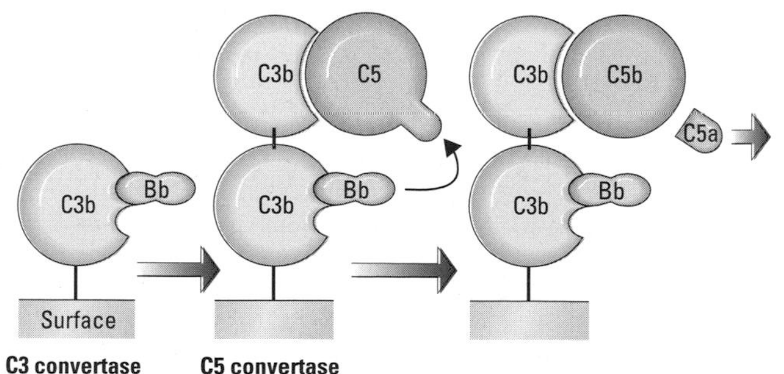

Figure 12.21 C5 convertase of the alternative pathway. The C3bBb complex (*C3 convertase*) binds covalently via its α′ chain to the C3b part of another C3 molecule that it has just activated. $(C3b)_2Bb$, or more generally the $(C3b)_nBb$ complex (*C5 convertase*), binds the C5 component via its extra C3b molecules and the Bb protease associated with the surface-bound C3b molecule clips off the C5a fragment, which leaves the complex. For the sake of simplicity, the properdin molecules that stabilize the C5 convertase are not shown.

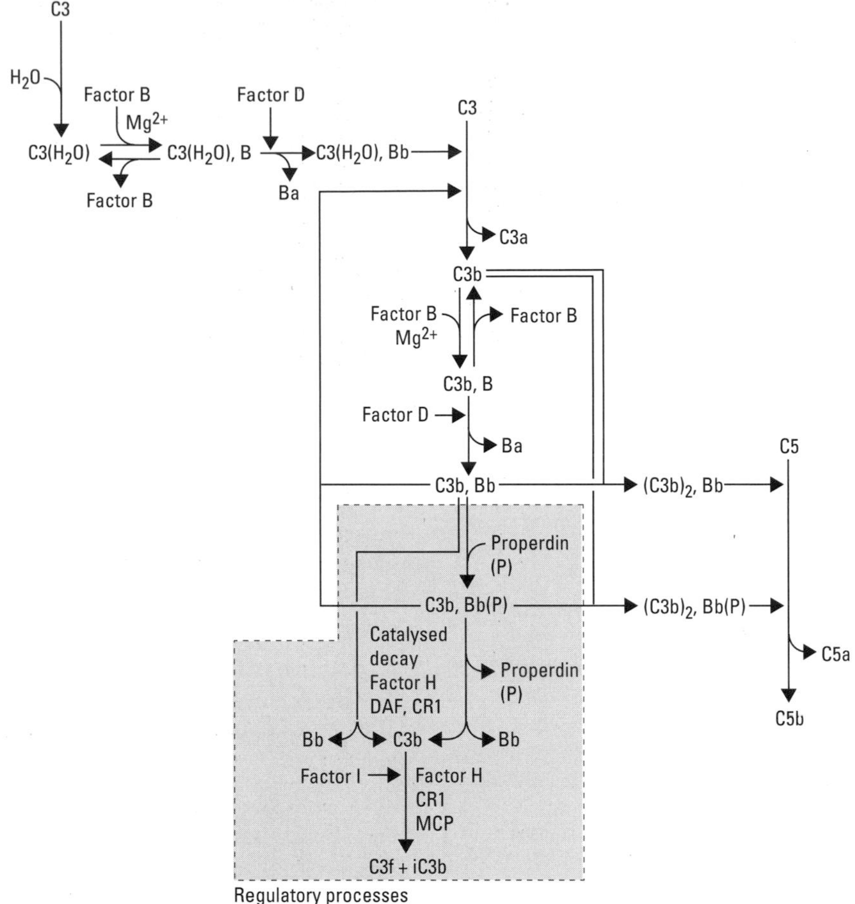

Figure 12.22 The alternative pathway of complement activation. The binding of water molecules to the native C3 molecule leads to spontaneous hydrolysis of the thioester bond in the latter. Hydrolysis exposes the binding site for factor B in the $C3(H_2O)$ molecule and reversible $C3(H_2O)B$ complex formation follows in the presence of magnesium cations. The bound factor B is cleaved by factor D, the Ba fragment is released and the Bb molecule of the $C3(H_2O)Bb$ complex (the initiating or fluid-phase convertase) proteolytically cleaves another C3 molecule, releasing the C3a fragment from it. The resulting C3b molecule must now attach itself to the surface of an activating agent via its thioester group. If this happens, the fixed C3b molecule binds (again reversibly and with the participation of magnesium cations) factor B, which is then cleaved by factor D. The surface-bound C3bBb complex is the *amplification C3 convertase*, which can act, via its Bb serine protease, on other C3 molecules and thus amplify the reaction. C3 convertase is stabilized by the association with properdin (P). The C3b molecule in C3bBb or the more stable C3bBb(P) complexes binds covalently another C3b molecule, and the $(C3b)_2Bb$ and $(C3b)_2Bb(P)$ complexes become *C5 convertases* capable of cleaving the C5 molecule into C5a and C5b fragments (where the enzymatic cleavage is catalysed by the Bb protease in the complex). The complexes ultimately dissociate into their individual components and the C3b molecules are inactivated and degraded by the action of factor I with the assistance of several co-factors (DAF, factor H, CR1 and MCP).

encounters C7, it attaches itself to the nearest cell and, upon binding C8 and C9, lyses it. This *reactive lysis* is minimized by the action of C5b67 inhibitors, such as the S-protein, clusterin and C8 (once C5b67 has bound C8 it can no longer bind to membrane) and lipoproteins. Better known under the name *vitronectin*, the *S-protein* shares some properties (including the binding motif RGD) with many adhesion molecules (Fig. 12.26). In the complement cascade, it functions as a scavenger of the C5b67 complexes from the fluid phase. By binding to the complex, it blocks the site by which the complex would otherwise attach to the membrane. *Clusterin* (*SP40,* complement cytolysis inhibitor, CLI) is a heterodimer of α and β chains with an M_r of 70 000. The two chains are produced by proteolysis of a single-chain precursor. Clusterin is found in the plasma and in the seminal fluid and is produced by Sertoli cells.

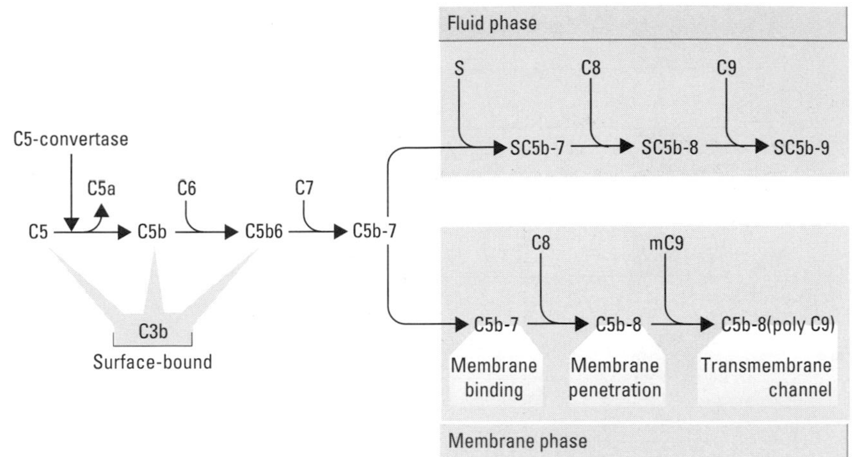

Figure 12.23 Steps involved in the assembly of the membrane-attack complex. From left to right: surface-bound C5 convertase (either from the classical or the alternative pathway) splits C5 into C5a (which diffuses away) and the metastable C5b (half-life 2.3 min at 37°C), which remains associated with C3b. C5b binds C6 and a stable C5b6 complex is created. The complex binds C7, which thus undergoes hydrophilic–amphiphilic transition and exposes a hydrophobic binding site. The C5b67 complex has two alternatives: either it binds via the hydrophobic site on C7 to the membrane, or it associates with the S protein in the fluid phase. The membrane-bound C5b67 complex binds C8, which thus undergoes hydrophilic–amphiphilic transition and its α chain enters the membrane. The C8 component then binds C9 and non-enzymatically catalyses its polymerization, during which C9 undergoes hydrophilic–amphiphilic transition and considerable molecular reorganization. Tubular poly-C9 forms, with C5b678, the polymerizing unit. The C5b6789 complex creates a large channel that lyses the cell (the C5b678 complex, in contrast, produces only a small membrane pore sufficient to lyse erythrocytes but usually not large enough to kill a nucleated cell). The fluid-phase SC5b67 complex binds C8 and C9 from hydrophilic SC5b6789 in which C9 does not polymerize. (Note that in the figure symbols such as C5b6789 are reduced to C5b–9.)

(Originally discovered in the rat testis, it was named *sulphated glycoprotein-2* or *SGP-2*.) It suppresses the cytolytic potential of nascent C5b67 complexes. In the male reproductive tract, it presumably protects sperm and epithelial cells against complement attack. Finally, *lipoproteins* apparently trick the released C5b67 complexes by disguising themselves as pieces of a membrane; the complexes are inserted into the lipoproteins and are thus no longer available for membrane insertion.

The C5b6 complexes that have encountered C7 while still attached to the membrane bind the *C7 component* and form a C5b67 complex, which detaches itself from the C5 convertase. The bound C7 undergoes a conformational alteration that exposes a previously hidden hydrophobic domain. The altered protein therefore has both hydrophilic and hydrophobic domains, i.e. it is *amphiphilic*. The *hydrophilic–amphiphilic transition* enables the forming complex to acquire affinity for membrane surfaces, to which it attaches via the hydrophobic part of the C7 component. If the complexed C7 finds no hydrophobic substrate, the complex is released into the fluid phase and presents a potential hazard for the host because it can then insert itself into the membranes of neighbouring cells. This *lysis of innocent bystander cells* is prevented by the regulatory plasma proteins described above.

Once bound to the membrane, the C5b67 complex expresses a stable binding site for *complement component 8*. In this molecule the α and γ chains are covalently linked by disulphide bonds and non-covalently associated with the β chain. All three chains have several hydrophobic regions by which they can interact with cell membranes. Upon binding to the C5b67 complex, the C8 component undergoes a conformational change that exposes the hidden hydrophobic domains in the α–γ dimer, i.e. the protein undergoes a hydrophilic–amphiphilic transition. The hydrophobic region inserts itself into the lipid bilayer and thus, in combination with one or more of the other C5b678 domains, creates a small membrane pore with a diameter of about 1 nm (Fig. 12.27). The plasma membrane of the target cell has been punctured.

The events that follow are merely a way of enlarging the hole. The attachment of C8 to the C5b67 complex exposes a binding site for C9 in the C8α chain. Upon its incorporation into the C5b678 complex, *component 9* undergoes a prominent conformational change that results in the insertion of its hydrophobic regions into the membrane interior,

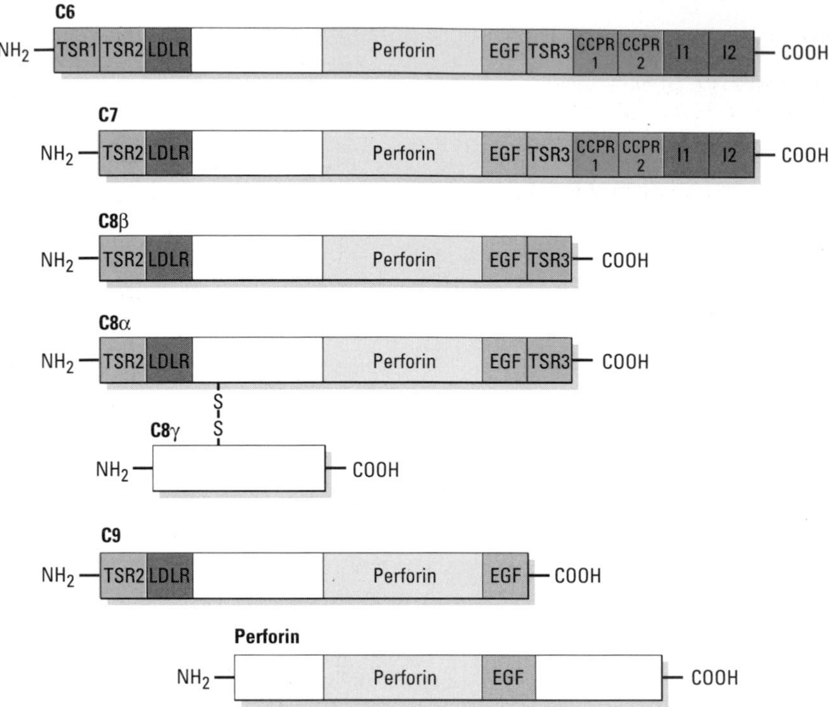

Figure 12.24 Components of the lytic complement pathway. The five polypeptide chains are all composed of modules that are also found in other proteins: the thrombospondin repeat (TSR), the perforin-like domain, the epidermal growth factor (EGF)-like module, the complement control protein repeat (CCPR) and the low-density lipoprotein receptor (LDLR) domain. The C6 and C7 proteins possess, in addition, a domain that they share with factor I (I/C6/C7) and each of the five proteins also has a unique region not homologous to any other known protein. The C8 component is a three-chain glycoprotein in which the α and γ chains are covalently linked via a disulphide bond and the β chain is non-covalently associated with them. The chains are encoded in three separate but closely linked loci. Perforin does not participate in the complement pathways; instead it is stored in granules of cytotoxic T lymphocytes and released upon cell activation to carry out a function similar to C9 (see Chapter 16).

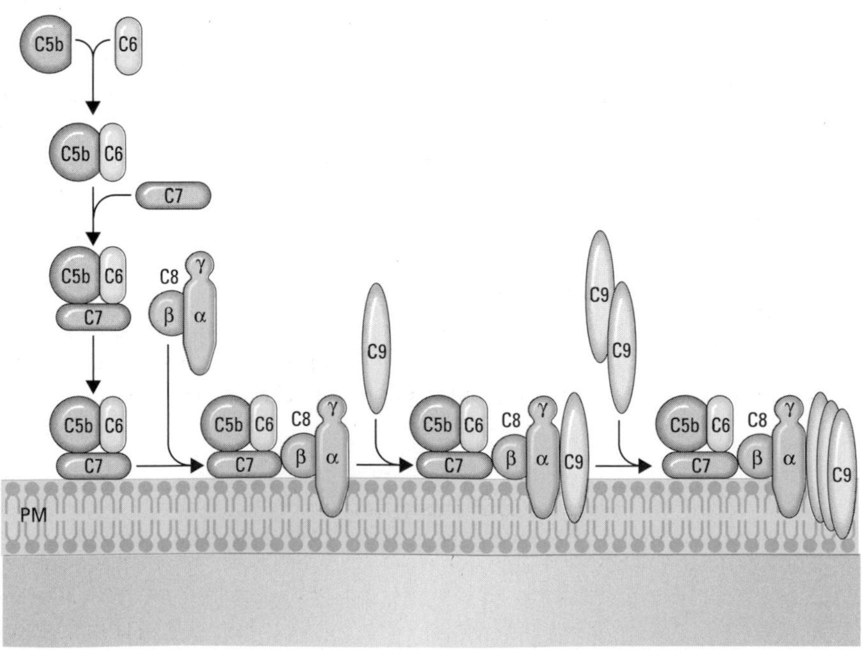

Figure 12.25 Lytic pathway: graphic depiction. Only the events leading to the assembly of the membrane-attack complex are shown. The scavenging regulatory pathway occurring in the fluid phase is omitted. PM, plasma membrane.

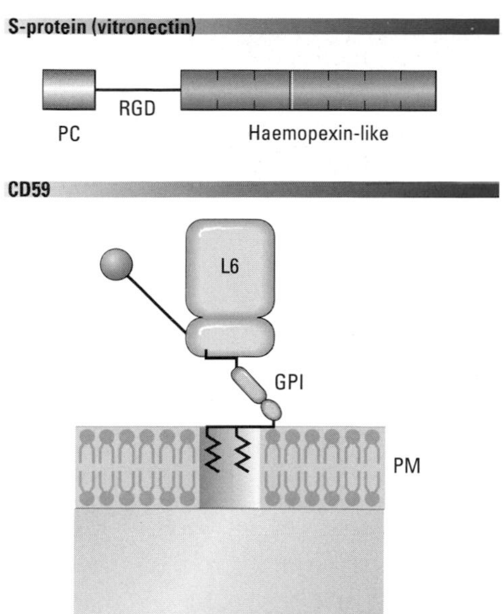

Figure 12.26 S-protein and CD59: two regulators of the lytic complement pathway. S-protein or vitronectin is a plasma protein consisting of either a single 459-residue chain or two disulphide-bonded chains that result from a proteolytic cleavage, probably intracellular, of the single chain. There are apparently two genetic variants of S-protein with a different residue near the cleavage site Arg 379–Ala 380, one variant subject to cleavage and the other not. The polypeptide contains three types of domains. The N-terminal cysteine-rich domain is homologous to modules present in the PC-1 glycoprotein of lymphocytes; the middle part is rich in acidic amino acid residues and includes the Arg-Gly-Asp or RGD motif shared by many adhesion molecules; and the C-terminal part contains two domains, each with two repeats homologous to those found in haemopexin, interstitial collagenase and stromelysin. S-protein functions by attaching itself to the exposed, metastable membrane-binding site of the C5b67 complex and thus prevents its binding to a membrane. The soluble SC5b67 complex contains three molecules of S-protein. It binds C8 and three molecules of C9, but because C9 does not polymerize, formation of the membrane-attack complex is prevented. S-protein thus serves as a scavenger of soluble C5b67 complexes. CD59 is a small glycoprotein (M_r 19 000; length of the single polypeptide chain 103 amino acid residues) attached to the cell surface via the glycosylphosphatidylinositol (GPI) anchor at position Gly 78. The extracellular domain is homologous to that found in the Ly6 family of proteins characterized by nine to ten conserved cysteine residues. The CD59 molecule contains a single *N*-linked carbohydrate and is expressed on leucocytes, vascular endothelium, epithelial cells and placenta. Its function is to block the assembly of the membrane-attack complex by binding the C8 and C9 components. PM, plasma membrane.

and expression of a binding site for another C9. In this manner, one C9 molecule after another enters the complex and assembles into a tubular structure, the MAC. The assembled MAC resembles a well, with a wall formed by the hydrophobic regions and with the rim on the membrane surface formed by the hydrophilic parts of the C9 molecule (Fig. 12.27). One MAC contains 12–19 C9 molecules.

The membrane pores allow the entry of calcium ions into the cell, which then indiscriminately activate a variety of intracellular pathways. The pathways, in turn, exhaust the supply of ATP and high-energy phosphates. Furthermore, the pores cause a breakdown of the membrane potential, as well as an efflux of potassium ions and an influx of sodium ions. The ions either leak through the hollow centre (*pre-formation* or *doughnut hypothesis*) or around the periphery (*leaky-patch hypothesis*) of the inserted MAC. Through the pores created by the MAC in the outer membrane of the bacteria, lysozyme gains access to the peptidoglycan layer and begins to degrade it. All these and other changes eventually lead to the death of the target cell. Since the concentration of proteins is higher inside the cell than outside, water begins to pour through the pores into the cell. As a result, the cell swells and the membrane becomes permeable for macromolecules. Proteins, nucleic acids and high-molecular-mass substances begin to leave the cell and the emptied cell is said to be *lysed*. Blood cells and vascular endothelial cells are protected from C9-mediated lysis by the CD59 molecules that they express on their surfaces. *CD59* (*protectin*, *HRF20*; see Fig. 12.26) is a glycoprotein, a member of the cardiotoxin protein superfamily, attached to the plasma membrane via a GPI anchor. It contains sites with affinity for specific segments of C8 and C9 exposed during the transition of these proteins from their soluble to membrane-inserted forms. CD59 molecules prevent binding of more than one C9 molecule to MAC, insertion of MAC into membranes and thus MAC assembly on the wrong cells. They provide an example of *homologous restriction*, the protection of an organism's own (i.e. homologous) cells against the effects of its own complement system. (Here 'homologous' has a different meaning from that used to compare proteins or genes.) Self cells can also rid themselves of MACs deposited on their surfaces by *vesiculation*, the removal of affected membranes in the form of vesicles.

Regulatory compartment

The complement cascade involves a series of regulatory steps that amplify, coordinate and confine the effects of its components. Since the system has to act quickly, small initial events must be *amplified* within a short time. In the

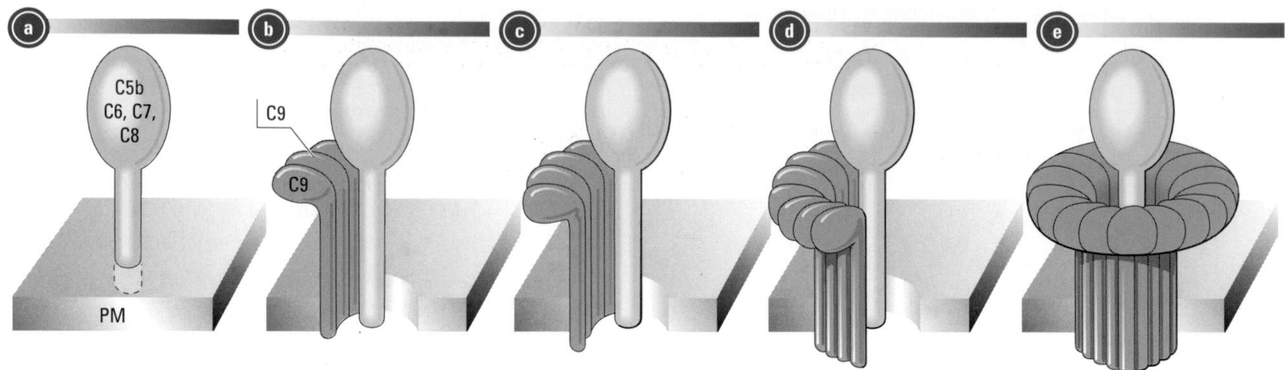

Figure 12.27 Assembly of the membrane-attack complex (MAC). (a) Anchoring of the C5b678 complex in the plasma membrane (PM) via the α chain of the C8 components. (b–e) Polymerization of C9 monomers and the formation of a transmembrane pore.

classical pathway, amplification occurs at two stages: the formation of bound C4 and the splitting of C3 by the C3 convertase. At each stage a single, enzymatically active molecule acts on multiple substrate molecules, which in turn act on their targets. In the alternative pathway, amplification is achieved primarily by stabilization of the C3 convertase, which then produces large quantities of C3b in a very short time. Amplification probably also occurs at other points in both pathways.

Coordination in the complement cascade is based on the relay race principle: most of the complement components exist in an inactive form and can be activated only by the activated component preceding them one step ahead in the pathway; in turn, they can activate a component following them but none other. Like team members in a relay race, the complement components all have their precisely defined position on the track and a set time in the sequence during which they can function.

Confinement of the damage to foreign particles is achieved mainly by the rapid inactivation of the activated complement components through spontaneous decay, stoichiometric inhibition and enzymatic degradation. *Spontaneous decay* influences the binding ability of C3 and C4. The binding site generated by the cleavage of the thioester bond is inactivated within a short time by the interaction with water molecules. *Stoichiometric inhibition* occurs by the interaction of the activated component with an inhibitor molecule in equivalent proportions without enzymatic cleavage. In *enzymatic degradation*, the activated component becomes the target of a specific enzyme that cleaves it into inactive fragments. The last two mechanisms require the participation of special regulatory components, which include C1-inhibitor, factor I, C4bBP, DAF, MCP, factor D, S-protein, clusterin, CD59, factor H and CR1. Factor H, MCP, CR1 and CR2, DAF and C4bBP are all members of one protein superfamily (Fig. 12.28). The characteristic feature of the superfamily is the CCPR (also referred to as *short consensus repeat*, SCR), which occurs in varying numbers in the different proteins. Regulatory interactions are summarized in Fig. 12.29.

Summary of the complement cascade

(Fig. 12.30)

Classical pathway

1 The heads of the C1q component attach to Fc regions of at least two IgG molecules or two sites on a single IgM molecule. The resulting conformational change of C1q activates one of the two C1q-associated C1r molecules without enzymatic cleavage. Activated C1r cleaves and activates the second C1r molecule, which in turn cleaves the first molecule. Activated C1r molecules cleave and thus activate the two C1q-associated C1s molecules.

2 C1s cleaves and activates the C4 molecule, and the C4b fragment attaches itself to a solid phase. The C2 proenzyme combines with the bound C4b fragment and is in turn cleaved by the neighbouring C1s. The C4bC2b complex, the C3 convertase, remains bound to the target surface.

3 The C4bC2b enzyme cleaves and activates C3, and the C3b fragment attaches itself to the solid surface. The C3b fragment binds C5, which is then cleaved by the catalytic site on C2b of the C4bC2bC3b complex, the C5 convertase.

Alternative pathway

1 The C3 components bind water molecules spontaneously

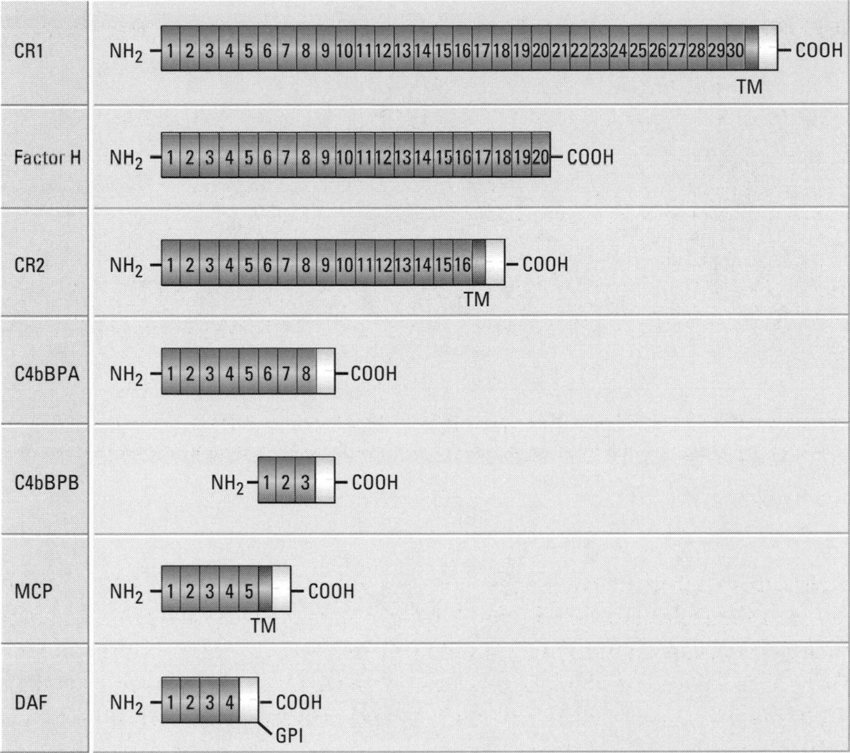

Figure 12.28 Complement control protein superfamily. All members of this group are modular proteins consisting of one type of domain only, the complement control protein repeat (CCPR). This domain is present in varying numbers in the different proteins, from three in C4bBPB to 30 in CR1 (the repeats are numbered consecutively from the N-terminus to the C-terminus). Each repeat is approximately 60 amino acid residues long and is presumably folded into a distinct domain stabilized by two disulphide bonds, one between the first and the third and the other between the second and the fourth cysteine residues. The individual repeats of the same protein, as well as of different members of the superfamily, show significant sequence similarity. Three members of the superfamily (CR1, CR2 and MCP) are integral membrane proteins attached to cell surfaces by distinct transmembrane regions and anchored in the cell interior by cytoplasmic tails. One member (DAF) is attached to the cell surface via a GPI anchor. All the other membranes are soluble proteins present in plasma. The proteins are *N*-glycosylated and bear variable numbers of carbohydrate moieties. The C4bBP, MCP and DAF components were described earlier; CR1 and CR2 will be described later. Human factor H is synthesized as a 1231-residue polypeptide chain from which signal peptidases subsequently remove 18 residues at the N-terminus and plasma proteases possibly remove two C-terminal residues, so that the mature protein is then 1211 residues long. It contains nine potential *N*-glycosylation sites. The chain is organized into 20 CCPR domains. Factor H functions as a co-factor in the cleavage of C3b by factor I in the alternative pathway. CR, complement receptor; C4bBP, C4b-binding protein (A and B); DAF, decay-accelerating factor; GPI, glycosylphosphatidylinositol (anchor); MCP, membrane co-factor protein; TM, transmembrane (region).

and the C3(H_2O) complexes associate with factor B. Factor D cleaves factor B in the C3(H_2O)B complex, producing the initiating C3 convertase, C3(H_2O)Bb.

2 C3 convertase cleaves C3 molecules and the C3b fragments associate with factor B, which in turn is cleaved by factor D to produce the amplification C3 convertase, C3bBb. Amplification only occurs, however, if the C3b fragments are deposited on the surface of foreign activator substances; fragments deposited on host surfaces are rapidly degraded.

3 C3bBb convertase is stabilized by interaction with factor P and cleaves additional C3 molecules, thus amplifying the effect.

4 The stabilized C3bBbP complex associates with additional C3b molecules and thus acquires the potential to cleave C5.

Lytic pathway

1 The C5b fragment remains bound to the C5 convertase and acts as an acceptor for the C6 component, which in turn binds C7.

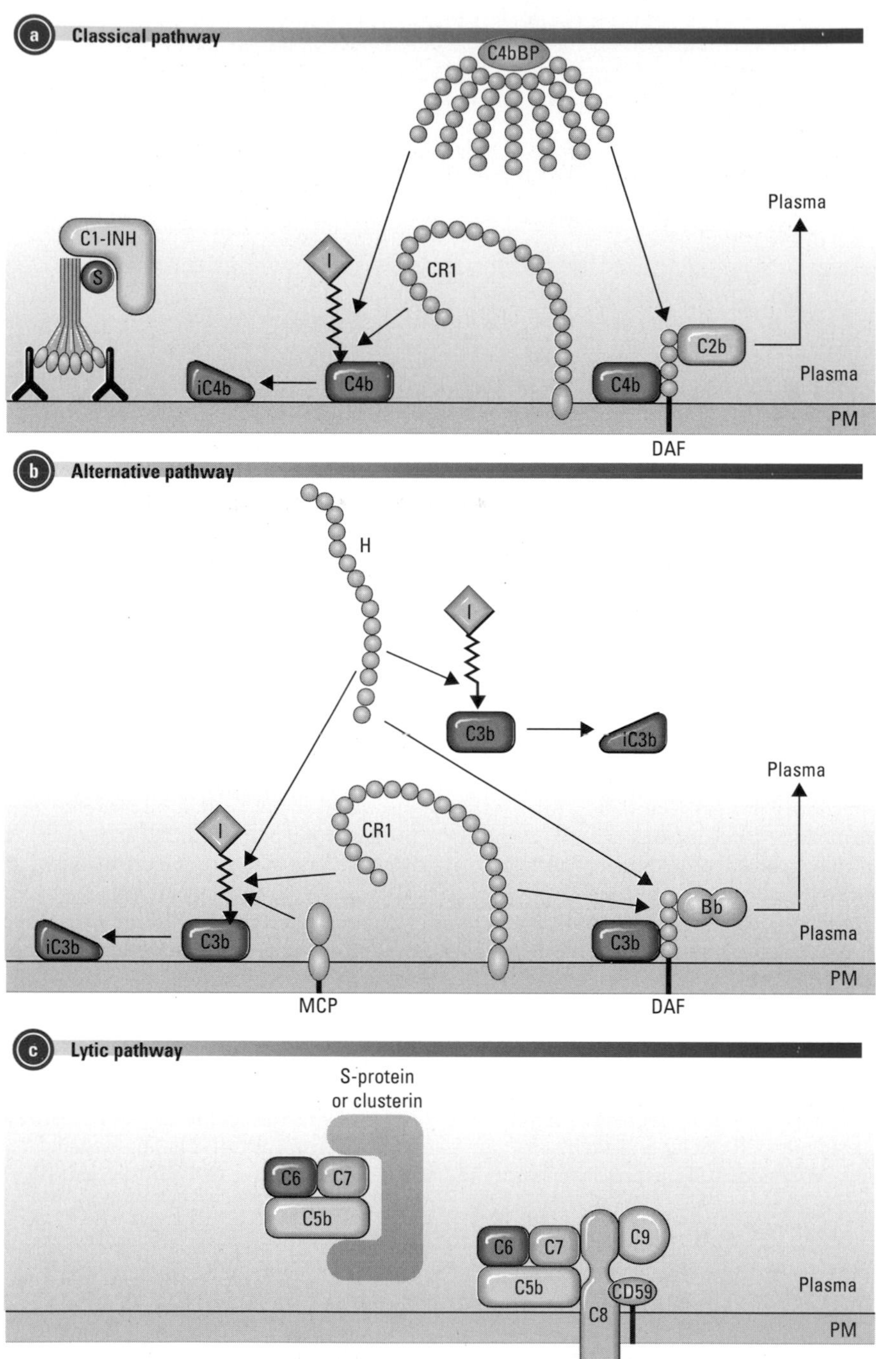

Figure 12.29 Summary of the regulatory processes. (a) In the *classical pathway* the C1-inhibitor (C1-INH) limits self-activation of C1 in the fluid phase by blocking the C1r and C1s components. The activity of C4b is restricted by factor I, which cleaves C4b into iC4b in the presence of C4b-binding protein (C4bBP) and with the participation of complement receptor type 1 (CR1). The classical pathway C3/C5 convertase is kept under control by the decay-accelerating factor (DAF) with the participation of C4bBP. (b) In the *alternative pathway*, C3b is inactivated (converted into iC3b) by the enzymatic action of factor I with the participation of CR1, factor H and membrane co-factor protein (MCP). The alternative pathway C3/C5 convertase, C3bBb, is inactivated by DAF with CR1 and factor H acting as co-factors. (c) In the *lytic pathway*, S-protein (vitronectin) or clusterin bind to C5b67 complexes in the fluid phase and thus prevent insertion of their complexes into the membrane. Assembly of the membrane-attack complex on the surface of a wrong cell is prevented by CD59, which inhibits C5b678-catalysed polymerization of C9. PM, plasma membrane. (From Jokiranta, T.S., Jokipii, L. & Meri, S. (1995) *Scandinavian Journal of Immunology*, **42**, 9.)

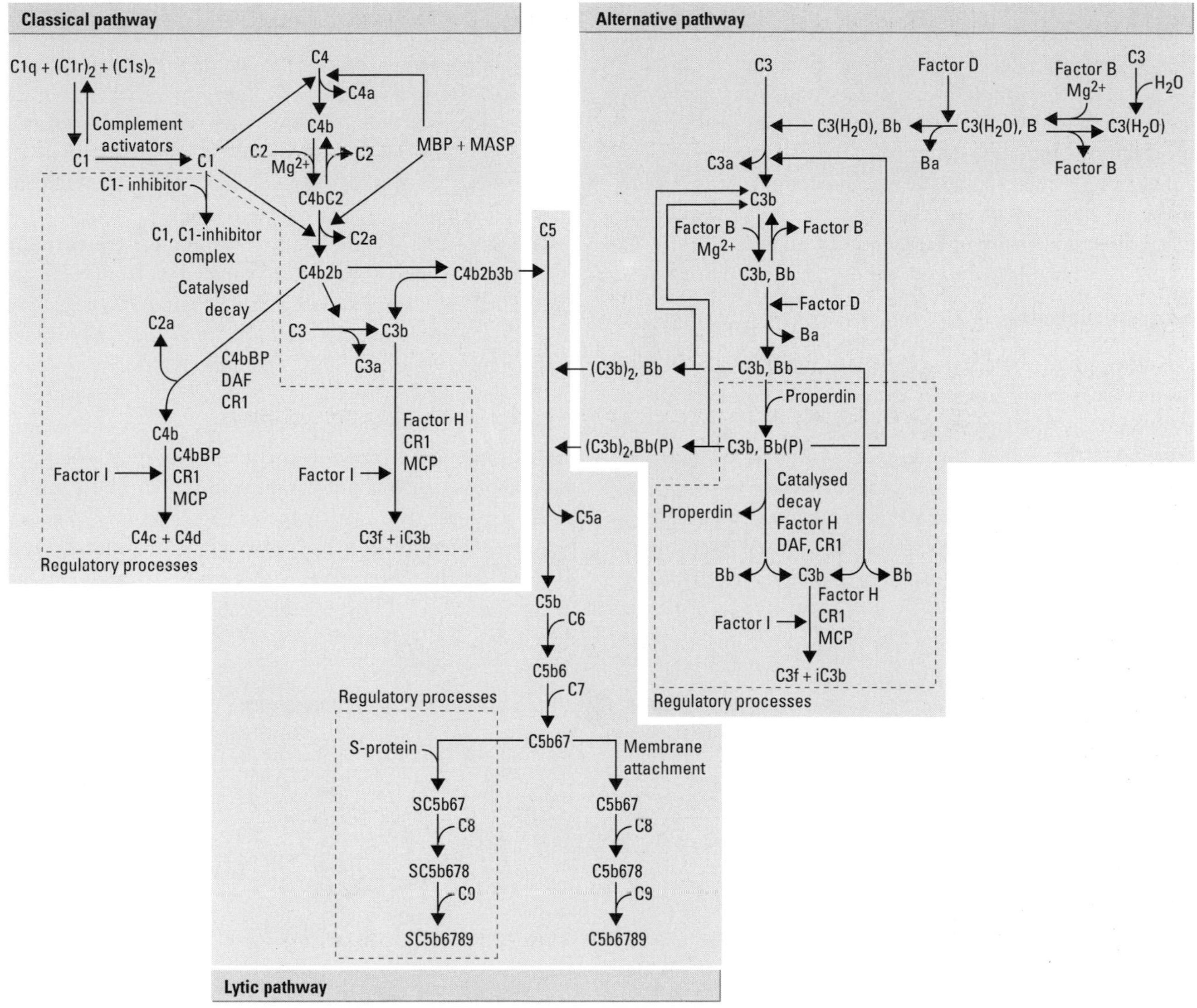

Figure 12.30 Summary of the complement cascade. The three pathways and their regulatory loops make use of seven functionally different classes of proteins: components binding to immunoglobulins in antigen–antibody complexes (C1q) or microbial carbohydrates (MBP); activating enzymes (C1r, C1s, MASP, C2b, Bb, D); membrane-binding proteins (C4b, C3b); membrane-attack proteins (C5b, C6, C7, C8, C9); regulatory proteins (C1-INH, C4bBP, CR1, MCP, DAF, H, P, CD59, clusterin, S-protein); complement receptors (CR1); and peptide mediators of inflammation (C5a, C3a, C4a). The functions of the individual components are as follows. In the *classical pathway*, MBP binds to carbohydrates on microbial cell surfaces; C1q binds to immunoglobulins in antigen–antibody complexes; C1r cleaves and activates C1s; C1s cleaves C4 and C2; C4b binds C2 and positions it for cleavage by C1s; C2b cleaves, as part of the C3/C5 convertase, C3 and C5; C3b binds C5 and positions it for cleavage by C2b. In the *alternative pathway*, C3b binds factor B and positions it for cleavage by factor D; Bb in the C3/C5 convertase cleaves C5; factor D cleaves factor B bound to C3b. In the *lytic (terminal) pathway*, C5b initiates the assembly of the membrane-attack complex; C6 binds to C5b and forms an acceptor for C7; C7 binds to C5b6 and attaches the complex to the plasma membrane; C8 binds to the C5b67 complex and initiates C9 polymerization; C9 forms a membrane-spanning channel and thus leads to cell lysis. (Adapted from Halkier, T. (1991) *Mechanisms in Blood Coagulation, Fibrinolysis and the Complement System*. Cambridge University Press, Cambridge.)

2 A conformational change in bound C7 unmasks hydrophobic regions by which the component attaches itself to the lipid bilayer of the plasma membrane.
3 The C5b67 complex binds C8 and thus unmasks hydrophobic regions in the latter, which then insert themselves into the lipid bilayer.
4 The pore is enlarged by the attachment of multiple units of the C9 component and the assembly of the membrane attack complex. Death of the target cell follows.

Anaphylatoxins

The cleavage of the complement components C3, C4 and C5 produces two fragments from each: a larger one that participates in the cascade and a smaller one that diffuses away and takes part in defence reactions outside the cascade. The smaller fragments are referred to as *anaphylatoxins* because they participate in *anaphylaxis*, a pathological immune response characterized by increased sensitivity immediately following exposure to an antigen (see Chapter 23). Anaphylatoxins can also be released in small amounts through limited proteolysis of C3, C4 and C5 by enzymes present in plasma in the absence of complement activation. The major non-complement enzyme that generates anaphylatoxins at inflammatory sites is believed to be neutrophil elastase. The elastase has been implicated in the pathogenesis of the adult respiratory distress syndrome characterized by poorly oxygenated lungs.

The three anaphylatoxins are similar in structure and function, although C5a differs somewhat from C3a and C4a. They are all single polypeptide chains, 77 (C3a, C4a) or 74 (C5a) amino acid residues long and have an M_r ranging from 9000 to 11 000. The anaphylatoxins represent the N-terminal portions of the α chains of their respective components. These short polypeptides are cross-linked by three disulphide bonds which confer stability to the molecules and they also contain a large number of basic amino acid residues; they are therefore positively charged (cationic) at neutral pH. The polypeptides are folded in such a way that the N-terminal and C-terminal segments are

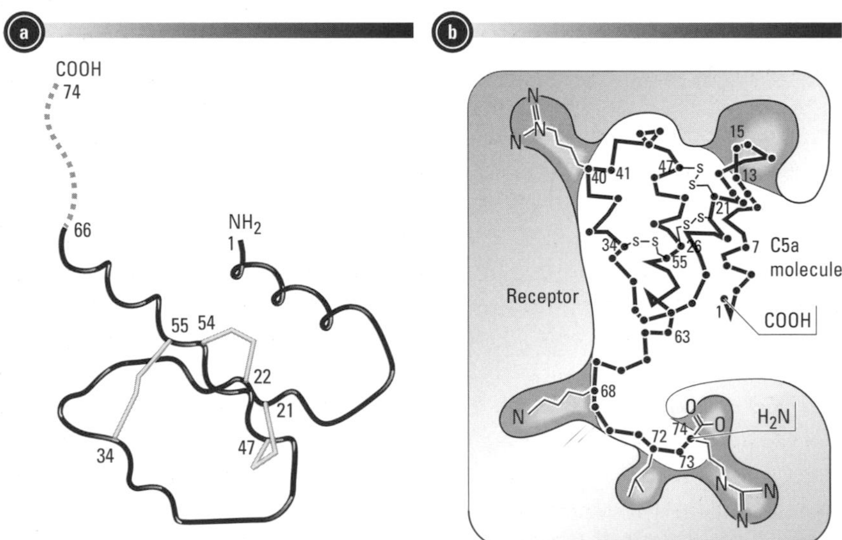

Figure 12.31 Anaphylatoxin C5a. (a) Three-dimensional structure. The molecule resembles a drumstick consisting of a central disulphide-linked knot looped around a long α-helical segment that takes up 40% of the C-terminal region. The last eight C-terminal residues of the 74-residue polypeptide have a disordered conformation in solution (indicated by the dotted line). The central knot contains three disulphide bonds between cysteine residues 21 and 47, 22 and 54, 34 and 55. A single carbohydrate moiety is attached to Asn 64 (not shown). The structure of C3a and C4a is similar to that of C5a. (b) Interaction of C5a with the C5a receptor. The anaphylatoxin is believed to contact its receptor in three regions: the C-terminus (via residues Lys 68, Leu 72 and Arg 74), the disulphide-linked knot (via Arg 40 Ile 41) and the loop region (via His 15) between the knot and the amino-terminal α-helix. The diagram shows the α-carbon skeleton of the C5a molecule and side-chains only at those positions believed to make contact with the receptor. The putative contact sites of the receptor are shaded. The C-terminal peptide MQLGR is indispensable but not sufficient for the biological activity of the C5a molecule. Binding of C5a to its receptor generates a signal that activates a variety of cellular processes resulting in the biological activities characteristic of the response to anaphylatoxin stimulation. (a, based on Protein Data Bank Swiss 3-D; b, slightly modified from Mollison, K.W. *et al.* (1989) *Proceedings of the National Academy of Sciences USA*, **86**, 292.)

largely α-helical, whereas the central, disulphide cross-linked portion is globular (Fig. 12.31). The C5a molecule has a large, complex oligosaccharide moiety attached to Asn at position 64; the C3a and C4a molecules are pure proteins.

All three anaphylatoxins induce smooth muscle contraction, increase the permeability of blood vessels and cause the release of histamine from mast cells and basophils. The C5a moiety, in addition, acts on neutrophils and monocytes by summoning them to a particular site (chemotactic migration), augmenting cell adherence, causing degranulation and the release of intracellular enzymes, enhancing arachidonic acid metabolism, stimulating the production of toxic oxygen metabolites, augmenting the expression of complement receptors and increasing the production of interleukin (IL)-1 by monocytes. The last two effects can lead to augmented immune responses, such as antibody production and T-cell proliferation *in vitro*; the remaining effects are part of the inflammatory response. The biological effects of C5a are the strongest of all three, followed by those of C3a and C4a. In terms of smooth muscle contraction, for example, C5a is 10–20 times more potent than C3a and 3000 times more potent than C4a. To effect all these biological activities, anaphylatoxins must bind to their corresponding receptors on the surface of target cells. The interaction of anaphylatoxin with the receptor generates a signal that initiates the intracellular reactions leading to the biological effect. C3a and C4a share the same receptor, whereas C5a acts via a different receptor which is described in the section that follows.

If unchecked, anaphylatoxins could cause considerable damage to the body. This is normally prevented by the action of plasma *carboxypeptidase N*, which removes the C-terminal arginyl residue from the anaphylatoxin molecule yielding the des-Arg derivative. Carboxypeptidase N is a tetrameric metalloprotease (a protein-cleaving, metal atom-containing enzyme) consisting of two identical heavy and two identical light chains. It inactivates not only anaphylatoxins but also bradykinin which, like anaphylatoxins, possesses a functionally essential C-terminal arginine residue.

Complement receptors

The system of complement components is supplemented by a set of *complement receptors*: a group of plasma-membrane structures capable of reacting specifically and reversibly with certain complement components or their fragments. Complement receptors should not be confused with the non-specific attachment sites to which complement components bind by their unstable binding sites, exposed for a fraction of a second immediately after activation. The attachment sites are not specialized structures; almost any protein in the membrane or in the fluid phase can function as a non-specific acceptor of an activated complement component, provided it possesses the right chemical group. Binding to the non-specific site does not stimulate any response in the target cell, whereas binding to a specific receptor often does.

At least nine complement receptors have been described (Table 12.2) of which only five have been characterized both structurally and functionally. They are the receptors CR1–CR4 and C5aR. *Complement receptor type 1* (*CR1*, CD35, C3bC4b receptor) binds fixed C3b and iC3b. The CR1-binding site is present in the C3c region of the α chain, but is normally hidden and is exposed only after rupture of the thioester bond. The CR1 molecule consists of a single glycoprotein chain known to exist in at least four variants (allotypes): type A (M_r 190 000), type B (M_r 220 000), type C (M_r 160 000) and type D (M_r 250 000). The four allotypes are controlled by alleles at a single locus. The extracellular part of the CR1 polypeptide chain consists of a series of CCPRs organized into four domains (A–D; Fig. 12.32). The four allotypes differ in that some of these repeats have been deleted from the molecules. The type A molecule contains 30 CCPRs, seven repeats in each of the four domains plus two extra ones (Fig. 12.32). The CR1 molecule is expressed ubiquitously. B cells begin to express CR1 at a very early stage in their development and then lose it prior to their differentiation into plasma cells. In the mouse, the time at which CR1-positive B lymphocytes appear after birth is controlled by two loci, one of which is linked to the major histocompatibility complex (*MHC*) gene. The function of CR1 is to bind C3b and C4b on foreign particles and thereby to stimulate phagocytosis; to accelerate the decay of C3b and C4b; and to accelerate clearance of immune complexes. The binding site for C4b is formed by the first four CCPRs of the CR1 molecule; one of the two binding sites for C3b is formed by repeats 8–11 and the other by repeats 15–18.

Complement receptor type 2 (*CR2*, CD21, C3d receptor, Epstein–Barr virus receptor) binds to a site in the C3dg region of the C3b fragment that becomes fully exposed after factor I has converted C3b into iC3b. The CR2 molecule is a single-chain glycoprotein with an M_r of 140 000 which, like CR1, consists of multiple CCPRs in its extracellular part (see Fig. 12.32). One form of the molecule has 16 CCPRs organized into four domains with four repeats per domain; another has 15 repeats. The molecule is expressed on 80–90% of all B lymphocytes, on follicular dendritic cells, pharyngeal and cervical epithelial cells and on a subset of thymocytes. In differentiating B cells it is expressed later than CR1 but, like CR1, it is lost when the lymphocytes dif-

Table 12.2 Characteristics of human complement receptors.

Receptor	Ligand	Structure ($M_r \times 10^3$)	Chromosomal localization	Cell distribution	Function
CR1 (CD35)	C3b, C4b, iC3b, iC4b	Single chain, four allotypes: 190 M_r, 220 M_r, 160 M_r, 250 M_r	1q32	Erythrocytes, monocytes/ macrophages, neutrophils, eosinophils, mast cells, B cells, some T cells, kidney podocytes, follicular dendritic cells	Phagocytosis, decay of C3b and C4b, clearance of immune complexes
CR2 (CD21)	iC3b, C3dg, C3d, EBV	Single chain, 140 M_r	1q32	B lymphocytes, follicular dendritic cells, pharyngeal and cervical epithelial cells, subset of thymocytes	B-cell co-receptor, EBV receptor
CR3 (CD11b/CD18)	iC3b, C3dg, C3d, *Staphylococcus epidermidis*, yeast, β-glucan	Two chains, 165 M_r α chain, 95 M_r β chain	16p11–13.1	Monocytes/macrophages, neutrophils, NK cells, some T lymphocytes	Phagocytosis, adhesion molecule
CR4 (CD11c/CD18)	iC3b, C3dg, C3d	Two chains, 150 M_r α chain, 95 M_r β chain	21q22.1 (CD18)	Monocytes/macrophages, neutrophils, NK cells, some T lymphocytes	Phagocytosis, adhesion molecule
CR5	C3d, iC3b, C3dg	Unknown	19	Neutrophils, platelets	Fluid phase scavenging of C3 fragments
fH-R	Factor H	Two or more subunits (M_r of subunit: 50)		B lymphocytes, neutrophils, monocytes	Regulation of alternative pathway?
C1q-R	Collagen-like portion of C1q	Single chain, M_r 65		B lymphocytes, neutrophils, monocytes, fibroblasts, platelets (low)	Binding of immune complexes to phagocytes
C3a/C4a-R	C3a, C4a	Seven transmembrane segment molecule		Mast cells (high), eosinophils (high), monocytes (low), neutrophils (low)	Mediation of leucocyte responses in inflammation
C5aR	C5a, des-Arg-C5a	Seven transmembrane segment molecule	19q13.3–13.4	Mast cells, neutrophils, monocytes, macrophages, eosinophils, basophils	Mediation of leucocyte responses in inflammation

C, complement; EBV, Epstein–Barr virus; f, factor; NK, natural killer; R, receptor.

ferentiate into plasma cells. CR2 is specific for the C3d portion of iC3b, C3dg and C3d. As part of the B-cell co-receptor it is involved in regulation of B-cell activation and proliferation. It also functions as an interferon-α receptor and an adhesion molecule (it binds CD23). It forms complexes with CD19, CD81 and other molecules. The Epstein–Barr virus (EBV) uses it as a receptor to gain entry into B cells and to cause virus infection (infectious mononucleosis) or malignant transformation of B lymphocytes (Burkitt's lymphoma) and epithelial cells (nasopharyngeal carcinoma). The binding sites for EBV and C3d are located in the first two N-terminal CCPRs.

Complement receptor type 3 (*CR3*, Mac-1, CD11b/CD18, αMβ2) has a high affinity for fixed iC3b and a much lower affinity for fixed C3dg and C3d. The binding requires the participation of calcium and magnesium cations. The receptor also binds, via a different site, β(1→3) glucan (zymosan) in the cell walls of yeasts and certain staphylococci, LPS, intercellular adhesion molecule-1 (ICAM-1), kininogen, as well as factor X and fibrinogen of the blood clotting cascade. The CR3 molecule, a member of the integrin family (see Chapter 10), consists of two non-covalently associated glycoprotein chains, α (M_r 165 000) and β (M_r 95 000) (see Fig. 12.32). The β chain is the same as that found in the CD11a/CD18 integrin (see Chapter 10) and CR4. CR3 is expressed on monocytes, macrophages, neutrophils, natural killer cells and cytotoxic T lymphocytes. The level of CR3 expression on peripheral blood

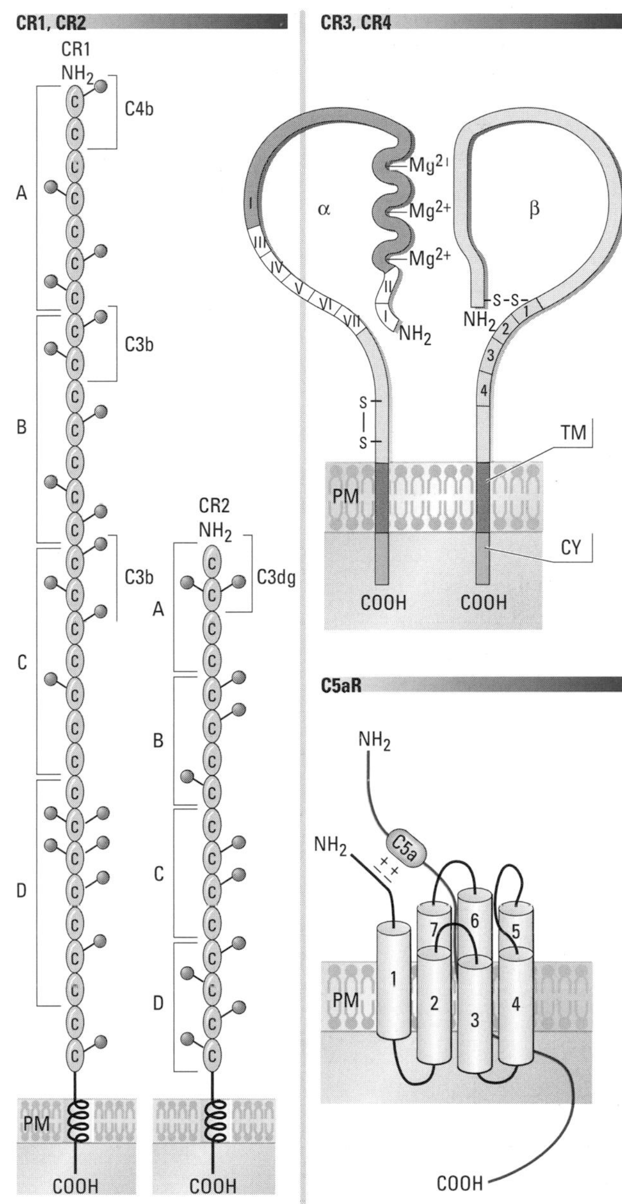

Figure 12.32 Complement receptors type 1, 2, 3, 4 and C5aR. *CR1* is a single polypeptide chain molecule with 20 *N*-glycosylation sites (⚲). It is anchored in the plasma membrane (PM) of erythrocytes, B lymphocytes, a subset of T lymphocytes, monocytes, macrophages, neutrophils, eosinophils and dendritic cells. Its extracellular part consists of 30 complement control protein repeats (CCPRs, here abbreviated to C), each repeat about 60 residues long. The repeats are organized into four domains (long homologous region, LHR, repeats A–D), each domain containing seven CCPRs. The sequence similarity of individual repeats within each LHR domain is greater than that between different LHR domains. Human CR1 occurs in four allotypic forms (A or F, B or S, C and D), which differ somewhat in their sequences and are controlled by alleles at one locus. Brackets indicate binding sites for C4b and C3b. Human *CR2* is also a single polypeptide with 11 *N*-glycosylation sites (⚲). It is an integral membrane glycoprotein of mature B lymphocytes, follicular dendritic cells, some epithelial cells and a subset of thymocytes. Its extracellular part consists of 15 or 16 CCPRs organized into four LHR domains, each domain consisting of four repeats. The extra repeat in the 16-repeat form is apparently the product of alternative splicing. The cytoplasmic domain contains potential protein kinase C and protein tyrosine kinase binding sites. The bracket indicates the binding site for C3dg. *CR3* and *CR4* are members of the integrin family of proteins. Each of them is a heterodimer of α and β chains. The extracellular part of the α chain contains seven internally homologous repeats (I–VII), each repeat about 25 residues long (see Fig. 9.6). Repeats II and III are separated by a 97-residue I (insertion) domain that contains sites for binding bivalent metal cations. The chain contains 19 potential *N*-glycosylation sites. The β chain of the mature human CR3 protein contains six potential *N*-glycosylation sites. Its extracellular part contains four cysteine-rich repeats (1–4). The same chain is also present in the CD11a/CD18 molecules (see Chapter 10). The structure of the human CR4 molecule is similar to that of CR3. S—S, disulphide bonds; TM, transmembrane region; CY, cytoplasmic domain. *C5aR* is a member of the G protein-coupled receptor superfamily. It consists of a single polypeptide chain that has seven transmembrane regions (barrels 1–7) connected by alternating intracellular and extracellular loops. It has a single *N*-glycosylation site in the N-terminal region. This region, which is highly acidic (it contains seven negatively charged amino acid residues), and the third extracellular loop are believed to be part of the region that interacts with C5a (see also Fig. 12.31b). The Ser/Thr-rich third intracellular region and the C-terminus are presumed to be the sites of G-protein binding and phosphorylation necessary for signal transduction. These parts are highly conserved among different species. The extracellular loops, on the other hand, are relatively divergent (about 68% sequence identity among different mammals), which is in line with the relative divergence of the ligands (60–70% sequence identity between C5a proteins of different mammals). The C5aR molecule is shown complexed with C5a; the strongly interacting sites are indicated by ±.

neutrophils and monocytes is greatly increased after stimulation with chemotactic factors. On the surface of neutrophils, monocytes and macrophages, CR3 interacts specifically with iC3b fixed to the surface of foreign particles; the interaction prepares these cells for efficient phagocytosis (it opsonizes them) and clearance of bacteria and yeasts. It also functions as an adhesion molecule that mediates neutrophil adherence to endothelial cells during the inflammatory response (see Chapters 10 & 21).

Complement receptor type 4 (*CR4*; CD11c/CD18; leucocyte adhesion receptor p150,95; LeuCAMc; αXb2) uses the same β chain as the CR3 receptor (and CD11a/CD18), which non-covalently combines with a different but related α chain (see Fig. 12.32; the α chains of the CR3 and CR4 molecules are identical in 87% of their amino acid sequence). The receptor has the same specificity as CR3, except that it does not bind zymosan. CR4 is strongly expressed on tissue macrophages but much less so on monocytes, neutrophils, cytotoxic T cells, natural killer cells and eosinophils. In the membrane, CR4 is less mobile than CR3 because it is more restrained by its interaction with elements of the cytoskeleton. This difference enables the CR3 and CR4 molecules to cooperate in the initiation of phagocytosis. The less numerous but more mobile CR3 molecules can aggregate rapidly at the initial site of contact with iC3b-coated particles and the more numerous but less mobile CR4 molecules can then initiate phagocytosis of the trapped particles.

The *C5a* and *C3a receptors* are members of the G-protein-coupled receptor family characterized by the presence of seven hydrophobic domains that span the plasma membrane (see Fig. 12.32). Other members of this family include receptors for the chemokines IL-8, macrophage inflammatory protein-1 (MIP-1) and platelet-activation factor (see Chapters 10 & 21). The receptor is expressed on neutrophils, mast cells, macrophages, eosinophils and basophils. It is specific for anaphylatoxin C5a. The receptor's affinity for C5a is very high ($K_d \sim 1$ nM) and the binding between the two molecules is virtually irreversible. The number of receptor molecules per cell is also high: some 200 000 molecules per leucocyte. Occupancy of the receptor by the ligand triggers a broad range of responses including, at subnanomolar to nanomolar levels of C5a, chemotaxis of neutrophils, eosinophils, basophils, macrophages and monocytes and an increase in vascular permeability markedly potentiated by prostaglandins. At higher C5a concentrations, it causes degranulation of leucocytes, production of activated oxygen and nitrogen-derived radicals (see Chapter 15) as well as smooth muscle contractions.

Some of the properties of the other complement receptors are summarized in Table 12.2.

Genetic control

Every complement component is encoded in at least one locus but some are encoded in several loci. Some of the complement loci are on the same chromosome (they are linked) while others are on different chromosomes. The complement gene cluster characterized in the greatest detail so far is that coding for components C4, C2 and factor B. This cluster resides in the middle of the *MHC* in all mammals studied. In humans, it is located between the class I and class II *HLA* loci on chromosome 6, with the order of loci being centromere . . . *HLA-DR* . . . *CYP21* . . . *C4B* . . . *CYP21P* . . . *C4A* . . . *BF* . . . *C2* . . . *HLA-B*, where *CYP21* is a locus coding for the enzyme 21-hydroxylase, *CYP21P* is a pseudogene, *C4A* and *C4B* are two loci coding for component 4 and BF is the locus coding for factor B. The number of *C4* loci in the cluster can vary from species to species and among individuals of a given species. Dogs have only one *C4* locus. Most mice have two or three, but the product of one locus (*C4-Slp*, for sex-limited protein) is inactive. Humans have two or three *C4* loci, but there is a functional difference between the products of the *C4A* and *C4B* loci. The cluster of *C4* loci expands and contracts by unequal crossing-over. The *C4* loci are evolutionarily related to the *C3* locus, which is on the same chromosome as *C4* in some species (e.g. the mouse) but some distance away from the latter; in other species C3 is on another chromosome (number 19 in humans). The *C2* and *BF* loci are related in origin and probably arose by duplication of a single ancestral locus.

The so-called *regulation of complement activation cluster* on the long arm of chromosome 1 is composed of *C4bBP*, *CR1*, *CR2*, *factor H*, MPC and *DAF* loci. The products of these loci are related in their function and evolution. They are proteins that regulate the activity of the C3 convertases in the classical and/or alternative pathways. They cause accelerated decay of these enzymes or serve as co-factors for factor I-mediated cleavage of C4b and/or C3b. Two of them, C4bBP and factor H, are plasma glycoproteins synthesized and secreted by hepatocytes, while CR1 and CR2 are membrane glycoproteins found in a variety of cells; DAF is a glycolipid-anchored glycoprotein. Despite these differences, the five loci seem to have a common origin, as indicated by the fact that their products contain a 60-residue repeat of high sequence similarity.

The short arm of human chromosome 1 also carries loci coding for two chains of the C8 component (*C8A* and *C8B*) and the three chains of the C1q component (*C1QA*, *C1QB* and *C1QC*). (The genes coding for the C1r and C1s components are on chromosome 12.) The *C6* and *C7* loci, which may have arisen by inverse gene duplication reside on chromosomes 5. In humans, there are single *C6* and *C7* loci, whereas *C6* is duplicated in dogs and mice, and *C7* is duplicated in Przewalski's horses. The properdin locus is on the X-chromosome and properdin is the only complement locus that shows X-linked deficiencies. Other complement-encoding loci are scattered throughout the human genome.

Many of the complement-encoding loci display a variation that can be detected by analysis of their products using electrophoresis or serological methods. The most variable of the loci is *C4*: 13 *C4A* alleles and 22 *C4B* alleles occur at appreciable frequencies in human populations and thus constitute genuine genetic polymorphism (Table 12.3; Fig. 12.33). Some of the electrophoretically defined allelic products are also distinguished by specific antibodies. In humans, two of the *C4* alleles were originally described as *Chido* and *Rodgers* blood groups (named after the original blood donors) and only later were these blood group antigens recognized for what they really were—C4d fragments deposited on erythrocyte surfaces. Rodgers and Chido are markers for the *C4A* and *C4B* loci, respectively. The Rodgers- and Chido-specific antibodies are produced by subjects who are *C4A*- and *C4B*-deficient, respectively.

The expression of complement genes has been studied by both *in vitro* and *in vivo* experiments. The former have revealed that macrophages and monocytes synthesize most complement components, including C1, C2, C3, C4, C5, factors B, D, P and I, as well as C1-inhibitor; neutrophils synthesize C3, C6 and C7. The *in vitro* studies can be somewhat misleading, however, since the complement-encoding genes do not seem to be repressed deeply and can be activated by the culture conditions. *In vivo* transplantation experiments have shown that hepatocytes synthesize the C3, C4, factor B, C6 and C8 components; liver macrophages synthesize the C7 component, and fat tissues, as well as nerves, synthesize factor D. The C1q subcomponent appears to be synthesized by epithelial cells of the small and large intestines. The C3, C4 and C5 components are synthesized as single polypeptide chains that are post-translationally cleaved into the corresponding number of chains: the human pro-C3 molecule is cleaved into α and β chains, the pro-C4 molecule is cleaved into α, β and γ chains and the pro-C5 molecule is cleaved into α and β chains. The three subcomponents of C1 are synthesized separately from different mRNA molecules. In some cases (e.g. C3), the precursor form is probably also present in plasma in a small amount.

The human fetus begins to synthesize complement components in the first 3 months of gestation. Placental transfer of complement occurs neither from mother to fetus nor vice versa. At birth, the plasma concentration of complement components is approximately half that of the maternal level; the concentration reaches adult levels at 6 months of age. Although colostrum contains significant amounts of C3, C4 and factor B, there is no evidence that any of these components reach the plasma of breast-fed infants.

Function

Parasites use all kinds of manoeuvres to breach the defence lines and invade the host (see Chapter 21). To counteract

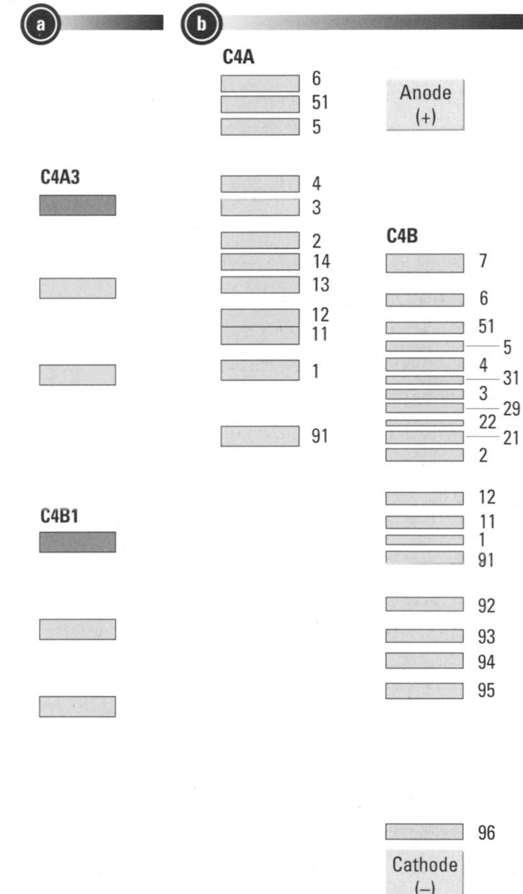

Figure 12.33 Polymorphism of human C4 molecules. (a) Example of a pattern of bands observed after electrophoresis of human serum from a *C4A3C4B1* individual. The bands were developed by a stain attached to C4-specific antibodies. (b) Diagrammatical summary of known C4A and C4B variants. Each variant may contain several bands, of which only the most anodal is shown. The bands were originally numbered from 1 to 6; when new bands, positioned between previously defined bands, were later discovered, they were assigned double-digit numbers (e.g. A12 and A13 are two bands between A1 and A2, the letter A referring to the *C4A* locus). (Based on Mauff, G. *et al.* (1983) *Immunobiology*, **164**, 184.)

Table 12.3 Frequencies of human *C4A* and *C4B* alleles in different races. (From Baur, M.P. *et al.* (1984) in *Histocompatibility Testing 1984* (Eds E.D. Albert *et al.*), p. 333. Springer-Verlag, Berlin.)

	Frequency in:				Frequency in:		
Allele	Caucasoids	Mongoloids	Negroids	Allele	Caucasoids	Mongoloids	Negroids
C4A1	0.3	0	3.7	*C4B1*	71.4	65.4	68.5
C4A2	6.4	1.9	6.2	*C4B2*	9.1	22.1	8.4
C4A3	70.2	67.0	71.2	*C4B3*	3.2	0.7	3.6
C4A4	6.1	7.7	1.2	*C4B4*	0.7	0	0
C4A6	3.8	1.3	1.2	*C4B5*	0.7	0	0
C4A12	0	12.2	0	*C4B6*	0.4	0	0
C4A13	0.5	0	0	*C4B7*	0.2	0	0
C4A51	0.2	0	4.9	*C4B11*	0.2	0	0
C4AQ0	12.5	9.9	11.6	*C4B12*	0.2	0.7	0
				C4B51	0.2	0	0
				C4BQ0	13.7	11.2	19.5
Sample size*	558	156	81		557	154	83

* Number of haplotypes counted.
Q0, quantity zero allele (either not expressed or detected as a weak band only). For explanation of the allelic designations, see Fig. 12.38.

these ploys, the defence system must be manifold and equipped to meet all variations of the attack. The complement system is a telling example of this versatility. Originally regarded as a system for the direct killing of microorganisms, it has since been shown to participate in many defence reactions: opsonization, neutralization of viruses, clearance of immune complexes, generation of specific immune responses and various aspects of the inflammatory reaction.

The *direct killing of microorganisms* depends on the insertion of the MAC into the lipid bilayer of the target cell or the virus particle. The presence of lipid layers is a prerequisite for lysis, and since many viruses and some cells do not have lipids exposed on the surface they cannot be killed by the complement system. Other microorganisms have evolved mechanisms that allow them to escape destruction by the complement system. *Neisseria gonorrhoeae*, for example, binds and activates complement and even develops lesions, yet the attacked bacteria somehow survive, possibly because the antibodies direct the complement components to the site in the membrane where the cell can repair the damage. Certain strains of *Salmonella* activate complement and allow the cascade to proceed all the way to the formation of the C5b67 complex, but then, when C8 is added, they dislodge the complex from the membrane and release it into the surrounding medium. Certain strains of *E. coli* harbour plasmids that somehow increase the resistance of the bacteria to complement-mediated killing. Thus, only certain bacteria and viruses are killed by complement. Nucleated cells are relatively resistant to complement-mediated killing, probably because they manage to remove the MAC from their surfaces by endocytosis. They are lysed only when a large number of MACs are deposited on them.

The *opsonizing function* of complement is mediated primarily by C3 and to a much lesser degree by C4 components. In the classical pathway, C3b attached to a target particle is rapidly converted into iC3b, which is then recognized by CR1 and CR3 on phagocytic cells. In the alternative pathway, only a portion (20–80%, depending on the bacterium) of the particle-attached C3b is converted into iC3b and then recognized by the phagocytic cells. Fixed C4b binds to the same receptors as C3b but with considerably lower affinity; fixed iC4b has very little or no opsonizing activity. Many different bacteria protect themselves against the opsonizing action of complement by surrounding themselves with a capsule that interferes with attachment to complement receptors.

Neutralization of viruses by complement is achieved in various ways. One is by depositing complement molecules on the surface of a virus and forming a thick protein coat that may mask structures required for the attachment of the virus particle to its target cell. Another way involves binding activated complement components to receptors on the viral particles, aggregating the particles and thus reducing the viral titre. A third mechanism depends on adherence of complement-coated viruses or virus-infected cells to lymphocytes, monocytes or leucocytes, followed by ingestion and destruction. Enveloped viruses can also be killed directly by activated complement components.

Clearance of immune complexes from the circulation is an important part of the body's normal physiology. Small immune complexes form continuously, but their level increases greatly during an infection. If not cleared, they are deposited in small blood vessels and in the kidneys and thus interfere with the function of the affected organs. Normally, immune complexes are cleared in two ways. The complexes can bind and activate complement, which is then recognized by CR1 on erythrocytes; the immune complex-coated erythrocytes are subsequently stripped of their coat by phagocytes of the reticuloendothelial system. Or, insoluble complexes are solubilized by the attachment of complement molecules (the insolubility of the complexes is determined by the stoichiometry of the participating components; see Chapter 14). The soluble complexes are then easier for the body to handle.

The *involvement of complement in the specific immune response*, in particular antibody formation, is still poorly understood. Experiments on animals have demonstrated that if a recipient is *decomplemented* (by the addition of cobra venom factor) it will, upon immunization, develop a normal primary antibody response but no secondary response. It has therefore been suggested that complement binds to immune complexes and thus helps to deliver them to the site of antibody formation in the germinal centres of lymph node follicles. On the other hand, it has also been demonstrated that patients lacking the C3 component are nevertheless able to mount normal secondary antibody responses.

The *effect of complement on inflammatory reactions* is mediated by anaphylatoxins, the small fragments cleaved off upon activation of the C3, C4 and C5 components. These fragments are biologically highly active and are responsible for some of the phenomena characterizing inflammation (see Chapter 21). Equally important, if not more so, are the reactions of bound C3 and C4 fragments with complement receptors.

Disturbances of complement function

Although carefully regulated, the complement system is none the less subject to disturbances that can result either in the elevation of one or more components to above-normal levels (*hypercomplementaemia*) or in the decrease in complement levels to below normal (*hypocomplementaemia*). The former condition is frequently associated with inflammatory reactions; the latter can result from increased consumption, increased catabolism or decreased production of complement components.

Increased consumption and *increased catabolism* of complement are the most frequent causes of hypocomplementaemia accompanying certain diseases (e.g. membranoproliferative glomerulonephritis, autoimmune haemolytic anaemia, leucopenia and thrombocytopenia; see Chapter 25). The decrease in complement level is presumably caused by excessive activation of the cascade or abnormally rapid degradation of complement components.

The *decreased production* of complement components can result from either environmental effects, such as malnutrition or hepatitis (both affecting the organ of complement synthesis, the liver), or hereditary deficiencies. *Hereditary complement deficiencies*, which usually affect one (rarely two) complement components, are caused by defects in the genes controlling complement synthesis. Complement deficiencies have been described in both humans and animals. Strains of guinea-pigs deficient in C4 or C2, of rabbits deficient in C6 and of mice deficient in C5 have been maintained in the laboratory for many years without showing any signs of ill health. In humans, deficiencies of almost all the complement components except factor B have been described (Table 12.4) and many of them are associated with serious diseases. The reason for this difference between humans and animals is not known; it is possible, however, that the animals were selected unwittingly by their breeders to compensate for the deficiency. Even in humans, it has been noted that some complement-deficient individuals enjoy good health their whole lifetime, while others become seriously ill. Obviously, factors other than the deficiency itself contribute to the development of the disease.

Diseases associated with complement deficiencies are characterized by frequent infections and immune complex formation. The most frequent infections in complement-deficient patients are those caused by pyogenic (pus-forming) bacteria, in particular *Neisseria*, which can lead to meningococcal meningitis and, less frequently, to disseminated gonococcal infections. Association with infection is particularly striking in deficiencies of the terminal components C5–C8. This is probably because granulocytes have difficulty in destroying *Neisseria* after phagocytosis and the main defence mechanism against these microorganisms is extracellular lysis by complement.

Most commonly, however, complement deficiencies, specifically those of the early components of the classical pathway, are associated with immune complex diseases, in particular systemic lupus erythematosus (SLE; see Chapter 25). Here again, only some patients with complement deficiency suffer from the disease, so the deficiency must be

Table 12.4 Human hereditary complement deficiencies.

Affected component	Frequency	Nature of defect	Defective function	Clinical manifestation
Classical pathway				
C1q	F	Absent or dysfunctional C1q	Haemolytic activity	SLE, glomerulonephritis, infections
C1r, C1s	I	Decreased concentration	Haemolytic activity	SLE, infections (meningitis), collagen disease
C4	I	Absence of C4; splicing defect	Haemolytic activity	SLE, collagen disease
C2	F	Absence of C2 mRNA	Haemolytic activity	Often none; SLE, discoid lupus erythematosus, juvenile rheumatoid arthritis glomerulonephritis
C1-INH	F	Decreased level of C1-INH mRNA or dysfunctional C1-INH	Uncontrolled complement activation	Hereditary angio-oedema, increased incidence of autoimmune diseases
C3 and alternative pathway				
C3	I	0.01% of normal C3 level, unstable gene product	Opsonization	Susceptibility to infection with pyogenic bacteria, glomerulonephritis, collagen diseases
D	I			Susceptibility to infection with pyogenic bacteria
P	I	Complete or partial deficiency	Opsonization	Recurrent pyogenic infections, meningitis, septicaemia
I	I	Absent factor I	Opsonization	Susceptibility to infection with pyogenic bacteria, meningitis
H	I	Decreased level	Haemolytic activity	Haemolytic uraemic syndrome, glomerulonephritis
Membrane attack complex				
C5	I	C5 undetectable	Bacteriolysis	Susceptibility to neisserial infection, recurrent meningitis, gonococcal arthritis
C6	I	C6 undetectable	Bacteriolysis	
C7	I	C7 undetectable	Bacteriolysis	
C8	I	γ–α chain decreased; β chain decreased or dysfunctional	Haemolytic activity	Recurrent disseminated neisserial infections
C9	HF	Decreased or absent C9		No symptoms
Receptors				
CR1		Decreased receptor number on erythrocytes, neutrophils and monocytes	Immune clearance	SLE
CR3		Decreased receptor number on neutrophils and monocytes	Phagocytosis and lysosomal enzyme activity	Susceptibility to infection with pyogenic bacteria, leucocytosis, delayed separation of umbilical cord

F, relatively frequent; HF, highly frequent; I, relatively infrequent; SLE, systemic lupus erythematosus.

regarded as a predisposing factor rather than the cause. The association is strongest in individuals with C3, C4 and C1 deficiencies. Virtually all patients deficient in C1q or in C1r/C1s develop the diseases. About 30% of all individuals homozygous for the C2 deficiency and more than 70% of individuals homozygous for the C4 deficiency develop SLE-like syndromes. C3-deficient subjects may develop an inflammation of skin arteries (cutaneous vasculitis), but do not get lupus. Occasionally even individuals with deficiencies in the late-acting complement components develop an immune complex disease.

The association between complement deficiencies and immune complex diseases may seem paradoxical. Since it is known that complement plays an important part in the damage caused by immune complexes (see Chapter 25), one might expect an absence of complement components, if anything, to alleviate the damage. However, an important mechanism believed to be responsible for the association is the failure to keep immune complexes soluble as they form, or to solubilize insoluble complexes in the absence of the critical complement component. Another mechanism responsible in particular for the association with C5–C8 deficiencies may be the failure to eliminate microorganisms that are not especially pathogenic but that can give rise to immune complex disease by virtue of their persistent production of antigenic material.

It will be recalled that in most individuals, the *C4* gene is present in two copies on each chromosome 6, but that in some it is present in three copies. Individuals with null alleles (*Q0*, quantity zero) at one but not the other of the two *C4* loci are not at all rare. For example, the *HLA* haplotype *A1,B8,DR3,BFS,C21* carries the *C4* allele *AQ0 B1*, although it is the most common of all Caucasoid haplotypes. On the other hand, double-null haplotypes, *C4AQ0–C4BQ0*, are extremely rare. In C4 deficiency, almost all homozygous *C4AQ0–C4BQ0* children are sick; sometimes, however, partially C4 deficient individuals are sick, too. Most of the *HLA* haplotypes associated with SLE carry null complement alleles at the *C4* or *C2* loci.

C2 deficiency is relatively common in Caucasoids, occurring with a frequency of about 1 in 10 000 individuals. Most of the deficiencies can be traced back to a single mutation present in the founder *HLA* haplotype *A10,B18,DR2,BFS,C4A,C4B2,C2Q0*. The relatively high frequency of this haplotype (about 1%) suggests that it may have some survival value despite the predisposition of the *C2Q0* allele to SLE or to juvenile rheumatoid arthritis.

At least two of the complement deficiencies are accompanied by such characteristic manifestations that they are considered as distinct diseases: hereditary angioneurotic oedema and paroxysmal nocturnal haemoglobinuria. *Hereditary angioneurotic oedema* is characterized by sporadic attacks of swelling, deep in the tissues, often starting around the mouth and spreading to the neck and face and sometimes also affecting the gut. It occurs in patients heterozygous for a deficiency of the C1-inhibitor. Since the patients have one normal and one defective C1-inhibitor gene they produce some of the factor, but usually its concentration in the blood is less than 35% of the normal level, and during attacks of angio-oedema it may fall to zero. The major predisposing cause of such an attack is trauma. (The original claim that the attacks often occur after excessive fatigue and mental stress – hence 'neurotic' in the designation – is disputed by some investigators.) The trauma-associated bleeding leads to local activation of the blood clotting cascade and the production of plasmin from its precursor, the plasminogen at the sites of blood vessel damage (see Chapter 21). Plasmin is an important consumer of the C1-inhibitor and the latter is, in turn, an important regulator of several blood and tissue enzymes, including kinin, components of the complement system and some components of the intrinsic blood clotting cascade (see Fig. 12.34). The released plasmin quickly exhausts the local supply of the C1-inhibitor and in the absence of the latter, all these enzymes autoactivate and trigger the attack. The activated kinin increases blood vessel permeability (hence 'angio' in the designation, from Greek *angeion*, vessel) and the escaped fluid causes local tissue swelling (Greek *oidema*). Swelling in the upper air passages puts the patient in danger of suffocating; swelling in the intestinal wall causes severe abdominal pain, diarrhoea and vomiting. Once the production of plasmin stops, the local supply of C1-inhibitor is regenerated, the inhibitor brings the enzymes under control and the attack ceases. Administration of drugs that inhibit plasminogen prevents the attack.

Genetic analysis has revealed two types of defects. In *type I hereditary angioneurotic oedema* the level of C1-inhibitor drops to approximately 15–30%, as measured by both functional and immunochemical tests. In *type II hereditary angioneurotic oedema* the level of C1-inhibitor is similarly decreased, as revealed by a functional test but is found to be normal when measured immunochemically. In both types, the patient has one functional copy of the C1-inhibitor gene; in type I the second copy is either absent or is present but does not encode a detectable product; in type II the second copy codes for a product that is non-functional. Most type I cases are the result of a partial or complete deletion of the second C1-inhibitor gene.

Type 2 oedema arises when point mutations change the active site of the enzyme. Recall that C1-inhibitor is a serine proteinase inhibitor that inactivates its target by pretending to be the protease's substrate. The deceived C1 component forms a complex with its serpin and attempts to cleave the peptide bond emanating from a particular residue (generally referred to as P1) of the 'substrate'. Instead the serpin itself cleaves the protease and thus inactivates it. Most type 2 mutations involve this essential P1 residue of the C1-inhibitor. The failure of C1 to recognize the P1 residue of C1-inhibitor results in the failure of the inhibitor to inactivate the C1 component. The P1-encoding codon contains the CpG dinucleotide which is known to be mutation-prone.

Paroxysmal nocturnal haemoglobinuria (PNH) is a condition that affects several proteins, including three complement components: DAF, CD59 and C8-binding protein. The effects on complement components, especially CD59, are to a large extent responsible for the symptoms of

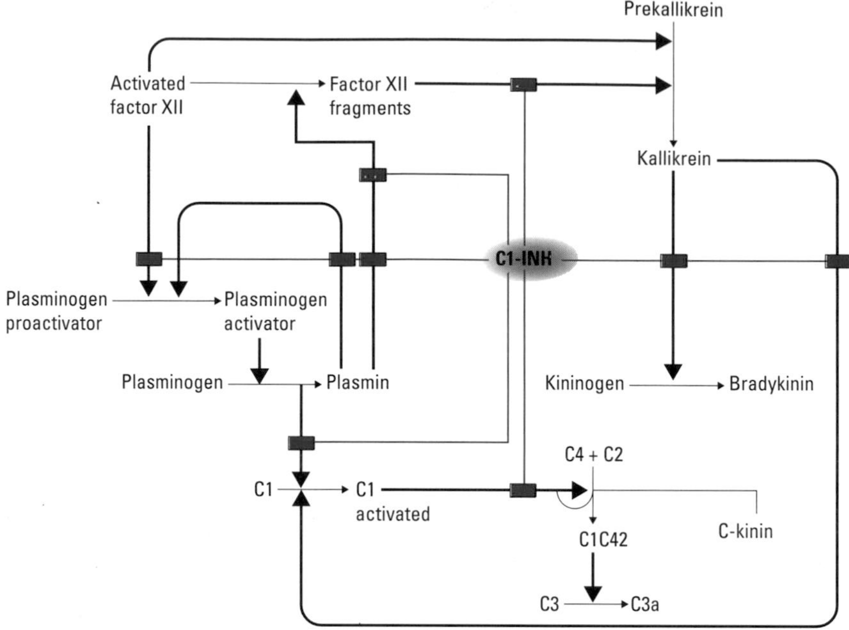

Figure 12.34 Possible mechanisms leading to angioneurotic oedema as a consequence of defective C1-inhibitor (C1-INH). Fine black arrows indicate conversion of one compound into another; thick black arrows indicate activation (catalysis); and red lines and rectangles signify blocking of the action indicated by the thick black arrows. Inactive factor XII binds to 'foreign' surfaces such as an exposed basement membrane, is thereby activated and initiates the coagulation cascade responsible for blood clotting (see Chapter 21). Activated factor XII converts prekallikrein to kallikrein in a reaction normally inhibited by C1-INH. Kallikrein can then participate in the activation of C1, and it can also convert kininogen to bradykinin. Both these reactions, too, are normally opposed by C1-INH. Activated C1 sets the classical complement pathway into motion, which leads to the production, among other compounds, of C-kinin and C3a anaphylatoxin. Inhibition of C1 activity is the main function of C1-INH. Activated factor XII also participates in the conversion of plasminogen proactivators to plasminogen activators, which then convert plasminogen to plasmin, a potent serine protease. Plasmin converts more plasminogen proactivator to plasminogen activator, participates in C1 activation and splits factor XII into active fragments. These three reactions are normally opposed by C1-INH. In the absence of C1-INH activity in a patient, conversion of kininogen to bradykinin, as well as the generation of C-kinin and C3a anaphylatoxin, are unregulated. Bradykinin, C-kinin and C3a anaphylatoxin accumulate and cause some of the effects characterizing angioneurotic oedema.

this condition, which include increased sensitivity to complement-mediated lysis of erythrocytes, formation of blood clots within blood vessels (thrombosis) at unusual sites (abdomen, liver, brain) and deficient haemopoiesis. The condition derives its name from the original observation that most of the haemolysis occurs suddenly (hence 'paroxysmal', from Greek *paroxyma*, to sharpen; here it refers to a sudden onset of symptoms) during sleep at night (hence 'nocturnal') and lead to the appearance of haemoglobin in urine (haemoglobinuria) in the morning. The proteins affected in PNH are unrelated to one another, but they all have one important feature in common: they are attached to the plasma membrane through the GPI anchor. We have mentioned GPI on several occasions already, but now we must acquaint ourselves with it in more detail.

GPI consists of three parts (Fig. 12.35): phosphatidylinositol (inositol being a derivative of glucose), glycan core (comprised of *N*-glucosamine and a string of three mannose molecules) and phosphoethanolamine. It is synthesized at the endoplasmic reticulum in three steps, depicted in Fig. 12.35, and when completed is attached to proteins containing characteristic sequences near their C-termini. The sequences include 11–15 hydrophobic residues, a shorter hydrophilic stretch and a position called ω, which can be occupied by certain residues only: serine > asparagine > glycine > alanine > aspartate > cysteine > leucine > valine > all others (the residues are arranged in the order of their readiness to mediate the attachment of GPI). As the protein nears the final phase of its synthesis, an enzyme (transamidase) cleaves it and attaches GPI to the residue at the ω

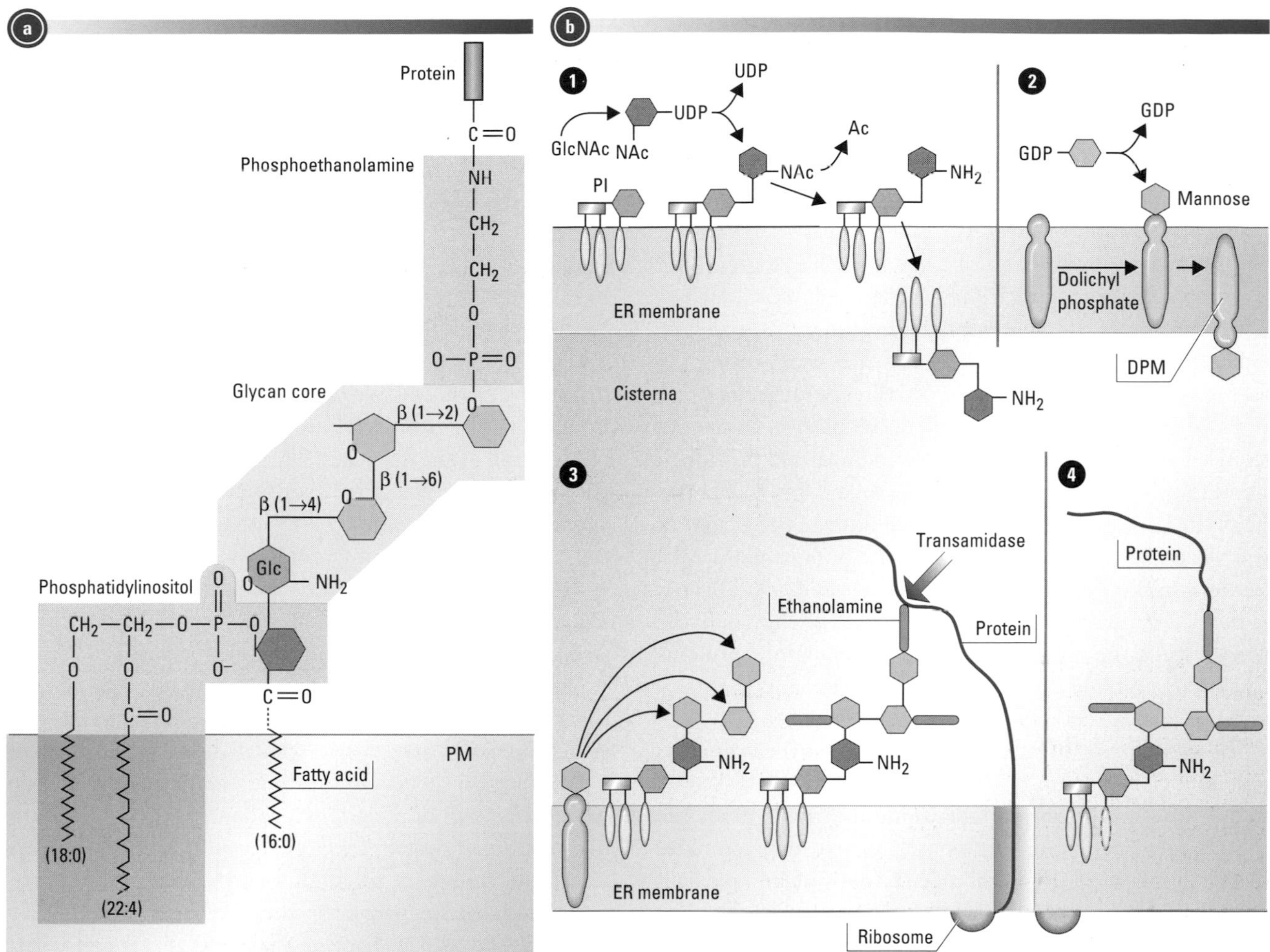

Figure 12.35 (a) Structure of the glycosylphosphatidylinositol (GPI) anchor. (b) Biosynthesis of the GPI anchor. Steps: (1) *N*-acetylglucosamine (GlcNAc) from uridine diphosphate-GlcNAc (UDP-GlcNAc) is transferred to phosphatidylinositol (PI) on the cytosolic surface of the endoplasmic reticulum (ER). GlcNAc is deacetylated and a palmitate or some other fatty acid is added to the inositol. The complex is then flipped to the luminal surface of the ER. (2) Mannose is added to dolichol phosphate on the cytosolic side of the ER. The resulting dolichol-phosphate mannose (DPM) is then flipped to the luminal side. (3) DPM acts as a donor of mannose for three mannosylation steps; ethanolamine is added to each mannose during this process. (4) Protein synthesized on the ER membrane is attacked in the lumen by transamidase; the enzyme joins the C-terminus of the cleaved protein with the terminal ethanolamine. GDP, guanosine diphosphate. PM, plasma membrane. (Slightly modified from Rosse, W.F. & Ware, R.E. (1995) *Blood*, **86**, 3277.)

position by a transamidation reaction, i.e. a reaction between the COOH group of the protein and NH_2 group of the ethanolamine in GPI. The various steps of the process are controlled by distinct genes presumably coding for the different enzymes catalysing these steps. The defects responsible for PNH occur always in the phosphatidylinositol glycan class A (*PiGA*) gene, which controls the first step in GPI synthesis, the transfer of *N*-acetylglucosamine (GlcNAc) from uridine diphosphate-GlcNAc to phosphatidylinositol (Fig. 12.35). The human *PiGA* gene is located on the X chromosome and hence is present in males in one copy only (there is no homologue of the gene on the Y chromosome). Although females have two copies of the *PiGA* gene, one of the copies is always inactivated by a process called *lyonization* (it was discovered by Mary F. Lyon). Hence, if the normally expressed copy of the *PiGA* gene is inactivated by a mutation, the patient, male or female, is left with no enzyme that could catalyse the first step in the formation of GPI. Since the same GPI is added to several different proteins (at least 18), most of these proteins fail to anchor themselves properly in the endoplasmic reticulum membrane and are subsequently degraded. (Some proteins, however, have a back-up system in the form of a transmembrane region that anchors them in the classical manner when the GPI system fails.) The multitude of proteins affected is undoubtedly the reason for the variation in PNH symptoms.

The inactivation of the *PiGA* gene occurs by mutation, most frequently by deletion of a single nucleotide resulting in a change of the reading frame. All the analysed mutations have been shown to have occurred in somatic, specifically haemopoietic, cells; a germ-line mutation inactivating the gene is apparently incompatible with life. Because the cause of PNH is a *somatic* mutation, the condition is always acquired and never congenital—it is not inherited. Although the mutation occurs in a single cell, for unknown reasons the progeny of this cell takes over the bone marrow so that in PNH patients more than 80% of the bone marrow cells are defective. The three complement components affected by the *PiGA* mutation are all normally GPI anchored. In the mutant cells, the absence of the three regulatory proteins leads to uncontrolled complement activation and haemolysis.

Another protein affected by the mutation is the *urokinase (plasminogen activator) receptor* (UPAR), which is normally expressed on the surface of monocytes. It binds the plasminogen activator, urokinase, which then initiates localized activation of plasminogen to plasmin and plasmin then cleaves fibrin, dissolving the clot (see Chapter 21). Absence of the urokinase receptor may stabilize the clot and thus promote thrombosis. Clot formation in PNH patients is also the result of increased generation of thrombin, which in turn is an indirect consequence of the absence of CD59 on platelets. (The unregulated formation of C9 complexes on the platelet membrane leads to the formation of small vesicles in which the complexes are gathered together and 'budded off' from the cell. These vesicles become sites that initiate prothrombinase complexes and these then generate thrombin.)

Evolution

Functional tests and cloning of complement genes provide evidence for the existence of the alternative pathway of complement activation in all extant vertebrate classes (Table 12.5). The classical pathway, on the other hand, may have arisen in jawed vertebrates, since jawless fish seem to lack it. Whether the alternative pathway also exists in some invertebrates is not known. The only direct indication that invertebrates may possess a form of complement pathway is the cloning of a gene in sea urchins that may be the ancestor of the *C3*, *C4* and *C5* genes. The emergence of the classical pathway seems to be closely connected to the appearance of adaptive immunity based on the molecular trio of MHC, T-cell receptor and immunoglobulin in jawed vertebrates.

Most of the complement components are modular proteins that have apparently been assembled from simpler structural units: domains and modules encoded by separate exons. The modularity of the proteins must have arisen through changes in the organization of the encoding genes that principally are of two kinds: duplications of exons within the same gene and shuffling of exons between genes. Intragenic exon duplications produce genes that code for homomodular proteins, i.e. polypeptide chains consisting of varying numbers of homologous repeats. This surely must explain the origin of the CCPR superfamily (see Figs 12.28 & 12.32). Each of these proteins is constructed from a single module repeated between three and thirty times. Because of the sequence similarity of the encoding exons, mispairing of the genes occurs frequently and produces (by unequal crossing-over) genes with different numbers of exons than the original genes. Potential therefore exists for continuing gene expansions and contractions and hence also for the creation of new proteins. Variation in

Table 12.5 Presence of complement components in representatives of vertebrate classes.

	C3	Bf	C1	C4	C2	C8	C9	C5	C6	C7	I/H	AP	CP
Jawless fish	*	*	ND	–	–	–	–	ND	ND	ND	–	+	–
Cartilaginous fish	+	+	+	+	–	+	+	ND	–	–	–	+	+
Bony fish	*	*	ND	ND	–	+	+	+	ND	ND	+	+	+
Amphibians	*	*	ND	*	–	+	+	ND	ND	ND	+	+	+
Reptiles	*	ND	ND	ND	–	+	+	ND	ND	ND	+	+	+
Birds	*	+	+	+	–	+	+	ND	ND	ND	+	+	+
Mammals	*	*	*	*	*	*	*	*	*	*	*	*	*

AP, alternative pathway; CP, classical pathway; +, presence shown by indirect methods; *, presence demonstrated by cloning; –, presumed absence; ND, not determined.

the number of repeats, combined with sequence divergence of individual repeats, provides suitable conditions for the assumption of new functions by the proteins.

Shuffling exons between loci creates genes that code for heteromodular proteins, i.e. polypeptides composed of very different domains. In the complement system, there are at least two prominent protein superfamilies that have arisen in this way. In the serine proteinase family, exons coding for serine protease domains have been hooked together with EGF, LDLR, von Willebrand factor type A, macrophage scavenging receptor, factors I, C6 and C7, factors C1r and C1s, as well as with CCPR exons to create the factor D, C1r, C1s, factor I, C2 and factor B encoding genes (see Fig. 12.29). In the perforin superfamily, the basic perforin gene segment has been connected with TSR, LDLR, EGF-like, CCPR and factor I exons to create the C6, C7, C8, C9 and perforin-encoding genes (see Fig. 12.24). Some of the exons in these genes have been duplicated either prior to being shuffled from one gene to another or after this event; the genes therefore now encode proteins that are both heteromodular and homomodular.

The second level of complement evolution entails the congregation of the individual components into a single, multicomponent, tightly regulated cooperative. The assembly of components into a pathway also involves at least two processes. The first is the recruitment of proteins that hitherto had carried out other functions and the delegation to them of an additional or exclusive function in the complement cascade. A serine protease that previously participated in attacks on foreign particles may, for example, be recruited to cleave the body's own protein when it is the latter's turn to be activated. The structure of the recruited component may have to be altered for the new function by natural selection, but usually the adjustments are only minor. The assembling system thus recruits prefabricated components and merely fine-tunes them.

The second process in the assembly of the cascade involved the duplication and divergence of the recruited genes. This process provided a means of expanding the cascade to deal with new, emerging situations. Thus the development of the classical pathway may have been made possible by the duplication of at least two genes: an ancestor of the *C3* and *C4* genes, as well as an ancestor of the *BF* and *C2* genes. The former probably arose itself by duplication from the same gene that gave rise to α_2-macroglobulin and C5 as depicted in Fig. 12.36. α_2-Macroglobulin (α2m) is a protein synthesized in the liver in response to infection and inflammation. Although it is not a member of the complement cascade, it is clearly related to C5, C3 and C4 in its structure, which includes the thioester site. A gene encoding an α2m-like protein may have been the ancestor of *C5*, *C3*

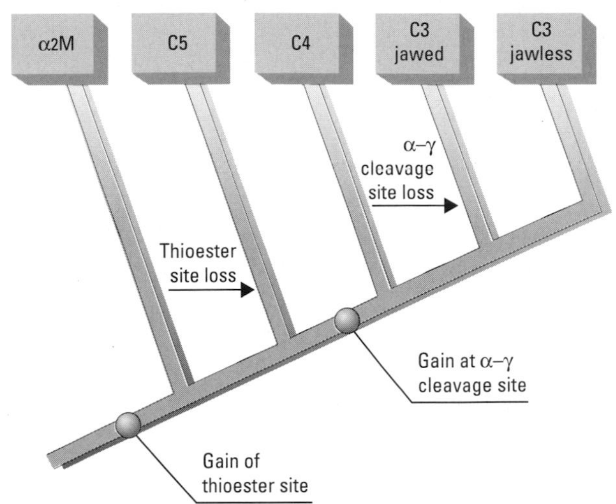

Figure 12.36 Postulated phylogenetic relationship of α_2-macroglobulin (α2M) and complement components C3, C4 and C5. The time of occurrence of some of the main events in the evolution of the proteins are indicated by arrows. (From Hughes, A.L. (1994) *Molecular Biology and Evolution*, **11**, 417.)

and *C4* genes. The similarity of C2 and factor B, a testimony to their origin from a common ancestor, is apparent from Fig. 12.13. To explain how the products of the duplicated genes may have contributed to the emergence of the classical pathway, we end this chapter by briefly describing how the complement system may have come into existence.

The oldest component of the cascade may have been C3-like, activated by proteases released at the site of infection and deposited on the surface of invading parasites. The fixed component was possibly bound by CR3-like receptors on phagocytic cells. (Recall that CR3 is a member of the integrin family and that similar proteins are known to exist in insects and other invertebrates.) At a later stage, the C3-like protein came to associate with a factor B-like protein, the two forming a primitive alternative pathway convertase. The gene for factor B probably originated from the fusion between a serum protease gene and another gene that provided the C3b-binding site. The association of the two proteins had the advantage that it localized the cleavage of C3 and the fixation of C3b to the area around a foreign particle. Subsequent involvement of other proteins provided a means of amplifying the primitive alternative pathway and increasing its specificity.

When immunoglobulins first appeared on the scene, perhaps in the ancestral jawed fishes, the opportunity arose for coupling the newly emerging system of adaptive immunity with the old C3-based defence. The link between C3 and immunoglobulins was provided by the ancestor of the C1q molecule. It may have resembled the mannan-binding protein that binds to C1q receptors on phagocytic cells and to carbohydrates on the surface of microbes. The acquisition of additional binding sites for immunoglobulins and the association of the ancestral C1q-like molecule with $C1r_2C1s_2$-like proteases created conditions for linking the complement system to adaptive immunity. The problem was, however, that the C3-like molecule targeted for providing the link was needed in the alternative pathway. Meddling with it would have endangered the molecule's function in the existing pathway. A way out of this dilemma was found when the gene for the C3-like molecule duplicated. One of the two resulting copies then remained active in the alternative pathway (the present *C3* gene) and the other, the present *C4* gene, was modified in such a way that its product became the substrate for the $C1r_2C1s_2$ proteases. Factor B probably first served the needs of both pathways but further specialization of the classical pathway later demanded the existence of its own counterpart of Bf. This became available after the ancestral *Bf*-like gene duplicated: of the two proteins encoded in the duplicated genes, one came to specialize in the alternative and the other in the classical pathway. The date of these duplications is uncertain. The *C3–C4* duplication, however, must have pre-dated the divergence of amphibians and mammals, whereas the *Bf–C2* duplication may even have occurred after the divergence of reptiles and mammals.

The original function of the complement cascade must have been the organization of foreign particles in preparation for efficient phagocytosis. Later, however, additional proteins became involved in the cascade that enabled an extension of the function to include killing of microorganisms by perforation of their membranes. The initial lytic pathway may have included only the C8 and C9 components; the C6 and C7 proteins were possibly added later to improve the efficiency of attaching the lytic complex to a membrane. The stage at which the C5 protein became part of the lytic pathway is unclear. Phylogenetic analysis (see Fig. 12.35) suggests that it diverged from C3 and C4 before these two components diverged from each other. Its appearance may therefore have preceded the emergence of C4. Yet, the lytic pathway seems to be absent in jawless fishes and present in a rudimentary form only in cartilaginous fishes. It is possible therefore that the ancestral C5 carried out some other function before becoming part of the lytic pathway.

Further reading

Colten, H.R. & Rosen, F. (1992) Complement deficiencies. *Annual Review of Immunology*, **10**, 809–834.

Dameran, B. (1987) Biological activities of complement-derived peptides. *Reviews of Physiology, Biochemistry and Pharmacology*, **108**, 151–206.

Davis, A.E. III (1988) C1 inhibitor and hereditary angioneurotic edema. *Annual Review of Immunology*, **6**, 595–628.

Davis, A.E. III, Bissler, J.J. & Aulak, K.S. (1993) Genetic defects in the C1 inhibitor gene. In *Complement Today. Complement Profiles* (Eds J.M. Cruse & R.E. Lewis Jr). Karger, Basel.

Esser, A.F. (1991) Big MAC attack: complement proteins cause leaky patches. *Immunology Today*, **12**, 316–317.

Farries, T.C. & Atkinson, J.P. (1991) Evolution of the complement system. *Immunology Today*, **12**, 295–300.

Frank, M.M. (1987) Complement in the pathophysiology of human disease. *New England Journal of Medicine*, **316**, 1525–1530.

Gerard, C. & Gerard, N.P. (1994) C5A anaphylatoxin and its seven transmembrane-segment receptors. *Annual Review of Immunology*, **12**, 775–808.

Halkier, T. (1991) *Mechanisms in Blood Coagulation, Fibrinolysis and the Complement System*. Cambridge University Press, Cambridge.

Hourcade, D., Holers, V.M. & Atkinson, J.P. (1989) The regulators of complement activation (RCA) gene cluster. *Advances in Immunology*, **45**, 381–416.

Lachmann, P.J. & Hobart, M.J. (1985) Genetics of complement. *Trends in Genetics*, **1**, 145–150.

Lambris, J.D. (1993) The chemistry, biology, and phylogeny of C3. In *Complement Today. Complement Profiles* (Eds J.M. Cruse & R.E. Lewis Jr). Karger, Basel.

Law, S.K. & Reid, K.B.M. (1988) *Complement*. IRL Press, Oxford.

Liszewski, M.K., Farries, T.C., Lublin, D.M., Rooney, I.A. & Atkinson, J.P. (1995) Control of the complement system. *Advances in Immunology*, **61**, 201–283.

Morgan, B.P. & Walport, M.J. (1991) Complement deficiency and disease. *Immunology Today*, **12**, 301–306.

Reid, K.B.M. (1986) Activation and control of the complement system. *Essays in Biochemistry*, **22**, 27–68.

Reid, K.B.M. & Day, A.J. (1989) Structure–function relationships of the complement components. *Immunology Today*, **10**, 177–180.

Ross, G.D. (Ed.) (1986) *Immunobiology of the Complement System. An Introduction for Research and Clinical Medicine*. Academic Press, Orlando.

Rosse, W.F. & Ware, R.E. (1995) The molecular basis of paroxysmal nocturnal haemoglobinuria. *Blood*, **86**, 3277–3286.

Volanakis, J.E. (1995) Transcriptional regulation of complement genes. *Annual Review of Immunology*, **13**, 277–305.

Whaley, K., Loos, M. & Weiler, J.M. (1993) *Complement in Health and Disease*. Kluwer Academic Publishers, London.

chapter 13 Antigens, superantigens and other lymphocyte-activating substances

If you ask an immunologist what an antigen is, it is like asking a physicist what 'matter' is, or a biologist what 'life' is. You can name one thing after another and the immunologist, the physicist and the biologist will tell you, most of the time without hesitation, whether it is an antigen or not, whether it is matter or not and whether it is alive or not. But they will be at a loss if you ask them for a definition of the broadest category dealt with in their disciplines. In Paul Ehrlich's time, *antigen* was defined as a substance that initiated antibody production (Greek *anti*, against; suffix *-gen*, producing), but we now know that this definition has at least three faults. First, it covers only the humoral arm of immunity and completely ignores cell-mediated reactions. Second, it applies to one aspect of the immune process (responsiveness) only and ignores the other (unresponsiveness). Finally, it is tautological, which means that it uses one term to explain another and then uses the second term to explain the first ('antigens are substances that induce antibody production; antibodies are substances induced by antigens').

Modern immunologists distinguish three not very precisely defined terms: antigen, immunogen and hapten. By *antigen* they usually mean the substance recognized by T- and B-cell receptors (i.e. by *immune receptors*); they designate as an *immunogen* a substance capable of eliciting immune response; and by *hapten* they mean substances of low molecular mass (less than 4000) that can bind antibodies but induce immune response only if covalently attached to a large *carrier* molecule (Fig. 13.1). Some immunologists also use the non-committal term *ligand* as a designation for molecules (haptens and antigens) that interact with antibodies.

In this text, we define *antigen* as *a substance that activates lymphocytes (positively or negatively) by interacting with the combining sites of T- or B-cell receptors. Positive activation leads to responsiveness, negative activation to unresponsiveness (tolerance)*. The term *immunogen* is superfluous in the light of this definition and we use it only when we want to emphasize the role of a given substance in the induction phase of lymphocyte activation. We use the

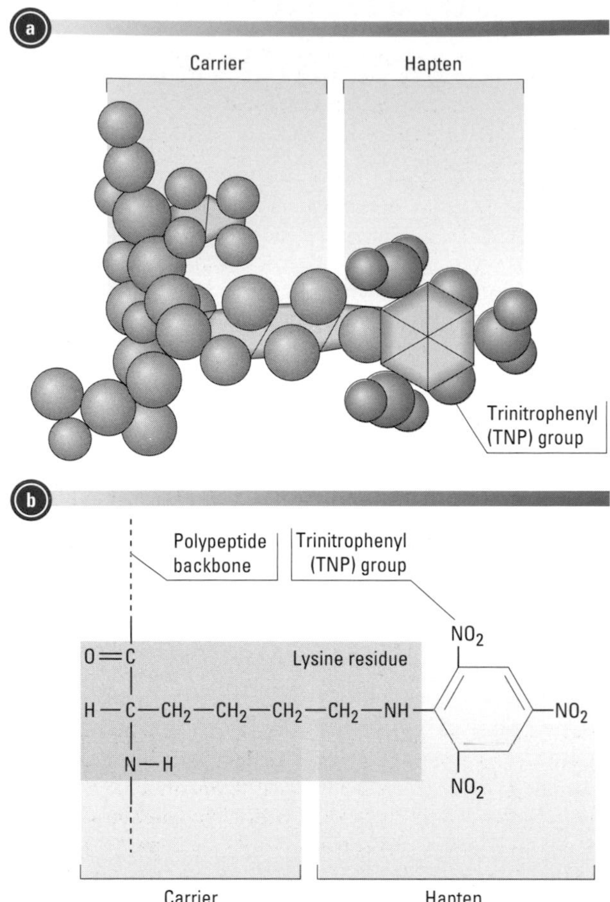

Figure 13.1 Hapten (trinitrophenyl, TNP) covalently coupled to a lysine residue of a carrier (bovine serum albumin). (a) Space-filling model. (b) Chemical formula.

terms *hapten*, *carrier* and *ligand* as defined above. Substances that enhance immune response non-specifically will be referred to as *adjuvants*.

What makes antigens antigenic?

There is no single property the possession of which would make a substance an antigen. In fact, so diverse are the substances called antigens that there is no simple answer to the question posed in the title of this section. The best we can do is to enumerate some of the properties that seem to be required, in certain circumstances at least, to make a substance antigenic.

Chemical nature

No inorganic substance has ever been found to activate lymphocytes by binding specifically with their T- or B-cell receptors (although lymphocytes can be activated by the attachment of certain inorganic molecules at sites other than immune receptors), and no one has ever produced antibodies to inorganic matter. Unresponsiveness to the inorganic world can be accounted for, partially at least, by the generally low molecular mass of inorganic substances. There must be other reasons, however, since not even large crystals, such as kidney stones, are able to induce an immune response. The T- and B-cell receptors are probably simply not constructed in such a way as to interact with inorganic substances. This specialization of receptors for the recognition of organic molecules undoubtedly has an evolutionary basis, for it is organic and not inorganic matter that poses the greatest danger to the integrity of an organism.

Many organic substances do not behave as antigens simply because they are too small. However, when attached to larger molecules (carriers), they can interact with immune receptors and activate lymphocytes. They thus behave as haptens that do not activate lymphocytes alone but do react with activated (immune) lymphocytes or immune molecules.

Among organic macromolecules, by far the most efficient antigens are *proteins*. Some immunologists believe that all proteins are antigenic, but such a notion is difficult to prove or disprove when one realizes how many proteins there are and how few have been tested. It is true, however, that all proteins that have been tested eventually proved to be antigenic. (Some proteins, such as collagen, were long thought to be non-antigenic, but eventually conditions were found in which even they behaved as antigens.) The antigenicity of proteins is not restricted to naturally occurring molecules; synthetic polypeptides produced by biochemists in a test tube can often be as effective antigenically as peptides or polypeptides extracted from living matter. Furthermore, peptides composed of D-amino acids that normally do not occur in living matter produce antibodies as well as (if not better than) L-amino acids. (D and L forms of a given amino acid are mirror images of each other.) However, antibodies produced against polypeptides composed of D-amino acids usually do not react with polypeptides composed of L-amino acids, and vice versa. The variation among proteins in the degree of antigenicity depends, to a certain extent, on their amino acid composition, and in particular on the ratio of aromatic and non-aromatic acids. Proteins containing a large proportion of aromatic amino acids, especially tyrosine, are often better antigens than proteins composed largely of non-aromatic amino acids. Moreover, weak antigens, such as collagen, can be turned into strong ones by attaching tyrosine residues to them.

In comparison to proteins, everything else is less antigenic, including *polysaccharides* (Fig. 13.2). Furthermore, proteins are the dominant (though not exclusive) initiators of T-cell responses; all other antigens activate predominantly B lymphocytes. Polysaccharides induce a strong antibody response in some species (e.g. human, mouse) and a poor response or no response at all in others (e.g. rabbit, guinea-pig). The reason for this difference is not known. It is extremely difficult to raise antibodies to some polysaccharides in all species.

Pure *lipids* usually do not activate lymphocytes, but when mixed with proteins they often function as haptens that bind antibodies produced with the help of the carrier molecule. An example of such a hapten is cardiolipin, the molecule detected by the Wassermann test for syphilis (Fig. 13.3).

Pure *nucleic acids*, like pure lipids, are probably incapable of inducing any form of specific immune response. However, antibodies to nucleic acids can be produced by immunization with nucleoproteins (complexes in which the proteins apparently function as carriers and the nucleic acids as haptens). Antibodies to nucleic acids also appear in the serum of patients with systemic lupus erythematosus, a connective tissue disease of autoimmune character. Some of the antibodies react best with denatured DNA, others with native DNA and others still with both native and denatured molecules. Antibodies to double-stranded RNA, or even to isolated nucleotide triplets (e.g. AAA, AAC or AUC), have also been obtained.

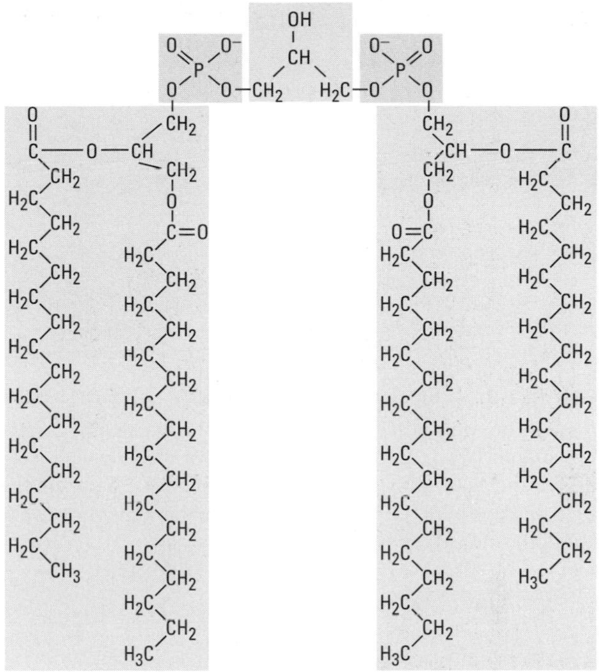

Figure 13.3 Cardiolipin as an example of a lipid antigen. The molecule consists of three glycerol residues joined together by two phosphate groups, with four fatty acid chains attached to the hydroxyl groups of the glycerols. Cardiolipin is obtained from beef heart muscle (hence the name) in which it is part of the mitochondrial membrane. It was once used as an antigen in tests for syphilis. *Treponema* infection leads to the release of cardiolipin into body fluids and to the production of autoantibodies. However, cardiolipin alone only binds antibodies, it does not stimulate their production (i.e. it behaves as a hapten). To become immunogenic, it must be attached to a protein carrier.

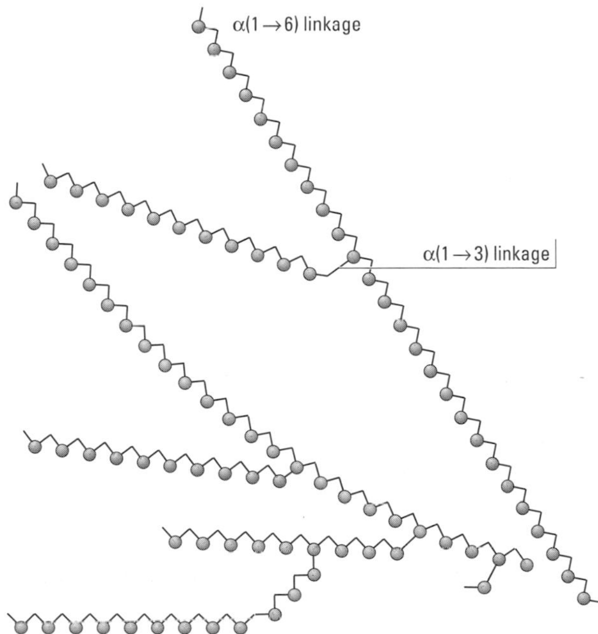

Figure 13.2 Dextran isolated from *Leoconostoc* bacteria as an example of a polysaccharide antigen. Dextran is a polymer of glucose (circles) formed by bacteria from sucrose. The glucose residues are α(1→6) linked, whereas the branching points are α(1→3) linked.

Chemical complexity

In general, the more complex a molecule, the better it functions as an antigen. A molecule composed of building blocks of one kind (such as an amino acid in a synthetic polypeptide; Fig. 13.4) either does not function as an antigen at all or activates lymphocytes poorly. The introduction of another kind of building block into a molecule usually improves antigenicity but a good antigen, as a rule, is composed of several different building blocks.

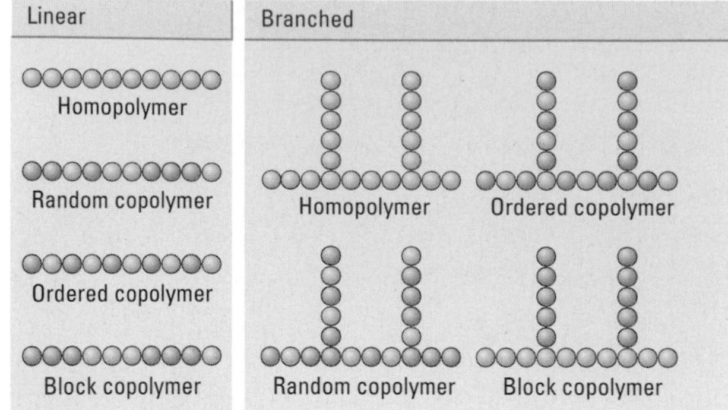

Figure 13.4 Types of synthetic polypeptides. Each circle represents one amino acid residue; different residues are differentiated by shading. The antigenicity of the polypeptides generally increases with their complexity. Synthetic polypeptides played an important part in the discovery of immune response (*Ir*) genes in the mouse and the guinea pig.

Molecular size

Unless coupled to large carriers, small molecules such as amino acids or monosaccharides usually do not activate lymphocytes at all. To serve as an antigen, a substance must have a relative molecular mass of at least 4000; to be a good antigen, it must have an M_r of more than 10 000; and the most potent antigens have an M_r greater than 100 000. However, there are exceptions to this rule.

Conformation

Change of conformation by denaturation, or unfolding of the molecule, results in a change in the antigenic properties of the compound, at least as far as B-cell responses are concerned. The denatured molecule does not cease to function as an antigen, but its antigenic properties often differ from those of the original molecule (some epitopes are lost and new ones appear). The way a molecule is folded and assembled thus determines what kind of antigen it is, again as far as B cells go.

Charge

Molecules need not be charged to function as antigens, and over a wide range the charge does not influence the amount of antibody elicited. However, an excessively high charge depresses the antibody response. Non-specific electrostatic interactions between the antigenic molecule and the cell surface may contribute to the selection of antigens by lymphocytes. These interactions may, in part at least, occur outside the combining site of the lymphocyte receptor and may also be one of the reasons for the inverse relationship observed between the net charge of the antigen and that of the antibody without any apparent change in antibody specificity.

Foreignness

Normally, an organism responds immunologically only to non-self substances, and the recognition of non-self is generally easier the more distinct non-self is from self. When a substance from one organism is introduced into another, the recipient's response often depends on the phylogenetic relationship between the two organisms. If the recipient possesses a substance similar to that introduced, the latter will act as a poor antigen, but if the introduced substance is unlike anything the host possesses, the response to this antigen will be vigorous. To give an example: collagens are poor antigens because they vary little from species to species; on the other hand, class I molecules controlled by the major histocompatibility complex (*MHC*) are generally good antigens because even individuals of the same species differ in these molecules.

Antigens can be divided into two broad categories, according to the genetic distance between the donor and the recipient: *alloantigens*, differentiating members of the same species; and *xenoantigens*, differentiating individuals of two different species (Fig. 13.5). There is also a third category, the so-called *autoantigens*, antigens present in the responder and eliciting immune response only in abnormal situations.

Mode of administration

Immunologists are able to predict the outcome of an experimental immunization with about the same accuracy as meteorologists predict the weather. The same substance may provoke a vigorous response when introduced in one way and no response when administered in another. The main variables are the route of antigen administration, antigen dose, immunization schedule and the time of testing the response. Normally, antigens are administered *parenterally*, i.e. by some means other than through the digestive tract (Greek *para*, alongside; *enteron*, intestine); *peroral* administration (Latin *per*, through; *os*, genitive *oris*, mouth) is used only rarely because the digestive enzymes of the stomach usually destroy potential antigens before they can be absorbed into the blood. For this reason, food (which contains many antigens) under normal circumstances does not immunize. Parenteral immunization can be carried out by injecting a substance into the skin

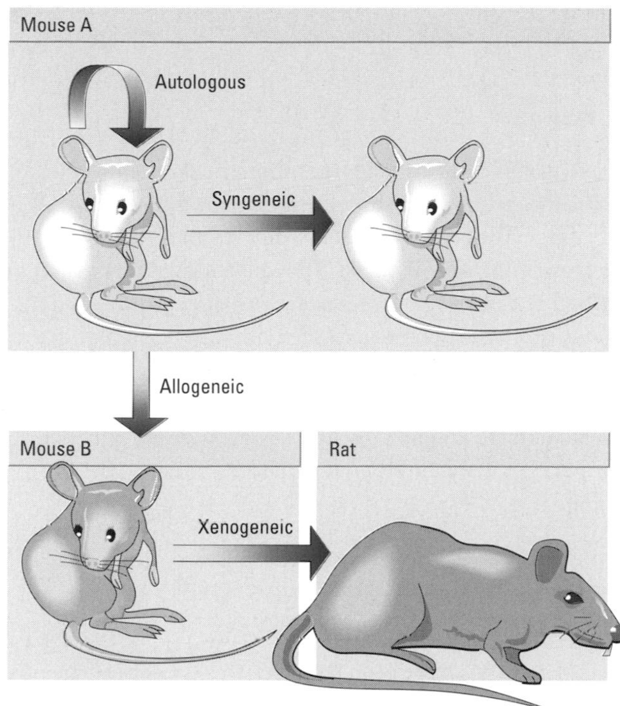

Figure 13.5 Types of immunization depending on the genetic relationship between the donor and the recipient. The two A mice are genetically identical (they belong to the same inbred strain A), whereas mouse B is different (it belongs to an inbred strain B). Antigens defined by autologous (syngeneic), allogeneic and xenogeneic immunization are autoantigens, alloantigens and xenoantigens, respectively. Autoantibodies, alloantibodies and xenoantibodies are defined similarly.

(*intradermally*; Greek *derma*, skin), beneath the skin (*subcutaneously*; Latin *cutis*, skin), into the muscle (*intramuscularly*), in the vein (*intravenously*) or into the peritoneal cavity (*intraperitoneally*). When administered by one of the first three of these routes, the antigen usually ends up in the regional lymph node; when administered intravenously or intraperitoneally, it accumulates predominantly in the spleen. The difference in the site at which the antigen is processed influences the type of ensuing response.

Each antigen has a certain optimal dose at which it produces the highest response: too low a dose fails to activate lymphocytes altogether; too high a dose may induce unresponsiveness. Some antigens induce an immune response after a single injection, but most must be administered repeatedly over prolonged periods before a response can be recorded. The number and temporal distribution of the individual injections must be determined empirically for each antigen. The time at which the assay is carried out should coincide with the peak of the response, which must also be determined by trial and error.

Genetic constitution of the immunized animal

The pathway leading to an immune response, from antigen entrance into the body to the appearance of immune lymphocytes or secretion of immune molecules, is a long one. Since several steps in this pathway are controlled by the recipient's genes, its genetic constitution influences not only the type of response but sometimes also whether or not the animal will respond at all. The best characterized of these *immune response genes* are those constituting the *MHC* (see Chapter 6) but there are also others that are not part of the *MHC*. The cause of unresponsiveness may lie in the hereditary absence of the lymphocyte receptors recognizing a particular antigen or in the failure of an antigen to be presented by a given MHC molecule.

Antigens activating T and B cells

The handling of antigen by T and B lymphocytes differs in several important aspects. A B lymphocyte is able to bind free antigen from the surrounding fluid; by contrast, most T lymphocytes interact only with processed antigen (peptide) presented by MHC molecules on the surface of another cell. B-cell receptors can focus on a small part of a large, intact molecule, whereas most T-cell receptors only recognize short peptides derived from large proteins by antigen processing. At the other extreme, BCRs are also able to bind simple chemical groups (haptens), whereas most TCRs do not recognize a peptide unless it is at least eight to nine amino acid residues long. The part recognized by a BCR can be made up of residues that are far apart from one another in the sequence but that come together into a circumscribed area by the folding of the molecule; the part recognized by a TCR is always a contiguous stretch of residues. BCRs can bind proteins, carbohydrates, nucleic acids and even, under certain circumstances, lipids. TCRs bind mostly peptides.

There are thus antigens that stimulate B lymphocytes but not T lymphocytes and others that do just the opposite. In a large protein molecule that, as a whole, stimulates both types of cells, there are areas that activate either T cells or B cells but not both. The parts of a protein to be recognized by the BCR will depend on the conformation of the molecule, its surface contours, the distribution of charges and other physicochemical characteristics. The part to be recognized by the TCR will be determined by the processing machinery, which produces some peptides but not others, as well as by the MHC molecules, which bind only a proportion of the

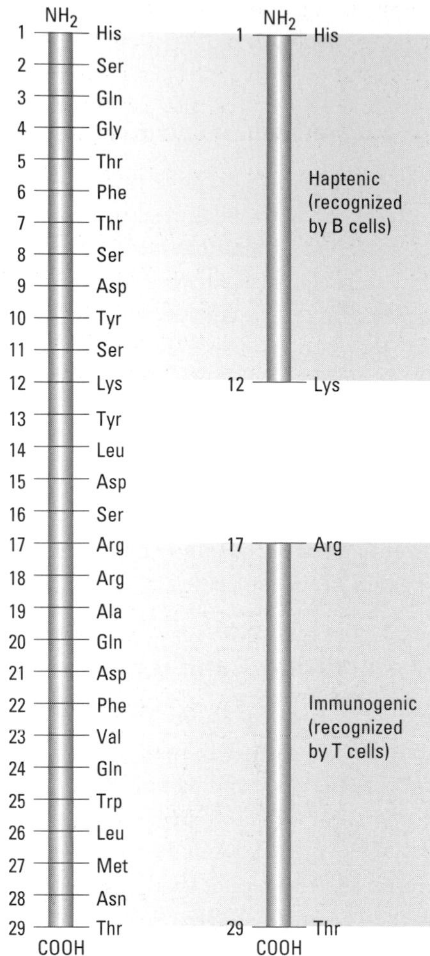

Figure 13.6 Glucagon, an example of a small antigen differentiated into regions recognized by B and T cells. (Based on Goodman, J.W. (1975), in *The Antigens* (Ed. M. Sela), vol. 3, p. 187. Academic Press, New York.)

produced peptides. A large antigenic molecule will therefore contain distinct B-cell and T-cell epitopes.

Such differentiation of epitopes even exists in relatively small molecules such as *glucagon*, a glycogenolysis-controlling hormone produced by the pancreas. The hormone, which consists of only 29 amino acids, carries two epitopes: a B cell-binding epitope in the N-terminal region, and a T cell-activating epitope in the C-terminal region (Fig. 13.6). The intact molecule therefore activates both B and T cells. However, the molecule can be broken into two fragments by trypsin: the N-terminal fragment, which combines with antibodies produced against the intact glucagon but is no longer able to stimulate antibody production; and the C-terminal fragment, which continues to activate T cells. The N-terminal portion of the molecule does not activate T cells, apparently because it is not loaded onto MHC molecules.

Epitopes

An antigen is often much larger than the combining site and sometimes even larger than the entire antigen receptor. With such large antigens, obviously only a small region fits into the combining site of the receptor. This region is called the *epitope* or the *antigenic determinant* (*site*). Some immunologists use these two terms indiscriminately; others draw a fine distinction between them: epitope is the part of an antigenic surface that fits into the combining site, whereas antigenic determinant is an abstract entity defined by the particular reactivity pattern of an antibody or a T lymphocyte.

Methods used to study antibody-defined protein epitopes

Several methods have been developed to determine the position of an epitope in the native protein and the epitope structure at the primary, secondary and tertiary levels. The most commonly used methods test which peptide fragments of the antigen bind to antibodies produced against the native protein. In earlier studies, peptides were generated by the enzymatic digestion of a protein, followed by chromatographic separation (Fig. 13.7). Later, the *natural peptides* were replaced almost entirely by synthetic ones, which can be made to order. Another advantage of using synthetic peptides is that each residue can be replaced by any of the

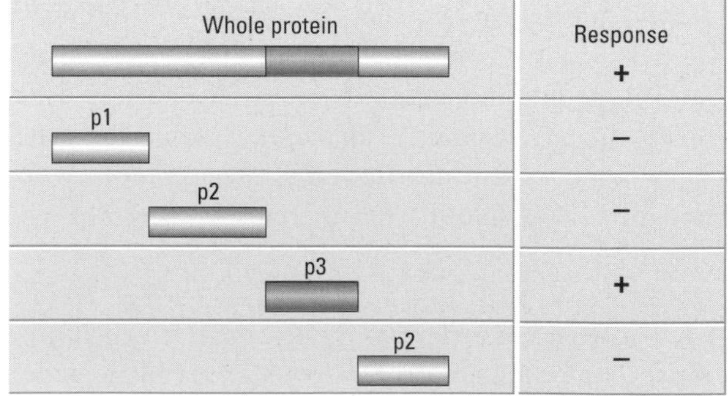

Figure 13.7 Mapping of an epitope by fragmentation of the antigen. Animals were immunized against the whole antigen and their immune cells then restimulated with the whole antigen or with peptides (p1–p4) synthesized to cover different regions of the polypeptide chain. Since only p3 of the four peptides elicited a response upon stimulation, it is assumed that the corresponding region of the polypeptide chain bears the epitope.

remaining 19 amino acids and the effect of the replacement on antibody binding can be assessed. Most recently, methods based on the use of peptides produced from cloned DNA have been introduced. *Synthetic peptides* (Fig. 13.8) can be used in a free form in solution, adsorbed to a solid phase such as the surface of a plastic dish or attached to a carrier. *Free peptides* are usually studied for their ability to inhibit the reaction between antibody and native protein. Reactivity of *solid phase-bound peptides* can be measured directly with labelled antibodies by one of the techniques described in Chapter 14. It must be kept in mind, however, that a significant portion of the surface of bound peptide may be unavailable for the interaction with antibody. This restriction applies also to *carrier-bound peptides*, which often react better with antibodies than solid phase-bound peptides, presumably because the carrier provides a micro-environment for the assumption of a peptide configuration suitable for interaction with antibody. Carrier-bound peptides are also more accessible to antibodies than peptides attached to a plastic dish.

Recombinant DNA techniques offer a number of innovative approaches to studying the relationship between peptides and protein epitopes. One of the simplest approaches is to splice a nucleotide sequence specifying the peptide under study into a gene encoding a vector protein and then to express the recombinant gene in a bacterial, insect or

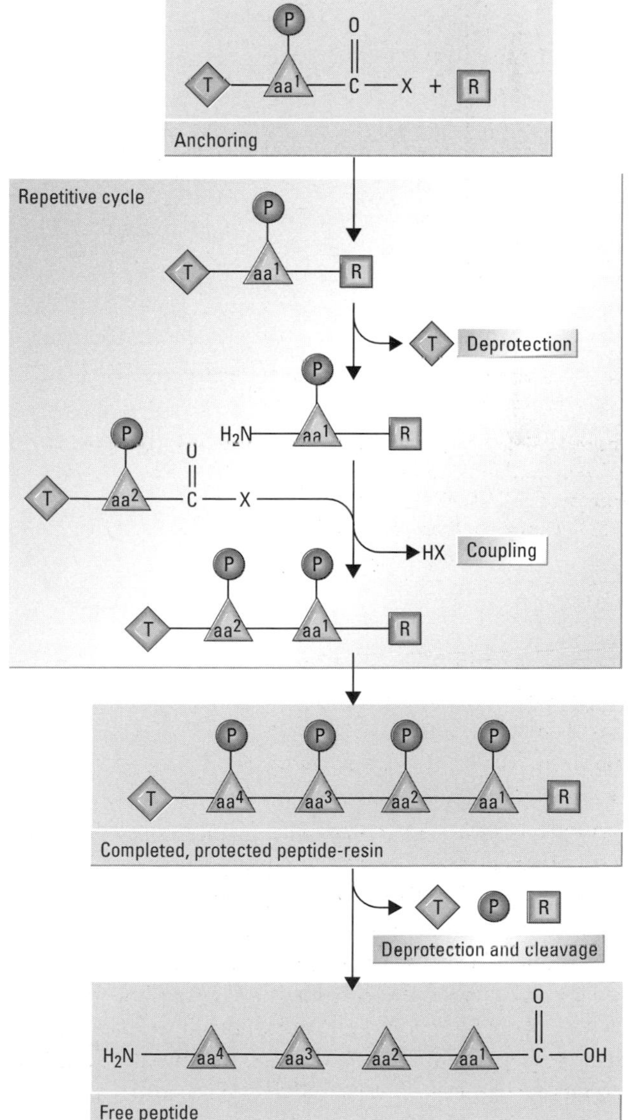

Figure 13.8 Synthesis of peptides by the solid-phase method. Peptides can be synthesized in solution (the classical method) or on a solid phase. The latter method is now commonly used in the production of peptides for research purposes. The growing peptide is anchored to an insoluble support or resin (R) via a chemical handle (X) that links the COOH group of the first amino acid residue (aa^1) to the support. Further amino acids (aa^2, aa^3, etc.) are then added, one at a time, until the growing chain reaches the desired length. Each new amino acid is linked to the preceding residue via a peptide bond between the free amino (NH_2) group of the residue already anchored and the activated carboxyl group (COOH) of the incoming amino acid in solution. Synthesis thus proceeds from the C- to the N-terminus, in the opposite direction to that in nature. To prevent unwanted reactions with reactive amino acid side-chains and between the incoming amino acids, the reactive groups must be blocked by protective chemical groups. Two types of blockers are used: the *temporary protecting groups* (T) block the amino group of the incoming amino acid until the latter is linked to the growing peptide and is itself ready to be linked to a new incoming amino acid; the *permanent protecting groups* (P) block the side-chains for the entire period of synthesis and are removed only when synthesis is completed. At the end of the synthesis, the peptide is cleaved off from the support and either left in a linear form or closed into a circle by linking the C- and N-terminal residues. This 'cyclization' stabilizes the secondary structure of the peptide. The advantage of the solid-phase method is that excess reagents and soluble reaction by-products can easily be removed by filtration and washing. (From Grant, G. A. (1995), in *Molecular Biology and Biotechnology. A Comprehensive Desk Reference* (Ed. R.A. Meyers), p. 654. VCH, New York.)

mammalian cell from which the recombinant protein can be extracted and purified. In this way the peptide can be either inserted into the protein or fused to the protein's N- or C-terminus. Depending on the choice of vector protein, the recombinant protein with the tested peptide can be expressed in the cytoplasm (e.g. bacterial β-galactosidase) or on the bacterial surface (e.g. LamB protein of *Escherichia coli*); it can be secreted into the medium (e.g. maltose-binding protein); or it can appear on the surface of virus particles (e.g. viral coat proteins).

A more sophisticated approach is the construction of *peptide libraries*, which contain all theoretically possible permutations of amino acid residues constituting peptide fragments of a given length displayed on the surface of bacteriophage particles (*phage display method*; Fig. 13.9). The libraries can then be screened with antibody, the reactive peptides identified and their sequence determined from the sequence of the oligonucleotide by which they are specified. The advantages of this approach are that the same library, once prepared, can be reused repeatedly for screening with different antibodies and that screening with the same antibody can yield all the peptides mimicking a given epitope.

In all the methods described thus far, antibodies raised against a native protein are used to test peptides. The proce-

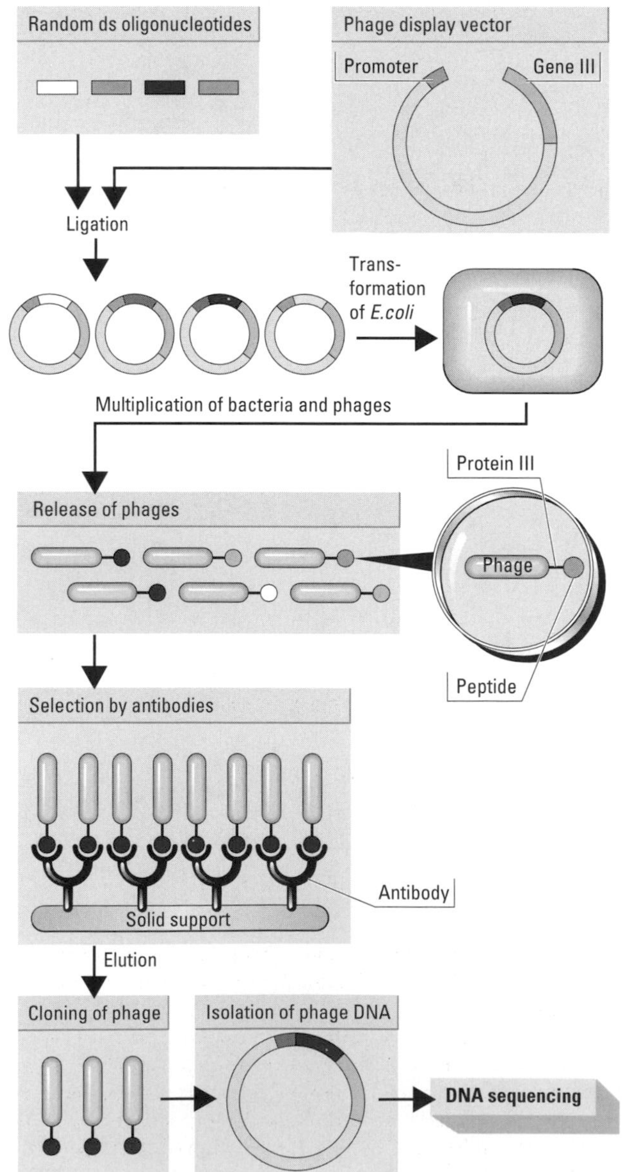

Figure 13.9 Preparation of peptide libraries. A large pool of double-stranded (ds) oligonucleotides differing in their sequence is synthesized. Ideally, the pool covers all possible permutations of amino acid residues in the peptides that the oligonucleotides code for. The oligonucleotides are ligated into an M13 phage vector, specifically into gene III, which codes for a minor coat protein expressed in the filaments on the surface of the phage. The oligonucleotides are inserted in such a way that they become part of gene III and the peptide they encode is displayed on the surface of the phage particle (*phage display*), each phage displaying a different peptide. The phages are used to transform *Escherichia coli* bacteria, allowed to multiply and more than 10^{11} different particles are harvested. The phages are incubated with monoclonal antibodies attached to a solid support and specific for a particular protein epitope. Particles that do not bind to the antibodies are removed and those that have attached via the displayed peptide to the antibody are eluted and cloned. They are then used to infect new bacteria and the procedure is repeated (not shown) to enrich for phages whose peptides are bound specifically by the antibody. The DNA of these phages is then isolated and sequenced. A peptide that is specifically bound by a particular antibody is thus identified. In its structure, the peptide is considered to resemble the epitope recognized by the antibody.

dure can also be reversed, however, and antibodies produced by immunization with synthetic peptides can be tested on native proteins. Reactivity of the peptide-specific antibodies with the protein is then taken as evidence that the peptide resembles the protein epitope. The initial claim that most peptide-specific antibodies bind to native proteins could not be substantiated. The proteins used in the earlier tests were apparently denatured by adsorption to the plastic dish in one step of the assay. Later studies revealed that the extent of cross-reactivity of peptide-specific antibodies with native proteins is actually rather limited.

If the sequence of a given antigenic protein is known to differ at various positions among different species, correlation between antibody reactivity and protein structure can be used to deduce the probable location of the epitope (Fig. 13.10). A modern alternative to this *phylogenetic approach* is to introduce a single amino acid replacement in a given protein by *site-directed mutagenesis* (see Fig. 7.32) of the encoding gene. Any change in antibody binding to the mutated protein in comparison with the wild-type protein is considered to be an indication that the particular residue is involved in the formation of the epitope. Specific residues can also be altered by *site-directed chemical modifications*. Single replacements or modifications of residues on the surface of a protein usually cause only local structural alterations; they can, however, alter the epitope indirectly by conformational changes in protein structure.

The relative position of epitopes on the surface of a protein can be studied by *competitive topographic mapping* using monoclonal antibodies. In these tests, a protein is coated with one antibody and a second antibody is then tested for its ability to bind to the protein under these conditions. Absence of second-antibody binding is interpreted as an indication that the two antibodies recognize either the

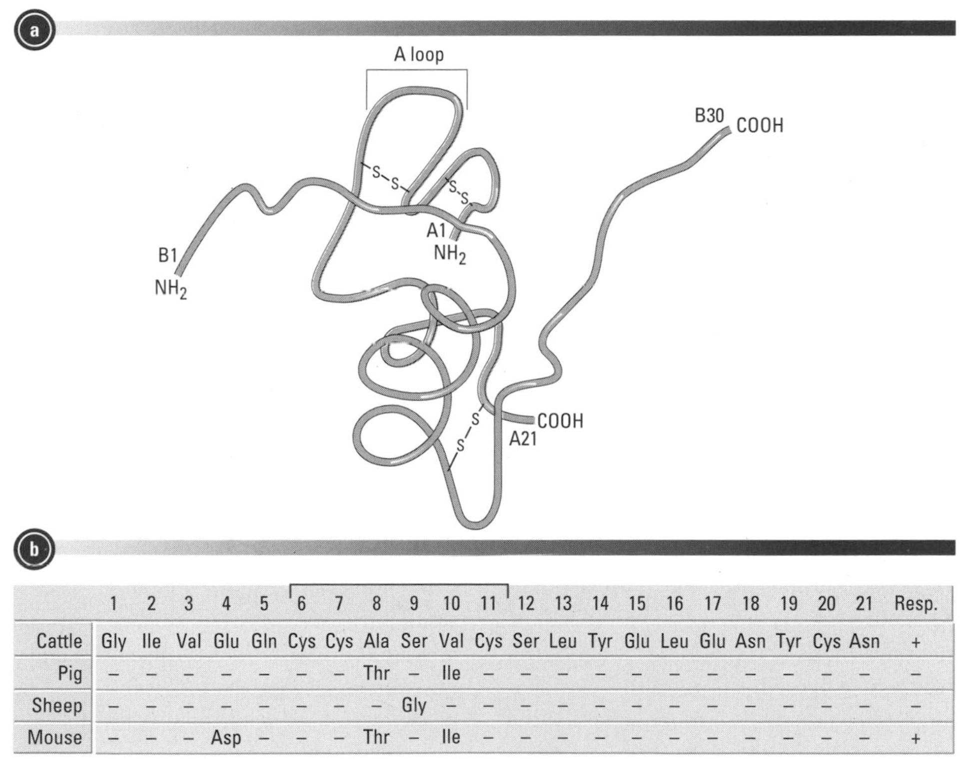

	1	2	3	4	5	6	7	8	9	10	11	12	13	14	15	16	17	18	19	20	21	Resp.
Cattle	Gly	Ile	Val	Glu	Gln	Cys	Cys	Ala	Ser	Val	Cys	Ser	Leu	Tyr	Glu	Leu	Glu	Asn	Tyr	Cys	Asn	+
Pig	–	–	–	–	–	–	–	Thr	–	Ile	–	–	–	–	–	–	–	–	–	–	–	–
Sheep	–	–	–	–	–	–	–	–	Gly	–	–	–	–	–	–	–	–	–	–	–	–	–
Mouse	–	–	–	Asp	–	–	–	Thr	–	Ile	–	–	–	–	–	–	–	–	–	–	–	+

Figure 13.10 Mapping of an epitope by restimulation with species variants of a protein. (a) Insulin, a hormone produced by the islets of Langerhans in the pancreas, is composed of two disulphide-bonded polypeptide chains, A and B. The A chain contains an intrachain disulphide bond (–S–S–) responsible for the formation of the characteristic A-chain loop that spans residues A6–A11. The amino acid sequence of the entire A chains of different species. (b) Dashes indicate identity with the top sequence. T cells from mice immunized against cattle insulin A chains respond to cattle and sheep but not to pig and mouse A chains. This pattern of responsiveness indicates that the T cells are specific for an epitope that includes Ala 8 and Val 10 in the A-chain loop. (Mouse and cattle A chains differ at positions 4, 8 and 9. The failure of pig A chains to restimulate the response indicates that the epitope does not include Glu 4, which cattle and pig share. The ability of sheep A chains to restimulate the response indicates that the epitope includes Ala 8 and Val 10, which cattle and sheep share.)

same epitope or two epitopes so close to each other on the protein's surface that when one binds, there is no room for the other. Binding of both antibodies indicates that the two antibodies bind to different epitopes far apart from each other and that there is no *steric hindrance* between the binding antibodies. In this way, an epitope map of the protein's surface can be constructed with a set of protein-specific monoclonal antibodies.

The most informative, but also the most time-consuming, method of epitope analysis is *X-ray crystallography* of antigen–antibody complexes. It not only defines the epitope precisely but also identifies the atomic contact sites between the epitope and its complementary region on the antibody molecule, the *paratope*.

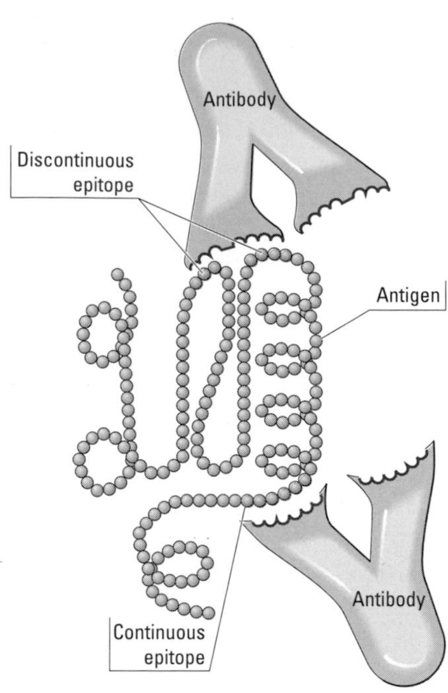

Figure 13.11 Continuous and discontinuous epitopes: a hypothetical example. In a continuous epitope, all the contributing amino acid residues form a single segment of the primary structure; in a discontinuous epitope, the contributing residues occur in different parts of the primary structure.

Nature of protein epitopes recognized by antibodies

In a protein, an epitope can be either continuous or discontinuous. In a *continuous epitope*, all participating amino acid residues are part of a single, uninterrupted sequence (other names for this type of epitope are 'sequential' or 'segmental'). A *discontinuous epitope*, on the other hand, consists of residues that are not contiguous in the primary structure but are brought together by folding of the polypeptide chain (Fig. 13.11). The epitope is sometimes also referred to as 'conformational' or 'topographical'. Most, if not all, epitopes recognized by antibodies produced by immunizing with native proteins are of the discontinuous type. This conclusion is based on both empirical observations and theoretical considerations. The theoreticians argue that proteins are so convoluted in their three-dimensional structure that there are virtually no contiguous regions on the molecular surface large enough to form an epitope. This argument, however, seems to ignore the fact that antibodies produced against native proteins often react with short peptides. The paradox has not been fully explained, but an obvious possibility is that the peptides represent only part of the epitope, the other part presumably being provided by another segment of the protein. The observation that peptides usually react less strongly with the antibody than the native protein supports this explanation. X-ray crystallographic data do indeed indicate that the actual epitopes are larger than has been deduced from peptide analysis (see next section).

Antibodies normally recognize epitopes on the surface of a protein. Amino acid residues hidden in the interior of the molecule are not recognized unless peptides are used for immunization. The extent to which a protein surface is antigenic for B lymphocytes is still being debated but the prevailing view is that virtually the entire accessible surface can combine with appropriate antibodies. The fact is, however, that immunization with a protein produces a predominance of antibodies against a limited number of epitopes. Persons exposed to influenza virus, for example, have antibodies in their sera specific for one of four main epitopes on the viral haemagglutinin molecule (Fig. 13.12). Antibodies specific for other regions of the molecule are either absent or are present in very low concentrations. Immunologists can elicit antibodies against these other regions, for example by immunization with the corresponding peptides, but exposure to the native molecule clearly focuses the response on small parts of the protein surface only. Although the surface may contain a number of potential epitopes, a certain low number of epitopes, usually not more than six, appears to be *immunodominant*.

Several explanations have been proposed for the observation that some regions of the protein surface are more immunogenic than others. The most likely one is that immunogenicity is determined in the first place by *accessibility of a region* to antibodies. In protein–protein interaction studies, one generally finds that the reactive receptor sites are concave and the corresponding ligand sites are convex. The combining site of the immunoglobulins is always concave and so the epitopes must be convex—they

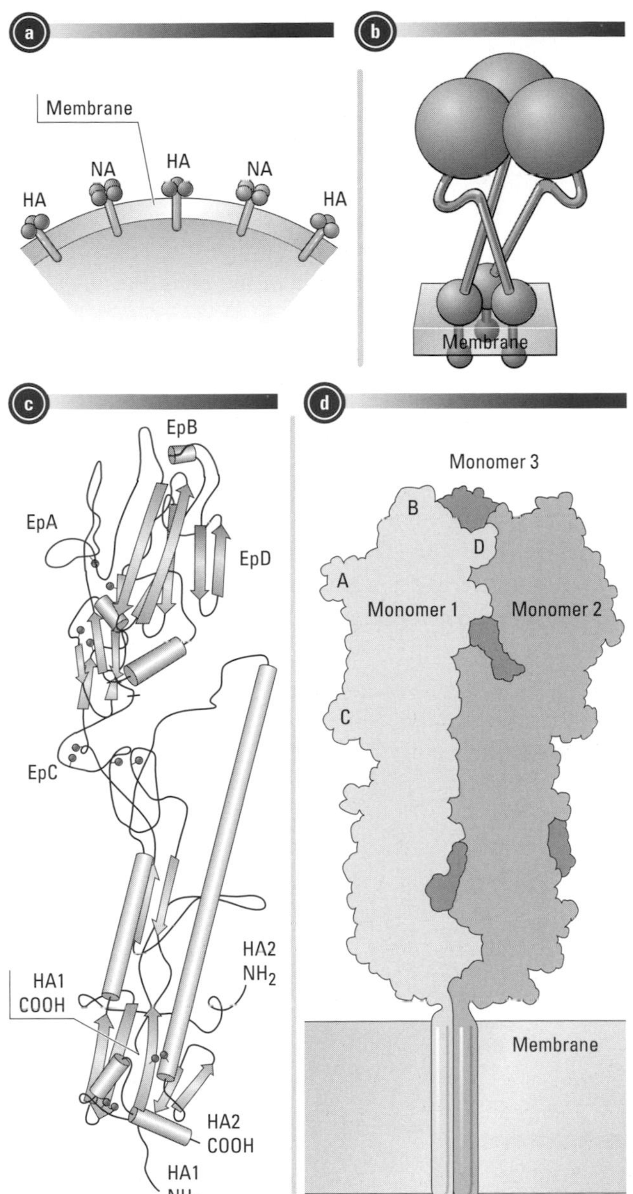

Figure 13.12 Main epitopes recognized by human antibodies on influenza virus haemagglutinin. (a) Part of the membrane enveloping the virus, with haemagglutinin (HA) and neuraminidase (NA) spikes protruding from the external surface. (b) The haemagglutinin molecule, which consists of three identical monomers. (c) The folding pattern of two polypeptide chains (HA1 and HA2) constituting one subunit of the haemagglutin complex. The globular head is formed by the HA1 chain, the stem structure is comprised of both chains. Arrows indicate β-strands; cylinders, α-helices and filled circles, disulphide bonds. Approximate positions of epitopes (EpA–EpD) are indicated. (d) Arrangement of the three monomers in the haemagglutinin trimer (the third monomer is at the back and hence hardly visible). Epitopes (A,B, D) on monomer I are indicated. (b and c, Based on Wilson, I. A. *et al.* (1981) *Nature*, **289**, 366; d, based on Wabuke-Bunoti, M.A.N. & Fan, D.P. (1983) *Journal of Immunology*, **130**, 2386.)

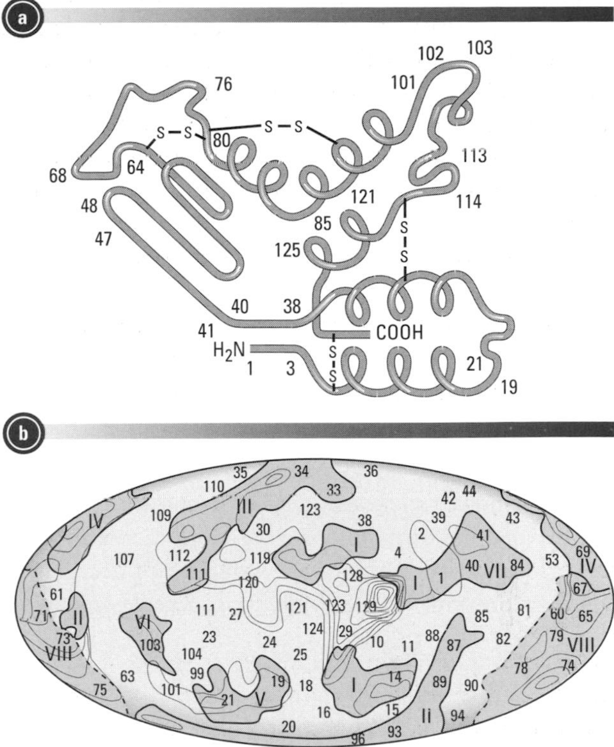

Figure 13.13 Correlation between surface accessibility and location of epitopes recognized by antibodies on the molecule of hen egg-white lysozyme (HEL). (a) Folding of the HEL polypeptide chain. Numbers indicate amino acid residues. (b) The so-called Mollweide projection of the molecular surface of HEL with contour interval ≥ 0.8 nm. The surface should be viewed as a topographical map in which points of the same height are always connected by a single line (numbers indicate residues). Superimposed on the projection are the antigenic sites recognized by antibodies. Site I, residues 5, 7, 13, 14 and 125; site II, residues 62, 87, 89, 93, 96 and 97; site III, residues 33, 34, 113, 114 and 116; site IV, residues 45–48 and 68; site V, residues 19 and 21; site VI, residues 102 and 103; site VII, residues 1, 41 and 84; site VIII, residues 64–80. Broken line indicates the position of the so-called loop determinant. (b, Modified from Novotny, J. *et al.* (1986) *Proceedings of the National Academy of Sciences USA*, **83**, 226.)

must protrude from the surface of the antigen. Indeed, molecular cartography studies, in which contour maps have been plotted analogous to terrain maps used to display the earth's surface, have shown that the epitopes usually coincide with the highest 'hills' of the protein surface (Fig. 13.13).

According to another explanation, antigenicity depends on *segmental mobility*. It is known that atoms in a molecule are not firmly fixed in their positions; they oscillate, some of them more than others, depending on the local environment. These motions are expressed in terms of *atomic temperature factors* (*B values* or Debye–Waller factors), which represent the mean-square displacement of each atom from an average position. When plotted against the residue number, temperature factors provide a graphic image of the degree of mobility along the polypeptide chain (Fig. 13.14). The plots show that certain surface segments are more mobile than others and that the distribution of mobile segments correlates with the distribution of epitopes. The rationale for the correlation theory is that mobility facilitates the ligand's adjustment to the combining site, which does not fit the antigenic surface exactly. Both the N- and C-termini of a protein often demonstrate a greater than average antigenicity, presumably because they are located on the surface and have a relatively high flexibility. Critics of this explanation have pointed out, however, that high-mobility regions are present mainly in surface projections such as loops and turns and that the correlation is therefore not so much with mobility as with surface accessibility. Moreover, the critics argue, when short peptides are used as probes, only those regions that correspond to mobile segments bind antibodies raised against the native protein; when longer, more rigid peptides are used, regions of low mobility are also found to be antigenic.

According to the third explanation, antigenicity is determined by the *relative hydrophilicity* of the different surface regions (Fig. 13.15). Regions that contain a high proportion of hydrophilic residues are thought to be better equipped to interact with the antibody-combining sites and are therefore more antigenic. Here, the critics have pointed out that in a globular protein hydrophilic residues tend to be surface oriented rather than buried inside the molecule and that the correlation between hydrophilicity and antigenicity once again reflects the more general correlation between surface accessibility and antigenicity. Moreover, hydrophobic and aromatic residues often do contribute to the construction of an epitope. Therefore, it is the topography of the molecular surface that determines which regions will be recognized by antibodies in the first place.

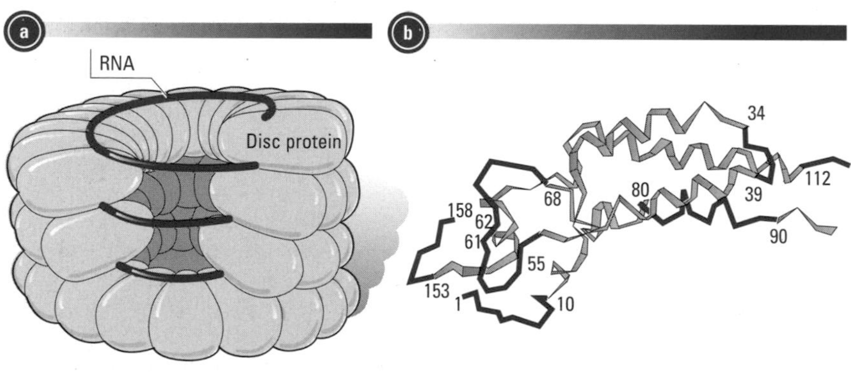

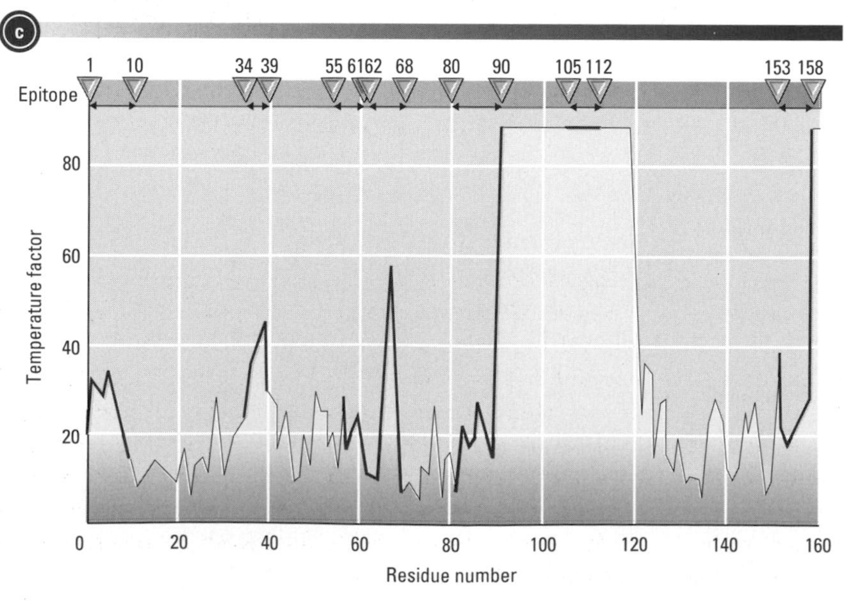

Figure 13.14 Correlation between mobility of main-chain atoms and antigenicity of the tobacco mosaic virus protein. (a) Part of the rod-like virus particle showing the helical array of protein subunits around a single-stranded RNA molecule. (b) α-Carbon polypeptide backbone of one protein subunit. All residues are shown (1–158) except for 94–106, which are omitted because this region has no specific conformation. The locations of seven continuous epitopes are indicated by red lines. (c) Atomic temperature factor of the main-chain atoms in each residue is plotted against residue number for the subunit protein. Positions of the seven antibody-defined epitopes are indicated in colour. (a, Modified from Hoppe, W. *et al.* (1977) *Biophysik*. Springer-Verlag, Berlin; b and c, modified from Westhof, E. *et al.* (1984) *Nature*, **311**, 123.)

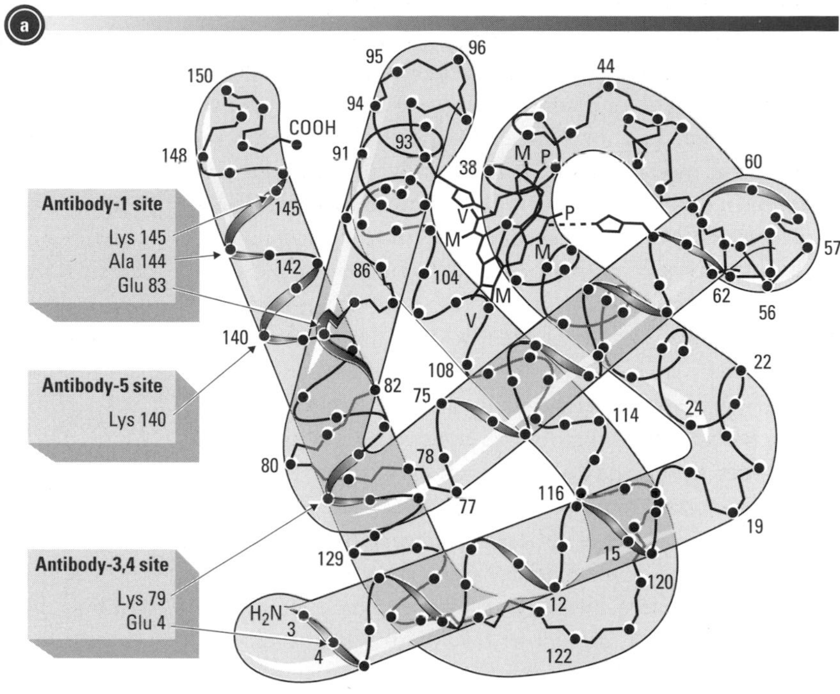

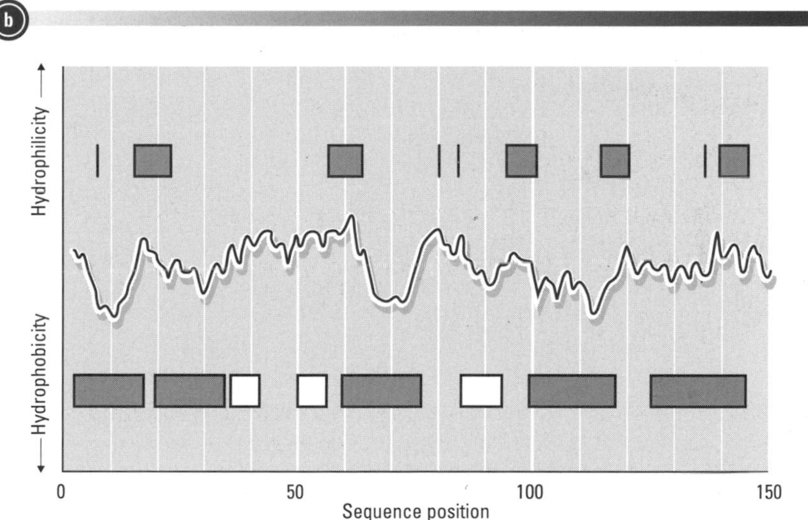

Figure 13.15 Correlation between relative hydrophobicity and antigenicity of sperm-whale myoglobin. (a) α-Chain carbon polypeptide backbone of the myoglobin molecule. Main epitopes are indicated in red. (b) Hydrophobicity profile of sperm-whale myoglobin. Bars above the profile indicate known major epitopes; vertical slashes represent single antigenic residues. Bars below the profile are helices. The larger helices that form the hydrophobic core of the molecule are represented by solid bars; open bars represent smaller, more exposed helices. The scale shows hydrophilicity at the top and hydrophobicity at the bottom. (a, Modified from Berzofsky, J.A. (1985) *Science*, **229**, 932 and Dickerson, R.E. (1964), in *The Proteins* (Ed. H. Neurath), 2nd edn, vol. 2, pp. 603–778. Academic Press, New York; b, modified from Hopp, T.P. (1986) *Journal of Immunological Methods*, 88, 1.)

An epitope was originally believed to consist of six to eight amino acid residues in a protein antigen and a similar number of monosaccharide units in a polysaccharide antigen. This estimate has been upgraded by subsequent X-ray crystallographic studies, which indicate that no less than 15 amino acid residues of an antigenic protein contact the combining site of an antibody. The shape of the epitope is highly irregular, covering an area of at least 7 nm². The same general area of the molecular surface is often recognized by several different antibodies, each antibody fitting into a different position from the previous one and covering a slightly different region;. the antigenic site can thus be viewed as a series of overlapping epitopes. Sometimes epitopes also fit into the combining sites of antibodies that they did not stimulate; the epitopes (and the corresponding antibodies) are then said to *cross-react*. A given antibody may also bind more strongly to epitopes other than the one against which it was raised. When this happens, the antibody is said to be *heteroclitic* (Greek *hetero*, other; *clitos*, a declivity, inclination).

Antigen–antibody complexes

When the paratope of an antibody finds a matching epitope of an antigen, the two combine into an *antigen–antibody complex*. Some two dozen such complexes have been crystallized and the nature of the interaction between the two partners in each pair has been determined by X-ray diffraction analysis. The antigens involved in the formation of the studied complexes range from small haptens to large molecules (in terms of M_r from 169 to 50 000). They include peptides, carbohydrates, nucleic acids and proteins. In the initial studies, myeloma proteins were used instead of antibodies because they were the only available source of pure, homogeneous immunoglobulins for crystallization at that time. Since the ligands of the myeloma proteins were not known, a large number of substances had to be screened to find one or two that were bound specifically by a given antibody. One such myeloma protein was found to precipitate pneumococcus C polysaccharide which contained *phosphocholine*, a derivative of a nitrogenous alcohol (Fig. 13.16). Phosphocholine (or phosphoryl choline in earlier literature) itself was found to bind to the particular myeloma protein and the phosphocholine–myeloma protein complex became the first immunoglobulin–hapten complex whose tertiary structure was determined (Fig. 13.16). Later, with the advent of monoclonal antibodies, the possibilities for crystallization of antigen–antibody complexes were greatly expanded and the number of complexes subjected to X-ray diffraction analysis increased considerably. In all the studies, Fab parts were used instead of the entire antibody molecules simply because it was easier to crystallize them.

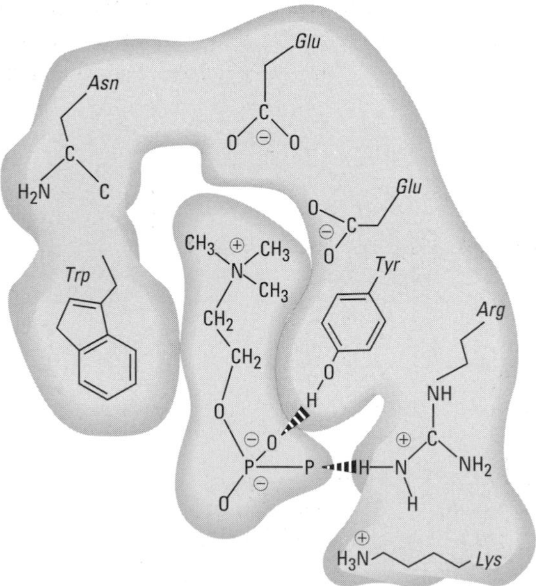

Figure 13.16 Interaction of phosphorylcholine (pink) with the mouse myeloma protein McPC603 (grey): a diagrammatic representation. The hapten is inserted into a crevice between the light and heavy chains. The choline part of the hapten is oriented towards the interior of the antibody molecule, whereas the phosphate group faces the surface. (Adapted from Padlan *et al.* (1976) *Immunochemistry*, 13, 945; Branden, C. & Tooze, J. (1991) *Introduction to Protein Structure*, p. 189. Garland Publishing, New York.)

The studies revealed that the combining site of the antibody (the paratope) is formed by the juxtaposition of six loops that connect the β-strands in the immunoglobulin variable domain, three provided by the heavy chain (loops H1, H2 and H3) and the other three by the light chain (loops L1, L2 and L3; see Chapter 8). The loops are also referred to as the *complementarity-determining regions* (CDRs). The L1 and L2 loops are encoded in the germ-line V_L gene segments; the H1 and H2 loops in the germ-line V_H gene segment. The L3 loop is formed by the joining of the V_L and J_L gene segments and the H3 loop by fusion of the V_H, D and J_H segments. The length of the CDRs varies from antibody to antibody. For the L1, L2, L3, H1, H2 and H3 loops, the ranges are 10–17, 7, 7–11, 5–7, 9–12 and 4–25 residues, respectively. Some antibodies use only four of the six hypervariable loops for contacting the antigen; others use all six (Table 13.1). The L3 and H3 loops are always used; the L2 loop is used only for binding of large antigens. Usually most of the antigen-contacting residues come from the heavy chain; fewer are from the light chain. In general, the latter seems to be less important for antigen binding than the heavy chain, since some antibodies that bind different proteins have almost identical light chains and certain heavy chains can be combined with different light chains while still retaining the ability to bind a given antigen.

The length of the CDRs determines to a large extent the shape of the combining site (Fig. 13.17). Some sites form a concave pocket that is able to bind only small antigens such as haptens, peptides, carbohydrates and nucleic acids (Fig. 13.17a). Other sites, such as those formed by lysozyme epitopes, are only slightly concave (Figs 13.17b & 13.18). The combining site for influenza neuraminidase (Fig. 13.19) is almost flat and the paratope for some other lysozyme epitopes actually protrudes into the active site of the lysozyme molecule.

When an antibody interacts with an antigen, part of its surface that was previously free becomes buried under the epitope and, similarly, part of the antigen surface becomes buried under the paratope. The size of the buried surface depends on the size of the antigen: the larger the antigen, the

Table 13.1 Hypervariable loops used by antibodies for antigen binding. (Adapted from Wilson, I.A. & Stanford, R.L. (1993) *Current Opinion in Structural Biology*, **3**, 113.)

		Light chain			Heavy chain			Contribution to antigen binding (%)	
Antibody	Antigen	CDR1	CDR2	CDR3	CDR1	CDR2	CDR3	V_L	V_H
B1312	Myohaemerythrin	+	–	+	+	+	+	22	78
17/19	Influenza haemagglutinin peptide	+	–	+	–	+	+	26	74
DB3	Progesterone	+	–	+	+	+	+	35	65
4-4-20	Fluorescein	+	–	+	+	+	+	40	60
Se155-4	Dodecasaccharide	+	–	+	+	+	+	40	60
HyHEL-5	Hen egg lysozyme	+	+	+	+	+	+	41	59
131	Angiotensin II	+	–	+	+	+	+	41	57
BV04	d(pT3)	+	+	+	+	+	+	43	57
HyHEL-10	Hen egg lysozyme	+	+	+	+	+	+	43	57
D1.3	Hen egg lysozyme	+	+	+	+	+	+	43	57
NC41	Influenza neuraminidase	–	+	+	+	+	+	46	54
McPC603	Phosphocholine	–	–	+	+	+	+	47	53
AN02	Dinitrophenyl spin-label	+	+	+	–	–	+	61	39
Total		11	6	13	11	12	13		

CDR, complementarity-determining region; +, at least one residue in the CDR loop is involved in binding antigen; –, no residue in the CDR loop is involved in binding. The percentage contribution of the variable light-chain (V_L) and heavy chain (V_H) domains to antigen binding was calculated from crystallographic data.

greater the area buried (Table 13.2). Initial studies seemed to indicate that the buried area was relatively small and that only a small part of the antigen penetrated deep into the combining site. But this impression proved to be false when the studies were extended from haptens to larger proteins. It is now known that the buried area can range from 1.6 nm^2 to over 9 nm^2 for both the antigen and the antibody (Fig. 13.18).

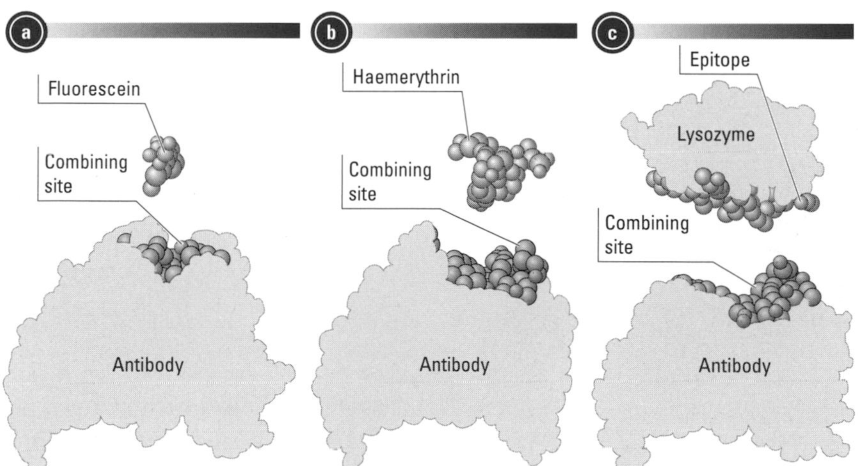

Figure 13.17 Three different shapes of antigen–antibody combining sites depicted on space-filling models (each sphere represents an atom). (a) Pocket (crevice)-shaped site that accommodates the hapten fluorescein. (b) Concave site capable of accommodating the peptide haemerythrin. (c) Flat site for one of the lysozyme epitopes. Antigen is shown at the top of the figure, antibody with highlighted combining site below it. (Based on Rees, A.R. *et al.* (1994), in *Immunochemistry* (Eds C.J. van Oss *et al.*), p. 615. Marcel Dekker, New York.)

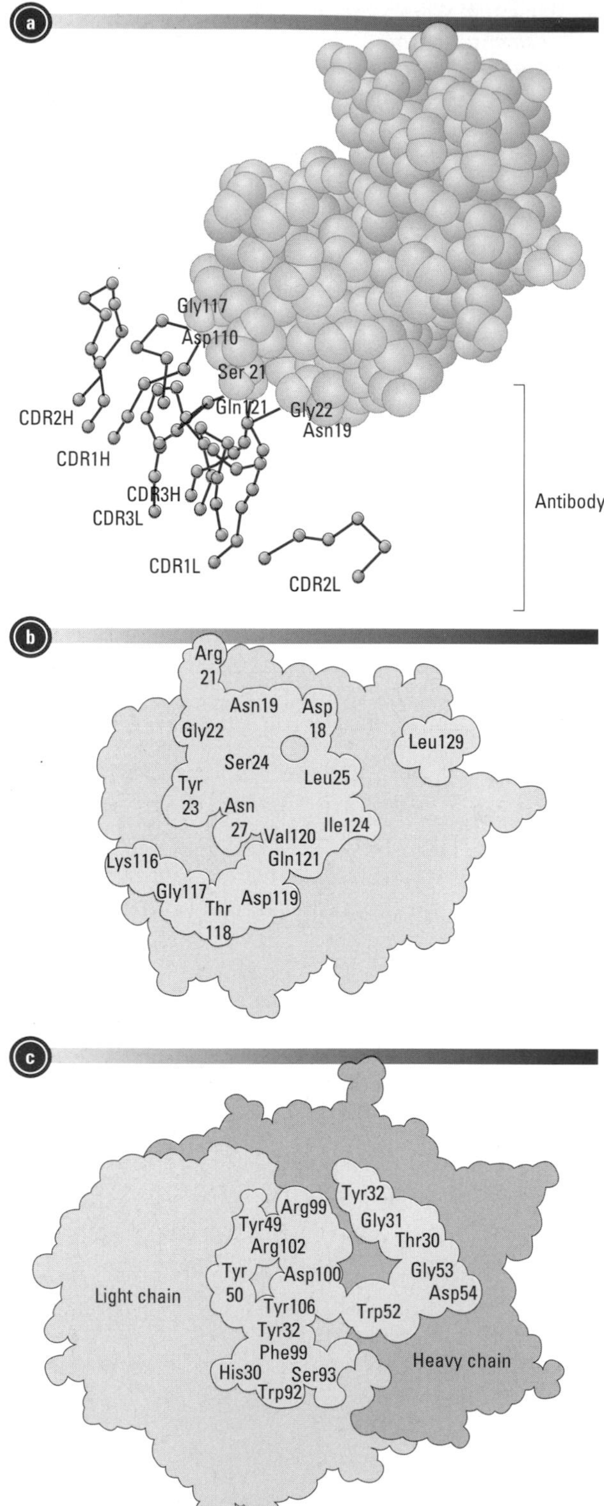

Figure 13.18 (*Left.*) Interaction between hen egg-white lysozyme (HEL) and an HEL-specific monoclonal antibody. (a) HEL–antibody complex. The antigen (HEL) is depicted in the form of a space-filling model with atoms shown as spheres. The combining site of the antibody is shown in the form of α-carbon backbones of the polypeptide segment. CDR, complementarity-determining residues in heavy (H) and light (L) chains. (b) End-on view of the lysozyme molecule in the region recognized by the antibody. The coloured (pink) part is the epitope with the indicated amino acid residues. (c) End-on view of the antibody-combining site (pink); the residues contacting the corresponding residues in the epitope are indicated. (a, Modified from Amit, A.G. *et al.* (1985) *Nature*, **313**, 156; b and c, based on Amit, A.C. *et al.* (1986) *Science*, **233**, 747.)

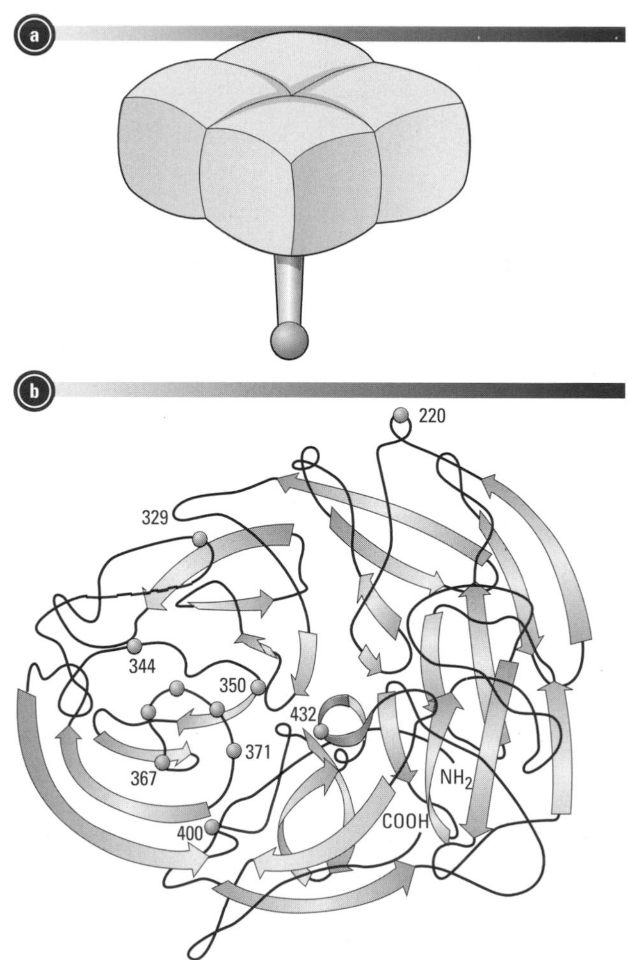

Figure 13.19 (*Above.*) Epitope recognized by antibodies on the neuraminidase (NA) molecule of influenza virus. (a) The NA tetramer with the cubical head region and the stalk by which the molecule is anchored in the virus envelope. (b) Folding of the polypeptide chain in one of the subunits of the head region. Numbers indicate amino acid residues. Coloured regions are part of the epitope. (a, Modified from Fields, B.N. *et al.* (Eds) (1985) *Virology.* Raven Press, New York; b, modified from Colman, P. M. *et al.* (1987) *Nature*, **326**, 358.)

Table 13.2 Physicochemical characteristics of antigen–antibody complexes analysed by X-ray crystallographic methods.

Antigen	Antibody	K_a (M)	Buried antigen surface area (nm2)	Antigen surface buried (%)	Buried Fab surface area (nm2)	Number of van der Waals' contacts	Number of hydrogen bonds	Number of electrostatic interactions	Reference
Haptens									
Phosphocholine	McPC603	1.7×10^5	1.37	81	1.61	30	2	3	1
Fluorescein	4-4-20	3.4×10^{10}	2.66	94	3.08	65	5	1	2
Peptides									
Myohaemerythrin	B1312		7.01	66	5.60				
Influenza haemagglutinin residues 100–108	17/9	5.0×10^7	4.36	59	4.68	74–81	13–15	1	3
Proteins									
Hen egg lysozyme	D1.3	1×10^9	6.80	12	6.90	75	15	0	4
Hen egg lysozyme	HyHel 10	5×10^9	7.74	14	7.21	111	14	1	5
Hen egg lysozyme	HyHel 5	2×10^{10}	7.50	14	7.46	74	10	3	6
Influenza neuraminidase	NC41		8.99	6	9.16	108	23	1	7
Immunoglobulin D1.3	anti-D1.3		8.00			100	9	1	8

K_a, association rate constant (see Chapter 14).

References: 1, Satow, Y. *et al.* (1986) *Journal of Molecular Biology* **190**, 593; 2, Herron, J. *et al.* (1989) *Proteins Structure, Function and Genetics* **5**, 271; 3, Stanfield R.L. *et al.* (1990) *Science* **248**, 712; 4, Schulze-Gahmen, U. *et al.* (1988) *Journal of Biological Chemistry* **263**, 17 100; 5, Amit, A.G. *et al.* (1986) *Science* **233**, 747; 6, Padlan, E.A. *et al.* (1989) *Proceedings of the National Academy of Sciences of United States of America (Washington DC)* **86**, 5938; 7, Sheriff, S. *et al.* (1987) *Proceedings of the National Academy of Sciences of United States of America (Washington DC)* **84**, 8075; 8, Tulip, W.R. *et al.* (1989) *Cold Spring Harbor Symposia on Quantitative Biology (Cold Spring Harbor NY)* **54**, 257; 9, Bentley, G.A. *et al.* (1990) *Nature* **348**, 254.

The number of residues in the epitope that contact the paratope ranges from 15 to 22 for proteins and from five to ten for peptides. All epitopes that have been characterized have proved to be discontinuous and to involve residues from two to five separate stretches. The contacts between epitope and paratope involve electrostatic interactions, hydrogen bonds and van der Waals' interactions (Table 13.2; see also Fig. 6.33). The last of these, named after the Dutch chemist Johannes Diderick van der Waals (1837–1923), occur between all atoms brought very close together (Fig. 13.20). The constant motion of the electrons of a normally non-polar atom cause it periodically to become fleetingly polar, i.e. to form a dipole, a structure having two equal but opposite charges. If an adjacent atom becomes distorted at the same moment, the opposite charges of the two atoms will produce an attractive force. Because the forces are very weak, they exert an effect only when atoms come very close together.

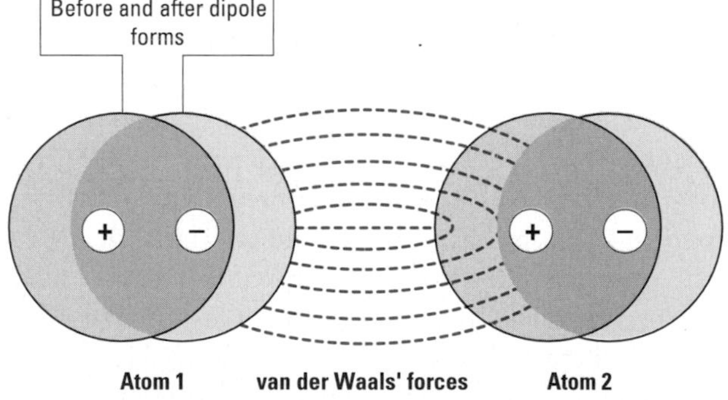

Figure 13.20 Principle of van der Waals' attraction. Atoms that are on average non-polar periodically become polar and thus exist as dipoles at these moments. A mutual attraction occurs between two rapidly fluctuating dipoles.

Contrary to a previously held notion that the paratope–epitope interaction requires expulsion of all water from the interface, water molecules have been found at several contact sites. It is believed that the molecules contribute to the stabilization of the interaction.

For many years, immunochemists have been debating whether the antigen–antibody interaction is accompanied by conformational changes in the participating molecules, whether the interaction is rigid, such as that between a lock and key, or whether the fit of the two molecules is induced to some degree. A resolution is now in sight. It has been observed that the antigen changes very little when it binds an antibody, whereas the latter may change considerably in some cases. Substantial rearrangements in the shape of the H3 loop occur in the antibody that binds influenza haemagglutinin. Significant changes take place also in the quaternary structure and arrangement of the L1 and H3 loops of the antibody that binds single-stranded DNA. Evidence is thus accumulating that *induced fit* does indeed contribute to antigen–antibody interaction.

Epitopes recognized by TCRs

Like BCRs (antibodies), TCRs focus on small, circumscribed areas of large antigenic molecules, i.e. they recognize *epitopes*. One can therefore speak of *T-cell epitopes* (an abbreviation for 'epitopes recognized by TCRs') and *B-cell epitopes*. There are, however, many differences between the two types of epitopes, of which one is cardinal: a B-cell epitope is a three-dimensional feature (usually a protrusion) on the surface of the antigenic molecule, whereas a T-cell epitope is in essence a two-dimensional string, a sequence of amino acid residues. Immunologists were aware of this difference for quite some time but began to understand its basis only recently. Numerous experiments have demonstrated that denaturation of a protein, unfolding of its secondary and tertiary structure, usually destroys, either entirely or partially, epitopes detected on an intact molecule by antibodies. In the cell-mediated immune response, on the other hand, T cells activated by immunization with native protein could be reactivated by reimmunization with denatured protein. The explanation of this difference is in the nature of antigen recognition by B and T lymphocytes. The BCR (antibody) binds an epitope on a native molecule or a molecular fragment on which the three-dimensional structure of the epitope has remained intact. The TCR, by contrast, normally does not come in contact with a native protein; instead it is presented with a small fragment (peptide) of the molecule only (exceptions to this rule exist; see Chapters 5, 7 & 21). Even when an immune T cell carries out its effector function, it does so through this fragment and not the whole antigen. Thus, when a cytotoxic T cell made immune to, say, influenza virus attacks a target, what it recognizes is not the virus itself, nor any of the components of the virus particle, not even a virus-encoded molecule on the surface of an infected cell. All it perceives is a peptide derived from one of the viral proteins and bound to the MHC molecule of the target cell.

All the other differences between T-cell and B-cell epitopes follow from this one cardinal distinction. Because BCRs and TCRs recognize native molecule and molecular fragments, respectively, B-cell epitopes are on the surface, whereas T-cell epitopes can be located anywhere in the molecule, even in its interior. For the same reason, B-cell epitopes are hydrophilic, mobile and usually non-contiguous, whereas T-cell epitopes are amphipathic, non-mobile and contiguous. Because the antigen-processing machinery is set up to deal with proteins and not other molecules, T-cell epitopes are, with some exceptions (see Chapter 21), peptidic in nature; B-cell epitopes, which do not require antigen processing prior to their presentation to BCRs, are not restricted to proteins but reside also on other molecules (carbohydrates, nucleic acids and lipids). For the same reason, again, a simple chemical group (hapten) attached to the surface of a large molecule may bind a BCR or an antibody if it finds one with a crevice deep enough to fit into and establish contacts that will hold it in place: it may become a B-cell epitope. By contrast, the likelihood is very small that the stretch of protein to which the hapten is attached will come through the antigen-processing machinery and be bound by an MHC molecule in such a way that the TCR will notice the difference between the modified and unmodified peptide. Finally, because the BCR recognizes *only* the epitope, whereas the TCR recognizes the peptide *and* part of the presenting MHC molecule, the concept of a T-cell epitope is inseparable from the MHC context. All in all, the concepts of B-cell and T-cell epitopes are very different from each other. A B-cell epitope is a physical entity, a feature on an antigenic surface. A T-cell epitope, on the other hand, is a mere label indicating where the peptide bound to an MHC molecule originated.

T-cell epitopes can be identified by the phylogenetic approach described earlier (see Fig. 13.10); by eluting the peptides bound to the MHC molecules, sequencing them and identifying their position in the protein from which they originated; or by measuring the peptide's ability to bind to a particular type of MHC molecule. In this last method, the peptides can be produced by proteolytic digestion of a protein (see Fig. 13.7) or synthesized chemically. The MHC-bound peptides can then be tested further for their ability to stimulate T lymphocytes in culture. Experiments of this type have shown that not all peptides capable of binding to MHC molecules are also capable of stimulating a T-cell response.

Superantigens

Antigens activate T lymphocytes by interacting with the peptide-binding groove of MHC molecules and the combining sites of the TCR. There is also a group of T-lymphocyte-activating substances, however, that act without engaging the peptide-binding or combining sites. The most potent among these are the *superantigens*. They are 'super' because they often stimulate a much more powerful response than conventional antigens. Immunologists have known about the existence of molecules now referred to as superantigens since the 1970s but the concept of superantigens only emerged in the last 6 years when pieces of seemingly unrelated information began to fall into place.

Superantigens are the products of microorganisms: viruses and bacteria. The viral and bacterial superantigens are structurally and functionally unrelated compounds united only by their mode of interaction with MHC and TCR molecules and the effect this interaction provokes. It is still not known how these very different compounds are able to act in such a similar way.

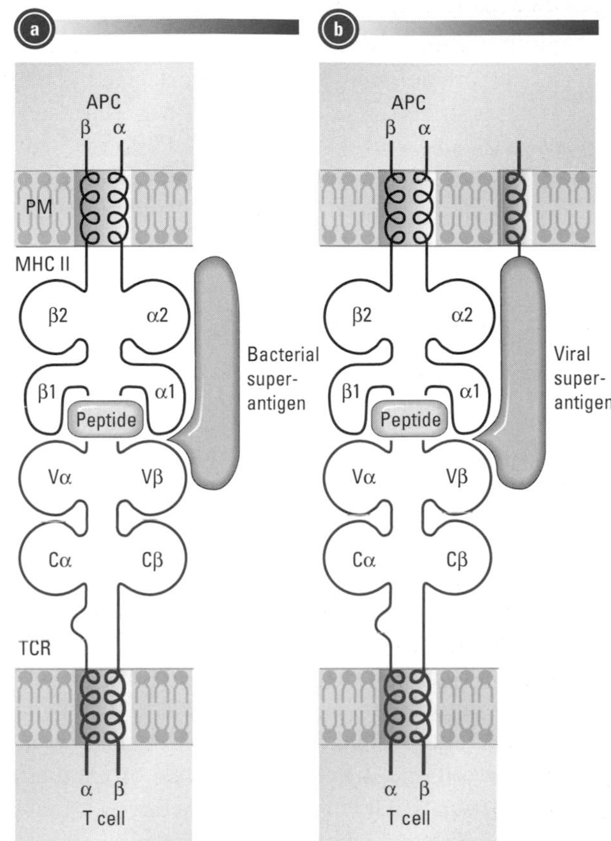

Figure 13.21 Interaction of bacterial (a) and viral (b) superantigens with the class II MHC molecule and the T-cell receptor (TCR). Bacterial superantigens are known to bind to the α1 domain of the class II molecule and to the Vβ domain of the TCR. Similar interactions presumably also take place between the viral superantigen, the class II MHC molecule and the TCR. Bacterial superantigen interacts in a soluble form, viral superantigen in a membrane-anchored form. APC, antigen-presenting cell; PM, plasma membrane.

Bacterial superantigens

Many bacteria secrete proteins that act adversely on the host and are therefore called *bacterial exotoxins* (see Chapter 21). Some bacteria produce only very few toxins while others secrete many. The best studied among the extracellular proteins are those produced by bacteria pathogenic to humans, particularly by staphylococci, streptococci, mycobacteria, *Mycoplasma* and *Yersinia*. They exert their toxic effects by blocking protein synthesis, inhibiting acetylcholine release in peripheral nerves, causing impairment of normal membrane permeability or by other mechanisms. Their action is an important part of pathogenesis in human infectious diseases such as cholera, diphtheria, anthrax, scarlet fever, pertussis, botulism, toxic shock syndrome and colitis. One group of exotoxins, the *superantigens*, has a dramatic effect on the host's immune system, causing massive proliferation of T lymphocytes and secretion of cytokines.

Bacterial superantigens are soluble globular proteins with an M_r between 25 000 and 80 000. They are relatively resistant to digestion by proteolytic enzymes, which is apparently an evolutionary adaptation to the environment in which many of them act (the intestine). All of them have a strong affinity for MHC class II molecules; none interact with class I molecules to any significant degree. In the mouse, they have a strong predilection towards association with the H2E molecule, the homologue of the human HLA-DR molecule. Some, however, bind also to the H2A molecule, the homologue of the human HLA-DQ molecule. Although the degree of association does vary between molecules encoded in allelic genes, this variation does not correlate with the specificity of the peptide-binding region (PBR). Indeed, it could be shown that the interaction between superantigens and class II MHC molecules takes place outside the PBR and that it does not require antigen processing; superantigens react with the MHC not as peptides but as molecules, as whole native proteins (Fig. 13.21).

The interaction of the superantigen with the MHC molecule, however, does not suffice for lymphocyte activation. The latter occurs only when the superantigen has simultaneously become bound to a TCR molecule. Superantigens bind almost exclusively to variable domains of the TCR β chain, largely ignoring the Vα domain. Some of the bacterial superantigens are related in their sequence while others are totally unrelated. Based on their sequences, they can be divided into several groups. Different groups of superantigens bind to different groups of TCR Vβ domains but each superantigen of a given group is capable of interacting with any member of a group of TCR Vβ sequences, regardless of the differences in the TCR's combining sites (Table 13.3).

Table 13.3 Bacterial superantigens and their specificity for TCR Vβ groups. (From Owen, P. & Meehan, M. (1994) in *Immunochemistry* (Eds C.J. van Oss & M.V.H. van Regenmortel), p. 393. Marcel Dekker, New York.)

Bacterium	Superantigen	M_r (× 10^3)	TCR Vβ specificity	Disease
Staphylococcus aureus	Enterotoxin A	26–28	?	Food poisoning, non-menstrual toxic shock
	Enterotoxin B	26–28	3, 12, 14, 15, 17, 20	Food poisoning, non-menstrual toxic shock
	Enterotoxin C1	26–28	12	Food poisoning, non-menstrual toxic shock
	Enterotoxin C2	26–28	12–15, 17, 20	Food poisoning, non-menstrual toxic shock
	Enterotoxin C3	26–28	5, 12	Food poisoning, non-menstrual toxic shock
	Enterotoxin D	26–28	5, 12	Food poisoning, non-menstrual toxic shock
	Enterotoxin E	26–28	5.1, 6.1, 6.3, 8, 18	Food poisoning, non-menstrual toxic shock
	TSST1	22	2	Toxic shock syndrome
Streptococcus pyogenes	Enterotoxin A	26	2, 12, 14, 15	Scarlet fever, psoriasis, toxic shock
	Enterotoxin B	29	8	Scarlet fever, psoriasis, toxic shock
	Enterotoxin C	24	1, 2, 5.1, 10	Scarlet fever, psoriasis, toxic shock
Group A streptococci	M protein (type 5)	40–80	2, 4, 8	Rheumatic fever and heart disease, glomerulonephritis

TSST1, toxic shock syndrome toxin 1.

The range of TCRs with which a given superantigen can interact is therefore much wider than that of a conventional antigen. While an antigen can bind to only 1 in 10^4 or 10^6 cells, a superantigen can bind to up to 40% of all T lymphocytes! A superantigen that has formed a bridge between the TCR of one cell and the class II molecule of another (see Fig. 13.21), usually a B lymphocyte, generates a signal that activates the T lymphocyte. A massive proliferation of T cells therefore follows an exposure to a superantigen. The advantage of such an exaggerated host T-cell response for the microbe is not clear. One possibility is that it leads to non-specific suppression of the immune system: by engaging so many cells that cannot harm the microorganism itself, the parasite draws attention away from its activities and uses this distraction to establish itself in the host. The activation of T cells is accompanied by the secretion of large quantities of cytokines and ends in the death of most of the proliferating cells. It may, therefore, represent part of the strategy by which the pathogen evades host immunity.

The tertiary structures of three bacterial superantigens have been resolved by X-ray diffraction analysis: the staphylococcal enterotoxin B (SEB) (Fig. 13.22), the staphylococcal enterotoxin A (SEA) and the toxic-shock syndrome toxin-1 (TSST1). The structures of SEB and TSST1 complexed with MHC class II molecules, as well as the structure of SEC superantigen with the TCRβ chain, have also been determined (Fig. 13.23). In the case of the SEC, the superantigen contacts the CDR1 (30%), CDR2 (47%), framework region 3 (13%), and the HV4 region (10%) of the TCRβ chain (the percentages relate to the total contact area of 1300 Å). The CDR3 and the entire variable region of the TCRα chain make no direct contact with the superantigen. The contact between the superantigen and the MHC class II molecule is restricted to the α chain of the latter. The superantigen wedges itself between the TCRβ chain and the MHCα chain, thus restricting the interaction between the TCR and MHC molecules and circumventing the normal mechanisms of T-cell activation by specific MHC/peptide assemblages.

Viral superantigens

Two types of viruses are known to manufacture superantigens: rhabdoviruses, exemplified by the causative agent of rabies; and the mouse mammary tumour virus (MMTV), a representative of the retrovirus category. As most of the work on viral superantigens has been carried out with the MMTV model, we limit our description to this virus.

Retroviruses are characterized by the possession of an enzyme, reverse transcriptase, that converts the RNA of their genome into DNA, the *provirus*. Integration of the provirus into the host cell chromosomes is an essential step in the life cycle of the retrovirus. Normally, the provirus integrates into the genome of the somatic cell, but from time to time it invades the chromosomes of a germ cell and is then perpetuated from generation to generation as if it were one of the host's own genes. At some point, it may lose its ability to instigate the formation of infectious virus particles and propagate itself merely as a piece of 'selfish DNA'. Its presence may go unnoticed by the host except in those cases in which the virus hitch-hikes a host's gene and turns it into a cancer-causing oncogene.

MMTV is a retrovirus whose infectious particles are transmitted via milk from mother to offspring and whose insertion into the genome causes, in some cases, cancer of the mammary gland in female mice. During the last 5–8

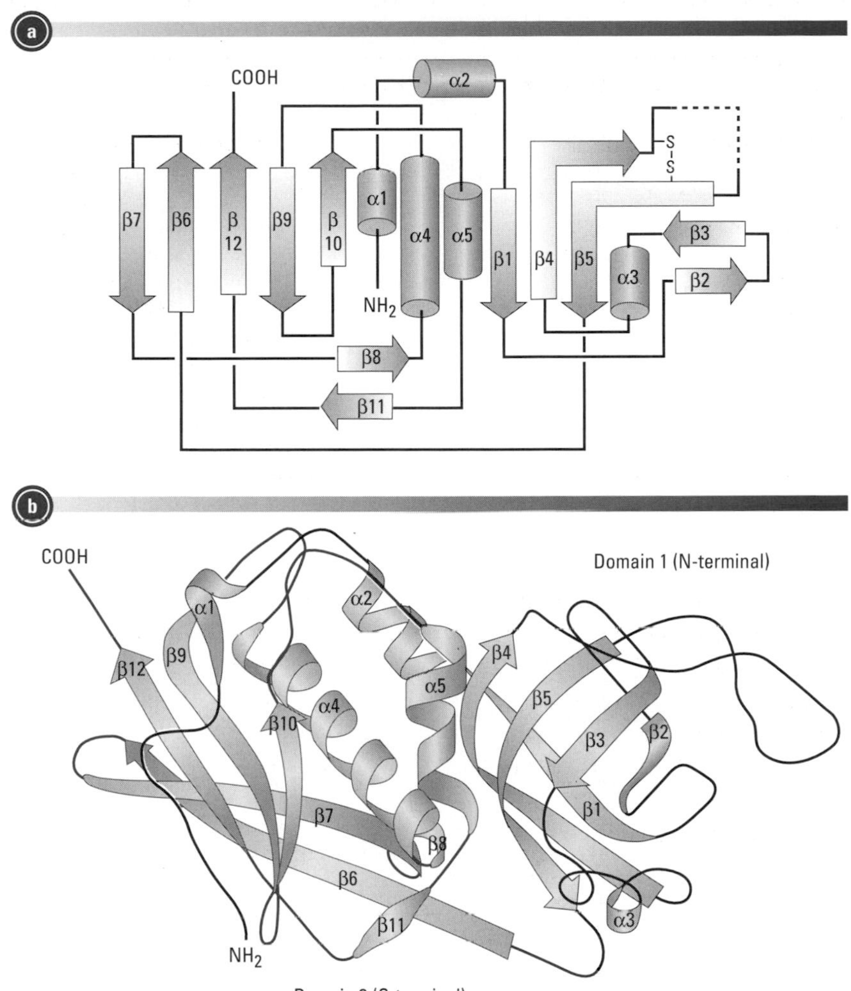

Figure 13.22 Structure of staphylococcal enterotoxin B (SEB). (a) Secondary structure. (b) Ribbon model of tertiary structure. The five known staphylococcal enterotoxins (A–E) are related but serologically distinct molecules secreted by various strains of *Staphylococcus aureus*. They cause food poisoning characterized by vomiting, diarrhoea and profound immune response. They act as superantigens by stimulating a large proportion of Vβ-bearing T lymphocytes. The SEB molecule consists of two domains, one comprising residues 1–120 and the other residues 127–239 with six residues forming a bridge between the two domains. Domain 1 contains two β-sheets, one formed by strands β1, β4 and β5, and the other by strands β2, β3, β4 and β5 (strands β4 and β5 curve around to form part of both strands). It also contains α-helices α1, α2 and α3 and one disulphide bond (S–S). The two sheets form a cylindrical barrel. Domain 2 consists of two parts. One part is comprised of α-helices α4 and α5 and of two very short strands, β8 and β11. The second part is comprised of strands β6, β7, β9, β10 and β12. The tertiary structure of staphylococcal enterotoxin A (SEA) is similar to that of SEB, even though there is only 36% sequence identity between the two proteins. The toxic shock syndrome toxin 1 (TSST1) molecule is smaller than either SEA or SEB and it lacks certain portions of the structure formed in these two molecules but otherwise the topologies of all three superantigens look alike. The TSST1-binding surface on the class II MHC molecule is extended, however, and also includes the peptide bound in the peptide-binding groove. The orientation of the TSST1 molecule in the complex with class II molecules, and presumably also in its interaction with the T-cell receptor, is somewhat different from that of the SEB molecule. (Adapted from Swaminathan, S. *et al.* (1992) *Nature*, 359, 801.)

million years, the mouse genome has been invaded on several occasions by MMTV proviral DNA. Both laboratory strains and wild mice carry MMTV proviral DNA at different sites referred to as *Mtv loci* and distinguished by numbers (*Mtv1–Mtv53*, with some gaps). Some of the *Mtv* loci are shared between strains while others differentiate various mouse groups. Each provirus is about 8.5 kb long and is flanked by *long terminal repeats* (LTR) generated

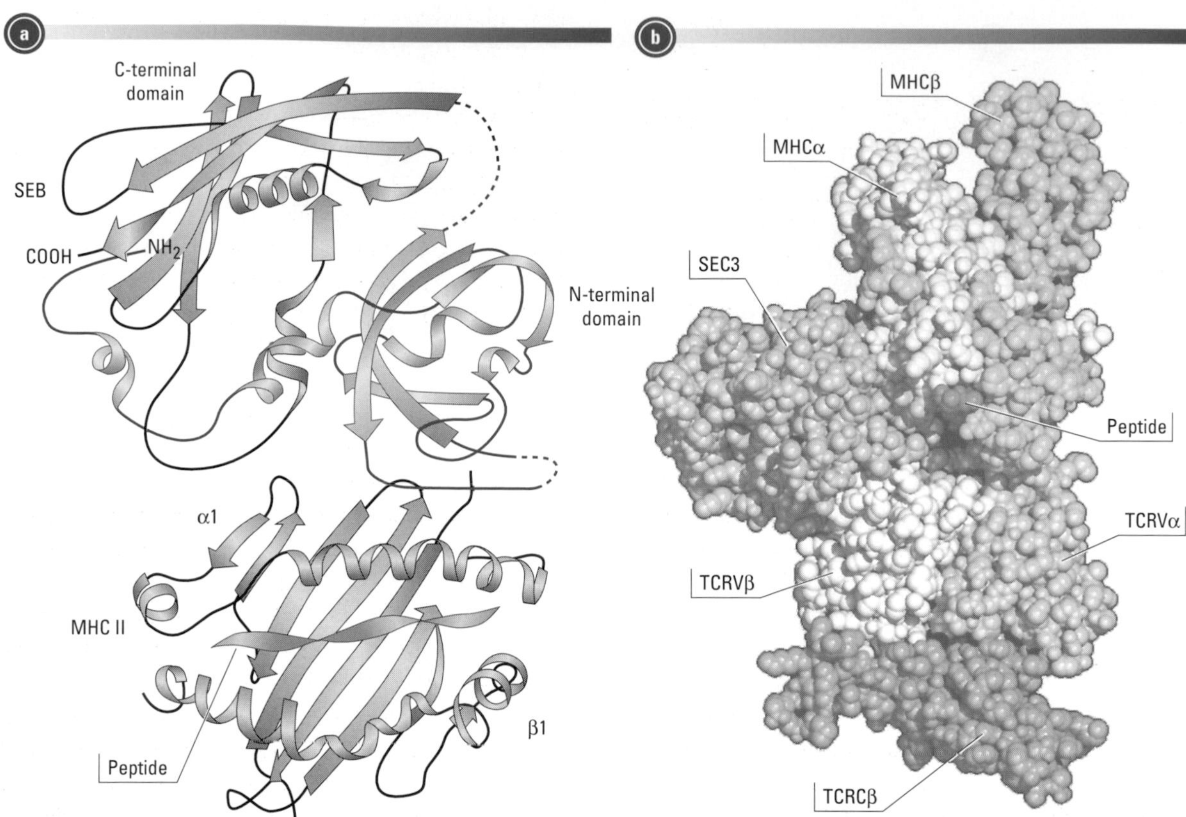

Figure 13.23 (a) The complex of the staphylococcal enterotoxin B (SEB) superantigen with an MHC class II (HLA-DR1) molecule. Interaction occurs between the α1 domain of the class II molecule and the N-terminal domain of the SEB molecule. The contact sites in the DR1 α1 domain are located on the first and third turns of the β-sheet (see Fig. 6.38) and in the N-terminal region of the α-helix. The contact residues form a deep, concave surface to one side of the peptide-binding groove. The contact sites in the SEB N-terminal domain are located in a turn between strands β1 and β2 and along strand β3 (see Fig. 13.22). The C-terminal SEB domain is oriented up and away from the class II molecule but three residues from the C-terminal helix α5 participate in the interaction with the class II molecule. The T-cell receptor (TCR)-binding region of the SEB molecule is believed to comprise a shallow cavity formed by residues from both domains (four residues from α2, one residue from β1, three residues from β4, two residues from β5, one residue from β10 and nine additional residues from interconnecting regions; see Fig. 13.22). (Adapted from Jardetzky, T.S. *et al.* (1994) *Nature*, **368**, 711.) (b) Space-filling model of a TCR: SEC3: peptide: MHC complex. Note how the superantigen (SEC3) is wedged between the α chain of the MHC and the Vβ chain of the TCR molecules. MHC, major histocompatibility complex; SEC3, *Staphylococcus aureus* enterotoxin C3; TCR, T-cell receptor. ((a) Based on B.A. Fields *et al.* (1996) *Nature*, **384**, 188, courtesy of Dr Roy A. Mariuzza.)

during the integration of the proviral DNA into the host chromosome (Fig. 13.24). Between the 5′ and 3′ LTR are the viral genes coding for the essential proteins needed for the propagation of the virus. But, as with many other retroviruses, most of the *Mtv* proviruses have lost their ability to produce infectious particles. Compared to other retroviruses, the 3′ LTR of the *Mtv* proviruses (and the corresponding region of the MMTV genome) is unusually long, containing an extra open-reading frame (ORF) of unknown origin. This ORF codes for a protein whose length can range from 323 to 330 residues, depending on which of the five available transcription initiation sites is used; it contains five potential *N*-linked glycosylation sites. The 5′ end of the nucleotide sequence specifying this protein overlaps with the 3′ end of the sequence coding for the envelope protein. The ORF element has its own promoter and several regulatory elements associated with it. The ORF-encoded protein, which has an M_r of about 45 000, integrates into the plasma membrane of B lymphocytes via a hydrophobic region near its N-terminus. It thus represents the so-called type II integral membrane protein which, in contrast to type I proteins, has its C-terminus on the outside and its N-

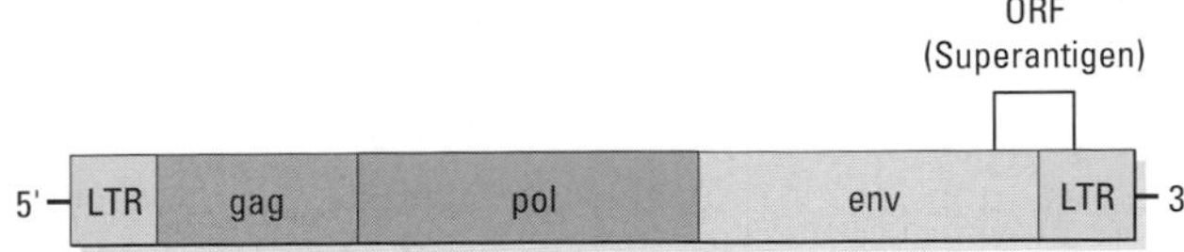

Figure 13.24 Mouse mammary tumour provirus (MMTV) genome. env, envelope (transmembrane glycoprotein); gag, group-specific antigen (core protein); LTR, long terminal repeat; ORF, open reading frame coding for the viral superantigen; pol, polymerase (reverse transcriptase).

terminus on the inside of the cell. However, the protein is easily cleaved by proteolytic enzymes and is released from the membrane in a soluble form. It is the membrane-bound form of the protein, however, that apparently functions as a viral superantigen.

MMTV superantigens produced by the various *Mtv* loci differ in sequence; in fact, their sequence identity can be as low as 85%. Most of the sequence differences are concentrated at the C-terminus, which contains a stretch of 21–38 highly variable amino acid residues. The various sequences can be classified into groups, each group capable of interacting with a particular set of TCR Vβ domains. In contrast to bacterial superantigens, viral superantigens interact with amino acid residues that are relatively distant from the peptide–MHC binding site of TCR molecules. The binding of MMTV superantigens to TCR and MHC molecules resembles that of bacterial superantigens, except that all three molecules are, in this case, membrane bound (see Fig. 13.21b). How the three molecules assemble to form the three-molecular complex is not known. The outcome of the interaction is similar to that involving bacterial superantigens (stimulation of the participating T cells), but the consequences are different.

MMTV requires epithelial cells of the mammary gland for the dissemination of its infectious particles. Epithelial cells, however, do not divide to a great extent and MMTV, like all retroviruses, can multiply only in dividing cells. MMTV has solved this dilemma in an interesting way. It initially infects B lymphocytes, inducing them to express viral superantigens on their surfaces. The superantigens interact with MHC class II molecules of the infected B cell and also with the TCR Vβ domains of helper (CD4+) T lymphocytes. The interaction of the three molecules activates both cells involved. The activated T cells produce cytokines that then trigger extensive B-cell proliferation, just what the virus needs for its multiplication! Moreover, the continuous activation ultimately exhausts the T cells and so lymphocytes that might have become involved in the immune response against the infectious virus particles are deleted from the T-cell repertoire.

Now, however, the virus faces another problem. The initial infection occurs when the young are still suckling. At this early age, the stomach is not yet acidified and the virus particles are therefore able to pass through it unharmed and reach the epithelium of the intestine before its replacement by a less supportive, adult epithelium. After crossing the epithelium, the virus is taken up by B cells of the underlying Peyer's patches and with the B cells is then delivered to the mammary gland. Once there, it is transferred in an unknown manner to the epithelial cells, where it completes its cycle. It thus uses the lymphocytes to multiply and to produce a large number of immature virus particles, as well as to transfer these particles to the mammary gland epithelium, where they mature and can be transmitted to the young in another infectious cycle.

The mouse, plagued by MMTV (in addition to having its immune system disturbed by the virus, it also runs a high risk, especially with increasing age, of being afflicted with a mammary carcinoma), may be searching for a way to strike back at the virus. As already mentioned, most of the *Mtv* loci are defective in the sense that they cannot initiate the production of infectious particles. However, they code for viral superantigens that, when expressed early in life in the thymus, cause the deletion of T lymphocytes with matching TCR Vβ domains. Some immunologists interpret this extensive purge of the mouse T-cell repertoire as an attempt on the part of the host to rid itself of the virus: in the absence of T lymphocytes, which the infected B lymphocyte would otherwise have stimulated via the viral superantigens, the B cells do not receive the signals necessary for their proliferation, without which MMTV cannot multiply. If this really is a measure to protect the mouse, it is a costly one because among the deleted T cells there undoubtedly must be many that the host could use for protection against other pathogens.

The superantigens encoded in the *Mtv* loci were identified many years before their real nature was recognized. As mentioned in Chapter 6, mixing of allogeneic lymphocytes in culture results in the proliferation of T cells. In most instances, proliferation can be observed only when the stimulating and the responding cells differ in their MHC, particularly class II molecules. In the mouse, however, it was also found to occur in certain strain combinations matched for their MHC loci. The molecules responsible for the stimulation were designated as *Mls antigens* (for *mixed lymphocyte stimulatory* or *minor lymphocyte stimulating*). The nature of the Mls antigens remained elusive until it was discovered that they are actually the products of the *Mtv* loci.

Adjuvants and immunostimulants

Definition and classification

Adjuvants (Latin *adjuvere*, to help) are substances that non-specifically augment the specific immune response to an antigen when mixed with the antigen prior to injection or when injected separately but into the same site. Substances that cause a transient general increase in immune response without having to be mixed with the antigen are referred to as *immunostimulants*. They differ from adjuvants in boosting the overall response rather than the response to a single antigen. The dividing line between the two groups of immunopotentiating substances, however, is not a sharp one.

The diverse and heterogeneous substances included in the adjuvant category can be loosely divided into six groups: oil adjuvants, mineral salts, synthetic polymers, liposomes, natural substances and others. The best-known representative of the *oil-adjuvant* category is *Freund's adjuvant* (named after the US immunologist Jules T. Freund (1890–1960)), which is used in one of two forms: complete or incomplete. *Complete Freund's adjuvant* is prepared by mixing mineral oil, heat-killed *Mycobacterium tuberculosis* and an emulsifying agent, such as lanolin (a fatty secretion of the sebaceous glands of the sheep) or Arlacel A (a complex mixture of neutral, moderately polar, predominantly carbohydrate polymers), adding a saline solution of the antigen to the above and emulsifying the mixture. The adjuvant then becomes a creamy emulsion, consisting of tiny drops of antigen surrounded by mineral oil; the bacilli stick to these droplets because of their lipophilic properties. *Incomplete Freund's adjuvant* is prepared in the same way but without the bacilli. Of the two, complete Freund's adjuvant is the more potent stimulator of immune response. For maximum effect, the adjuvant must be injected subcutaneously or intradermally. Another oil used as adjuvant is *Bayol F*, composed of paraffin (43.5%), monocyclic naphthalene (31.4%) and polycyclic naphthalene (26.1%).

The best-known representative of the *mineral salt adjuvants* is *aluminium sulphate* with K^+, Na^+ or NH_4^+ ions. Its formula is $AlK(SO_4)_2·12H_2O$, $AlNa(SO_4)_2·12H_2O$ or $AlNH_4(SO_4)_2·12H_2O$. When added to a solution, the salt precipitates the antigen and the precipitate can then be injected into the animal. Because of their excellent safety record, aluminium compounds are the most commonly used adjuvants in humans. Other mineral substances with an adjuvant effect are silica, kaolin and carbon.

The group of *synthetic polymers* includes synthetic polyribonucleotides, such as polyinosinic–polycytidilic (poly IC) and polyadenylic–polyuridylic (poly AU) acids, as well as non-ionic polymer surfactants, in particular pluronic polyol compounds composed of co-polymers of hydrophilic polyoxyethylene and hydrophobic polyoxypropylene in different proportions. (*Surfactants* are substances that reduce the surface tension of a liquid; they include detergents and emulsifiers.)

Liposomes are small vesicles that form spontaneously when phospholipids are placed in water. The phospholipids form two layers resembling the bilayer of biological membranes, with the hydrophobic tails oriented internally and the hydrophilic heads facing the aqueous phase (Fig. 13.25). A liposome can consist of one such bilayer (*unilaminar liposome*) or several, concentrically organized bilayers (*multilaminar liposome*). Antigens trapped within artificial liposomes often stimulate higher responses than antigens inoculated in aqueous solutions.

Natural substances that act as adjuvants are produced by fungi, parasites and especially by bacteria. The best-known representative is *wax D*, extracted by chloroform from *M. tuberculosis*. It is composed of glycolipids and peptidoglycolipids; the minimal structure required for activity is *N*-acetyl-muramyl-L-alanyl-D-isoglutamine (muramyldipeptide or MDP; Fig. 13.26). Muramyldipeptide is the main active principle of complete Freund's adjuvant. Other active substances are present in *Bordetella pertussis*, *Salmonella typhimurium* and in bacteria of the *Brucella* group. *Bordetella pertussis* is the small, non-motile, Gram-negative aerobic bacillus that causes whooping cough. The cell possesses several substances that act synergistically to enhance the immune response. The main adjuvant components are lipopolysaccharide (LPS) and pertussis toxin (PT). LPS is mentioned briefly in Chapter 12; PT is an exotoxin with the ability to activate adenylate cyclase in the cells of the bronchial epithelium. It potentiates immune response by altering the recirculation of T lymphocytes. *Salmonella typhimurium* is one of the most common types of salmonellae found in humans; it causes disease in mice and other animals. Its adjuvant activity is mediated principally by LPS, specifically by the *lipid A* portion of the molecule (see Chapter 21).

The remaining group includes all adjuvant substances that do not fit into any of the previous groups. Examples are vitamin A and tapioca (starch from the root of the tropical American plant, *Janipha manihot*).

Mechanism of action

The augmentation of the immune response by adjuvants is

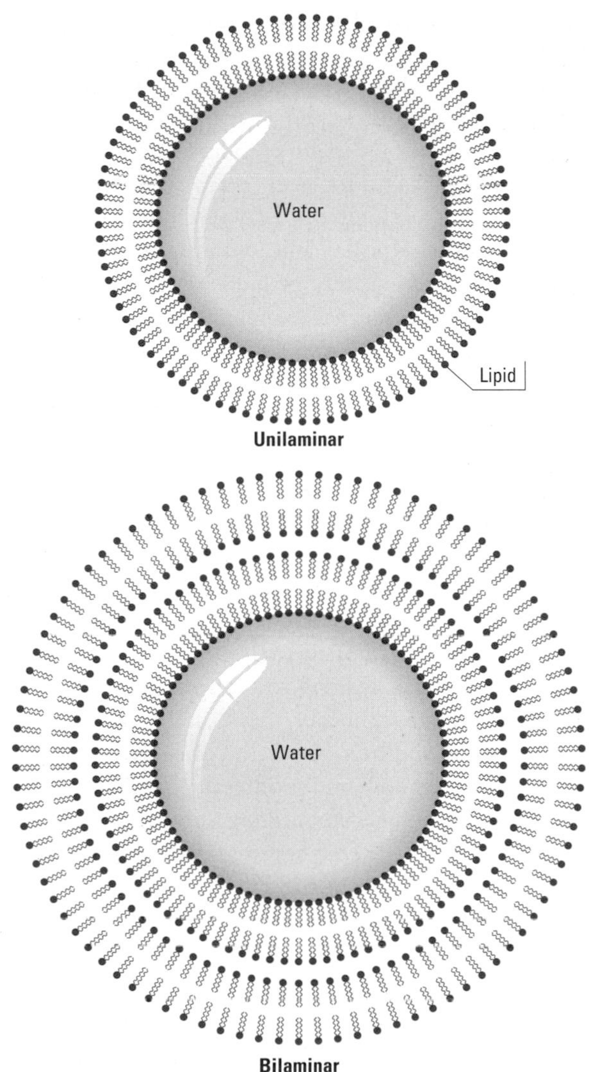

Figure 13.25 Liposomes consisting of one lipid bilayer (unilaminar liposome) or two concentrically arranged bilayers (bilaminar liposome). Each lipid consists of a polar head oriented towards the surface and two fatty acid chains oriented towards the interior of the bilayer.

the result of the combined effect of several factors, some of which are enumerated below.

1 Adjuvants trap the antigen and cause the formation of depots from which the antigen is released slowly over a prolonged period. The destruction of the antigen is thus delayed and the organism's exposure to the antigen lengthened.

2 Adjuvants stimulate non-specific migration of cells to the site of antigen injection and thus increase the probability of cell–antigen interaction. Often a dense, granular mass of cells, a *granuloma*, develops at the site of adjuvant injection.

3 Adjuvants increase antigen dispersion in the recipient's body by continually delivering the antigen in small droplets from the injection site to the regional lymph nodes or spleen.

4 Some adjuvants have a mitogenic effect: they stimulate lymphocyte proliferation non-specifically.

5 Some adjuvants (e.g. synthetic polyribonucleotides) help to stimulate lymphocytes by activating adenylate cyclase and other chemical messengers.

6 Adjuvants may increase the probability of contacts between T cells, B cells, macrophages and antigen through activation of lymphocyte-trapping mechanisms.

7 Adjuvants may tip the balance between tolerance and immunity in favour of the latter.

Some adjuvants act predominantly on T cells, others on B cells and others still on both T and B cells. Since purified antigens are often weak immunogens, adjuvants must be added to vaccines that contain synthetic peptides.

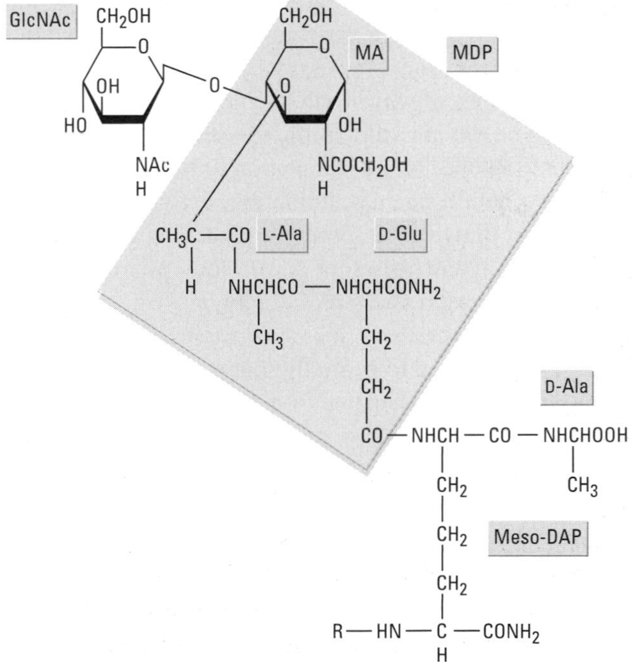

Figure 13.26 Structure of murein (peptidoglycan), the basic unit of mycobacterial cell walls. It consists of *N*-acetylglucosamine (GlcNAc), muramic acid (MA), L-alanine (L-Ala), D-glutamic acid (D-Glu), *meso*-diaminopimelic acid (Meso-DAP) and D-alanine (D-Ala). R indicates the connection to another such unit. Muramyl dipeptide (MDP) is the active component of Freund's adjuvant. (Modified from Barksdale, L. & Kim, S.-S. (1977) *Bacteriological Reviews*, **41**, 217.)

Unfortunately, the most potent adjuvants are also the most toxic.

Immunostimulants

Only two examples of these substances will be given here, BCG and *Corynebacterium parvum*. BCG is the abbreviation for *bacille bilié de Calmette–Guérin*, an attenuated strain of *M. tuberculosis* named after the French bacteriologists Léon C.A. Calmette (1863–1933) and Camille Guérin (1872–1961). BCG vaccination results in generalized enhancement of immune response, characterized by increased antigen clearance and phagocytosis, enhanced humoral immunity, accelerated graft rejection, increased resistance to infection and augmented tumour immunity. *Corynebacterium parvum* is a Gram-negative bacterium that, when given in a non-viable form, stimulates primarily macrophage functions and acts as an antitumour agent.

Lectins

Lectins (Latin *legere*, to select or choose, in reference to the ability of these substances to choose between different blood groups) are a heterogeneous group of compounds that have no structural features in common except that they are all proteins. They are characterized by the following three properties, of which only the first is mandatory for a protein to be classified as a lectin: specific binding to sugars, agglutination of cells and stimulation of lymphocytes.

Extracts with haemagglutinating activity have been obtained from over 800 species of plants, numerous invertebrates (snails and horseshoe crabs), some microorganisms (e.g. *Pseudomonas*) and a few vertebrates (e.g. the rabbit). Among plants, the main source of lectins is legumes, the family characterized by butterfly-shaped flowers; but agglutinins have also been isolated from pokeweed, castor beans, wheat, potatoes and many other species. Most lectins are found in the seeds, but some are also present in other parts of plants, such as roots, leaves and bark. Plant lectins are sometimes referred to as *plant haemagglutinins*, *phytohaemagglutinins* (Greek *phyton*, a plant) or *phytomitogens*. Of the large number of lectins, only about 50 have been isolated in a pure form.

All lectins bind sugars, but with varying specificity. Most lectins interact preferentially with a single sugar, such as galactose or fucose, but some have a broader specificity, reacting with a number of closely related sugars (e.g. mannose, glucose and arabinose); others still interact only with complex carbohydrates, such as those present in glycoproteins on the cell surface. The carbohydrate specificity and other properties of the common lectins are given in Table 13.4.

The interaction between lectins and cells occurs via a binding site of the former and a receptor of the latter. The binding site is specific for the carbohydrate carried by the receptor. A single lectin molecule often contains more than one binding site; a single cell may carry some 10^7 lectin-binding receptors. Normal cells, with the exception of erythrocytes, bind lectins only at high lectin concentrations. The earlier observation that malignant cells and cells transformed in culture are better at binding lectins than the corresponding normal cells raised hopes for using lectin binding as a marker for malignancy and transformation; however, subsequent studies have blurred the originally sharp dividing line between malignant and normal cells.

In some instances, lectin binding leads to cell agglutination; in others, agglutination does not occur, even though lectin attachment to the cell surface can be demonstrated. The mechanism of lectin-mediated cell agglutination is not yet fully understood, but the process apparently involves complex interactions leading to the formation of multiple bridges between adjacent cells.

Following the addition of a lectin, non-dividing lymphocytes grow, differentiate and proliferate; in other words, the lectin acts as a mitosis-stimulating substance or *mitogen* (see also Chapter 16). Lectin-stimulated lymphocytes display the same spectrum of functional characteristics as do lymphocytes stimulated by antigens: stimulated B lymphocytes differentiate into immunoglobulin-secreting plasma cells, whereas stimulated T lymphocytes produce cytokines and act as cytotoxic cells. The difference between antigen activation and lectin activation is in the number of activated lymphocyte clones: while an antigen activates only those T- or B-cell clones bearing the corresponding receptors (usually only about 0.02–0.1% of the cells), lectins activate many clones that carry receptors with different antigen-binding specificity, often as many as 30–60%. (For this reason, lectins are sometimes referred to as *polyclonal activators*.) However, lectins never activate *all* lymphocyte subsets (T or B cells) and even in each subset they activate only about one-third of the cells. The reason for this restricted activation is not clear, but the restriction is definitely not caused by the absence of lectin receptors: when cross-linked or bound to Sepharose beads, even lectins normally specific for T cells will activate B cells. The mitogenic effect is not common to all lectins; some lectins do not stimulate lymphocytes at all.

Several lectins (e.g. ricin and abrin) are highly toxic for mammalian cells. Once taken up by these cells, they inhibit protein synthesis by interfering with polypeptide-chain

Table 13.4 Lectins used in immunological research. (Adapted and modified from Kabat, E. (1976) *Structural Concepts in Immunology and Immunochemistry*, 2nd edn. Holt, Rinehart & Winston, New York.)

Lectin	Source	Specificity: Sugar	Specificity: Human blood group	M_r ($\times 10^3$)	Number of subunits	Association constant (number of binding sites)	Metalloprotein	Biological properties
Concanavalin A	*Canavalia ensiformis* (jack bean)	D-Manα1$\rightarrow$	A, B, O, AB (weakly)	102	4 (α4)	1.4×10^4 (4)	Mn^{2+} Ca^{2+}	Mitogen for T cells; B cells if aggregated
Ricin RCA I	*Ricinus communis*	D-Galβ1$\rightarrow$	None	118–120	4 (α2β2)			Low toxicity
Ricin RCA II		D-Galβ1$\rightarrow$	None	60–65	2 ($\alpha\beta'$)			Toxic
Soybean	*Glycine max*	D-GalNAcα1$\rightarrow$ 3-D-Galβ1$\rightarrow$ 3-D-GlcNAc	None	120	4 (α4)	3×10^4 (2)		
Wheat germ	*Triticum vulgaris*	D-GlcNAcβ1$\rightarrow$ 4-D-GlcNAcβ1$\rightarrow$ 4-D-GlcNAc	None	23	1			
Pokeweed	*Phytolacca americana*		A, B, O, AB	32	1			Mitogen for T and B cells
Phytohaemagglutinin E-PHA	*Phaseolus vulgaris* (kidney bean)	D-GalNAcα1$\rightarrow$	A, B, O, AB	140	4 (α2β2)			Mitogen for T cells (α subunit)
L-PHA		D-GalNAcα1$\rightarrow$	None	140	4 (α4)			Mitogen for T cells (α subunit)
Sponge agglutinin	*Axinella polypoides*	D-Galβ1$\rightarrow$6	None					
Sponge agglutinin (Aaptos lectin I)	*Aaptos papillata*	D-GlcNAcβ1$\rightarrow$ 4-D-GlcNAcβ1$\rightarrow$ 4-D-GlcNAcβ1$\rightarrow$ 4-D-GlcNAc	None					
Limulus haemagglutinin	*Limulus polyphemus*	*N*-acetylneuraminic acid	A, B, O, AB	400	18		Ca^{2+}	

elongation on polyribosomes. Many other lectins (for example, those commonly used in immunological studies) are also toxic, but at least 1000 times less so than ricin and abrin. Some lectins preferentially kill cells that have undergone malignant transformation.

The function of lectins in the life of a plant is not known, but several possibilities have been suggested: defence against soil bacteria, phytopathogens and insect predators; transport and storage of sugars; mediation of enzyme attachment in multienzyme systems; regulation of development, cell differentiation and cell adhesion; binding of nitrogen-fixing bacteria; and regulation of plant cell-wall extension.

Immunologists, cell biologists and biochemists have found a variety of uses for lectins. These include the generation of dividing lymphocytes for chromosome analysis, the separation and differentiation of cell subsets, the isolation of glycoproteins, the study of lymphocyte activation and the analysis of membrane fluidity.

The three lectins most frequently used in immunology are concanavalin A, phytohaemagglutinin and pokeweed mitogen. *Concanavalin A (Con A)*, one of the most extensively studied lectins and one of the most specific T-cell mitogens, is present in extracts from the jack bean, *Canavalia ensiformis* (Fig. 13.27). It is a pure polypeptide that constitutes about 15% of the total jack bean seed protein. It binds to sugars containing α-D-mannose or α-D-glucose residues in either the terminal or internal positions. The Con A molecule (M_r 102 000) consists of four identical subunits (monomers), each composed of one 237-residue polypeptide chain (M_r 30 500). Isolated Con A spontaneously forms dimers or high-molecular-mass aggregates, depending on the pH. The helmet-shaped monomers are paired, base to base, to form dimers and the dimers are then

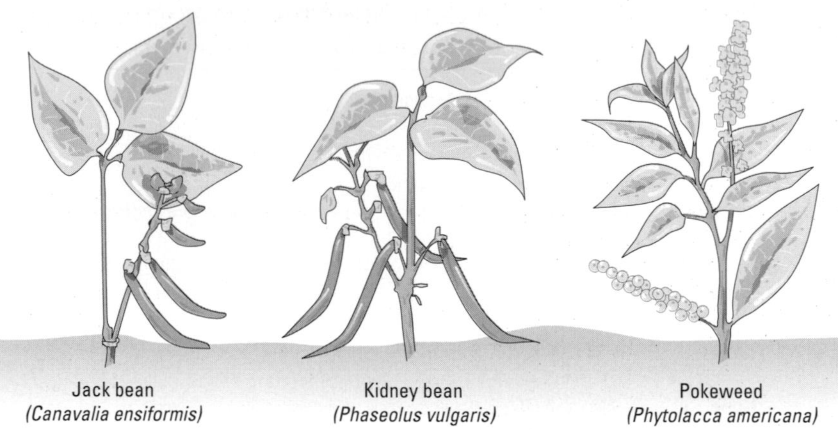

Figure 13.27 Plants from which the three commonly used lectins are extracted: jack bean, the source of concanavalin A (Con A); kidney bean, the source of phytohaemagglutinin (PHA); and pokeweed, the source of pokeweed mitogen (PM). (From Klein, J. (1982) *Immunology: The Science of Self–Nonself Discrimination*. John Wiley & Sons, New York.)

paired at right-angles to form tetramers (Fig. 13.28). Part of the polypeptide chain in the monomer is arranged into two antiparallel, β-pleated sheets, while the rest forms a random coil (Fig. 13.29). Each monomer has one carbohydrate binding site and one binding site for each of the Ca^{2+} and Mn^{2+} ions needed for interaction with the carbohydrate.

Phytohaemagglutinin (PHA) is the lectin (haemagglutinin) from the kidney bean (see Fig. 13.27); however, the designation is sometimes used as a generic name for haemagglutinins of plant origin. Like Con A, PHA (M_r 140 000) is a tetramer but, unlike Con A, it is composed of two kinds of subunits, L and R. The L form agglutinates leucocytes (hence the designation), but no erythrocytes, and is mitogenic; the R form agglutinates red blood cells but has no mitogenic activity. The tetramers are composed of one of five possible monomeric combinations: L_4, L_3R, L_2R_2, LR_3 and R_4. Mixtures of L_4 and L_3R molecules agglutinate leucocytes and are therefore referred to as L-PHA; mixtures of L_2R_2 and LR_3 (H-PHA) agglutinate both leucocytes and erythrocytes; and R_4 molecules agglutinate erythrocytes

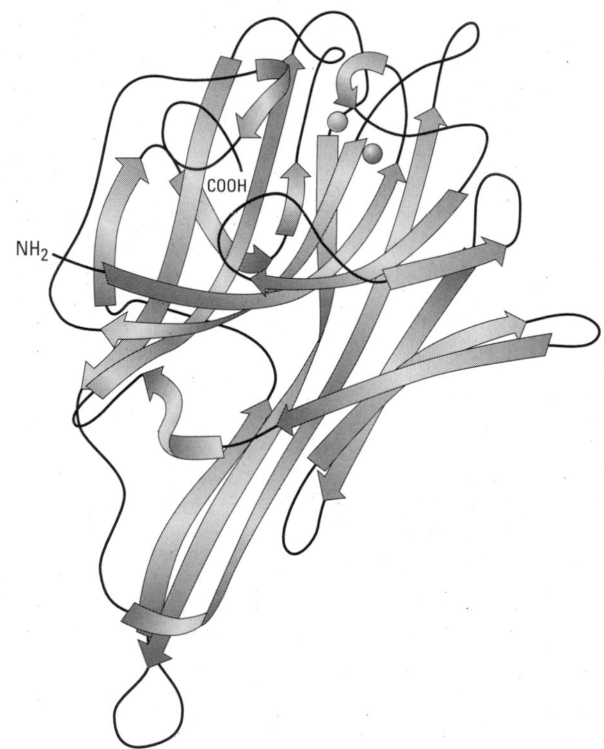

Figure 13.29 Tertiary structure of concanavalin A subunit: ribbon model. Spheres are calcium and manganese cations. (From Protein Data Bank Swiss 3-D; based on data from Becker, J.W. *et al.* (1975) *Journal of Biological Chemistry*, **250**, 1513.)

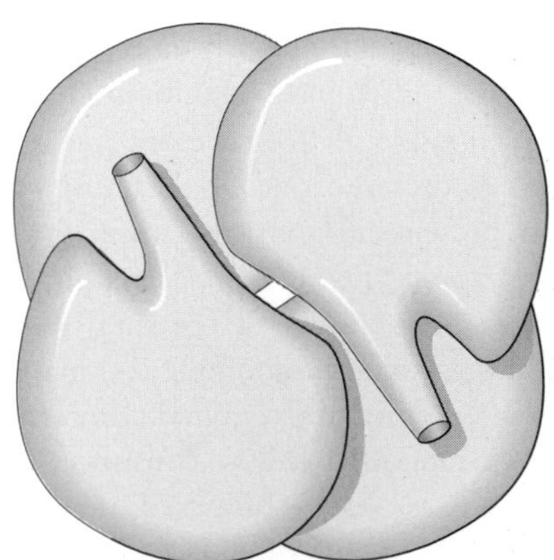

Figure 13.28 Arrangement of monomers in the tetrameric molecule of concanavalin A. (From Klein, J. (1982) *Immunology: The Science of Self–Nonself Discrimination*. John Wiley & Sons, New York.)

but, in contrast to the other two PHA preparations, do not possess mitogenic activity. Commercially available PHA is a mixture of these various forms. The R and L monomers are homologous in structure and probably related in their origin. PHA is a T-cell mitogen specific for complex polysaccharide.

Pokeweed mitogen (PWM) is found in the roots of pokeweed, *Phytolacca americana* (see Fig. 13.27). It is a mixture of at least five mitogenic proteins, one of which is a polymer, mitogenic for both T and B lymphocytes, while the other four are T-cell mitogens. PWM binds to di-*N*-acetylchitobiose.

Other lymphocyte-activating substances

Lymphocytes can be activated by a variety of substances in addition to antigens and lectins. The most important of these are lipopolysaccharides and immunoglobulin- or TCR-specific antibodies. Lipopolysaccharides are described in Chapter 21. Antibodies to immunoglobulins or TCRs can be class specific, allotype specific or idiotype specific. Immunoglobulin-specific antibodies activate B lymphocytes but not T lymphocytes, whereas TCR-specific antibodies activate T but not B lymphocytes. A number of other antibodies specific for various cell-surface antigens can also activate lymphocytes, either alone or in conjunction with certain other lymphocyte stimuli.

Further lymphocyte-activating substances include certain cytokines, periodate, zinc ions, mercury, proteolytic enzymes (trypsin, chymotrypsin), polyanions (dextran sulphate, polynucleotides) and agents that cause the formation of aldehyde groups on the lymphocyte surface. Mild activation can also be accomplished by physical agents, such as heat, cold and ultrasonication. The mechanisms responsible for the activation are not understood; in some instances at least, the agents may be acting indirectly by changing the surface properties of lymphocytes, allowing other agents to become involved.

Further reading

Abrahmsén, L. (1995) Superantigen engineering. *Current Opinion in Structural Biology*, 5, 464–470.

Acha-Orbea, H. & MacDonald, H.R. (1995) Superantigens of mouse mammary tumor virus. *Annual Review of Immunology*, **13**, 459–486.

Davies, D.R., Padlan, E.A. & Sheriff, S. (1990) Antibody–antigen complexes. *Annual Review of Biochemistry*, **59**, 439–473.

Dyson, H.J. & Wright, P.E. (1995) Antigenic peptides. *FASEB Journal*, 9, 37–42.

Grey, H.M., Sette, A. & Buus, S. (1989) How T cells see antigen. *Scientific American*, **261**, 38–46.

Herman, A., Kappler, J.W., Marrack, P. & Pullen, A.M. (1991) Superantigens: mechanism of T-cell stimulation and role in immune responses. *Annual Review of Immunology*, **9**, 745–772.

Hopp, T.P. (1986) Protein surface analysis. Methods for identifying antigenic determinants and other interaction sites. *Journal of Immunological Methods*, **88**, 1–18

Laver, W.G., Air, G.M., Webster, R.G. & Smith-Gill, S.J. (1990) Epitopes on protein antigens: misconceptions and realities. *Cell*, **61**, 553–556.

Livingstone, A.M. & Fathman, C.G. (1987) The structure of T-cell epitopes. *Annual Review of Immunology*, **5**, 477–501.

Novotny, J., Handschumacher, M. & Bruccoleri, R.E. (1987) Protein antigenicity: a static surface property. *Immunology Today*, 8, 26–31.

Rothbard, J.B. & Gefter, M.L. (1991) Interactions between immunogenic peptides and MHC proteins. *Annual Review of Immunology*, 9, 527–565.

Sela, M. (Ed.) (1973–1987) *The Antigens*, Vols 1–7. Academic Press, New York.

Thibodeau, J. & Sékaly, R.-P. (Eds) (1995) *Bacterial Superantigens: Structure, Function and Therapeutic Potential*. R.G. Landes, Austin, TX.

Van Oss, C.J. & van Regenmortel, M.V.H. (Eds) (1994) *Immunochemistry*. Marcel Dekker, New York.

Warren, H.S., Vogel, F.R. & Chedid, L.A. (1986) Current status of immunological adjuvants. *Annual Review of Immunology*, **4**, 369–388.

Wilson, I.A. & Stanfield, R.L. (1993) Antibody–antigen interactions. *Current Opinion in Structural Biology*, **3**, 113–118.

chapter 14 Measurement of antigen–antibody interactions

Molecules of liquids are in constant motion: they bump into each other like balls, bounce apart, collide with other molecules, rebound, collide again, and so on. If one of the colliding molecules is an antigen (hapten) and the other happens to be the corresponding antibody, the molecules may not rebound after the collision; instead, the epitope may slip into the combining site and the two may stick together. The reason why the two molecules do not recoil from the collision is because at the same moment as their complementary surfaces come into contact, weak binding forces glue them together. These forces are the same as those governing protein-to-protein interactions in general: hydrogen bonds, ionic bonds, van der Waals' bonds and hydrophobic interactions. The bond holding the molecules together may be stronger in some cases and weaker in others, depending on how well the epitopes fit into the combining sites and the strength of the forces that develop between the molecules.

Law of mass action

The binding of an antigen to an antibody is not irreversible, however. No matter how perfect the fit between the two, sooner or later they will separate again. The reasons for the dissociation are slight conformational changes induced by the interaction and thermal motion of molecules: other molecules collide with the antigen–antibody complexes and during each collision some energy is passed onto the complexes, making them less stable. The dissociated molecules can then reassociate or associate with other molecules and so the process continues, a constant joining and parting. This situation can be expressed in the form of an equation:

$$\mathrm{Ag} + \mathrm{Ab} \rightleftarrows \mathrm{AgAb} \qquad (14.1)$$

where Ag represents the antigen, Ab the antibody and AgAb the antigen–antibody complex. (For easier reference, equations in this section will be numbered.)

According to the physicochemical law known as the *law of mass action*, the association rate (i.e. the rate at which antigen–antibody complexes form) is proportional to the concentration of antigen and antibody, and can thus be expressed as k_1[Ag][Ab], where k_1 is the *association rate constant* and the brackets indicate concentrations. Similarly, the dissociation rate of the antigen–antibody complexes is equal to k_2[AgAb], where k_2 is the *dissociation rate constant*. After the mixing of an antigen with an antibody, the solution eventually reaches equilibrium, in which the association rate equals the dissociation rate:

$$k_1[\mathrm{Ag}][\mathrm{Ab}] = k_2[\mathrm{AgAb}] \tag{14.2}$$

The k_1/k_2 quotient, the ratio of complexed to free reactants at equilibrium, is known as the *equilibrium constant*, K:

$$K = \frac{k_1}{k_2} = \frac{[\mathrm{AgAb}]}{[\mathrm{Ag}][\mathrm{Ab}]} \tag{14.3}$$

This equation can also be written:

$$K[\mathrm{Ag}][\mathrm{Ab}] = [\mathrm{AgAb}] \tag{14.4}$$

Let us first consider a situation in which each antibody possesses only one combining site and each antigen molecule only one epitope. The total concentration of antibody molecules $[\mathrm{Ab_t}]$ equals the sum of concentrations of free antibodies $[\mathrm{Ab_0}]$ and those bound to the antigen $[\mathrm{Ab_b}]$, where $[\mathrm{Ab_b}] = [\mathrm{AgAb}]$:

$$[\mathrm{Ab_t}] = [\mathrm{Ab_0}] + [\mathrm{Ab_b}] \tag{14.5}$$

The concentration of free antibodies is thus:

$$[\mathrm{Ab_0}] = [\mathrm{Ab_t}] - [\mathrm{Ab_b}] \tag{14.6}$$

If we now introduce the Ab value from eqn 14.6 into eqn 14.4, we obtain:

$$K[\mathrm{Ag}]([\mathrm{Ab_t}] - [\mathrm{Ab_b}]) = [\mathrm{AgAb}] \tag{14.7}$$

After multiplying out the left-hand side of eqn 14.7 and rearranging the values, we obtain:

$$K[\mathrm{Ag}][\mathrm{Ab_t}] = [\mathrm{AgAb}](1 + K[\mathrm{Ag}]) \tag{14.8}$$

and after dividing both sides of eqn 14.8 by $[\mathrm{Ab_b}](1 + K[\mathrm{Ag}])$, we obtain:

$$\frac{[\mathrm{AgAb}]}{[\mathrm{Ab_t}]} = \frac{K[\mathrm{Ag}]}{1 + K[\mathrm{Ag}]} \tag{14.9}$$

The ratio $[\mathrm{AgAb}]/[\mathrm{Ab_t}]$, which we designate as r, is the fraction of antibody molecules bound to the antigen (number of molecules of bound antigen per antibody molecule). Equation 14.9 thus becomes:

$$r = \frac{K[\mathrm{Ag}]}{1 + K[\mathrm{Ag}]} \tag{14.10}$$

If we now consider, instead of monovalent antibodies, identical (homogeneous) antibodies with n number of combining sites (n is the valency of the antibody), we can write eqn 14.10 as:

$$r = \frac{nK[\mathrm{Ag}]}{1 + K[\mathrm{Ag}]} \tag{14.11}$$

After multiplying both sides of this equation by $(1 + K[\mathrm{Ag}])$, and rearranging the values, we obtain:

$$r = nK[\mathrm{Ag}] - rK[\mathrm{Ag}] \tag{14.12}$$

and after dividing by [Ag], we obtain:

$$\frac{r}{[\mathrm{Ag}]} = nK - rK \tag{14.13}$$

or, if we designate [Ag] as c (the concentration of free antigen), we obtain:

$$\frac{r}{c} = nK - rK \tag{14.14}$$

When one has a set of values for r and c over a range of antigen concentrations available, one can plot r/c vs. r. This so-called *Scatchard plot* (developed by G. Scatchard in 1949; Fig. 14.1) should, theoretically, give a straight line of slope K (provided that all antibody-combining sites are identical and independent). The x (abscissa) intercept of this line gives the n, and the y (ordinate) intercept gives the nK value.

To calculate K and n from eqn 14.14, we must know $[\mathrm{Ab_t}]$, the total concentration of antibody molecules, [AgAb], the concentration of antigen bound by the antibody, and [Ag], the concentration of free antigen. However, the determination of total antibody concentration is possible only when one works with a pure antibody preparation. To avoid the pure-antibody requirement, one can use

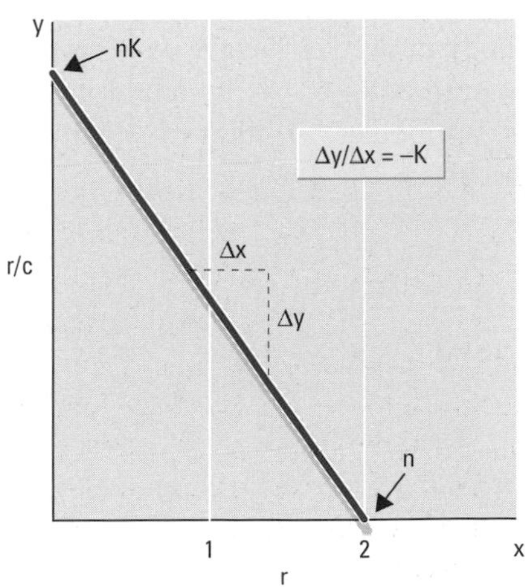

Figure 14.1 Scatchard plot of an antigen interacting with a homogeneous antibody. Explanation in the text. (Modified from Pickard, R.N. & Weir, D.M. (1973), in *Handbook of Experimental Immunology* (Ed. D.M. Weir), 2nd edn, p. 161. Blackwell Scientific Publications, Oxford.)

an alternative method for calculating K, a method in which one needs to know only the concentration of the free and bound antigen. In this method, one derives K for the antibody-combining site rather than for the antibody molecule and thus eliminates the n from consideration. Up to eqn 14.9, the derivation proceeds in the same way as in the preceding method, with the exception that the symbol Ab now means antibody-combining site. If we take the reciprocal of eqn 14.9, we have:

$$\frac{[Ab_t]}{[AgAb]} = \frac{1+K[Ag]}{K[Ag]} \qquad (14.15)$$

Dividing both sides of eqn 14.15 by $[Ab_t]$ produces:

$$\frac{1}{[AgAb]} = \frac{1+K[Ag]}{[Ab_t]K[Ag]} \qquad (14.16)$$

Expanding the right-hand portion of eqn 14.16, we obtain:

$$\frac{1}{[AgAb]} = \frac{1}{[Ab_t]K[Ag]} + \frac{1}{[Ab_t]} \qquad (14.17)$$

By plotting 1/[AgAb] against 1/[Ag], we obtain a straight line, with slope $1/K[Ab_t]$ and y intercept $1/[Ab_t]$.

Average association constant

One of the conditions in the preceding discussion was monovalency of antibodies: we assumed that each antibody had only one combining site, although we know that it normally has at least two. To take the bivalency into account, we can calculate K from a point on the straight line where, on average, each antibody reacts with only one instead of two epitopes (haptens); in other words, a concentration at which antibody molecules behave as if monovalent. Since for bivalent antibodies $r = 2$, it should be equal to 1 for monovalent antibodies, so that if r and $n = 2$, then eqn 14.14 becomes:

$$\frac{1}{c} = 2K - 1K \qquad (14.18)$$

or

$$\frac{1}{c} = K \qquad (14.19)$$

When defined this way, K is referred to as the *average association constant* and designated K_0. The *average association constant* is thus the reciprocal of free-antigen concentration. It is obtained by reading the r/c value from the straight line at $r = 1$. Concentration, c, is expressed in moles per litre and r/c (K_0) in litre moles.

Affinity and avidity

The strength of a reaction between monovalent antigen (hapten) and monovalent antibody (combining site) is referred to as *affinity*. Antibodies that combine loosely with antigens and dissociate readily are said to have low affinity, while those that bind tightly are said to have high affinity. Antibody affinity is influenced by many factors, which include the degree of stereochemical fit between the combining site and the epitope and the size of the region over which attractive or repulsive forces act. A measure of affinity is the equilibrium constant, K. The binding strength of a heterogeneous mixture of antibodies with diverse equilibrium constants is referred to as *average affinity*; the measure of average affinity is the average equilibrium constant, K_0.

Affinity must be distinguished from *avidity*, a term introduced at the end of the nineteenth century to explain the observation that antitoxin content ('antitoxin' being an antiserum against a bacterial toxin) does not always correlate with the protective ability of the antiserum. The observation was explained by the postulate that the protective ability depended on the antibody's binding power or avidity. Contemporary immunologists use the term 'avidity' to describe the overall tendency of antibodies to combine with antigens, particularly antibodies with multiple combining sites and antigens with multiple epitopes. Hence, affinity is a more precise, and avidity a more nebulous, designation for the rate of antigen–antibody reaction. Just to complicate matters, some immunologists use avidity synonymously with affinity, and others reverse the terms to mean exactly the opposite. Avidity is expressed in terms of *titre*, the last serial dilution of antibodies that still gives a measurable reaction with the antigen. Avidity is influenced by affinity, valency of antigens and antibodies and composition of antibodies

Methods of measuring equilibrium constants

A chemical reaction cannot proceed faster than the speed with which molecules meet by diffusion; since the antigen–antibody reactions approach this limit, the majority of collisions between antigens and antibody molecules result in bond formation. The antigen–antibody interaction is thus one of the fastest chemical reactions known. In comparison, interactions leading to covalent bond formation have an association rate one million times lower. Such fast reactions are difficult to study and it has been necessary to devise special techniques in order to measure them.

Several methods are available for determining the

value of the equilibrium constant, K, for a given antigen (hapten)–antibody reaction: equilibrium dialysis, fluorescent quenching, hapten inhibition of precipitation and ultracentrifuge measurement. In reality, however, all the methods are calibrated against the values determined by equilibrium dialysis.

Equilibrium dialysis

To calculate K, it is necessary to know the concentrations of free and bound hapten (antigen) after the hapten–antibody equilibrium has been established. To determine these two values, a dialysis cell is used, consisting of two compartments separated by a semi-permeable membrane. A known amount of the low-molecular-mass, radioactively labelled hapten is placed in one compartment and the high-molecular-mass antibody in the other, and then the solution in the antibody compartment is sampled periodically. The pores in the membrane are too small for the antibodies to move out of the compartment but large enough for the hapten molecules to move into it, thus allowing the hapten to diffuse into the antibody compartment until its concentration in both compartments is the same. However, some of the diffusing hapten will react with the antibody, so that at equilibrium the amount of *free* hapten will be the same in both compartments. But since the bound hapten does not 'count', the concentration of *total* hapten will be greater in the antibody compartment than in the hapten compartment (Fig. 14.2). The difference in the total hapten concentration between the two compartments indicates the amount of hapten bound to the antibody.

Fluorescent quenching

Tryptophan residues in a protein such as the antibody absorb ultraviolet (UV) light with a wavelength of 280 nm and emit fluorescent light with a wavelength of 330–350 nm. When an antibody reacts with an antigen, some of the energy that would normally be emitted is transferred to the bound molecules and dissipated. Binding of antigens to antibodies thus extinguishes or quenches the fluorescence of UV-irradiated molecules. Since the degree of fluorescent quenching is proportional to the number of antibody-combining sites interacting with the antigen, by measuring the fluorescence of an antibody solution during the gradual addition of small amounts of antigen the amount of bound antigen can be determined.

Inhibition of precipitation by a hapten

After a monovalent hapten has bound to an antibody-combining site, this site is no longer available for subsequent binding of bivalent antigens; since bivalent antigens are needed for the precipitation of antigen–antibody complexes to occur, the addition of a hapten inhibits antigen precipitation. Furthermore, since the more hapten that has been added, the greater the inhibition, one can determine the amount of free hapten using this assay.

Ultracentrifuge measurements

In this assay, the hapten reacts with antibody and the

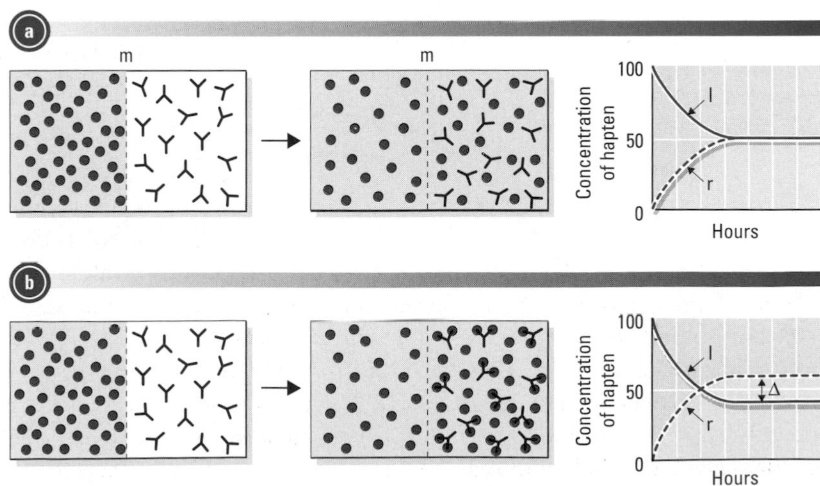

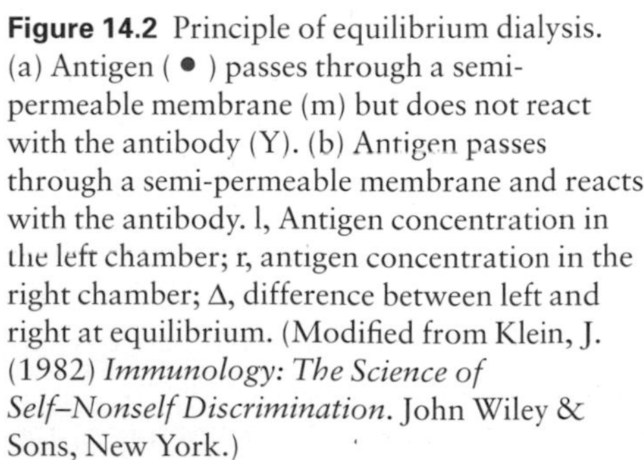

Figure 14.2 Principle of equilibrium dialysis. (a) Antigen (●) passes through a semi-permeable membrane (m) but does not react with the antibody (Y). (b) Antigen passes through a semi-permeable membrane and reacts with the antibody. l, Antigen concentration in the left chamber; r, antigen concentration in the right chamber; Δ, difference between left and right at equilibrium. (Modified from Klein, J. (1982) *Immunology: The Science of Self–Nonself Discrimination*. John Wiley & Sons, New York.)

mixture is then spun in an ultracentrifuge. Since free hapten sediments at a slower rate than hapten–antibody complexes, the two components can be separated and the concentration of free hapten determined.

Following this general introduction to antigen–antibody reactions, two specific forms by which the reactions manifest themselves, precipitation and agglutination, are now described. We begin with precipitation.

Precipitation

Assay

When a small molecule, such as a hapten, combines with an antibody, the resulting antigen–antibody complex remains soluble, and is thus invisible to the immunologist's eye; but when a macromolecule enters the reaction, the soluble antigen–antibody complexes fall out (*precipitate*) of the solution in a visible form. To measure the precipitin reaction, one sets up a series of tubes, adds a constant amount of antibody to each and then adds a progressively increasing amount of antigen to the tubes. After incubation in the refrigerator for at least 24 hours, one centrifuges the tubes, separates the precipitate from the supernatant and determines the amount of precipitate (antigen–antibody complexes), the amount of antigen and antibody in the precipitate and the presence or absence of antigen and antibody in the supernatant.

The amount of precipitate formed is measured by spectrophotometric methods based on the absorption of UV light. Sometimes it suffices to know only the amount of the precipitated antigen or of the precipitated antibody. To determine these values, one can use radioactively labelled reagents, either antigens or antibodies.

The determination of antigen and antibody content in the precipitate is closely connected with the determination of antigen and antibodies in the supernatant (see below). For the tubes in which the supernatant does not contain any demonstrable antigen after the reaction has taken place, it is assumed that all of the antigen has entered the precipitate. In this case, the amount of antigen in the precipitate equals the amount of antigen added to the tube, and the amount of antibody equals the total amount of precipitated protein minus the amount of antigen. In tubes in which some antigen remains in the supernatant even after the completion of the reaction, one must determine how much of the antigen is left behind and subtract this value from the total amount of antigen added to obtain the amount of antigen in the precipitate.

The data can be expressed in the form of a graph by plotting the values of total protein (or antibody) precipitated on the ordinate and the amount of antigen added on the abscissa (Fig. 14.3).

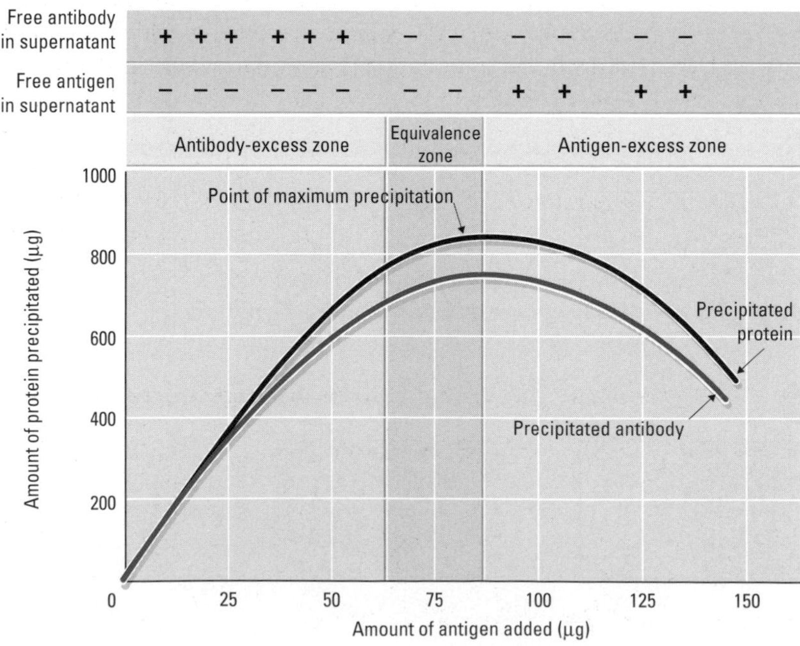

Figure 14.3 Precipitin curve. Quantitative precipitin reaction between ovalbumin and rabbit ovalbumin-specific antibody. (Based on data from Heidelberger, M. & Kendall, F.E. (1935) *Journal of Experimental Medicine*, **62**, 697.)

Precipitin curve

Figure 14.3 shows a typical plot of a quantitative precipitin reaction. It can be seen that, with the addition of increasing amounts of antigen, the amount of precipitate rises until it reaches a *point of maximum precipitation* and then declines. This particular precipitation curve starts at the 0 value on the abscissa; other curves, however, may start at some positive value and, instead of having the parabolic shape shown, may be bell-shaped. The shape of the curve depends to a large degree on the predominant class of antibody in the antiserum and on the solubility of the antigen–antibody complexes in the region of antibody excess.

Based on the results of supernatant testing, the curve can be divided into three zones: the *antibody-excess zone (prozone)*, characterized by the presence of free antibody and the absence of free antigen in the supernatant; the *equivalence zone*, characterized by the absence in the supernatant of both antigen and antibody; and the *antigen-excess zone*, characterized by the presence of free antigen and absence of free antibody (Fig. 14.3). The point of maximum precipitation usually lies in the equivalence zone or in the zone of slight antigen excess. The portion of the antigen-excess zone in which the quantity of antigen–antibody precipitate decreases is called the *inhibition zone*. In Fig. 14.3, the antigen-excess and inhibition zones overlap, but in the case of some other antisera the curve levels off in the antigen-excess zone before it starts to decline, and in such instances the inhibition zone constitutes only part of the antigen-excess zone; some immunologists even divide this zone further into zones of complete and partial inhibition.

With monospecific antisera (i.e. antisera reactive with a single epitope), the supernatants in individual test tubes are Ag^-Ab^+, Ag^-Ab^- or Ag^+Ab^-, but never Ag^+Ab^+. With polyspecific antisera (i.e. antisera containing a mixture of antibodies reactive with different epitopes), on the other hand, Ag^+Ab^+ supernatants may occur, and can be explained by different equivalence zones of the two or more antibodies involved: the doubly positive supernatants probably represent an $Ag_1{}^+Ag_2{}^-Ab_1{}^-Ab_2{}^+$ situation, in which Ag_1, Ag_2 and Ab_1, Ab_2 are two different kinds of antigen and antibody, respectively (the antigen-excess zone of one antigen overlaps the antibody-excess zone of the other). The occurrence of doubly positive supernatants thus provides a simple means of detecting polyspecificity of antisera in the precipitation test.

Lattice theory

The molecular composition of antigen–antibody complexes in the different zones of the precipitin curve influences the size and thus the solubility (or precipitability) of these complexes. In the antibody-excess zone, virtually every antigenic molecule is complexed with an antibody, but since there is not enough antigen to bind all antibody molecules some of these remain free. Furthermore, because of the relatively small number of antigenic molecules, there is only a low probability that a single antibody molecule will bind two antigenic molecules simultaneously, so that the predominant type of complexes consists of one antigen molecule surrounded by several antibody molecules. (The number of the latter depends among other things on the valency of the particular molecule; Fig. 14.4). Since small complexes are soluble and there is only a low probability that large, insoluble complexes will form, only a small amount of precipitate falls out of the solution. However, as the amount of added antigen increases, more antibody molecules cross-link individual antigen molecules and form a reasonably stable network, or lattice, of alternating antigen and antibody molecules (Fig. 14.4b). This lattice is most intricate in the equivalence zone, in which almost all antigen and antibody molecules participate in the formation of relatively large complexes. Then, as the concentration of antigen continues to increase, many antigen molecules surround each individual antibody molecule, separating it from the other antibody molecules and thus preventing lattice formation. This *lattice theory* explains why antigen–antibody complexing, unlike other

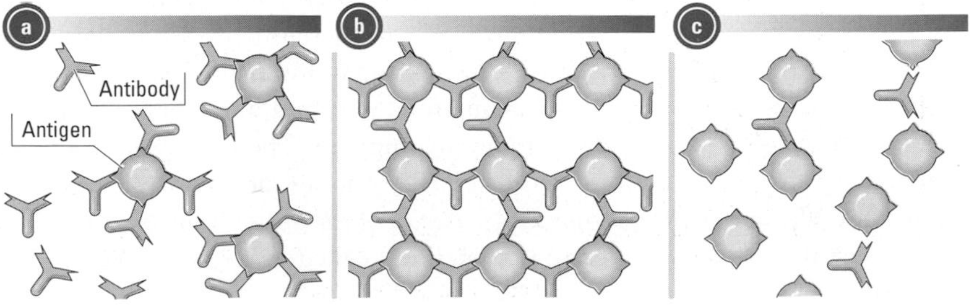

Figure 14.4 Predominant types of antigen–antibody complexes present in (a) antibody excess, (b) equivalence zone and (c) antigen excess.

biochemical reactions, reaches a maximum and then declines. The lattice theory, however, fails to take into account the interactions that take place outside the combining site of the antibody (e.g. interactions via the Fc regions).

An alternative to the lattice theory is the *two-stage model of immune precipitation*. In stage one of this model, antibodies interact with their corresponding antigens via combining sites and form complexes that can be either insoluble or soluble. In stage two, the insoluble complexes form the core of the precipitate to which the otherwise soluble complexes bind via portions of the antibody molecule outside the combining site.

Non-precipitating antibodies

In some instances, no visible precipitation occurs, although one can prove by other means that an antigen–antibody reaction is taking place and even though the same antigen tested with other antibodies precipitates normally. It must be the antibodies, therefore, that are responsible for the absence of precipitation. Originally, immunologists believed that the reason why some antibodies did not precipitate was their monovalency and hence their inability to cross-link the antigen, but we know now that all antibodies are at least bivalent. A more likely explanation is that non-precipitating antibodies are of low affinity and antigen must therefore be added in relatively high concentrations to sway the reaction in favour of antigen–antibody complex formation. However, since in the antigen-excess zone only small, soluble complexes form, no precipitate is discernible. Another interpretation assumes that the non-precipitating antibodies bind with both their combining sites to epitopes on the same antigenic molecule, rather than on different molecules. This type of *monogamous binding* precludes cross-linking of the antigen and so prevents lattice formation. The precipitating and non-precipitating antibodies may also differ in their rigidity: the more rigid antibodies do not precipitate well.

To detect non-precipitating antibody, one uses a trick introduced by R.S. Farr. The *Farr assay* is based on the observation that 50% saturation of a serum with ammonium sulphate results in the precipitation of immunoglobulins but not, for example, of albumin. One can therefore add radioactively labelled antigen to a constant amount of serially diluted antiserum and, after incubation, precipitate the globulin in each tube with ammonium sulphate. The radioactivity of the precipitate indicates the amount of antigen bound, i.e. the *antigen-binding capacity* of the antiserum. (For this reason, the assay is sometimes called the *ABC test*.)

Agglutination

The only principal difference between precipitation and agglutination is in the size of the antigen: in the former, the antigen is a soluble macromolecule; in the latter, a microscopic particle (a bacterium or an erythrocyte). Agglutination (clumping) results from the cross-linking of particles (cells) by antibodies (agglutinins) specific for antigen (agglutinogens) on the particle's surface. For agglutination to occur, a multivalent antibody must bind to an antigen on one particle with one combining site, and to an antigen on another particle with the other combining site, thus forming a lattice similar to that in the equivalence zone of the precipitin reaction. In the zone of antibody or antigen excess, antibodies bind to particles but do not cross-link (and hence agglutinate) them. For this reason, agglutinins often display a *prozone*, i.e. absence of agglutination at highest antibody concentrations. This fact must be kept in mind when testing agglutinating antisera because false-negative results may be obtained when an antiserum is not diluted sufficiently. Agglutination is strongly influenced by the ionic strength of the medium in which the clumping takes place. At neutral pH, bacterial cells and erythrocytes have a strong negative charge that normally keeps them at a distance and prevents their bridging by antibodies.

Methods for the detection of antigen–antibody reactions

Immunodiffusion tests

To observe *precipitation in liquid medium*, antiserum is dispensed into small tubes and carefully overlaid with an antigen-containing solution so that the two do not mix. Usually the amount of antiserum per tube is constant, whereas the antigen concentration increases from tube to tube. The precipitate produced at the interface of the antigen–antibody solution forms an opaque, clearly visible band or ring and for this reason the method is referred to as the *ring test*.

To observe *precipitation in semi-solid medium*, one (*simple* or *single diffusion method*) or both (*double diffusion method*) of the two immune reagents (antigens and antibodies) are allowed to diffuse through a gel (usually agar) and to form precipitin bands at the site where the two reagents meet. The agar gel can form either a column (*one-dimensional method*) or a plate (*two-dimensional method*). In the simple (single) diffusion in one dimension (*Oudin technique*), the antiserum is incorporated in the melted agar and the antibody–agar mixture is poured into tubes and allowed to form a gel (Fig. 14.5a). The antigen solution is

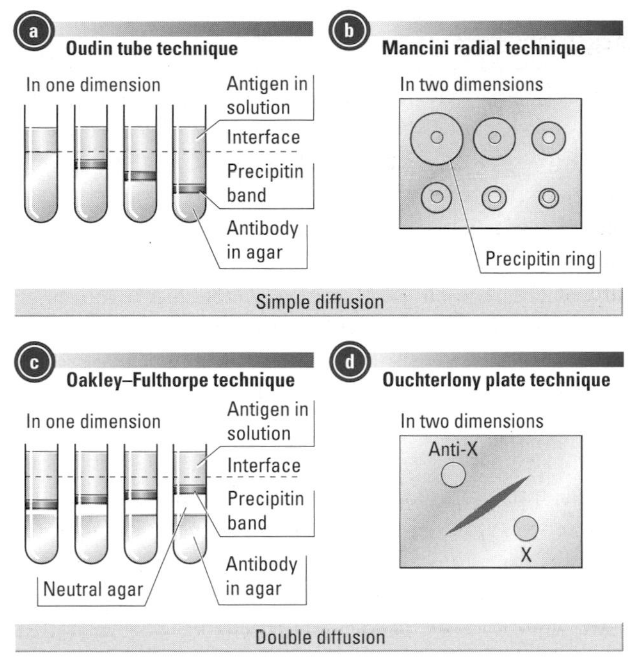

Figure 14.5 Types of precipitin (immunodiffusion) assay *in vitro*. X, antigen. (a) The antibody is incorporated in the melted agar in a test tube. The antigen is added on top of the vertical gel. The diffusing antigen forms a precipitin band in the equivalence zone. (b) Melted antibody-containing agar is spread on a slide and serially diluted antigen is placed into the punched-out wells. A growing circle of precipitate forms as the antigen diffuses radially through the agar. The area of the ring is proportional to the concentration of the antigen. (c) The antibody is incorporated in the melted agar in a test tube. Fresh agar (without antibody) is poured on top and the antibody from the lower agar layer is permitted to diffuse into it. Serially diluted antigen is then added on top of the neutral agar; as it enters the neutral agar it forms a precipitate at a decreasing distance from the interface depending on its concentration. (d) Wells are punched out on an agar plate and filled with antigen or antibodies. Precipitin lines form where the diffusing antigen and antibody meet. (Modified from Klein, J. (1982) *Immunology: The Science of Self–Nonself Discrimination*. John Wiley & Sons, New York.)

then added to the top of the vertical gel column and the tube is sealed to prevent evaporation. The antigen diffuses downwards into the gel, creating a concentration gradient that decreases from top to bottom. The diffusing antigen reacts with the antibody present in the gel, forming antigen–antibody complexes. In the region of the gradient where the concentration of the diffusing antigen is equivalent to that of the antibody, the complexes form a lattice of visible precipitate. Behind the moving front, the antigen concentration becomes too high relative to the concentration of the antibody and the formed precipitate dissolves again, just as in the antigen-excess zone of the precipitin curve. The precipitate thus forms a narrow band that moves down the tube with the front of the antigen concentration gradient. The speed of the downward movement depends on the speed of antigen diffusion, which in turn depends on the size and shape of the antigen molecules and on the antiserum concentration in the upper reservoir. If the reservoir contains several antigens, each with a different molecular mass, the antigens diffuse with different speeds and each forms a distinct precipitin band. Other versions of the immunodiffusion technique are depicted and described in Fig. 14.5b–d.

Immunodiffusion tests can be used to establish the identity of antigens. Consider, as an example, a situation in which an antiserum gives a single precipitin line when tested separately with two antigens: are the two antigens identical or does the antiserum contain two antibodies, one reacting with the first antigen and the other with the second? To answer this question, three triangularly arranged holes are made in an agar plate (Fig. 14.6), the antiserum is placed in one well and the two antigens are each placed in one of the other wells. Lines now form between the antiserum well and the two antigen wells. If the two antigens share epitopes, the two lines fuse smoothly (*line of identity*; Fig. 14.6a). If the antigens carry different epitopes, the two lines cross each other (*lines of non-identity*; Fig. 14.6b). If the antiserum contains antibodies to two different epitopes, both of which are present on one antigen and only one of which is present on the second, one of the two lines fuses with the other line but the second line forms a spur over the first (*lines of partial identity*; Fig. 14.6c). Finally, if one antigenic preparation contains a mixture of two antigens and the other preparation only contains one of these antigens, one line of identity plus a second line appear after the reaction with the mixture of X- and Y-specific antibodies (Fig. 14.6d). More complex patterns of lines form with multi-epitope antigens and multicomponent mixtures. How the different line patterns arise is explained in Fig. 14.7.

Immunoelectrophoresis

This technique is a combination of gel electrophoresis and immunodiffusion. There are many variants of the immunoelectrophoretic method. In the *standard immunoelectrophoresis (Grabar–Williams) technique*, melted agar is poured onto a glass plate and allowed to gel. A hole is then punched out in the agar and filled with the antigen solution and the antigens are separated by electrophoresis (see Fig. 6.16). Following this separation, the plate is removed from the electrophoresis apparatus, a longitudinal trough is cut in the gel, the trough is filled with antiserum and the plate is incubated to allow diffusion to take place. Where

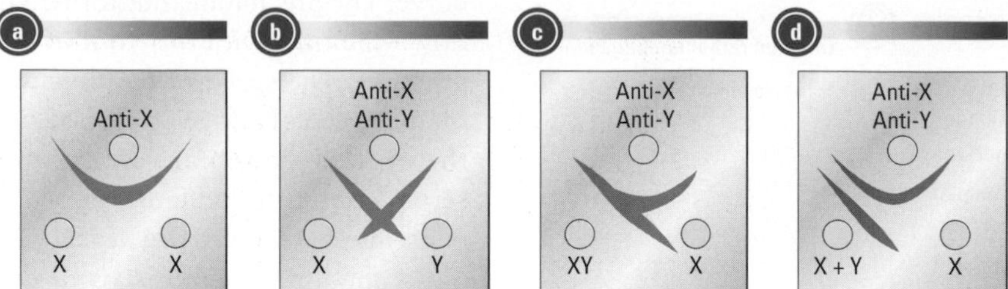

Figure 14.6 Precipitin lines formed by diffusion of antibodies (anti-X, anti-Y) and antigens (X and Y) from wells (circles) in agar gel. (a) Line of identity formed by antigens bearing the same epitope X and diffusing from two different wells against anti-X from a third well. (b) Lines of non-identity formed by epitopes X and Y on separate molecules diffusing against a mixture of anti-X and anti-Y. (c) Line of partial identity formed by antigenic molecules bearing epitopes X and Y and molecules bearing only epitope X. The two types of molecules are diffusing against a mixture of anti-X and anti-Y. (d) Lines formed when one well contains a mixture of molecules bearing X and molecules bearing Y epitopes, while the other well contains only molecules with the X epitope. The third well contains a mixture of anti-X and anti-Y.

the diffusing antigens meet the corresponding diffusing antibodies, characteristic arcs of precipitate form, one arc for each antigen–antibody system (Fig. 14.8). Other versions of the immunoelectrophoresis technique are shown in Fig. 14.9.

Methods based on agglutination

Agglutination assays are extremely versatile. One can agglutinate bacteria, erythrocytes, spermatozoa or even polystyrene particles; one can carry out the assay on a microscopic slide, in a test tube or in wells of a plastic tray; the diluent can be physiological salt solution, normal serum albumin, dextran or polyvinyl pyrrolidone; and one can score the result from the shape of the sediment, from shaking the tubes and counting the number of pieces the clump breaks into, from flushing the sediment with fluid or from observing the clustering of cells with the aid of a microscope. The scores are usually expressed semi-quantitatively in numbers of plus signs ('4+' indicating the strongest reaction and '–' standing for the absence of agglutination) and the overall result in titre (or the reciprocal thereof). The assay is thus rather imprecise, but this disadvantage is offset by its high sensitivity.

There are two principal forms of the agglutination assay, active and passive (Fig. 14.10). In the *active agglutination*

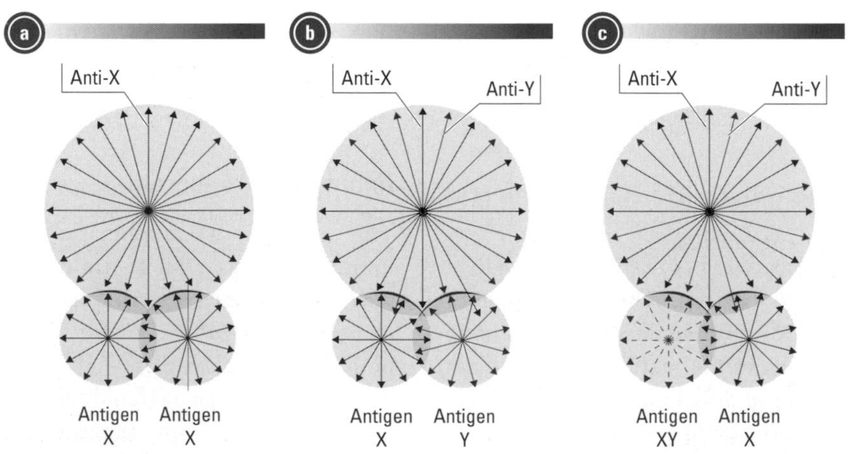

Figure 14.7 Formation of a line of identity (a), lines of non-identity (b) and lines of partial identity (c) in the double immunodiffusion technique. In (a) neither the antigen nor the antibody diffuses beyond the precipitin line. In (b), anti-Y diffuses beyond the X anti-X precipitin line and anti-X diffuses past the Y anti-Y line. In (c), neither anti-X nor anti-Y diffuses beyond the XY anti-X, anti-Y line, but anti-Y diffuses past the X anti-X line.

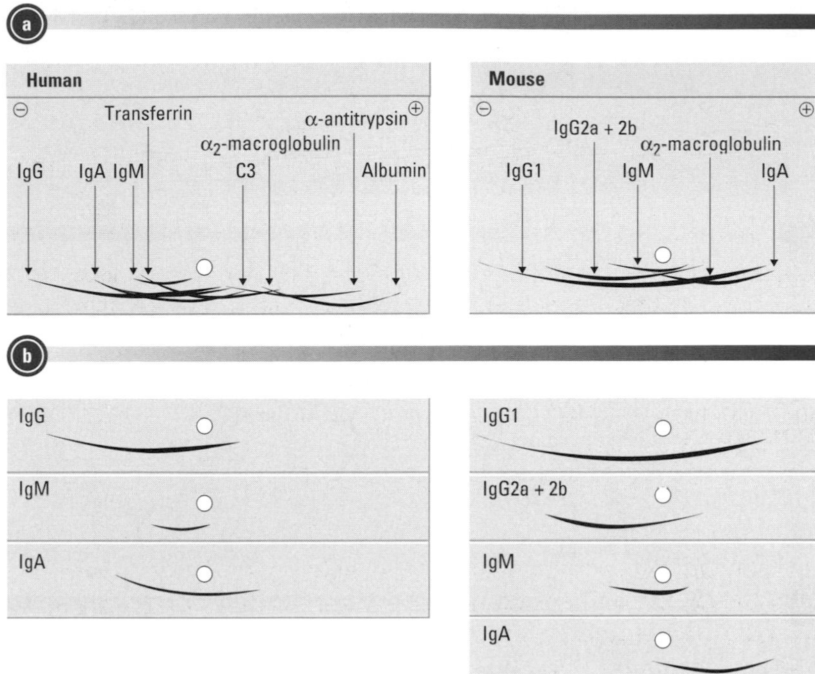

Figure 14.8 Immunoelectrophoresis of human and mouse normal sera. (a) Plates developed with antiserum made against the whole serum. (b) Plates developed with antisera specific for indicated immunoglobulin classes. (Modified from Klein, J. (1982) *Immunology: The Science of Self–Nonself Discrimination.* John Wiley & Sons, New York.)

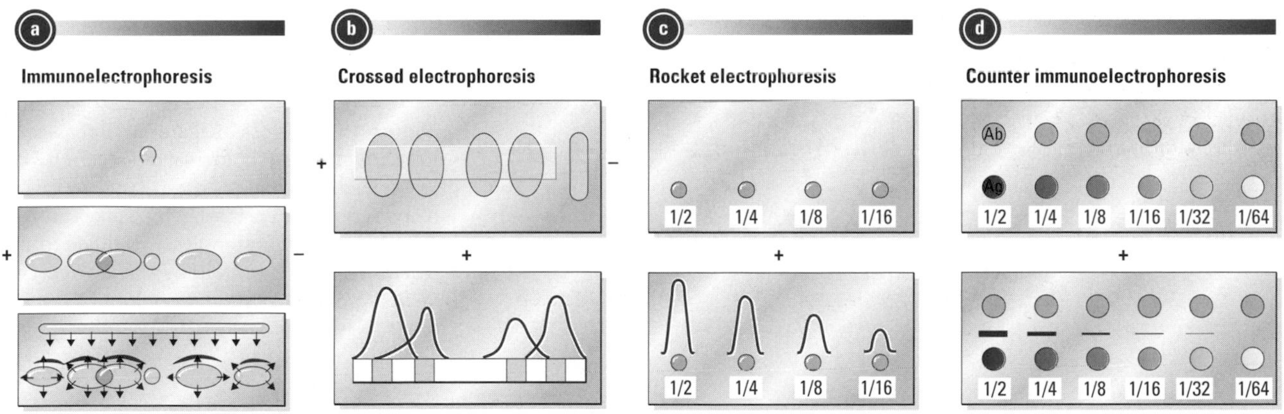

Figure 14.9 Types of electrophoresis. (a) *Immunoelectrophoresis.* Melted agar is poured onto a glass plate (top), a hole is punched out in the gel and the well is filled with antigen solution. The proteins in the solution are separated by electric current (middle). A longitudinal trough is cut in the gel and filled with antiserum. Where the diffusing antigens meet with the corresponding diffusing antibodies, characteristic arcs of precipitate form (bottom). (b) *Crossed electrophoresis.* A transverse slit cut in gel on a plate is filled with antigen and the individual proteins are separated by electric current. A longitudinal strip containing the separated bands is then cut out from the middle of the gel and laid on another plate; there it is overlaid with antibody-containing gel and an electric current is introduced in a direction perpendicular to the original direction. The diffusing antigens form a series of peaks, the height of which is proportional to antigen concentration. (c) *Rocket electrophoresis.* A series of holes cut along the edge of the agar-coated plate are filled with antigen at increasing dilution. Since the agar is soaked with antibodies, rocket-shaped peaks of precipitin develop when an electric current is introduced perpendicular to the row of holes. (d) *Counter immunoelectrophoresis.* Two rows of wells are cut out in the gel; wells of one row are filled with antibody and wells in the second row are filled with serial dilutions of the antigen. An electric current is then introduced making the antigen and antibodies travel against each other (this can happen, however, only when the two bear opposite charges). The technique is thus analogous to one-dimensional diffusion with the difference that the reactants are brought together by means of electrophoresis. (Modified from Klein, J. (1982) *Immunology: The Science of Self–Nonself Discrimination.* John Wiley & Sons, New York.)

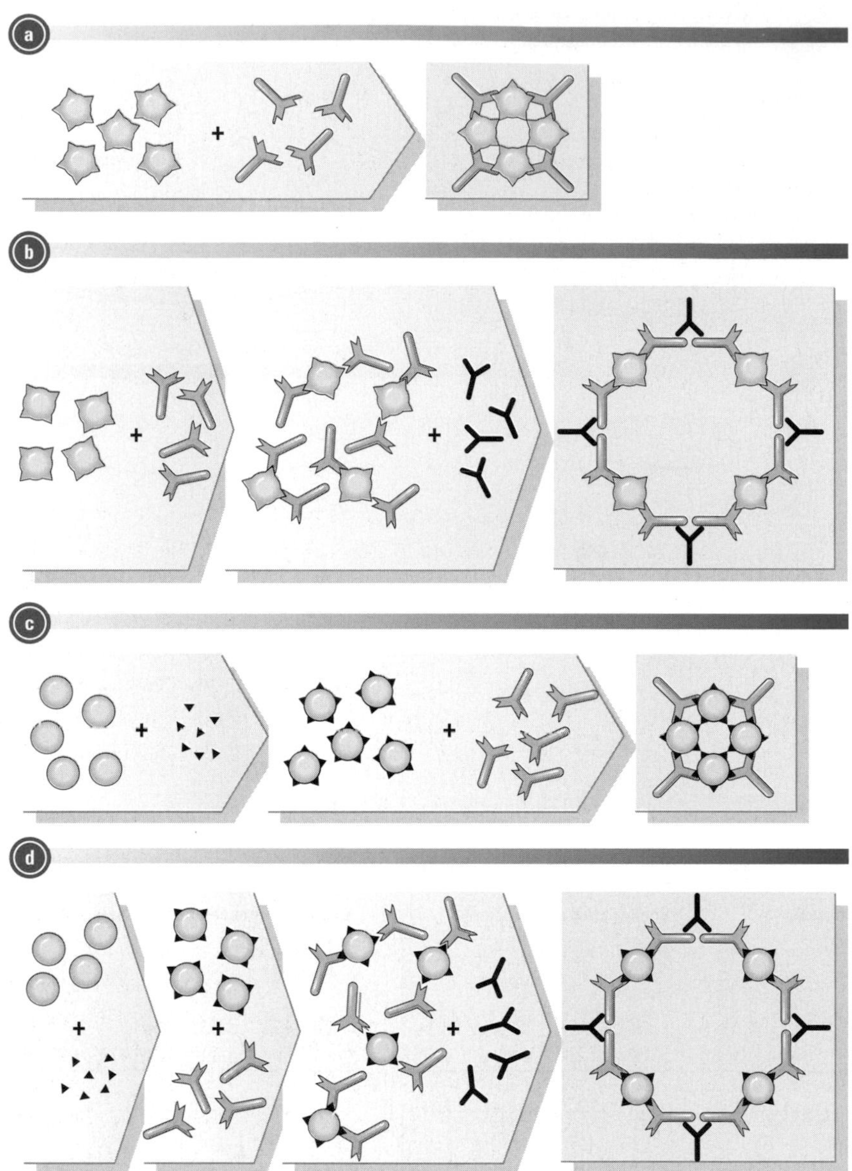

Figure 14.10 Types of agglutination assay: (a) active, direct; (b) active, indirect; (c) passive, direct; and (d) passive, indirect. Circles represent erythrocytes, spikes antigen, Y-shaped forms antibodies. (Modified from Klein, J. (1982) *Immunology: The Science of Self–Nonself Discrimination*. John Wiley & Sons, New York.)

assay, the antigen is indigenous to the particles and one can therefore achieve agglutination simply by mixing the particles with the antiserum. The active test can be either direct or indirect. In the *direct agglutination test* (Fig. 14.10a), particles are agglutinated by antibodies directed against antigens on the particles' surface. In the *indirect agglutination assay* (Fig. 14.10b), particles carrying antigen X are first allowed to react with anti-X (which alone is unable to agglutinate the particles) and then xenogeneic antiserum against anti-X is added to the mixture. The xenogeneic antibodies combine with the coating antibodies and bridge the particles. Because of the use of anti-immunoglobulin reagents, the system is also referred to as the *antiglobulin test* or, after the scientist who developed it, the *Coombs' test*.

In the *passive agglutination assay*, the antigen is attached to the particle's surface in one of two ways: via noncovalent bonds (e.g. erythrocytes spontaneously adsorb certain lipopolysaccharides of Gram-negative bacteria); or via special linkers and covalent bonding. Commonly used linkers are *bis*-diazotized benzidine and glutaraldehyde. As in active agglutination, the passive reaction can also be either direct (mediated solely by antibodies to the antigen; Fig. 14.10c) or indirect (mediated by anti-immunoglobulin serum directed against the coating antibody; Fig. 14.10d).

The principle of competitive inhibition, which is described later in this chapter, forms the basis of the *agglutination inhibition assay*. Here, soluble antigens are added to the agglutination system, and as their concentration increases they occupy more and more of the antibody-combining sites, making them unavailable for particle agglutination. A special case of agglutination inhibition occurs with certain viruses that bind directly to erythrocytes via cell-surface receptors. The resulting erythrocyte clumping can be inhibited by the addition of antibodies that react with the viruses, rendering them incapable of attaching themselves to the red-cell receptors.

Methods requiring complement participation

These assays can also be either direct or indirect. In the *direct assays*, activation of the complement cascade results in the lysis of cells, be they bacteria (*bacteriolytic tests*), erythrocytes (*haemolytic tests*) or nucleated cells (*cytotoxic tests)*. The dead cells can be identified by their changed morphology, altered light transmission properties, release of haemoglobin, uptake of vital stains such as trypan blue or eosin, or release of ^{51}Cr previously fixed to cytoplasmic components. In the *indirect (complement fixation) test*, an indication that the antigen–antibody reaction has taken place is the disappearance of complement (its fixation to the antigen–antibody complexes) from the mixture, as measured by a special indicator system (see Chapter 12). A variant of the complement fixation test is the *conglutination complement adsorption test*. *Conglutinin*[1] (Latin *conglutino*, to glue together) is a protein in the serum of cattle and other ruminants that adsorbs to erythrocyte–antibody–complement complexes and agglutinates the red cells (in systems in which the antibody alone is unable to effect agglutination). The protein is not an immunoglobulin and its level does not increase after immunization; it binds certain sugars of the C3 complement component (in the presence of Ca^{2+}). In the conglutination complement adsorption test, conglutinin is used as an indicator system to test whether complement has been fixed: if an antigen–antibody reaction has consumed all free C3, antibody-coated erythrocytes are not agglutinated by the addition of conglutinin.

[1] Conglutinin must not be confused with *immune conglutinin*, or immunoconglutinin, which is an IgM autoantibody specific for activated C3 or C4 components. Immune conglutinin is present at low levels in most normal sera but its concentration increases after various infections and after immunization with many antigens; animals are not tolerant of the epitopes detected by immunoconglutinins because these are normally hidden in the molecule and become exposed only after C3 or C4 activation.

Methods based on neutralization of biological activities

Many biologically active agents are inactivated when they combine with antibodies. Loss of biological activity in these situations is an indication that antigen–antibody reaction has taken place. The commonly used agents are toxins, viruses, bacteriophages and enzymes.

Fluorescent antibody techniques

One can visualize the antigen–antibody reaction by attaching a tag to the antibody or the antigen. The tag is a molecule with a special property such as emission of light (fluorescent antibody techniques), enzymatic activity (enzyme immunoassays), high electron-scattering capacity (the immunoferritin method) or radioactivity (radioimmunoassays). Procedures based on the use of tagged antibodies are called *immunocytochemical* or *immunohistochemical*.

When a photon (a quantum of light) strikes an atom, some of the electrons absorb energy and the atoms enters an energy-rich, excited state. Excited atoms are unstable and quickly return to their original, low-energy ground state. This return is accompanied by the release of energy in the form of a chemical reaction, heat or visible light. The form in which the energy is released depends on the structure of the molecule containing the atom. For example, molecules with freely rotating bonds, such as those in the aliphatic saturated compounds, dissipate the absorbed energy in rotational movement, whereas structurally rigid molecules release energy in the form of light. The emission of absorbed light is called *fluorescence* and the structurally rigid molecules capable of fluorescence are *fluorochromes*. The emitted light has a lower energy (a longer wavelength) than the absorbed light and fluorescence can be observed when the former is in the visible and the latter in the invisible, UV range.

A fluorochrome attached to an antibody molecule enables identification of the latter through its fluorescence. The two fluorochromes commonly used in immunology are *fluorescein* and *rhodamine disulphonic acid* (lissamine rhodamine B200, tetramethylrhodamine isothiocyanate; Fig. 14.11). Before they can be conjugated to proteins (antibodies) fluorescein and rhodamine must first be converted into isothiocyanates, which provide the reactive group for interaction with the amino groups of the protein. The

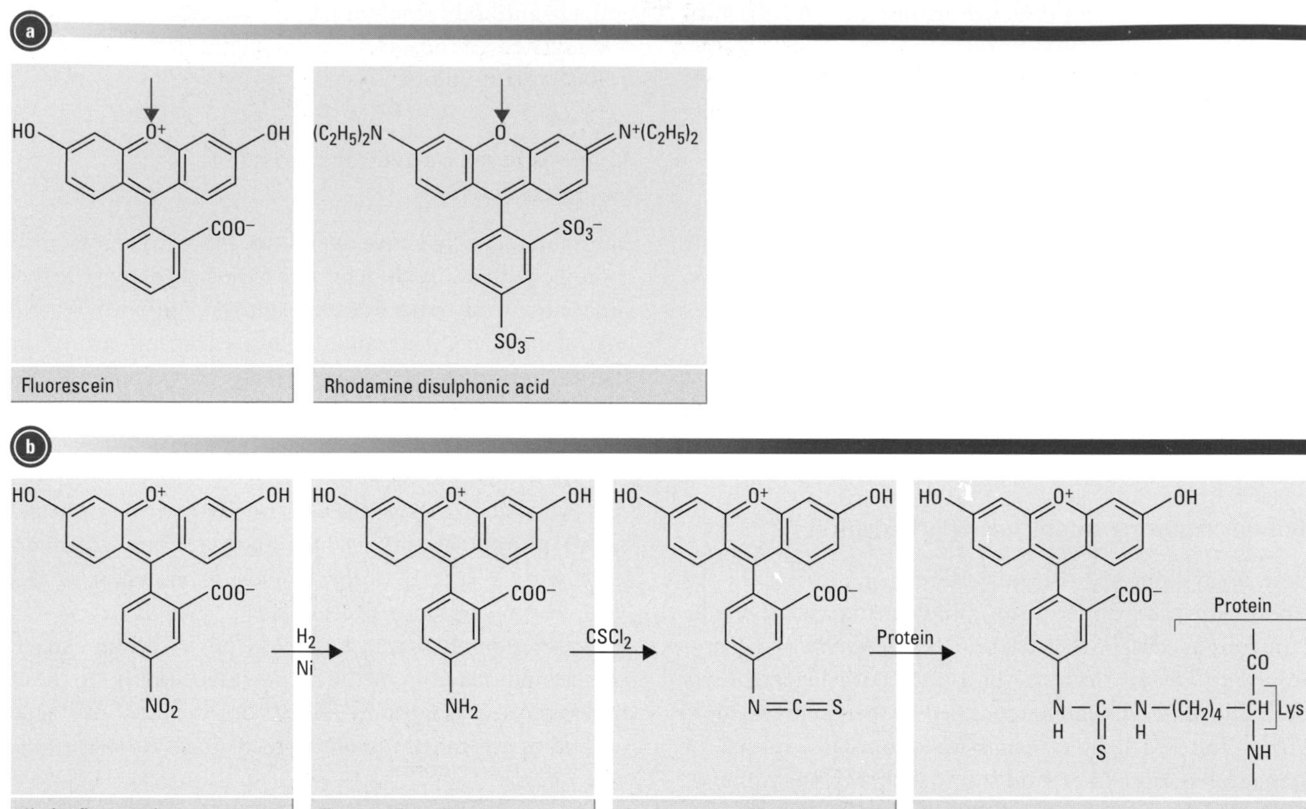

Figure 14.11 (a) Two fluorochromes frequently used in immunology. Red arrows point to the relatively rigid part of the molecule. (b) Synthesis of fluorescein isothiocyanate (FITC) from 4′-nitrofluorescein and conjugation of FITC with the NH_2 group of a lysine in a protein. Nitrofluorescein is produced by condensation of 4-nitrophthalic anhydride with two equivalents of resorcinol. Nitrofluorescein diacetate is converted into fluorescein amine by hydrogenation with Raney nickel. Fluorescein amine is turned into FITC by thiophosgene ($CsCl_2$) treatment.

fluoresceinated (or rhodaminated) antibodies are then allowed to bind to cellular antigens, the unbound proteins are removed by washing and the cells are examined under a fluorescence microscope. The actual test can be carried out in one of three ways (Fig. 14.12a–c): in the *direct test*, cells are coated with fluorochrome-tagged antibodies specific for cell-surface antigens; in the *indirect test*, cells are first coated with a specific, unconjugated antibody, which is then reacted with a fluorochrome-tagged xenogeneic anti-immunoglobulin reagent; in the *sandwich test*, an antigen is allowed to attach to cell-surface immunoglobulin (B-cell receptor) and then a tagged antibody is reacted with the bound antigen (the antigen is thus sandwiched between two antibodies). The sandwich technique can be used to detect antigen-specific B cells. Fluorescent antibodies are also the principal component of flow cytometry techniques, described in Chapter 5 (see Fig. 5.9).

Enzyme immunoassays

In these tests, an enzyme rather than a fluorochrome is attached to antibodies and enzymatic activity of the antigen–antibody complexes is measured after the addition of the specific enzyme substrate. There are only a few enzymes suitable for this form of antibody tagging; they include horseradish peroxidase, alkaline phosphatase and *p*-nitrophenylphosphatase. *Horseradish peroxidase* can be attached to a protein via bifunctional agents such as 4,4′-difluoro-3,3′-dinitro-phenylsulphone (Fig. 14.13). The conjugated antibodies are then reacted with antigens, unbound antibodies are removed by washing and the enzyme is allowed to convert its substrate, hydrogen peroxide (H_2O_2), to water:

$$2H_2O_2 \xrightarrow{4H} 4H_2O$$

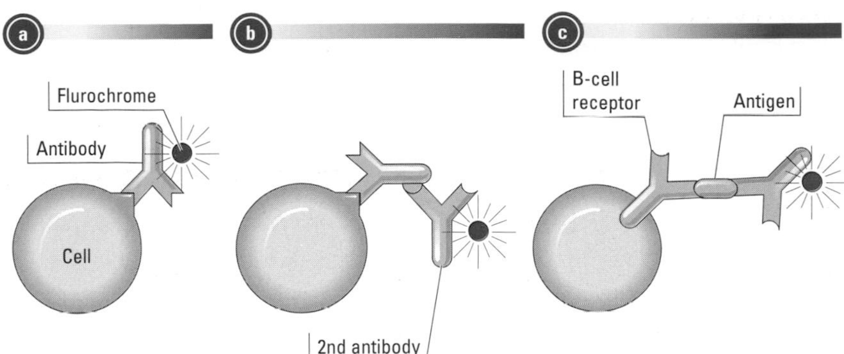

Figure 14.12 Types of fluorescent antibody assays: (a) direct; (b) indirect; (c) sandwich. (Modified from Klein, J. (1982) *Immunology: The Science of Self–Nonself Discrimination*. John Wiley & Sons, New York.)

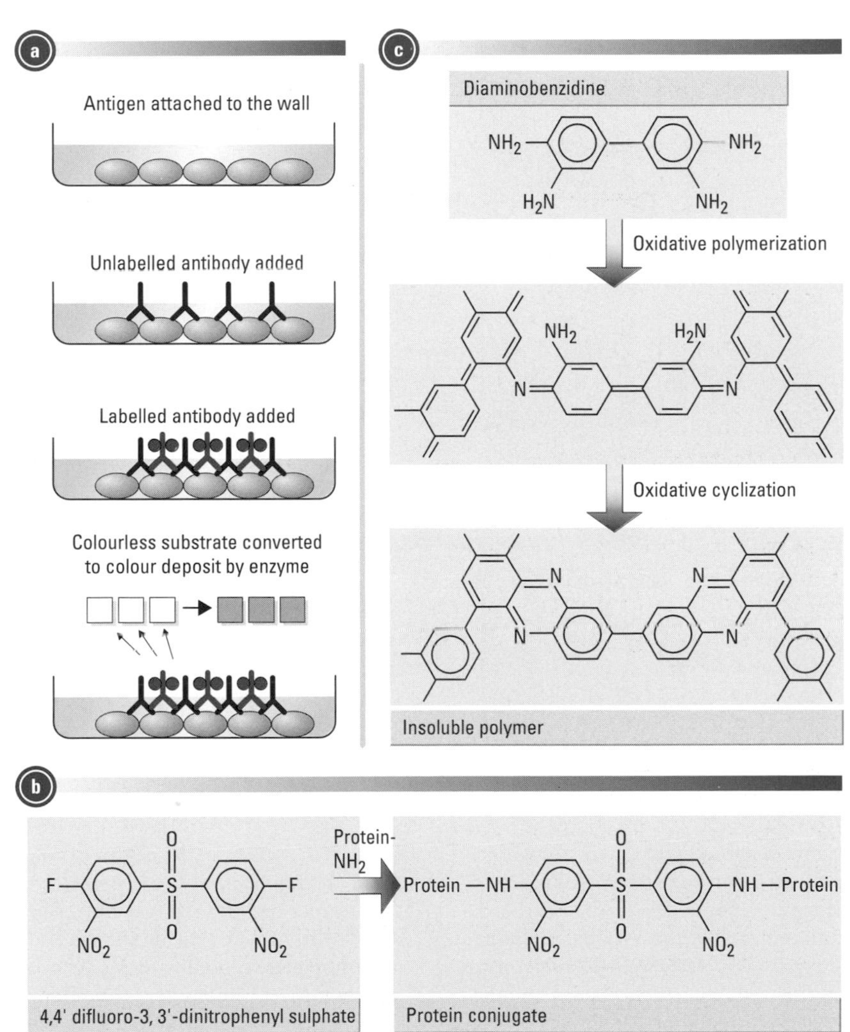

Figure 14.13 Enzyme-linked immunosorbent assay (ELISA). (a) The principle of the test. In one version of this assay, the antigen (a protein or a cell) is attached non-covalently to each well of a plastic microtitre plate and the unattached antigen is washed off. Most antigens stick non-specifically to the plastic, but to obtain a better coating the wells can be precoated with poly-L-lysine (PLL), a synthetic polypeptide that imparts a positive charge on the dish surface and thus entices negatively charged cells or molecules to bind. To block the unoccupied binding sites, the wells are incubated with an albumin solution. The test antibody is then added to the well and unbound antibody is removed at the end of the incubation period by washing. In the final step, enzyme-labelled antibodies specific for the first antibody are added, the excess antibodies are washed off, the substrate for the enzyme is added and the reaction revealed by the conversion of colourless substrate to coloured substance is scored. (b) One of the coupling reagents used to conjugate an enzyme to an antibody. (c) Conversion of a colourless substrate to a coloured precipitate in the peroxidase-catalysed reaction.

The reaction can take place only in the presence of electron donors such as diaminobenzidine, which are thereby oxidized. The oxidation products rapidly polymerize into an amorphous, insoluble, brown substance deposited at the site of antibody binding and visible in a light microscope. In other versions of the assay, the action of the enzyme turns the *substrate* into a coloured, *soluble* substance and the intensity of the solution's colouring can be quantitated spectrophotometrically. There are three principal variants of this *enzyme-linked immunosorbent assay* (ELISA): indirect, sandwich and competitive (Fig. 14.14). The first variant is used to detect the presence of antibodies in a tested sample

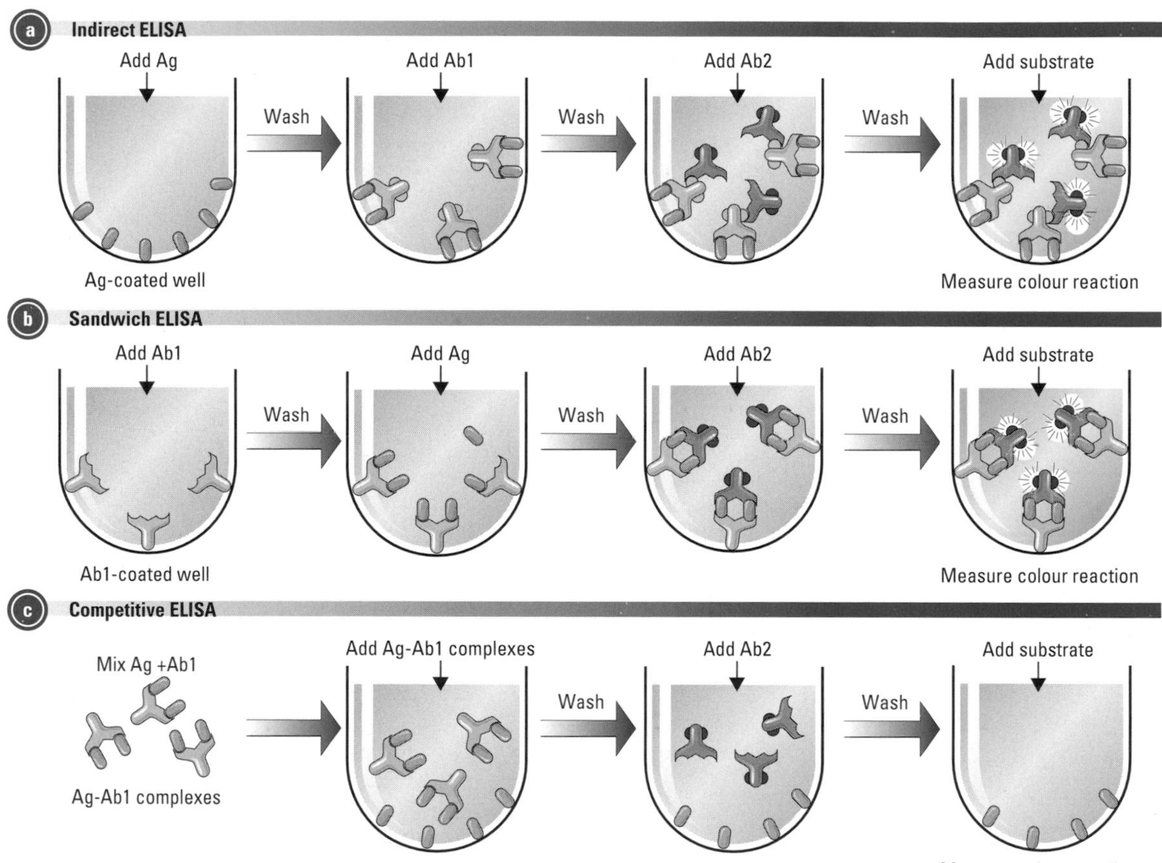

Figure 14.14 Principal variants of enzyme-linked immunosorbent assay (ELISA). In all three variants, two antibodies are used: Ab1 is specific for the antigen (Ag) and is not labelled; Ab2 is either specific for Ab1 or for Ag and is tagged by the enzyme. (a) *Indirect ELISA* is the type shown in Fig. 14.13. Here, wells of a microtitre plate are coated with Ag, unattached Ag is washed away and the attached Ag is allowed to react with added Ab1. Free Ab1 is washed away and Ab1 in the Ag–Ab1 complexes attached to the wall is allowed to react with Ab2, which is specific for Ab1. Unbound Ab2 is washed away, the enzyme's substrate is added and the colour reaction is measured spectrophotometrically (i.e. it is determined how much light passing through the solution the coloured substance absorbs). (b) *Sandwich ELISA* is used to detect the presence of Ag in a test sample. Here, the wells are coated with Ab1, excess of Ab1 is washed away, the attached Ab1 is allowed to react with Ag, unbound Ag is removed by washing and bound Ag is allowed to react with added Ab2, which is specific for another epitope of the antigen. After washing and addition of substrate, the degree of colouring is measured spectrophotometrically. (c) *Competitive ELISA* is also a test for the presence of Ag in a test sample. The Ag-containing sample is mixed with Ab1 and the mixture is added to the wells of a microtitre plate coated with Ag. After an incubation period, the unbound Ag–Ab1 complexes and free Ab1 are washed away, and Ab2 specific for Ab1 is added. If the test sample contained Ag, Ab1 will have been bound into Ag–Ab1 complexes and the amount of Ab1 available for interaction with Ag attached to the surface of the well will be reduced. At a certain concentration, the Ag in the solution will have bound *all* Ab1 so that none is left to interact with the surface-adsorbed Ag. In this case, too, no Ab1 is left to react with Ab1-specific Ab2, so that after washing away unbound Ab2 no colour reaction develops following addition of the substrate. If in the initial mixture only part of Ab1 became bound in Ag–Ab1 complexes, some colour reaction will develop following the addition of Ab2. The colour intensity will be inversely proportional to the concentration of Ag.

(e.g. HIV-specific antibodies in human serum); the second and third variants are used to detect the presence of the antigen in the test sample. All three variants can be used either qualitatively or quantitatively. In the latter case, the degree of colouring after the addition of the enzyme substrate is compared with standard curves obtained in reactions containing increasing, known concentrations of antibody and antigen. All three variants have two antibodies: an antibody that is specific for the antigen (Ab1) and another (Ab2) that is specific either for Ab1 (indirect and competitive ELISA) or for another epitope of the antigen (sandwich ELISA). The principles of the three assays are explained in Fig. 14.14.

Avidin–biotin immunoassay

Biotin (vitamin H, co-enzyme R) is a low-molecular-mass (M_r 244) water-soluble substance that is a member of the vitamin B complex (Fig. 14.15a). It functions as a co-enzyme for a number of enzymes in a variety of organisms. It binds two proteins very strongly, avidin and streptavidin. *Avidin* is an egg-white protein responsible for human biotin deficiency in persons who have consumed large numbers of raw eggs: avidin binds biotin so tightly as to prevent its intestinal absorption. The function of avidin in the egg is believed to be prevention of bacterial growth. *Streptavidin* is a bacterial protein with M_r of 66 000. It is made up of four identical subunits, each containing a high-affinity binding site for biotin. Streptavidin is preferred over avidin in the biotin-based techniques because it displays less non-specific binding. The dissociation constant (K_d) of the biotin–streptavidin complex is 10^{-15} M, which makes the interaction one of the strongest known (almost irreversible). Biotin can be chemically attached to a variety of substances, including proteins and nucleic acids. In preparation for the attachment, biotin is modified by the addition of reactive groups (e.g. amino, phenol, imidazol, aldehyde, carboxyl and thiol groups) capable of interacting with the substance to be biotinylated. Protein biotinylation is usually carried out with biotinyl-*N*-hydroxysuccinimide ester (Fig. 14.15b). Biotinylated protein, such as an antibody, can then be visualized (detected) by labelling either the biotin or the streptavidin and allowing the streptavidin to bind the biotin. The label can be a fluorochrome, a metal such as gold or an enzyme such as that used in the ELISA. The biotin–streptavidin technique exists in many variants, four of which are shown in Fig. 14.16.

Immunoferritin techniques

Ferritin is a protein containing about 20% iron in the form of a ferric hydroxyphosphate complex. Each ferritin molecule has a protein shell enveloping an inner core of four iron micelles, which have a high electron-scattering capacity. Ferritin molecules can be attached to antibodies either chemically or immunologically. The chemical attachment in the *direct ferritin-labelling technique* proceeds in two steps (Fig. 14.17). In the first, ferritin molecules are treated with a coupling agent, such as toluene-2,4-diisocyanate, and in the second step, the resulting complex is conjugated with antibody molecules. The ferritin-labelled antibodies are then applied directly to cells and the specimens are prepared for electron microscopy. In the *indirect ferritin-labelling technique*, ferritin is coupled to xenogeneic antibodies specific for alloantibodies that, in turn, are specific for an antigen on the cell surface.

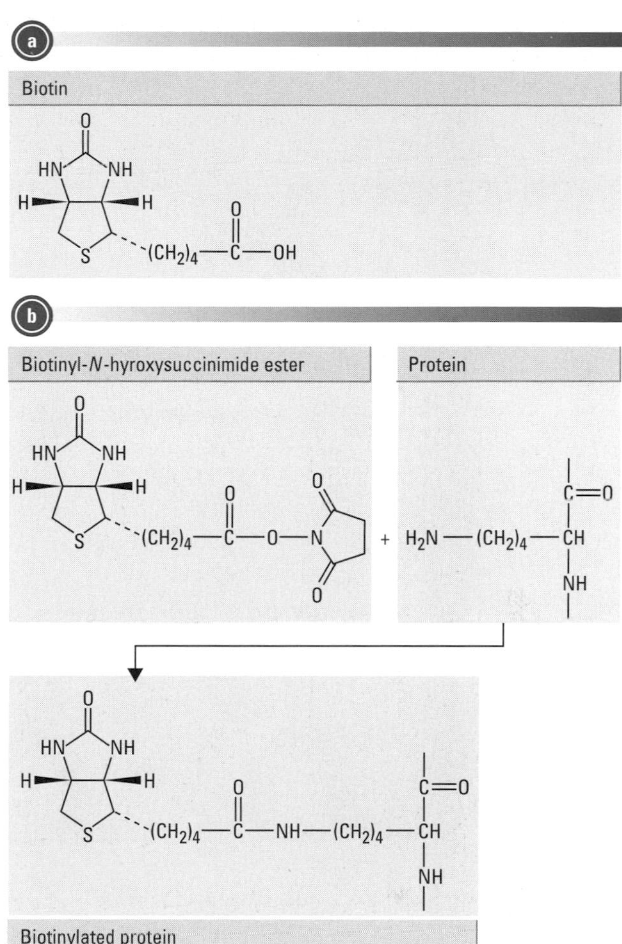

Figure 14.15 (a) Chemical formula of biotin. (b) Attachment of biotin to a protein (biotinylation of the protein).

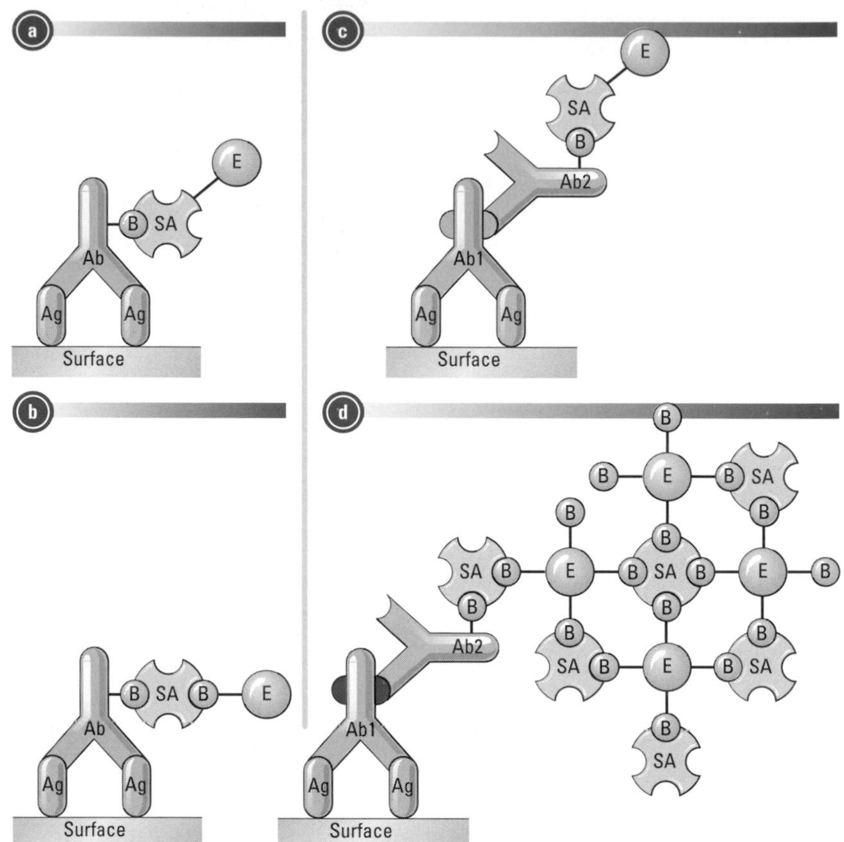

Figure 14.16 Four variants of biotin–streptavidin-based techniques for the measurement of antibody reaction with antigen. (a) Surface-bound antigen (Ag) is reacted with biotinylated (B) antibody (Ab) and the biotin is then reacted with enzyme (e.g. horseradish peroxidase)-conjugated streptavidin (SA). Addition of substrate to the complex leads to a measurable colour reaction. The procedure is otherwise carried out as described for the ELISA in Fig. 14.14. (b) In this variant, the enzyme is not conjugated to the streptavidin molecules but rather biotinylated. The set-up is otherwise the same as in (a). (c) Antigen is reacted with antigen-specific antibody (Ab1), and a biotinylated second antibody (Ab2) reacting with Ab1 is then added. The reaction is completed by the addition of enzymatically labelled streptavidin. (d) A preformed complex of streptavidin and biotinylated enzyme is added to the Ag–Ab1–biotinylated Ab2 complex (see c). Because each streptavidin molecule has four biotin-binding sites, the interacting molecules form a lattice that attaches to the biotin on Ab2 with the remaining free binding sites. This arrangement intensifies the signal emanating from the marker (here the enzyme) attached to the biotin. E, enzyme.

Radioimmunoassay (RIA)

In the simplest version of this method, the antigen is labelled with a radioactive isotope and an unlabelled (cold) test antigen is used to compete with the 'hot' antigen for combining sites on the antibody (Figs 14.18 & 14.19). Lowering of the radioactivity of the antigen–antibody complexes in the presence of the test antigen is an indication that the test antigen has reacted with the antibody. The degree of inhibition by the cold antigen can be used to calculate the content of the hot antigen. In an alternative to RIA, it is the antigen that is labelled rather than the antibody.

The soluble antigen–antibody complexes can be separated from the free antigen by an antiglobulin serum, chromatography, gel diffusion or electrophoresis, or one can attach the antibodies to a solid surface, wash off the free antigen and determine the radioactivity of this surface. RIAs can detect extremely small amounts of antigen and are thus among the most sensitive methods at the immunologist's disposal.

Western blotting

In molecular biology, 'blotting' refers to the transfer of macromolecules (nucleic acids or proteins) from one solid

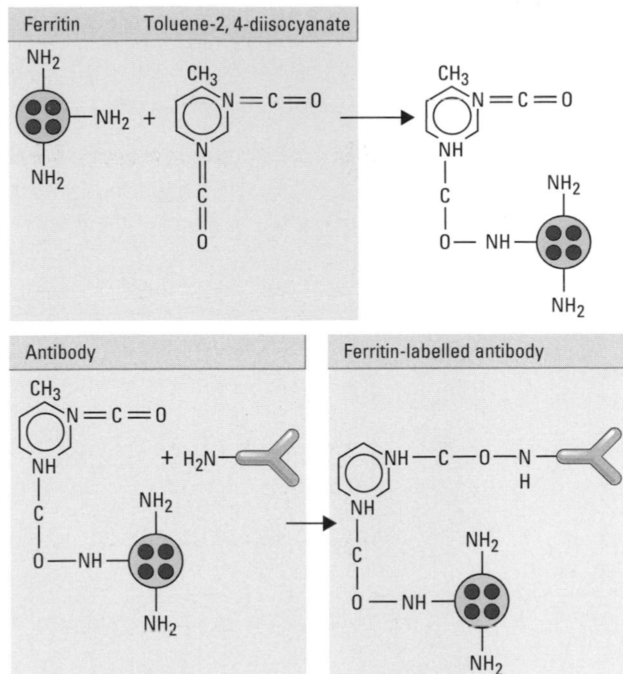

Figure 14.17 Conjugation of ferritin to antibodies. Ferritin-labelled antibodies can then be used to visualize the antigen on cells or tissues by electron microscopy.

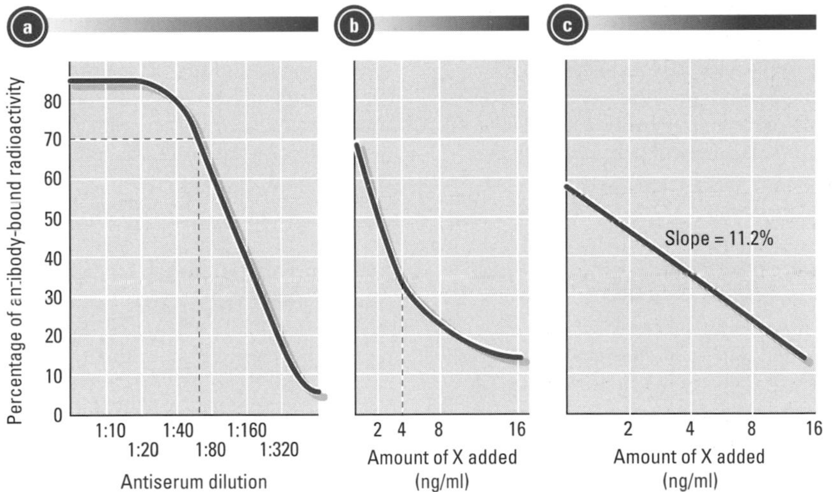

Figure 14.18 Radioimmunoassay (RIA). The assay is carried out in the following steps. (1) Antibody against antigen X is produced. (2) Antigen X is radiolabelled. (3) A constant amount of the labelled antigen (X*) is mixed and incubated with different dilutions of anti-X and the antigen–antibody complexes are precipitated with a xenogeneic antiserum specific for anti-X. (The amount of X* is chosen empirically so that the reaction occurs in great antibody excess in which only soluble antigen–antibody complexes form.) The precipitate is separated, the radioactivity of the precipitate and the remaining free X* determined, the ratio of the two values (the percentage of X* bound by the antibody) calculated and the percentage plotted against the antiserum dilution (a). For further experimentation, an antiserum dilution is chosen that binds 70% of X* (a point on the titration curve where the straight region begins and where the assay is most sensitive). (4) Diluted anti-X is distributed in aliquots into several tubes containing constant amounts of X*. Known increasing amounts of X (unlabelled antigen) are added to the individual tubes, the antigen–antibody complexes are precipitated with the xenogeneic antiserum and the radioactivity of these complexes is plotted against the amount of X added (b and c). (5) A standard curve (c) is then used to determine the amount of X in a test sample. To this end, the test sample is mixed with the same amount of anti-X and X* as was used in the preceding step, radioactivity of the precipitate and of free X* is determined, the percentage of X* bound by anti-X is calculated and the concentration of X in the test sample is read off from the standard curve. In our example, the test sample reduced the percentage of antibody-bound radioactivity from 70% (absence of unlabelled X) to 35%; this value corresponds to 5 ng of X per 1 ml.

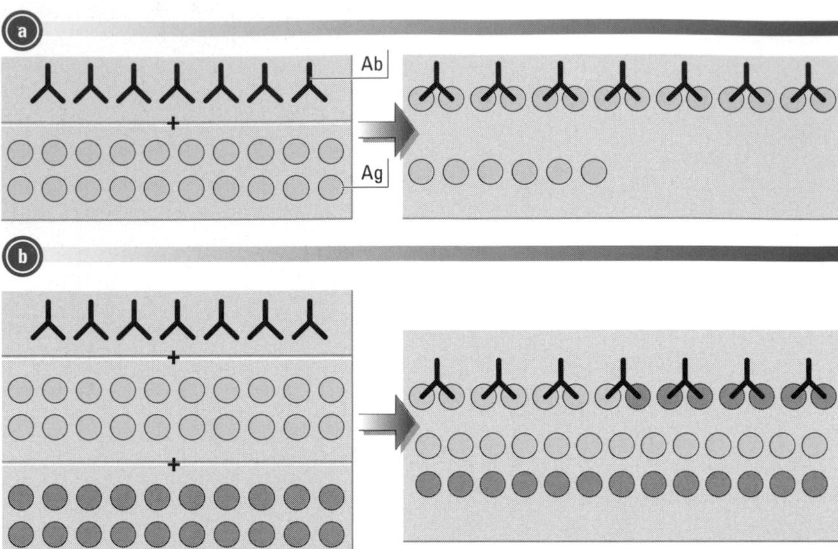

Figure 14.19 Principle of competitive inhibition on which the radioimmunoassay is based. Consider a mixture of seven bivalent antibody molecules and 20 molecules of labelled antigen (a). If all the antibody-combining sites react with the antigen, 14/20 or 70% of the antigen molecules become antibody bound and will be brought down with the precipitate. Consider another mixture consisting of seven antibody molecules, 20 labelled and 20 unlabelled antigen molecules (b). Both the labelled and unlabelled antigens have an equal chance of combining with antibodies, so that probably half the bound molecules will be labelled. In this case, only 7/20 or 35% of the labelled antigen molecules will be precipitated out of the solution; the rest of the combining sites will be occupied by unlabelled antigen molecules. Thus, by competition the unlabelled molecules inhibit the binding of the labelled ones and this inhibition is greater the more unlabelled molecules one adds to the mixture. If one knows that the 35% reduction of antibody-bound radioactivity is brought about by 20 unlabelled antigen molecules, one can conclude that any unknown sample causing this much reduction must contain 20 antigen molecules. Ab, anibody; Ag, antigen.

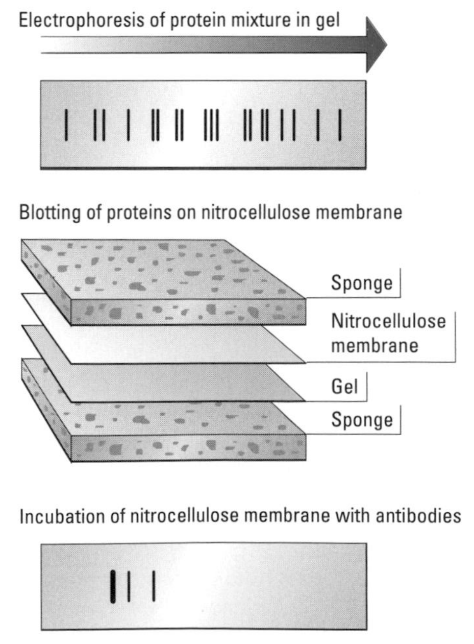

Figure 14.20 Principle of western blotting. For explanation, see text.

or semi-solid medium to another, usually from a gel to a filter paper. Depending on the macromolecules that are being transferred, there is Southern blotting (DNA transfer), northern blotting (RNA transfer) and western blotting (protein transfer). Southern blotting, the first of this sort of transfer technique developed, is named after the investigator who introduced this method; northern and western blotting are terms inspired by Dr Southern's name. *Western blotting* is a method of finding a particular antigen in a complex mixture of proteins. To this end, the proteins in the mixture are separated by gel electrophoresis and the gel is covered with a nitrocellulose membrane and sandwiched between buffer-saturated sponges. The proteins in the gel are transferred into the nitrocellulose membrane by electric currents passed between the sponges (Fig. 14.20). The membrane with the proteins non-covalently but firmly attached to it is then incubated with a radioactively or enzymatically labelled antibody specific for the particular antigen in a direct test, or an unlabelled first antibody and a labelled second antibody in an indirect test. After developing the enzymatic or radioactivity label the antigen band becomes visible while all the other protein bands remain invisible.

Further reading

Absolom, D.R. (1986) The nature of the antigen–antibody bond and the factors affecting its association and dissociation. *CRC Critical Reviews in Immunology*, 6, 1–46.

Campbell, D.H., Garvey, J.S., Cremer, N.E. & Sussdorf, D.H. (1970) *Methods in Immunology*, 2nd edn. Benjamin, New York.

Day, E.D. (1990) *Advanced Immunochemistry*, 2nd edn. Wiley-Liss, New York.

Lefkovits, I. & Pernis, B. (Eds) (1979) *Immunological Methods*. Academic Press, New York.

Steensgaard, J. (1984) The mechanism of immune precipitation. *Immunology Today*, 5, 7–10.

Van Oss, C.J. & van Regenmortel, M.H.V. (Eds) (1994) *Immunochemistry*. Marcel Dekker, New York.

Weir, D.M. (1986) *Handbook of Experimental Immunology*, 3rd edn, Vols. 1–4. Blackwell Scientific Publications, Oxford.

Williams, C.A. & Chase, M.W. (Eds) (1967–1976) *Methods in Imunology and Immunochemistry*, Vols. I–V. Academic Press, New York.

chapter 15 Defence reactions mediated by phagocytes

Having completed the description of the organs, tissues, cells and molecules involved in vertebrate (human) immunity, we now discuss how the elements of the immune system act to protect the body from the threats of the hostile environment. We begin with reactions mediated by phagocytes.

What are phagocytes?

A foreign element that has managed to break through the body's bulwarks, for example via a wound or an abrasion, and has entered the tissues underlying the surface layers, encounters the second line of defence, the phagocytes. These cells are either encamped behind the bulwarks or circulate with the body fluids, ready to leave the circulation and attack the intruder in any place at any time. Their methods of combat are manifold, but their main way is simply to devour the intruder, which is why they are called *phagocytes*, 'cells that eat'. Many other cells 'eat' and 'drink', but they can only ingest small particles, molecules or droplets of fluid. Phagocytes, on the other hand, ingest large particles (1 µm or more in diameter) and have a special way of accomplishing this.

Phagocytes are sometimes divided into professional and non-professional. *Professional phagocytes* are neutrophils, eosinophils, monocytes and macrophages; *non-professional phagocytes* include epithelial cells of the various mucous membranes, lymphocytes, platelets, mast cells and fibroblasts. In reality, however, there is only one group of phagocytes and that is the professional group. These cells have eating and drinking as their main occupation related to the body's defence. Non-professional phagocytes do occasionally ingest larger particles, but their primary function is different and ingestion is not followed by the response that accompanies phagocytosis. In particular, the particles ingested by non-professional phagocytes are not digested; instead, they are often expelled from the cell by exocytosis into intercellular spaces, where they are attacked by professional phagocytes. A special case is the dendritic cells. Their phagocytic abilities are limited, but as major antigen-presenting cells (see Chapter 16) they engulf antigenic particles by *macropinocytosis*, a process resembling phagocytosis in some respects. From now on, whenever we mention 'phagocytes' we will always be referring to the professional ones.

A common misconception is that *macrophages* are the

main killers of microorganisms. They are not. Although they are often the first cells of the immune system to encounter the invader, and although they may also ingest it, intracellular killing is not their forte. Instead, they act as sentries, sounding the alarm that the enemy is *ante portas*, at the gate. Upon ingesting a particle, macrophages secrete a variety of soluble substances, some of which may, by diffusing out, summon the real killers to the site of an attack; others may participate in the attack extracellularly. Normally, however, during peacetime, their voracious appetite serves a scavenging function: they filtrate blood and lymph and engulf worn-out cells or cellular debris; macrophages in the human liver remove about 10^{11} senescent erythrocytes from the circulation every day. When they do turn into killers, they kill by mechanisms other than those used by, for example, neutrophils. However, 'macrophages' are merely one extreme of a continuum that is sometimes referred to as *mononuclear phagocytes*. At the other end of the continuum are the bone marrow precursors of monocytes, while in the middle are the blood monocytes. Macrophages themselves may acquire distinct structural and functional characteristics depending on their location and state of activation (discussed later). Bone marrow promonocytes and blood monocytes are usually somewhat better equipped for intracellular digestion than macrophages.

The number one professional killer of invading microorganisms is the *neutrophil*, which has highly developed mechanisms for intracellular digestion of ingested particles. Patients with severe neutropenia, a decrease of 90% or more in the normal number of neutrophils, are in grave danger of succumbing to a microbial infection. *Eosinophils* are also efficient killers but even though they are capable of bona fide phagocytosis they actually specialize in the extracellular killing of larger invaders, such as multicellular parasites. *Basophils* are probably not capable of phagocytosis to any significant degree.

The phagocyte that is not fighting invaders or scavenging the body is said to be in a *resting state*. Its metabolism is at a basal level; it may move around, passively or actively, but otherwise does little else. However, it is responsive to a variety of stimuli that can initiate its transformation into an *activated state*. The stimuli are received by receptors on the outer surface of the plasma membrane and translated into signals. The latter cross the membrane, enter the cytoplasm, as well as the nucleus, and initiate the responses characterizing the activated state. The stimuli can be quite diverse; in the macrophage alone, over 50 stimuli acting via different receptors have been identified (for example immune complexes, microbial surface carbohydrates, cytokines, hormones, anaphylatoxins). Some of the stimuli and their receptors are shared by different phagocytes, while others are specific for the particular cell type. Some of them initiate certain responses, which are not initiated by other stimuli, but many initiate a similar plethora of responses. Only eosinophils appear to be chronically agitated and to exert a low level of response that in other phagocytes would require stimulation for its initiation. Upon receiving a stimulus, eosinophils respond by increased activity, but the increase is generally lower than that found in other stimulated phagocytes. Macrophages are unusual in that they can be found at three levels of activity: resting, primed and activated. There is a certain terminological confusion regarding the different activation states. Here, we refer to macrophages stimulated via their Fc receptors, by contact with microbial surface carbohydrates, anaphylatoxins and many other stimuli as *primed*, and to macrophages stimulated by T_H1 (T helper) cells and cytokines [interferon γ (IFN-γ), tumour necrosis factor α (TNF-α)] as *activated*. The primed state is sometimes also called 'stimulated', 'elicited' or 'activated' and the 'activated' state (in our sense) 'hyperactivated'. Activated macrophages can carry out functions, such as the killing of tumour cells, which the primed (not to mention resting) macrophages cannot.

Stimulation of phagocytes via various surface receptors leads mainly to activation of the following functions:

- phagocytosis;
- production of bactericidal reactive oxygen compounds derived from the superoxide anion radical;
- release of the contents of cytoplasmic granules into the phagosome or to the exterior (degranulation, exocytosis);
- secretion of cytokines and other regulatory intermediates attracting other cells to the site of infection and activating them;
- crossing the blood vessel endothelia, penetration into the inflamed tissue (extravasation) and active movement in the tissue towards the source of infection or inflammation (chemotaxis);
- the distinctive feature of activated macrophages is the production of bactericidal nitric oxide and its derivatives.

More detailed discussion of these phagocyte functions and the molecular mechanisms triggering them follows.

Phagocytosis

Attachment phase

A basic decision that has to be made by phagocytes is what to devour and what not; in other words, they must be able to distinguish foreign intruders or damaged self cells from healthy components of the body. This distinction is achieved in two ways. First, phagocytes have *pattern receptors* on their surface that recognize structures characteristic of various pathogens or abnormal cells but absent from healthy self cells. Second, they carry receptors for *opsonins*: immunoglobulins and complement fragments that bind to the pathogen's surface and thus mark it as foreign.

Two major classes of pattern receptors on the phagocyte surface are:

- surface lectins that recognize carbohydrate structures present on the surface of various bacteria, yeasts and senescent cells;
- scavenger receptors that recognize anionic polymers present on microbial surfaces but also on the surface of worn-out or dying cells.

These receptors are found mainly on the surface of macrophages. Perhaps best known of the surface lectins is the *mannose-specific macrophage receptor* (*surface lectin*; Fig. 15.1a), which binds avidly to mannose and fucose residues on microbial surfaces. The extracellular part of this receptor (relative molecular mass, M_r 180 000) consists of eight lectin-domain repeats with slightly different carbohydrate-binding sites. A similar receptor on dendritic cells has 10 such mannose-binding domains. The two receptors belong to a large family of C-type lectins. Among the other members of this family are several adhesion molecules present on leucocytes and other cell types. They include selectins (CD62L, CD62E and CD62P), CD23, CD69, CD72 and a family of natural killer (NK) cell receptors.

Macrophages also possess another receptor structurally similar to the mannose-specific lectin but which recognizes galactose and *N*-acetylgalactosamine instead of mannose residues. This *galactose-specific lectin* is used mainly by liver macrophages (Kupffer cells) for the recognition of senescent erythrocytes that have lost the terminal sialic acid residues from the saccharide chains of their glycoproteins and thus reveal the penultimate galactose residues. Yet another macrophage surface lectin, *β-glucan receptor*, binds polymers of glucose or *glucans*. It is identical to the complement type 3 receptor and the adhesion molecule Mac-1 (the αMβ2 integrin; see Chapters 9 & 12).

There are several well-characterized, structurally related *scavenger receptors*. They have a remarkably broad binding specificity, which includes oxidized lipoproteins, polyribonucleotides, anionic polysaccharides, asbestos and bacterial lipopolysaccharides. The receptors are probably involved mainly in the recognition of senescent cells and cells undergoing apoptosis. A characteristic feature of apoptotic cells is the appearance of anionic phospholipids on their surface that in normal cells are sequestered strictly to the inner, cytoplasmic leaflet of the plasma membrane. The major scavenger receptor (see Fig. 15.1b) is a trimeric membrane glycoprotein whose extracellular part consists of three modules. The C-terminal module contains three cysteine-rich domains connected by a long fibrous stalk formed by the collagen-like and α-coiled-coil modules to the transmembrane domain.

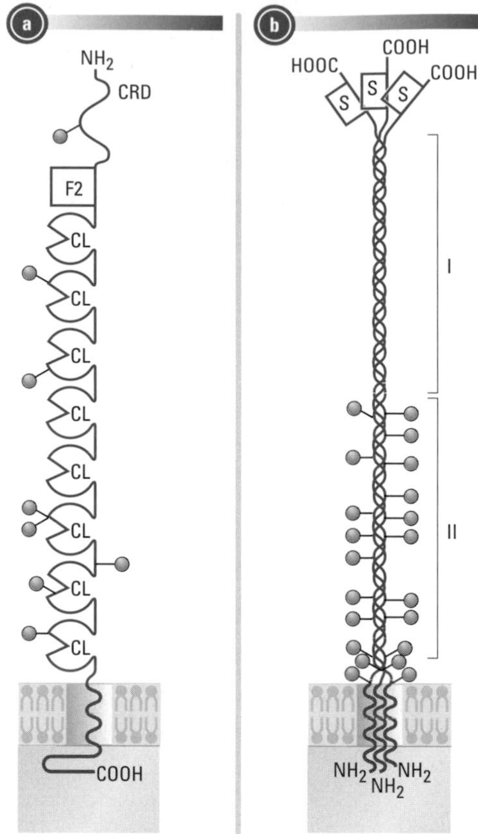

Figure 15.1 Diagrammatic models of (a) mannose-specific macrophage receptor and (b) type I scavenger receptor. The extracellular part of the mannose-specific macrophage receptor molecule consists of a short N-terminal cysteine-rich domain (CRD), a fibronectin type II (F2) domain and eight C-type lectin (CL) domains. The extracellular parts of the trimeric type I scavenger receptor chains consist of a C-terminal scavenger receptor (S) domain (rich in cysteine residues), a collagen-like (I) and α-helical coiled-coil (II) domains. ●–, *N*-linked oligosaccharides. (Based on Barclay, A. N. *et al.* (1993) *The Leucocyte Antigen Facts Book*. Academic Press, London.)

Engagement of the membrane lectins and scavenger receptors elicits signals for phagocytic engulfment that are not yet fully elucidated and causes other effects characteristic of activated phagocytes.

Recognition by opsonin receptors

'The phagocytes won't eat the microbes unless the microbes are nicely buttered for them' is a famous line from *The Doctor's Dilemma* by George Bernard Shaw, the 'butter' being *opsonin*, a substance that facilitates phagocytosis. The two main classes of opsonin are IgG and IgA antibodies and the third component of complement, or rather fragments thereof. Opsonins bind to the surface of the phagocytosed particle with one end and, via specific receptors, to the phagocyte with the other end. There are two main classes of phagocyte receptors corresponding to the two classes of opsonin: Fc receptors specific for the Fc region of IgG, IgA and IgE antibodies; and complement receptors specific for C3b fragments.

Phagocytes express several kinds of *Fc receptors* (FcR): FcγRI (CD64), FcγRII (CD32), FcγRIII (CD16), FcαR (CD89), FcεRI and FcεRII (CD23; see Chapter 8). FcγRI is expressed on monocytes, FcγRIIa on all major types of phagocytes, FcγRIIIb (CD16b) on neutrophils and FcαR on monocytes, macrophages and neutrophils. Upon binding of immune complexes containing the antibodies of appropriate isotypes these receptors induce phagocytosis and other activating reactions in phagocytes.

There are at least three classes of complement receptors (CR) on the phagocyte surface: CR1 (CD35), CR3 (CD11b/CD18) and CR4 (CD11c/CD18; see Chapter 11). They promote phagocytosis, but only if a second signal is provided either by phagocyte attachment to a component of intracellular matrix, fibronectin, or by simultaneous binding via Fc receptors.

The dependence of phagocytosis on opsonins seems to contradict the participation of phagocytes in the early stages of infection. If phagocytes rely on the presence of antibodies, how can they defend the body before antibodies have been formed against the invader? The most likely explanation is that at an early stage of infection, phagocytes rely on a set of alternative mechanisms. First of all, phagocytes recognize microorganisms directly via surface lectins and probably other pattern receptors. Further, some microorganisms activate the alternative pathway of complement in the absence of antibodies and the generated C3 fragments exert an opsonizing effect almost immediately after infection. Finally, immediate opsonization can also occur by *natural antibodies* present in the plasma of most individuals. Such antibodies are generated because of continual exposure of the host to a variety of pathogenic and non-pathogenic microorganisms (see Chapter 21). The attachment of these natural antibodies to the microbial surface initiates the classical pathway of complement activation and the resulting C3 fragments further enhance opsonization. The complement pathway can also be activated by two other factors: the *mannose-binding protein* (MBP) and the *C-reactive protein* (CRP) (see Chapter 12).

All these mechanisms result in the attachment of phagocytes to their targets and in the commencement of ingestion almost immediately after the infection. While the immediate reactions are taking place, antigens of the invading microorganisms are presented to cells of the adaptive immune system, antibodies are produced within a few days, and these then opsonize the invaders more efficiently. They also activate the classical pathway of complement and the large quantity of the C3b fragment produced further increases opsonization and consequently the efficiency of phagocytosis.

Ingestion phase

After its attachment to the phagocyte, a particle is engulfed. Outwardly, one can see projections rising from the cell surface in the region where the particle has touched it and pseudopodia forming a cup-like structure around the particle (Fig. 15.2). The rim of the cup rises gradually, adhering closely to the surface of the particle, until the advancing pseudopods meet at a single point at which the membrane fuses. The region requiring membrane fusion is very small, no greater than in pinocytosis. After the cup-like structure

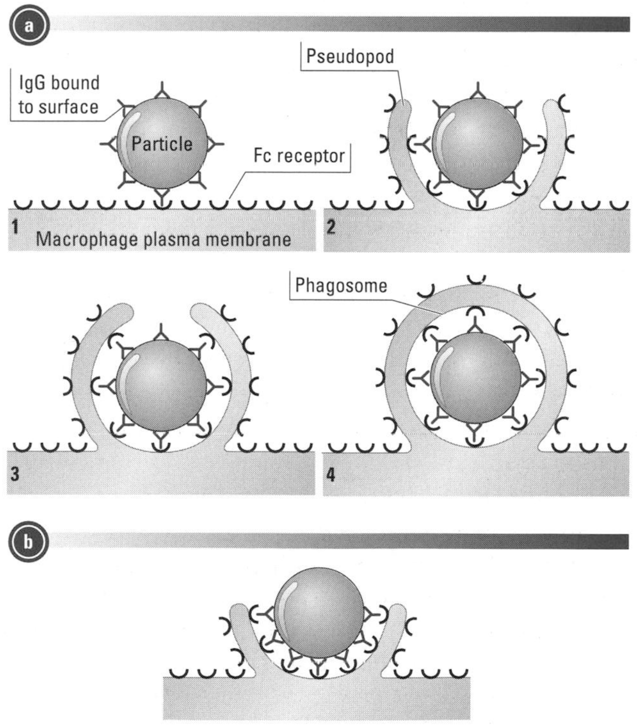

Figure 15.2 Ingestion of an opsonized particle by a phagocyte. (a) Ingestion of a particle coated with antibodies on the entire surface. Individual stages: attachment of the particle; formation of pseudopodia and a cup-like structure surrounding the particle; closing over the particle; formation of a phagosome. (b) Ingestion of a partially coated particle: only the part coated with antibodies is engulfed by pseudopodia; the non-coated part remains free.

has closed, the particle finds itself in a vesicle, the *phagosome*, which then begins to move from the surface toward the cell's interior. The phagosome is lined by what used to be the plasma membrane and is now almost fully occupied by the ingested particle with very little fluid between the particle and the membrane.

The mechanism of engulfment is still a matter of conjecture. Rim formation is believed to occur by the same mechanism as the formation of pseudopodia during the movement of an amoeba. Engulfment of particles by amoeba, however, clearly differs from phagocytosis. When an amoeba touches a particle that lies in its path, it forms pseudopodia that surround but hardly touch the particle's surface. Pseudopod formation is triggered by the first contact with the particle but it is not directed any further by contact with the increasing area of the particle's surface. In phagocytosis, on the other hand, the extending pseudopod is in continuous contact with the microbial surface and its growth is led by additional points of contact. This pattern is aptly called the *zippering mechanism*. Particles that have half of their surface covered by IgG are only semi-engulfed: the phagocytic cup formation stops when the pseudopod arrives at the boundary between the coated and non-coated halves of the particle. Engagement of the phagocyte receptors apparently provides signals to a circumscribed area of the membrane and cytoplasm and elicits changes resulting in local pseudopod extension. The process is fundamentally dependent on the induced assembly of actin microfilaments. Electron microscopic observations show bundles of actin filaments accumulating in the phagocytic cup and providing mechanical support to it (Fig. 15.3). Cytochalasins, substances that depolymerize actin filaments, block phagocytosis efficiently. We return to the underlying signalling mechanisms in the second part of this chapter.

Another process, *macropinocytosis*, resembles phagocytosis in some respects. It is used by dendritic cells to capture antigenic particles, such as fragments of microorganisms, non-specifically. In this process, relatively large vesicles (about 1 μm in diameter) are formed by a similar mechanism as phagosomes: pseudopodia dependent on actin microfilament meshwork arise, surround a certain volume of external liquid and close to form the macropinocytic vesicle. This process appears to be indiscriminate, yet it is nevertheless very efficient. Its efficiency increases by the adsorption of some microbial polysaccharides to the mannose receptor of dendritic cells, which is distinct from the macrophage mannose receptor.

The ingestion process is very rapid. Within 30 min, a macrophage can engulf sufficient particles to cause the interiorization of some 50% of the particle's surface, a feat made possible only by the cell's possession of large internal stores of plasma membrane.

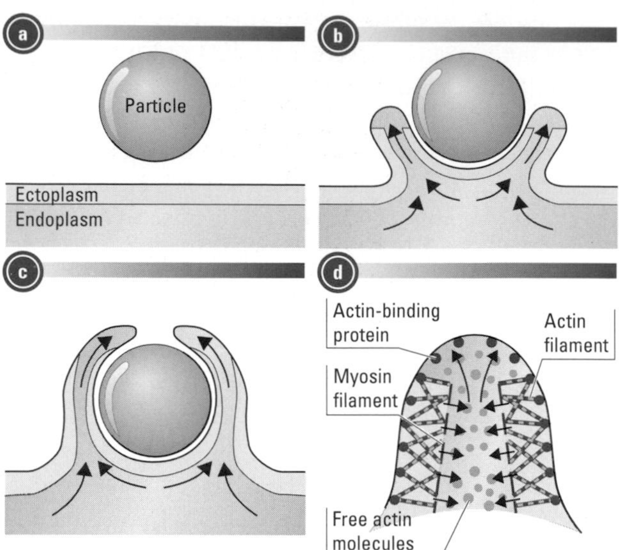

Figure 15.3 Hypothetical mechanism of particle engulfment during phagocytosis. (a) Cytoplasm of a phagocyte is differentiated into outer, gel-like ectoplasm and inner, sol-like endoplasm. (b) Upon the attachment of a particle, pseudopodia are formed. Endoplasm streams into the tips of the pseudopodia and converts the gel into sol. (c) Streaming extends the pseudopodia further, with cytoplasm in the tips remaining in the more fluid sol state. (d) Pseudopod. Ectoplasm is believed to consist of membrane-attached actin-binding proteins that polymerize actin molecules into filaments. These criss-cross the ectoplasmic layer and attach to myosin filaments. Contraction of myosin squeezes the layer and causes streaming of the endoplasm into the tip of the pseudopod. In the endoplasm the actin molecules depolymerize and thus allow its increased fluidity. The membrane receptors that contact the particle are omitted for simplicity.

Digestion phase

The cytoplasm of a neutrophil or a macrophage is full of small, membrane-lined bags filled with an assortment of enzymes and other molecules (Fig. 15.4). In macrophages, most of the bags are *lysosomes*, which contain mainly hydrolytic enzymes. In granulocytes they are the *granules*, which are more heterogeneous. The two basic types are the *primary* or *azurophilic granules* (specialized lysosomes) and *secondary* or *specific granules*; two additional forms that are similar to secondary granules but distinguishable from them by their composition and density are the *secretory vesicles* and *gelatinase granules*, which are discussed later in this chapter. The signals generated by the recognition of the

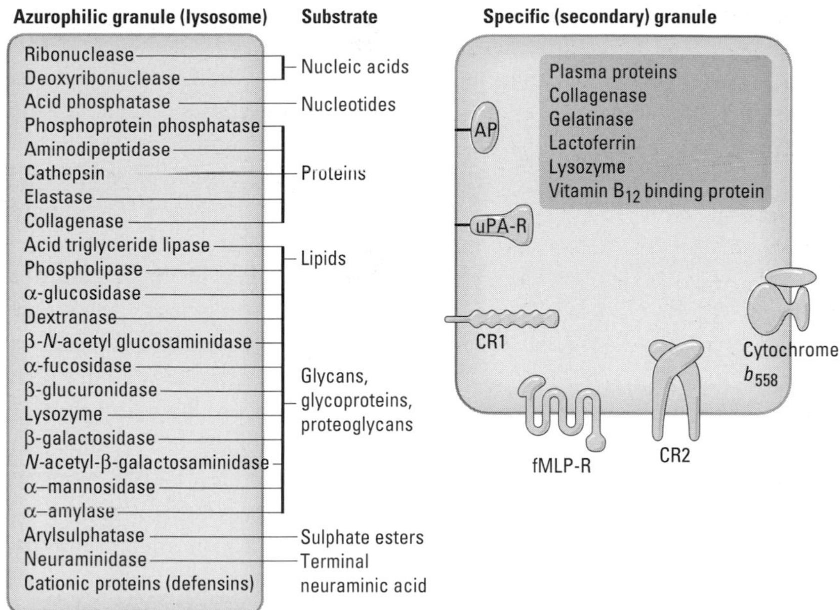

Figure 15.4 Contents of primary and secondary granules found in neutrophils. When discharged (degranulated), the enzymes act on their indicated substrates and thus contribute to the digestion of the ingested particles in the phagosome. Other components (defensins) kill ingested microbes by creating lytic pores in their membranes. Two other types of granules (secretory vesicles and gelatinase granules) similar to secondary granules are not shown here. In the case of secondary granules, examples of membrane proteins residing in them are shown: CR1, complement receptor type 1 (CD35); CR3, complement receptor type 3 (CD11b/CD18); uPA-R, urokinase plasminogen activator receptor (CD87); alkaline phosphatase (AP); cytochrome b_{558}. After fusion of the granule with the plasma membrane these receptors will appear on the cell surface. Note that some of these are transmembrane proteins while others (AP, uPA-R) are anchored in the membrane via a glycolipid tail. The membranes of the azurophilic granules also contain integral membrane proteins (not shown here) such as CD63, lysosome-associated membrane protein 1 (LAMP-1; CD107a) and LAMP-2 (CD107b). These heavily glycosylated proteins protect the lysosomal membrane from destruction by lysosomal hydrolases.

particle cause lysosomes (azurophilic granules) to fuse with the phagosome and empty their content into it. The lysosomes adhere to the phagosome membrane and the membranes fuse and dissolve, forming an opening through which the content of the granule passes into the vacuole. The undissolved granule membrane becomes an integral part of the vacuole membrane so that with each fusion the vacuole (now referred to as a *phagocytic lysosome* or *phagolysosome*) increases in size. This emptying process is most striking in neutrophils, in which the cytoplasm gradually becomes (and remains) granule-free, or *degranulated*, as a result.

The emptying of granules into the phagocytic vacuole actually begins while the vacuole is still open, through a membrane channel to the cell exterior, and for this reason some of the granule's contents may be discharged to the outside. Extracellular enzyme release may also occur under other circumstances, most notably when the cell dies, whether before, during or after phagocytosis. Lysosome contents can be also discharged to the outside when the phagocyte attempts to devour an object that is too large, e.g. a multicellular parasite or an antibody-coated glass bead presented by an immunologist in the laboratory. The enzymes and other active substances released by extracellular degranulation are responsible for the tissue injury associated with a variety of immunological reactions. In many instances, the effect of these enzymes is probably similar to that occurring during intracellular degranulation.

One of the consequences of degranulation is *acidification* of the phagosome, which can even begin before the first lysosome or granule has fused with the phagocytic vacuole. Within a few minutes of particle ingestion, the pH in the phagosome begins to drop until it reaches a value of 4 or lower. The reason for this initial drop is the accumulation of lactic acid and hydrogen ions produced by glycolysis during the respiratory burst (another microbicidal mechanism described later). Further decrease in pH occurs when acidic lysosomes and granules empty their contents into the

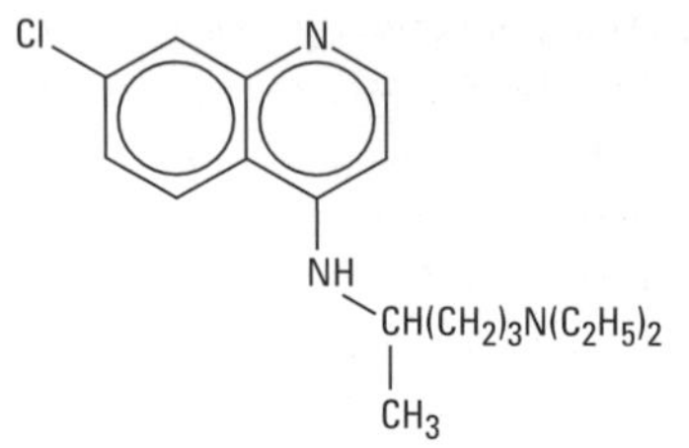

Figure 15.5 Structural formula of chloroquine.

phagosome. The acidification of the phagosome facilitates the killing of ingested microorganisms in at least two ways. First, few bacteria can live at low pH and those that do cannot multiply. Second, many enzymes contained in the granules function best at an acid pH.

Lysosomes achieve their acidity by pumping in hydrogen cations (H^+, protons) with the help of specialized ATP-driven proton pumps. The function of lysosomes can be blocked by weak bases such as ammonium chloride or *chloroquine* (Fig. 15.5). In their uncharged lipophilic form, these substances readily cross membranes and home in on lysosomes. Once in the lysosomes, they bind H^+ ions (they are protonated) and thus become trapped because in this charged form they are unable to cross the membranes again. The trapped protons cause the pH to rise and the lysosomal enzymes that require an acidic environment become inactive. The digestion of ingested material then slows down or stops completely. (The well-known therapeutic effect of chloroquine on malaria can be explained on the same principle: the accumulation of chloroquine in the lysosomes of the parasite blocks the digestion of haemoglobin, the parasite's main source of nutrients.)

Azurophilic granules contain several antibiotic peptides and proteins, such as bacterial permeability increasing factor (BPI), lysozyme, lactoferrin, the peptides bactenecins, protegrins and indolicidin, a group of small basic proteins (defensins) and serine protease homologues (serprocidins). BPI is a membrane-associated protein of M_r 55 000. Its very basic N-terminal half has a strong affinity for the negatively charged lipopolysaccharides of the Gram-negative bacterial envelope. The binding of BPI to the bacterial envelope perturbs its organization, resulting in increased permeability and loss of intracellular components. *Lysozyme* is an enzyme (muramidase) that hydrolyses polysaccharides of bacterial cell walls. *Lactoferrin* binds iron ions very tightly, sequestering them effectively and thus preventing their utilization by microorganisms.

Defensins are among the major components of azurophilic granules: they make up 18% of the total protein in rabbit granulocytes. Ten defensins from various species have been described in detail; their molecules consist of 29–43 mostly basic amino acid residues and contain three characteristic intramolecular disulphide bonds (Fig. 15.6). Human neutrophils contain four structurally similar defensins, the *human neutrophil protein (HNP)-1, -2, -3* and *-4*; HNP-1, -2 and -3 differ from one another in one amino acid residue only. Mouse neutrophils lack defensins but defensin-like proteins, *cryptdins,* are present in mouse Paneth cells, specialized epithelial cells of the small intestine that are part of the antimicrobial barrier in the small bowel mucosa. Defensins are mainly active in combating Gram-negative bacteria, fungi and enveloped viruses. Their molecules have two faces, one cationic and the other hydrophobic. They attach to the negatively charged microbial surface polymers by the cationic face and then insert themselves into the membrane via the hydrophobic face. Oligomers of such membrane-inserted defensin molecules form lytic, permeable channels in the membrane, similar to those formed by the complement membrane attack complex. In addition to their bacteriolytic activity, defensins also have chemotactic effects on leucocytes. Defensins may be evolutionarily very old. They are part of the antimicrobial defence system of insect haemolymph (see Chapter 1) and similar protective peptides occur in plants as well. However, it is not quite clear whether vertebrate and invertebrate defensins are evolutionarily related or rather products of convergent evolution.

Serprocidins are a group of cationic glycoproteins with M_r 25 000–29 000. They include the proteolytic enzymes *cathepsin G, elastase* and *proteinase-3 (PR-3)*. Their abundance in azurophilic granules of neutrophils matches that of

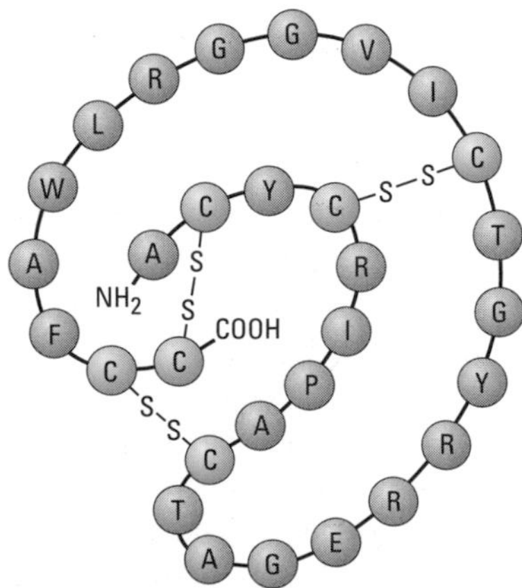

Figure 15.6 Primary structure of the human defensin HNP-1 (human neutrophil protein 1). Note the three disulphide bonds that influence tertiary structure of the molecule. Amino acid residues are given in the one-letter code. (See appendix 1.)

defensins but they are also present in lower amounts in monocytes and macrophages. One member of this group, *azurocidin*, is structurally similar to the other, enzymatically active serprocidins, but it has no enzymatic activity. It is a 'sterile enzyme' because of two amino acid substitutions (His→Ser, Ser→Gly) in the region corresponding to the catalytic site. Azurocidin is especially active against Gram-negative bacteria. In contrast to defensins, which are most efficient on actively growing microorganisms at neutral pH, azurocidin functions best at low pH irrespective of the metabolic state of the attacked microbe. The cationic azurocidin seems to act by binding to the anionic lipopolysaccharide (LPS) of Gram-negative bacteria. Azurocidin is also a potent chemotactic agent for monocytes and therefore an important inflammation-inducing factor.

The formation of the phagosome and the phagolysosome is somewhat more complicated than described here. In reality, the composition of the phagosome membrane (which was originally part of the plasma membrane) is considerably modified before it fuses with azurophilic granules. During this process of *phagosome maturation* some proteins are removed from the membrane and recycled back to the cell surface, while others are added by fusion with small vesicles originating from other intracellular membraneous compartments such as the Golgi apparatus and endosomes.

Disposal phase

The Czech poet, Jan Neruda, once wrote an essay entitled 'Whither with it?', in which he described his trials and tribulations in trying to get rid of a straw mattress in nineteenth-century Prague. 'Whither with it?' is also the problem a phagocyte faces once it has digested foreign material. Instead of a mattress, 'it' refers in this case to the leftovers of digestion. Many substances are digested right back to their building blocks (amino acids, sugars, lipids and nucleotides) but the remainder often prove to be indigestible. The building blocks may cross the membranes to be reutilized in the cell's metabolism, but the 'indigestibles' are difficult to dispose of. The phagocyte, theoretically, has three choices: defecation, indigestion or death. It can discharge the contents of old lysosomes into the surrounding medium by exocytosis. However, this solution means that hydrolytic enzymes are released from the bag and could damage extracellular structures. Alternatively, the phagocyte can store the indigestible material within the lysosomes, fusing them into ever greater vesicles filled with wastage. By opting for this solution, the phagocyte may become chronically constipated, which is not good for the body either. Finally, the phagocyte may simply continue accumulating the wastage until it is full, gobbling up as many particles as it can before it dies and is ejected from the body, for example with the sputum. It seems that this third possibility, the least harmful for the body, is the one that phagocytes most frequently use.

Under normal conditions the phagocytes (mainly granulocytes) die by apoptosis, which does not lead to the release of dangerous lysosomal components. Instead, the cytoplasm becomes highly cross-linked and the cell partially disintegrates into *apoptotic bodies* in which the cellular contents are safely contained. Granulocytes succumbing to apoptosis and the apoptotic bodies themselves can then be removed by macrophages or ejected from the body.

In certain pathological conditions, the constraints on unloading lysosomal contents into extracellular spaces may break down and the released enzymes may erode the tissues. This seems to happen, for example, in rheumatoid arthritis, when phagocytes fail to digest the masses of immune complexes and begin to pour hydrolases into phagosomes while these are still open to the extracellular spaces. Part of the damage to the joint tissue, which is characteristic of rheumatoid arthritis, may be caused by this uncontrolled, extracellular spillage of hydrolases.

Damage by phagocytes also appears to contribute significantly to the development of *atherosclerosis*, specifically to the appearance of *atherosclerotic plaques* in arterial walls. Precursors of the plaques are the 'fatty streaks', macroscopically distinguishable white spots formed mainly by *foam cells*. The latter are monocytes that have engulfed large amounts of fatty droplets consisting of the major blood lipoprotein, low-density lipoprotein (LDL). According to one hypothesis, LDL particles modified by oxidation are deposited on arterial walls and recognized by the scavenger receptors on monocyte and macrophage surfaces. Macrophages adhering to the arterial wall and stimulated via their scavenger receptors may release toxic substances from their primary granules and reactive oxygen intermediates during their attempts to phagocytose the lipoprotein particles firmly attached to the vessel walls. The result is direct tissue damage and development of local chronic inflammation, which aggravates the situation and may finally lead to irreversible necrotic changes. An alternative hypothesis suggests that the primary injury is caused in sites subject to increased haemodynamic stress due to high blood pressure, smoking or hypercholesterolaemia. The injured endothelial cells may expose their *stress proteins* (heat-shock proteins) that are presumably recognized by a subset of T cells. Activation of these T cells could be the primary cause of local inflammation accompanied by infiltration of the chronically stimulated macrophages and monocytes.

Respiratory burst

An important mechanism contributing to the killing of phagocytosed microorganisms is the *respiratory burst*, in which oxygen metabolites are produced that are toxic to the microbes. Resting neutrophils and monocytes consume little oxygen, since they derive most of their energy from the enzymatic degradation of glucose occurring in the absence of oxygen (anaerobic glycolysis). Upon stimulation of both neutrophils and macrophages, oxygen uptake markedly increases above the baseline level. The increase is more pronounced for neutrophils than for other phagocytes, it occurs rapidly and is accompanied by other metabolic changes usually associated with respiration, hence the name *respiratory (metabolic, oxidative) burst.* The metabolic changes usually accompany, and are actually part of, phagocytosis but they can be separated from the ingestion process. For example, the mould metabolite cytochalasin B, an inhibitor of actin polymerization, inhibits the ingestion but not the digestion of particles.

While respiration is normally carried out by enzymes in the mitochondrial membranes, the respiratory burst clearly has nothing to do with these organelles. Agents such as azides and cyanides, which block the mitochondrial enzymes, have no effect on the respiratory burst. Instead, the latter involves a complex enzyme, *nicotinamide adenine dinucleotidephosphate (NADPH) oxidase*, in the plasma and the phagosomal membranes. The enzyme catalyses the reaction:

$$2O_2 + \text{NADPH} \rightarrow 2O_2^- + \text{NADP}^+ + H^+$$

The principle of this reaction is reduction (addition of an electron) of molecular oxygen, O_2, to *superoxide anion*, O_2^-. Superoxide, which is a *radical* because it contains an unpaired electron, is then converted spontaneously and enzymatically into other products described below.

The electrons required for the $O_2 \rightarrow O_2^-$ conversion are donated by NADPH (Fig. 15.7), a universal, soluble reduction agent used by cells in many synthetic reactions. NADPH is produced in the cytoplasm by the *pentose phosphate pathway*, also called the *pentose shunt* or *hexose monophosphate pathway (shunt).* The pathway is a sequence of enzymatic chemical reactions in which glucose (a hexose) is first converted into glucose 6-phosphate, which is then converted, via 6-phosphogluconate, into ribose 5-phosphate (a pentose). This conversion requires the participation of NADP^+ as an electron acceptor, which is thereby converted to NADPH. The latter is then used in the respiratory burst. Ribose 5-phosphate is further degraded in a series of steps into CO_2; during this process, 24 equivalents of hydrogen atoms are obtained in the form of reduced NADPH.

The NADPH $\rightarrow$ NADP^+ reaction during the respiratory burst generates large amounts of NADP^+; additional NADP^+ is also released during the subsequent reduction of superoxide, as discussed later. The accumulation of NADP^+ stimulates the pentose phosphate pathway, which regenerates NADPH from NADP^+. The subsequent increased flow of glucose through this pathway is one of the hallmarks of the respiratory burst. Further characteristics are associated with the processing of superoxide generated in the first stage of the burst.

The redox reaction[1] yielding the superoxide radical anion is somewhat more complicated than the summary reaction given above might seem to indicate. A central role in the NADPH oxidase is played by cytochrome b_{558}, which binds NADPH and another redox intermediate, flavin adenine dinucleotide (FAD; Fig. 15.7). In the course of the enzymatic reaction, NADPH first converts FAD into its reduced form, FADH_2, and the latter in turn passes the electrons on to the iron (Fe^{3+}) ions of the haem prosthetic group of cytochrome *b* (Fig. 15.8). The reduced cytochrome *b* then transfers an electron on to the O_2 molecule turning it into the superoxide radical anion O_2^-. The electrons thus pass from one electron carrier to the next.

Assembly and regulation of NADPH oxidase

NADPH oxidase is a multicomponent structure that is assembled and activated only when the superoxide and other reactive oxidative intermediates are required (Fig. 15.9). The core of the enzyme complex is cytochrome b_{558}, which is composed of two transmembrane subunits, an α subunit (p21phox; M_r 21 000 phagocyte oxidase factor) and a β subunit (gp91phox) of M_r 91 000. The β subunit is heavily glycosylated and contains binding sites in its cytoplasmic domain for both FAD and NADPH. The haem group seems to be located in the α subunit. Cytoplasmic components of the NADPH oxidase complex include two proteins, p47phox and p67phox, and a GTP-binding protein (G-protein), Rac-2, with M_r 21 000. After activation, these three proteins move from the cytoplasm to the membrane, associate with the cytochrome and change its conformation in such a way that it becomes capable of catalysing the formation of superoxide. A fully functional enzyme is assembled within 2 s after stimulation. The signals responsible for the regulated activation of

1 Redox, or oxidation–reduction reaction, is generally any reaction in which one partner is oxidized and the other reduced.

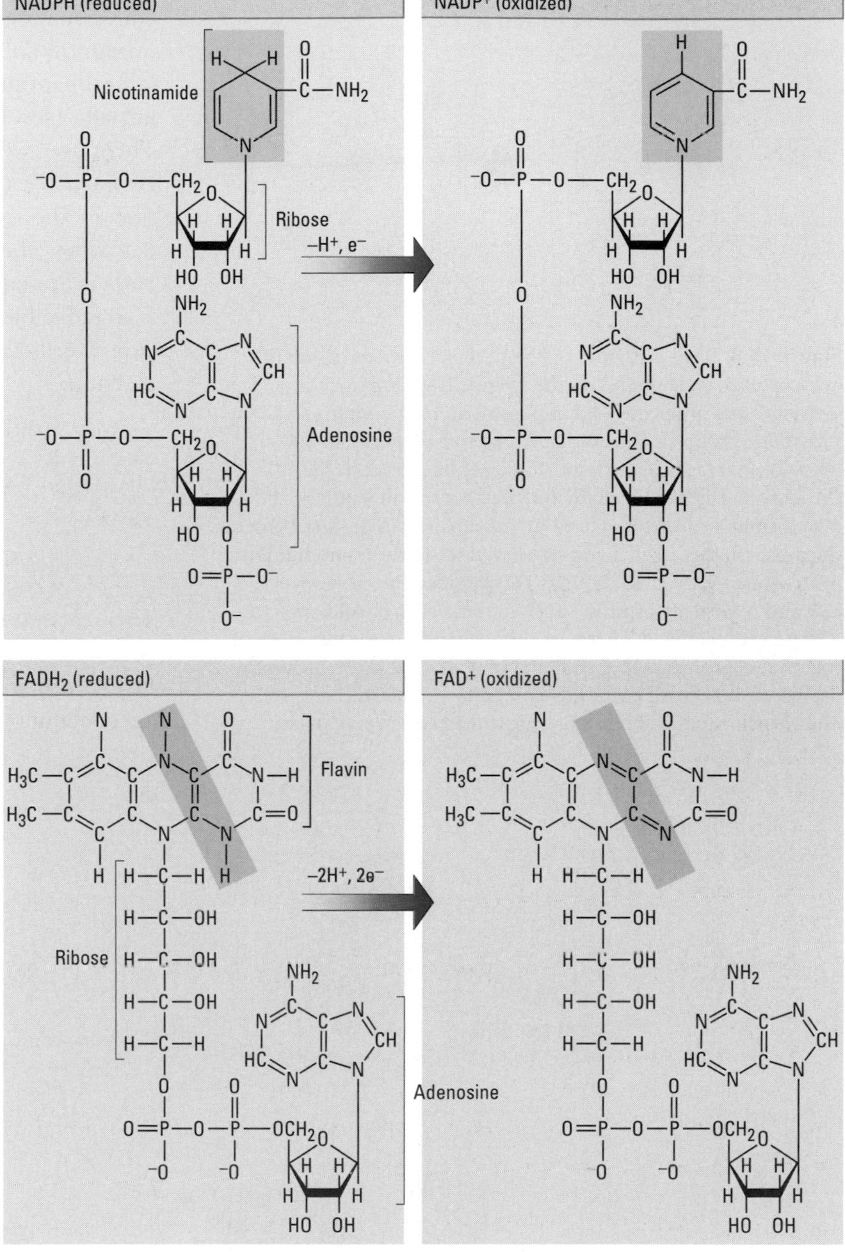

Figure 15.7 Structures of NADPH, NADP+, $FADH_2$ and FAD^+. NADPH, reduced form of nicotinamide adenine dinucleotide phosphate; $NADP^+$, oxidized form thereof; $FADH_2$, reduced form of flavine adenine dinucleotide; FAD^+, oxidized form thereof.

NADPH oxidase complex are discussed later in this chapter.

Production of other reactive oxygen intermediates from superoxide

Superoxide anions are quite unstable in aqueous solutions, particularly at acid pH. They dissociate spontaneously (i.e. without the participation of enzymes or other catalysts) into hydrogen peroxide, H_2O_2, and molecular oxygen, O_2:

$$2O_2^- + 2H^+ \rightarrow H_2O_2 + O_2$$

Some 80% of O_2^- generated during the respiratory burst undergoes spontaneous dismutation (Greek *dis*, two; Latin *muto*, change; a reaction in which two molecules of a similar kind interact in such a way that one is oxidized and the other reduced) at the cell surface or in the acidic phagosome. The rest may diffuse across the membrane and into the cytosol, where it can be converted into harmful substances. To prevent this from happening, the escaped super-

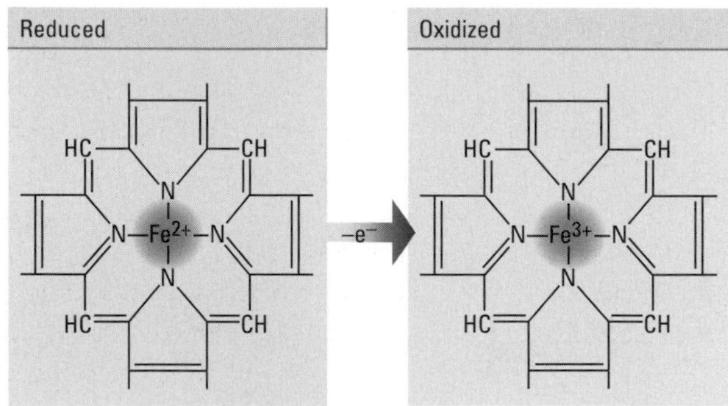

Figure 15.8 Basic structure of haem, the prosthetic group of cytochromes (side-chains on the pyrrole rings are not shown). Cytochromes are proteins that possess an iron-containing haem prosthetic group similar to that found in haemoglobin and myoglobin. Haem imparts a colour, generally red, to the cytochrome, as well as characteristic absorption bands to the cytochrome's spectrum. Based on the position in the spectrum of the most characteristic bands observed when the compounds are in a reduced state, cytochromes are classified into three types, *a*, *b* and *c*, with absorption bands in the region of 600, 555 and 550 nm, respectively. The types differ slightly in the structure of their haem groups. The iron in the centre of the haem group can oscillate between an oxidized (Fe^{3+}) and a reduced (Fe^{2+}) state, and cytochromes can therefore function as electron carriers.

oxide must be neutralized by conversion into water. The conversion occurs by dismutation catalysed by *superoxide dismutase* (SOD) in the cytosol. The enzyme is present in large quantities in all organisms that require oxygen for growth (aerobes); anaerobes contain little or no SOD. There are two kinds of SOD, one containing copper and zinc and the other containing manganese. It is the former that in the cytosol of neutrophils and other phagocytes detoxifies the superoxide anion; manganese-containing SOD is present in the mitochondria. In macrophages, SOD is an inducible enzyme, its activity being promoted by exposure of cells to high oxygen concentrations. It catalyses the reaction:

$$2O_2^- + 2H^+ \rightarrow H_2O_2 + O_2$$

Hydrogen peroxide is then converted into water and oxygen:

$$2H_2O_2 \rightarrow 2H_2O + O_2$$

This reaction is accelerated by *catalase*, a cytosolic enzyme with four haem groups. An alternative way of converting H_2O_2 into water involves glutathione (GSH), a reducing agent commonly used by eukaryotic cells:

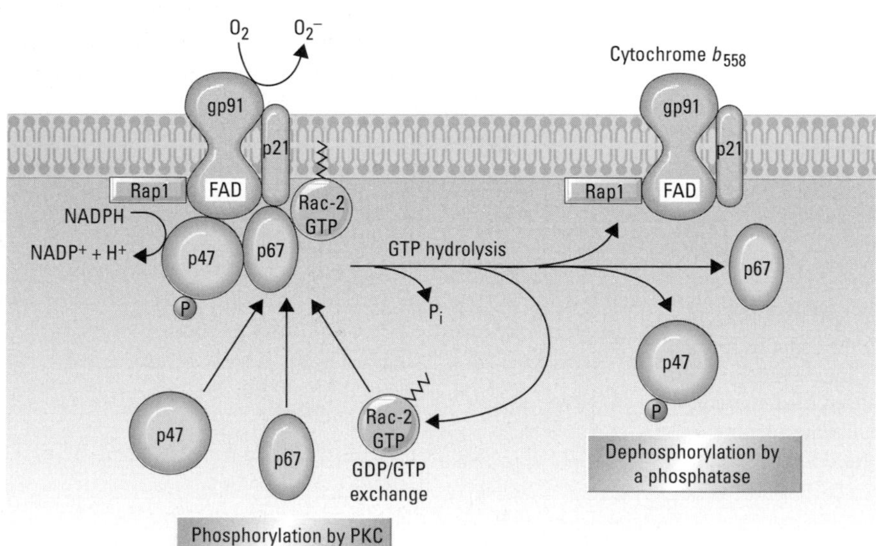

Figure 15.9 Activation of NADPH oxidase. Cytochrome b_{558} is an integral membrane protein consisting of two subunits, gp91phox (gp91) and p21phox (p21) constitutively associated with a small G-protein Rap1a, whose function is not known. The glycosylation site of the cytochrome is on the exterior and the flavine adenine dinucleotide (FAD) and nicotinamide adenine dinucleotide phosphate (NADPH) binding sites are on the interior of the plasma membrane. On activation (initiated by signals from Fc receptors, chemotactic receptors, etc.; see Fig. 15.1), cytosolic constituents p47phox (p47), p67phox (p67) and Rac-2 are translocated to the plasma membrane, where they bind to the cytochrome and initiate superoxide formation. This process involves phosphorylation of p47 by protein kinase C (PKC) and exchange of guanosine diphosphate (GDP) for guanosine triphosphate (GTP) on Rac-2. The latter is also regulated by phosphorylation of regulatory proteins not shown here. The G-protein Rac-2 is covalently modified by isoprenylation, which is necessary for membrane attachment. Rac-2 itself has GTPase activity, which causes GTP hydrolysis into GDP and phosphate (P_i) and leads to disassembly of the active complex. (Modified from Bastian, N. R. & Hibbs Jr, J. B. (1994) *Current Opinion in Immunology*, **6**, 131.)

$$H_2O_2 + 2GSH \rightarrow 2H_2O + GSSG$$

where GSH is the reduced and GSSG the oxidized form of glutathione (the latter is a Glu-Cys-Gly tripeptide; Fig. 15.10). The reaction is catalysed by the selenium-containing enzyme *glutathione peroxidase*. GSSG is then converted back into GSH by reduction with NADPH:

$$GSSG + 2NADPH \rightarrow 2GSH + 2NADP^+$$

This conversion is catalysed by the enzyme *glutathione reductase*. The $NADP^+$ generated in this reaction enters, together with $NADP^+$ generated by the action of NADPH oxidase, the pentose monophosphate pathway. The reactions of the respiratory burst are summarized in Fig. 15.11.

The respiratory burst generates two other oxygen species, hydroxyl radical and singlet oxygen, in addition to the superoxide anion and the peroxide anion. *Hydroxyl radical*, ·OH, forms when an electron is added to hydrogen peroxide. This can happen by reaction of superoxide with hydrogen peroxide:

$$O_2^- + H_2O_2 \rightarrow O_2 + OH^- + {}^{\cdot}OH$$

Singlet oxygen, $^1O_2$, can theoretically be formed in several chemical reactions, for example by spontaneous dismutation:

$$2O_2^- + 2H^+ \rightarrow {}^1O_2 + H_2O_2$$

The difference between this and the earlier reaction ($2O_2^- + 2H^+ \rightarrow H_2O_2 + O_2$) lies in the type of oxygen produced, either ground-state or singlet. Both have the same number of electrons but one of the unpaired electrons in the singlet oxygen has been altered. In the ground-state oxygen, the unpaired valence electrons spin in separate orbits in the same direction, whereas in the singlet oxygen they spin in opposite directions. Singlet oxygen is inherently unstable and returns to the ground state spontaneously within a short time, a process that is accompanied by the release of photons. Light production during a chemical reaction, or *chemiluminescence*, is one of the characteristics of the respiratory burst. Light production by neutrophils reaches a maximum about 15 min after ingestion of microorganisms. The flashes of light are too weak to be seen with the naked eye, but they can be recorded by a scintillation counter.

Toxicity of oxygen radicals

The four oxygen derivatives generated during the respiratory burst, superoxide anion, hydrogen peroxide, hydroxyl radical and singlet oxygen, are highly reactive. In most biological systems, these four act as oxidants by accepting electrons from a variety of compounds. In doing so, they change the properties of these compounds and thus interfere with their normal function; in other words, they are toxic. As the oxygen consumption occurs in the region of

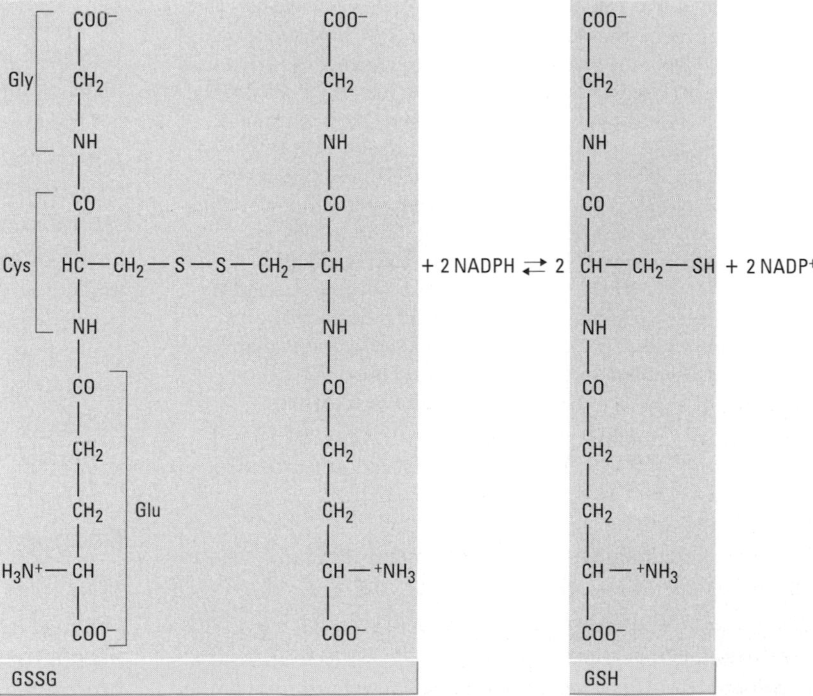

Figure 15.10 Interconversions of the oxidized (GSSG) and reduced (GSH) forms of glutathione.

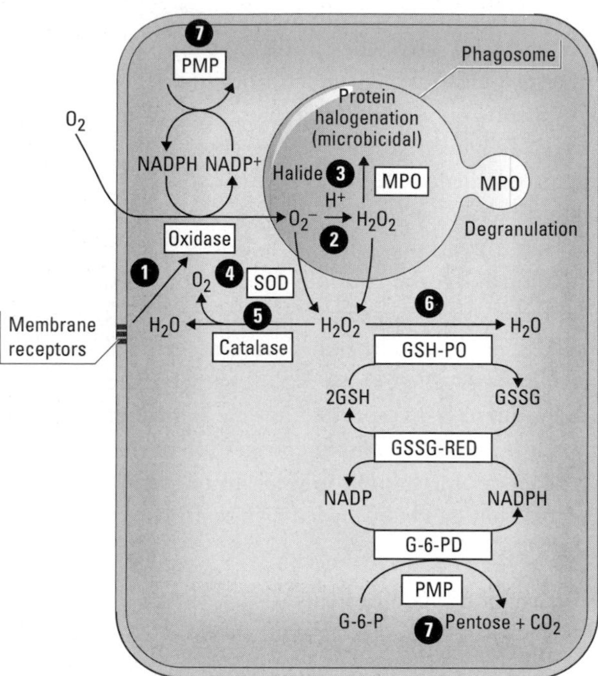

Figure 15.11 Some of the reactions occurring during the respiratory burst in the neutrophil. (1) Signal received by a receptor on the outer surface of the plasma membrane is transmitted to nicotinamide adenine dinucleotide phosphate (NADPH) oxidase, which converts molecular oxygen (O_2) into superoxide (O_2^-) with the help of NADPH provided by the pentose monophosphate (PMP) pathway. (2) Superoxide in the phagosome is further reduced by spontaneous dismutation to hydrogen peroxide (H_2O_2). (3) Myeloperoxidase (MPO), discharged into the phagosome from granules, uses H_2O_2 together with halide ions as substrate and catalyses halogenation of bacterial proteins, thus killing the invaders. (4) Superoxide that has escaped from the phagosome is reduced further to peroxide in a reaction catalysed by the enzyme superoxide dismutase (SOD). (5) Peroxide is reduced further to O_2 and H_2O in a reaction catalysed by the enzyme catalase. Some of the O_2 may be reused and again converted into superoxide. (6) Peroxide oxidizes glutathione (GSH) in a reaction catalysed by glutathione peroxidase (GSH-PO). The oxidized glutathione (GSSG) is reduced with the aid of NADPH and the enzyme glutathione reductase (GSSG-RED). (7) NADPH is provided by the pentose monophosphate pathway in which glucose is degraded into simpler molecules. The pathway is stimulated by the availability of NADP+ generated during the respiratory burst in reactions catalysed by NADPH oxidase and glutathione reductase. (Modified from Root, R. K. & Cohen, M. S. (1981) *Reviews of Infectious Diseases*, 3, 565.)

particle attachment to the plasma membrane and then on the inner surface of the phagosome, the reactive oxygen species, almost all of which are short-lived, attack the particle during its ingestion.

Superoxide anion itself does not seem to participate in the attack because it is almost immediately converted into other reactive oxygen derivatives. Hydrogen peroxide is a well-known germicidal agent, whose activity is greatly enhanced by peroxidase and halides. The interaction with a chloride, for example, produces hypochlorous acid:

$$H_2O_2 + Cl^- + H^+ \rightarrow H_2O + HOCl$$

The reaction is catalysed by the enzyme *myeloperoxidase* (MPO), which the phagosome receives from the lysosomes (granules). Hypochlorous acid can react with chloride to form chlorine:

$$HOCl + Cl^- \rightarrow Cl_2 + OH^-$$

HOCl and Cl_2 are highly reactive agents that can chlorinate and oxidize a large number of compounds. (Chlorine derivatives are widely used as disinfectants.) The myeloperoxidase–H_2O_2–halide system has been shown to kill a variety of bacteria, fungi, viruses, mycoplasmas, protozoa such as *Leishmania* and *Trypanosoma*, multicellular organisms such as schistosomula of *Schistosoma mansoni* and tumour cells. MPO is present primarily in the granules of resting neutrophils and increases in amount after stimulation. Eosinophils contain another enzyme in their granules, *eosinophil peroxidase* (EPO), which seems to act by a similar mechanism to MPO. EPO is a strongly basic protein that binds firmly to negatively charged surfaces such as those of *Staphylococcus aureus*. The binding concentrates the reaction directly on the microorganism. Promonocytes and monocytes contain MPO-positive granules, but macrophages generally lose their granular peroxidase during maturation in tissues, which is one of the reasons why mature macrophages are not very good at killing ingested microorganisms.

Other reactive oxygen derivatives such as the hydroxyl radical and singlet oxygen can also attack biopolymers of the microorganism. They can break double bonds in unsaturated fatty acids of the membrane, produce carbonyl groups in proteins, which can then react with amino groups and cause protein cross-linking, and oxidize thiol groups in the active sites of many enzymes. The hydroxyl radical may break both hydrogen bonds and polynucleotide chains and degrade purine and pyrimidine bases in nucleic acids. The end result of these and many other changes is the cessation of normal function in ingested microorganisms.

Phagocyte secretions

Primary (azurophilic) granules (lysosomes) are used by neutrophils to kill phagocytosed microbes. Secondary (specific) phagocyte granules contain various plasma proteins and proteolytic enzymes which, after their release, contribute to the digestion of the extracellular matrix and thus facilitate movement of the stimulated phagocytes through the tissues towards the source of infection. The membranes of these granules contain large numbers of various receptors and adhesion molecules (see Fig. 15.4). Fusion of the granules with the plasma membrane greatly increases the number of these molecules on the cell surface, where they are needed following activation of the phagocyte. This is a rapid process (it takes place within minutes after stimulation) because it is not dependent on *de novo* synthesis of proteins. Intracellular granules thus serve as storage containers for proteins that can rapidly (within minutes after stimulation) be delivered to the cell surface.

Granulocyte *secondary (specific) granules* are the major source of soluble enzymes that include collagenase, plasminogen activator, part of the membrane-bound CR3 and urokinase plasminogen activator receptor (uPAR; CD87).

Secretory vesicles contain soluble plasma proteins and membrane-bound CR1, as well as membrane-bound enzymes such as alkaline phosphatase and cytochrome b_{558} (the core part of NADPH oxidase). They are the most easily mobilized type of cytoplasmic granules because they fuse with the plasma membrane in response to minor stimuli, sometimes even as insignificant as manipulation of neutrophils during their isolation (centrifugation, washing, incubation in physiological solution).

Gelatinase granules are the main reservoir of gelatinase, another protease that efficiently digests the extracellular matrix, and of several previously mentioned membrane proteins, such as the receptor of chemotactic bacterial peptides (fMLP receptor), cytochrome b_{558} and CR3. In most cases, there is no absolute segregation of proteins among the different cytoplasmic granules (vesicles); most of the granules contain certain amounts of all the proteins, but in different proportions.

Granulocytes, as terminally differentiated, metabolically not very active cells of short lifespan, are rather limited in their ability to secrete large amounts of soluble proteins or other substances continuously. Their main strength in this respect is the possession of large supplies of preformed molecules stored in the granules. After activation, however, neutrophils *are* capable of increased protein synthesis and secretion of freshly made proteins, including several cytokines (interleukin (IL)-1β, IL-8, TNF-α, IL-1 receptor antagonist and others) and products of arachidonic acid metabolism (see Chapter 11).

Macrophages are able to produce and secrete many products, such as complement components of the classical and alternative pathways, clotting factors, cytokines, many hydrolytic enzymes such as most of those contained in lysosomes (see Fig. 15.4), blood plasma proteins (e.g. transferrin, transcobalamin II, fibronectin, thrombospondin), enzyme inhibitors (plasmin inhibitor, α_2-macroglobulin, α_1-antitrypsin), nucleotide metabolites, steroid hormones and arachidonic acid derivatives (prostaglandins, prostacyclin, thromboxanes; see Chapter 11). A few products are secreted constitutively whereas others require selective induction via cell-surface receptors. The occupancy of some of these receptors, for example Fc receptors, triggers a widespread secretory response; the occupancy of others results in a more restricted response. Some receptors, such as the complement receptors, do not initiate any secretory response at all. The mere clustering of Fc receptors on the cell surface by multivalent ligands, without internalization, is sufficient to initiate release of some of the products.

The extensive biological potential of the secreted products is described in more detail in Chapter 21.

Chemotaxis and extravasation

The battle between invaders and defenders in the afflicted host tissues can be recognized by the 'smoke' rising above the battlefield, which is made up of many substances that diffuse into the surrounding tissues. The concentration of these substances is highest at the actual site of invasion and decreases gradually with distance: there is a chemical *concentration gradient* emanating from the battlefield. Phagocytes in the surrounding tissues, and particularly in the local blood vessels, recognize some of the substances in the gradient and respond to them. As if beckoned by an invisible signal, they stop their random browsing or passive flow with the bloodstream, choose their direction and head straight towards the battlefield. This directed movement of cells in response to a signal is called *chemotaxis* (Greek *chemos*, juice, liquid; *taxis*, an arrangement, also movement). Chemotaxis is, of course, not restricted to phagocytes; it is also exerted by lymphocytes, fibroblasts, melanoblasts, plant spermatozoa or bacteria, but few other cells can respond to such a variety of *chemotactic factors (signals)* as phagocytes. The signals may be generated by numerous different processes taking place during the invasion.

If mechanical injury accompanies the invasion, the damaged cells release a number of substances, some of which act as chemotactic factors. Proteases released from these cells or from activated phagocytes act on complement component 5, splitting off the C5a fragment from it and thus generating one of the most powerful chemotactic factors known. The C5a fragment is, of course, also released during activation of the complement pathway, either directly by bacteria (in the alternative pathway) or by MBP and immune complexes (in the classical pathway).

The fragment is rapidly converted to C5a-des-Arg, which has little inherent chemotactic activity but which combines with an anionic molecule in the serum and thereby regains this activity. Damage to the basement membrane or collagen in the affected tissues leads to the activation of coagulation factor XII, which then converts prekallikrein into kallikrein, another strong chemoattractant (see Chapter 21). Phagocytosis by cells that have already encountered the invader results in the activation of arachidonic acid metabolism and some of the generated metabolites, for example leukotriene B_4, display chemotactic activity. Activated macrophages, neutrophils and lymphocytes also release IL-8 and several related chemokines, all of which are known to stimulate chemotactic behaviour when bound by other macrophages or neutrophils. Chemokines are SOS signals sent out by the succumbing warriors and answered by other warriors. In the later stage of the response, when lymphocytes and mast cells also become involved, they too begin to secrete chemotactic factors. Finally, the invaders themselves become a source of chemotactic activity as described in Chapter 21. All in all, there are many possibilities for an invasion to produce not just one but a whole plethora of factors that attract additional phagocytes to the site of injury or infection. Although some of the accumulating phagocytes are derived from local, proliferating macrophages, the majority are immigrants from other sites, in particular from the blood.

Upon receiving a chemotactic signal, the phagocyte first orients itself in the gradient in such a way that the pseudopod faces the source of the chemoattractant; the cell then begins a directed movement towards the source. How the cells perceive the gradient is not clear. One possibility is that the phagocyte is able to tell the difference between the concentration of the chemoattractant at its front (the pseudopod) and at its tail, and that the cytoplasm always streams in the direction of higher concentration. Evidence is indeed available that phagocytes can distinguish differences in concentration of as little as 0.1% across the cell. Another possibility is that the phagocyte detects differences in concentration at different points in time. It registers the concentration at one point, moves in one direction and then registers the difference in concentration in comparison to the previous point. It continues in this direction only when its 'senses' inform it that the concentration is higher at the second than at the first point. Such temporal 'sensing' might be related to the forward movement of the chemotactic receptors with the extending pseudopod.

Like many other biological processes, chemotaxis, if not stopped when it is no longer needed, may cease to be beneficial and indeed begin to harm the body. Excessive chemotaxis is prevented by a series of control mechanisms that operate according to one of two principles: inactivation of the chemotactic factors or halting of their production. A number of agents that inhibit chemotaxis by one or the other mechanism have been identified. Examples of factor inactivators are the various regulatory proteins associated with the complement cascade and with other activation systems in the plasma. Among the agents that decrease chemotactic responses are cyclic nucleotides; a neutrophil-immobilizing factor extracted from human polymorphonuclear cells and mononuclear leucocytes; a number of pharmacologically active substances such as hydrocortisone, cyclophosphamide and aspirin; certain bacterial products such as *Staphylococcus* cell-wall peptidoglycan and streptolysin O; plasma esterase inhibitors; tuftsin (the phagocytosis-enhancing tetrapeptide, Thr-Lys-Pro-Arg); and alterations in the physicochemical environment such as changes in pH, osmolarity and temperature. Phagocytes that sense the chemotactic signals from the injured site leave the blood circulation, cross the endothelia and enter the tissue by the process of extravasation, as described in Chapter 9.

Macrophage activation

As mentioned earlier, macrophages differ from other phagocytes in that they exist not in two, but in three different states: resting, primed and activated. *Activated macrophages* differ from resting and primed macrophages morphologically, biochemically and functionally. They are larger, they attach more rapidly to glass and plastic and spread more extensively on the support; they display a characteristic undulating (ruffled) plasma membrane; they contain a greater number of mitochondria, lysosomes and ribosomes and a more extensive Golgi apparatus; they exhibit an increased rate and speed of phagocytosis; and they display increased total protein synthesis, increased ATP, lysosomal enzyme and pentose monophosphate pathway activity and increased oxygen consumption. The functional change in activated macrophages manifests itself in their strongly increased ability to destroy microorganisms intracellularly. So conspicuous is the change that immunologists, who are not profuse with hyperbole, refer to these cells as 'angry' or even 'bloodthirsty'!

The transition from resting to primed and from primed to activated macrophage is initiated by different stimuli. Resting macrophages are stimulated by the binding of opsonized particles, various mediators of inflammation and by cytokines, certain bacterial components, synthetic polyanionic co-polymers or muramyl dipeptide (Table 15.1). Primed macrophages secrete a large number of regulatory and effector substances described earlier.

Table 15.1 Selected agents that augment macrophage functional activities.* (From Reiner, N.E. (1994) *Immunology Today*, 15, 374.)

Agent	Response or altered phenotype
Exogenous agents	
Lipopolysaccharide (lipid A)	Y-P, ↑ microbicidal and tumoricidal activities, ↑ cytokine production
fMLP	Oxidative burst, chemotaxis, ↑ cytokine production
Muramyl dipeptide	↑ Tumoricidal and antimicrobial activities, ↑ cytokine production
Zymosan	Y-P, oxidative burst, ↑ arachidonate metabolism and cytokine production
Bacterial exotoxins (e.g. staphylococcal and streptococcal)	↑ Cytokine production
Peptidoglycans	↑ Cytokine production
Endogenous mediators	
Cytokines and growth factors	
Interferon-γ	Y-P, ↑ expression of MHC class I and class II molecules, ↑ tumoricidal and microbicidal activities, priming for cytokine production
Interferon-α, interferon-β	Induction of antiviral and tumoricidal activities
Granulocyte–macrophage colony-stimulating factor	Y-P, priming for oxidative burst, ↑ antimicrobial and tumoricidal activities
Colony-stimulating factor 1	Y-P, priming for oxidative burst, ↑ tumoricidal activities
Tumour necrosis factor	↑ Microbicidal and tumoricidal activities, ↑ MHC class II antigen expression and antigen presentation, chemotaxis
Interleukin-2	↑ Microbicidal and tumoricidal activities
Miscellaneous	
Platelet-activating factor	↑ Arachidonate metabolism and cytokine production
Leukotriene B_4	Chemotaxis, ↑ adhesion, IL-6 production and AP-1 transcription factor activity
Antigen–antibody complexes	Y-P, ↑ cytokine production

* Unless otherwise stated, cytokine production refers to IL-1 and/or TNF. Arrows indicate increase of the activities.
AP-1, activator protein 1 family of transcription factors; fMLP, *N*-formyl-methionyl-leucyl-phenylanine; MHC, major histocompatibility complex; Y-P, tyrosine phosphorylation.

Macrophages are activated mainly by their interaction with T_H1 helper cells (inflammatory T cells). This interaction, described in greater detail in the following chapter, involves mutual stimulation of the two cells. On its surface, the macrophage presents peptide fragments of the ingested microorganism associated with major histocompatibility complex (MHC) class II glycoproteins to the precursor of the T_H1 cell and secretes stimulatory cytokines such as IL-1 and IL-12. The cytokines, especially IL-12, activate the T cell, which starts to produce several cytokines of its own, among others IFN-γ, a powerful macrophage activator. A positive feedback loop thus exists in which IL-12 secreted by macrophages stimulates T_H1 cells, which secrete IFN-γ. Another cell type that may under some circumstances activate macrophages is the NK cell which, like the T_H1 cell, is stimulated by macrophage-produced IL-12 to secrete IFN-γ. Activated macrophages kill intracellular and large extracellular parasites as well as cancer cells by means of reactive oxygen and nitrogen intermediates. Reactive oxygen is described earlier in this chapter; the description of nitrogen intermediates follows.

Nitric oxide and other reactive nitrogen intermediates

Nitric oxide (NO) is a highly reactive molecule with many biological effects. It is produced from the amino acid L-arginine and oxygen in a reaction catalysed by the cytosolic enzyme nitric oxide synthase (NOS):

$$\text{L-arginine} + O_2 \xrightarrow{\text{NOS}} \text{L-citrulline} + \text{NO}^{\bullet}$$

The other product of the reaction, citrulline, is an amino acid not present in proteins. There are at least three different forms of NOS. One of them is present in endothelial cells, in which it produces small amounts of NO upon stimulation in short pulses. The latter binds to the prosthetic haem groups of the enzyme guanylyl cyclase, the activated enzyme catalyses the production of cyclic guanosine monophosphate (GMP) and the cyclic GMP becomes involved in the relaxation of smooth muscle cells and thus in vasodilation. Another form of NOS is expressed in neurons, in which NO serves as an important modulator of synaptic function. The third form of this enzyme, *immune* or *inflammatory NOS* (*iNOS*), is induced in activated macrophages, in which NO and its reaction products contribute to the killing of intracellular parasites (in particular mycobacteria) and to the inhibition of viruses such as ectromelia, vaccinia and herpes simplex 1 residing in mouse macrophages. Inhibition of iNOS causes a fatal mousepox in animals infected with ectromelia virus. The enzyme can also be induced in other infected cells, such as hepatocytes

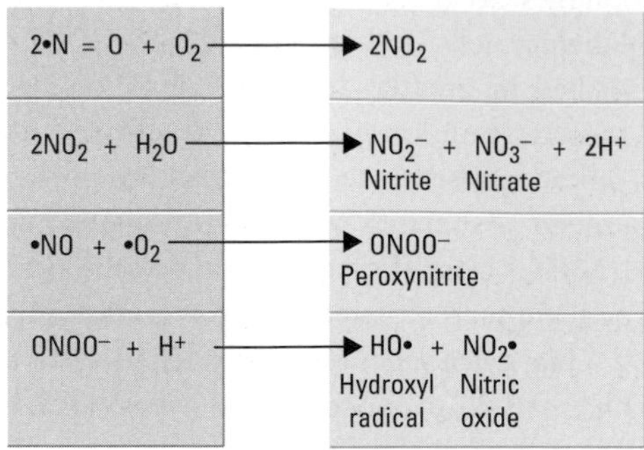

Figure 15.12 Reactions yielding reactive nitrogen intermediates in activated macrophages.

or endothelial cells. Knock-out mice with both copies of their *iNOS* gene disrupted by homologous recombination are highly susceptible to the intracellular parasite *Leishmania major* and to the above-mentioned viruses.

Like superoxide, NO is a radical (it has a free electron) and therefore a very reactive molecule. It can react with ubiquitous molecular oxygen to produce nitrogen dioxide, NO_2, or with superoxide to form peroxynitrite, $ONOO^-$ (Fig. 15.12). These reactive compounds chemically modify functionally important amino, hydroxyl, phenyl and thiol groups in structural proteins and enzymes and irreversibly inhibit their function. NO binds avidly to Fe^{2+} ions in the haem or FeS prosthetic groups of enzymes such as the mitochondrial cytochromes. Inactivation of these enzymes blocks respiration. NO may also impair DNA replication by directly attacking the DNA and by inhibiting enzymes involved in DNA repair. Finally, NO seems to inhibit the development of T_H1 cells and thus prevent overexpansion of these cells.

Regulation of NO production

The iNOS contains binding sites for co-factors NADPH, FAD and FMN (flavin mononucleotide) in its C-terminal haem group. It seems to be structurally related to a haemoprotein, cytochrome P_{450}, which is involved in the hydroxylation of various chemicals that are foreign to the body (xenobiotics). Closely associated with the enzyme is the coenzyme tetrahydrobiopterin and calmodulin. The former is a reduced form of a low-molecular-mass heterocyclic compound; the latter is a cytosolic Ca^{2+}-binding protein that regulates many cytoplasmic enzymes. Obviously, iNOS is a complex structure and the catalytic reaction occurs in several steps, each step involving different parts of the complex.

Production of NO is regulated by two signals that control the transcription of the *iNOS* gene. The first ('priming') signal is provided by IFN-γ and then by TNF-α or bacterial surface components such as LPS, muramyl dipeptide and lipoteichoic acid. Biosynthesis of NO is inhibited by several cytokines such as IL-10, IL-4 or transforming growth factor β, and NO in turn inhibits iNOS; this inhibition is an example of negative feedback regulation. Syntheses of O_2^- and NO are separately regulated and cells avoid the simultaneous production of these potentially self-damaging products and their dangerous derivatives.

Signalling in phagocytes

Earlier in this chapter we described several processes by which phagocytes respond either to an encounter with a microbe or to various other stimuli. These processes are phagocytosis, respiratory burst, exocytosis and degranulation, extravasation, chemotaxis and general activation leading to the secretion of cytokines and various mediators. Each of these responses begins by the interaction of a surface receptor with its ligand (ligation of the receptor), followed by the transmission of the information on this event to the cell interior (signal transduction) and by the triggering of the effector mechanisms (Fig. 15.13). Now we scrutinize signalling mechanisms in some detail (for general aspects of receptor signalling, see Chapter 10).

Signalling in phagocytosis

The signalling involves both constitutively active receptors (such as the mannose receptor and Fc receptors) and receptors activated by various mediators of inflammation. Usually, several receptor types are simultaneously engaged and generate an array of signals and a variety of responses to them. The best characterized is signalling via the Fc and complement receptors. The interaction between Fc receptor and opsonized particle leads to receptor clustering, which brings together protein tyrosine kinases (PTK) bound to the cytoplasmic regions of the Fc receptor-associated γ (and in some Fc receptors also β) chains (Fig. 15.14). These PTK (mainly Lyn, Fgr and Hck), which belong to the Src family (see Chapter 10), phosphorylate each other on the critical tyrosine residues. Phosphorylation activates these enzymes, which in turn phosphorylate the immunoreceptor tyrosine activation motifs (ITAM) in the cytoplasmic regions of the Fc receptor-associated γ and β chains. Phosphorylated ITAM can bind proteins possessing SH2 domains; these include the Src family PTK themselves as well as a more distantly related PTK, Syk. The clustered Fc receptors thus become associated with a group of activated PTK that

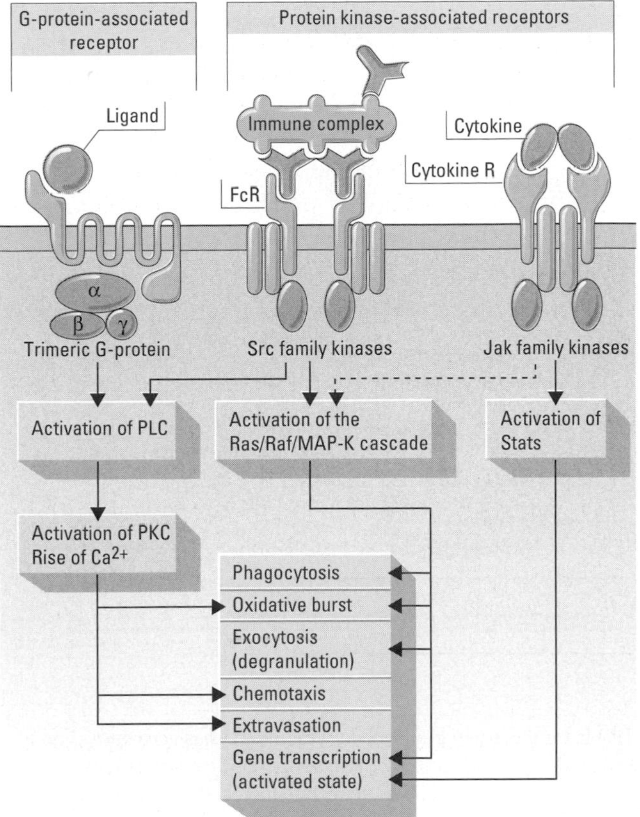

Figure 15.13 Simplified scheme of phagocyte stimulation. Stimulatory ligands can bind to two main types of receptors: those associated with trimeric G-proteins or those associated with protein kinases. The principles of signalling through these two types of receptors are described in Chapter 10 (see Figs 10.23 & 10.27). Among the G-protein-associated receptors are those for interleukin (IL)-8 and other chemokines, anaphylatoxins C3a and C5a, leukotrienes, platelet-activating factor (PAF) and chemotactic bacterial peptides (fMLP). Fc receptors (FcR) and receptors for phagocyte-stimulatory cytokines (e.g. interferon (IFN)-γR) belong to the group of protein kinase-associated receptors: the former are associated with Src family kinases and the latter with Jak family kinases. Signalling via Fc receptors is described in more detail in Fig. 15.14; molecular details of respiratory burst activation are shown in Fig. 15.9; signalling via the IFN-γ receptor is discussed later in this chapter and more generally in Chapter 10. MAP-K, mitogen-activated protein kinase; PKC, protein kinase C, PLC, phospholipase C isoenzymes.

are able to further phosphorylate intracellular substrates, some of which are enzymes (other kinases, phosphatases, phospholipases) or proteins regulating the activity of other enzymes. In this way, a complex interconnected network of phosphorylation-based cascade activations is initiated that triggers various effector mechanisms, including actin filament assembly, pseudopod formation and phagocytosis. The exact nature of the pathway from initial Fc receptor ligation-induced Src kinase activation to actin polymerization is not known. Signals emanating from ligated Fc receptors are somehow able to produce 'nucleation foci' for actin polymerization, probably by changing the structures of certain cytoplasmic actin-binding proteins. The affinity of several of these actin-binding proteins towards actin is modulated by membrane lipids, phosphoinositides, which are in turn modified by the enzyme phosphatidylinositol 3-kinase (PI3-K). The activity of this enzyme is regulated by tyrosine phosphorylation carried out by the Syk kinase. Other intracellular components probably participating in rearrangement of the actin cytoskeleton include the SH2 domain-containing adaptor proteins Shc and Grb2 (see Chapter 10). These proteins cooperate with the small GTP-binding proteins Ras and Rac to modify the activity of several enzymes, including PI3-K (see Fig. 15.14).

CR3 (identical to αMβ2 or CD11a/CD18 integrin) collaborates with the Fc receptor to enhance the intensity of phagocytosis. Some CR3 molecules at least are constitutively associated with the cytoskeleton and their association facilitates the reorganization of actin filaments necessary for phagocytosis. The functional cooperation between Fc receptor and CR3 is aided by the close physical association of these two types of receptors on the phagocyte surface. The importance of CR3 in phagocytosis is demonstrated by the existence of leucocyte adhesion deficiency syndrome in patients who carry a defective gene that normally codes for the β2 integrin subunit of the receptor. Phagocytes of these patients bind to IgG-opsonized targets normally but fail to ingest the particles.

Phagocytosis also involves the β1 family of integrins, which are receptors for various components of the extracellular matrix: large proteins such as fibronectin, vitronectin, entactin, collagens, thrombospondin, von Willebrand factor or laminin (see Chapter 9). Ligation of these components is a signal to the phagocytes, informing them that they are no longer in the bloodstream but in a tissue and that they should get ready for fulfilling their mission. Interaction of at least three integrin receptors (α3β1, α6β1 and an incompletely characterized molecule called *leucocyte response integrin*, LRI) with the extracellular matrix leads to activation of intracellular enzymes, such as phospholipase C and protein kinase C, and to effects on the cytoskeleton synergistic with the effects elicited via the Fc receptor and CR3.

Signalling in the generation of the respiratory burst

Engagement of Fc receptors, complement receptors, scavenger receptors, chemotactic receptors and receptors for

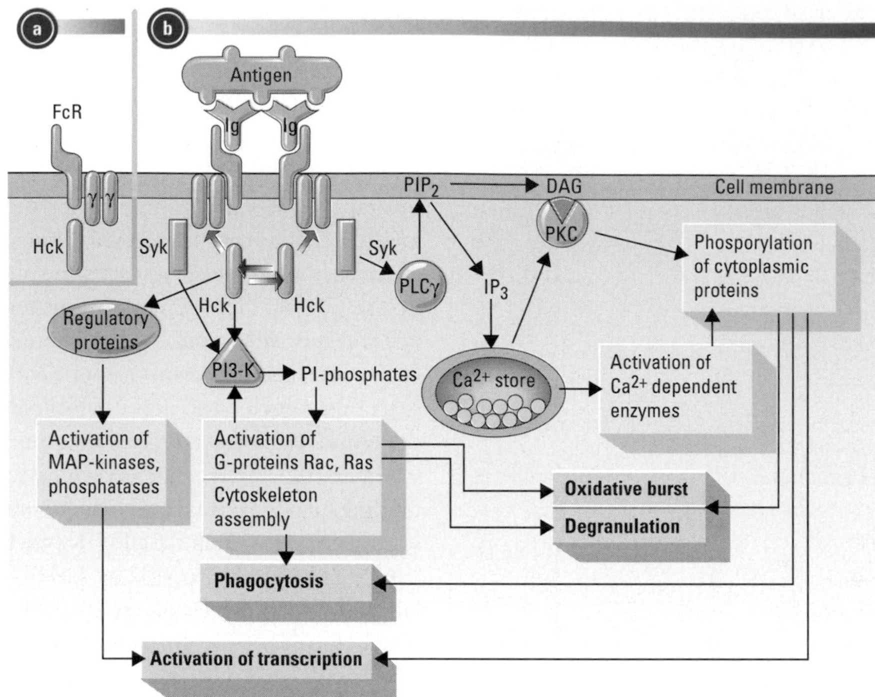

Figure 15.14 Fc receptor signalling. Fc receptors are linked with dimers of γ chains carrying the immunoreceptor tyrosine-based activation motifs (ITAMs; see Fig. 7.30) and associated with Src family protein tyrosine kinases such as Hck, Lyn or Fgr (a). After binding to immune complexes containing multiple IgG molecules (b), several Fc receptor complexes aggregate. The associated Src-family kinases phosphorylate (red arrows) and thereby activate each other. The activated kinases phosphorylate the ITAM sequences of the γ chains (grey arrows). The phosphorylated ITAMs bind protein kinase Syk, which becomes activated. The activated Src-family and Syk kinases phosphorylate several cytoplasmic substrates, which initiate intracellular signalling cascades as generally described in Chapter 10 (see Fig. 10.27). PLCγ, phospholipase Cγ; PIP_2, phosphatidylinositol bisphosphate; DAG, diacylglycerol; IP_3, inositol trisphosphate; PI3-K, phosphatidylinositol 3-kinase; PI, phosphatidylinositol; PKC, protein kinase C.

platelet-activating factor and leukotriene B_4 (LTB_4) triggers the rapid assembly of functional NADPH oxidase in the phagocyte plasma membrane. Assembly is achieved by the translocation of p40phox, p47phox, p67phox and Rac from the cytoplasm to the membrane and the association of these components with cytochrome b_{558}. It is also induced by agents activating protein kinase C (phorbol esters, diacylglycerols) or calcium ionophores (which induce an influx of Ca^{2+} into the cytoplasm), but in these cases the response is much slower compared with physiological stimuli. Fc receptors induce these effects via signals based on the activation of PTK associated with them. Chemotactic receptors, on the other hand, are typical G-protein-associated receptors that function according to a different principle: whereas the PTK-associated receptors activate specific intracellular signalling proteins by phosphorylation, the α-subunits of activated (GTP-bound) G-proteins form complexes with them that exhibit changed enzymatic or binding activities (see Figs 10.23 & 15.1). Both types of receptors indirectly activate several cytoplasmic protein kinases, some of which phosphorylate, among other substrates, p47phox (see Fig. 15.9). Phosphorylation changes the conformation of p47phox and uncovers its regulatory SH3 domains, making them available for interactions with proline-rich sequences in the cytoplasmic tail of p22phox. Simultaneously, the SH3 domain of another protein, p67, is uncovered by an unknown mechanism, and then binds the proline-rich sequence of p47phox. The last component that attaches to the assembling NADPH oxidase complex is a small G-protein, Rac-2 (for classification and description of basic properties of G-proteins, see Chapter 10). It probably binds directly to cytochrome b_{558} and partially also to p67phox, thus modifying both the conformation and enzymatic activity of the whole assembly (see Fig. 15.9). Like other G-proteins, Rac-2 exists in two forms: GTP bound and GDP bound. The ratio between the two forms seems to be critical for the control NADPH oxidase activity because the fully active NADPH oxidase requires the presence of

GTP-bound Rac-2. The oscillation of Rac-2 between the GTP- and GDP-bound forms is regulated by several proteins. One of them, the GTPase-activating protein (GAP), stimulates hydrolysis of GTP into GDP and phosphate by Rac-2 itself (Rac-2, as a typical G-protein, has a rather low intrinsic GTPase activity that can, however, be increased by interaction with GAP). Another regulator protein, guanine nucleotide dissociation inhibitor (GDI), stabilizes the Rac–GDP or Rac–GTP complexes and another still, the guanine nucleotide exchange factor (GEF), enhances the rate of GDP exchange for GTP. The activities of some of these regulatory proteins are controlled by phosphorylation. There is also another small G-protein, Rap1a, which is constitutively associated with cytochrome b_{558}, but its function in the complex is not known. Disengagement of NADPH oxidase must involve the enzymatic dephosphorylation of p47phox (and probably also several other components such as the regulators of Rac-2) by phosphatases that have thus far not been identified.

It is difficult to determine experimentally which phagocyte surface receptors provide signals initiating the oxidative burst (or any other phagocyte responses) because the natural ligands, such as immune complexes or opsonized microorganisms, interact simultaneously with several receptors. To dissect the signalling roles of individual receptor types, immunologists often use simpler, better defined ligands that are highly specific for some of the receptors only, and record the phagocyte response. Among the artificial ligands that mimic the natural ones, the most widely used are monoclonal antibodies or $F(ab)'_2$ fragments specific for particular receptors. (The potentially phagocyte-binding Fc parts of the antibodies must be removed enzymatically before use.) The interaction of $F(ab)'_2$ with one or two binding sites of the macrophage surface receptors is usually not sufficient to aggregate the receptors. To achieve activation, it is necessary to cross-link these primary antibodies with secondary antibodies, such as polyclonal sheep or goat antibodies to mouse $F(ab)'_2$ (most of the monoclonal antibodies are of mouse origin). $F(ab)'_2$ can be bound to the surface of small inert particles or to the surface of plastic dishes. The contact of phagocytes with antibody-coated surfaces mimics their contact with the opsonized antigenic particle. To study the possible cooperation between different types of receptors, mixtures of monoclonal antibodies to these receptors are used and the primary antibodies are cross-linked by the secondary antibody. Using these methods it can be demonstrated that cross-linking of each of the three Fcγ receptors stimulates respiratory burst, that cross-linking of FcγRII and FcγRIII provides a stronger signal than cross-linking of each receptor type alone and that CR3 cooperates with Fc receptors. Moreover, cross-linking of several other phagocyte surface receptors, such as the LPS receptor CD14, also stimulates respiratory burst.

The FcγRIIIb (CD16b) and the LPS receptor (CD14) are anchored in the membrane via a glycosylphosphatidylinositol (GPI) lipidic tail (see Fig. 12.16). Since these molecules have no intracellular parts, their interaction with the intracellular molecules responsible for signal initiation and propagation was difficult to comprehend. We now know, however, that the GPI-anchored proteins are sequestered into small areas of the membrane that differ from the rest of the membrane in their specific lipid composition (higher glycosphingolipid and cholesterol content). These membrane microdomains contain only very few transmembrane proteins but they do accumulate certain proteins, including Src-family protein kinases, on their cytoplasmic side. Perturbation of the GPI microdomains by cross-linking antibodies or by natural ligands would seem to cause redistribution of the associated protein kinases and their activation, thus triggering the signalling cascade. However, some GPI-anchored receptors may also initiate signalling via transmembrane proteins associated with them. Thus, two important GPI-anchored phagocyte receptors, CD16b (FcγRIIIb) and CD87 (receptor for the protease plasminogen activator), are known to be associated with CR3, which they use for signal transmission.

Signalling for chemotaxis, extravasation and exocytosis

Most phagocyte receptors for chemotactic substances (e.g. bacterial chemotactic peptides, anaphylatoxins C5a and C3a, IL-8, LTB_4) have a similar structure: they are proteins whose polypeptide chains cross the membrane seven times in a snake-like fashion (serpentine or seven-span receptors; see Fig. 15.13) and their intracellular parts are firmly associated with trimeric G-proteins (see Chapter 10, Fig. 10.23).

The steps that follow ligand binding to the receptor and activation of the associated G-protein are largely unknown but the signalling cascade must ultimately effect changes in actin microfilaments necessary for pseudopod formation and chemotactic locomotion. The mechanisms underlying these processes are probably similar to those operating in phagocytosis. The signals initiated by chemotactic substances also effect the respiratory burst and stimulate adhesion of phagocytes to endothelial cells and extravasation.

Signals for extravasation seem to depend mainly on several adhesion molecules (such as selectins, integrins and CD44; see Chapter 9). Ligation of the selectins and chemotactic receptors generates signals that induce a conformational change in the β2 integrins resulting in higher affinity of binding to their ligands. The nature of these signals and the nature of the conformational change, however, remain obscure; the signals could be transmitted via the associated cytoplasmic protein kinases and G-proteins.

The signals that lead to phagocytosis stimulate concomitantly exocytosis. This process requires the directed movement of granules to the phagosome, membrane fusion and regulated actin filament assembly and disassembly. Here again, the steps leading to these effects are largely unknown. They seem to involve small cytoplasmic G-proteins of the Rho and Rab families that somehow participate in oriented movement of the cytoplasmic vesicles and in regulation of actin polymerization.

Signalling for secretion of cytokines and mediators

These signalling pathways apparently operate on the same principles as signalling via growth factor receptors or antigen-specific receptors. Here, ligation of an Fc receptor, complement receptor or chemotactic receptor initiates activation of receptor-associated protein kinase (or a G-protein), which triggers a cascade of enzymatic reactions involving cytoplasmic kinases and phosphatases. The enzymes ultimately modify transcription factors (or proteins regulating them) and the activated transcription factors then initiate transcription of genes coding for cytokines or enzymes involved in the synthesis of soluble mediators such as leukotrienes. Alternatively, the receptor-activated protein kinases or G-proteins directly activate cytoplasmic enzymes capable of synthesizing soluble mediators. For example, phospholipase A_2, an enzyme initiating the cascade of reactions leading to synthesis of leukotrienes and other arachidonic acid-derived mediators (see Chapter 11), is activated by interaction with receptor-regulated G-proteins and by phosphorylation.

Signals leading to the activated macrophage phenotype

The cytokine that brings macrophages to the fully activated state is IFN-γ, produced by T_H1 cells, and the signals that initiate this marked phenotypic change emanate from the IFN-γ receptor. The latter is a typical cytokine receptor consisting of two subunits: α, which binds IFN-γ with medium affinity; and β, which increases the strength of binding and is essential in signal transduction. The signalling mechanisms used by this receptor, based mainly on the associated Jak kinases, are described in Chapter 10. The genes whose transcription is strongly enhanced as a result of IFN-γ receptor-triggered signals include those encoding the subunits of the inducible NOS, genes of the *MHC* complex and many others.

Phagocytic defects

In a system as vital as phagocytosis, malfunctions can be expected to have serious consequences. They occur when one of the genes that controls phagocytosis becomes defective as a result of mutation. Several such defects have been described both in humans and animals. Here we briefly mention those that are relatively well characterized: neutrophil specific granule deficiency, Chédiak–Higashi syndrome, hyperimmunoglobulin E (Job's) syndrome, chronic granulomatous disease and myeloperoxidase deficiency. Most of these defects are inherited as autosomal recessive traits, which means that their effect on the progeny is not influenced by the sex of the parent and that two faulty genes must meet in an individual for expression of the disease.

Neutrophil specific granule deficiency results from a defect in granule genesis. The patients either lack specific granules altogether or have 'empty' granules devoid of their normal content. The peripheral white blood cell count is usually normal, but visualized with Wright's stain the neutrophils appear to lack granules. The normal constituents of specific granules, such as lactoferrin, vitamin B_{12}-binding protein and cytochrome *b*, are either absent or markedly reduced and the cells are deficient in the plasma-membrane marker alkaline phosphatase. Since specific granules are preferentially released during diapedesis and migration into tissues and since degranulation is essential for monocyte recruitment, it is not surprising that this last function is defective in patients suffering from specific granule deficiency. Failure of monocyte recruitment leads to a deficient release of monocyte chemoattractants or factors capable of generating chemoattractants in serum. Impairment of chemotaxis is accompanied by deficient respiratory burst, impaired bacterial killing and increased susceptibility to recurrent bacterial infections.

Chédiak–Higashi syndrome (CHS), named after the Frenchman Moisés Chédiak and the Japanese physician Ototaka Higashi, is caused by a mutation in one of the genes controlling the formation and packaging of membrane vesicles, such as the lysosomal granules in granulocytes and the melanosomes (pigment granules) in melanocytes. The defective vesicles fail to segregate the contents of the azurophilic and specific granules and enlarge to an abnormal size, making the cell more rigid and slowing down its locomotion. The abnormal neutrophils are slow in carrying out their normal function, i.e. chemotaxis, phagolysosomal fusion and killing of phagocytosed microorganisms. The abnormal melanocyte granules are responsible for the partial albinism (fair skin, silvery hair and abnormal sensitivity to light) of CHS patients. Another characteristic of CHS, the profoundly depressed NK-cell activity and defective antibody-dependent cell-mediated cytotoxicity, may be responsible for the lymphoproliferative disorder accompanying this syndrome. CHS patients either die of microbial infection or succumb to lymphoreticular tumours. A defect resembling CHS has been described in Aleutian mink, partial albino Hereford cattle, albino whales and beige mice.

In *hyperimmunoglobulin E (Job's) syndrome*, the primary defect may not be in any of the phagocytic functions but rather in the production of IgE antibodies. Patients with Job's syndrome suffer from recurrent infections of skin, sinuses, ear and lungs with *S. aureus*, *Haemophilus influenzae* and *Candida albicans*. The skin infections are usually 'cold', which means that they lack the typical signs of inflammation. The infections are, for unknown reasons, accompanied by high serum levels of IgE antibodies specific for the infecting organism. The specific antibody is believed to cause a release of histamine from mast cells and to suppress the migration of leucocytes, the main reason why Job's syndrome is listed as a phagocytic defect. One of the characteristics of the disease is coarse facial expression and scarring from the skin infection. The name of the syndrome does not refer to a Dr Job, but to the biblical patriarch who endured disfiguration as a test of his faith.

Various forms of *chronic granulomatous disease* (CGD) are caused by mutations in genes encoding any of the four basic components of NADPH oxidase (p21, gp91, p47 and p67). These mutations prevent the expression of these proteins and thereby lead to impairment of the respiratory burst and inability to generate toxic oxygen derivatives necessary to kill microorganisms. In some cases the mutations lead to expression of only partially defective NADPH oxidase components. The seriousness of the condition varies depending on the affected gene. Patients with the 'classic' (X chromosome-linked) form of CGD, in which the gene encoding the gp91 subunit of the enzyme is affected, develop life-threatening infections early in life, usually within the first year. Manifestations of the disease include lung abscesses, skin and soft-tissue infections, inflammation and enlargement of lymph nodes (lymphadenitis and lymphadenopathy), inflammation of the marrow (osteomyelitis) in small bones of the hand and feet, liver abscesses, multiplication of microorganisms in the bloodstream (septicaemia), inflammation of the brain and spinal cord membranes (meningitis), brain abscesses and infections of the gastrointestinal and genitourinary tracts. CGD patients are particularly susceptible to catalase-positive microorganisms such as *S. aureus*, *Aspergillus*, *Chromobacterium violaceum* and *Acremonium strictum*, which destroy their own hydrogen peroxide. Catalase-negative microorganisms, which do not destroy the patient's endogenous hydrogen peroxide, when phagocytosed presumably supply the deficient host phagocytes with toxic oxygen derivatives. The disease is readily diagnosed by a defect in the ability of phagocytes to reduce the dye nitroblue tetrazolium or by other tests of respiratory burst.

Myeloperoxidase deficiency is a relatively common disorder affecting approximately 1 in 2000 individuals. It is caused by mutations in the gene coding for the enzyme myeloperoxidase, normally present in azurophilic granules. Depending on the particular mutation, the enzyme might be completely absent (which is the case in some 50% of patients) or it may be merely reduced in quantity. In some patients at least the enzyme is produced but is apparently not processed post-translationally and is therefore not packaged into the granules. Myeloperoxidase deficiency is usually not a life-threatening condition and most patients do not run the risk of serious infections. The bactericidal activity of their neutrophils is usually normal but the ability to handle fungal, especially *Candida*, infections may be moderately to severely impaired.

A different type of phagocyte deficiency is caused by defects in the genes coding for the adhesion molecules of these cells, the leucocyte integrins (see Chapter 9). This *leucocyte adhesion deficiency (LAD) syndrome* is caused by loss of the β2 subunit (CD18) shared by all leucocyte integrins, which are involved in phagocyte extravasation (LFA-1, CR3 and CR4) and in the recognition of opsonized microorganisms (CR3 and CR4). In patients with LAD syndrome, phagocytes and other leucocytes do not immigrate properly into the inflamed tissue and this causes recurrent bacterial infections characterized by abscesses with unusual absence of pus formation. The patients have marked leucocytosis, an increased number of blood leucocytes (mainly granulocytes), because these cells are unable to leave the circulation and to enter tissues. The defects are caused by point mutations in the *CD18* gene, which in some cases prevent its expression altogether and in milder cases allow the gene to be expressed at least partially. Another type of LAD syndrome (LAD-2) is caused by a defect in the gene encoding the α1,2-fucosyltransferase, one of the glycosyltransferase enzymes involved in the biosynthesis of the sialyl-Lewis^x oligosaccharide ligand of selectins (see Chapter 9). Immunological defects in these patients are similar to those seen in LAD.

Further reading

Allen, L.A.H. & Aderem, A. (1996) Mechanisms of phagocytosis. *Current Opinion in Immunology*, **8**, 36–40.

Badway, J.A. & Karnovsky, M.L. (1980) Active oxygen species and the functions of phagocytic leukocytes. *Annual Review of Biochemistry*, **49**, 695–726.

Bastian, N.R. & Hibbs, J.B. Jr (1994) Assembly and regulation of NADPH oxidase and nitric oxide synthase. *Current Opinion in Immunology*, **6**, 131–139.

Berón, W., Alvarez-Dominguez, C., Mayorga, L. & Stahl, P.D. (1995) Membrane trafficking along the phagocytic pathway. *Trends in Cell Biology*, **5**, 100–104.

Bokoch, G.M. (1995) Regulation of the phagocyte respiratory burst by small GTP-binding proteins. *Trends in Cell Biology*, **5**, 109–113.

Boman, H.G. (1995) Peptide antibiotics and their role in innate immunity. *Annual Review of Immunology*, **13**, 61–92.

Brown, E.J. (1995) Phagocytosis. *BioEssays*, **17**, 109–117.

Cassatella, M.A. (1995) The production of cytokines by polymorphonuclear neutrophils. *Immunology Today*, **16**, 21–26.

Downey, G.P. (1994) Mechanisms of leukocyte mobility and chemotaxis. *Current Opinion in Immunology*, **6**, 113–124.

Gabay, J.E. & Almeida, R.P. (1993) Antibiotic peptides and serine protease homologs in human polymorphonuclear leukocytes: defensins and azurocidin. *Current Opinion in Immunology*, **5**, 97–102.

Ganz, T. & Lehrer, R.I. (1994) Defensins. *Current Opinion in Immunology*, **6**, 584–589.

Gordon, S., Clarke, S., Greaves, D. & Doyle, A. (1995) Molecular immunobiology of macrophages: recent progress. *Current Opinion in Immunology*, **7**, 24–33.

Gordon, S., Fraser, I., Nath, D., Hughes, D. & Clarke, S. (1992) Macrophages in tissues and *in vitro*. *Current Opinion in Immunology*, **4**, 25–32.

Greenberg, S. (1995) Signal transduction of phagocytosis. *Trends in Cell Biology*, **5**, 93–99.

Hallet, M.B. & Lloyds, D. (1995) Neutrophil priming: the cellular signals that say 'amber' but not 'green'. *Immunology Today*, **16**, 264–268.

Hulett, M.D. & Hogarth, P.M. (1994) Molecular basis of Fc receptor function. *Advances in Immunology*, **57**, 1–127.

Lehrer, R.I., Lichtenstein, A.K. & Ganz, T. (1993) Defensins: antimicrobial and cytotoxic peptides of mammalian cells. *Annual Review of Immunology*, **11**, 105–128.

Lloyd, A.R. & Oppenheim, J.J. (1992) Poly's lament: the neglected role of the polymorphonuclear neutrophil in the afferent limb of the immune response. *Immunology Today*, **13**, 169–172.

Nathan, C. & Xie, Q.-W. (1994) Nitric oxide synthesis: roles, tolls, and controls. *Cell*, **78**, 915–918.

Pearson, A.M. (1996) Scavenger receptors in innate immunity. *Current Opinion in Immunology*, **8**, 20–28.

Petty, H.R. & Todd III, R.F. (1996) Integrins as promiscuous signal transduction devices. *Immunology Today*, **17**, 209–212.

Ravetch, J.V. (1994) Fc receptors: rubor redux. *Cell*, **78**, 553–560.

Rietschel, E.T. & Brade, H. (1992) Bacterial endotoxins. *Scientific American*, **267**(2), 54–61.

Rotrosen, D. & Gallin, J.I. (1987) Disorders of phagocyte function. *Annual Review of Immunology*, **5**, 127–150.

Savill, J., Fadok, V., Henson, P. & Haslett, C. (1993) Phagocyte recognition of cells undergoing apoptosis. *Immunology Today*, **14**, 131–136.

Selsted, M.E. & Ouellette, A.J. (1995) Defensins in granules of phagocytic and non-phagocytic cells. *Trends in Cell Biology*, **5**, 114–119.

Stahl, P.D. (1992) The mannose receptor and other macrophage lectins. *Current Opinion in Immunology*, **4**, 49–52.

Swanson, J.A. & Baer, S.C. (1995) Phagocytosis by zippers and triggers. *Trends in Cell Biology*, **5**, 89–93.

Ulevitch, R.J. (1993) Recognition of bacterial endotoxins by receptor-dependent mechanisms. *Advances in Immunology*, **53**, 267–289.

van Oss, C.J. (1986) Phagocytosis: an overview. *Methods in Enzymology*, **132**, 3–15.

van de Winkel, J.G.J. & Capel, P.J.A. (1993) Human IgG Fc receptor heterogeneity: molecular aspects and clinical implications. *Immunology Today*, **14**, 215–221.

chapter 16 T-lymphocyte and natural killer cell responses

The phagocyte activities described in the preceding chapter are part of the *non-adaptive immune response*, which is characterized by an early and rapid onset, relative non-specificity (different stimuli activate the same cells) and non-clonality (all cells of a given type express the same receptors). Almost simultaneously with the non-adaptive response, the *adaptive immune response* develops. The latter is dominated by the activities of lymphocytes, takes somewhat longer to develop and is characterized by specificity (different antigens activate different cells) and clonality (the lymphocyte pool consists of a large number of clones, where cells of the same clone express the same receptors but cells of different clones express different receptors). The adaptive response involves both T and B lymphocytes; for convenience and clarity, however, the activities of these two cell types are dealt with separately. Here we describe T-lymphocyte activities, which often slightly precede B-lymphocyte responses.

T lymphocytes recognize an antigen only when it is presented to them in the form of small fragments bound to major histocompatibility complex (MHC) molecules on the surface of another cell (possible exceptions are discussed later; see Fig. 16.1). They ignore antigens in solution or on cells, such as bacteria, that lack MHC molecules. Any cell expressing MHC molecules associated with antigen fragments on its surface may be regarded as an *antigen-presenting cell* (APC). In most situations, however, more than the mere display of an MHC-bound antigen fragment on a cell surface is required to activate a T lymphocyte. In addition to the signal delivered via the T-cell receptor (TCR) engaged by MHC molecule plus antigen, the T cell must also receive co-stimulatory signals from the APC. Only then does it become fully activated and is able to proliferate and differentiate into an effector cell. Two kinds of APC can thus be distinguished: *non-professional*, capable of delivering one signal only (via TCR); and *professional*, capable of delivering all signals necessary for T-cell activation, proliferation and differentiation. In this book, the term 'APC' always refers to a professional antigen-presenting cell.

Although the various T-cell (and B-cell) responses form a highly interconnected network, they can nevertheless be divided into two major pathways that correspond to the two main T-cell subsets, the T_H (helper) and T_C (cytotoxic) lymphocytes. The T_H pathways branch out into two sub-pathways, one delivering help to B lymphocytes and the other to macrophages. The three pathways can be summarized thus:

Antigen → Professional APC → T_H lymphocyte → B lymphocyte → Antibodies

Antigen (intracellular parasite) → Macrophage → T_H1 lymphocyte → Activated macrophage

Antigen → APC → Precursor T_C cell + T_H cell → Effector T_C cell

This chapter is organized according to these pathways. We begin with the description of antigen presentation and T-cell activation and then move on to the various forms of T_H-cell responses followed by T_C-cell responses. Finally, we deal with natural killer (NK) cell responses and unusual or atypical T-cell responses.

Antigen presentation

To initiate adaptive responses an infectious agent must encounter an APC, i.e. a dendritic cell, macrophage or activated B lymphocyte. Tissue *dendritic cells*, the best studied of which are the epidermal Langerhans' cells, ingest microbial fragments by macropinocytosis and rush with the ingested and partially digested prey to the nearby lymph node. Once in the lymph node, they profoundly change their properties and turn into professional APCs. The hallmark of this change is an increase in the number of MHC molecules on their surface, accompanied by the expression of several adhesion molecules and the co-stimulatory molecules CD80 (B7/BB1) and CD86 (B7.2). After this metamorphosis, lymphoid dendritic cells, now called *interdigitating cells*, display on their surface MHC–antigen assemblies, as well as co-stimulatory and adhesion molecules necessary for making contact with T cells (Fig. 16.1). *B lymphocytes*, found mainly in the follicles of lymph nodes and other secondary lymphoid organs, are well suited for capturing and concentrating soluble antigens such as bacterial toxins by virtue of their antigen-specific receptors. After binding an antigen, the receptor–antigen complex is internalized by receptor-mediated endocytosis, the antigen is processed into peptides, the antigenic fragments are associated with MHC class II molecules and the peptide–MHC class II molecular assemblies (see Chapter 6) are displayed on the cell surface (Fig. 16.2). To act as a professional APC, however, the resting B cell must first be activated, for example by bacterial lipopolysaccharide. The resulting activated *blast cell* expresses CD80 and CD86 on its surface, an increased level of MHC class II molecules and adhesion molecules, all of which are required for effective antigen presentation.

Naive (i.e. unstimulated) T lymphocytes can recognize peptides bound to MHC molecules on both non-professional and professional APCs, but the outcome of such recognition varies between these two situations (Fig. 16.3). While an encounter with a professional APC activates the T cell and sends it on a path towards prolifera-

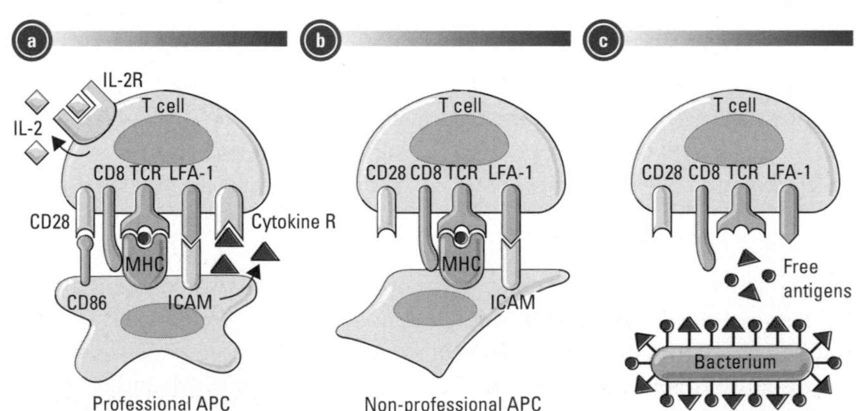

Figure 16.1 Recognition of antigen by T cells. (a) The interaction of a T cell with the antigen (peptide bound by the MHC glycoprotein) on the surface of a professional antigen-presenting cell (APC) provides the first signal via the T-cell receptor (TCR), followed by a set of secondary (accessory) signals via CD28 and probably also via other adhesion molecules such as LFA-1, as well as via cytokine receptors. These signals lead to the production of autocrine cytokines (e.g. IL-2), proliferation and differentiation into mature helper or cytotoxic T cells. (b) If a naive T cell encounters the antigen on the surface of cells that do not possess co-stimulatory molecules (e.g. CD80 and CD86 ligands of CD28), the signal via the TCR leads to unresponsiveness or even apoptosis. (c) The TCR is usually unable to recognize soluble or cell-surface antigens alone; it recognizes exclusively peptides bound to MHC molecules.

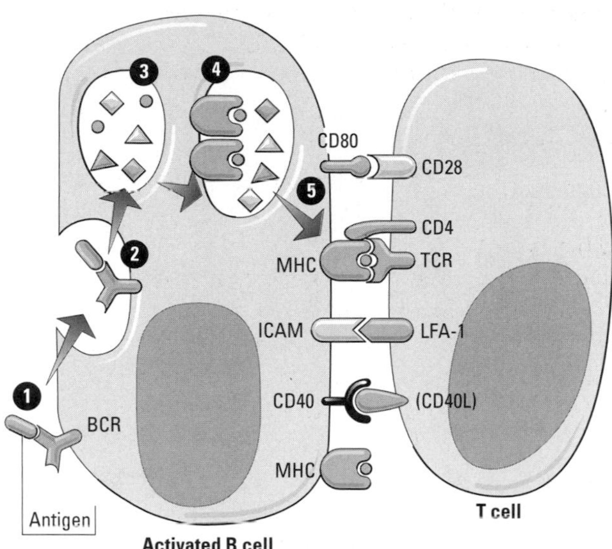

Figure 16.2 Activated B cell (B blast) as a professional antigen-presenting cell. The activated B cell binds the antigen via its B-cell receptor (BCR) (1), internalizes it (2) and cleaves it (and also the BCR) into peptides (3), some of which bind to MHC class II molecules (4). The peptide–MHC assemblies are displayed on the cell surface (5) where they are recognized by the TCR of a helper T cell precursor. Activated B cells (in contrast to resting B cells) possess adhesion (ICAM-1) and co-stimulatory (CD80, CD86) molecules on their surface. After activation, the T cell expresses the CD40 ligand (CD40L) on its surface, which binds to the CD40 receptor on the B cell and contributes to further stimulation of the B cell. Expression of CD40L on the activated but not resting (naive) T cell is shown by parentheses. Additional activation antigens expressed on the activated T-cell surface (e.g. IL-2 receptor, CTLA-4, CD69) are not shown.

tion and differentiation, an encounter with a non-professional APC *in*activates the T lymphocyte for an extended period (see Chapter 20).

Processing and presentation of exogenous antigens by MHC class II molecules

Microbes engulfed by dendritic cells are contained in endosomes. These then fuse with specialized lysosome-like organelles that contain a mixture of hydrolytic enzymes in an acidic sap (with a pH of approximately 5). The acidic endosomes fuse with vesicles derived from the Golgi apparatus that carry MHC class II molecules complexed with the invariant chain (see Chapter 6). In the acidic endosomes the invariant chain is destroyed by proteolysis except for the class II-associated invariant chain peptide (CLIP), which remains associated with the peptide-binding groove of the MHC class II molecules. After the arrival of DM molecules into the vesicle, the CLIP is also removed and exchanged for peptides in the vesicle, some of which are derived from the engulfed antigen. The vesicles then return to the surface of the APC and fuse with the plasma membrane. The MHC class II molecules loaded with peptides thus become available for recognition by T lymphocytes. A fraction of the MHC class II molecules on the cell surface either remains 'empty' or associated with suboptimal peptides, which can be exchanged for other peptides that bind with a higher affinity. This supplementary mechanism thus makes use of peptides generated from antigens trapped on the cell surface. Surface proteases can trim the protruding ends of peptides bound to MHC class II molecules.

Presentation of endogenous antigens by MHC class I molecules

Antigens in the cytosol are digested in *proteasomes* and the resulting peptides are transported from the cytosol into the lumen of the endoplasmic reticulum, where they are loaded onto the class I MHC molecules. The peptide–MHC class I molecule assemblies are then transported via the Golgi apparatus to the cell surface (see Chapter 6). Most of the peptides bound to the MHC class I molecules originate from the cell's own endogenous proteins. However, if the cell is infected by a virus or some other parasite living in the

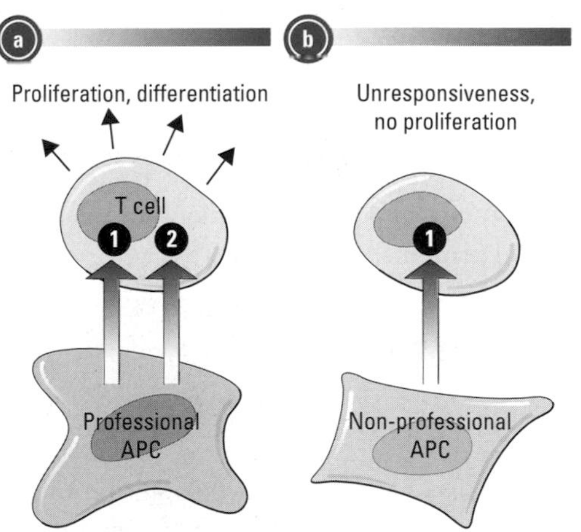

Figure 16.3 Difference between the presentation of antigen on the surface of a professional (a) and non-professional (b) antigen-presenting cell (APC). Cooperation of signals 1 (T-cell receptor) and 2 (CD28 and possibly other receptors) leads to positive stimulation, proliferation and differentiation. Delivery of signal 1 alone leads to unresponsiveness. A negative signal may also be given when the first signal is incomplete (e.g. when co-receptor molecules CD4 or CD8 are prevented from binding to MHC molecules or when the TCR contacts structurally modified peptides bound to MHC molecules).

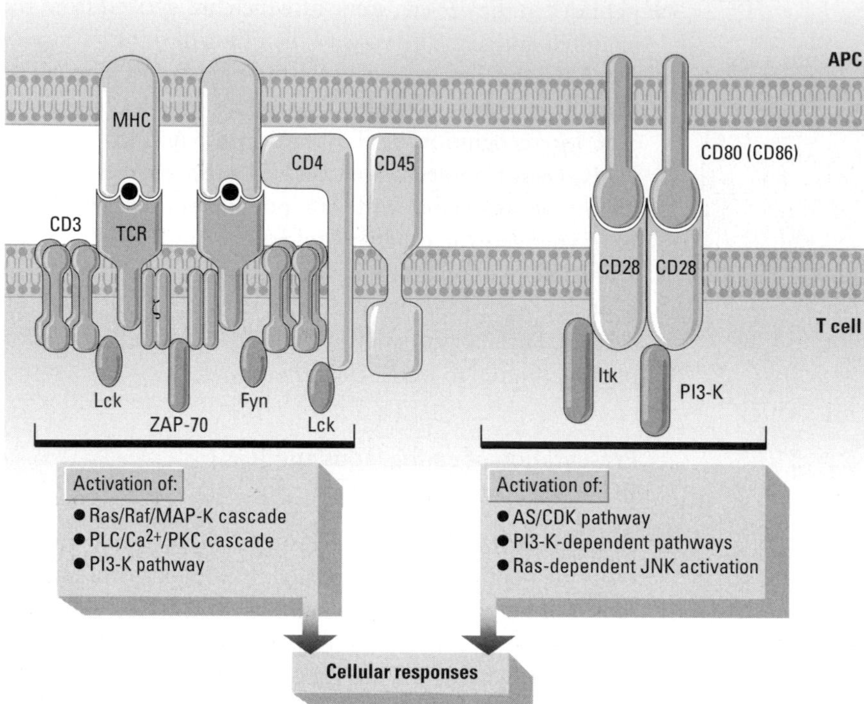

Figure 16.4 Signalling pathways initiated by T-cell receptor (TCR) ligation and clustering and CD28 ligation. For description see text. APC, antigen-presenting cell; AS, acidic sphingomyelinase; CDK, ceramide-dependent kinase; PLC, phospholipase C; PI3-K, phosphatidylinositol 3-kinase; MAP-K, mitogen-activated protein kinase.

cytoplasm, some of the parasite's peptides will also bind to MHC class I molecules and appear on the cell surface. The mechanism by which professional APCs acquire antigen for processing and presentation by class I molecules in cases in which they themselves are not infected remains obscure. There is good evidence, however, that part of the exogenous proteins engulfed by APCs can 'leak' into the cytoplasm, be fragmented by proteasomes and the resulting fragments then pumped into endoplasmic reticulum to associate with MHC class I proteins.

Activation of T cells

Signalling through the TCR

The TCR consists of the antigen-recognition module, composed of the α and β or γ and δ chains, and the CD3 complex, composed of the γε, δε and ζζ pairs (see Chapter 7). In some TCR complexes the ζζ dimer is replaced by ζη or ηη dimers. In some T cells the ζζ dimer is substituted by a structurally closely related γγ dimer[1].

[1] Note that there are, unfortunately, three different molecules relevant to the TCR, all called γ: one of them is the γ chain of the γ:δ TCR proper; the second one is the CD3 γ chain; and the third one is the ζ-like γ chain, which is usually the component of Fc receptor complexes.

The CD3 chains link the TCR complex to the intracellular signalling molecules, protein tyrosine kinases Fyn and Lck of the Src family (see Chapter 10). The complex is weakly associated with other T-cell surface molecules, especially the co-receptors CD4 or CD8 whose intracellular domains are in turn associated with the Lck kinase.

T-cell activation is triggered by ligation of the TCR with the peptide–MHC molecule assemblies on the surface of the APC. Ligation presumably induces aggregation of TCR complexes and thus brings together the intracellular CD3-associated protein kinases, enabling them to phosphorylate each other as well as the intracellular domains of the ζ chains (Fig. 16.4). Simultaneously, co-ligation of the co-receptors CD4 or CD8 (depending on the nature of the MHC molecule involved) results in the phosphorylation of the co-receptor-associated Lck kinases.

Subsequently, another protein tyrosine kinase, ZAP-70 (zeta-associated protein; relative molecular mass (M_r) 70 000) binds to the phosphorylated ζ chain of the TCR complex and is thereby activated. By now, the intracellular part of the TCR complex contains at least three activated protein tyrosine kinases, which can phosphorylate a number of intracellular proteins. The signalling pathways initiated by ligation of the TCR complex are essentially identical to those shown generally in Fig. 10.27 and need not be repeated here. An important point is regulation of

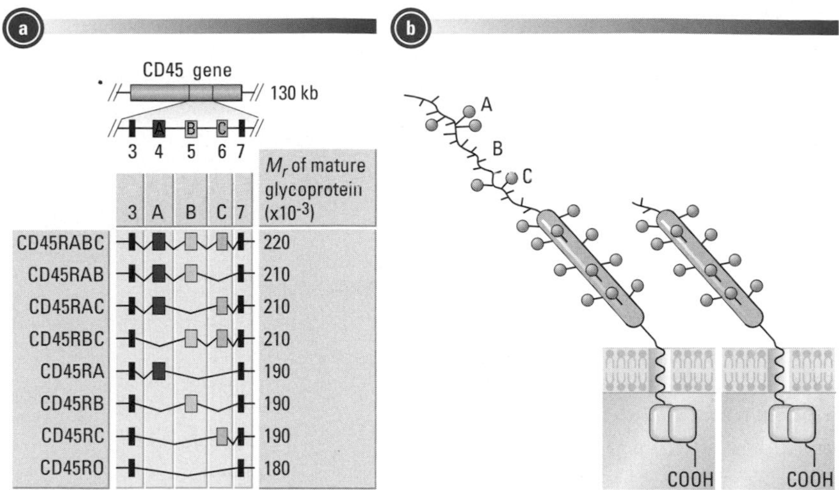

Figure 16.5 Major leucocyte membrane tyrosine phosphatase CD45. (a) The gene encoding the CD45 protein (1268 amino acids) stretches over 130 kb on human chromosome 1q31–32 and consists of 30 exons. Alternative splicing of three of them, which are located at the 5′ end of the translated part of the gene and denoted as exons 4, 5 and 6, gives rise to eight mRNA species. Individual alternative forms differ by combinations of the segments encoded in exons 4, 5 and 6 (the corresponding segments in the protein molecules are called A, B and C, respectively, their length being 66, 47 and 48 amino acid residues). All of them are richly *O*-glycosylated. Strictly speaking, the different CD45 forms should be given the same designations as in this figure, i.e. according to the combinations of A, B and C segments present in them. However, because of practical difficulties in distinguishing between the variants of similar size, the CD45 protein forms are often called CD45RA, RB, RC and RO, indicating only the presence of segments A, B and C, respectively, and disregarding any other segments they may contain; this nomenclature is obviously ambiguous. (b) Schematic representation of the largest (CD45RABC) and smallest (CD45RO) forms in the membrane. Short bars branching out of the polypeptide chain represent *O*-linked ( ) and *N*-linked ( ) oligosaccharide chains. The membrane-proximal domain of the extracellular part is identical in all forms. The intracellular part of the CD45 molecule (705 amino acid residues) consists of two similar domains, one of which has tyrosine-phosphatase activity. CD45 is expressed on all leucocytes but on no other cells (it is a *pan-leucocyte marker*). The expression of the various CD45 forms is tightly regulated: B cells and naive T cells express the long forms containing the A segment; activated and memory T cells replace these forms by the CD45RO form. All forms have the same tyrosine-phosphatase activity. The reason for variability in expression of the various CD45 forms as well as the functions of the extracellular domains of CD45 molecules are unknown. The major intracellular function of CD45 is to dephosphorylate the phosphotyrosine residue at the C-terminus of Src kinases and thus activate them (see Fig. 10.29). Part (a) modified from Rogers, P.R. *et al.* (1992) *Journal of Immunology*, **148**, 4054. Part (b) modified from Barclay, A.N. *et al.* (1993) *The Leucocyte Antigen Facts Book*. Academic Press, London.

activity of the primary TCR-signalling devices, the Src-family kinases. This was shown in Fig. 10.29; some details on the positive regulatory phosphatase, CD45, are given in Fig. 16.5.

To prevent an over-reaction, the activation cascade must be regulated: when it reaches a point at which it is no longer needed, it must be halted and the cell brought back into the resting stage. The mechanisms that put the brakes on TCR-triggered activation are mainly based on the activities of numerous intracellular protein phosphatases. The activity of Src-family kinases is also negatively regulated by another protein kinase called Csk (C-terminal Src kinase), which phosphorylates a regulatory tyrosine residue near the C-terminus of Src kinases (see Fig. 10.29).

Signalling induced by agonists, partial agonists and antagonists of the TCR

Immunologists used to consider the TCR as a simple switching device: either it binds with an above-threshold affinity to the peptide–MHC molecule assembly and the signalling cascade is triggered with all its consequences; or the affinity is too low for binding and nothing happens. In reality, the TCR is a much more sophisticated switch. Minor changes in the peptide bound to the MHC molecule may not affect the affinity of the peptide–MHC molecule interaction, yet they may generate *partial signals* that lead to a *halfway response* characterized by proliferation and secretion of only a fraction of the cytokines produced during a full T-cell response. Some modified peptides may even block proliferation and cytokine secretion altogether and induce a state of T-cell anergy or unresponsiveness. There are thus three different types of peptides: *agonist* (those that stimulate a full response), *partial agonist* (those that stimulate a partial response) and *antagonist* (those that induce unresponsiveness). When a single APC presents a mixture of an agonist and an antagonist on its surface, the negative effect of the latter can overcome the positive effect of the former, even if the antagonist is present in much smaller amounts than the agonist. Some viruses seem to use mutations in their proteins to produce antagonist peptides capable of suppressing the activity of the T-cell clones that recognize agonist peptides derived from the original wild-type virus.

The molecular mechanisms underlying these differential responses remain largely obscure. The low affinity of TCR–ligand interaction may shorten the duration of the intermolecular contacts, induce the formation of only small TCR aggregates and thus lower the opportunities for mutual phosphorylation of the associated kinases. The short duration of the contacts may also be insufficient for the proper attachment of the CD4 and CD8 co-receptor molecules to the transient complex and thus affect the outcome of the initial phosphorylation.

As a result of its low affinity, an antagonist ligand may serially engage many more TCRs than the agonist ligand present on the same APC and thus effectively inactivate them by making them inaccessible for the agonist ligand. This might explain the surprising ability of antagonist ligands to overcome the positive stimulation by agonists even at low concentrations. One clear difference between the signalling initiated by an agonist and that initiated by an antagonist is in the distinctive patterns of phosphorylation of the ζ chain (phosphorylation on different tyrosine residues) and the lack of ZAP-70 activation in the case of interaction with the antagonist.

Co-stimulatory receptors

Activation of a naive T cell by TCR stimulation alone is not sufficient for the initiation of an immune response; co-stimulatory signals provided by several adhesion/signalling molecular pairs on the surfaces of T cells and APCs are also necessary (Fig. 16.6). The major co-stimulatory receptor on the T-cell surface is the CD28 glycoprotein, which binds glycoprotein ligands CD80 and CD86 on the APC surface. The CD80 and CD86 molecules are not simply redundant, functionally equivalent ligands of CD28. They differ markedly in the pattern of their expression, CD86 being more strongly expressed on dendritic cells and monocytes

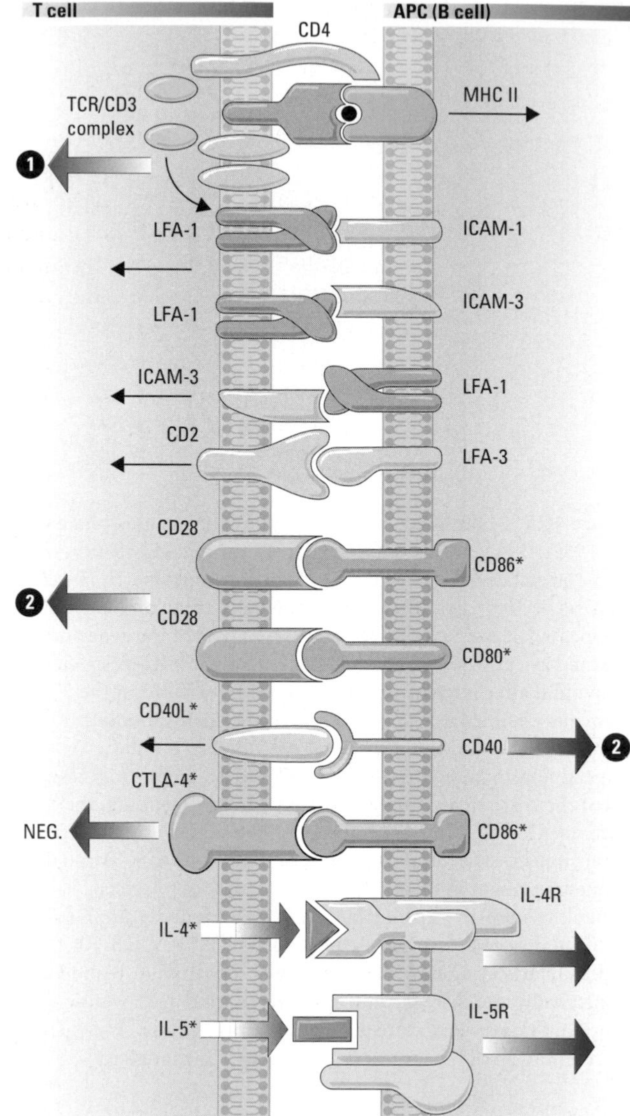

Figure 16.6 Cell-surface adhesion and signalling molecules participating in contacts between T cell and antigen-presenting cell (APC; here, an activated B cell). Proteins newly expressed by activated cells are shown with asterisks. Thick red arrows represent critically important signals emanating from the particular receptors. Signal 1 on the T-cell side represents the first activating signal provided via the T-cell receptor (TCR) complex. The number 2 on both sides designates the co-stimulatory signal provided to the T cell via the CD28 receptor and to the B cell via the CD40 receptor. Thin arrows represent signals that are probably of minor significance. The arrow pointing down from the TCR complex to LFA-1 indicates the signal that causes transition of the LFA-1 molecule to a high-affinity state. The negative signal provided by ligation of the CTLA-4 receptor is indicated (NEG.). Grey arrows indicate secretion of soluble cytokines. Several other pairs of interacting molecules are not shown (e.g. CD30–CD30L, CD27–CD70, CD5–CD72, CD22–CD45).

and appearing more rapidly on activated B cells than CD80. The final outcome of T-cell activation may therefore be different depending on whether the CD28 receptor binds mainly to CD86 or CD80.

Molecular mechanisms of signal transduction via the CD28 receptor are only partially understood (see Fig. 16.4). The intracellular part of the CD28 molecule is associated with phosphatidylinositol 3-kinase (PI3K) which, on activation by receptor ligation, can phosphorylate the membrane lipid phosphatidylinositol and probably also some proteins. Another signalling molecule associated with the intracellular domain of CD28 is the tyrosine kinase Itk (interleukin-2-dependent kinase; M_r 72 000). This enzyme, too, becomes activated after CD28 engagement. CD28 also associates during the activation process with the adaptor molecule Grb-2, which provides a link to activation of the small G-protein Ras. The associations probably trigger multiple pathways that lead to the stimulation of other intracellular protein kinases and activation of a specific phospholipase, acidic sphingomyelinase. The latter produces a lipidic second messenger, ceramide, by the cleavage of the membrane lipid sphingomyelin and the ceramide then activates ceramide-dependent protein kinases.

One part of the signalling pathway triggered by CD28 involves the serine/threonine kinase JNK (Jun N-terminal kinase), which also participates in the terminal part of the TCR-induced signalling pathway. This enzyme phosphorylates the c-Jun subunit of the transcription factor AP-1 and probably also regulates the activity of another transcription factor NF-κB (see Fig. 10.27). The TCR-induced and CD28-induced pathways appear to coalesce at this point to produce sufficient amounts of AP-1 and NF-κB to bind to regulatory regions of several genes, including the *IL-2* gene. Engagement of these transcription factors greatly increases expression of the genes necessary for full T-cell activation and proliferation. The CD28-induced signalling pathway also stabilizes mRNA molecules encoding several cytokines and thus increases the levels of cytokine secretion.

One further receptor, CTLA-4 (cytotoxic lymphocyte antigen-4, structurally similar to CD28), is rapidly expressed on activated T cells and binds CD80 and CD86 ligands with a much higher affinity than CD28. In contrast to CD28, CTLA-4 is a *negative* signalling receptor, participating in the deceleration of the activation process. The molecular mechanism of this inhibitory effect is based on association of the CTLA-4 cytoplasmic domain with a protein tyrosine phosphatase.

Signals provided by the engagement of other adhesion/signalling molecules on the T-cell surface are probably necessary for optimal T-cell activation, proliferation and terminal differentiation (see Fig. 16.6). One such stimulatory molecule is the adhesion receptor CD2, which binds LFA-3 (CD58) (see Chapter 9). However, mouse mutants with 'knocked-out' *CD2* genes are immunologically normal, suggesting that the CD2 molecule is possibly redundant and dispensable or has a special function not manifested in the experiments carried out with these mice.

Similarly, interleukin (IL)-1 produced by some APCs was originally considered to be an important co-stimulatory molecule for T-cell activation but this involvement is now controversial. However, IL-1 does seem to play a supportive part, especially in the activation of memory cells by suboptimal APCs.

Outcome of T-cell activation

The changes initiated by the TCR in the first few minutes to hours of activation lead to transition of the cell from the G_0 to G_1 phase of the cell cycle. Several hours after stimulation the T cell begins to express IL-2 and high-affinity IL-2 receptor. *IL2* gene expression is effected by a set of transcription factors that are activated by the converging signalling pathways triggered by the ligation of TCR, CD28 and possibly other T-cell surface molecules.

The transcription factors also induce expression of the *CD25* gene, which encodes the α-subunit of the high-affinity IL-2 receptor. The interaction of IL-2 with the high-affinity receptor initiates signalling pathways (see Chapter 10) that cause the T cell to transit from the G_1 to the S phase of the cell cycle and progress to cell division. The signalling pathways control the expression and activity of several key proteins necessary for cell division. Some of these are also activated directly by TCR- and CD28-dependent signals, while others are energized only by signals provided via the IL-2 receptor. Among the IL-2-regulated molecules are c-Jun and c-Fos (the subunits of the AP-1 transcription factor), the transcription regulator c-Myc and the protein Bcl-2, which prevents apoptosis. These proteins regulate the expression of many other genes, the products of which are necessary for cell proliferation.

The stimulated T cell undergoes a sequence of phenotypic changes beginning with its progression from the resting state to mitosis and later to differentiation into effector and memory cells. Among the *earliest* (*immediate*) *changes*, observable within 15–30 min of stimulation, are the expression of genes encoding transcription factors such as c-Fos, NF-AT, c-Myc and NF-κB, protein kinases such as Jak-3 and protein phosphatases such as Pac-1. The subsequent *early changes*, occurring within several hours of stimulation, mark the beginning of the expression of genes encoding *activation antigens*. These include several cytokines (IL-2 and others), IL-2 receptor subunit α (CD25), insulin receptor, transferrin receptor and several other surface molecules such as CD26, CD30, CD54, CD69 and CD70, most of which are receptors or adhesion molecules. Activation antigens reach a maximum level of expression just before the first division, 24 hours after stimulation. During this period the level of expression of several other molecules already expressed on resting T cells (such as CD2, CD27 or CD44) increases. In some of these molecules, novel activation-related epitopes appear probably on account of differences in glycosylation or associations with other membrane molecules. One example is the CD2R form ($T11_3$ epitope) of the adhesion receptor CD2. Expression of a few T-cell surface molecules is transiently decreased upon activation; among these are the TCR–CD3 complex, CD4, CD8 and CD62L (L-selectin).

At a later point, some days after activation commenced, *late activation antigens* become expressed on the T cells. These include MHC class II molecules (in humans but not in the mouse) and several members of the β1 integrin family (VLA-1–VLA-5; see Chapter 10). One of the late effects involves a change in expression of the alternative form of the major leucocyte surface glycoprotein CD45: the longer form, CD45RA, is replaced by the shortest form, CD45RO (see Fig. 16.5). Expression of late activation antigens marks the differentiation of the activated cell into effector or memory T cells.

Negative regulation of T-cell activation

The process of T-cell activation and proliferation obviously has to be kept under strict control to prevent self-damaging over-reactions and excessive proliferation. Control is achieved at several levels. As already mentioned, the positive activation mediated by phosphorylation of multiple enzymes and regulatory proteins is constantly held in balance by dephosphorylation executed by a number of phosphatases. One of the key phosphatases, Pac-1 (which inactivates the mitogen activated protein (MAP) kinase), is a protein whose expression is rapidly upregulated during T-cell activation. Thus the activity of any phosphorylation-dependent enzyme is at all times determined by the mutually opposed effects of protein kinases and phosphatases.

Another level of negative regulation involves the expression of specific inhibitors of transcription factors. An example is IκB-α, a protein that binds to the general transcription factor, NF-κB, and thus prevents its interaction with DNA. The production of IκB-α is strongly upregulated in the earliest phases of T-cell activation.

The activation process is negatively regulated also by mechanisms leading to the self-destruction of activated effector T cells. The activated cells express a surface protein, the Fas ligand (FasL), which is structurally similar to tumour necrosis factor α (TNF-α). Interaction of FasL with its receptor, Fas (CD95), leads to the induction of apoptotic death. This mechanism thus limits the lifespan of an activated effector cell following its encounter with antigen. The fate of the effector T cell resembles that of a bee, which dies after using its sting.

T-cell memory

Most of the effector T cells that arise via the activation process die by apoptosis within a few days after the infection has been successfully warded off and they are no longer required. Some of the activated T cells, however, turn into *memory cells*, which the body retains to fight future infections by the same parasite. (Alternatively, memory T cells may arise directly from naive cells.) It is usually the T cells with highest affinity towards the antigen that turn into memory cells. This is probably because these high-affinity cells have a chance to experience protracted contact with the sparse antigen and the signals resulting from this contact overcome the apoptotic mechanisms that otherwise automatically liquidate the effector cells carrying TCR of lower affinity.

It has proved difficult to distinguish memory cells unequivocally from recently activated T cells and effector cells. In contrast to memory B cells (see Chapter 17), memory T cells are not marked by somatic mutations and isotype switching. A consensus view is that memory T cells are long-lived (although they seem to have a shorter lifespan than resting T cells) and that they express a characteristic set of surface molecules, primarily various adhesion receptors. In contrast to effector cells, memory cells neither secrete large amounts of cytokines (as do T_H cells) nor are they able to kill target cells immediately (as do T_C cells). The surface molecules characteristic for memory T cells are the adhesion receptor β1 integrins (VLA antigens), CD44 and the CD45RO isoform. The expression of adhesion molecules reflects a homing behaviour that differs from that of naive cells. Memory T cells do not tend to leave the blood circulation in the postcapillary venules of lymph nodes but rather extravasate into the skin or gut mucosa. Separate subpopulations of memory T cells with specific affinity for the skin or intestinal blood vessel endothelium can be distinguished. Their tissue-homing specificity is due to the expression of additional adhesion molecules, such as the glycoprotein ligand for E-selectin (CD62E) found on endothelial cells of inflamed skin and the α4β7 integrin that recognizes the MadCAM-1 glycoprotein expressed on mucosal endothelium. The length of time necessary to activate memory T cells and turn them into effector cells is somewhat shorter than in the case of naive cells. The functional properties of both primary and secondary effector cells (the latter being derived from memory cells), however, seem to be similar. Hence the major benefit to the body from the existence of memory cells is the increase in frequency of antigen-specific cells and their accentuated readiness to migrate to inflamed tissues.

How the memory cells are maintained in the body and whether they require periodical contact with small amounts of antigen is still a matter of controversy. Minute amounts of antigen (persisting in the form of immune complexes on follicular dendritic cells (see Chapter 17) or in certain chronically infected cells for example) markedly enhance T-cell memory. On the other hand, some experiments suggest that restimulation of memory T cells may, to a large extent, depend on the recognition of cross-reactive antigens, either foreign or autoantigens. Memory T cells may have a shorter lifespan than an individual but they perpetuate themselves by dividing from time to time in response to a low level of antigenic stimulation.

Collaboration of T_H cells with B lymphocytes in the initiation of antibody response

Differentiated T_H cells provide accessory signals to B lymphocytes that received the first signal by binding of antigen to their surface immunoglobulin (B-cell receptor, BCR). The precursors of T_H cells are distinguished by the presence of the CD4 co-receptor molecule on their surface (see Chapter 5). Activation, proliferation and terminal differentiation of these precursors into mature helpers, the T_H2 cells, is initiated by the interaction with professional APCs, either macrophages, dendritic cells or B-cell blasts (see Fig. 16.2). If a macrophage or a dendritic cell is the APC, the cooperation of three cells is required (T cell, APC, B cell; Fig. 16.7);

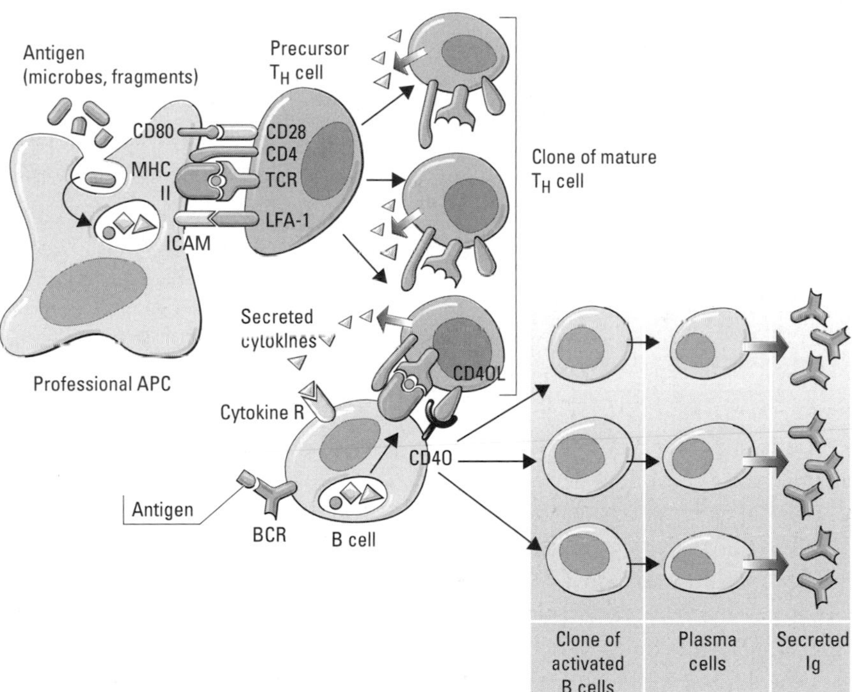

Figure 16.7 Overview of the steps leading to antibody production. Antigen is internalized by a professional antigen-presenting cell (APC) and degraded into fragments, some of which bind to MHC class II molecules and are displayed on the APC surface. The MHC–peptide complexes are recognized by a precursor helper T (T_H) cell, which receives co-stimulatory signals via CD28 and other receptors. A clone of mature T_H cells arises from the activated T_H precursor and is poised to interact with B cells that received the first signal via their B-cell receptor (BCR) and that express assemblies of MHC class II molecules with the same peptides as those recognized originally on the APC. The T_H cell provides secondary signals to the B cell via cytokine (IL-4, IL-5) and CD40 receptors. The cytokines are secreted in a highly oriented way into the narrow cleft between the two cells. The B cell proliferates into a clone. Most of the activated B cells differentiate into plasma cells that secrete large amounts of antibodies but some of them turn into memory B cells (not shown). For the sake of simplicity, a number of interacting molecules are not shown. For more details on the development of activated B cells see Chapter 17. Black arrows indicate proliferation and differentiation of cells from precursors; arrows within the cells indicate transport, processing and re-expression of antigen fragments in the APC. Red arrows indicate secretion of cytokines or antibodies.

if the B-cell blast serves as an APC, the minimal cooperation of two cells (T cell and B cell) is sufficient. Phagocytic APCs are necessary when large antigenic particles, such as bacteria, are involved. In the case of relatively small, easily endocytosed antigenic molecules, such as soluble proteins secreted by a microbe or released from a lysed microorganism, B-cell blasts (activated B cells) are the APCs of choice. The latter, in contrast to other APCs, are able to selectively concentrate the antigen because they are equipped with the antigen-specific BCR.

The encounter between naive T lymphocytes and APCs occurs in the lymph node parenchyma. If the T cell discovers an APC expressing a peptide–MHC molecule assembly that matches its antigen-specific receptor, it stops wandering, becomes activated and gives rise to a clone of mature T_H2 cells distinguished by the production of cytokines such as IL-4, IL-5, IL-6, IL-10 and IL-13. Mature T_H2 cells then provide two types of accessory signals to B cells stimulated by antigen recognition. First, they supply them with cytokines such as IL-4, IL-5, IL-6 and IL-13. Local concentrations of the cytokines are very high as they are secreted in an oriented way nearly exclusively into the narrow cleft between the adhering T_H and B cells. Second, they express the membrane-bound cytokine CD40L on their surface (see Table 10.2), which is the ligand for the B-cell surface receptor CD40 (see Fig. 16.2). Interaction between CD40 and CD40L is necessary for the initiation of the last phase of B-cell development, characterized by somatic hypermutation and immunoglobulin class switching (see Chapter 17).

Collaboration of T_H lymphocytes with macrophages in the inflammatory response

Activated macrophages are essential for combating intracellular parasites and large parasites that cannot be phagocytosed. When a precursor of a T_H cell encounters a peptide–MHC class II molecule assembly on the macrophage surface, it begins to proliferate and then differentiates into a mature T_H1 cell with the help of co-stimulatory signals provided by the macrophage (Fig. 16.8). Mature T_H1 cells produce multiple soluble or membrane-bound cytokines, two of which (soluble interferon-γ (IFN-γ) and membrane-bound tumour necrosis factor (TNF-α)) become essential for inducing the activated state in macrophages. These and other products of mature T_H1 cells also contribute to the develop-ment of local inflammation and stimulation of immune responses. First, IFN-γ and TNF-α are potent inducers of MHC class II expression on macrophages as well as other cells that normally do not express these molecules. This process transforms macrophages into better APCs that can stimulate more T cells. Second, several

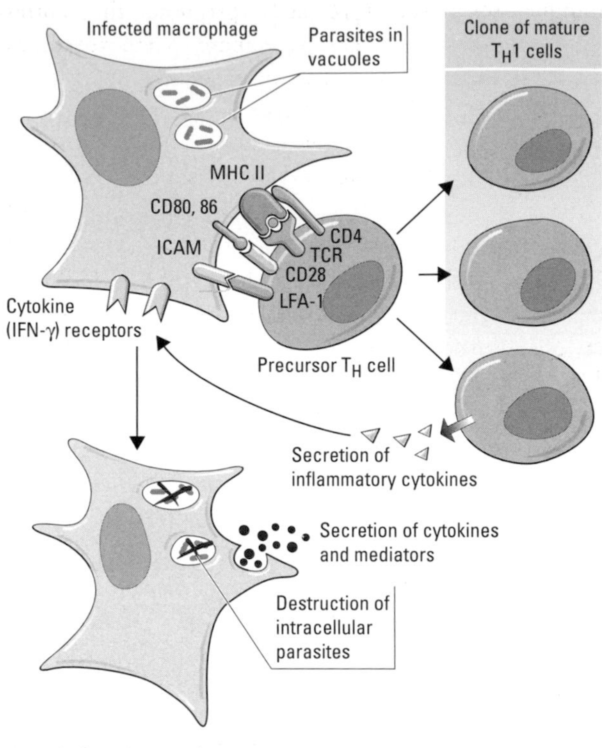

Figure 16.8 Schematic view of the interactions leading to macrophage activation. An infected macrophage expresses MHC class II molecules charged with parasite-derived peptides on its surface. These complexes are recognized by the helper T (T_H1) cell precursor, which also receives co-stimulatory signals (via CD28 and possibly other adhesion and cytokine receptors). The T_H1 cell proliferates and differentiates into mature T_H1 cells that activate the macrophage via interferon-γ (IFN-γ) and other cytokines. The activated macrophages acquire mechanisms capable of intracellular parasite destruction and secrete inflammatory cytokines and mediators.

of the cytokines produced by T_H1 cells attract even more phagocytes to the site of inflammation and stimulate endothelial cells to express adhesion molecules that are essential for both the attachment of phagocytes to the blood vessel walls and emigra-tion to the tissue. While IFN-γ stimulates the transition of macrophages into the activated state, other cytokines such as IL-4, IL-10, IL-13 and TGF-β have opposing, deactivating effects. They act either directly on macrophages or indirectly by suppressing IFN-γ production by T_H1 cells. When these mechanisms fail to eliminate the infection, the inflammation may become chronic, accompanied by various types of local tissue damage.

Development of T_H1 vs. T_H2 cells

Two distinct types of T_H cell participate in antigen-specific immune response: T_H2 cells promote the antibody response, while T_H1 cells participate in the development of the inflammatory response based on activated macrophages. T_H1 and T_H2 cells develop from a common precursor: naive CD4+ T cells. It is therefore important that the immune system makes the right choice when it is faced with the decision as to which T_H cell type should develop in a particular situation. To give an example, *Mycobacterium leprae*, the causative agent of leprosy, grows inside macrophage vesicles. If the inflammatory branch of the immune response based on the collaboration of T_H1 cells and macrophages is initiated, the *tuberculoid type* of the disease develops, which progresses very slowly and is accompanied by skin and other tissue damage caused by intense inflammation. However, when the antibody response (dependent on T_H2 cells) is launched, the disease develops into the much more deadly *lepromatous form*, in which the pathogen grows extensively in macrophages, well hidden from the abundantly produced antibodies.

An important feature of T_H-lymphocyte development is that the cytokines produced by one subset (T_H1 or T_H2 cells) stimulate (in an autocrine way) development of the same subset but suppress development of the other. Thus, T_H1 and T_H2 cells act as mutual adversaries or antagonists. When the decision T_H1 vs. T_H2 is made, the pathway tends to stabilize itself and prevents the parallel development of the other. The factors determining which differentiation pathway is to be taken appear to be the cytokines produced by cells of the non-adaptive immune system. Some micro-organisms, especially intracellular bacteria and viruses, stimulate macrophages to produce IL-12, which selectively stimulates development of T_H1 cells. IL-12 also stimulates NK cells to produce IFN-γ, which suppresses the development of T_H2 cells and further stimulates macrophages.

The reason why IFN-γ inhibits the development of T_H2 but not T_H1 cells is that T_H2 cells express the two-chain, high-affinity IFN-γ receptor (IFN-γR) on their surface, whereas T_H1 cells lack one of the receptor subunits, IFN-γRβ. Interaction of IFN-γ with the complete, but not incomplete, receptor generates an antiproliferative signal.

In situations in which IL-4 rather then IL-12 predominates in the vicinity of the precursor T_H cell, the cytokine induces the development of T_H2 cells and inhibits the development of T_H1 cells. Possible early sources of IL-4 could be mast cells and basophils stimulated by the encounter with antigen in immune complexes or CD1-restricted NK-like T cells, described later in this chapter.

Another factor that influences the T_H1 vs. T_H2 response appears to be the density of antigenic peptides presented by MHC class II molecules on the surface of the APC. When the peptides bind with low affinity to MHC molecules, the density of the complexes on the APC surface is low and naive lymphocytes recognizing such complexes tend to develop into T_H2 cells. Naive CD4+ T cells that encounter a high density of peptides bound to MHC class II molecules preferentially develop into T_H1 cells. As far as the nature of the signal is concerned, it would seem to make a difference whether 100 or 1000 TCRs become engaged simultaneously.

The nature of the secondary signals provided by the different APC types also plays a role. T_H1 cells seem to be less dependent on the co-stimulatory signal provided via the CD28 receptor than T_H2 cells, so that APCs relatively low in CD80 and CD86 may preferentially stimulate the development of T_H1 responses.

The division of T_H lymphocytes into T_H1 and T_H2 cells may, however, be an oversimplification, especially in humans. A continuous range of T_H-cell clones may exist that differ in the spectrum of cytokines they produce; in this case, the typical T_H1 and T_H2 clones would merely represent the two extremes of this spectrum.

Cytotoxic responses

Most T_C lymphocytes are distinguished by the presence of the co-receptor molecule CD8 (and absence of CD4) on their surface. Their major task is to seek out cells infected by viruses or other intracellular parasites and to kill them, thus eliminating the source of further infection. T_C cells develop from naive CD8+ precursors which recognize peptidic fragments of viral proteins complexed to MHC class I proteins on the surface of professional APCs capable of providing co-stimulatory signals, primarily via the CD28 receptor. If the first encounter of the cytotoxic precursor happens to be with the surface of some other cell that is unable to provide the co-stimulatory signals, the precursor becomes unresponsive to further stimulation or even dies (see Fig. 16.1).

Many *in vitro* experiments have indicated that the assistance of CD4+ T_H cells is necessary for efficient development of T_C cells. It seems, however, that T_H cells also function indirectly by stimulating the APC to express more co-stimulatory surface molecules such as CD80 or CD86 and T-cell stimulatory cytokines such as IL-1 or IL-12. Mature T_C cells no longer require accessory second signals: the signal provided via their TCRs is sufficient to activate the effector mechanisms. They are therefore able to kill any type of infected cells regardless whether these express co-stimulatory surface molecules or not.

Some CD4+ T_C cells are able to kill MHC class II-positive cells. Their function in the immune response, however, is not known, nor their relationship to other T_H subsets. They could specialize in the destruction of infected MHC class II-positive cells or in the regulation of the number of APCs and thus abrogation of the immune response.

CD8+ T cells not only kill but also secrete a number of cytokines and thus contribute to regulation of the immune response. Subpopulations of CD8+ T cells also seem to exist that differ in the spectrum of cytokines produced. It is not clear, however, how the two functions of the CD8+ cells (cytotoxicity and cytokine secretion) are related: whether the CD8+ precursors can differentiate into either killers or cytokine secretors or whether these two functions are executed by the same cell.

Mature, functionally fully competent T_C cells, also called *armed* T_C or *cytolytic T lymphocytes* (CTL), express a high level of adhesion molecules such as LFA-1 and CD2 necessary for the attachment to target cells. The cytoplasm of T_C cells contains secretory granules (a specialized form of lysosomes) loaded with proteins that participate in cell killing. One of the proteins is *perforin*, which is structurally related to the C9 component of complement; others are serine proteases called *granzymes*. The human perforin (pore-forming protein or cytolysin) molecule consists of 534 amino acid residues. The sequence contains two potential *N*-glycosylation sites and the mature molecule has an M_r of 70 000. The amino acid sequences of human, mouse and rat perforins are 70–85% identical. The middle part of the perforin polypeptide chain (residues 100–400) exhibits about 20% sequence identity with the complement proteins C6–C9. Human perforin is encoded in a gene on chromosome 10 that is specifically expressed in CTL and NK cells. The most important granzymes are *granzyme A* and *granzyme B* encoded in closely linked genes on human chromosome 5q11–q12. The former is a homodimer with a subunit size of M_r 30 000, the latter a monomer of similar size. Granzyme A cleaves peptide bonds between arginine and lysine residues while granzyme B cleaves peptide bonds between aspartic acid and glutamic acid (this substrate specificity is rather unique: the only other eukaryotic protease with a similar specificity is *interleukin-1β converting enzyme* (ICE), which is, however, a cysteine protease).

T_C cells contact cells in tissues via their adhesion molecules. If within a short time their TCRs do not find a matching peptide–MHC molecule assembly, T_C cells detach

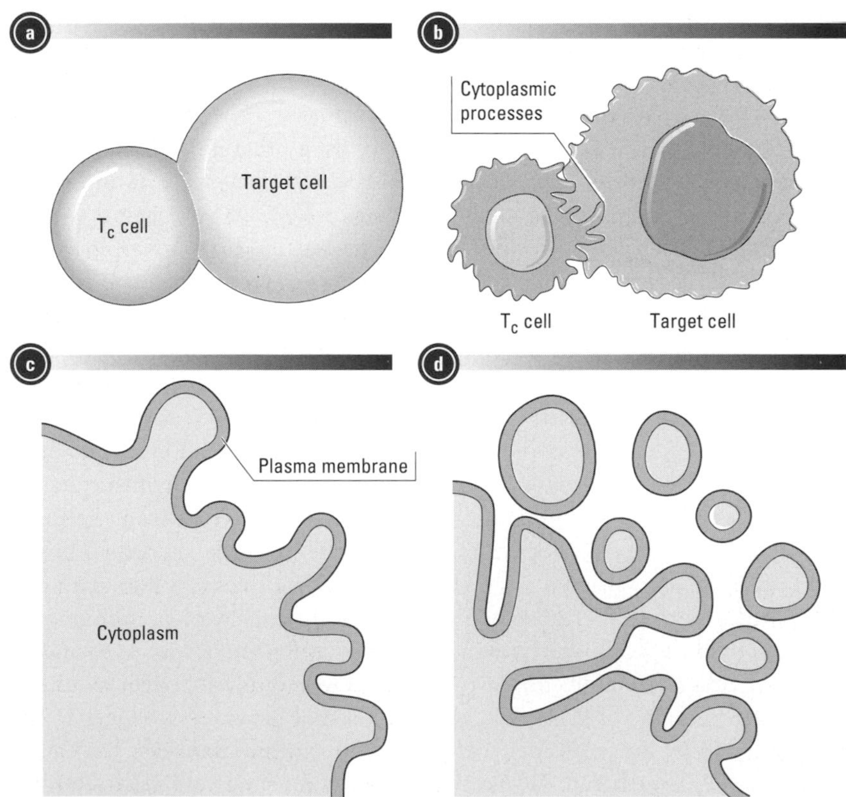

Figure 16.9 Cell-mediated lymphocytotoxicity. (a) Broad contact between the cytotoxic T (T_C) cell on the left and the target cell on the right is established. (b) Cytoplasmic processes of the T_C cell invade the target cell and deliver the lethal hit. (c) The plasma membrane of the target cell appears to 'boil'. (d) Plasma membrane and cytoplasm become fragmented as the cell dies by apoptosis or in some cases by lysis. (Modified from Klein, J. (1986) *Natural History of the Major Histocompatibility Complex*. John Wiley & Sons, New York.)

themselves and move on to the next cell; the mechanism of detachment is not known. When the TCR finds a matching ligand on the contacted cell, the LFA-1 molecule acquires a high-affinity conformation as a result of signals delivered via the TCR, thus strengthening the bond between the two cells (Fig. 16.9). The exocytic granules then move rapidly (about 1.2 μm/s) along microtubules towards the site of T_C cell–target cell contact, fuse with the T_C cell membrane and their contents are discharged into the narrow cleft between the two cells. In the presence of Ca^{2+} ions, perforin monomers released from the cytotoxic granules undergo conformational changes, bind to phospholipids of the target cell membrane, insert into it and subsequently aggregate to form homopolymeric pores containing 3–20 monomers (Fig. 16.10). Within the polyperforin pores, the hydrophobic amino acid residues of the monomers probably face the acyl chains of the membrane lipids, while the hydrophilic residues line the interior of the pore, the diameter of which ranges from 5 to 20 nm depending on the number of monomers involved. The pores resemble those formed by the membrane-attack complex of complement (see Chapter 12). Large perforin-based pores seem to damage the integrity of the membrane and thus lead to rapid osmotic lysis of the target cell. Under physiological conditions, however, smaller pores are probably formed predominantly and these enable penetration of other components of the cytotoxic granules, including granzymes, through the membrane. Alternatively, perturbation of the membrane by perforin oligomers may induce target cell reactions including enhanced endocytosis, a process that can also transport granzymes inside the cell.

Granzymes, especially granzyme B, that penetrate into

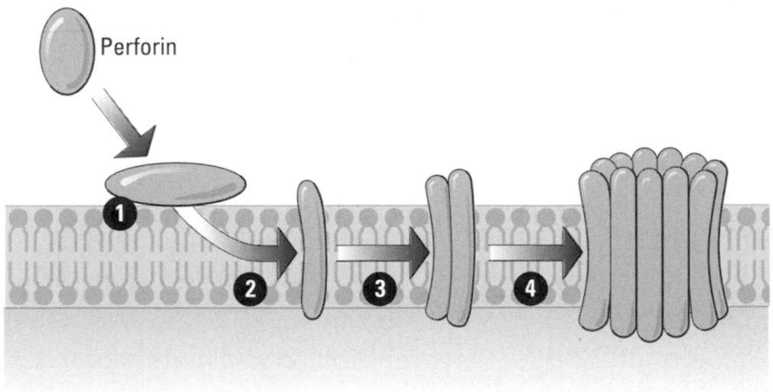

Figure 16.10 Postulated mechanism of perforin action. In the presence of Ca^{2+}, perforin monomers undergo conformational changes and bind to membrane phospholipids (1), are inserted into the membrane (2) and subsequently aggregate to form homooligomeric pore structures (3 and 4). These pores perturb membrane permeability and result in osmotic lysis or uptake of granzymes. (Modified from Liu, C.-C. *et al.* (1995) *Immunology Today*, **16**, 194.)

the target cell cleave a cytoplasmic protein (or proteins) that has not been characterized to any significant degree. The products of this cleavage induce apoptotic mechanisms including cross-linking of cytoplasmic proteins, membrane disorganization, fragmentation of the nucleus and finally breakdown of the cell into a number of small apoptotic bodies that are cleared by macrophages. After delivering the lethal blow, the T_C lymphocyte detaches itself from the target cell and moves on to the next cell. A single T_C lymphocyte can therefore serially kill many infected target cells, a process requiring the continuous synthesis of cytotoxic granules and of their contents.

The cytotoxic mechanism employed by T_C lymphocytes probably makes use of the suicidal machinery inherent in any cell type. Cells can produce their own suicidal proteases that, upon proper activation, initiate the apoptotic process. These proteases are similar to ICE, which cleaves the precursor of IL-1β into the mature cytokine. Since granzyme A has a similar substrate specificity (it also cleaves the IL-1β precursor), it is believed to function by initiating the same reaction cascade that is otherwise activated via endogenous ICE-like proteases in response to natural apoptotic stimuli.

The cytotoxic mechanism based on exocytic granules, perforin and granzymes is not the only weapon T_C cells possess. Another is the *Fas ligand* (*FasL*), a cell-surface cytokine of the TNF family that can specifically bind to the widely distributed *Fas (CD95)* receptor. The receptor belongs to the TNFR superfamily (see Chapter 10). Engagement of the Fas receptor also induces apoptosis, independently of perforin-mediated lysis (Fig. 16.11). Different cell types also differ in their sensitivity to perforin/granzymes and Fas engagement, so that these two mechanisms complement each other. Most of the FasL is stored in the membranes of the exocytic granules and appears on the surface only upon their contact-induced fusion with the plasma membrane.

The mechanism by which T_C lymphocytes avoid self-destruction by the cytotoxic substances they excrete remains obscure. The lymphocytes are not intrinsically resistant to the killing since it can be demonstrated experimentally that one T_C cell can kill another (but not itself). One possibility is that the exocytic vesicles actually fuse with the target cell membrane, thus avoiding any spillage of their contents on to the killer cell itself.

Some of the cytokines produced by T_C lymphocytes may also contribute to the effector mechanisms. Thus, IFN-γ induces expression of MHC glycoproteins in the target cell, making it a better target for the T_C lymphocyte. This cytokine also inhibits viral replication in the infected cell. Similarly, an uncharacterized factor produced by $CD8^+$ T cells appears to inhibit replication of human immunodefi-

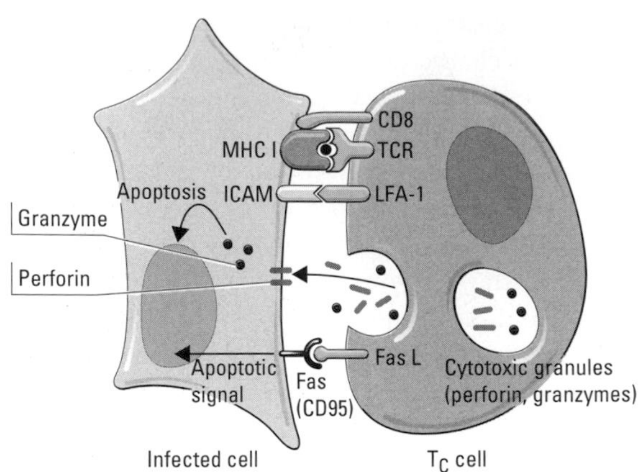

Figure 16.11 Cytotoxic mechanisms used by T_C cells. The mature T_C cell recognizes the antigen (MHC class I protein loaded with a viral peptide) on the surface of an infected cell. The cells firmly adhere to each other via several pairs of adhesion molecules such as ICAM-1–LFA-1. T-cell receptor (TCR) engagement generates a signal that triggers degranulation (release of the granular contents into the cleft between the two cells). One of the granule's components, perforin, inserts itself into the membrane of the attacked cell and creates pores that facilitate the delivery of the granzyme molecules. These act on intracellular targets and thus initiate programmed cell death (apoptosis). Massive perforation of the membrane can also lead to osmotic lysis (rupture of the membrane). In addition, a T_C cell-surface protein, FasL, binds to the Fas receptor on the surface of the target cell and this interaction, too, generates an apoptotic signal.

ciency virus (HIV) in infected CD4+ T lymphocytes. This raises the possibility that, in some instances at least, T_C lymphocytes may not kill but rather cure the infected cell. Other cytokines, such as TNF-α and lymphotoxin, contribute to the killing. By binding to their receptors on the target cells they induce apoptosis in a similar manner to that of the Fas pathway (recall that FasL is actually similar to TNF-α and that, furthermore, membrane-bound forms of TNF-α exist).

T_C cells are a powerful tool of defence but they also exemplify the proverbial double-edged sword of the immune system. By attacking infected host cells, they can sometimes cause more harm than good. Such a situation can occur when the infected host cells perform an essential function in the body and when the infecting pathogen is not particularly dangerous. A good example is the lymphocytic choriomeningitis virus (LCMV) in the mouse. It normally infects a variety of tissues without causing disease, but if it gains access to the brain (which usually only happens when the experimenter injects it there) it infects brain cells, which are then attacked by T_C lymphocytes. The attack mobilizes many elements of the non-adaptive defence system and leads to inflammation of the meninges (the membranes enclosing the brain), cellular infiltration of the ependyma (the membrane lining the ventricles of the brain and the central canal of the spinal cord) and to serious neurological impairment. Similar damage is inflicted in the case of human hepatitis B virus infection in which the infected hepatocytes are attacked by T_C lymphocytes. It is also likely that destruction of HIV-infected CD4+ T cells by T_C lymphocytes contributes to the pathology of AIDS. In most situations, however, the immune system manages to avoid such adverse consequences of T_C cell attack and uses these cells for the benefit of the body only.

In addition to the cytotoxic mechanisms directed against infected cells, T cells (and NK cells) also appear to be able to kill or inhibit certain fungi, bacteria and multicellular parasites directly. To do so, T cells must first be activated by antigens, mitogens or cytokines. They then adhere to the microbe surface via unidentified surface receptors and discharge the contents of their cytotoxic granules on to it. This mechanism resembles in some aspects that used by phagocytes (although T cells and NK cells are not capable of true phagocytosis). Direct killing mechanisms have been observed *in vitro*; their physiological importance *in vivo* remains undocumented.

NK-cell cytotoxicity

NK cells to some extent resemble T_C lymphocytes. Like T_C cells, they have exocytic granules containing perforin and granzymes and use them in a similar way. They may also use other killing mechanisms based on interactions of their surface-bound or secreted cytokines with apoptotic receptors, such as Fas, of target cells. There are, however, two major differences between NK and T_C cells. First, NK cells do not use receptors similar to the TCR and, second, they do not require sensitization by antigen and differentiation from precursors to become efficient killers. Instead, NK cells are always ready for use and kill sensitive targets immediately upon recognition. However, NK-cell killing activity can be increased by exposure to cytokines such as IFN-α, IL-2 or IL-12.

NK cells detect and kill cells that have lost their MHC class I molecules. Any healthy human cell expresses certain amounts of the three classical MHC class I molecules, HLA-A, -B and -C. An infection by particular viruses or malignant transformation may decrease the expression of all or some of the molecules substantially. Such cells then become the main target of NK cells (see Chapter 7). Like T cells, NK cells use adhesion receptors such as CD2 or LFA-1 to establish initial contact with their target cells. Some of the adhesion molecules (e.g. CD56 and CD57) are more or less specific for NK cells, while others are expressed on other cells as well. The adhesive interactions probably contribute to the generation of a positive, stimulatory signal. However, the major stimulatory signals are delivered via the NK receptors of the stimulatory type (see Chapter 7).

The different NK cell clones of an individual express various combinations and different levels of inhibitory NK receptors recognizing MHC molecules (see Chapter 7). Any NK cell must possess enough inhibitory receptors to override positive stimulatory signals generated upon contact with a normal self cell. When the expression of at least one MHC class I type or allelic form is substantially decreased, at least some NK cells detect this anomaly and kill the target cell because signals from the stimulatory receptors are insufficiently counteracted by signals from the inhibitory receptors. A cell that has shut off the expression of most or all MHC class I molecules becomes vulnerable to attack by most NK cells. Because the NK-cell inhibitory receptors probably recognize a region of the MHC class I molecules close to the peptide-binding site, it is possible that certain peptides derived from the infecting pathogen alter the conformation of the MHC molecule to the extent that it is no longer properly recognized by the NK-cell inhibitory receptors. In this way, NK cells might be able to recognize some infected cells even if they have not downregulated MHC expression.

This system obviously requires a finely tuned balance between the effects of stimulatory and inhibitory receptors. It must avoid autoreactivity (which could occur if the inhibitory branch were too weak and thus unable to buffer the effects of insignificant physiological variation in MHC expression) but on the other hand it must be sensitive enough to detect anomalous cells. The tuning probably requires positive and negative selection analogous to some extent to that used by T cells. The mechanisms of these presumed selection processes remain undetermined, and hardly anything is known about the mechanisms responsible for transduction of either inhibitory or stimulatory signals by NK-cell receptors.

NK cells also have an alternative recognition system to detect and kill infected cells. They have a low-affinity Fc receptor (FcγRIIIa, CD16a) on their surfaces, which enables them to bind to cells coated by IgG antibodies. Cross-linking of these receptors on the NK-cell surface generates an activating signal that triggers the release of exocytic granules and leads to killing of the infected cell (Fig. 16.12). This process, referred to as *antibody-dependent cellular cytotoxicity (ADCC)*, has been well documented *in vitro* but its significance *in vivo* is uncertain.

NK cells probably also exert regulatory effects on both adaptive and non-adaptive immune responses and on haemopoiesis. Some immunologists even believe that these

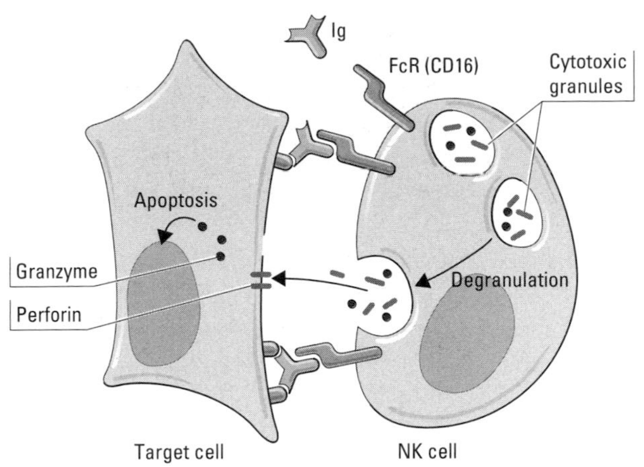

Figure 16.12 Activation of natural killer (NK)-cell killing by antibody-dependent cellular cytotoxicity. Antibodies bind to antigens on the target cell surface and their Fc portions bind to the Fc receptors (CD16) on the surface of NK cells. The interaction initiates degranulation and killing by the perforin–granzyme based mechanisms (see Fig. 16.11).

regulatory functions of NK cells are more important than their cytotoxic effects. The functions are mediated by various cytokines, such as IL-3, TNF-α, granulocyte monocyte colony stimulating factor (GM-CSF), IFN-γ and others, which NK cells produce. The rapid production of IFN-γ during early phases of infection may in particular be important for the stimulation of macrophages and for preferential induction of T_H1 cell differentiation. In contrast to cytokine production by T cells, cytokine production by NK cells is rapid, does not require prior activation, is induced by non-specific stimuli (surface structures of target cells, immune complexes) and may involve large numbers of NK cells simultaneously.

Function of γ:δ and other unusual T cells

γ:δ T cells

The T cells discussed so far have been those carrying TCRs composed of α and β chains. These α:β T cells undergo thymic development and maturation into two major subsets, T_H and T_C cells (see Chapter 7), but there is another, less well characterized T-cell subpopulation carrying TCRs composed of γ and δ chains. These γ:δ T cells exhibit several unique features: they arise early in ontogeny in the thymus but their maturation appears to be thymus independent and they usually do not express CD4 or CD8 co-receptors. (In ruminants, however, γ:δ T cells specifically express a WC1 family of membrane proteins of so far unknown function that might serve as co-receptors.) At least some $\gamma{:}\delta$ T cells secrete a range of cytokines and have cytotoxic properties similar to T_C or NK cells.

Most of the $\gamma{:}\delta$ T cells do not recognize complexes of MHC molecules with peptides but rather certain specific antigens alone, in a manner similar to B lymphocytes. They seem to be preoccupied mainly with the recognition of mycobacterial fragments containing phosphorylated carbohydrates and compounds like alkylphosphates, unprocessed viral proteins and possibly also highly conserved stress proteins. A significant subpopulation of $\gamma{:}\delta$ T cells resides in the epithelia. These cells have a dendritic appearance, are fixed between keratinocytes in the epidermis and have very uniform TCRs. They probably recognize a component of stressed self cells, possibly stress proteins. They seem to function as guardians of epithelial integrity because upon detecting a defective epithelium they become activated and secrete cytokines, such as keratinocyte growth factor, which help to repair the damage. As such, $\gamma{:}\delta$ T cells may be considered as part of the non-adaptive immune system. The $\gamma{:}\delta$ T cells in the submucosal layer possibly act as sentries that recognize invading microorganisms and contribute to local inflammatory defence.

Atypical $\alpha{:}\beta$ T cells

In addition to typical $\alpha{:}\beta$ T cells (either $CD4^+$ or $CD8^+$) there is a bewildering collection of less well characterized $\alpha{:}\beta$ T cells that are unusual in several respects. Among them are $CD4^-CD8^-$ cells, NK-like T cells (expressing some of the receptors otherwise characteristic for NK cells) and T cells expressing the CD8$\alpha\alpha$ homodimer instead of the usual CD8$\alpha\beta$ heterodimer (see Chapter 7).

A number of these unusual T cells do not depend on the thymus for their development and some have a somewhat altered TCR/CD3 complex, using the γ chains otherwise found in Fc-receptor complexes instead of the ζ and η chains. Many of these T cells appear to recognize MHC class Ib molecules (human HLA-E, -F and -G, mouse H2-M, -Q and -T) complexed with peptides or the MHC class I-like CD1 molecules complexed with non-peptide ligands such as mycobacterial glycolipids and fragments of lipopolysaccharides.

A striking feature of CD1-restricted NK-like T cells (either $CD4^-CD8^-$ or $CD4^+CD8^-$) is their very limited repertoire of V_α and V_β segments: nearly all mouse cells of this kind possess TCRs composed almost exclusively of α chains containing $V_\alpha14$ and $J_\alpha281$ segments and β chains containing mainly $V_\beta8$ segments (human NK-like T cells have a similarly restricted α-chain repertoire using $V_\alpha24$ and $J_\alpha Q$ segments). These atypical T cells are found usually in small numbers (1–2%) in the blood and most secondary lymphoid organs, but they are associated primarily with the mucosal immune system. NK-like T cells develop in the thymus and possibly undergo positive and negative selection on CD1-expressing immature thymocytes. In the mouse, they represent 10–20% of all mature (medullary) thymocytes. A conspicuous feature of NK-like T cells is that after contact with antigen they rapidly (within 30–90 min) produce large amounts of IL-4 and some other cytokines. They may therefore be the major early source of IL-4 necessary for the differentiation of T_H2 cells. It has been suggested that parasitic worms induce expression of CD1 molecules on local mucosa, which are recognized by NK-like T cells and stimulate them to IL-4 production. IL-4 then triggers the T_H2-dependent humoral response dominated by IgE, which is protective in this situation (see Chapters 18 & 21). NK-like T cells are probably also precursors of the majority of *lymphokine-activated killer* (*LAK*) cells that arise by *in vitro* cultivation of peripheral lymphocytes with IL-2 and which are thought to play a part in defence against tumours (see Chapter 22).

Intraepithelial T lymphocytes (IEL) are found in mucosal epithelia (see Chapters 18 & 21). Thcy are phenotypically heterogeneous but all have specific adhesion molecules in common: two integrins of the $\beta7$ family, $\alpha4\beta7$ (LPAM-1) and $\alpha E\beta7$ (HML-1). The adhesion receptors recognize ligands present on the surface of mucosal blood vessel endothelial cells and on the epithelial surface and are thus responsible for the specific mucosal homing of IEL (see Chapter 9). Another speciality of IEL T cells is that many of them possess an unusual form of the CD8 co-receptor (a dimer of CD8α chains rath er than the usual CD8$\alpha\beta$ heterodimer). Others co-express CD8α and CD4 molecules. TCR complexes of IEL T cells, especially those expressing CD8α homodimers, do not contain the associated ζ chains but structurally similar γ-chain dimers instead, which are otherwise regular components of Fc-receptor complexes.

The function of IEL is not known. Some of them could participate in establishing a proper balance between tolerance towards harmless antigens such as food components and immunity against pathogens using mucosal surfaces for entry into the body (see Chapter 18). Others may be part of the non-adaptive mechanisms by specializing in the recognition of relatively invariant bacterial components bound to MHC class Ib molecules or to CD1 molecules. In this respect they may complement the activities of intraepithelial $\gamma{:}\delta$ T cells. The IEL secrete a spectrum of cytokines following stimulation by antigen and some of them may therefore act as helpers for those B cells that produce antibodies to non-protein antigens.

Further reading

Allison, J.P. (1994) CD28–B7 interactions in T-cell activation. *Current Opinion in Immunology*, **6**, 414–419.

Bendelac, A. (1995) CD1: presenting unusual antigens to unusual T lymphocytes. *Science*, **269**, 185–186.

Bennett, M., Yu, Y.Y.L., Stoneman, E. *et al.* (1995) Hybrid resistance: 'negative' and 'positive' signaling of murine natural killer cells. *Seminars in Immunology*, **7**, 121–127.

Berke, G. (1994) The binding and lysis by cytotoxic lymphocytes: molecular and cellular aspects. *Annual Review of Immunology*, **12**, 737–773.

Croft, M. (1994) Activation of naive, memory and effector T cells. *Current Opinion in Immunology*, **6**, 431–437.

DeFranco, A.L. (1995) Transmembrane signaling by antigen receptors of B and T lymphocytes. *Current Opinion in Cell Biology*, **7**, 163–175.

de Vries, J.E., Carballido, J.M., Sornasse, T. & Yssel, H. (1995) Antagonizing the differentiation and functions of human T helper type 2 cells. *Current Opinion in Immunology*, **7**, 771–778.

Germain, R.N., Levine, E.H. & Madrenas, J. (1995) The T-cell receptor as a diverse signal transduction machine. *Immunologist*, **3**, 113–121.

Gray, D. (1994) Regulation of immunological memory. *Current Opinion in Immunology*, **6**, 425–430.

Havran, W.L. & Boismenu, R. (1994) Activation and function of γδ T cells. *Current Opinion in Immunology*, **6**, 442–446.

Henkart, P.A. (1994) Lymphocyte-mediated cytotoxicity: Two pathways and multiple effector molecules. *Immunity*, **1**, 343–346.

Howard, J.C. (1995) Supply and transport of peptides presented by class I MHC molecules. *Current Opinion in Immunology*, **7**, 69–76.

Izquierdo Pastor, M., Reif, K. & Cantrell, D. (1995) The regulation and function of $p21^{ras}$ during T-cell activation and growth. *Immunology Today*, **16**, 159–164.

Jameson, S.C. & Bevan, M.J. (1995) T cell receptor antagonists and partial agonists. *Immunity*, **2**, 1–11.

Jenkins, M.K. (1994) The ups and downs of T cell costimulation. *Immunity*, **1**, 443–446.

Jenkins, M.K. & Johnson, J.G. (1993) Molecules involved in T-cell costimulation. *Current Opinion in Immunology*, **5**, 361–367.

Kaufmann, S.H.E. (1995) Immunity to intracellular microbial pathogens. *Immunology Today*, **16**, 338–342.

Klein, J.R. (1995) Advances in intestinal T-cell development and function. *Immunology Today*, **16**, 322–324.

Lanier, L.L. & Phillips, J.H. (1996) Inhibitory MHC class I receptors on NK cells and T cells. *Immunology Today*, **17**, 86–91.

Lanzavecchia, A. (1990) Receptor-mediated antigen uptake and its effect on antigen presentation to class II-restricted T lymphocytes. *Annual Review of Immunology*, **8**, 773–793.

Levitz, S.M., Mathews, H.L. & Murphy, J.W. (1995) Direct antimicrobial activity of T cells. *Immunology Today*, **16**, 387–391.

Linsley, P.S. & Golstein, P. (1996) T-cell regulation by CTLA-4. *Current Biology*, **6**, 398–400.

Liu, C.-C., Walsh, C. M. & Young, J.D.-E. (1995) Perforin: structure and function. *Immunology Today*, **16**, 194–201.

Minami, Y. & Taniguchi, T. (1995) IL-2 signalling: recruitment and activation of multiple protein tyrosine kinases by the components of the IL-2 receptor. *Current Opinion in Cell Biology*, **7**, 156–162.

Moretta, L., Ciccone, E., Mingari, M.C., Biassoni, R. & Moretta, A. (1994) Human natural killer cells: origin, clonality, specificity, and receptors. *Advances in Immunology*, **55**, 341–380.

Mosmann, T.R. & Sad, S. (1996) The expanding universe of T-cell subsets: Th1, Th2 and more. *Immunology Today*, **17**, 138–146.

Poussier, P. & Julius, M. (1994) Thymus-independent T cell development and selection in the intestinal epithelium. *Annual Review of Immunology*, **12**, 521–553.

Raulet, D.H., Correa, I., Corral, L., Dorfman, J. & Wu, M.-F. (1995) Inhibitory effects of class I molecules on murine NK cells: speculations on function, specificity and self tolerance. *Seminars in Immunology*, **7**, 103–107.

Robey, E. & Allison, J.P. (1995) T-cell activation: integration of signals from the antigen receptor and costimulatory molecules. *Immunology Today*, **7**, 306–310.

Sette, A., Alexander, J., Ruppert, J. *et al.* (1994) Antigen analogs/MHC complexes as specific T cell receptor antagonists. *Annual Review of Immunology*, **12**, 413–431.

Sim, G.-K. (1995) Intraepithelial lymphocytes and the immune system. *Advances in Immunology*, **58**, 297–343.

Smyth, M.J. & Trapani, J.A. (1995) Granzymes: exogenous proteinases that induce target cell apoptosis. *Immunology Today*, **16**, 202–206.

Steinman, R.M. (1991) The dendritic cell system and its role in immunogenicity. *Annual Review of Immunology*, **9**, 271–296.

Swain, S.L. (1993) Polarized patterns of cytokine secretion. *Current Biology*, **3**, 115–117.

Thomas, M.L. (1994) The regulation of B- and T-lymphocyte activation by the transmembrane protein tyrosine phosphatase CD45. *Current Opinion in Cell Biology*, **6**, 247–252.

Thompson, C.B. (1995) Distinct roles for the costimulatory ligands B7-1 and B7-2 in T helper cell differentiation? *Cell*, **81**, 979–982.

Trinchieri, G. (1995) Natural killer cells wear different hats: effector cells of innate resistance and regulatory cells of adaptive immunity and of hematopoiesis. *Seminars in Immunology*, 7, 83–88.

Valitutti, S. & Lanzavecchia, A. (1995) A serial triggering model of TcR activation. *Immunologist*, **3**, 122–124.

Vicari, A.P. & Zlotnik, A. (1996) Mouse NK1.1+ T cells: a new family of T cells. *Immunology Today*, **17**, 71–76.

Weiss, A. & Littman, D.R. (1994) Signal transduction by lymphocyte antigen receptors. *Cell*, **76**, 263–274.

Yokoyama, W.M. (1995) Natural killer receptors. *Current Opinion in Immunology*, 7, 110–120.

chapter 17 B-lymphocyte responses

Like T lymphocytes, B lymphocytes are able to recognize antigens specifically by means of the antigen-specific receptors residing on their surfaces. The structure of the B-cell antigen receptor (BCR, surface immunoglobulin) and the genetic mechanisms responsible for generation of its clonal diversity are very similar to those of the T-cell receptor (TCR) (see Chapter 8). In contrast to T cells, B lymphocytes recognize by means of their BCR certain structural features on the surface of an antigen itself and they produce soluble forms of their antigen-specific receptors, the secreted immunoglobulins (antibodies).

Many points relevant to B lymphocytes and the production and properties of different isotypes of antibodies have already been discussed in Chapters 8, 14 and 16. In this chapter, we concentrate on more specific aspects.

Antigen recognition by B lymphocytes

The BCR binds proteins, carbohydrates, lipids or synthetic chemicals of virtually every structure and the antigens can be soluble or bound to the cell surface. The interaction of the BCR with the antigen provides the B cell with the first signal necessary for proliferation and differentiation into antibody-secreting plasma cells. In most cases, however, this signal is insufficient and must be followed within a short time by co-stimulatory signals provided by T_H lymphocytes, as discussed in the previous chapter. If this help is not provided, signalling by the BCR has a negative effect and the cell becomes unresponsive or may even die by apoptosis. This negative signalling is a mechanism preventing the production of potentially harmful antibodies directed at autoantigens. If a B cell has a BCR that binds to a self molecule, it will not receive help because T cells recognizing fragments of self proteins associated with MHC molecules were eliminated during thymic development. B cells are prone to this type of autoantigen-induced elimination mainly in the late stage of their maturation, when they express only the BCR of the IgM isotype.

Signalling through the BCR

The mechanisms of signalling via the BCR are similar to those used by the TCR and by Fc receptors. Like the TCR, the BCR complex consists of an antigen-recognition module, membrane immunoglobulin, and an associated signalling module composed of at least two membrane proteins, CD79α (Igα) and CD79β (Igβ), functional analogues of the CD3 proteins (see Chapter 8). In their intracellular domains, the CD79 proteins have the immunoreceptor tyrosine-based activation motifs (ITAM) required for non-covalent association with intracellular protein tyrosine kinases of the Src family (Lyn, Blk, Fyn, Lck) and, after activation, also with the Syk kinase (similar to the ZAP-70 kinase participating in TCR signalling). The BCR complex is associated with further molecules still, the *BCR-associated proteins* (BAP). At least four of these molecules have been identified, called BAP29, BAP31, BAP32 and BAP37, as their relative molecular masses (M_r)are 29 000, 31 000, 32 000 and 37 000, respectively. All of them are structurally related, evolutionarily highly conserved, non-glycosylated membrane proteins. Their role is not known but they are probably involved in fine tuning the receptor signalling that is dependent on the BCR isotype. The BCR of the IgM isotype is associated with BAP32 and BAP37, whereas the BCR of the IgD isotype is associated with the similar yet distinct BAP29 and BAP31. This difference may be responsible for the fact that interaction of an antigen with the IgD BCR results in a more protracted activation of the associated protein tyrosine kinases as compared with the IgM BCR, and thus leads to stronger B-cell stimulation. BAP may also play a role in internalization of the BCR–antigen complex.

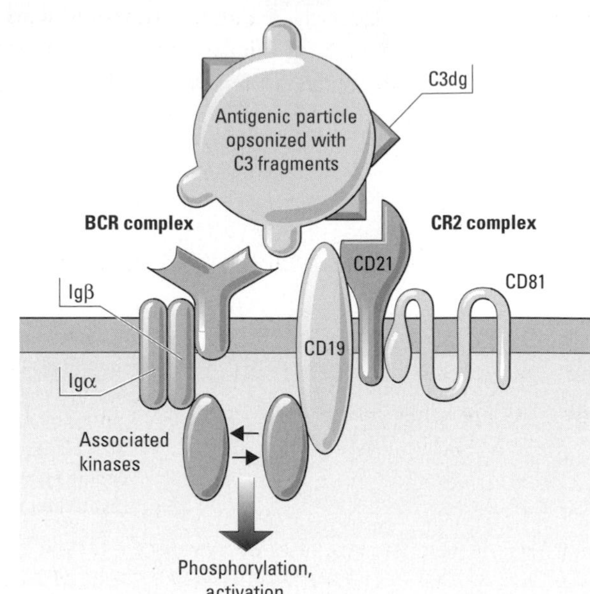

Figure 17.1 Cross-linking of the B-cell receptor (BCR) complex with the CR2 complex by means of immune complexes containing C3dg fragments. The CR2 complex consists of the CR2 (CD21) receptor itself, CD19, TAPA-1 (CD81) and probably other molecules. The BCR complex (Igα/Igβ proteins) and CD19 are associated with protein kinases that, upon clustering of both receptor complexes, phosphorylate (arrows) and thereby activate each other. This triggers signalling cascades leading to B-cell activation.

Other B-cell surface molecules involved in BCR signalling

Important components of the TCR complex are the co-receptors CD4 and CD8. In B cells, a similar auxiliary role in antigen recognition and signalling is played by the complement receptor type 2 (CR2) complex (see Chapter 12). This co-receptor becomes involved when the BCR recognizes an immune complex containing covalently attached C3d or C3dg complement fragments. These fragments are recognized by CR2 (CD21); simultaneous binding of an antigen epitope by the BCR then brings the BCR and CR2 complexes together (Fig. 17.1). The CD19 glycoprotein tightly linked to CR2 is associated with the protein tyrosine kinase Lyn and also with phosphatidylinositol 3-kinase (PI3-K) in its intracellular domain. The cross-linking of these two receptor complexes brings their associated kinases into close proximity and they activate each other by mutual phosphorylation. The engagement of BCR with CR2 decreases the threshold of B-cell stimulation 100-fold (i.e. 100-fold higher antigen concentrations are required if the CR2 complex does not participate). Another B-cell surface protein with a co-receptor function is the membrane lectin CD22 (see Chapter 9). Small amounts of this adhesion receptor appear to be associated with the BCR and rapidly become tyrosine phosphorylated upon BCR engagement. B-cell mutants lacking CD22 molecules cannot signal via the BCR. The phosphorylated intracellular tail of the CD22 molecule helps to recruit some of the intracellular signalling proteins (such as protein tyrosine kinases, PI3K and phospholipase Cγ) as well as negative regulators of activation (protein tyrosine phosphatases; see below) to the proximity of the BCR complex. Just as in the case of the TCR, the BCR-associated Src-family protein kinases are positively regulated by the transmembrane protein tyrosine phosphatase CD45, which counteracts the negative regulation by the kinase Csk (see Figs 10.29 & 16.5). The BCR and the CR2 complex are also associated with another B-cell surface protein, CD38. This membrane enzyme catalyses the conversion of nicotinamide adenine dinucleotide (NAD^+) into cyclic ADP-ribose (cADPR) and its subsequent hydrolysis to ADP-ribose (ADPR). Cyclic ADP-ribose is involved in the regulation of intracellular Ca^{2+} levels and thus may participate in some aspects of BCR-mediated signalling.

BCR signalling is also affected by the major histocompatibility complex (MHC) class II proteins. In resting B cells, the engagement of MHC class II molecules is accompanied by cyclic AMP generation and nuclear translocation of protein kinase C, which inhibits cell activation or even leads to apoptosis. In contrast, ligation of MHC class II molecules on B cells preactivated by cross-linking of the BCR in the presence of interleukin (IL)-4 has marked co-stimulatory effects.

Signalling pathways initiated by BCR engagement

Aggregation of BCR or co-aggregation with the CR2 complex leads to mutual phosphorylation of the associated Src-family protein kinases, which are thereby activated to phosphorylate other protein substrates such as CD79 and CD19. This enables the subsequent interactions of various SH2 domain-containing proteins (see Chapter 10) with these tyrosine-phosphorylated sequences. In this way, additional Src-family kinases, another tyrosine kinase Syk, linker proteins Grb and Shc and others may bind to the phosphorylated components of the activated receptor complex. New potential substrates are then brought into the proximity of the activated receptor-associated protein kinases, some of which are enzymes or regulatory proteins whose activities change upon phosphorylation. Intracellular signalling cascades are thus initiated that apparently resemble those described for the TCR (see Chapter 16). Just as in the case of the TCR, signalling through the BCR also leads to activation of the small G-protein Ras, which regulates the MAP-kinase pathway. Other signalling pathways triggered via both the BCR and TCR are based on phospholipase Cγ and the production of second messengers diacylglycerol (DAG) and inositol trisphosphate (IP_3), and on activation of PI3-K (see the general scheme in Fig. 10.27). All these pathways ultimately lead to the activation of transcription factors and the modification of cytoskeletal and other cytoplasmic proteins. The final outcome of these signals substantially depends on the interaction with signals provided simultaneously by other receptors (co-stimulatory receptors, cytokine receptors).

Negative signalling due to joint cross-linking of BCR and FcγRII

B-cell activation must be regulated to limit and ultimately terminate the production of specific antibodies. One such mechanism of negative feedback is based on joint cross-linking of the BCR with FcγRII (CD32). As soon as IgG antibodies are produced against an antigen, immune complexes are formed that can bind simultaneously to the BCR (via the antigen epitope) and to the Fc receptor (via the Fc parts of the antibodies present in the immune complex). This brings the BCR and Fc receptor complexes, including their associated intracellular components, into close proximity. The intracellular part of FcγRII is associated with a protein tyrosine phosphatase called SHP (SH2 domain-containing phosphatase) or PTP-1C (protein tyrosine phosphatase 1C), which dephosphorylates various cytoplasmic tyrosine-phosphorylated proteins and thus counteracts the action of BCR-associated protein tyrosine kinases and inhibits B-cell activation (Fig. 17.2). Thus, immune complexes can, depending on their composition, either enhance (Fig. 17.1) or suppress (Fig. 17.2) B-cell activation. The regulatory properties of immune complexes are dependent on the isotypes of the antibodies produced: isotypes other than IgG do not bind to FcγRII, whereas IgM activates the complement cascade and thereby tends to produce co-stimulatory immune complexes containing C3dg fragments.

The negative regulator of BCR signalling, PTP-1C, may also be brought into the proximity of the BCR complex by carrier molecules other than FcγRII. One of them is the membrane lectin CD22 whose intracellular domain

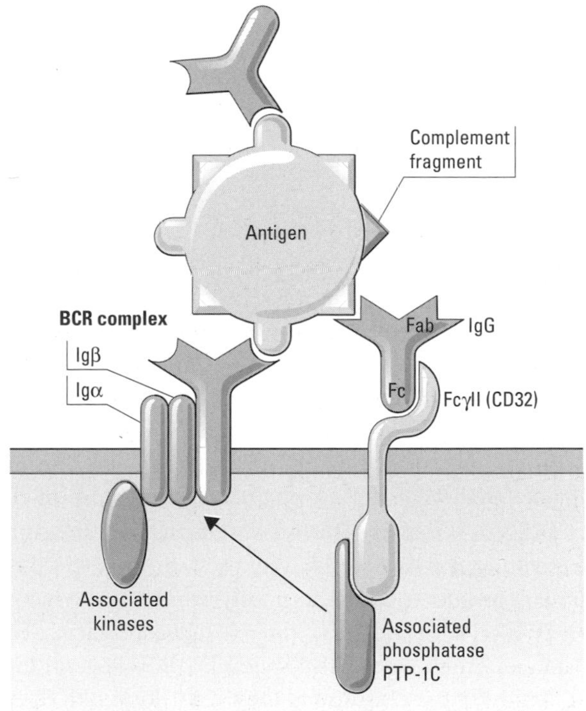

Figure 17.2 Inhibition of B-cell activation by cross-linking of the B-cell receptor (BCR) complex and FcγRII (CD32) on the B-cell surface by an immune complex containing IgG antibodies. The Fc receptor-associated protein tyrosine phosphatase PTP-1C dephosphorylates the phosphotyrosine residues on the BCR-associated protein tyrosine kinases (arrow) and in the cytoplasmic domains of the Igα and Igβ chains, which blocks further B-cell activation via the BCR complex.

associates with this regulatory phosphatase after BCR cross-linking. Small amounts of PTP-1C seem to be associated with the BCR in resting B cells and thus prevent the BCR from being triggered too easily. The physiological importance of PTP-1C phosphatase is revealed by the finding that mouse mutants with a defective *PTP-1C* gene have, among other immunological disorders, greatly increased numbers of B1 ($CD5^+$) lymphocytes, which are constitutively activated and produce large amounts of autoantibodies.

Thymus-independent responses

If neonatal removal of the thymus abolishes the ability of B lymphocytes to respond to an antigen, such responses are said to be *thymus dependent*; B-cell responses that occur even in the absence of the thymus are referred to as *thymus independent*. The latter are induced by a group of substances known as *thymus-independent* (*TI*) *antigens*. Immunologists use different criteria for including an antigen in this group: the ability of the antigen to induce an antibody response in congenitally athymic animals (for example *nude* mice, which are born without a thymus); the ability to stimulate antibody production in animals that have been thymectomized at birth and later lethally irradiated but treated by an inoculation of bone marrow cells; or the ability to produce antibodies in T-cell depleted cultures. These three criteria may not always define the same category of TI antigens.

There are two types of TI antigens, TI.1 and TI.2. *Type 1* (*TI.1*) *antigens* induce antibody response in the total absence of accessory cells such as macrophages and in newborn mice as well as in the immunodeficient strain of mice CBA/N. Antibodies induced by TI.1 antigens are predominantly of the IgM, IgG2 or IgG3 class. Examples of TI.1 antigens are trinitrophenylated lipopolysaccharide (TNP-LPS), trinitrophenylated *Brucella abortus* and trinitrophenylated Sephadex. A characteristic feature of these TI.1 antigens is that at high concentrations they are capable of activating B cells polyclonally: they can non-specifically stimulate proliferation and antibody production in many or even all B cells, regardless of their antigen specificity. These substances are therefore also called *B-cell mitogens*. However, at lower concentrations they only stimulate those B cells carrying the BCR that specifically recognizes them because these cells alone can concentrate sufficient amounts of such TI.1 antigens on their surface.

The *type 2* (*TI.2*) *antigens* are not entirely T-cell independent because extensive T-cell depletion significantly reduces or even abolishes the *in vitro* responses to these antigens. The addition of small numbers of T lymphocytes to the cultures restores the response. Macrophages are required for the responses to occur and newborn mice, as well as the immunodeficient CBA/N mice, fail to mount responses to these antigens. The predominant antibodies produced upon stimulation with TI.2 antigens are of the IgM or IgG3 class. The antigens are normally large, polymeric molecules with repeating epitopes. Many of the antigens are relatively resistant to degradation and hence persist in the body for a prolonged time. Responses to TI.2 antigens *in vitro* are weaker than the responses to thymus-dependent antigens and they peak a day or two earlier (Fig. 17.3). TI.2 antigens appear to stimulate B lymphocytes by extensive cross-linking of their BCRs, which may provide a qualitatively different signal compensating in some way for the lack of co-stimulatory signals from T_H cells. TI.2 antigens, in contrast to TI.1, stimulate mature B cells and inactivate immature B cells. Examples of TI.2 antigens include type III pneumococcal polysaccharide, polyvinylpyrrolidone (PVP), polyriboinosinic-polyribocytidylic acid, dextran (poly-D-glucose), levan (poly-D-fructose), poly-D-amino acids, polymeric bacterial flagellin (monomeric flagellin is a T-dependent antigen; Fig. 17.4) and lipopolysaccharide. B-cell responses to the TI.2 antigen are dependent on cytokines provided by either T cells or NK cells. The most powerful cytokine combinations supporting TI.2 responses are IL-2 + interferon-γ (IFN-γ) or IL-2 + IL-3 + GM-CSF (granulocyte-monocyte colony stimulating factor). The basic difference between TI.2 responses and T-dependent B-cell responses is that the former do not require direct T_H cell–B cell contact but merely the soluble cytokines, which may be provided in part by NK cells. NK cells may be stimulated to cytokine secretion by some of the TI.2 polysaccharide antigens via their multiple surface lectins. The ability of B cells (mainly B1 cells distinguished by the expression of the surface receptor

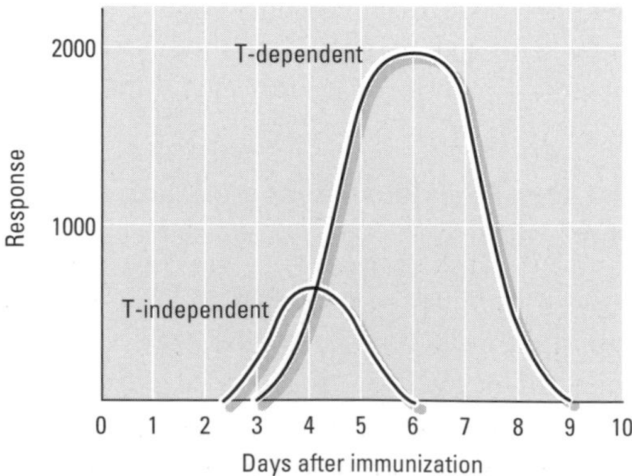

Figure 17.3 Difference in the primary B-cell response to T-dependent and T-independent antigens. The response can be measured, for example, in terms of the number of antibody-producing B cells per 10^6 cells.

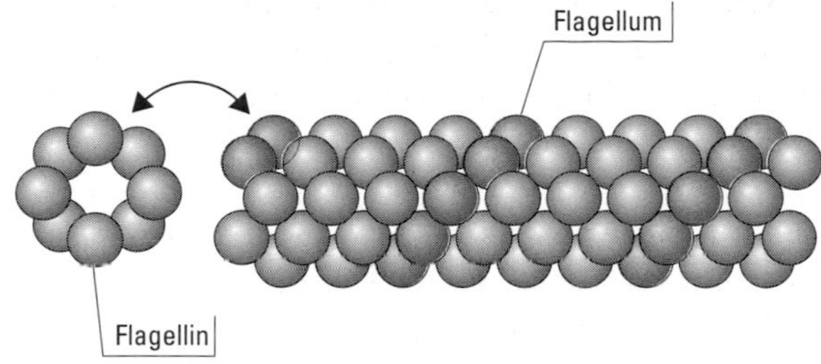

Figure 17.4 An example of a T-independent (TI.2) antigen: *Salmonella* flagellin. Monomeric flagellin is a protein that assembles into large fibrillar structures, the bacterial flagella. Polymeric flagellin is a T-independent antigen, while monomeric flagellin is a T-dependent antigen.

CD5; see Chapter 5) to respond to TI.2 antigens makes possible the production of antibodies to antigens such as bacterial surface polysaccharides, which do not evoke T-cell help because their fragments do not bind to MHC molecules. Most bacterial, viral and fungal pathogens have antigens with TI.2 characteristics on their surface. Humoral responses against them represent a rapidly activated first line of defence, but they produce little or no memory. For unknown reasons, the immature immune system of neonates is unable to mount TI.2 responses and has to rely in this respect on maternal antibodies obtained transplacentally or from milk (see Chapter 18). TI antigens are a small minority in the antigenic universe; most antigens are T-cell dependent, which means that they are only able to stimulate B cells with the help of T_H lymphocytes.

T-cell dependent responses

Primary antibody response

During an infection, the pathogen is captured by tissue dendritic cells, ingested and digested, and delivered to the nearest lymph node. There the dendritic cells express large numbers of MHC class II (but also class I) molecules, some of which are loaded with peptide fragments derived from the pathogen. Alternatively, the pathogen or its fragments can be phagocytosed by macrophages in the lymphoid organs, its peptides loaded on to MHC class II molecules and the molecules expressed on the cell surface. The complexes on the surface of the professional antigen-presenting cell (APC) can be recognized by T_H precursors, which are thereby stimulated to proliferate and develop into mature effector T_H cells ready to help the B cells (see Chapter 16, Fig. 16.7).

B cells receive the first essential signal when their BCRs bind to an antigenic molecule of the pathogen. This can happen anywhere in the periphery, in the lymph nodes or in other secondary lymphoid organs, to which antigens are being continuously delivered and captured mainly in the form of immune complexes. The B cell internalizes the antigen, cleaves it into peptidic fragments and displays some of them on its surface in association with MHC class II proteins. These events take place when the antigen is small enough to be engulfed by receptor-mediated endocytosis, but not when the antigen is part of a large particle such as a whole microorganism. In any case, the B cell must now meet the right T_H cell, a meeting that takes place most efficiently in the specialized microenvironment of the lymphoid tissue, i.e. the T-cell areas of lymphoid tissues (lymph nodes, spleen, gut-associated lymphoid tissue). The T cells are either already in a mature state induced by professional APCs or they are T_H precursors stimulated to proliferation and maturation by contact with the B cell acting as an APC. A naive B cell that has received only the first signal by recognition of an antigen via the BCR is not an efficient APC. The co-stimulatory molecules CD80 and CD86 are absent on its surface and the B cell therefore cannot stimulate the precursors of T_H cells. On the other hand, B cells activated by an antigen plus another stimulus, such as bacterial lipopolysaccharide, or B cells fully activated by an antigen and T_H cells express the CD80 and CD86 co-stimulatory ligands and therefore function as professional APCs.

The T_H cell physically contacts the B cell sensitized by initial recognition of the antigen via the BCR. Several adhesion and signalling molecules participate in this contact (see Fig. 16.6). Thus, the TCR of the T_H lymphocyte binds to the peptide–MHC class II molecule assembly, the T-cell adhesion receptor CD2 binds to its ligand LFA-3 (CD58) and another adhesion receptor, LFA-1 (present on both the T and B cell), binds to its broadly expressed ligands (ICAM-1, ICAM-2, ICAM-3). These interactions provide signals to both partners: they instruct the T_H cell to secrete stimulatory cytokines and they contribute to stimulation of the B cell. Two types of signals from T_H cells are required by the B cell: first, those mediated by soluble cytokines such as IL-4, IL-5 and IL-6 secreted by the T_H cell; second, the signal provided by CD40L (CD40 ligand), the surface molecule (membrane cytokine) of activated T_H cells, which binds to the B-cell surface receptor CD40.[1] The soluble cytokines secreted by T_H cells also act via specific receptors on the B-

[1] The function of the CD40 receptor is not limited to B cells. It is present also on monocytes, follicular dendritic cells, some epithelial cells and carcinomas. The CD40–CD40L interaction seems to provide signals not only to the cells carrying CD40 receptors (mainly B cells) but also to activated T cells. CD40L-mediated signals contribute to the process of T-cell activation and may also play a role in thymic maturation.

cell surface (see Chapter 10). They are secreted by T_H cells in a highly oriented way within the area of close contact between the T_H cell and the B cell. B cells stimulated by contact with the antigen and with the T_H cell proliferate and most of them differentiate into plasma cells secreting large amounts of mostly IgM antibodies of relatively low affinity. Some of these activated B cells, however, enter lymphoid follicles in the cortical area of lymph nodes where they initiate a *germinal centre reaction*. The reaction provides the basis of the secondary antibody response producing a new wave of antibodies with increased affinity for the antigen and of a different isotype.

Germinal centre reaction, secondary antibody responses, affinity maturation and class switching

Activated B cells that crossed the T-cell zone and entered the primary follicles in the cortical region of lymph nodes give rise to *germinal centres*. These are foci for intense B-cell proliferation, extensive mutations of immunoglobulin genes and selection of variants carrying high-affinity BCRs — the *centrocytes*. This process of *affinity maturation* is dependent on the contact of activated B cells with T_H cells that have arisen during the first phase of antibody response and with a dense network of *follicular dendritic cells* (FDC; see Chapter 4), which concentrate and store immune complexes on their surfaces for a long time. Here, the antigen molecules can be recognized by the BCRs of mutated centrocytes. Some of the antigen can be taken up by the activated B cells and processed into peptides that are exhibited on the surface for recognition by T_H cells. As the amount of antigen is limited, only mutants possessing BCRs with the highest affinity will bind it for a sufficiently long time to receive further positive signals that save them from death. The variants with low-affinity BCRs die by apoptosis in the germinal centre. As the antibody response proceeds, larger and larger amounts of secreted antibodies accumulate in the centre, which compete for binding the antigen. Thus the selection pressure regulating the quality (high affinity) of the BCR on B cells undergoing the process of affinity maturation becomes ever stronger. This process leads ultimately to the selection of B-cell variants carrying high-affinity BCRs and capable of secreting high-affinity antibodies.

In addition to affinity maturation, *isotype switching* (rearrangement of gene segments coding for the constant parts of the immunoglobulin heavy chain) also occurs during this phase of B-cell maturation (see Chapter 8). Isotype switching is regulated primarily by soluble cytokines: in mouse B cells, IL-4 and IL-13 mainly induce the switch to IgG1 and IgE, while transforming growth factor (TGF)-β induces the switch to IgA and IgG2b, and IFN-γ to IgG3 and IgG2a. Therefore, the type of T_H cell providing the help (and the cytokine environment in general) determines which of the isotypes will prevail. An essential signal for germinal centre formation, affinity maturation and isotype switching is provided by the T_H cell via the B-cell receptor CD40. Mutations causing defects in the CD40 receptor or in its ligand CD40L lead to immunodeficiencies characterized by the lack of germinal centres and the production of large amounts of relatively low-affinity IgM antibodies but very few high-affinity antibodies of other isotypes. The affected individuals also completely lack B-cell memory (see Chapter 26).

B cells that survived the selection in the germinal centres are destined to become either short-lived plasma cells or long-lived memory cells. Plasma cells are highly specialized, terminally differentiated cells that secrete soluble immunoglobulins at a high rate and die after a few days (see Chapter 5). Most of the plasma cells arising in the germinal centres migrate to the bone marrow and the antibodies they produce appear in the blood and lymph.

B lymphocytes selected in the germinal centre to become memory cells initiate, upon subsequent encounter with the same antigen, a *secondary response*. It is much quicker and more efficient than the primary response because it relies on a pool of high-affinity B cells that do not have to go through the lengthy process of affinity maturation (which nevertheless also occurs during the secondary response and may lead to further improvement of the antibodies produced). The presence of memory T_H cells, which can be rapidly activated by APCs expressing antigen fragments, further accelerates the response. The major factor determining whether a B cell will become a plasma cell or a memory cell is probably the duration of B-cell stimulation via the CD40 receptor: prolonged engagement of this receptor with its ligand CD40L induces memory-cell development.

Specific T_H cell–B cell interactions vs. bystander help

So far we have assumed that all T_H cell–B cell interactions during the development of a humoral response are *specific*; in other words, the T_H cell recognizes the B cell that should receive help by binding the specific peptide–MHC class II molecule assembly on its surface. However, *in vitro* experiments indicate that mature T_H cells can also provide help, via both cell-to-cell contact and oriented cytokine secretion, to *bystander B cells* primed by recognition of unrelated antigens (Fig. 17.5). At present, the significance of bystander help under physiological conditions is not known. Its role may be important, however, considering how densely packed the cells are in lymphoid organs.

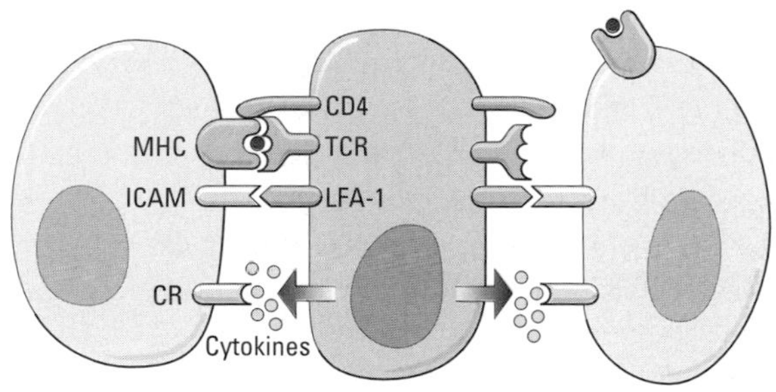

Figure 17.5 Specific and bystander stimulation of B cells by helper T (T_H) cells. Specific stimulation of a B cell (left) is provided by a T_H cell that recognizes a peptide–MHC protein assembly on the B-cell surface and secretes cytokines binding to cytokine receptors (CR) on the B-cell surface. The B cell on the right does not express a ligand on its surface (peptide–MHC protein assembly) recognizable by the T-cell receptor (TCR) of the particular T_H cell. The T_H cell and the bystander B cell (which may have received the first signal through its B-cell receptor by recognition of an unrelated antigen) interact via adhesion molecules (e.g. LFA-1–ICAM-1). For the sake of simplicity, other relevant molecules (BCR, CD40, CD40L) are not shown. Red arrows indicate the secretion of cytokines.

Haptens, carriers and T cell–B cell collaboration

It may be useful at this point to remind ourselves of some relevant classical immunological concepts formulated long before the molecular mechanisms of T cell–B cell collaboration were discovered. *Haptens*, it will be recalled, are small molecules that induce antibody formation only when attached to a large protein *carrier*. To study haptens and carriers, immunologists construct chimeric molecules in which a chemical group such as trinitrophenyl (TNP), dinitrophenyl (DNP), or 4-hydroxy-3-iodo-5-nitrophenyl acetic acid (NIP) is chemically attached to a natural protein such as bovine serum albumin (BSA), bovine gamma globulin (BGG) or ovalbumin (OA). The chemical group represents the hapten and the large protein the carrier. In more natural situations, the hapten is a small part of a larger molecule, e.g. the side-chain of an amino acid residue in a polypeptide, a monosaccharide or disaccharide in a complex carbohydrate or a nucleotide in a nucleic acid; the carrier is always a stretch of amino acid residues in a protein. The artificial attachment of a hapten to a protein carrier is merely a convenient way of distinguishing the two. An animal immunized against the hapten H1 attached to the carrier C1 can be restimulated with either H1–C2 or H2–C1 and the anti-hapten can thus be separated from the anti-carrier response. Obviously, any response in an animal immunized against H1–C1 and then restimulated with H1–C2 must be hapten specific, whereas the response after restimulation with H2–C1 must be carrier specific. In carrying out such experiments, immunologists noted that an augmented antibody response to the second injection of a hapten occurred only when the hapten was presented on the same carrier in both the first and second injections. In other words, an animal immunized with H1–C1 produced high levels of H1-specific antibody only when immunized a second time with H1–C1; neither H1–C2, nor C1 alone sufficed (Fig. 17.6). This phenomenon is referred to as the *carrier effect*.

Further analysis of the carrier effect revealed that during the immune response, the hapten and carrier are recognized by different cells: the hapten by the B lymphocyte and the carrier by the T lymphocyte. This fact can be verified by immunizing one animal against H1–C1 and another against C2. If B cells from the first animal are then mixed with T cells from the second, and the mixture is restimulated with H1–C2, an augmented antibody response against H1 will occur (Fig. 17.7). (The cells must be injected into a recipient

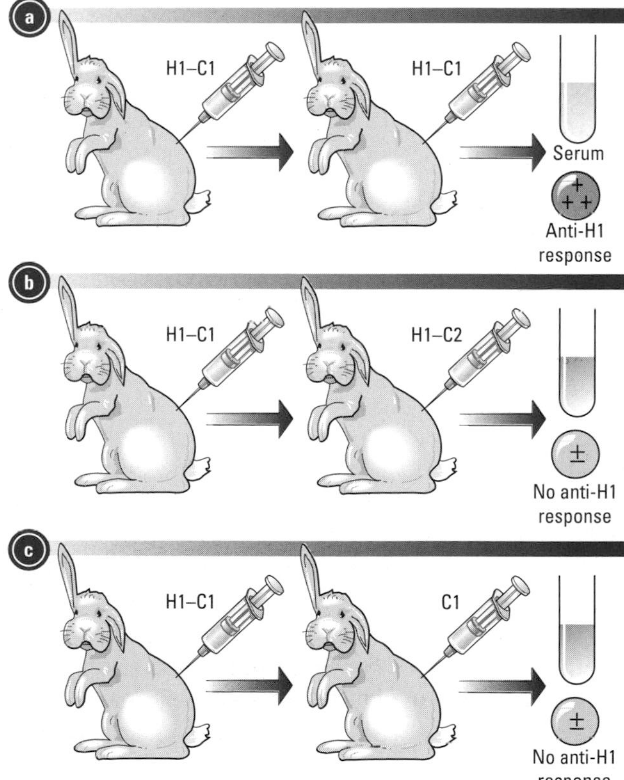

Figure 17.6 Experiment demonstrating the carrier effect. (a) A rabbit immunized against the hapten H1–carrier C1 complex and then rechallenged with the same complex produces a high titre of H1-specific antibodies. (b) A rabbit immunized against H1 on one carrier and rechallenged with H1 on another carrier does not give a secondary anti-H1 response; (c) neither does a rabbit immunized against H1–C1 and rechallenged with the carrier alone.

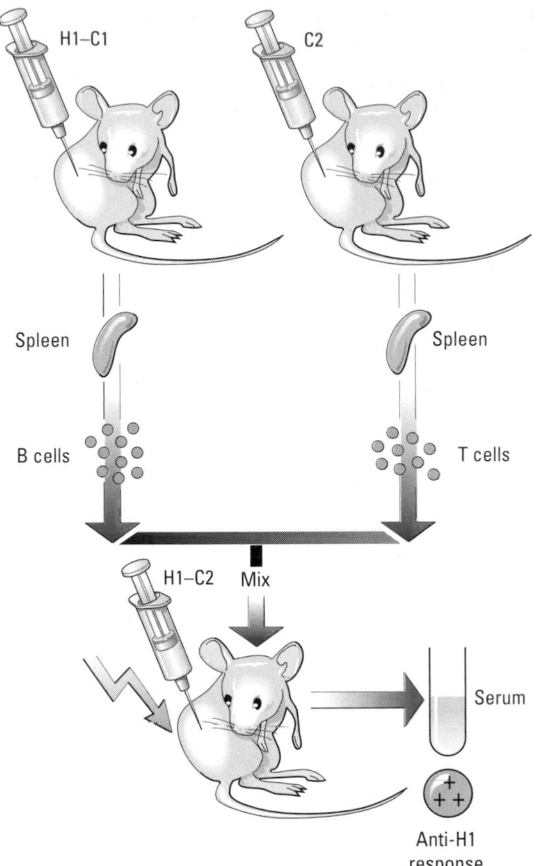

Figure 17.7 Experiment demonstrating that B cells from a mouse immunized against hapten H1 on carrier C2 collaborate with T cells from a mouse immunized against carrier C2, provided that the cell mixture is rechallenged with H1 coupled to C2. The mixture was transferred into a new recipient that was irradiated ( ) to make space for the new cells. H1-specific antibodies were then measured in the serum of this recipient.

genetically identical with the donor and the recipient must be irradiated to kill its own lymphocytes. The inoculation of immune cells into a new recipient is referred to as *adoptive transfer*.) The reciprocal experiment does not function: B lymphocytes from an animal immunized against C2 and mixed with T cells from an animal immunized against H1–C1 do not produce a high level of H1-specific antibodies when restimulated with H1–C2. The experiment also reveals that B lymphocytes *collaborate* with T lymphocytes in producing antibodies to a particular antigen. The B cells produce the antibody, but to do so T_H cells are necessary to activate them and to supply them with growth and differentiation factors. Collaboration involves the recognition of the hapten by B lymphocytes and the recognition of the carrier by T lymphocytes. In the artificial situation of the experiment, the hapten and carrier differ in size, if nothing else; in natural situations, this difference may be non-existent. As discussed in Chapter 14, X-ray crystallographic studies reveal that combining sites of antibodies that recognize proteins such as lysozyme interact with a substantial area of the protein surface. Here the 'hapten' and the 'carrier' may not differ to any great extent from each other in size.

The experiment just discussed could be extended: instead of restimulating the mixture of T and B lymphocytes with the H1–C2 complex, restimulation with a mixture of free H1 and free C2 or a mixture of H1–C1 and C2 could be attempted. Failure to obtain an augmented anti-H1 response in such an experiment indicates that the hapten recognized by the B cells and the carrier recognized by the T cells must be physically linked; they must be part of the same molecule or at least the same cell. The reason for this becomes clear when we remind ourselves of the way in which collaboration between the two cells is achieved (see Fig. 16.2). A B cell carrying the BCR capable of hapten recognition binds the hapten–carrier conjugate, endocytoses it and cleaves the carrier into peptides, some of which bind to MHC class II molecules. These complexes reappear on the cell's surface, where they are recognized by T_H cells, which then provide the necessary help to the B cell. Help is most efficient when the B and T_H cells are in close contact with each other and thus can interact via their peptide–MHC molecules and TCRs. This scenario remains basically unchanged even if the primary stimulation of the specific T_H clone occurs with a professional APC other than the B cell; after some delay the mature T_H cell finds a B cell possessing the specific peptide originating from the carrier on its surface.

The collaboration mechanisms ensure that the same B cell can receive help from many T_H cells of different specificity, recognizing different antigenic peptides. The antigen recognized by the B cell through a relatively simple epitope may be quite complex. It may be composed of several non-covalently associated components of different nature (proteins, complex carbohydrates, lipids, nucleic acids), some of which can be recognized by BCRs but which do not produce peptide fragments recognizable by T_H cells. This *intermolecular help* enables efficient humoral responses to non-protein antigens. Just as a single B cell can receive help from many different T_H cells, the reverse is also true: the same T_H cell can provide help to many B cells of different specificity as long as they express the 'right' peptide–MHC class II molecule assemblies on their surface.

Kinetics of antibody production

The antibodies produced by plasma cells are collected by

the lymph and blood and then circulate through the body, the concentration of the antibody increasing with time. Immunologists measure this increase by sampling the blood and testing the serum for reactivity with the immunizing antigen. They refer to a serum that shows antibody reactivity as *antiserum*. The first exposure of an individual to an antigen, referred to as *priming*, results in the *primary response*; the second exposure, sometimes called *boosting* or *rechallenging*, leads to the *anamnestic* or *secondary response* (Greek *anamnesis*, recollection); subsequent responses are tertiary, quaternary and so forth. The kinetics of the primary and secondary responses differ from each other.

Primary response

By plotting the antibody concentration against the time following the first antigen exposure, one obtains a curve resembling that of bacterial growth. The curve can be divided into four (not always easily discernible) phases known by names originally used by bacteriologists (Fig. 17.8). The *lag (latent) phase* is the period between antigen administration and the appearance of detectable serum antibody. Its length is influenced by the antigen, the route of injection, the type of adjuvant used and the recipient. It can be as short as 3 hours and as long as several weeks. The *log (logarithmic, exponential growth) phase* is the period during which antibody concentration increases at an exponential rate (the curve forms a straight line in this region when the antibody concentration is plotted on a logarithmic scale). The *doubling time*, the time necessary for a twofold increase in antibody concentration, determines the slope of the curve; it depends on the antigen dose and the type of antigen injected, as well as many other factors. The *steady-state (plateau) phase* is the period in which no net increase or decrease in serum antibody level can be observed. The time required to reach it, its height and its length vary, depending again on the antigen used. The phase may be missing in some responses, while in others it may last for several weeks. The *decline (decreasing) phase* covers the time in which the immunoglobulin degradation rate begins to prevail over the synthetic rate and the serum antibody concentration progressively drops. The length of this phase, once again depending on the circumstances, may range from a few days to several weeks.

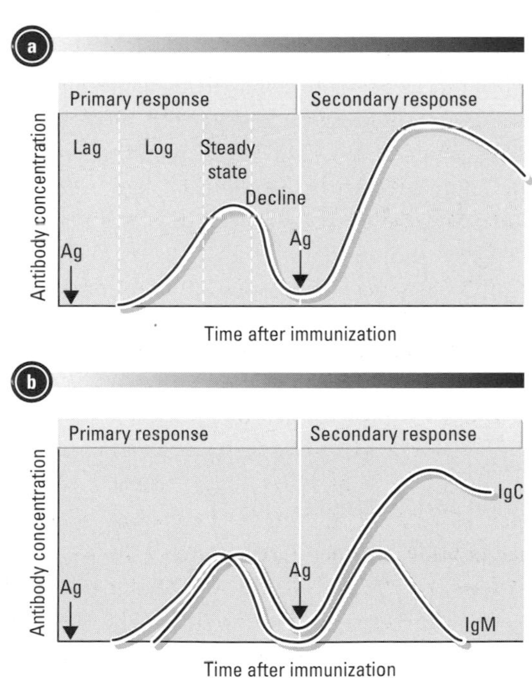

Figure 17.8 Kinetics of antibody production during primary and secondary B-cell response. (a) Total antibody. (b) IgM and IgG antibody. Ag, antigen. Time and concentration units are left unspecified to indicate the variability encountered with different antigens. (Modified from Klein, J. (1982) *Immunology: The Science of Self–Nonself Discrimination*. John Wiley & Sons, New York.)

Secondary response

The second exposure to antigen elicits a reaction that differs from the primary response in several aspects (see Fig. 17.8): it has a shorter lag phase (about half that of the primary response); more rapid increase in antibody concentration (the increase is still exponential but the curve is steeper); earlier attainment, greater height and greater length of the steady-state phases; longer persistence of the decline phase (longer persistence of antibody synthesis); lower antigen dose eliciting a detectable response; prevalence of IgG over IgM response; and higher affinity as well as higher homogeneity of antibody affinity. The magnitude of the secondary response depends on the interval between the two injections. The response is low when this interval is short (the still-present antibody binds with the antigen and the resulting antigen–antibody complexes are rapidly cleared) or long (although the memory cells are long-lived, they are not immortal and the memory eventually fades away).

The capacity for a secondary response may persist for many months or years, long after the last of the antibodies in the blood has vanished. It is this capacity that provides animals with long-lasting protection against an infection once withstood. There is also a difference between primary and secondary response in the requirement for concomitant administration of an adjuvant: a significant primary response to many protein antigens can be induced only when the antigen is injected in an emulsified form in an adjuvant, while boosting can be achieved with aqueous antigen solution. Furthermore, primed cells respond to lower antigen concentrations more strongly than unprimed cells, suggesting that memory B-cells have greater affinity.

Changes in immunoglobulin class

A simple test for determining the immunoglobulin class during antibody response involves the treatment of a serum with reducing agents such as 2-mercaptoethanol. Pentameric IgM antibodies are much more efficient than IgG in agglutinating cells or mediating cell lysis by complement, but when dissociated by 2-mercaptoethanol into their 7S subunits they have roughly the same activity as IgG antibodies. Therefore, when an antiserum containing predominantly IgM antibodies is treated with 2-mercaptoethanol, its activity is greatly reduced; in contrast, treatment of IgG-dominated antiserum has little effect on the reactivity of the antiserum.

IgM and IgG are usually produced during both the primary and secondary responses, but IgG production in the primary response starts later than IgM production and the secondary response is dominated by IgG production (see Fig. 17.8b). In both responses, the concentration of IgM in the serum declines rapidly and the antibody ceases to be detectable after 1 or 2 weeks; IgG antibodies, on the other hand, persist in the serum for a long time. As mentioned earlier, however, the so-called TI antigens often stimulate predominantly or exclusively IgM responses.

The reason why IgM is detected earlier than IgG in the primary response is that secretion of IgM starts earlier than secretion of IgG because activated IgM-producing cells later switch to IgG production (see Chapter 8).

B-cell memory

B cells, like T cells, possess memory. In one experiment, for example, rabbits were immunized against DNP–BGG and rechallenged 1 year later. They responded in a characteristic secondary fashion, indicating that in this instance the memory was stored in the DNP (hapten)-recognizing B cells. However, since the secondary response largely affects IgG antibodies and IgG production is T-cell dependent, the secondary antibody response usually involves both memory B and memory T cells.

It is not quite clear what mechanisms maintain memory B cells. Is the persistence of minute amounts of the antigen necessary to constantly restimulate them? Or are some memory cells so long-lived that they do not need antigen restimulation? Is weak restimulation of memory cells by partially cross-reactive antigens (foreign or autoantigens) the most important factor? These questions have still to be answered, although the last possibility appears to be most likely at present.

A discussion of B-cell memory would be incomplete without mentioning the so-called *original antigenic sin*. Adult humans vaccinated against an influenza virus strain produce antibodies of high titre against antigenic determinants that are common to those present in the virus strain encountered during childhood but not against other antigenic determinants that are unique for the new strain. It is as if humans live with an immunological memory of experiences acquired in the age of innocence, just as humankind is supposed to live under the burden of Adam's original sin. This original antigenic sin has been reproduced in laboratory animals and demonstrated to occur with several different antigens. In influenza research, however, original antigenic sin has been used to define serotypes of extinct viruses from past epidemics.

The phenomenon can be explained by assuming that memory cells elicited by the original antigen persist in the body and are restimulated by the new antigen, which cross-reacts with the original one. *Cross-stimulation* then results in augmented production of antibodies specific for the original antigen. The production of antibodies against the novel determinants appears to be actively suppressed in some way, as if at the expense of enhanced production of antibodies against the previously experienced determinants. The suppression is caused by the presence of small amounts of antibodies against the 'old' determinants, which form immune complexes with the antigen. The immune complexes act differently on memory B cells and naive B cells: while co-cross-linking of the BCR with FcγRII on the surface of a naive B cell provides an inhibitory signal preventing the initiation of B-cell activation, memory B cells are not affected by such a negative signal (see Fig. 17.2).

B-cell repertoire

Formation and dynamics

The assembly of all B-lymphocyte clones expressing different BCRs is the *B-cell repertoire*. The main difference between B- and T-cell repertoires is that the former is less stable and more dynamic than the latter. In the T-cell compartment, the output of lymphocytes from the thymus gradually declines in an adult individual, and ultimately may stop altogether. In the B-cell compartment, new lymphocytes are continuously being generated from stem cells in the bone marrow and released into the periphery at a steady rate. The B-cell repertoire, like the T-cell repertoire, is primarily formed by the mechanisms responsible for creating antigen-receptor variability: *V(D)J* rearrangements, junctional diversification and combinatorial heavy–light chain pairing (see Chapter 8). The repertoire in both the T- and B-cell compartment is then shaped by elimination of autoreactive cells. In the case of B cells, an additional major factor continuously shaping the repertoire is the selection of high-affinity variants in the germinal centre reaction.

Early steps of B-cell repertoire formation take place in the bone marrow. There the developing B cells go through several checkpoints at which they have to demonstrate that productive rearrangement of their immunoglobulin genes has taken place (see Chapter 8). Immature B cells that encountered an autoantigen in the bone marrow are arrested in their development and make a final attempt to avoid elimination by reactivating the recombination machinery and changing their BCR specificity (receptor editing). It is estimated that around 60–70% of immature B cells die in the bone marrow as a result of apoptosis (see Chapter 8). An adult mouse produces about 10^7 mature B cells daily, which are exported from the bone marrow to the periphery. Most of these young B cells are captured in the spleen within 30 min, primarily in the T-cell zones of the white pulp and in the red pulp. A large majority of the cells die within a few days by apoptosis, probably as a result of encounter with an autoantigen. These cells represent the so-called *short-lived (transient) pool of B cells*. A minority of about 5% of B cells that do not carry potentially autoreactive BCRs enter primary follicles and receive unidentified rescue signals that save them from death. The B cells that previously recognized an autoantigen are somehow prevented from entering primary follicles and receiving the survival impulse. The rescued B cells thus comprise the majority of the *stable pool of B lymphocytes* with a lifespan of 3 weeks to a few months. During this time, they constantly recirculate, dividing their time between blood (lymphatic) circulation, lymphoid follicles and T-cell zones of secondary lymphoid organs. In the latter, the recirculating follicular B cells wait for a possible encounter with the antigen and with appropriate T_H cells. The other major part of the stable pool are *non-recirculating B cells of the marginal zones*, which are recruited from the recirculating follicular B-cell pool. The stable pool of B cells consists mainly of resting (G_0 stage) virgin B cells and a minority of resting memory B cells. For unexplained reasons, about once every second a B cell in the stable pool is activated, proliferates and forms a small clone of immunoglobulin-secreting cells that then rapidly decay. About 10^5 of these incipient clones arise every day and contribute a lion's share to the pool of approximately 10^6 immunoglobulin-secreting cells present in an adult mouse.

The B cells that encounter antigen and receive all the necessary signals proliferate to yield a clone of short-lived plasma cells and small numbers of long-lived memory cells that join the stable pool. As a result of the germinal centre reaction, new clones of B cells carrying mutant BCRs appear and the system gradually becomes enriched in the clones producing antibodies of higher affinity toward the antigen.

An adult mouse has approximately 3×10^8 small lymphocytes (excluding those in the thymus and bone marrow), of which approximately 2×10^8 are T lymphocytes and 10^8 are B lymphocytes. If we disregard the division into transient and stable pools, we can estimate the maximum number of different B-cell clones in the mouse B-cell repertoire to be 10^8, in which case each clone would consist of a single cell. If there were 10 cells per clone, the maximum size of the B-cell repertoire would be 10^7 different clones, which is approximately the number of possible combinations of genetic elements from which the BCR is assembled. According to these calculations approximately 1 in 500 B cells should express a particular V_H gene, which has indeed proved to be the case. There are, however, different means of repertoire diversification other than combinatorial (junctional diversification, somatic mutations) and, furthermore, many of the B-cell clones consist of more than 10 cells. Also, individual mice differ in the germ-line genes they carry. All these facts indicate that the B-cell repertoire is probably not the same in all mice at any time. It may fluctuate as a result of the dynamics of B-cell generation, differential exposure to environmental antigens, the process of somatic diversification or even the genetic make-up of the individual. This last effect may be responsible for genetic differences between individuals in their capacity to mount certain B-cell responses. In general, however, these differences are much less pronounced than those found in T-cell responses. The fluctuations of the B-cell repertoire are largely stochastic and they probably do not matter much because the response is degenerate, so that even when certain *V(D)J* combinations are transiently missing from the repertoire, there is enough cross-reactivity among the BCRs for other *V(D)J* combinations to substitute for them. In the long run, however, there is probably selection during the evolution of a species for certain *V*, *D* and *J* gene segments that provide the best protection against the prevailing parasites.

Clonal selection from preimmune repertoire

When an antigen enters the immune system, it binds the BCR of certain B-cell clones. The binding occurs with different affinities depending on the degree of complementarity between the epitopes and the combining sites, and when it reaches a certain level it leads to the stimulation of B lymphocytes. The number of B-cell clones to which an antigen binds initially has not been determined. There are, however, instances in which the binding of a particular antigen by a B cell is determined by V_H and V_κ genes alone, while the contribution of the *D* and *J* segments to the binding is minimal. In such situations it is conceivable that the antigen binds initially to more than 100 B-cell clones (4 $J_H \times 11\ D \times 4\ J_\kappa$); theoretically the number would increase by two orders of magnitude if it were only a particular V_H needed for the binding, as has been suggested for some simple antigens.

To measure the number of B-lymphocyte clones that are actually *stimulated*, immunologists obtain B cells from immunized animals at a particular time after antigen inoculation, fuse them with plasma-cell tumours and determine which immunoglobulin gene segments in the resulting hybridomas have been assembled for antibody production. Using this approach, the B-cell response to haptens such as 2-phenyl-5-oxazolone, 4-hydroxy-3-nitrophenylacetyl, *p*-azophenylarsonate and phosphorylcholine, as well as to complex antigens such as influenza virus haemagglutinin, have been studied. We illustrate the conclusions drawn from these studies using the example of the response to oxazolone (Fig. 17.9).

Seven days after the single injection of the antigen, eight different types of oxazolone-specific antibodies were detected by one group of investigators and 14 types by another, giving a total of 20 antibody types because two types were found in both studies. Slightly less than one-half of these antibodies were of the IgM class; the rest were of the IgG1 subclass, with one exception that was of the IgG2a subclass. All of the antibodies had the κ light chain. Since the constant region does not contribute to the specificity of the antibody, isotypic differences among the antibodies can be ignored and so we end up with 16 different antibodies derived from seven different V_H genes and five different germ-line V_κ genes. Certain V_H and V_κ genes are clearly preferred over other genes in the generation of oxazolone-specific antibodies: $V_H Ox1$ from the V_H2 family has been used by some 70% of hybridomas tested and an additional 10% of hybridomas have used a gene closely related to, but nevertheless different from, *Ox1*. Hence, altogether some 80% of the B cells that produce oxazolone-specific antibodies use the same or related V_H genes. Similarly, some 76% of the B lymphocytes use the same or related $V_\kappa Ox$ gene. At day 7 therefore most of the antibody-secreting cells express a combination of heavy and light chains encoded in

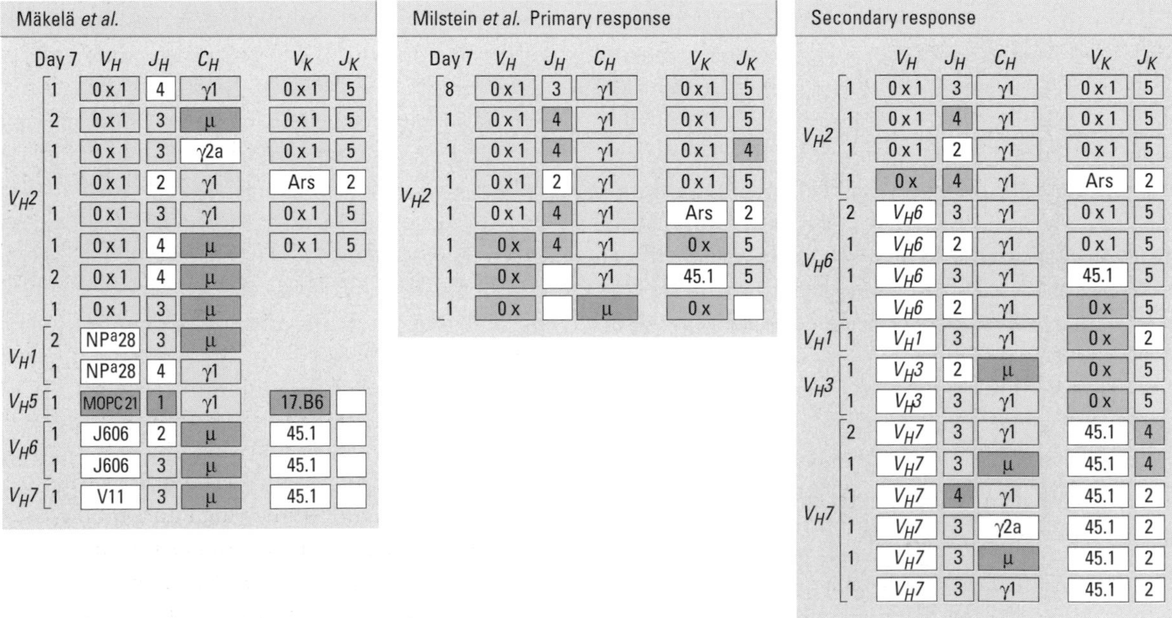

Figure 17.9 Repertoire of B-cell response to a hapten. In these two experiments, one carried out by Cesar Milstein and his colleagues and the other by Oli Mäkelä and his associates, mice were first immunized against oxazolone. Seven days after immunization, B cells producing oxazolone-specific antibodies were immortalized (by fusing them with myeloma cells) and the gene segments contributing to the construction of these antibodies were subsequently identified by sequencing. In a similar manner, Milstein and his colleagues also analysed the B cells stimulated after a secondary immunization. Each group of rectangles indicates the identity of the gene segments (V_H and V_L) for each type of antibody found. The number preceding the group is the number of times a given type occurred in the set. The brackets indicate the gene families to which individual types belong. (Based on Berek, C. & Milstein, C. (1987) *Immunological Reviews*, **96**, 23.)

a single pair of germ-line genes, $V_H Ox1$ and $V_\kappa Ox1$. These genes have combined with different *D* and *J* segments, although certain restrictions on the usage of these segments seem to exist. For example, the V_HOx1 polypeptide is consistently joined to a D segment that is three amino acid residues in length, and to a J_H segment that is shorter than its germ-line counterpart. In the light chains there is a strong preference for the use of $J_\kappa 5$ and an absolute conservation of a leucine residue at position 96, where sequence variation is often introduced during *V–J* recombination. Whenever genes other than $V_H Ox1$ are used, the overall length of the V_H chain is always conserved, even when the genes originate from different V_H families.

The repeated occurrence of hybridomas with an identical $V_H D J_H$ and $V_\kappa J_\kappa$ combination could indicate either that the clone expressing this combination was of a much larger size in the preimmune repertoire than other clones or that it was preferentially expanded by the antigen after immunization. In the absence of any knowledge concerning the preimmune repertoire, it is difficult to decide between these two possibilities; they may, in fact, both apply. However, the existence of the repeats does indicate that either not all B-cell clones capable of binding the antigen are stimulated or, if they are stimulated, not all are expanded to a detectable level. In the initial phase of the response, antigen may bind to a large number of B-cell clones and even stimulate many of them, but competition among the clones then results in the preferential expansion of only some of them. The advantages that one clone might have over the rest are a larger initial size and a higher binding affinity for a given antigen. Although the initial response is heterogeneous, it does not exhaust the entire potential of the B-cell repertoire for heterogeneity. Certain clones may dominate the response because of a combination of genetic and environmental factors. The dominance provides an explanation for the relatively homogeneous antibody responses to certain antigens in animal strains and the prevalence of certain idiotypes in such antibodies.

Clonal shifts and affinity maturation during secondary response

Let us now return to Fig. 17.9 and inspect the composition of B-cell clones after the second inoculation of oxazolone into the same mice. The picture has now changed somewhat. Although some B-cell clones still express the $V_H Ox1$ combination, the frequency of these clones has dropped to less than 23%. Instead, new clones appear expressing V_H or V_κ genes not encountered during the primary response, as well as new combinations of V_H and V_κ genes. Some of these clones appear to be replacing the ones that dominated the primary response. These *shifts in the composition of the responding clones* after the secondary immunization are obviously caused by somatic mutations in the *V* genes, which accompany the late phases of primary response (or more precisely the secondary response immediately following the primary response; see Chapter 8).

The increase in antibody affinity in relation to the increasing number of accumulated mutations (*affinity maturation*) is striking. High affinity is an essential feature of antibodies because these proteins are often used to neutralize molecules such as toxins that can inflict harm on the body at very low concentrations. Somatic diversification focuses the response on a few, well-adapted clones that are then stored in the B-cell memory for an encounter of the second kind.

Since the mutations are essentially random, they sometimes improve the fit between the antibody-combining site and the epitope and at other times worsen it. The former antibodies are selected for and the latter are selected against, with the result that only cells with improved affinity are propagated further and expanded. This selection is the basis for affinity maturation. The *V* genes, however, are not equal in their ability to sustain random mutations. The nucleotide sequence of some of these genes might be such that most random mutations will quickly lead to a loss of binding ability in the corresponding antibody, whereas that of other genes may provide a more favourable playground for the mutations to experiment on. The former genes thus have a lower *adaptability* than the latter. A given *V* gene may have high affinity and low adaptability, high affinity and high adaptability or low affinity and high adaptability (Fig. 17.10). At the beginning of the response, when there is plenty of antigen available for all the receptors (even those with low affinity) low adaptability has no effect on B-cell stimulation. Later, however, when antigen becomes scarce, low adaptability becomes a disadvantage. Many mutations lower the affinity of such clones, which subsequently cannot compete successfully with the high-affinity clones and drop out of the race. On the other hand, clones with low initial affinity but high adaptability have a good chance of improving their affinity through somatic mutations. At the beginning of the response, at the time of antigen plenty, they manage to survive and later begin to compete with other clones. The high-affinity–high-adaptability clones do well during the entire response but they must compete with the upstarts in the later phase of the response. Because of competition among the clones during the response, the composition of the responding clones changes, leading to the shifts documented in experimental situations.

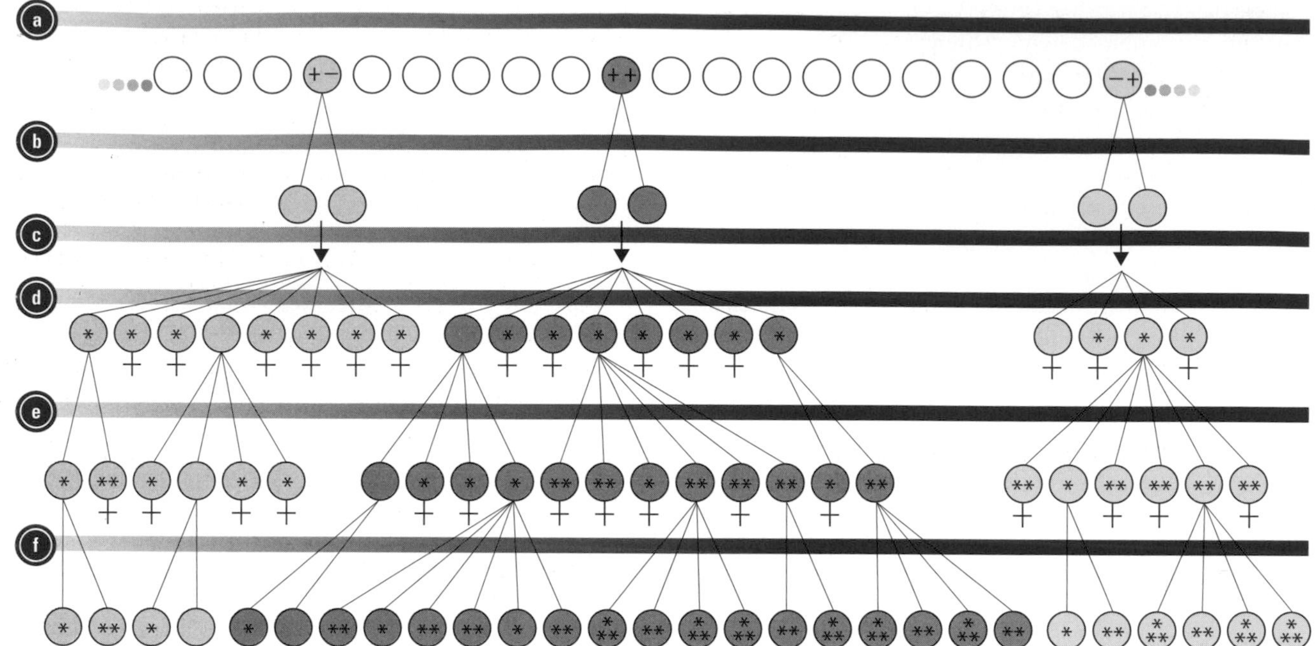

Figure 17.10 Antigen-driven expansion of B-cell clones. (a) Antigen stimulates three B cells (clones) of the preimmune repertoire. The pink clone (+−) has high affinity for antigen but low adaptability (ability to sustain somatic mutations without loss of antigen specificity); the red clone (++) has high affinity and high adaptability; and the grey clone (−+) has low affinity and high adaptability. (b) When the antigen is in excess, all three clones are expanded equally. (c) As antigen concentration becomes a limiting factor and (d) somatic mutations (indicated by asterisks) begin to accumulate in the *V* segments, the pink and red clones expand more than the grey clone. (e) Somatic mutations continue to accumulate and result in loss of antigen specificity of some of the clones, which thus cease to expand (+). (f) Because of its low adaptability, the pink clone decreases in size, whereas the red and grey clones expand. (Modified from Manser, T. *et al.* (1985) *Immunology Today*, **6**, 94.)

Antibody formation *in vitro*

The obvious advantage in studying antibody formation in tissue culture is that the conditions are simpler and more amenable to manipulation than in the whole animal. Several *in vitro* techniques of antibody production have been developed and named after their inventors: the *Mishell–Dutton assay* (Fig. 17.11a), the *Marbrook assay* (Fig. 17.11b) and the *Jerne plaque assay* (Fig. 17.12). These 'classical' assays are used to study *in vitro* model responses to the surface antigens of sheep red blood cells.

Assay systems for more complete study of *in vitro* antibody formation, including broader range of antigens, somatic mutation and the memory element, were developed after the essential role of the signals provided through the CD40 receptor was recognized. By using monoclonal antibodies to the CD40 receptor that were immobilized on Fc receptor-expressing fibroblasts and upon addition of IL-4, it was possible to grow normal human B cells for extended periods of time. Improved results were achieved when the recombinant CD40L, expressed at high density in cell membranes, was used to stimulate B-cell cultures *in vitro*.

A modern variant of the plaque assay (Fig. 17.12) is the ELISPOT technique. Its use is not limited to surface antigens of red blood cells or antigens that can be coupled to them. In this method, the antigen is adsorbed onto a nitrocellulose membrane that is spread over the agarose medium in which the B-cell single-cell suspension is cultivated. The antibodies produced, for example by mouse cells, diffuse to the antigen-coated nitrocellulose membrane and adsorb to it. The spots on the membrane containing the bound antibodies are then visualized by incubation of the membrane with a solution of an antibody against mouse immunoglobulins conjugated with an enzyme (peroxidase or alkaline phosphatase) followed by exposure to a solution of a suitable chromogenic substrate of the enzyme. The result is a pattern of fine coloured spots on the nitrocellulose membrane visible under the microscope, each corresponding to a single B cell producing the specific antibody. These spots therefore correspond to the haemolytic plaques in the Jerne technique. One advantage of this method is that it is possible to enumerate the cells producing antibodies of a given isotype (e.g. IgM, IgG1, IgG2a, etc.) by using enzyme-conjugated isotype-specific antibodies for detection.

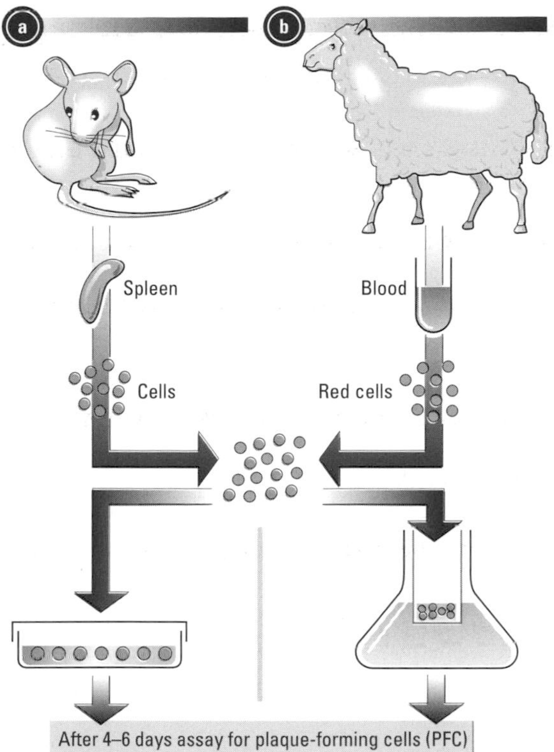

Figure 17.11 Two assays for measuring antibody production *in vitro*. (a) In the Mishell–Dutton assay, a cell suspension is prepared from spleens of non-immunized mice, mixed with sheep red blood cells, placed in a small Petri dish and grown for 4–6 days in culture medium containing fetal bovine serum, under low oxygen tension with gentle agitation. At the end of the culture period, the cells are harvested and tested for antibody production to sheep red blood cells in the haemolytic plaque assay (see below). The number of antibody-forming cells rises above the background level at 2 days and peaks at 4–6 days of culture, at which time the culture contains about 10^3 antibody-forming cells per 10^6 spleen cells. Antibody formation in Mishell–Dutton cultures cannot be regarded as a fully fledged immune response, comparable to that occurring *in vivo*. For one thing, sheep red blood cells are virtually the only antigen against which these cultures produce antibodies, while most other antigens stimulate a meagre, poorly reproducible response. Further, IgM is virtually the only antibody class produced in the cultures; IgG antibodies are either not produced at all or produced in small quantities only. Finally, the addition of fresh sheep red blood cells to the culture after 6 days of incubation fails to induce a secondary response; instead, the ongoing response wanes and cells in the culture die. However, secondary antibody response can be induced *in vitro* by antigen stimulation of cells from an animal immunized to sheep red blood cells *in vivo*. Despite these imperfections, however, the Mishell–Dutton culture system has been an extremely useful tool for studying a host of questions related to the interplay of cells and factors in the antibody response. Why sheep red blood cells are so unique in stimulating *in vitro* responses is not known. They may possess intrinsic mitogenic and other stimulatory properties that make up for the deficiencies of the *in vitro* system. Alternatively, the precursors of B lymphocytes that respond to sheep red blood cells might already be presensitized or preconditioned for the response in some other way. At least three cell types interact in the Mishell–Dutton system to produce sheep red blood cell-reactive antibodies. These include B lymphocytes, as precursors of antibody-forming cells; T lymphocytes, providing help in B-cell differentiation; and macrophages, providing conditions necessary for the growth of cells and for T cell–B cell interaction. The observation that the addition of IL-5 (see Chapter 10) to the culture suffices for antibody production points to a relative T-cell independence of the response's early phase, since IL-5 is thought to act only in the final stages of B-cell development. This relative T-cell independence of antigen recognition is another property distinguishing the Mishell–Dutton system from many of the *in vivo* responses. Normal mouse spleen cells can be separated into two populations, one adhering to glass or plastic surfaces, the other non-adherent. Neither population, when stimulated *in vitro* with sheep red blood cells, was able to give rise to antibody-forming cells, but when the two were recombined a good response comparable to that of an unseparated spleen-cell population ensued. Later studies demonstrated that the non-adherent population contained the actual antibody-forming cells, whereas the adherent population played an accessory role in the response. Later still, the *adherent* or *accessory cells* were identified as macrophages. The fact that they can be replaced by 2-mercaptoethanol or other thiols suggests a non-immunological role of macrophages pertaining to general cell survival in the culture. (b) The *Marbrook assay* is a variant of the Mishell–Dutton system in which the mixture of spleen cells and sheep red blood cells is first placed into a glass tube with a dialysis membrane at one end and the tube is then immersed in the medium in a larger flask. After 4–6 days of incubation, the suspension in the tube is tested for the presence of cells producing antibodies to sheep red blood cells. In this arrangement, the nutrients of the medium can diffuse freely to the cells and the metabolites can diffuse away from the cells into the medium. Antibodies produced by the cultured cells are secreted into the medium in the tube and one can detect their presence by one of the serological methods described in Chapter 14. However, one can also test *in vitro* antibody synthesis by assaying directly for antibody-producing cells. The test used to identify such cells is the Jerne plaque assay. (Modified from Klein, J. (1982) *Immunology: The Science of Self–Nonself Discrimination*. John Wiley & Sons, New York.)

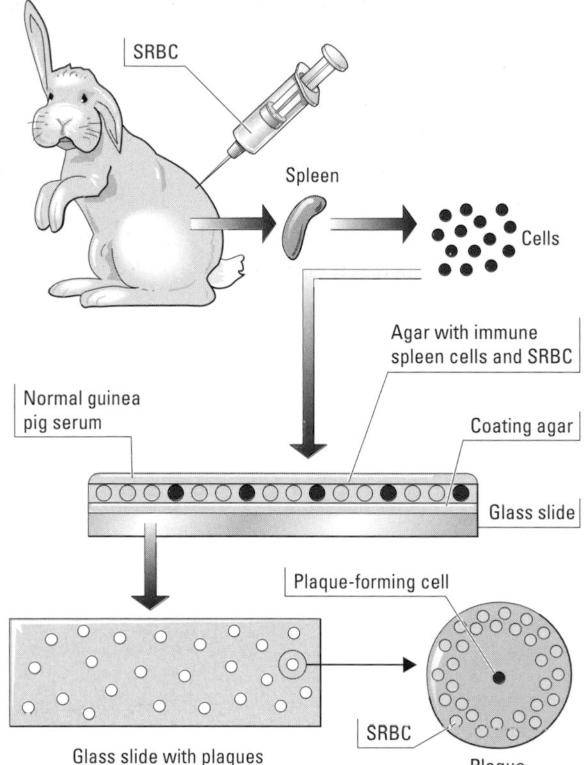

Figure 17.12 Jerne plaque assay for measuring antibody production *in vitro*. Cells obtained from culture or from an immunized animal and producing antibodies to sheep red blood cells are mixed with an excess of sheep erythrocytes in warm agar and a thin layer of the agar is then poured onto a glass slide or into a Petri dish, the surface of which has been precoated with a supporting agar layer. The agar is then allowed to solidify and the slide is incubated for 1 hour at 37 °C. The immune cells in the suspension continue to produce antibodies, which diffuse through the agar and bind to the surrounding sheep red blood cells. After incubation, the top of the agar layer is covered with complement (normal guinea-pig serum) and the slide is incubated for about 40 min. As the complement diffuses through the agar, it binds to antibodies coating the erythrocytes and lyses the latter. As a result, a clear area (plaque) forms around each antibody-producing cell, now referred to as a *plaque-forming cell* (PFC). Since, at a certain low density of spleen cells, one plaque corresponds to one PFC, one can estimate the number of antibody-producing cells in the suspension by counting the plaques. In this *direct plaque assay*, the only antibodies detected are of the IgM type, since IgG antibodies are not efficient enough in complement binding to mediate cell lysis under these experimental conditions. To detect IgG antibodies one must resort to the *indirect plaque assay*, in which one incubates the agar plate, prior to the addition of complement, with a xenogeneic antiserum specific for the coating antibodies (e.g. rabbit anti-mouse IgG serum if the coating antibodies are of mouse origin). The xenogeneic immunoglobulin molecules cross-link the coating antibodies and generate conditions for efficient complement binding and hence for cell lysis. SRBC, sheep red blood cells. (Modified from Klein, J. (1982) *Immunology: The Science of Self–Nonself Discrimination*. John Wiley & Sons, New York.)

Further reading

Armitage, R.J. & Alderson, M.R. (1995) B-cell stimulation. *Current Opinion in Immunology*, 7, 243–247.

Arpin, C., Déchanet, J., Van Kooten, C. *et al.* (1995) Generation of memory B cells and plasma cells *in vitro*. *Science*, **268**, 720–722.

Czerkinsky, C. & Sedgwick, J. (1993) Enzyme-linked immunospot (ELISPOT) assays for detection of specific antibody-secreting cells. In *Methods of Immunological Analysis* (Eds R. Masseyeff, W.H. Albert & N.A. Staines), Vol. 3, pp. 504–540. VCH, Weinheim.

Dutton, R.W. (1993) How does the immune system remember? *Current Biology*, 3, 901–903.

Germain, R.N. & Margulies, D.H. (1993) The biochemistry and cell biology of antigen processing and presentation. *Annual Review of Immunology*, **11**, 403–450.

Clark, E.A. & Ledbetter, J.A. (1994) How B and T cells talk to each other. *Nature*, **367**, 425–428.

DeFranco, A.L. (1995) Transmembrane signaling by antigen receptors of B and T lymphocytes. *Current Opinion in Cell Biology*, 7, 163–175.

Gold, M.R. & DeFranco, A.L. (1994) Biochemistry of B lymphocyte activation. *Advances in Immunology*, **55**, 221–295.

Gray, D. (1993) Immunological memory. *Annual Review of Immunology*, **11**, 49–77.

Gray, D., Siepmann, K. & Wohlleben, G. (1994) CD40 ligation in B cell activation, isotype switching and memory development. *Seminars in Immunology*, **6**, 303–310.

Harnett, M.M. (1994) Antigen receptor signalling: from the membrane to the nucleus. *Immunology Today*, **15**, P1–P3.

Hodgkin, P.D. & Basten, A. (1995) B cell activation, tolerance and antigen-presenting function. *Current Opinion in Immunology*, 7, 121–129.

Kehry, M.R. & Castle, B.E. (1994) Regulation of CD40 ligand expression and use of recombinant CD40 ligand for studying B cell growth and differentiation. *Seminars in Immunology*, **6**, 287–294.

Kim, K.-M., Adachi, T., Nielsen, P.J. *et al.* (1994) Two new proteins preferentially associated with membrane immunoglobulin D. *EMBO Journal*, **13**, 3793–3800.

MacLennan, I.C.M. (1994) Germinal centers. *Annual Review of Immunology*, **12**, 117–139.

MacLennan, I.C.M. (1995) Deletion of autoreactive B cells. *Current Biology*, **5**, 103–106.

MacLennan, I. & Chan, E. (1993) The dynamic relationship between B-cell populations in adults. *Immunology Today*, **14**, 29–34.

Mond, J.J., Vos, Q., Lees, A. & Snapper, C.M. (1995) T cell independent antigens. *Current Opinion in Immunology*, 7, 349–354.

Möller, G. (Ed.) (1986) Population Dynamics of Lymphocytes. *Immunological Reviews*, **91**, entire volume.

Neuberger, M.S. & Milstein, C. (1995) Somatic hypermutation. *Current Opinion in Immunology*, 7, 248–253.

Nossal, G.J.V. (1994) Differentiation of the secondary B-lymphocyte repertoire: the germinal center reaction. *Immunological Reviews*, **137**, 173–183.

Parker, D.C. (1993) T cell-dependent B-cell activation. *Annual Review of Immunology*, **11**, 331–360.

Schriever, F. & Nadler, L.M. (1992) The central role of follicular dendritic cells in lymphoid tissues. *Advances in Immunology*, **51**, 243–284.

Silverman, G.J. (1994) Superantigens and the spectrum of unconventional B-cell antigens. *Immunologist*, **2**, 51–57.

Thomas, M.L. (1995) Of ITAMs and ITIMs: turning on and off the B cell antigen receptor. *Journal of Experimental Medicine*, **181**, 1953–1956.

van Noesel, C.J.M., Lankester, A.C. & van Lier, R.A.W. (1993) Dual antigen recognition by B-cells. *Immunology Today*, **14**, 8–11.

chapter 18 Systemic and regional immune responses

Systemic immune response

Antigen handling by the body

Now that we know in general how T and B lymphocytes respond to antigenic stimuli, let us turn to the two main forms of immune response: *systemic immunity*, which involves most of the body, and *regional* or *local immunity*, which is largely confined to one particular part. The former usually concerns the spleen, major lymph nodes, blood and lymph. The latter mainly relates to lymphoid tissues underlying body surfaces, i.e. the skin and the mucosa. This division is not sharp, however, since systemic immunity may begin regionally and regional immunity usually involves communication between different parts of the body.

A decisive factor in determining the form of response is the manner of exposure to the antigen. To initiate a systemic response involving the spleen, the antigen must enter the bloodstream, since blood vessels provide the only afferent connection to this organ. However, not all of the antigen that has entered the bloodstream reaches the spleen. Most of it is degraded in the plasma and removed by *natural clearance* from the body. The degradation process is threefold (Fig. 18.1). In the *equilibrium phase*, the soluble (but not particulate) antigen diffuses from the plasma into extravascular spaces and its initially high concentration drops rapidly. In the *metabolic decay phase*, the circulating antigen is gradually degraded enzymatically and cleared by phagocytic cells so that its concentration declines slowly. Phagocytic traps are set up for blood-borne antigen throughout the reticuloendothelial system, especially in the spleen, liver, bone marrow, lymph nodes and kidney. In these organs, while passing from arteries to veins, the antigen is forced through narrow sinusoids lined with phagocytic cells. The *immune elimination phase* begins as soon as antibodies against the antigen are formed. They bind the antigen and the ensuing soluble antigen–antibody complexes are taken up and digested by monocytes and neutrophils. If antibodies are already present in the plasma at the time of antigen exposure, the antigen concentration declines rapidly from the beginning without a discernible metabolic decay phase.

Immune response histology in the spleen

Antigen is brought into the spleen along with arterial blood, is spilled over the marginal zone and is delivered by the arterial capillaries to the marginal sinus (see Chapter 3). From the marginal zone it is transported by lymphocytes and macrophages to the lymphoid follicle of the white pulp, where it remains for some time. At least three kinds of macrophage have been identified in this region: marginal-zone macrophages in the marginal zone itself; standard macrophages scattered through all spleen compartments; and marginal metallophils in the outermost layers of the follicles and in the periarteriolar lymphoid sheath (PALS) adjacent to the inner border of the marginal zone. Other, and probably the most important, antigen-presenting cells

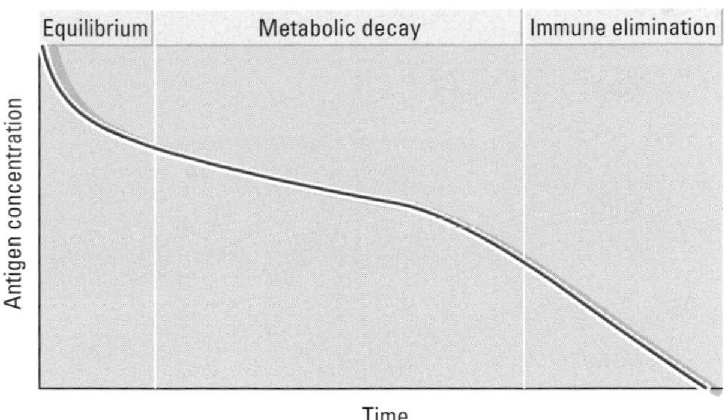

Figure 18.1 Three phases of antigen degradation in the plasma. Time and antigen concentration units are left unspecified to indicate the variability encountered with different antigens under different conditions. (Modified from Klein, J. (1982) *Immunology: The Science of Self–Nonself Discrimination.* John Wiley & Sons, New York.)

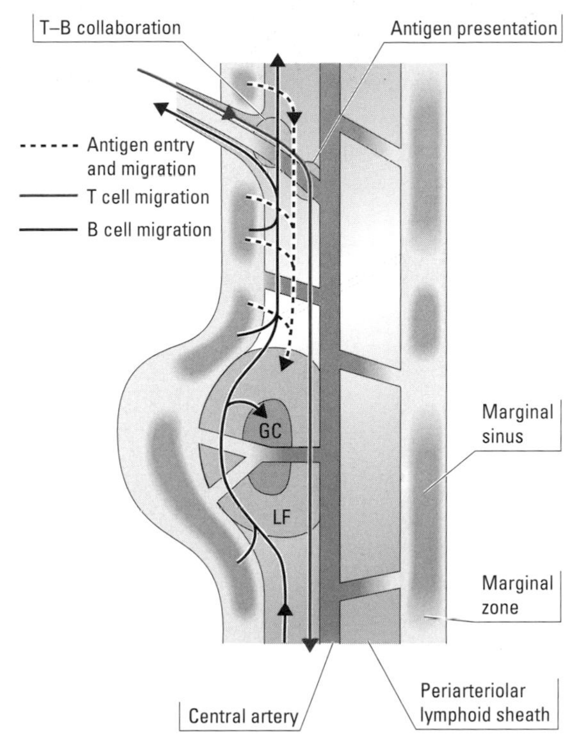

Figure 18.2 Initiation of immune response in the spleen showing the entry and presumed route of migration for the antigen, T cells and B cells, as well as the probable sites of antigen presentation and of collaboration between T and B lymphocytes. For the sake of simplicity, migration routes are shown on one side of the diagram only and antigen–T cell and T cell–B cell sites of interaction are restricted to single regions. GC, germinal centre; LF, lymphoid follicle.

(APCs) in this region are the interdigitating dendritic cells in the central PALS. Actual antigen presentation very likely takes place in the T-cell-rich area of the PALS, where close contact between T lymphocytes and interdigitating dendritic cells has been observed. (Recall that the inner PALS mainly contains T cells, the outer PALS a majority of T cells and a minority of B cells, the follicles mostly B lymphocytes, the marginal zone mainly macrophages and some B cells, and the lymphoid sheaths around the terminal arterioles contain primarily T lymphocytes and only a small number of B cells.) Stimulated T cells proliferate in the PALS and collaborate with B cells, probably in the outer PALS or in the sheath of lymphoid tissue surrounding the terminal arterioles. These areas represent the borders between T- and B-cell domains, and B lymphocytes cross them when they migrate from the marginal zone to the lymphoid tissues around the terminal arterioles. Stimulated B lymphocytes follow the same route, migrating along the border of the PALS and marginal zone and through the base of the lymphoid follicle (Fig. 18.2). Some of the B cells enter the mantle and even the germinal centre of the follicle, while others follow the sheath of the terminal arterioles, then enter the arterioles and are delivered by them into the red pulp. They differentiate along the way into antibody-producing B cells and ultimately into plasma cells, which are then collected from the red-pulp sinuses by the trabecular and splenic veins. Circulating plasma cells continue to secrete antibodies at a high rate, generating a systemic response.

Some B lymphocytes that enter lymphoid follicles turn into memory cells that are activated upon a second exposure to the same antigen. Increased numbers of proliferating cells are indeed seen in the follicles and outer PALS during the secondary response. One of the factors that turns activated B lymphocytes into memory cells might be the high concentration of antigen–antibody complexes around and in the follicle. These complexes may become trapped by follicular dendritic cells, which then provide the transforming stimulus.

Antigen ends up in the spleen when it is injected directly into the veins (*intravenous injection*), by an immunologist or by a biting insect. This organ is probably also the main delivery site for antigens injected into the peritoneum[1], an unnatural port of entry for an antigen and largely confined to experimental situations. One immunologist compared the *intraperitoneal injection* to a bull's horns piercing the flanks of a toreador's horse. The inoculated antigen is taken up with the peritoneal fluid by broad, flattened lacunae

[1] *Peritoneum* (Greek *peritonaion*, something that is streched over) is the membrane lining the walls of the abdominal and pelvic cavities, and covering the viscera, the organs within these cavities.

('stomata') located beneath the peritoneum of the diaphragm, the membrane dividing the lungs from the stomach. The lacunae are the beginnings of draining lymphatics that connect with collecting lymphatics beneath the pleura of the diaphragm. From there, the antigen-containing fluid is carried by the lymphatic trunks to the right lymphatic duct or the thoracic duct, and ultimately into the bloodstream and spleen. On its way to the ducts, however, the lymph is filtered through the superior mediastinal lymph nodes, in which an immune response may be initiated in addition to that elicited in the spleen.

Immune response histology in the lymph node

Antigen injected into the skin (*intradermal injection*) or under the skin (*subcutaneous injection*) arrives in the lymph and is delivered by afferent lymphatics into the nearest *draining (regional) lymph nodes*. It enters the subcapsular sinus of the node and then percolates with the lymph through the cortex towards the medulla (Fig. 18.3). On its way, the antigen may encounter several types of APC. In the inner cortex, it is likely to come in contact with *interdigitating cells*, which are in close apposition to T lymphocytes and may represent the main APCs of the lymph node. The antigen might also encounter *macrophages*, which are scattered through all compartments in the lymph node. A special subpopulation of macrophages seems to form the 'subsinus layer' immediately beneath the subcapsular sinus and in the internodular zone of the outer cortex; it may correspond to the macrophage layers in the marginal zone of the spleen. Finally, in the germinal centres of the follicles, the antigen may encounter *follicular dendritic cells*, which have affinity for antigen–antibody complexes and retain these on their processes for a long time.

Prominent antigen transporters and presenters in the lymph nodes are probably the epidermal Langerhans' cells. These cells take up antigen by endocytosis or macropinocytosis and while processing it they transform into *veiled cells*, which then migrate via afferent lymphatics to the regional lymph node. There they again become interdigitating dendritic cells, which are excellent APCs because they express large amounts of major histocompatibility complex (MHC) class II glycoproteins and all necessary adhesion and co-stimulatory molecules on their surfaces.

The APCs present the antigen to helper T (T_H) cells when these pass through the lymph node as part of their regular migratory circuit. Antigen-reactive T cells become activated, interrupt their migration and settle down. They are thus rapidly removed from circulation and the individual goes through a period in which it has almost no T cells reactive with a given antigen in the circulating lymph: all

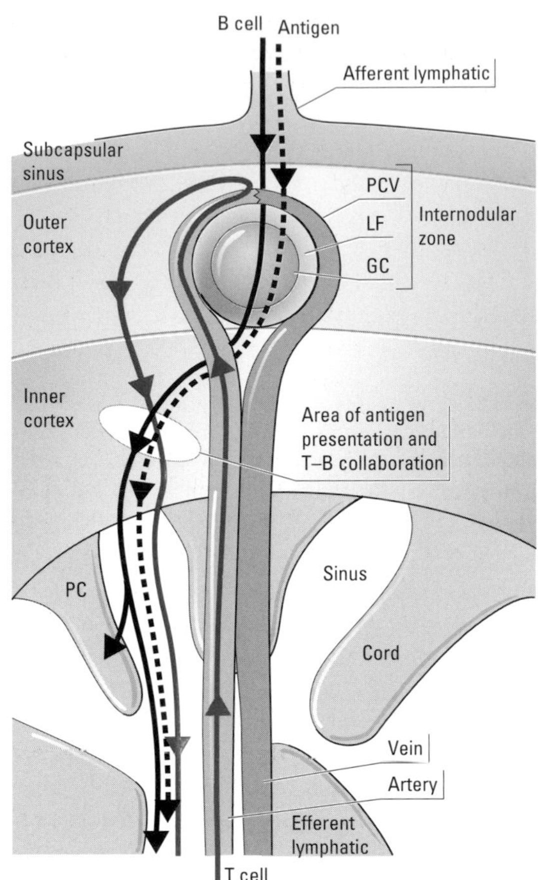

Figure 18.3 Initiation of immune response in the lymph node showing the entry and routes of migration for the antigen, T cells and B cells, as well as the probable sites of antigen presentation and collaboration between T cells and B cells. GC, germinal centre; LF, lymphoid follicle; PC, plasma cell; PCV, postcapillary venule.

the cells are either in the lymph nodes or in the spleen. Lymphocytes enter the lymph nodes through postcapillary venules or via afferent lymphatics, and upon encountering antigen-charged APCs in the cortex (a T-cell domain) they become blast cells, divide and form clones of effector and memory cells. Activated T_H cells interact with B lymphocytes, probably at the border between the T- and B-cell areas, and particularly at the border between the internodular zone of the outer and inner cortex. Being more sedentary than T cells, B lymphocytes show no pronounced withdrawal from circulation after antigen stimulation; most are already in the lymph node, waiting for the antigen. The majority of the newly arriving B lymphocytes reach the lymph node via the afferent lymphatics. After stimulation by the antigen and by T_H cells, B cells also transform into blasts and begin to divide. Stimulated memory B cells enter the follicle and establish the germinal centre. The appearance of the germinal centre 4–5 days after antigen injection transforms the primary follicle into the secondary follicle. The germinal centres remain prominent for several days and then disappear. The progeny of the activated mature B cells differentiate into plasma cells and memory cells, both of which leave the follicle and descend towards the medulla. Some plasma cells are retained in the lymph node, settle down between the sinuses, in medullary cords, and secrete antibodies. Memory T cells, some memory B cells and some plasma cells enter the efferent lymph and are carried via the major lymphatic ducts into the bloodstream and to other lymphoid tissues. A considerable number of plasma cells settle in the bone marrow.

Activated T cells in the lymph node secrete cytokines, some of which cause local vessel dilatation and so allow leakage (transudation) of plasma from vessels into extravascular spaces. Other cytokines attract macrophages and granulocytes to the node and these then plug some of the medullary sinuses, causing lymph drainage into efferent lymphatics to slow down. Fluid and cell accumulation is responsible for the lymph node enlargement characteristic of an infection. Gradually, however, when most of the antigen supply is exhausted, the lymph nodes return to their normal size.

Secreted antibodies are transported via efferent lymphatics into the venous system and circulate with blood through the body. Antibodies of the IgG class can traverse blood vessel walls and enter extravascular tissue spaces. Normally, IgG is divided about half and half between blood and extravascular body fluids. Antibodies of the IgM (and also IgA, IgE and IgD) class, on the other hand, usually cannot cross blood vessel walls and so are largely confined to the bloodstream and to a few other sites. Circulating antibodies bind the offending antigens and participate in several other effector functions.

Regional (local), mucosal and secretory immunity

The systemic immune response involves lymphoid tissues organized into organs—spleen and lymph nodes. Regional responses, on the other hand, rely on lymphoid tissue associated mainly with body surfaces. All body surfaces are protected by a special tissue having two main components, the outer *epithelium* and the inner *connective tissue* (Fig. 18.4). The epithelium covering *outer (dry) body surfaces* is called *epidermis*, the underlying connective tissue is the *dermis*, and both components together form the *skin*. The outer epithelium of *inner (wet) body surfaces* retains the name *epithelium*, the underlying connective tissue is the *lamina propria*, and the combination of the two tissues is the

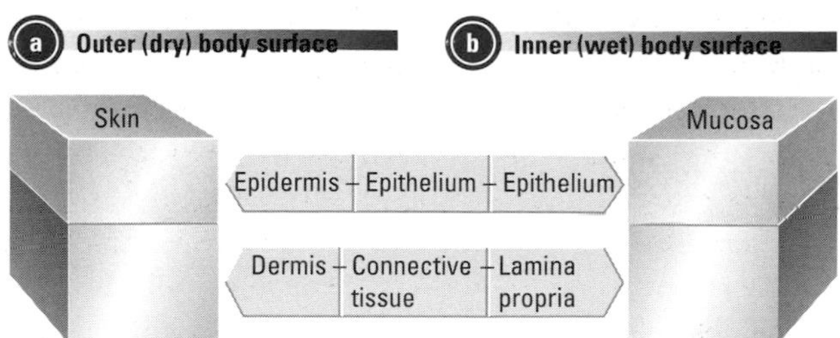

Figure 18.4 Two types of body surface.

mucosa or the *mucosal membrane*. Most of the surface tissues contain *glands*, groups of cells specializing in the production of secretory products. Because these glands release their products to the outside they are referred to as *exocrine*, in contrast to endocrine glands that release their products into the bloodstream. The products of exocrine glands (*secretions*) can be of two kinds: *external*, which contain the products of exocrine glands only; and *internal*, which are mixed with *exudate*, the fluid seeping from blood and lymph vessels into tissues and from there into internal body cavities (Latin *ex*, out; *sudare*, to sweat). External secretions are saliva and tears, as well as nasal, tracheobronchial, intestinal and genitourinary secretions. Internal secretions are the fluids filling the anterior chamber of the eye (aqueous humour), bathing the brain and spinal cord (cerebrospinal fluid, CSF), filling the joint cavity (synovial fluid), bathing the lungs (pleural fluid), bathing the jaws and gums (gingival fluid), filling the abdominal cavity (peritoneal fluid) and surrounding the fetus (amniotic fluid).

Non-systemic immunity is called *regional* or *local* because it affects only parts of the body; it is referred to as *mucosal* because it is most frequently effected by the lymphoid system associated with the mucosa; and it is called *secretory* because its elements (antibodies, immune cells) are often found in secretions, mainly external. All these designations are more or less synonymous. We have chosen the term 'regional' because that is the name of a journal devoted to this subspeciality of immunology. Lymphoid tissues associated with the individual body parts and responsible for the particular form of regional immunity have their own names and acronyms: SALT is the skin-associated lymphoid tissue and MALT is the mucosa-associated lymphoid tissue. The specific forms of MALT are GALT, the gut-associated lymphoid tissue, and BALT, the bronchus-associated lymphoid tissue; special designations are usually not used for lymphoid tissues associated with other mucosas, i.e. those of the mammary gland, conjunctiva, salivary gland, oral cavity, genitourinary tract and the middle ear. A discussion of the individual forms of regional immunity follows.

Skin-associated immunity

Pathogenic microorganisms that have managed to penetrate the deeper layers of the skin are dealt with by the SALT and the *skin's immune system* (SIS). The SIS is composed of APCs, T lymphocytes, keratinocytes, neutrophils, mast cells and vascular as well as lymphatic endothelial cells. The most prominent among the APCs are the *Langerhans' cells*, scattered in the stratified squamous epithelium (the spinal cell layer) of the epidermis (Fig. 18.5). Large numbers of Langerhans' cells form a regular network through their dendritic processes. The cells are derived from bone marrow stem cells, remain in the skin for about 3 weeks (at least in the mouse) and then leave the epidermis, perhaps via lymphatics. The characteristics of Langerhans' cells include expression of CD1 molecules, otherwise found on maturing thymocytes (once T lymphocytes leave the thymus, they cease to express CD1), class II MHC molecules, a small number of CD4 molecules, surface receptors for C3 and for the Fc part of IgG, and synthesis of interleukin (IL)-1. The *Granstein cells* (named after Richard D. Granstein) resemble Langerhans' cells but are resistant to irradiation with ultraviolet light and are claimed to activate preferentially suppressor cells rather than T_H cells. The *indeterminate cells* found in the papillary dermis express the CD1 antigen like Langerhans' cells. The *interdigitating cells* occur only in the inflamed skin of patients with psoriasis, leprosy, atopic dermatitis and pityriasis rosea, often in juxtaposition with T lymphocytes (*peripolesis*). The *veiled*

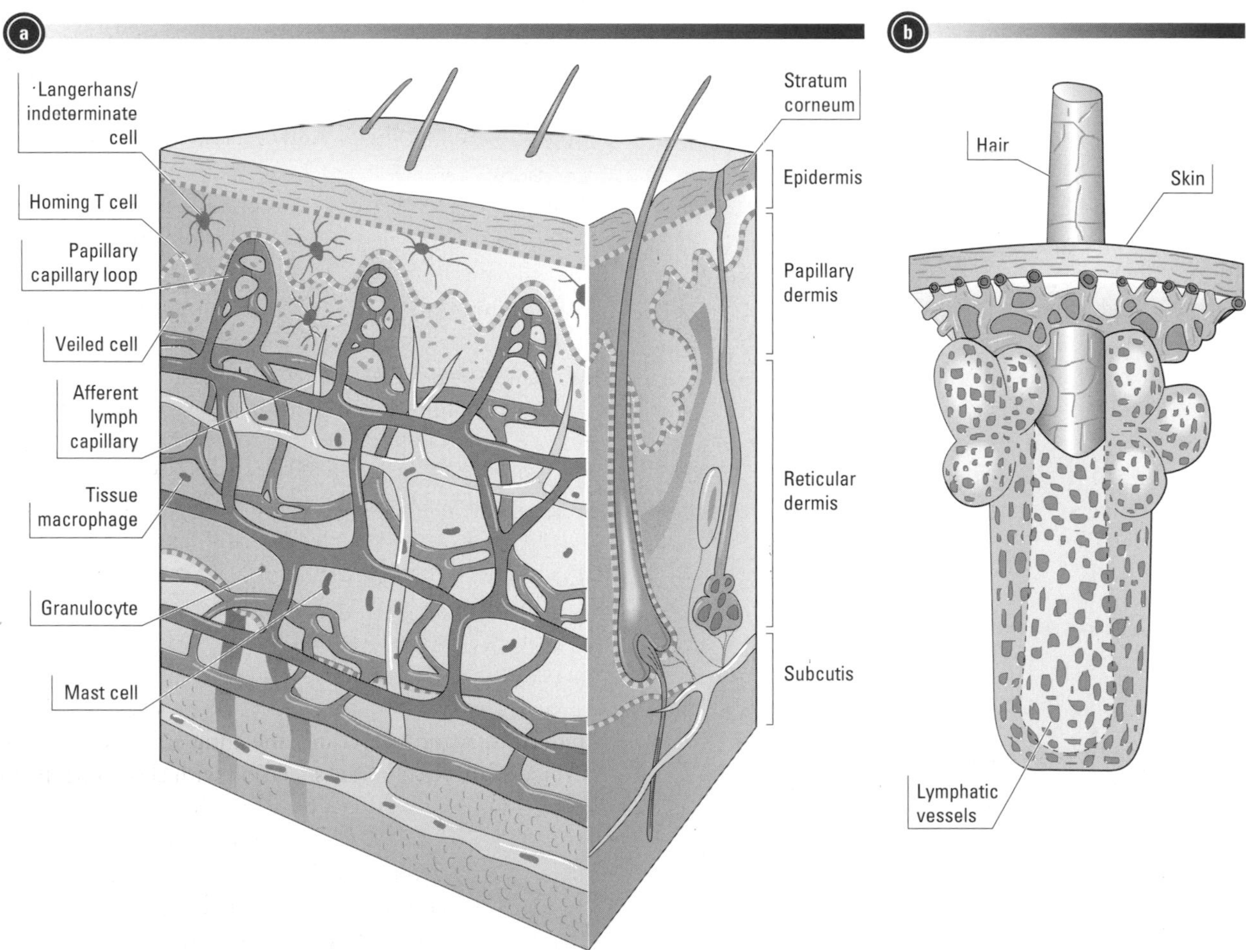

Figure 18.5 Histology of human skin. (a) Diagrammatic representation of main cells and tissue types, including cells of the skin immune system (SIS). (b) Network of lymphatic vessels and capillaries surrounding a hair follicle of the skin. (a, Modified from Bos, J. D. & Kapsenberg, M. L. (1986) *Immunology Today*, 7, 235; b, modified from Kahn, F. (1965) *The Human Body*. Random House, New York.)

cells are present in the lymph of the lymphatics that drain the skin. All these cells are presumably derived from the bone marrow and all express class II MHC molecules. Their possible interrelationships are shown in Fig. 18.6. The skin, like most other organs, also contains *macrophages* (histiocytes), which can present antigen to T cells in certain situations. However, they normally function as scavengers of debris.

The *T lymphocytes* of the skin appear to represent a subset that homes specifically to the skin (*epidermotropic T cells*). They are normally scattered throughout the skin, particularly around and above the superficial vein knots. Epidermotropism is especially pronounced in skin diseases, from the rare cutaneous lymphomas to common benign inflammatory diseases, such as eczema and psoriasis.

A special subpopulation of mouse skin T lymphocytes is associated with keratinocytes. These cells express γ:δ T-cell receptors (TCRs) that are essentially homogeneous: (i.e. TCRs with little or no clonal diversity in their variable regions), have a dendritic appearance and seem to recognize autoantigens from stressed keratinocytes in an MHC-independent way. Upon activation they secrete keratinocyte growth factor. They probably function by detecting early signs of skin damage or infection, initiating wound repair and local inflammation.

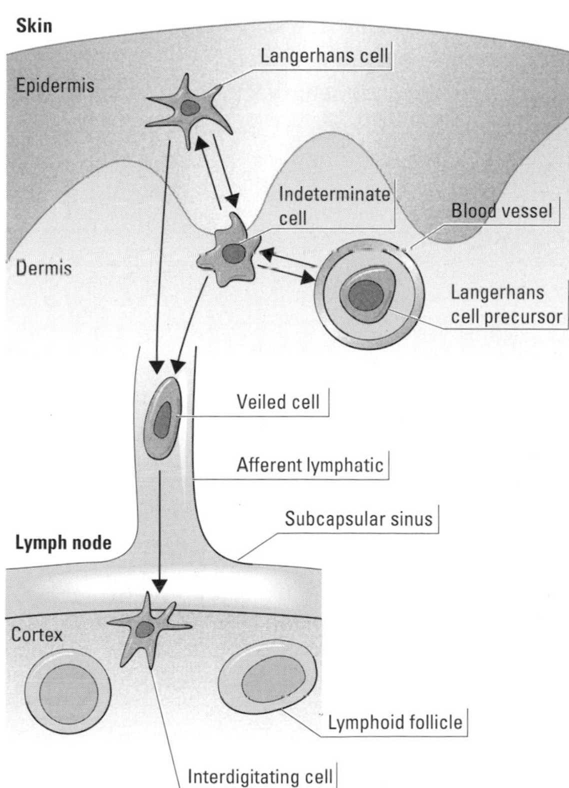

Figure 18.6 Presumed migration patterns and relationships among various subsets of dendritic cells present in the skin. (Modified from Bos, J. D. & Kapsenberg, M. L. (1986) *Immunology Today*, 7, 235.)

Keratinocytes are the main cells of the epidermis. They synthesize keratin, the primary structural protein of the skin's outer layer and of hair. They also synthesize and secrete several cytokines and can be induced to express class II MHC molecules. Skin epithelium appears to be structurally similar to thymic cortical epithelium: thymic epithelial cells contain granules apparently identical to the keratohyaline granules of keratinocytes; at least three surface-marker molecules of thymic epithelial cells are also present on the surface of keratinocytes from the basal layer of the human epidermis; and the co-culture of immature thymocytes with keratinocytes induces expression of terminal deoxynucleotidyltransferase in the former. Certain malignant T lymphocytes seem to have a high affinity for the skin; virtually all lymphocytic malignancies in which there is widespread infiltration of the skin are of T-cell origin, while most of those in which the skin is unaffected are of B-cell origin. Finally, the fact that a single mutation can apparently affect thymus and skin (the *nude* gene in the mouse is responsible for hairlessness *and* the failure of the thymus to develop) also points to a possible connection between these two organs. Some immunologists speculate that the skin, like the thymus, might be a site in which certain types of T cells undergo maturation, and that keratinocytes in the skin may have some influence on post-thymic stages in T-cell maturation.

Of the other SIS cells, *mast cells* may be involved in regulating skin vasculature and perhaps even T-cell migration patterns. The most important function of extravascular *neutrophils* may be phagocytic, in particular with respect to the clearance of large antigen–antibody complexes. *Endothelial cells* in the lymphatic and blood vessels may function as non-professional APCs (they are class II MHC positive but do not express co-stimulatory molecules).

Antigen that has penetrated the skin is picked up by one of the types of APC, most often by Langerhans' cells in the epidermis. After processing, the antigen is displayed on the surface of these cells in association with class II MHC molecules. The Langerhans' cells then either present the antigen to T_H cells in the skin or migrate with it to the draining lymph nodes. Skin lymphatics start with open ends within the papillary dermis and transport lymph in one direction only, towards the skin-associated lymph nodes. The latter are particularly prominent in the body folds such as elbows and knees, as well as the cervical, axillary and inguinal regions. If Langerhans' cells are damaged by ultraviolet irradiation, the antigen is picked up instead by Granstein cells or by interdigitating cells derived from them, which then possibly activate different T-cell subsets than Langerhans' cells. If the presentation by Langerhans' cells takes place directly in the skin, keratinocytes may become involved. If viruses are present during the challenge and stimulate the production of interferon-γ (IFN-γ), the latter may induce keratinocytes to express class II MHC molecules and thus enable them to function as APCs. The antigen delivered to the draining lymph nodes is handled there in the manner described earlier for the systemic response.

Mucosal immune system

General characteristics

The mucosal epithelium in an adult individual covers an area of about 400 m^2. Mucosal surfaces are the major sites of the body's encounters with antigen and they are continuously bombarded by antigens, be they ingested food particles, microbes, toxins, parasites or allergens. Most infectious diseases begin on mucosal surfaces and many are limited to these sites. To cope with this constant threat, vertebrates have developed a complex *mucosal immune system* (MIS), whose delicate task is to limit infections without interfering with the function of the fragile mucosal tissue. (At least some of these functions depend on the presence of non-pathogenic microorganisms, which the immune system must therefore learn to disregard (see Chapter 21).)

The main structural component of the MIS is the specialized MALT, which is present beneath all mucosal surfaces except the uterus, fallopian tubes and the cervix. The total mass of the MALT exceeds that of all the lymphoid organs combined. The MALT expands after the birth of an individual, probably stimulated by antigen encounters. In most species it persists throughout adult life, but in some, such as the sheep, it involutes with age. The lymphoid tissue can be either dispersed or organized into aggregates of lymphoid follicles, the prevailing form depending on the specific location. The tissue surrounding and overlying the follicles often assumes special properties that enable it to participate in the immune response. The spectrum of the immune responses that the MALT can mount varies, depending on the particular region, but in general it includes both humoral and cellular immunity, as well as a variety of non-adaptive defence mechanisms.

Antigen presentation

To stimulate regional immunity, an antigen must reach the particular mucosal surface, traverse the epithelium and be picked up by macrophages in the subepithelial layer. The passage is unlikely to involve the whole microorganism. It is more probable that the destroyed particles are partially degraded by agents in the secretions and that some of the degradation products travel across the barrier. The manner of crossing apparently determines whether an antigen will induce regional immunity, systemic immunity, or both.

On some mucosal surfaces, crossing is effected by specialized cells overlying the lymphoid follicles. In the gut, and probably also the respiratory system, the crossing is the function of *M cells*, so called because they have microfolds (irregular ridges) instead of microvilli, or because they are flattened ('membranous') while adjacent cells are columnar. On the luminal side of the gut M cells are easily recognized, being somewhat smoother than the cells of the absorptive epithelium: they stand out like windows in a brick wall (Fig. 18.7). On the side opposite the luminal surface, lymphocytes attach themselves closely to M cells and sometimes even bulge into them. M cells are attached to the absorptive epithelium via tight junctions so that no material can pass between the cells. However, M cells bind antigen on the luminal side, endocytose it, transport the endocytic vesicles to the opposite side and exocytose them, releasing the antigen. The passage across the cell apparently does not harm the antigen: it emerges intact.

M cells can bind (probably via polyvalent adhesions) and endocytose a diverse array of material, soluble as well as particulate. However, they do discriminate among the materials to some degree, e.g. they do not take up commensal microorganisms residing in the gut. This selectivity is

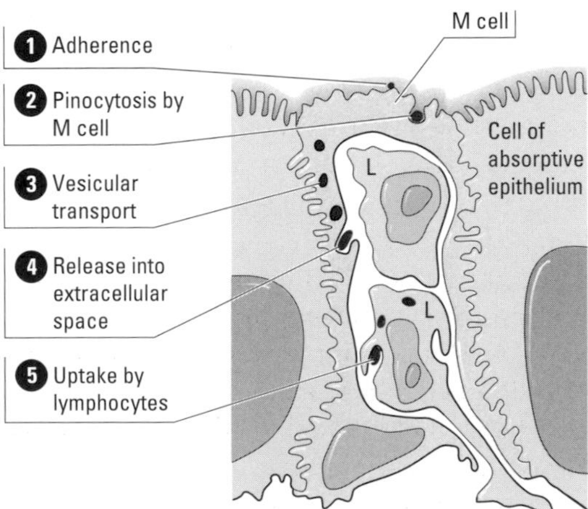

Figure 18.7 Crossing of material through intestinal M cells. A particle is shown passing from the intestinal surface towards lymphoid tissue underlying the epithelium (various stages of the crossing are shown) and two lymphocytes (L) are shown moving in the opposite direction. (Modified from Owen, R. L. (1977) *Gastroenterology*, 72, 440.)

probably based on differential binding: an antigen must attach to the M-cell surface, and commensal microorganisms either lack the necessary attachment molecules or their attachment may be blocked by antibodies. The latter mechanism may provide a way of regulating the size of the resident population and of keeping it from overexpanding. The transport of non-commensal microorganisms to the subepithelial lymphoid tissue is normally a mechanism that enables the immune system to liquidate the invaders. Some invasive pathogens, however, have apparently usurped it to their own advantage, as a way of getting across the mucosa and into the body. Since they have also learned how to avoid macrophage and lymphocyte attack once in the body, they are on the winning side, temporarily at least, in the evolutionary race between the host and its parasites.

M cells transport material in both directions. Lymphocytes, for example, have been seen moving through M cells by diapedesis and then entering the lumen of the gut. Most of the lymphocytes found on the luminal surface of the gut mucosa might have reached their destination in this manner. The lymphoid tissue may also interact with M cells in at least one other way. Since M cells originate from epithelial cell precursors that migrate from the crypts to the dome area and differentiate on the way, it has been suggested that the stimulus inducing differentiation is provided by the lymphoid follicle.

Antigen uptake via M cells is the physiological way of initiating an immune response. It is influenced by a variety of factors: hormones in some species (e.g. adrenal corticosteroids can 'close' the intestinal epithelium in some circumstances); the relative digestibility of the antigen during its passage through the stomach; the chemical nature of the antigen; vitamin A and bile salts (presumably through their ability to influence membrane activity); and by the local microflora. Under pathological conditions, antigens can also enter the body through or between the epithelial cells, and through villous extrusions from epithelial cells.

M cells deliver antigen to lymphocytes but are unable to present it (they lack class II MHC molecules and are incapable of processing the antigen). Some other MALT cells, probably dendritic, must therefore carry out this latter function. Presentation probably occurs both in the MALT and in the draining lymph nodes. Dendritic cells may present antigen to lymphocytes juxtaposed to M cells, or they may migrate with it to the lymph nodes and present the antigen there in the manner described earlier. The antigen is presented to T lymphocytes but is also picked up by B cells, so that both cellular and humoral responses are initiated.

Intestinal epithelial cells, too, may serve as efficient APCs for intraepithelial lymphocytes. They express MHC class I and class II molecules, the MHC class I-like CD1d protein and can be stimulated by cytokines such as granulocyte-monocyte colony stimulating factor (GM-CSF) to express the co-stimulatory molecule CD80. IFN-γ stimulates increased MHC class II expression in these cells, making them better APCs. Intestinal epithelial cells also produce IL-7, a growth factor for intraepithelial lymphocytes.

Humoral immune response

The basic features of humoral responses in the MALT are essentially the same as those described in Chapter 17. The antigen is taken up by APCs and its fragments are loaded on to MHC class II molecules and presented to specific T_H cells. The activated T_H cells proliferate and differentiate into a clone of mature T_H effectors which help antigen-specific B cells to differentiate into plasma cells. A major specific feature of the mucosal humoral response is its striking predilection for the production of IgA.

The collaboration of T_H cells with B lymphocytes may occur in the MALT or in the draining lymph nodes. B cells that have encountered antigen and received the necessary help leave the MALT with efferent lymph (recall that no afferent lymphatics supply this tissue) without producing antibodies. They migrate to the draining lymph nodes, where they complete their development and begin to secrete antibodies. Antibody-producing B cells (blast cells), plasma cells, as well as T_H and memory cells leave the draining lymph nodes via efferent lymphatics and enter the thoracic duct and bloodstream, which then disseminates them throughout the body (Fig. 18.8). They then leave the blood and enter the various MALTs. Homing to the MALT is determined by expression on their surface of β7 integrins. The latter serve as homing receptors that recognize specific ligands (addressins) on the surface of venular endothelial cells in the MALT (see Chapter 9).

MALT-specific B and T_H cells discriminate partially between various MALTs, which means that there is a certain degree of subcompartmentalization within the MIS. For example, oral immunization may induce strong IgA antibody responses in the small intestine, the ascending colon and mammary and salivary glands, and a much weaker response in the distal segments of the large intestine, the tonsils or the female genital tract mucosa. Similarly, intranasal immunization results in IgA production in mucosa of the upper respiratory tract but not in the gut. These differences are probably based on specific homing behaviour of activated B or T_H cells; the molecular basis of this behaviour, however, is not known. At any rate, the homing specificity is not absolute: T_H and B lymphocytes stimulated at a particular MALT site seed many other MALT locations, where they initiate IgA production

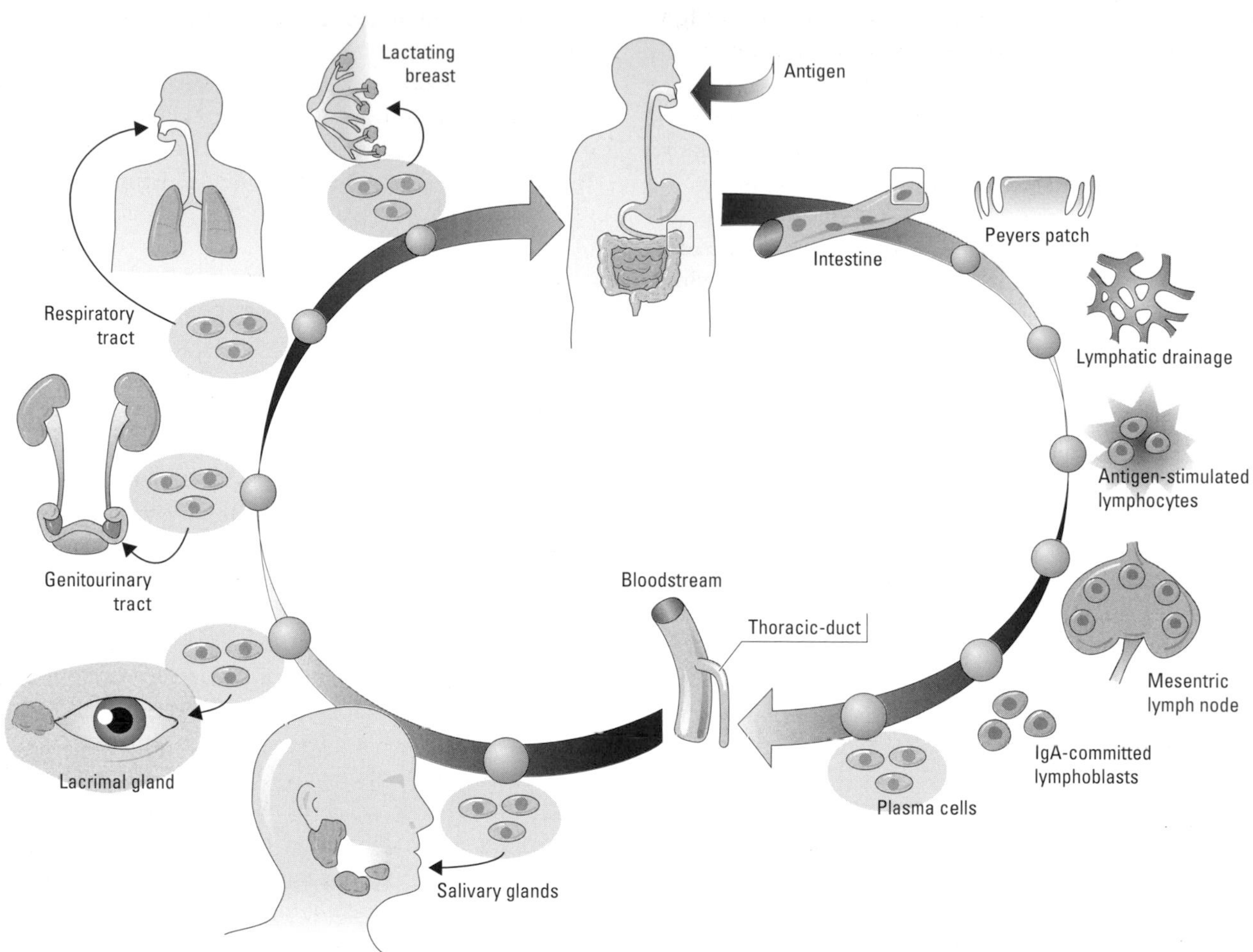

Figure 18.8 Secretory immune system. Antigen enters the system through the mouth and the specialized epithelium (M cells) of the Peyer's patches in the lumen of the gut. It stimulates B and T lymphocytes in the lymphoid tissue underlying the Peyer's patch; antigen-stimulated B cells leave the tissue with lymph of the draining lymphatics and enter the mesenteric lymph nodes where they proliferate and differentiate. (Alternatively, antigen may be brought into mesenteric lymph nodes and stimulate T and B lymphocytes there.) Lymphoblasts committed to IgA synthesis leave the nodes with efferent lymph, enter the blood circulation via the thoracic duct, and on their way differentiate into plasma cells. Blood then distributes plasma cells to the specific organs and tissues of the secretory immune system, where they settle down and begin to manufacture IgA.

immediately. In this way, the various MALTs communicate with one another so that immunization on one mucosal surface leads to the production of antibodies with the same specificity on other surfaces. The adaptive advantage of such an intercommunicating system is that newborns of many species receive stimulated antibody-producing cells with the colostrum and milk. The cells seeding the gut of the newborn are those that it needs most, i.e. cells sensitized to antigens of the gut flora, the antigens it is first likely to encounter. Seeding is also advantageous in situations in which a single microorganism infects two sites simultaneously (for example, *Neisseria gonorrhoeae* affects the pharynx and the genital tract); here, seeding ensures the simultaneous production of antibodies at both sites.

Homing of B lymphocytes to the various MALTs is one characteristic of the MIS; another is the dominance of IgA-producing B cells over any other B lymphocytes. This dominance is caused by a specific mucosal cytokine environment. B cells can be prompted to switch to IgA production by the combined effect of transforming growth factor-β (TGF-β), IL-10 and IL-4, TGF-β being the most important component in this cocktail. All these cytokines are produced by mucosal T_H2 cells. The major source of TGF-β and IL-10 are epithelial intestinal cells. Thus cooperation between lymphocytes and epithelial cells in the mucosal microenvironment is essential for the preferential maturation of IgA-committed B cells. The hallmark of mucosal B lymphocytes, regardless of the immunoglobulin isotype they produce, is their expression of the J chain needed for the assembly of oligomeric IgA and IgM molecules. The cytokines responsible for the IgA switch probably also regulate J-chain expression.

The IgA produced in the lamina propria has to traverse the epithelial cell layer to reach the mucosal surface, where it can carry out its function. Crossing represents transcellular transport, during which the dimeric IgA binds to a specialized receptor on the laminal (sub-mucosal) surface of epithelial cells, the complex is endocytosed and the endocytic vesicle is moved across the cell and opened on the opposite side, the luminal surface of the cell (see Chapter 8 for a more detailed description of *transcytosis*; Fig. 8.45). The IgA is then released from the receptor, of which it retains a fragment (the secretory component). The transport receptor is not recycled and so must be continuously synthesized. In some species, such as rabbit and rat, the transport receptor is also expressed on liver parenchymal cells, thus allowing recovery of dimeric IgA from blood and its redirection into the bile and ultimately the intestine. The transport receptor also accepts dimeric IgA with antigen bound to it, an arrangement that has two advantages: it provides the MIS with a mechanism by which it can remove excess antigen and it spreads the antigen to other mucosal surfaces.

Plasma cells residing in the lamina propria produce the bulk of the IgA that appears in secretions (sIgA); the IgA produced in lymphoid tissues of non-secretory organs is discharged into the bloodstream and becomes part of systemic immunity. Some of the IgA produced in the mucosa is transported across the epithelial cells and ends up as sIgA in secretions; the rest forms dimers that are released via the lymphatics and the thoracic duct into the systemic circulation and may be brought secondarily into the secretory organs. The significantly higher concentration of IgA in secretions compared with plasma is probably due to rapid IgA clearance in the latter. In rodents this function is carried out by hepatocytes; in some other mammals, dimeric IgA may be transferred from plasma to secretions in certain epithelia such as the salivary and mammary glands.

Little is known about the *kinetics of the IgA response*, except that in the primary response the antibodies are produced after IgM. In the secondary response, the behaviour of IgA is intermediate between IgM and IgG: although IgA is produced at higher concentrations, its level never approaches that of IgG. Also, the duration of IgA memory appears to be generally shorter than that of IgG (a few weeks to a few months), although instances have been reported in humans in which the memory lasted for several years.

The main functions of IgA antibodies in the *newborn* are the establishment of a balanced normal bacterial flora and protection from pathogenic microorganisms. At birth, mammals are virtually free of microorganisms; however, within a matter of hours the newborn begins to be colonized by many species and strains of bacteria, particularly in the gastrointestinal section of the digestive tract. Only some bacteria entering the digestive tract, those that are either harmless or beneficial to the host, are allowed to colonize it. Selection of the colonizing bacteria is influenced by many factors, including sIgA, which is known to prevent the growth of certain microorganisms.

Some mammals, e.g. cattle and sheep, are born without any antibodies because in these species immunoglobulins cannot pass through the placenta. In other mammals (e.g. humans), some antibodies pass transplacentally to the fetus from the mother, but the immunoglobulin concentration is not sufficient to protect the newborn from infection. In both groups, additional protection is provided by secretory immunoglobulins, particularly sIgA, present in the mother's colostrum (the milk secreted at the termination of pregnancy). The requirement for sIgA in this phase of life is evident from the observation that if colostrum is withheld from calves, many succumb to infection within a short time. Colostrum contains about the same level of sIgA as other external secretions and the predominance of IgA persists even after colostrum has been replaced by milk. However, the longer the mother nurses the young, the more other immunoglobulins appear in the milk.

In many species, the gastrointestinal tract of the newborn is highly permeable to ingested macromolecules. Each species has a characteristic period of high permeability, which can vary from 2–3 days, as in cattle, to 18–20 days, as in mice and rats. The permeability of the tract then gradually decreases with age. In some species, humans for example, the gastrointestinal tract is already largely impermeable at birth. Free passage of macromolecules through the gastrointestinal wall in this critical period is prevented by a number of mechanisms, including the mechanical barrier formed by the mucous coating, degradation of ingested particles by proteolytic enzymes and binding of antigens to IgA. Some of the mechanisms by which IgA and other secretory immunoglobulins protect the adult organism from colonization of the mucosa by pathogenic viruses and bacteria are enumerated below.

To colonize a mucosal membrane, a microorganism must attach itself to the membrane's epithelial cells. IgA may prevent this either by *coating the interaction sites* or by *inhibiting the growth* of the pathogen once attached. The latter is probably accomplished with the help of ancillary factors such as lysozyme or lactoferrin. By binding to the microorganism, IgA may *facilitate its entrapment* in the mucus, or it may *block* some essential step in the reproductive cycle of the microorganism. Direct *killing* of microorganisms requires the participation of complement, but IgA is not able to fix components of the classical complement pathway. To *facilitate phagocytosis*, immunoglobulins must bind to Fc receptors. An IgA receptor (CD89) has indeed been found on monocytes, macrophages and granulocytes. Bacteriolysis and opsonization can be mediated by other antibodies present in the secretion, for example IgG.

sIgA is relatively resistant to proteolysis by intestinal enzymes. However, some pathogens, such as meningococci, gonococci, *Streptococcus pneumoniae* and *Haemophilus influenzae*, secrete a protease capable of selectively cleaving molecules of the IgA1 subclass. Molecules of the IgA2 subclass, on the other hand, lack a sensitive site in the α-chain hinge region, and may therefore represent a form of evolutionary adaptation developed to counter these pathogens. IgA-deficient individuals are generally healthy, however, although they may show increased susceptibility to mucosal infections, certain allergies and autoimmune diseases. Although IgA is apparently not absolutely necessary for survival, as part of the multicomponent MIS it does contribute to the overall fitness of an individual.

IgA molecules are not the only antibodies produced by the MIS. IgM-, IgG- and IgE-producing plasma cells are normally present in the lamina propria and display the same selective localization to mucosal tissues as observed with IgA-producing cells. In persons with selective IgA deficiency, large numbers of IgM plasma cells populate the lamina and sIgM becomes the predominant immunoglobulin class in secretions. In ruminants, IgG-producing cells dominate the lamina and IgG is present in secretions, including milk. Most serum IgE is produced by plasma cells in the mucosal lamina propria and in the draining lymph nodes. IgE is present in secretions of several mucosal tissues such as those of the nose, eye, bronchi and gut. The function of IgM, IgG and IgE antibodies in secretions is unclear. They are not transported nearly as effectively across epithelia as IgA and they are much less resistant to proteolysis, suggesting that they probably play only an auxiliary part in regional immunity.

Cellular immunity

Compared with humoral immunity, much less is known about cellular immunity on mucosal surfaces. The MALT contains lymphocytes, natural killer (NK) cells, macrophages, mast cells and eosinophils. At least some of the lymphocytes, the *intraepithelial lymphocytes* (IEL), seem to be a speciality of mucosae. They are a heterogeneous population containing several types of T cells and NK cells. Many of the IEL T cells express the γ:δ TCR (the proportion of these cells to α:β TCR-bearing cells is species dependent and they appear to be independent of the thymus in their development). Another subpopulation of IEL T cells express the conventional α:β TCR but are phenotypically and functionally different from conventional α:β T cells (see Chapter 16).

The lamina propria contains conventional *lymphocytes*, both T and B cells. Some of the T lymphocytes are helper cells and others are cytotoxic cells. The T_H cells are involved in collaboration with B lymphocytes and probably also with T_C cells. Cytotoxic responses are mounted in the lamina propria against viruses and perhaps also against emerging tumour cells.

Large numbers of *macrophages* are found in many of the mucosal tissues, especially in the lungs and gut. Whether they are in any way specialized and whether they specifically home to these tissues remains unclear. However, they are also found in draining lymph and apparently reach other sites as well. Their ability to present antigen is a matter of contention.

The mucosa contains special *mucosal mast cells*, which differ from connective-tissue mast cells in their histochemical properties, density of Fcε receptors, responses to various antiallergic compounds, their enzyme and proteoglycan content, and in mediators released upon degranulation. The number of mucosal mast cells increases dramatically during nematode infections and during inflammatory bowel disease. The mucosa apparently contains a large number of precursors that can differentiate into mast cells when prompted to do so by inflammatory stimuli. In addition to these cells, the mucosal lamina propria also contains a small number of *eosinophils*. Both mast cells and eosinophils are believed to be involved in the expulsion of parasites from mucosae.

The mediators released by degranulation of stimulated mast cells and eosinophils (mainly histamine and serotonin) cause local increase in blood flow, increased vascular permeability and smooth muscle contraction. These changes lead to fluid accumulation in the surrounding tissue and to an influx of phagocytes and lymphocytes, which then participate in local defence reactions. These reactions may cause diarrhoea or vomiting in the digestive tract, mucus secretion and coughing in the airways, and may contribute to the mechanical expulsion of parasites from mucosal surfaces. The same responses also bring about the allergic reactions described in Chapter 23.

Both the humoral and cellular immune responses

mounted by the MALT are influenced by a number of factors. In addition to those already mentioned (antigen dose, adjuvant, route of antigen administration, nature of the antigen, the affinity of the antigen for certain cells), nutrition, infections, genetic constitution, age, drugs, permeability of the epithelium and the neuroendocrine system also have an effect on mucosal immunity.

Mucosal immune response regulation

A characteristic feature of mucosal exposure to antigens (by ingestion or inhalation) is that it may result in the development of a state of peripheral immunological tolerance. Animals fed or having inhaled antigen do not respond (or their response is much diminished) to the same antigen when it is introduced by the systemic route. This effect is most pronounced for T-cell-mediated responses, especially those of the T_H1 (inflammatory) type. It seems to be an important physiological mechanism by which inflammatory responses against many ingested food proteins are avoided.

Although details of the mechanism are not available, it seems that its critical components are the same T_H cells that govern IgA-based humoral responses. The cytokines produced by these cells (especially IL-4, IL-10 and TGF-β) not only induce IgA switching but also suppress T_H1 cell development. It seems that some of the T_H cells stimulated in the MALT migrate to secondary lymphoid organs outside the MALT where they effectively suppress, upon encounter with antigen, T_H1 responses that would otherwise develop. There are also some indications that IgA antibodies themselves may in some way contribute to the suppression. These conclusions are supported by the observation that mice with 'knocked-out' genes for IL-10 or TGF-β develop inflammatory bowel disease and systemic multifocal inflammatory reactions.

Immunological relationships between mother and fetus (infant)

Fetus tolerance

The immunological fetal–maternal relationship has two aspects: the non-responsiveness of the mother's immune system to antigens borne by the fetus, and the protection of the infant during the time in which its immune system is not fully developed. Since the fetus inherits genes from both parents, it will express antigens that the mother lacks. The question that has long puzzled immunologists is: Why does the mother not react immunologically against the fetus? At least four answers have been proposed. First, it is known that sites in the body exist that are protected from the host's immune attack; when foreign tissues are transplanted into them, the tissues are not rejected (see Chapter 24). It has been suggested that the uterus is one such *immunologically privileged site*. Second, it has also been speculated that the embryo lowers the mother's immunological responsiveness. The lowering could be either specific, affecting only responsiveness to paternal antigens, or non-specific, affecting general immune responsiveness. Third, to avoid the rejection of the fetus, it would suffice if it, or at least the tissue in which the maternal and fetal circulatory systems intercommunicate, did not express any histocompatibility antigens, in particular MHC antigens. Finally, it is possible that the fetus is separated from the mother by a protective barrier that blocks off the mother's immune system. Evidence for all four possibilities has been reported.

From the earliest stage, the embryo is separated from the mother by special tissues that may shield it from an immune attack by the mother's defence mechanisms (Fig. 18.9). In the primary follicles of the ovary, the maturing ovum is surrounded by follicular cells that secrete a thick, translucent, extracellular glycosaminoglycan and proteoglycan coat, the *zona pellucida* (Latin *pellucidus*, translucent; Fig. 18.9a). The ovum remains enveloped in the zona when it leaves the follicle and the ovary; during fertilization, the sperm must first penetrate this protective layer before it can reach the ovum. The zona is shed shortly before implantation of the embryo. It is possible that one of the zona's functions is to shield the antigens of the embryo until further protective layers develop. Supporting this notion is the observation that an embryo that has lost the zona pellucida prematurely becomes susceptible to an immune attack.

At implantation, the embryo acquires a new protective layer. At this stage, the uterine wall consists of two main layers: the thick layer of muscles, or *myometrium* (Greek *mys*, muscle; *metra*, uterus), and the inner mucous membrane, the *endometrium* (Greek *endon*, within). Within a few hours after the embryo has contacted the uterine surface, the epithelial cells at the implantation site begin to loosen and degenerate. At the same time, active growth commences in the mucosa and shortly afterwards an appreciable swelling develops. The swollen mucosa is referred to as *decidua* because it is eventually shed again (Latin *decidus*, falling off). The thick decidual coating of the maternal uterus may act as a temporary immunological barrier during the time of implantation. If it does, the protective action must be limited to the embryo, since other grafts transplanted onto the decidua are apparently rejected.

When it reaches the uterine cavity, the embryo has the appearance of a hollow sphere (blastocyst), differentiated

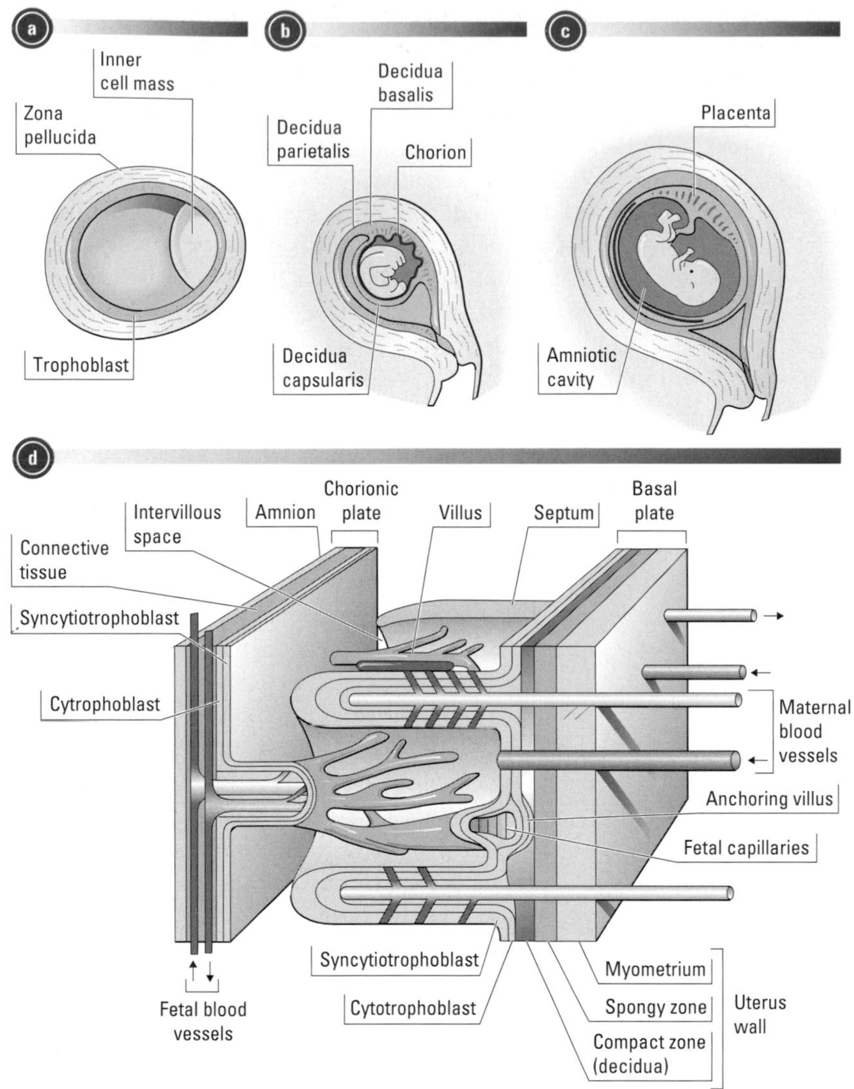

Figure 18.9 Membranes presumably protecting the embryo and fetus from an attack by the mother's immune system. (a) Blastocyst with zona pellucida and trophoblast. (b) Development of the chorion and decidua. (c) Development of the placenta. (d) Contact area between fetal and maternal tissues.

into a knot of cells (inner cell mass) at one pole, with a layer of *trophoblast cells* making up the rest of the sphere's wall (Fig. 18.9a). As the trophoblast contacts the uterine cell wall, the trophoblastic cells proliferate rapidly and form a multinucleate mass in which no cell boundaries are discernible. As the embryo sinks into the uterine wall, it is completely enclosed by the trophoblast, which forms an interface between the maternal and embryonic tissues. The trophoblast is uniquely qualified by its location to act as an anatomical barrier between the mother and the conceptus, provided that it is non-antigenic to the mother itself.

Human trophoblast expresses very few, if any, classical MHC class I and class II molecules. However, it does express a non-classical MHC class I protein, HLA-G, which, as far as is known, is unable to present peptides to T_C lymphocytes but which confers resistance to NK cells (as noted in Chapter 16, NK cells attack cells lacking MHC class I molecules). Interestingly, NK cells have been implicated in some cases of spontaneous abortion.

In the later stages of embryonic development, the outermost fetal membranes (trophoblast, chorion, allantois; Fig. 18.9b) fuse with part of the uterine mucosa to form an organ of metabolic exchange between fetus and mother, the *placenta* (the Latin name for a cake, used in reference to the organ's characteristic shape; Fig. 18.9c). In the placenta, fetal and maternal blood vessels are apposed, yet clearly separated: fetal and maternal blood do not mix (Fig. 18.9d). Electron microscopic studies reveal that many cells on the fetal side of the placenta, particularly the giant trophoblastic cells, are surrounded by a layer of amorphous, electron-dense *fibrinoid material*, varying in thickness from 0.1 to 2 µm and composed of glycosaminoglycans and proteoglycans rich in hyaluronic and sialic acids. Some immunologists believe that the fibrinoid layer of the placenta masks histocompatibility antigens of the embryo, preventing their recognition by maternal immune cells. Supporting this interpretation is the observation that dissolution of the fibrinoid by neuraminidase increases the antigenicity of trophoblastic cells. Additional isolation is provided by the absence of classical MHC molecules on the surfaces of the trophoblast and the placenta, which are directly exposed to maternal blood. However, the barrier between the fetus and the mother is not impenetrable. Using chromosomal markers or radioactively labelled cells, investigators have repeatedly demonstrated the presence of fetal cells in the mother's blood and in some cases also of maternal cells in the fetal circulation; some limited exchange of cells, particularly blood elements (erythrocytes, leucocytes and platelets), must therefore occur across the placenta. Additional evidence for the exchange of cells is the fact that the serum of multiparous women often contains antibodies to red blood cell (Rh) and leucocyte (HLA) antigens. The production of such antibodies is presumably induced by cells or cell fragments that originate in the fetus and are brought by blood into the mother's lymphoid organs.

Some insight into the mechanisms suppressing an attack by the maternal immune system against the fetus was obtained in experiments with transgenic mice. These were females naturally expressing H2-K^k MHC molecules on their cells and genetically manipulated by gene transfer to express, on all their T lymphocytes, homogeneous TCRs specifically recognizing the H2-K^k protein loaded with a peptide derived from the H2-K^b molecule. Since nearly all T cells of the transgenic female were directed against a potential paternal alloantigen, the effects of pregnancy on the T cells could easily be followed. This is obviously not possible in non-transgenic females, in which only a small fraction of all T cells recognize paternal alloantigens. The transgenic females that were mated with H2-K^b males and therefore carried H2-K^b-expressing fetuses strongly downregulated expression of TCRs by mid-gestation and lost expression of the CD8 co-receptor on most T cells. By contrast, TCR-transgenic females mated either to syngeneic (H2-K^k) or 'third party' (H2-K^s) males showed no such changes in their T-cell phenotype. TCR and CD8 expression returned to normal levels in the postpartum period, indicating that these effects were reversibly regulated. The results indicated that the maternal immune system is not isolated from the fetal antigens but is aware of the presence of the allogeneic fetus. However, this awareness does not lead to attempts to destroy the foreign tissues but rather to specific reversible switching-off of the T cells potentially harmful to the fetus. In these experiments, small amounts of fetal cells could be detected in the maternal circulation (these presumably induced the effects observed) but no maternal cells could be found in the fetus. The molecular mechanism of this pregnancy-specific immunosuppression is not known.

Yet another factor potentially contributing to the suppression of an attack on the embryo by the maternal immune system is the immunosuppressive protein *fetuin*, which substitutes for structurally similar serum albumin in the fetal blood. The mechanism of this immunosuppressive activity is not known.

Protection of the newborn by the maternal immune system

In mammals, the mother can provide immunological protection for her developing offspring in two ways: through the placenta, when the fetus is still in her body, or with colostrum and milk after birth. The relative importance of these two systems varies from species to species and is determined by a variety of factors, one of the most important of which is the structure of the placenta, in particular the number of placental membranes. In mammals with a large number of membranes (e.g. the horse), there is very little, if any, transfer of immune elements across the placenta and protection is provided by the colostrum. In species with fewer placental membranes (e.g. primates and rodents), the placental route of transfer is more important than the colostral. In species with an intermediate number of membranes (e.g. cat and dog), both routes contribute significantly to the immunological protection of the fetus and newborn.

Transfer across the placenta concerns almost exclusively immunoglobulin molecules. The fetus is normally protected from antigenic stimuli while in the uterus and so the transfer of antibodies from maternal to fetal circulation must be regarded as preparation for life after birth. (The fetus will respond by antibody production, however, if the mother is infected with an agent such as rubella virus, cytomegalovirus or *Toxoplasma* that can cross the placenta.) The type of antibodies that cross the placenta depends on a number of factors, in particular the quantity and quality of the antibodies themselves. In humans, for example, antibodies against diphtheria toxin, tetanus toxin, erythrogenic toxin, staphylococci, flagellar antigens of *Salmonella*, streptolysin, and viruses such as rubeola, rubella, mumps and polio cross the placental wall easily. On the other hand, antibodies against *H. influenzae*, *Bordetella pertussis*, *Shigella flexneri* and certain streptococci cross the placenta poorly. No transplacental transfer has been demonstrated for antibodies against *Escherichia coli* and syphilis. The feasibility of transplacental transfer, however, also means that not only protective but also harmful autoantibodies find their way into the fetal circulation and damage the embryo. Generally, only certain subclasses of IgG antibodies can cross the placenta.

Colostrum and milk provide the infant with sIgA antibodies, in addition to other protective molecules and cells. Most of the IgA antibodies that the suckling receives are directed against intestinal microorganisms and antigens. Resistance to the action of proteolytic enzymes allows IgA antibodies to pass unharmed through the infant's entire digestive system and to reach their destination in the intestine. The immediate availability of IgA antibodies may be one of the factors explaining the lower incidence of enteric and respiratory infections, as well as the significantly diminished colonization of the intestine by *E. coli* in breast-fed vs. bottle-fed infants. Whether the cells of the colostrum and milk can also survive passage through the stomach and thus transfer cellular immunity to the infant is not known.

Further reading

Dunkley, M., Pabst, R. & Cripps, A. (1995) An important role for intestinally derived T cells in respiratory defence. *Immunology Today*, **16**, 231–236.

Erle, D.J. (1995) Scratching the surface. *Current Biology*, **5**, 252–254.

Hunt, J.S. (1992) Immunobiology of pregnancy. *Current Opinion in Immunology*, **4**, 591–596.

Lefrancois, L. & Puddington, L. (1995) Extrathymic intestinal T-cell development: virtual reality? *Immunology Today*, **16**, 16–21.

Mostov, K.E. (1994) Transepithelial transport of immunoglobulins. *Annual Review of Immunology*, **12**, 63–84.

Ogra, P.L., Mestecky, J., Lamm, M.E., Strober, W., McGhee, J. R. & Bienenstock, J. (Eds) (1994) *Handbook of Mucosal Immunity*. Academic Press, San Diego, CA.

Poussier, P. & Julius, M. (1994) Intestinal intraepithelial lymphocytes: the plot thickens. *Journal of Experimental Medicine*, **180**, 1185–1189.

Sim, G.-K. (1995) Intraepithelial lymphocytes and the immune system. *Advances in Immunology*, **58**, 297–344.

Simpson, E. (1996) Why the baby isn't thrown out . . . *Current Biology*, **6**, 43–44.

Staats, H.F., Jackson, R.J., Marinaro, M., Takahashi, I., Kiyono, H. & McGhee, J.R. (1994) Mucosal immunity to infection with implications for vaccine development. *Current Opinion in Immunology*, **6**, 572–583.

Steinman, R.M. (1991) The dendritic cell system and its role in immunogenicity. *Annual Review of Immunology*, **9**, 271–296.

chapter 19 Immune response regulation

One of the main features of the adaptive immune response is its capacity for rapid amplification. Because it is clonal, the response nearly always begins modestly but advances rapidly to involve a large number of cells and molecules. The ability to amplify, however, brings with it the danger of over-reaction. Like milk in a saucepan, the immune system can easily boil over. Expansion of the stimulated clones may not stop in time, secretion of soluble substances may continue unchecked and large numbers of cells may be dispatched to the wrong places. On the other hand, the system must not under-react either because then the response might not be adequate to deal with the stimulus. Since both over-reaction and under-reaction may have catastrophic consequences, the immune system needs to be tightly controlled to provide an adequate response at all times. Not one but several *regulatory mechanisms* control the immune response. Some of these have already been mentioned in the preceding chapters; others are discussed here.

Antigen regulation

Lymphocytes removed from an immunized individual and placed in a culture dish that contains everything the cells need for their growth will proliferate for only as long as the immunizing antigen is present. Withdraw the antigen from the culture and the divisions stop; add it again and proliferation resumes. T lymphocytes can be cycled in this manner for a long time and used to establish long-term cell lines or clones. Establishing long-term cultures of B lymphocytes is more difficult but presumably only because the right ingredients necessary for B-cell growth have not yet been concocted.

A similar process of cycling presumably also occurs in the body. As long as antigen is available, a response is mounted; when the supply is exhausted, the response stops. The antigen is therefore the primary regulator of the adaptive response for both T and B lymphocytes. This makes sense, since the antigen provides the first signal in the lymphocyte activation process and without the antigen lymphocytes normally are not stimulated.

It must be remembered, however, that the whole system changes profoundly through exposure to the antigen: memory T and B cells remain in the body after the antigen has disappeared (or only traces of it remain) and the immune reactions have waned. Thus memory cells govern any subsequent responses to the reappearance of the antigen.

Cytokine and cell–cell contact regulation

In addition to antigen, lymphocytes need various soluble or membrane-bound cytokines as well as direct contact with other cells for their activation and proliferation. For example, helper T (T_H) cells must receive additional signals from antigen-presenting cells (APCs) and from cytokines produced by activated T_H cells themselves. B lymphocytes must receive accessory signals from T_H (and probably also from follicular dendritic) cells. A cytokine can have both a stimulatory and an inhibitory effect, depending on the target cell. For example, interleukin (IL)-4, transforming growth factor β (TGF-β) and IL-10 produced by T_H2 cells inhibit the development of T_H1 but not T_H2 cells; interferon γ (IFN-γ) produced by T_H1 cells, on the other hand, inhibits the development of T_H2 but not T_H1 cells. These differential regulatory effects of cytokines seem to determine which kind of immune response will be used to deal effectively with a particular pathogen (see Chapters 16 & 17).

An important form of negative regulation is the self-destruction of cytotoxic T (T_C) cells. One of their weapons, the surface cytokine-like glycoprotein FasL, interacts with the 'death receptor' Fas on the same cell or on another T_C cell and delivers an apoptotic signal that brings to an end the T_C cell's short life (see Chapter 16).

Antibody regulation

Mechanism

Some of the most efficient regulatory elements of the humoral immune response are the antibodies themselves. They regulate via the mechanism of feedback, by which they can either downregulate (dampen) or upregulate (enhance) the response. *Downregulation* can be demonstrated by inoculating antibodies into an animal that is actively producing antibodies of the same specificity. Administration of antibodies prior to, at the time of or after inoculation of the antigen suppresses the humoral response. Administration later than 24 hours after immunization has little effect on the primary IgM response, although the IgG secondary response may be suppressed. The duration of suppression depends on the biological half-life, amount and class of the injected antibodies. Both IgM and IgG can suppress antibody response, although IgM can sometimes have the opposite effect: it may increase the response of mice to suboptimal doses of sheep erythrocytes. Enhancement, rather than suppression, has also been noted in several other systems, and the effect of the antibodies has been found to depend on the circumstances of the response (the particular antigen, antibody, presence of antigen–antibody complexes and so on). *Upregulation* of the response can be demonstrated by replacing the plasma of animals producing antibodies at a high rate by plasma of non-immunized individuals. The reduction of antibody concentration promptly increases the rate of antibody synthesis.

Suppression of antibody production occurs by one of at least two mechanisms: antigen blocking and receptor cross-linking (Fig. 19.1). *Antigen blocking* occurs as a result of competition between antibodies and the B-cell receptor (BCR). Antibodies bind to the antigen, masking its epitopes and making them unavailable to the BCR, and hence lowering the B-cell response. Antigen blocking occurs at high antibody concentration and does not require the participation of the Fc regions. *Receptor cross-linking* occurs when an antibody binds with its Fc region to the Fc receptor on the B cell and with its combining site to the antigen; the same antigen then binds with another epitope to the BCR on the same B cell. The cross-linking of the Fc and immunoglobulin receptors by immune complexes brings the tyrosine phosphatase PTP-1C associated with the Fc receptor CD32 to the vicinity of the BCR, which counteracts the activating effects of the tyrosine kinases associated with the cytoplasmic domain of the BCR complex (see Chapter 17, Fig. 17.2). Antibodies also regulate an important phase of the antibody response by driving affinity maturation in germinal centres: the antibody binds the antigen, thus lowering its concentration. As a result only BCRs with the highest affinity can compete with the free immunoglobulin molecules (see Chapter 17).

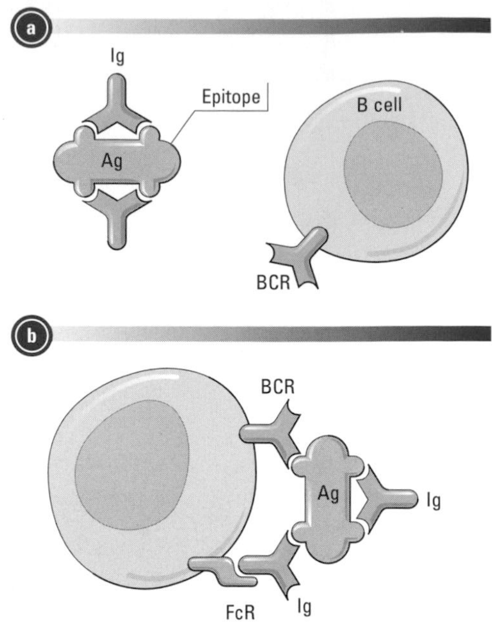

Figure 19.1 Regulation of B-cell response by antibodies. In *antigen blocking* (a), all the epitopes on the antigen (Ag) are occupied by antibodies so that fresh B cells have nothing to bind to. In *receptor cross-linking* (b), each B cell binds antigen (in the form of an immune complex) via its B-cell receptor (BCR) as well as via its Fc receptors (FcR). This joint cross-linking generates a negative signal blocking proliferation (see also Fig. 17.2).

Idiotype-specific antibody regulation

Idiotypes are the epitopes of the V region on BCRs, free immunoglobulin or T-cell receptors (TCRs) (see Chapter 8). Here the discussion is limited to idiotypes of antibodies, but much of it also applies to BCR and TCR molecules.

Consider an antigen, or more generally a ligand and an antibody against this ligand (*antibody 1*; Fig. 19.2a).

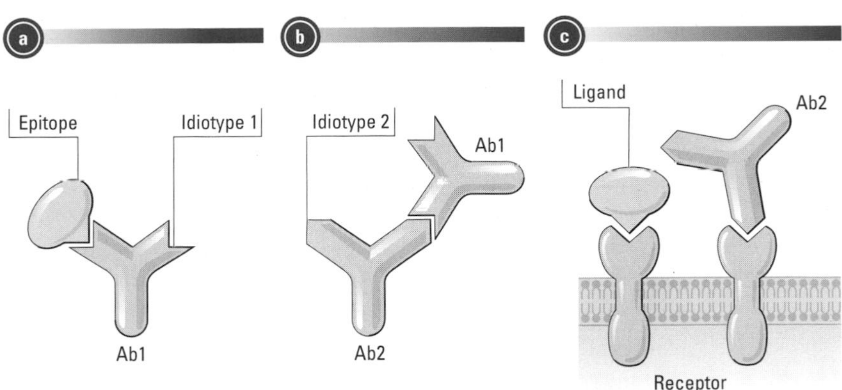

Figure 19.2 Idiotype-specific antibodies mimicking antigenic epitopes. For explanation see text. Ab, antibody.

Consider further an antibody against antibody 1, which we shall call *antibody 2* (Fig. 19.2b). The combining site of antibody 1 is complementary to a structure (epitope) on the immunizing antigen (ligand). The combining site of antibody 2, in turn, is complementary to a portion of the combining site of antibody 1. Therefore, the combining site of antibody 2 should resemble the epitope of the immunizing antigen. Antibody 2 can be said to carry an *internal image* of the external antigen and thus masquerades as antigen. It does not mean, of course, that all type 2 antibodies will resemble the immunizing antigen, but some should, and indeed they do. Many examples have been described in which an antibody can replace a receptor's ligand in its physiological action (Fig. 19.2c).

One of the first such examples reported involved insulin. Antibodies were produced against insulin and used to produce type 2 (idiotype-specific) antibodies. The latter antibodies were shown to be able to bind to insulin receptors (and hence mimic the ligand, insulin) and even to stimulate glycolysis by activating the receptor-bearing cells. Similar experiments have been carried out with thyroid-stimulating hormone, prolactin, glucocorticoids, vasopressin, glucagon, acetylcholine, endorphins, catecholamines, dopamine, retrovirus and retinol-binding protein. In all these instances, the idiotypic antibodies were shown to act on the corresponding receptors and to mediate specific physiological effects normally initiated by the ligands. The retrovirus haemagglutinin is a particularly telling example of ligand mimicry. It has been shown that the haemagglutinin has a region in which the amino acid sequence closely resembles a sequence in the V_L region of the idiotype-specific antibody.

This aspect of idiotype research is expected to have considerable clinical relevance in providing a new method of immunization: instead of immunizing with a microbial antigen, one might be able to immunize with an idiotype-specific antibody. The advantages of such *surrogate vaccines* are that the vaccine does not contain the pathogen itself, a highly effective monoclonal antibody can be produced in large quantities, and the vaccine can be aimed at selected epitopes (e.g. epitopes shared by various viral strains that often do not produce effective immunity themselves). The feasibility of this approach has been demonstrated in experimental animals. For example, chimpanzees have been immunized against rabbit antibodies specific for idiotypes on human antibodies, which were specific for surface antigens of the hepatitis B virus. Immunization resulted in protection of the chimpanzees against subsequent infection with the virus. Less spectacular results were obtained when idiotype-specific antibodies were used to control the growth of B cell tumours. Here, the main problem is that while the antibody may prevent the growth or even eliminate B cells bearing the idiotype, the population of tumour cells contains variants that have lost the particular idiotype on their BCR and these rapidly take over. Another problem, which concerns all clinical applications of idiotypic antibodies, is how to avoid the patient's immune response against the idiotype-specific antibodies, which generally have to be obtained from an animal. This problem could be overcome, however, by some of the new methods of antibody engineering described in Chapter 8.

The degree to which idiotype-specific antibodies regulate specific immune response remains an open question. Such antibodies have been reported to stimulate B lymphocytes in some situations and yet inhibit them in others, without the participation of antigen. Inoculations of idiotype-specific antibodies into animals, particularly newborns, have been reported to cause either suppression or enhancement of antibody response to an antigen that the idiotype-bearing antibody normally recognizes. These antibodies have also been claimed to recognize idiotypes on the TCR and to activate T lymphocytes.

Network hypothesis

It can be imagined that idiotopes of the idiotype-specific antibodies can again elicit the production of another generation of antibodies, which produce yet another generation and so forth. This line of thought has led to the formulation of the *network hypothesis*, which postulates that idiotype-specific interactions are of key importance in the development and regulation of the immune system. The hypothesis has stimulated a great deal of theoretical work. Sophisticated mathematical models have been developed describing the immune system as a regulated network of idiotypic interactions. Depending on the adjustment of initial parameters defining the functional effects of these interactions, these models strive to describe how the immune system ought to behave. However, the initial enthusiasm of some immunologists as regards the potential of these models seems to have waned for two reasons. First, great progress has been made in the elucidation of other, more direct regulatory mechanisms (cytokines and their receptors, adhesion and signalling membrane molecules, intercellular interactions). Second, it has been extremely difficult to design unambiguous experiments that would test the network hypothesis. At present, this ambitious hypothesis is not much more than an interesting theoretical possibility, whose explanatory value for real-life phenomena remains dubious.

Antigenic competition

Normally, an individual is capable of responding simultaneously to many different antigens. There are some situations, however, in which the response to one antigen influences the response to another. For example, rabbits immunized against a foreign serum produce antibodies against globulins but not against albumins, although both proteins are present in the inoculum. To obtain albumin-specific antibodies, the rabbits must be immunized against albumin alone. This phenomenon, in which the response to one *dominant antigen* (globulin) inhibits the response to a *suppressed antigen* (albumin), has been termed *antigenic competition*. There are two principal kinds of antigenic competition, intermolecular and intramolecular.

In *intermolecular competition*, the two competing antigens are present on two different molecules. In *sequential competition*, the animal responds to the first antigen administered but not to the second. *Intramolecular competition* occurs when the two competing epitopes are carried by the same molecule.

Antigenic competition can be explained by interference at the level of antigen processing and presentation. The peptides produced in the APC from one protein or from different proteins may bind with different affinity to major histocompatibility complex (MHC) class II molecules. Competition between the peptides for binding to MHC molecules may result in different densities of the various peptide–MHC molecule assemblies. Since the density of the complexes may be critical in the stimulation of T_H1 or T_H2 cells, the humoral response to a particular antigen may be either stimulated or suppressed. Only a few useful peptides are produced by the APC from any antigen and their size and yield can be profoundly influenced by several factors, such as the type of APC, the form of antigen used for immunization, the simultaneous presence of other antigens in the APC, and the agonistic vs. antagonistic character of the peptides (see Chapter 16).

Immune suppression

To *suppress* means to keep from appearing, to restrain or to subdue. It implies the existence of latency, a potential that is prevented from expression by an active process. Immunologists speak of suppression each time an immune response does not appear when, in theory, it should. Suppression is therefore a broad term that can be applied to a number of different situations and to a variety of mechanisms.

The ability to suppress immune responses has been ascribed to three major members of the immune system: B lymphocytes, macrophages and T lymphocytes. Suppression by *B lymphocytes* may occur, for example, when antibodies produced by one set of B cells coat the antigen and thus make it unavailable for other B cells. The lymphocytes in the second set then fail to respond to the masked antigen: they appear to be suppressed, although in reality their unresponsiveness is simply due to the lack of antigen in an appropriate form. This example illustrates that, superficially, a phenomenon may be interpreted as suppression when in fact it is nothing of the sort. Suppression by *macrophages*, on the other hand, could be a true subduing of a response, in certain situations at least. Activated macrophages are known to produce substances such as thymidine, polyamine oxidase, complement components, prostaglandins, cyclic AMP and various cytokines including IFN-α, all of which can have, under certain circumstances, an inhibitory effect on the immune response. Each of the substances inhibits the response by a different mechanism. *Thymidine*, for example, is produced when macrophages ingest and degrade large amounts of DNA from dying cells. At high concentrations, thymidine is incorporated into the cells and inhibits their proliferation. *Polyamine oxidase* acts on the polyamines spermine and spermidine normally present in fetal and neoplastic tissue, converting them into aminoaldehydes that inhibit the growth of a wide variety of cells. *Complement components* may, upon activation, lyse immune cells. *Prostaglandins, cyclic AMP* and *IFN-α* may interfere with the activation of lymphocytes and of other cells, each in its own way.

When immunologists discuss suppression, however, they usually mean inhibition of the immune response by *T lymphocytes*. Many functional tests over the past 30 years have indicated that some T cells enhance while others suppress the immune response (Fig. 19.3). The helper cells were usually found to be present in the fraction of T lymphocytes carrying the CD4 marker, while the suppressor cells were present in the fraction of lymphocytes carrying the CD8 marker. These observations were interpreted to

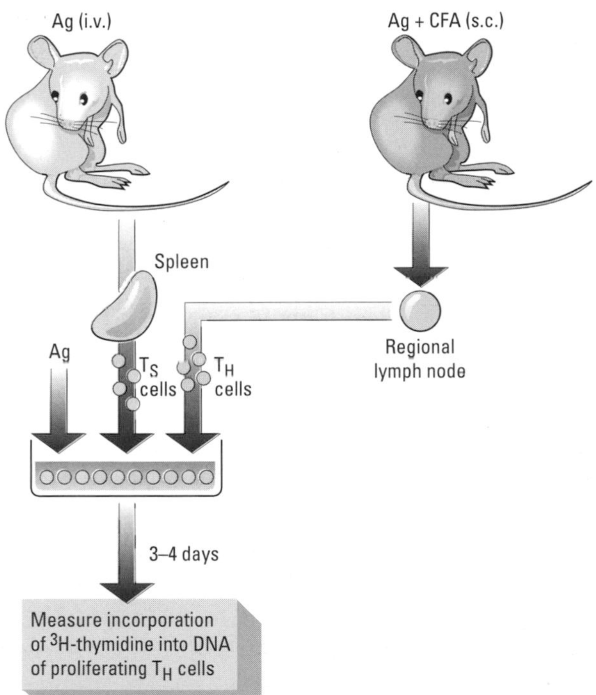

Figure 19.3 Functional assay used to demonstrate the presence of suppressor T (T_S) lymphocytes. Two different immunization protocols are applied to recipient mice: one, in which the antigen (Ag) in physiological salt solution is introduced intravenously (i.v.), is believed to activate preferentially T_S cells; the other, in which antigen is administered in complete Freund's adjuvant (CFA) subcutaneously (s.c.), is known to activate proliferation of helper T (T_H) cells. The mixture of lymphocytes obtained from these two donors is cultured for 3–4 days and the proliferation of T_H cells measured. Lowering of the proliferative response in comparison with a culture of T_H cells without T_S cells is taken as evidence for suppression.

mean that there were two types of regulatory T cells, T_H (CD4+) and T_S (CD8+). Further studies of CD4+ cells led to elucidation of their helper mechanisms: these cells were demonstrated to recognize, via their TCRs, MHC class II molecules loaded with antigenic peptides and then to send stimulatory signals via soluble cytokines and membrane-bound proteins. By contrast, it has proved much more difficult to elucidate the molecular mechanisms responsible for the suppressive effects of CD8+ T cells. The problem was to find cell-surface markers that would distinguish T_S from T_C cells. Although several markers have been *claimed* to be T_S-cell specific, none of these claims has been substantiated. The best known among the presumed T_S-cell markers was the *J* (or *I-J*) *antigen* in the mouse. The antigen was claimed to be controlled by a separate locus within the *H2* complex, the mouse *MHC*, specifically in the region between the *Ab* and *Eb* loci (the 'J' designation was used as the next available letter of the alphabet to name what was then believed to be a new region of the complex). However, molecular biologists have failed to find any coding sequence in the *J* region, and biochemists have failed to isolate and characterize any product using antibodies believed to be specific for the antigen. (The antibodies were produced by cross-immunization between mouse strains thought to be genetically identical except for a difference at the *J* locus. Here again, however, molecular biologists failed to find any difference between these strains.)

Two kinds of T-cell-mediated suppression have been described, non-specific and specific. *Non-specific suppression* occurs when T cells stimulated by one antigen inhibit the response of lymphocytes to this and virtually any other antigen. This form of suppression is based on the fact that certain T lymphocytes probably produce soluble factors that shut off other cells. Among these are cytokines (IL-10, TGF-β), prostaglandins, cyclic AMP, or some similar substances already implicated in suppression by macrophages. It is the specific suppression that remains the bone of contention.

Specific suppression occurs when T_S cells activated by a particular antigen inhibit the response of other T cells to this and no other antigen. Specific T_S cells were supposed to act by way of *soluble specific suppressor factors* (T_SF). Several such factors have been described for responses to different antigens, but their nature, and indeed their existence, remains doubtful. T_SF have been claimed to bind the antigen or hapten specifically, the response to which they suppress, and to be structurally related to the TCR. T_S cells have been hypothesized to act mainly on T_H cells, but the proposed mechanisms remain speculative.

In spite of the inability to demonstrate convincingly the existence of T_S cells as a specific, separate T-cell lineage and despite ambiguities in the interpretation of their activities, suppression mediated by CD8+ T cells appears to be real: purified CD8+ T cells from animals that have been rendered unresponsive (tolerant) to an antigen by a specific immunization protocol can suppress the *in vitro* or *in vivo* immune response in other, genetically identical animals; in other words the unresponsiveness can be adoptively transferred (see Fig. 19.3). Depletion of CD8+ T cells prevents induction of oral tolerance and leads to more severe disease in some autoimmune disorders. CD8+ T cells are responsible for the pathologically low T_H1 response in some leprosy patients. How can all these reproducible observations be explained?

One possibility is that T_S cells are not fundamentally different from T_C cells. T_C cells may suppress immune responses by killing either antigen-specific T_H cells or APCs exhibiting antigenic fragments on their surface. In the former case, peptides derived from the variable region of the TCR bound to MHC class I molecules could be recognized by T_S cells on the surface of specific T_H cells. (This situation would be somewhat similar to the idiotype-specific regulatory interactions of B cells.) Another possibility is that activated T_H cells may pick up and internalize antigenic fragments recognized on APCs and re-express them on their own surfaces where they might be recognized by other T cells. Activated human T cells do indeed express large numbers of MHC class II molecules whose function remains unclear.

Yet another possibility is that T_S cells are in fact the T_C cell precursors that were made unresponsive by the recognition of antigenic fragments on cells other than professional APCs. Such cells may exert their suppressive activity by competing with properly activated T_C cells for the available antigen or by secretion of inhibitory cytokines and other mediators. There is good evidence that subsets of CD8+ T_C cells analogous to CD4+ T_H1 and T_H2 cells exist that differ in the cytokines produced. Antigen-specific clones of CD8+ T cells that secreted TGF-β and inhibited the development of T_H1 cells have been obtained from patients with lepromatous leprosy. Furthermore, the mechanism of oral tolerance may be based on intestinal CD8+ T cells which, after recognition of the antigen in the mucosa-associated lymphoid tissue, become stimulated to secrete suppressive cytokines, migrate to lymph nodes and block the development of T_H cells.

Immune system–neuroendocrine regulation

In addition to regulatory mechanisms inherent in the immune system itself, there are also regulatory interactions between the neural, endocrine and immune systems. These interactions occur at several levels. Lymphoid organs are richly innervated so that a direct contact exists between neurons and leucocytes. Neurotransmitters, especially noradrenaline, secreted by nerve endings bind to receptors expressed at low levels on leucocyte surfaces and in this way initiate signalling in these cells. Direct interactions between the various types of leucocytes and neurons are possible because both cell types have in common several surface receptors for cytokines and neuropeptides in common. Leucocytes also express receptors for several hormones produced by endocrine glands. Among the best-known examples are corticosteroids, products of the adrenal gland, which have marked immunosuppressive properties. They are used therapeutically to suppress the rejection of transplanted organs or to mitigate autoimmune diseases (see Chapter 24). Corticosteroids are known to induce apoptosis in thymocytes and to inhibit activation of mature T cells; CD4+ T cells are more sensitive to them than CD8+ T cells. The anti-inflammatory effects of corticosteroids can be explained by the inhibitory activity on T_H1 cells. Corticosteroids are also known to influence the migratory behaviour of lymphocytes, mainly their interactions with endothelial cells. Since the production of corticosteroids by the adrenal gland is regulated by a pituitary gland hormone (adrenocorticotropic hormone, ACTH), the production of which is in turn regulated by hypothalamic releasing factors, the immune system can be partially regulated by the brain.

A number of other hormones and neuropeptides are known to act via specific receptors on the cells of the immune system. They include endorphins, growth hormone, thyroid hormones, substance P and ACTH (see Chapter 21). Some of these hormones also appear to regulate indirectly the development of thymocytes by influencing the secretion of thymic peptide hormones, such as thymulin, produced by thymic epithelial cells. The size and activity of the thymus is also influenced by sex hormones. Elevation of circulating oestrogens causes thymic atrophy; age-related involution of the thymus can be partially reversed by castration; and marked transient involution of the thymus occurs during pregnancy and is reversed when lactation ceases. Similarly, production of B cells in the bone marrow is inhibited during pregnancy. These observations may explain the dependence of some autoimmune diseases on the sex and age of afflicted individuals. Regulatory effects of neuropeptides on the immune system are exploited by some parasites: the hookworm *Schistosoma mansoni* produces proopiomelanocortin-derived peptides that have immunosuppressive effects.

Influences in the opposite direction, from the immune to the neuroendocrine system, also occur. Many cytokines and other soluble products of leucocytes can act on neurons and endocrine glands. The most striking example is the action of IL-1, tumour necrosis factor α (TNF-α) and IL-6 on hypothalamic neurons and pituitary cells. These cytokines induce the secretion of releasing factors for pituitary hormones such as ACTH. IL-1 and IL-6 also regulate body temperature via brain receptors (see Chapter 21). Leukaemia inhibitory factor (LIF) mediates local neurotransmitter switching in nerve endings. Finally, many endocrine hormones and neuropeptides (endorphins, ACTH, thyroid stimulating hormone, growth hormone, substance P, vasoactive intestinal peptide, oxytocin) are actually produced in small amounts by the cells of the immune system.

Several important surface molecules, mainly adhesion receptors, are shared by neurons and leucocytes. The Thy-1 glycoprotein is an abundant neuronal molecule in many species and a major T-cell surface marker in rodents (but not in humans). A form of the neuronal cell adhesion molecule N-CAM, called CD56, is present on natural killer cells; the CD4 co-receptor molecule of T cells is expressed at a low level in the brain. Interestingly, all these molecules are members of the immunoglobulin superfamily.

These regulatory relationships have been claimed to underlie the mental effects on the resistance of the organism to infections. Various types of stress, including emotional stress, are known to affect immunological parameters such as the ratio of lymphocyte subsets in circulation or phagocytic activity of macrophages. The mainly negative effects on immunity can be explained by stimulation of the hypothalamic–pituitary–adrenal axis resulting in increased concentration of immunosuppressive corticosteroids. Claims that concentration of 'mental energy' or 'positive thinking' can positively contribute to defence of the organism against disease are hard to take seriously.

Further reading

Blalock, J. E. (1994) The immune system—our sixth sense. *Immunologist*, **2**, 8–15.

Bloom, B.R., Modlin, R.L. & Salgame, P. (1992) Stigma variations: observations on suppressor T cells and leprosy. *Annual Review of Immunology*, **10**, 453–488.

Bloom, B.R., Salgame, P. & Diamond, B. (1992) Revisiting and revising suppressor T cells. *Immunology Today*, **13**, 131–136.

Franco, A., Ishioka, G.Y., Adorini, L. *et al.* (1994) MHC blockade and T-cell receptor antagonisms. Strategies for immunomodulation. *Immunologist*, **2**, 97–102.

Hayday, A. (1995) Is antigen-specific suppression now unsuppressed? *Current Biology*, **5**, 47–50.

Immunology Today, vol. 15, no. 11 (1994) Immune–neuroendocrinology special issue.

Jameson, S.C. & Bevan, M.J. (1995) T cell receptor antagonists and partial agonists. *Immunity*, **2**, 1–11.

Kemeny, D.M., Noble, A., Holmes, B.J. & Diaz-Sanchez, D. (1994) Immune regulation: a new role for the CD8+ T cell. *Immunology Today*, **15**, 107–110.

Kos, F.J. & Engleman, E.G. (1996) Immune regulation: a critical link between NK cells and CTLs. *Immunology Today*, **17**, 174–176.

Lombardi, G., Sidhu, S., Batchelor, R. & Lechler, R. (1994) Anergic T cells as suppressor cells *in vitro*. *Science*, **264**, 1587–1589.

Perelson, A.S. (1989) Immune network theory. *Immunological Reviews*, **110**, 5–36.

Seder, R.A. & Paul, W.E. (1994) Acquisition of lymphokine-producing phenotype by CD4+ T cells. *Annual Review of Immunology*, **12**, 635–674.

Wilder, R.L. (1995) Neuroendocrine–immune system interactions and autoimmunity. *Annual Review of Immunology*, **13**, 307–338.

chapter 20 Immunological tolerance

Concept

The vertebrate immune system anticipates (theoretically at least) *all* possible epitopes, even those borne by the body's own molecules. Cells capable of recognizing these self epitopes must be purged from the repertoire or silenced to avoid an attack on self tissues (Fig. 20.1). After purging, individuals become *immunologically unresponsive* to or *tolerant* of self components. *Immunological tolerance* is thus the lack of ability to mount an immune response to epitopes to which an individual has the potential to respond. In most natural situations, immunological tolerance concerns self molecules: an individual that expresses receptors for self epitopes normally never uses them to mount an immune response. In experimental situations, however, the immune system can be fooled into regarding foreign antigens as self and hence into becoming tolerant of non-self epitopes. Most past inquiries into the nature of immunological tolerance have, in fact, been carried out by inducing unresponsiveness to foreign molecules. Underlying these studies has been the assumption that the mechanism of self tolerance is the same as that of induced tolerance. In recent years, however, methods for studying self tolerance have become available and insights into this process have been obtained.

Experimental observations

Experimental studies have shown that certain conditions favour tolerance induction, while others lead to immunity. A brief description of these conditions follows.

State of lymphoid system

It is easier to induce tolerance in animals with an immature lymphoid system or with a lymphoid system damaged by irradiation, drugs, thoracic duct drainage or antilymphocytic serum treatment compared with untreated mature animals. As we discussed in Chapter 3, the lymphoid system matures over a period of time, which varies from species to species. The more mature the system, the more difficult it is to render unresponsive. Fully mature animals *can* be made tolerant, however, provided that one of two conditions is fulfilled. First, the animal's immunocompetence has to be inhibited temporarily by one of the treatments that damage the lymphoid system, and antigen has to be given during that time; when treatment has been discontinued, the system has recovered and full immunocompetence has been regained, the animal remains unresponsive to the administered antigen. Second, the antigen must be given in either a non-immunogenic form or by a non-immunizing route (see below).

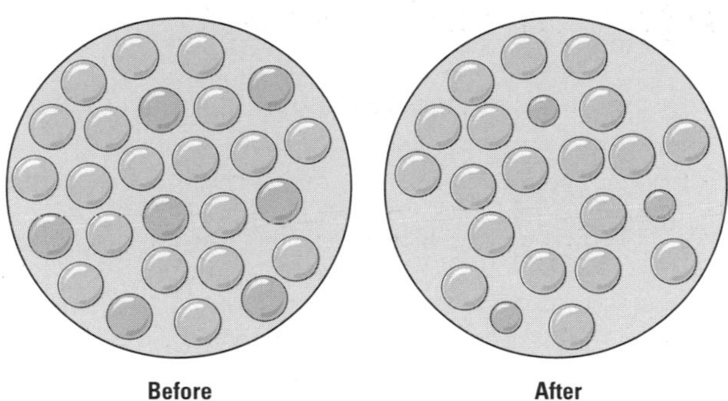

Figure 20.1 Principle of immunological tolerance. *Before* tolerance is induced, the lymphocyte repertoire of an individual (large circle) contains clones with receptors for foreign antigens (small pink circles) but also clones with receptors for self molecules (small grey circles). *After* tolerance is induced, the repertoire is purged of self-reactive clones either by physical elimination of some of them or by incapacitation of others (the smaller grey circles).

Physicochemical properties of antigen

An important feature determining whether a given antigen will induce responsiveness or unresponsiveness is the size of the molecule. The effect of size is particularly conspicuous with antigens that occur in both polymeric and monomeric forms and with antigens that form aggregates. An example of the former is flagellin from *Salmonella adelaide* (see Chapter 13). Polymerized flagellin (POL), which has a relative molecular mass (M_r) of 10^7, is a potent immunogen, inducing T-independent responses almost exclusively. Monomeric flagellin (MON), which has an M_r of 40 000, induces responsiveness when administered at low doses and unresponsiveness when administered at high doses. Fragment A, which is obtained by cyanogen bromide cleavage of MON and has an M_r of 18 000, is tolerogenic at all doses. The difference between the three forms is not that they present the host with different epitopes, since all three forms consist of the same repeating subunits, but exclusively in the size of the molecule.

Many serum proteins (e.g. albumin or γ-globulin) form aggregates spontaneously when left in an aqueous solution, and the speed of aggregation is increased by heating. The aggregates can be removed by ultracentrifugation so that two forms of the protein can be obtained: aggregated and deaggregated. The two forms have different effects on the immune system: aggregated proteins are strongly immunogenic, whereas deaggregated proteins promote the induction of tolerance. Previously immunized animals, however, respond equally well to aggregated and deaggregated proteins, and an immunogenic dose of aggregated protein can be prevented from immunizing an animal when administered simultaneously with a large dose of deaggregated protein. On the other hand, deaggregated proteins can be made immunogenic by incorporation into adjuvants.

Certain compounds are by nature strong *tolerogens*, substances capable of inducing tolerance. A good example is provided by the D-amino acid polymers, which induce tolerance over a wide range of doses, in contrast to L-amino acid polymers, which are immunogenic at these same doses. Furthermore, pretreatment of animals with the tolerogenic form often prevents the formation of antibodies to haptens presented on an immunogenic carrier. For instance, mice given an injection of dinitrophenyl conjugated to a polymer of D-glutamic acid and D-lysine (DNP-D-GL) fail to make antibodies to DNP when subsequently given an injection of DNP conjugated to the immunogenic carrier, keyhole limpet haemocyanin. A slight modification of a molecule may often convert it from an immunogen to a tolerogen. For example, following acetoacetylation MON becomes tolerogenic, even at doses that normally induce immunity.

Epitope density

Variation in the number of epitopes on a molecule may sway lymphocytes from one state to another. For example, when DNP-POL is added to spleen cells in culture, the response of the lymphocytes will depend on the number of DNP groups per flagellin molecule. At a density of about 0.7 DNP groups per molecule, a good anti-DNP response is observed over a wide range of antigen concentrations; at a density of about 2.7 DNP groups per molecule, a good antibody response is observed at intermediate concentrations; and finally, at a density of 3.8 DNP groups per molecule, all antigen concentrations induce tolerance.

Antigen dose

Low antigen doses often induce tolerance, intermediate doses induce immunity and high doses induce tolerance (Fig. 20.2). There are thus two kinds of tolerance, low-zone and high-zone; some investigators also distinguish an ultra-low-zone tolerance, induced by minute quantities of antigen. *Low-zone tolerance* can be induced by frequent inoculation of subimmunogenic doses of antigen over long periods of time. In the original demonstration of low-zone tolerance, bovine serum albumin was inoculated into mice three times a week for up to 16 weeks. In newborns, low-zone tolerance can be induced by a wide variety of antigens, whereas in the adult only a few antigens are known to work. However, low-zone tolerance to many antigens can be induced in adults that have been irradiated, thymectomized or otherwise compromised immunologically. Low-

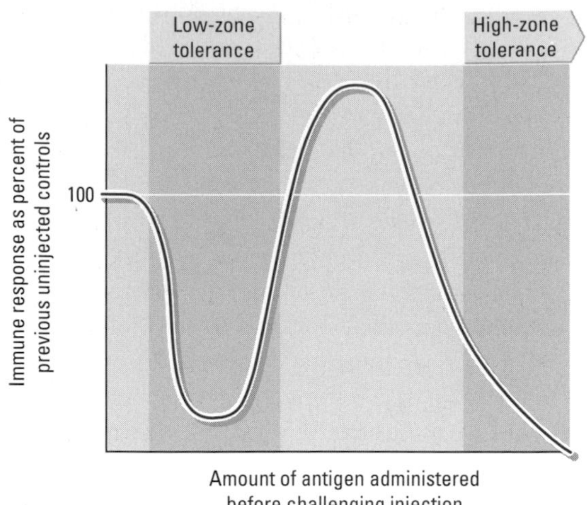

Figure 20.2 Effect of antigen dose on the induction of tolerance (dark grey region) or immunity (light grey region). The antigen dose and the level of response are not specified.

zone tolerance is probably a T-cell phenomenon, since T cells are apparently more susceptible to tolerization by low antigen doses than are B cells. We return to this point later.

Mode of antigen presentation

The route of antigen administration is probably more important with adult animals than with newborns. The route of injection determines accessibility of the antigen to antigen-presenting cells (APCs) which, as has already been mentioned, is one of the major factors influencing the choice between tolerance and immunity. Macrophage-bound antigen is highly immunogenic: for example, only about one-thousandth as much macrophage-bound bovine serum albumin as unbound antigen is required to immunize a mouse. Removal or paralysis of macrophages often facilitates tolerance induction. A change in the route of administration may sometimes convert an immunogen into a tolerogen. For example, when aggregated serum proteins, which are normally immunogenic, are injected into the hepatic portal vein, they are quickly brought into the liver; there the aggregates are removed by Kupffer cells and the rest of the antigen passes in an aggregate-free form into the circulation, where it induces tolerance. An example of how certain routes of antigen administration preferentially lead to unresponsiveness is *oral tolerance* (see Chapter 19). Feeding an animal with an antigen induces unresponsiveness to subsequent challenge by the same antigen given intravenously or by other routes.

Genetic make-up of the recipient

The genetic influence on the ease of tolerance induction is exemplified by the inbred mouse strains BALB/c and C57BL/10. The former strain is relatively resistant to tolerance induction by xenogeneic γ-globulin; the latter is relatively easy to make tolerant. In crosses between BALB/c and C57BL/10, tolerogenicity segregates among the offspring, indicating that it is genetically controlled.

Experimental T- and B-cell tolerance

The principle of tolerance is that lymphocytes that would normally recognize a particular antigen and mount a response are prevented from doing so. Since two types of lymphocytes recognize antigen, we must ask: Can both T and B lymphocytes be made tolerant? A simple experiment answers this question. Neither T nor B lymphocytes from a tolerant animal are capable of collaborating with their non-tolerant opposites when transferred into irradiated recipients (Fig. 20.3). Therefore, in an experimental situation at least, tolerance affects both T and B cells. However, there are certain differences in the way these two cell types respond to tolerization. T lymphocytes are tolerized almost instantaneously after the administration of tolerogen, and

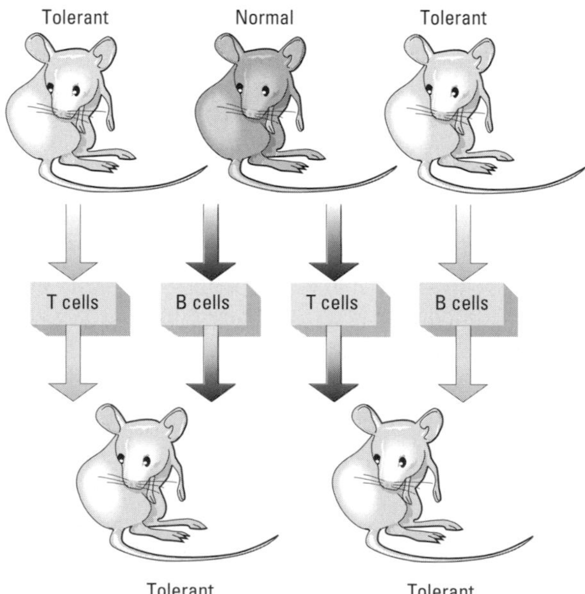

Figure 20.3 Experiment demonstrating the existence of both T-cell and B-cell tolerance. Neither T nor B cells from tolerant mice are capable of collaborating with T or B cells from a non-tolerant mouse, when the cell mixture is inoculated into lethally irradiated recipients and then challenged with the antigen (tolerogen).

certainly no later than within a few hours, whereas tolerization of B lymphocytes takes at least a day or two. There is also a difference in the tolerogenic dose between the two lymphocyte types: 100–1000 times higher doses of tolerogen are generally required to tolerize B cells than to tolerize T cells. High-zone tolerance can therefore be both a T- and B-cell affair, whereas low-zone tolerance affects T lymphocytes only. Even so, T-cell tolerance is of much longer duration, lasting for months, than B-cell tolerance, which lasts several weeks only. This last difference can probably be explained by the more rapid renewal of B lymphocytes compared with T cells. As soon as the tolerogen is cleared from the body, newly generated B lymphocytes are no longer tolerized, and the animal gradually regains its ability to respond immunologically to the antigen. Even at the highest doses of administered tolerogen, B cells are often not fully tolerized, probably because the bone marrow continuously generates B lymphocytes with the potential of responding to the antigen.

One way of demonstrating absence of B-cell tolerance is by showing that B cells from a tolerant animal can collaborate with non-tolerant T cells. Another way is to stimulate the B cells with either a mitogen, such as lipopolysaccharide (LPS), or with a T-independent antigen. It could be shown, for example, that mice tolerant of DNP conjugated to human γ-globulin (HGG) do not respond to subsequent injections of DNP-HGG, but do form DNP-specific antibodies when challenged with DNP-POL. In this situation, B cells have apparently recovered from tolerance and helper T (T_H) cells have not, but the latter are replaced in their helper effect by the T-independent antigen.

Tolerance completeness and termination

Experimentally induced tolerance is seldom complete, in particular as far as the B-cell compartment is concerned. Tolerant animals often produce small amounts of antibody, especially if the tolerogen is a complex molecule. If one tolerizes with a mixture of proteins (e.g. normal serum) in which some proteins are present in a higher concentration than others, tolerance to some components of the mixture and immunity to others may be induced. However, even a single epitope is not recognized by one lymphocyte clone, but by several clones bearing receptors with different affinities. Since affinity of receptor–antigen binding probably influences tolerance induction, some of the clones might become tolerant and others not. The completeness of tolerance will then depend on the proportion of tolerant and non-tolerant clones.

When tolerance is measured simultaneously by a number of parameters, it can sometimes be detected by one assay but not another. Such a *split tolerance* has been observed, for example, upon the injection of tuberculin followed by the injection of the bacillus Calmette–Guérin into guinea-pigs. The animals are tolerant when tested by the delayed-type hypersensitivity assay (see Chapter 23) but they produce antibodies to the tuberculin. Split tolerance sometimes also occurs in regard to different immunoglobulin classes. In some cases, split tolerance can be explained by differential regulation of the immune response leading, for example, to a shift from predominantly T_H1 to predominantly T_H2 response.

Induced tolerance is not permanent. After induction it gradually wanes and, if the animal lives long enough, is eventually lost. The duration of tolerance depends on many factors, one of the most important of which is the continual presence of the tolerogen. Although a single dose of serum protein may render newborn mice tolerant for several months, the tolerance eventually terminates spontaneously. To prolong the duration of the tolerant state, one must repeatedly rechallenge the animal with the tolerogenic form of the antigen. Replicating antigens such as the cell-surface alloantigens on proliferating cells in lymphoid chimeras may induce lifelong tolerance.

Tolerance can also be terminated experimentally, most commonly by the injection of an antigen that cross-reacts with the antigen to which the host is tolerant. For example, if bovine serum albumin (BSA) is injected into newborn rabbits and human serum albumin (HSA) inoculated into the tolerant animals some time later (HSA is known to cross-react with BSA to a small extent), the rabbits produce antibodies to HSA. If the animals are now challenged with BSA, they will also produce BSA-reactive antibodies, although before the injection of HSA they produced none (Fig. 20.4). The BSA-reactive antibodies are directed against epitopes shared between BSA and HSA. Since the animal produced no BSA antibodies before HSA was injected (it was tolerant of all epitopes, including the shared ones), the administration of HSA must have partially terminated tolerance of BSA. However, the animal remains tolerant of BSA-specific epitopes, even when repeatedly challenged with BSA. In fact, the production of antibodies to the shared epitopes gradually decreases, and eventually the animal returns to a state of full unresponsiveness to all BSA epitopes. The mechanism of termination of partial tolerance is not known. Administration of HSA seems to lead to the bypassing of the T-cell block, which is responsible for the absence of help necessary for B-cell stimulation.

Cross-reactive antigens can also induce termination of natural tolerance of the body's own molecules. An example

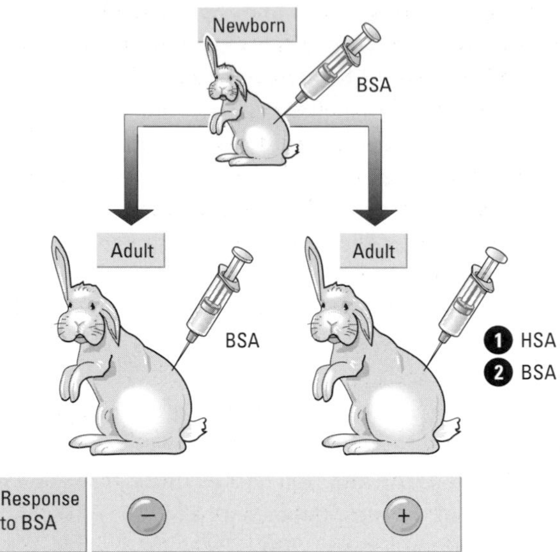

Figure 20.4. Termination of tolerance by inoculation with a cross-reactive antigen. Rabbits made tolerant of bovine serum albumin (BSA) will respond to this antigen if they are later challenged with a dose of human serum albumin (HSA) before the inoculation with BSA. The response to BSA is directed against epitopes this antigen shares with HSA.

of this is the induction of antibodies to thyroglobulin, a hormone produced by the thyroid. When thyroglobulin of one species is injected into an animal of another species, the latter begins to produce antibodies to epitopes shared by the two thyroglobulins and hence, in fact, against self molecules.

Tolerance can also be terminated by the administration of chemically altered antigens or by non-specific stimulation accomplished by the administration of lectins, antigen–antibody complexes (e.g. tolerogen combined with xenogeneic antibodies to a cross-reactive antigen) and allogeneic cells capable of inducing graft-vs-host reaction (see Chapter 24). The non-specific stimulants probably activate T_H cells, which then provide non-specific help to immunocompetent B cells. For example, when mice are made tolerant of HGG and then 90 days later, at the time when T cells are still tolerant of HGG but B cells are not, HGG and LPS (a B-cell mitogen that replaces T-cell help) are injected into the recipients, the animals begin to produce HGG-specific antibodies (Fig. 20.5). Injection of either HGG or LPS alone has no effect on the tolerance status of the animals.

Experimental observations on self tolerance

Is the immune system normally non-reactive to an individual's own components simply because the potentially self-reactive clones of B and T lymphocytes have been eliminated? Or are the self-reactive clones present but suppressed and hence unable to respond?

Immunologists have probed the tolerant vs. non-tolerant status of B lymphocytes using at least three methods. First, they tested the sera of healthy, not intentionally immunized animals for the presence of autoreactive antibodies (i.e. immunoglobulins that react with self components) and invariably found them. Mouse serum, for example, was shown to contain antibodies reacting with mouse thyroglobulin, α-fetoprotein, complement component 5, serum albumin, actin, tubulin, myoglobin, fetuin, transferrin, cytochrome *c*, collagen and DNA, as well as those reacting with mouse erythrocytes, thymus cells, brain extracts, skin extracts and stomach cells. Autoantibodies have been found for virtually every self component tested. They occur at such a low concentration, however, that they

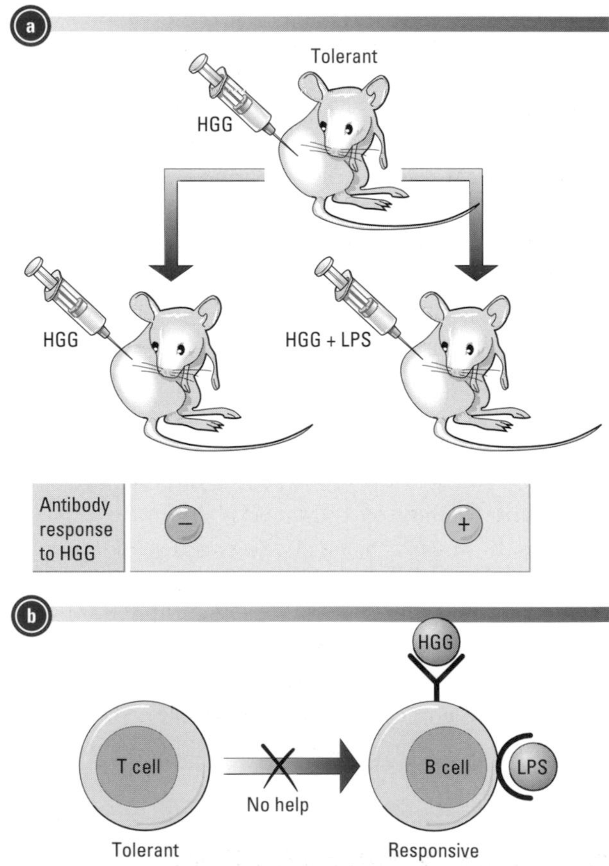

Figure 20.5 Termination of tolerance by inoculation with bacterial lipopolysaccharide (LPS) along with the antigen (human γ-globulin, HGG). (a) Experimental protocol. (b) Mechanism. At the time when B cells are no longer tolerant (but T cells are), LPS, together with the antigen, provides the signals necessary to activate the B cell in the absence of help from T cells.

cause no harm and in fact may be beneficial, for example in the clearance of ageing and decaying self components.

In the second method, B lymphocytes were distributed into the wells of a plastic plate in such a way that each well contained only one cell (while some contained, in these *limiting dilution conditions*, no cells at all), expanded into a clone by the addition of a mitogen such as LPS, and the receptor specificity of the clone was then tested. These experiments have revealed that individuals not only possess B lymphocytes specific for self antigens, such as albumin or myosin, but also that the frequency of such cells is not significantly lower than that of B cells with receptors for foreign forms of these components (e.g. a mouse has about the same number of B cells with receptors for mouse serum albumin as it does for rabbit serum albumin).

The third method of examining B-cell tolerance consisted of stimulating B lymphocytes with a mitogen, fusing the activated cells with an appropriate tumour cell and screening the produced hybridomas for secretion of autoreactive antibodies. This approach has also demonstrated the presence in healthy individuals of B lymphocytes capable of producing antibodies against self components.

At first glance, these observations seem to indicate that self-reactive B lymphocytes are not eliminated from the immune system. Nevertheless, as we discuss later, these findings may have other explanations.

As far as T lymphocytes are concerned, immunologists agree that they must become tolerant of self, but it is still not known whether this applies to all or only some T lymphocytes. The presence in healthy individuals of T cells capable of being stimulated by self molecules such as thyroglobulin, collagen and myelin basic protein has been demonstrated. However, these proteins are relatively sequestered in the tissues and are present in the circulation only in very low concentrations. Nobody has succeeded in demonstrating the presence of T cells that could be activated by self proteins such as serum albumin or γ-globulin, which are present at high concentrations. These observations suggest that although some T_H cells may not be tolerant of self (or their tolerance state can easily be overcome), many T_H cells have either been eliminated by the tolerance-induction process or are in a state in which they cannot be activated.

Mechanisms of natural (self) and experimentally induced tolerance

Considerable light has been shed on the mechanism of tolerance by experiments involving transgenic mice. Two types of transgenic mice have been used, distinguished by the nature of the transgenes. In one type, the transgene encoded antigen-specific receptors (T-cell receptor (TCR) or B-cell receptor (BCR)) of known specificity; in the other, it coded for a well-defined protein antigen such as hen egg lysozyme or ovalbumin. The transgenes contained promoters that ensured expression in selected tissues only. Thus, the TCR transgene was expressed in T cells only, the BCR transgene in B cells and the ovalbumin transgene in either liver, thymus or pancreatic β cells. The intensity of transgene expression was regulated by the type of promoter used, so that the animal would express ovalbumin in the liver in either massive or trace amounts. Moreover, double transgenic mice, expressing ovalbumin and TCR specific for an ovalbumin peptide for example, have also been produced.

Experiments with transgenic as well as with more conventional animal models have identified several factors involved in the maintenance of self tolerance and of experimentally induced tolerance of foreign antigens. A brief description of these factors follows.

Limited access of the immune system to some autoantigens

Some components of the body are shielded from the immune system by an anatomical barrier so that lymphocytes normally never reach them. One example is the *blood–testis barrier* in the male reproductive organs (Fig. 20.6). The testis is covered by a connective tissue capsule and is divided by partitions projecting from this capsule into 200–400 wedge-shaped lobes. Within each lobe there are from three to ten coiled seminiferous tubules, which produce the germ cells. The spaces between the tubules are filled with connective tissue, blood vessels and a network of thin-walled lymphatic capillaries. Each tubule is surrounded by a basement membrane that, together with the layer of nursing (Sertoli) cells on the luminal side, forms a barrier that prevents the penetration of cells and large molecules from blood. When testicular tissue is injected into an animal or when the testis is damaged by inflammation, the immune system does not recognize it as self and attacks it.

Another example is the *blood–brain barrier* formed by the walls of brain capillaries (Fig. 20.7). These walls lack the openings present in other capillaries, their endothelial cells overlap so that in some places the wall is two cells thick and the capillary is surrounded by a basement membrane as well as by cytoplasmic extensions of astrocytes. The walls are impassable not only for cells but also for many large molecules and the free exchange that exists in other tissues between capillaries and the surrounding fluid is extremely limited in the brain.

Other self components occur in such small amounts

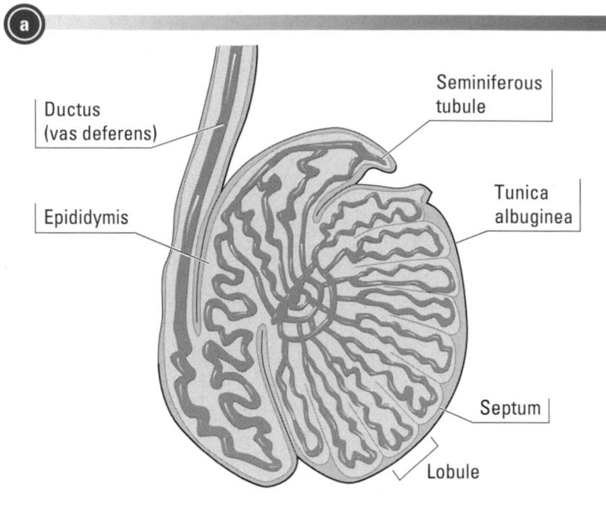

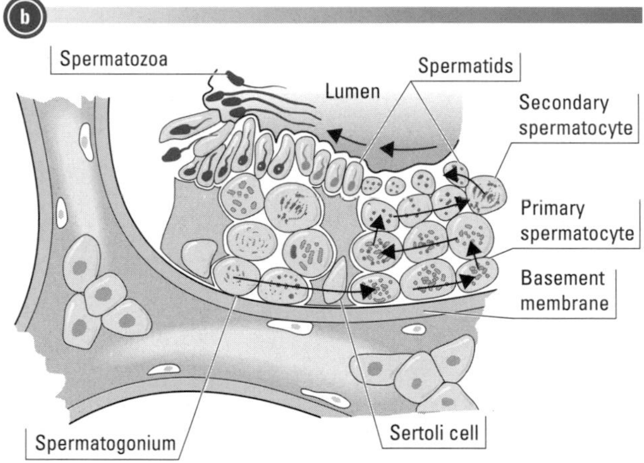

Figure 20.6 Blood–testis barrier. (a) Anatomy of the testis. (b) Cross-section through a portion of a seminiferous tubule. The blood–testis barrier, which is formed by the basement membrane and the tight apposition of Sertoli cells, isolates the developing spermatozoa from the cells of the immune system.

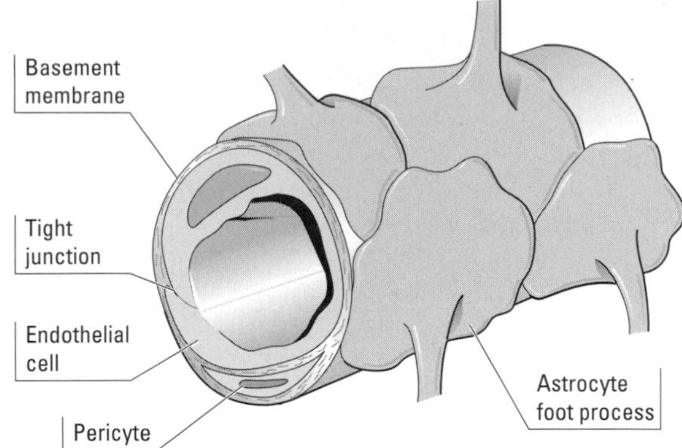

Figure 20.7 Blood–brain barrier. The brain capillary is surrounded by foot processes of astrocytes (supporting cells of the nervous tissues). The pericyte is a contractile, elongated cell wrapped around precapillary arterioles. The endothelial cells of the capillary are the main barrier to free passage of cells from the capillary into the surrounding tissue of the brain.

that they are all but ignored by the immune system. Lymphocytes can be activated only when a threshold concentration of antigen is reached. The concentration of certain self components may simply be too low for lymphocyte stimulation. An example is provided by thyroglobulin, a large glycoprotein that serves as a carrier of the hormones thyroxine and triiodothyronine in the thyroid gland. The main structural components of the gland are the numerous tiny sacs or follicles (Fig. 20.8). The wall of each follicle consists of cells closely packed together and surrounded on the outside by a thin membrane and a dense network of blood capillaries. The cells produce hormones that bind thyroglobulin in the viscous fluid inside the follicle. When the need for the hormones arises, the follicular cells ingest tiny droplets of the fluid, degrade the thyroglobulin into component amino acid residues and release the small hormone molecules into the bloodstream. Thyroglobulin is therefore largely confined to the interior of the thyroid gland follicles and is thus inaccessible to the immune system. Although the sequestration is not complete, the level of thyroglobulin in the bloodstream is far too low to elicit an immune response. It may not be a coincidence, however, that when something goes wrong with tolerance of self, the thyroid, more specifically thyroglobulin, is frequently the target of an attack.

Similarly, when only minute amounts of a foreign protein are produced by a transgenic mouse, this protein is ignored by the immune system. The immune system therefore contains a number of potentially self-reactive lymphocyte clones against inaccessible or rare autoantigens. Activation of these clones under special conditions is the most frequent cause of autoimmune diseases (Chapter 25).

Elimination and inactivation of self-reactive lymphocytes during their development

Most thymocytes expressing TCRs that recognize self peptides bound to major histocompatibility complex (MHC) proteins on the surface of thymic epithelial and dendritic cells are eliminated during development in the thymus via the process of negative selection (see Chapter 5). In this way the immune system rids itself of most precursors of potentially autoreactive cytotoxic T (T_C) and T_H1 cells and precursors of those T_H2 cells that could help B lymphocytes

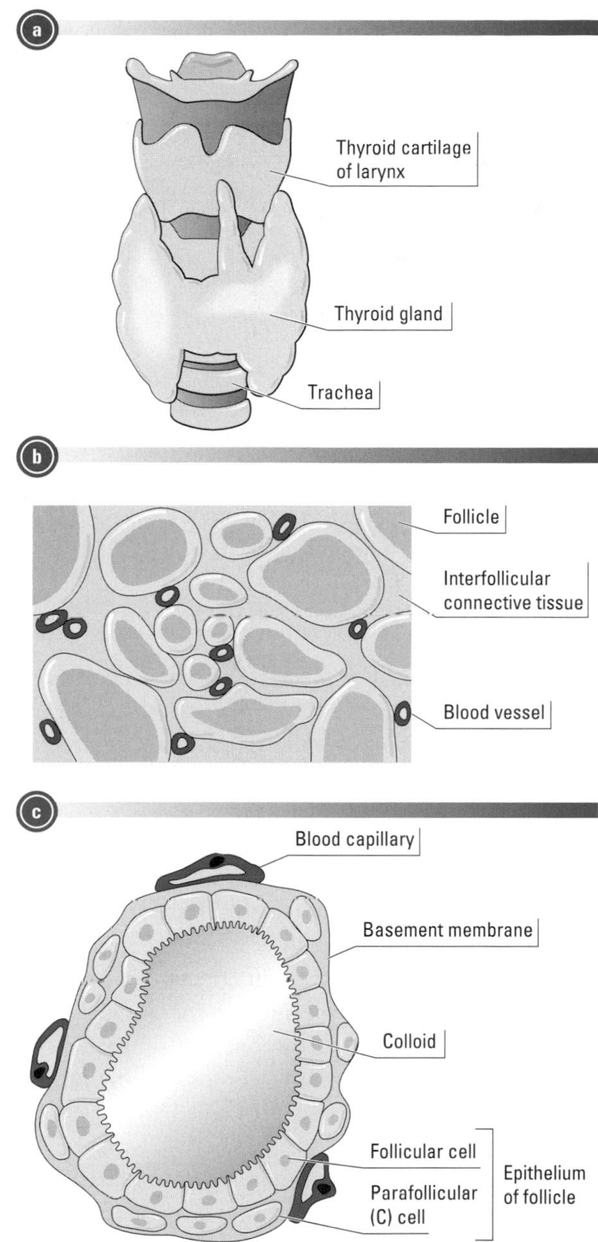

Figure 20.8 Thyroid gland. (a) Location. (b) Section through the gland. (c) Single thyroid follicle.

recognize ubiquitous autoantigens. Potentially autoreactive T cells that have escaped elimination in the thymus mainly because they recognize peptides poorly represented in this organ, and presumably also T cells that mature extrathymically (the γ:δ T cells, some intestinal epithelial T cells), are functionally inactivated (anergized) by contact with non-professional APCs lacking the necessary co-stimulatory molecules.

Most self-reactive B cells are inactivated or physically eliminated by apoptosis after recognition of autoantigens in the absence of co-stimulation by specific T_H cells, which have been eliminated in the thymus. B cells are especially prone to inactivation during the early stages of their development, when they express the BCR of the IgM isotype only. A B-cell's encounter with any substance that can bind strongly to its BCR during this stage either induces apoptotic suicide or anergy. The need for help from antigen-specific T_H cells is another safeguard against inappropriate activation of autoreactive B cells. Thus both T and B cells are eliminated when they recognize substances during their early stages of development and both are rendered anergic when they do not receive second signals—B cells from T_H cells and T cells from professional APCs.

B cells that have encountered a self component are also excluded from homing into lymphoid follicles, which are essential for their expansion and differentiation. Ligation of BCRs by self components in the absence of help from T_H cells seems to alter the B-cell surface (perhaps the expression of some adhesion molecules), which handicaps these cells in competition with other B cells for the limited space in lymphoid follicles. As a result, these autoreactive B cells do not receive the required survival signals and die.

Inactivation of mature T cells

To be stimulated, precursors of T_C and T_H cells must encounter antigen on the surface of professional APCs expressing CD80 (B7), CD86 and possibly other co-stimulatory molecules. If the precursor T cells encounter antigens on the surface of other cells, they will become non-reactive (anergic) and sometimes die by apoptosis. This is probably the major mechanism responsible for the experimental induction of tolerance by administration of the antigen in specific tolerogenic ways and for the extrathymic inactivation of T cells that recognize tissue-specific antigens not available in the thymus. For example, if a small amount of soluble, deaggregated foreign antigen is administered to a mouse intravenously, it is bound and internalized by naive antigen-specific B lymphocytes. These subsequently internalize the BCR–antigen complex, digest it into peptides and re-express some of the peptides on the cell surface bound to MHC class II molecules. The complexes are recognized by precursors of T_H cells and provide a negative signal because of a lack of co-stimulatory molecules on the B-cell surface. By contrast, an aggregated antigen or an antigen in an emulsion with adjuvant is taken up mainly by professional APCs, which provide all the positive co-stimulatory signals necessary for the proliferation and differentiation of T_H

cells. Some cancer cells may express antigens that could be potentially recognized by T cells (see Chapter 22), but since they do not have the co-stimulatory properties of professional APCs they do not stimulate the development of mature effector T_C or T_H cells: instead they paralyse the T-cell precursor.

The anergy caused by T-cell stimulation without co-stimulatory receptor engagement can be partially reversed by the addition of exogenous interleukin (IL)-2. Anergic T cells themselves are not necessarily inactive. They may secrete cytokines such as IL-4 after receiving only one of the necessary two signals.

The absence of co-stimulatory signals from the CD28 receptor is not the only method of delivering an incomplete, tolerogenic signal to a T cell. Others include blocking of the CD4 or CD8 co-receptor molecules and interaction with antagonistic rather than agonistic peptide–MHC assemblies (see Chapter 16).

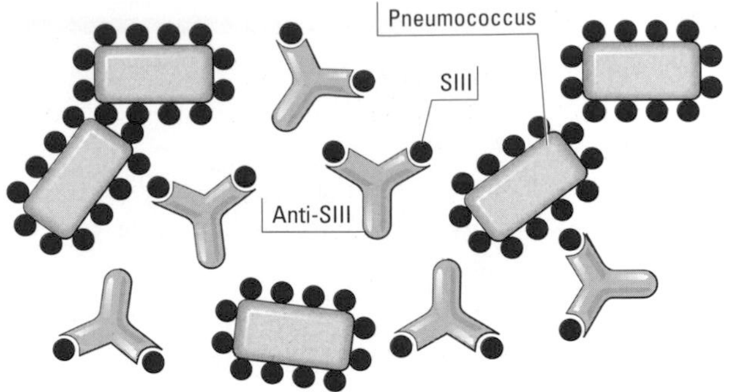

Figure 20.9 Immunological paralysis. In this special case of immunological unresponsiveness, the organism is flooded with such a high dose of the antigen (pneumococcal polysaccharide type III, SIII) that all the antibodies produced against it are busy clearing it and very few are left to deal with the inoculated bacteria (pneumococci). The bacteria multiply unopposed and the animal succumbs to the infection.

Other tolerance mechanisms

T cells that become anergic as a result of their encounter with antigen on cells other than professional APCs may have a regulatory function. They may compete for the antigen on the APC surface with cells of similar specificity and they may produce suppressive cytokines. They can therefore be responsible, at least in part, for the observed antigen-specific suppression.

Mice that receive a single injection of antibodies specific for the CD4 and CD8 co-receptor molecules and simultaneously receive either a skin graft from a genetically different strain or a protein antigen become tolerant of the antigen: they fail to reject the skin graft or to produce antibody against the protein antigen. If T cells from an untreated animal are then injected into a tolerant recipient, they not only do not cause rejection of the graft (i.e. they are 'overcome' by the suppressors) but gradually become suppressors themselves, as if suppression were contagious. This phenomenon, referred to as *infectious tolerance*, is highly specific for the original antigen used for the immunization. Its mechanism is not known, but one possibility is that blocking of the CD4 or CD8 co-receptor interaction with MHC molecules results in incomplete signalling and leads to T-cell anergy. The latter is accompanied by the production of suppressive cytokines that stimulate the development of anergic T cells in their vicinity. These may then be responsible for the spreading of the antigen-specific tolerance in the recipient that has received T cells from the untreated donor.

There are several experimental situations in which a certain treatment renders an animal unresponsive to the administered antigen, but the mechanism is probably different from that involved in tolerance of self components. These forms of unresponsiveness are sometimes referred to as *pseudotolerance*. Two examples are exhaustive immunization and immunological paralysis.

In *exhaustive immunization*, the antigen challenge is so great that all B cells capable of recognizing the particular antigen may be stimulated to differentiate into end-stage antibody-producing cells without the generation of memory cells. Such differentiation effectively exhausts the supply of B lymphocytes specific for the antigen, so that there is no memory and no response to subsequent challenges with this same antigen. Unresponsiveness caused by clonal exhaustion has been described for certain T-independent antigens.

A classical example of *immunological paralysis* is the lack of protection against pneumococci in the mouse, observed upon injection of high doses (180 mg/mouse) of pneumococcal polysaccharide type III (SIII; Fig. 20.9). However, the recipients are only outwardly unresponsive; in reality, they produce antibodies that combine immediately with the persistent non-degradable polysaccharide, thus failing to protect the animal. The paralysed animals have the same frequency of antibody-forming cells as animals into which a low dose of SIII is inoculated and which are protected against the bacteria. Immunological paralysis can be turned into high-zone tolerance, however, if the antigen dose is increased to 250 mg/mouse. After such treatment, SIII-reactive antibody-forming cells are no longer detected in the spleen of the immunized animals.

Further reading

Charlton, B., Auchincloss Jr, H. & Fathman, C.G. (1994) Mechanisms of transplantation tolerance. *Annual Review of Immunology*, **12**, 707–734.

Cornall, R.J., Goodnow, C.C. & Cyster, J.G. (1995) The regulation of self-reactive B cells. *Current Opinion in Immunology*, 7, 804–811.

Goodnow, C.C. (1992) Transgenic mice and analysis of B-cell tolerance. *Annual Review of Immunology*, **10**, 489–518.

Kroemer, G. & Martínez, C. (1992) Mechanisms of self tolerance. *Immunology Today*, **13**, 401–404.

Lenschow, D.J. & Bluestone, J.A. (1993) T cell co-stimulation and *in vivo* tolerance. *Current Opinion in Immunology*, 5, 747–752.

MacLennan, I.C.M. (1995) Deletion of autoreactive B cells. *Current Biology*, 5, 103–106.

Matzinger, P. (1994) Tolerance, danger, and the extended family. *Annual Review of Immunology*, **12**, 991–1046.

Miller, J.F.A.P. & Morahan, G. (1992) Peripheral T cell tolerance. *Annual Review of Immunology*, **10**, 51–69.

Möller, G. (Ed.) (1993) Peripheral T-cell immunological tolerance. *Immunological Reviews*, 133, entire volume.

Nossal, G.J.V. (1994) How to stop bad B cells. *Nature*, **371**, 375–376.

Scott, D.W. (1993) Analysis of B cell tolerance *in vitro*. *Advances in Immunology*, **54**, 393–425.

Waldmann, H. & Cobbold, S. (1993) Monoclonal antibodies for the induction of transplantation tolerance. *Current Opinion in Immunology*, 5, 753–756.

Weiner, H.L. (1994) Oral tolerance. *Proceedings of the National Academy of Sciences USA*, **91**, 10762–10765.

Weiner, H.L., Friedman, A., Miller, A. *et al.* (1994) Oral tolerance: immunologic mechanisms and treatment of animal and human organ-specific autoimmune diseases by oral administration of autoantigens. *Annual Review of Immunology*, **12**, 809–838.

chapter 21 Defence against invaders

Interactions between hosts and their invaders

To smaller life forms (*microorganisms*, *microbes*), and to some larger ones as well, the vertebrate body must appear as a richly prepared banquet table at which food is up for grabs. Many forms, irresistibly drawn to this bountiful supply of nutrients, invade vertebrate bodies and attempt to colonize them. Most of the attempts miscarry, either because the invaders are unable to adapt evolutionarily to the microenvironment of the body or because the host's immune system prevents them from establishing a foothold on the body's surfaces. During the long course of evolution, however, some microorganisms, mainly bacteria and fungi, have succeeded in adapting themselves gradually to the microenvironment and have become *commensals*, literally guests 'eating at the same table'. Commensals are constituents of the *normal microbial flora*, the relatively stable, total microbial population of a localized region such as the skin or the intestinal tract. Some commensal microorganisms live together with their hosts, with neither harm nor benefit to either; others actually aid the host, either by producing nutrients or by protecting the host from other, harmful organisms. The coexistence of the normal microbial flora with the host is a fragile and precarious affair. It does not take much to transform a microbe from harmless to harmful. Moreover, it is not very likely that microbes will observe the 'house regulations' voluntarily; more probably they are kept in line by the immune system, which has them under constant surveillance. How essential the immune system is for keeping the normal microbial flora under control becomes apparent when the system is compromised either because of a genetic defect or by the action of biological, chemical or physical agents. In such situations, components of the flora often turn on and kill the host.

Invaders that obtain their nutrients from the host and harm it in the process are called *parasites*: microparasites when they are small (viruses, bacteria, fungi and protozoa) and macroparasites when they are multicellular (helminths and arthropods). *Microparasites* reproduce directly within the host, usually at very high rates; they have a short generation time; their association with a given host is of short duration relative to the host's lifespan; and they induce long-lasting immunity in hosts that have recovered from the invasion. *Macroparasites*, for the most part, do not reproduce directly within the definitive host; they have a much longer generation time than microparasites; and they induce immunity of short duration and reinvade the same host continually.

The entrenchment of a parasite in the body of a host is called *infection*; the outward manifestations of damage caused by a parasite are referred to as *symptoms*. The condition that produces symptoms is called *(infectious) disease*, the disease-causing organisms *pathogens* (a term more or less synonymous with 'parasite') and the origination and development of a disease *pathogenesis*. The ability of a parasite to cause a disease is referred to as *virulence* or *pathogenicity*. The last two terms are usually used synonymously, but sometimes 'pathogenicity' is used in reference to parasite species, whereas 'virulence' is used in reference to strains within a species. Thus, for example, *Bacillus anthracis* is said to be more pathogenic than *Bacillus subtilis*, but the Vollum strain of *B. anthracis* is said to be more virulent than the Sterne strain. Another distinction between the two terms is that 'pathogenicity' is sometimes used in reference to the capacity of a parasite to cause a disease, whereas 'virulence' is used in reference to variations in the degree of disease. A host that has recovered from an infectious disease may serve as a *carrier* of the parasite for some time afterwards, spreading the parasite to other individuals. Sometimes hosts may remain infected by parasites for a prolonged period without showing any signs of disease. This status is referred to as *asymptomatic carriage* or *asymptomatic infection*.

All parasites, with the exception of viruses, derive ultimately from free-living, non-parasitic forms. Transition from the free-living to the parasitic state involves two major changes: adaptation to the environment of the host body and acquisition of virulence factors, i.e. the elements responsible for disease induction. *Adaptation to the host* must be the most difficult part of the transition; it probably occurs gradually over millions of years and involves many genetic alterations. To appreciate the extent of genetic modification an organism must undergo to adapt itself to a host, consider the simple case of a bacterium that lives in a puddle but attempts to establish itself in the intestine of a mammal. Suppose that when lapped up with the water, it somehow survives the acid bath in the mammal's stomach, which one researcher has compared to 'the hot oil and pitch that was dumped on raiders of mediaeval castles', and that it ends up unharmed in the intestine. To successfully colonize this new niche, it must undergo the following modifications: produce molecules that will enable it to adhere to the intestinal wall; alter its metabolism so that it can function at a higher temperature, higher osmotic pressure and higher pH than it was exposed to in the water; find a way of resisting the high concentrations of membrane-disrupting bile salts; adjust to anaerobic conditions; learn to use an entirely new set of nutrients and a new source of iron; come up with a strategy of out-competing microorganisms already established in the intestine; and, finally, devise a method of escaping the attention of the host's immune system. Obviously, these adaptations cannot occur in a single step. They can be implemented gradually and this takes time, even in the case of a rapidly multiplying organism such as a bacterium. (Incidentally, some bacteria, for example *Vibrio cholerae*, have adapted to the transition so successfully that they now alternate between living in water for a period and then in the intestine.)

The adaptation of a bacterium to a single host is complex enough; it is still relatively simple, however, compared with the adaptation of an invader whose life cycle includes a free-living as well as a host-borne stage, an intermediate and a definitive host or even several intermediate hosts belonging to different phyla. The genetic alterations underlying such adaptations must take a very long time to evolve.

The adapted invader may first become a commensal and only later turn into a parasite. The emergence of a parasite is characterized by the acquisition of *virulence*, the appearance of effects that harm the host. Virulence is a complex trait that consists of several components, *virulence factors*, controlled by different genes. Depending on the number and type of factors a parasite has acquired, its virulence may vary in degree. A parasite that has lost its virulence is said to be *avirulent* or *attenuated* ('weakened'), but between avirulence and high virulence there can be various intermediate degrees.

However, virulence has two aspects: harming the host is one, benefiting the parasite is the other. The actual purpose of virulence is to make the invader a better parasite, i.e. one that can exploit the host most efficiently and thus achieve a higher reproductive success, a higher *evolutionary fitness*. Unfortunately, what benefits the parasite is nearly always detrimental to the host: the fitness of the parasite and the host are like water levels in the two arms of a U-tube—when one rises, the other falls and vice versa.

Evolutionary fitness of a parasite can be increased by perfecting its ability to utilize the host's resources in one or all stages of the parasite's life cycle. The stages include *colonization* of the host (*adhesion* of the parasite to host cells and *invasion* of the parasite into host tissues or cells), *multiplication* in host tissues and *transmission* to new hosts. A genetic change that enables the parasite to improve its success in any of these stages becomes a virulence factor; the harmful effects on the host are a consequence of this improvement. Because of its two-sidedness, virulence can be discussed in terms of either infectivity (the changes benefitting the parasite in regard to colonization, multiplication and transmission) or disease severity (the changes detrimental to the host). Selected examples of both types of change follow: first, those relating to improved *infectivity* and then those responsible for *disease severity*. It must be remembered, however, that both are expressions of the same phenomenon and that only the emphasis changes: in the first case, it is parasite fitness and in the other, host fitness. Most of the examples are drawn from the study of parasitic bacteria, in which significant progress has been made in recent years towards the elucidation of pathogenicity.

A number of parasitic bacteria produce *pilins*, proteins that assemble into rod-like structures on the bacterial cell surface, the *pili* or *fimbriae*. These, or specialized sets of proteins at their tips, mediate attachment of bacteria to host-cell receptors, usually the carbohydrate parts of cell-surface glycoproteins or glycolipids. The normal function of the receptors is to anchor cells at their ultimate destination in the body, mediate cell–cell contacts and transmit signals from the surface to the cell interior. The parasite usurps the receptors for its own purpose. Pili occur in *V. cholerae*, *Escherichia coli*, *Neisseria gonorrhoeae*, *Pseudomonas aeruginosa* and other bacteria.

Some parasitic bacteria possess, in addition to pili, *afimbrial adhesins*, single proteins scattered over bacterial surfaces. Adhesins, which do not assemble into pili-like structures, bind tightly to host cells following the initial pili-mediated attachment. Afimbrial adhesins have been demonstrated in *Bordetella pertussis* and *Clostridium difficile*.

The invasion of host tissues by bacteria is facilitated by a variety of molecules. Some bacteria (e.g. *Yersinia enterocolitica*, *Yersinia pseudotuberculosis*, *Salmonella typhi*) synthesize *invasins*, cell-surface proteins that bind to integrins of host-cell membranes and then induce reorganization of the underlying cytoskeleton, including polymerization and depolymerization of actin molecules. The rearrangements of actin lead to the formation of pseudopodia around the bacterium and ultimately to its engulfment. The bacterium thus forces a normally non-phagocytic host cell to become phagocytic in order to enter it.

Multiplication of bacteria that have invaded host tissues depends on an adequate supply of nutrients, first and foremost *iron*. Because most iron in the body is bound to proteins such as lactoferrin, transferrin, ferritin and haemin and is thus normally inaccessible to bacteria, iron deficiency is one of the major factors limiting bacterial growth. By solving the iron problem, bacteria come one step closer to becoming successful parasites. Parasitic bacteria have gained access to iron in a variety of ways, of which only two are mentioned here. Some bacteria excrete *siderophores* into their surroundings, which are low-molecular-mass compounds with a high affinity for free iron. The same bacteria also produce receptors that bind iron–siderophore complexes (including those containing siderophores produced by other organisms) and deliver them into the cell where the iron is released. Other bacteria have learned how to extract iron from lactoferrin, transferrin, ferritin and haemin.

Of the many examples of parasites influencing their own mode of *transmission*, none are more spectacular than those in which the parasite alters the behaviour of the host. Perhaps the most celebrated of these is the case of the worm *Leucochloridium paradoxum*. The worm has two hosts, a snail of the genus *Succinea* and a snail-eating bird. The parasite develops from eggs distributed by the birds in their droppings and picked up by the snail. In the final stage of their development, the maturing worms gather in large numbers on the snail's eyestalks, acquire brilliant colours and cause the eyestalks to look like caterpillars. The mimicry is so good that birds fall for it and eat the snails along with their parasites. In the bird's digestive tract, the parasites complete their maturation and release eggs that are then disseminated with the bird's droppings.

Infectivity-associated virulence harms the host indirectly by increasing the number of parasites that colonize the host and multiply in it. Virulence factors associated with disease severity, on the other hand, harm the host directly. Among the best characterized of the various disease-causing virulence factors are bacterial *exotoxins*, proteins secreted or otherwise released by bacteria, which adversely affect host cells. Some exotoxins (e.g. those of *Corynebacterium diphtheriae*) block protein synthesis; others (e.g. those of *Bordetella pertussis* and *V. cholerae*) ADP-ribosylate G-proteins and thus disrupt the function of ion pumps via deregulation of cyclic AMP (cAMP); others still cleave neurotransmitters (e.g. the exotoxins of *Clostridium botulinum*) or create holes in host-cell membranes (e.g. exotoxins of *E. coli* and *Streptococcus pyogenes*).

It is not always clear how the parasite benefits from harming the host. In fact, in some cases it does not. For example, *C. botulinum* is a bacterium that normally grows in the soil or in lake sediments but is unable to grow in the human colon at densities high enough to cause disease. However, its spores can contaminate food sealed in jars with little oxygen, germinate and produce *botulinal toxin*. When ingested with food, the toxin is absorbed by the stomach, enters the bloodstream, binds to neurons and stops nerve transmission. Lack of muscle stimulation by the nerves then leads to generalized paralysis, which is of no consequence to the bacterium that produced the toxin.

In those instances in which the benefits of harming the host are known, the injury is a mere side-effect. Three examples follow. First, it has been observed that some exotoxins are produced only when the level of iron available in the host is low. It is therefore believed that exotoxin-mediated host-cell killing is the bacterium's way of releasing ferritin- and haem-bound iron from intracellular stores. Second, the adherence of *V. cholerae* to the lining of the small intestine triggers the excretion of cholera exotoxin, which disrupts the function of ion pumps in the mucosal cells. The result is a decreased net flow of sodium into tissue, a net flow of chloride (and water) out of tissues and massive diarrhoea. The alkaline, salty fluid in the lumen of the intestine favours the growth of *V. cholerae* over competing bacteria, which are thus flushed out. Here, diarrhoea benefits the bacteria by providing them with a competitive edge over the microorganisms of the normal flora. Third, various *Shigella* bacteria use invasins and induced phagocytosis to enter cells of the colonic mucosa. Inside the cell they escape from the phagocytic vesicle into the cytoplasm, where they use the host's actin molecules to propel themselves and to invade adjacent cells. In this manner, they spread from one cell to another, killing the invaded cells in the process, either by disrupting their metabolism or by prompting them to commit suicide. Destruction of the intestinal mucosa is the main cause of diarrhoea associated with *Shigella* infections, but also the bacterium's way of reaching new cells in the same host, as well as new hosts: the diarrhoeal flow washes out the multiplying bacteria and contaminates water, which then becomes the source of new infections.

In addition to the aforementioned virulence factors associated with infectivity and disease severity, there is also a large category of factors that benefit the parasite by enabling it to evade the barrier a host has erected for its own defence, or to escape an attack by the host's immune system. These are described later in this chapter.

We see, then, that virulence is advantageous for the parasite, but generally deleterious for the host. The parasite thus faces an evolutionary dilemma: on one hand, it is driven by natural selection to further increase its reproductive rate; on the other, the more virulent it becomes the more it damages the host and the fewer are its chances for transmission to new hosts. Natural selection apparently solves this conflict by striking a balance between parasite virulence and host survival. It favours less virulent parasites that allow the host to stay alive during infection and hence to pass the parasite's progeny on to new hosts. At the same time, however, it favours virulent over avirulent strains because the former produce more progeny than the latter. A compromise is thus reached by which the parasite produces maximum progeny under conditions that do not endanger parasite transmission by overexploitation of the host. The dynamics of the interaction between the parasite and its host become more complex in the presence of multiple parasites or if multiple strains of the same parasite are present in a host population. In such instances, apparently, both the more virulent and the less virulent forms may persist in the population, the former because they are more successful reproductively and the latter because they have a higher transmission probability due to the survival of infected hosts.

But how do hosts become parasitized in the first place? To answer this question, evolutionary biologists have produced phylogenetic trees based on nucleotide sequences of groups of related parasites and compared them with trees based on nucleotide sequences of the hosts of these parasites. In some instances they found the parasite and the host trees to be completely concordant (Fig. 21.1). In these cases, the parasites have co-evolved with their hosts and the host–parasite associations have lasted for many millions of years. Figure 21.1 shows the members of the papovavirus group comprising human *pa*pilloma virus, which causes warts or papillomas, mouse *po*lyoma virus, which produces several types of neoplasia in newborns, and simian *va*cuolating virus 40 (SV-40), which causes neoplastic transformation of monkey cells. The three members of the papovavirus groups diverged more than 80 million years ago and evolved along the same lines as their hosts. In certain other instances, the host and parasite trees

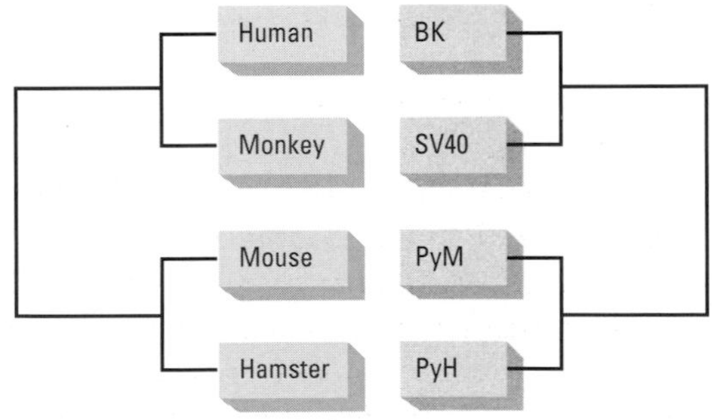

Figure 21.1 Phylogenetic trees showing the relationships of four mammalian species (left) and of four viruses that parasitize them (right). BK, SV40, PyM and PyH are human, monkey, mouse and hamster viruses, respectively. The mammalian species tree is based on palaeontological data, as well as on DNA sequences. The virus tree is based on DNA sequences. (Based on data from Soeda, E. *et al.* (1980) *Nature*, **285**, 166 and Shadan, F. F. & Villarreal, L. P. (1993) *Proceedings of the National Academy of Sciences USA*, **90**, 4117.)

coincide only partially. Thus, for example, the blood flukes of the genus *Schistosoma* (former name *Bilharzia*; Platyhelminthes: Trematoda) are parasites of many rodents and ungulates but not of primates, except humans; all have freshwater amphibious snails as intermediate hosts. Mitochondrial DNA sequence comparisons indicate that of the species parasitic to humans, *S. haematobium* and *S. intercalatum* are closely related to ungulate parasites such as *S. bovis* of cattle, whereas *S. mansoni* is closely related to rodent parasites such as *S. rodhaini* of the rat (Fig. 21.2). It is therefore believed that humans acquired their schistosomal parasites from ungulates and rodents at the time their ancestors invaded the African savannah some 5 million years ago. (The origin of another human species, *S. japonicum*, which also parasitizes a number of animals, is unclear.) Thus human schistosomes are examples of *lateral transfers* of parasites between unrelated host species. (However, parasites can also be transferred laterally between related species such as humans and apes.) There are many other examples of lateral transfers (influenza virus from ducks, *Yersinia pestis* from rats and fleas, African trypanosomes from ungulates, to name just a few), several of which have occurred in historical times, some of them quite recently (e.g. human immunodeficiency virus (HIV) was apparently transferred to humans from Old World monkeys in the 1970s). The recent invaders of human populations are sometimes referred to as *emerging parasites (pathogens)*; they include viruses (Table 21.1) and bacteria (e.g. *Borrellia burgdorferi*, the causative agent of Lyme disease, originated from the white-footed mouse and was apparently transmitted to humans by ticks). The emergence of new parasite-caused diseases is often associated with changes in the ecology and behaviour of the human species.

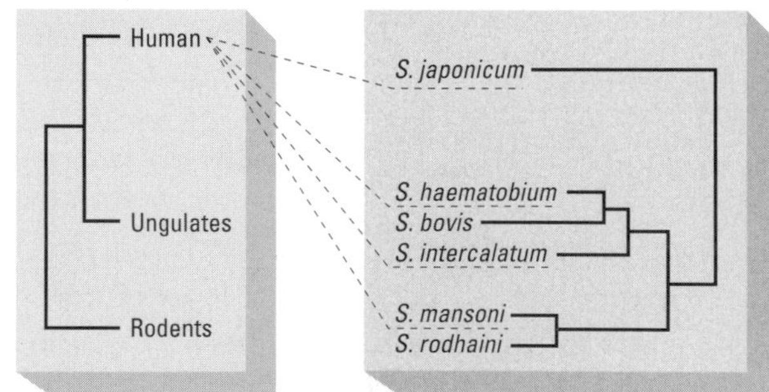

Figure 21.2 Phylogenetic trees showing the relationships of three mammalian orders (left, humans representing primates) and six species of *Schistosoma* (right). The broken lines indicate presumed lateral transfers of ungulate parasites (*S. haematobium* and *S. intercalatum*), a rodent parasite (*S. mansoni*) and a parasite from an unidentified host (*S. japonicum*) to humans; *S. bovis* and *S. rodhaini* are cattle and rat parasites, respectively. (Based on data from Despres, L. *et al.* (1992) *Molecular Phylogenetics and Evolution*, **1**, 295.)

Normal microbial flora is also a potential source of pathogenic forms. We have mentioned already that some of the commensals turn into parasites in immunocompromised individuals; these are then referred to as *opportunistic parasites (pathogens)*. For example, the protozoan *Pneumocystis carinii* is widely distributed in the lungs of rats, mice, rabbits, sheep, goats, horses, monkeys and apparently also humans. In healthy persons, the protozoan remains dormant or at least kept in check by the immune system. However, when the immune system is damaged, as happens for example in AIDS patients, the organism multiplies, fills the alveolar spaces, impairs ventilation and causes shortness of breath and ultimately death. Sometimes innocuous (avirulent) bacterial strains acquire virulence factors and convert into parasites that can attack even fully immunocompetent individuals. Thus, *E. coli* is a common commensal of the human large intestine and, as such, entirely harmless. When it acquires virulence factors, however, it can cause a wide variety of diseases, including diarrhoea, dysentery, haemolytic uraemic syndrome (acute kidney failure accompanied by haemolytic anaemia), bladder and kidney infections, septicaemia (blood poisoning, the presence of microorganisms or their toxic products in the blood), pneumonia and meningitis (inflammation of the meninges, the three membranes that envelop the brain). The type of disease the converted *E. coli* bacteria cause is determined by the virulence factors they have acquired. This example illustrates that it is not the species or the genus that makes a microorganism a parasite but the set of virulence factors it carries.

Although occasionally a microbial strain may become virulent by a mutation in a single gene, more commonly several genes are involved. Even then, conversion to virulence can be a single-step process because many of the virulence genes occur in blocks, often on plasmids that can be transferred from one bacterium to another during conjugation. Blocks of virulence genes can also be transduced into bacterial strains by bacteriophages. In all these instances, however, the invader is already adapted to life in the vertebrate body and the acquisition of virulence factors merely changes its behaviour in the body: it turns it into a parasite.

Defence at body surfaces

The initial encounter between the vertebrate body and its invaders occurs at the body's surface. Generally, invaders that manage to colonize the surface without penetrating the

Table 21.1 Examples of emerging viruses. (From Morse, S. S. & Schleuderberg, A. (1990) *Journal of Infectious Diseases*, **162**, 1–7.)

Virus	Signs/symptoms	Distribution	Natural host
Family: Orthomyxoviridae (RNA, 8 segments)			
Influenza	Respiratory	Worldwide (often from China)	Fowl (and pigs)
Family: Bunyaviridae (RNA, 3 segments)			
Hantaan, Seoul, etc.	Haemorrhagic fever with renal syndrome	Asia, Europe, USA	Rodent (e.g. *Apodemus*)
Rift Valley Fever*	Fever ± haemorrhage	Africa	Mosquito; ungulates
Oropouche*	Fever	Brazil, Trinidad, Panama	Midge
Family: Togaviridae (Alphavirus genus, RNA)			
O'nyong-nyong*	Arthritis, rash	Africa	Mosquito
Sindbis*	Arthritis, rash	Africa, Europe, Asia	Mosquito, birds
Family: Flaviviridae (RNA)			
Yellow fever*	Fever, jaundice	Africa, South America	Mosquito, monkey
Dengue*	Fever ± haemorrhage	Asia, Africa, South America, Caribbean	Mosquito, human/monkey
Rocio*	Encephalitis	Brazil	Mosquito, birds
Kyasanur Forest*	Encephalitis	India	Tick, rodent
Family: Arenaviridae (RNA, 2 segments)			
Junin (Argentine HF)	Fever, haemorrhage	South America	*Calomys musculinus*
Machupo (Bolivian HF)	Fever, haemorrhage	South America	*Calomys callosus*
Lassa fever	Fever, haemorrhage	West Africa	*Mastomys natalensis*
Family: Filoviridae (RNA)			
Marburg, Ebola	Fever, haemorrhage	Africa	Unknown
Family: Retroviridae (RNA + reverse transcriptase)			
HIV	AIDS	Worldwide	Human virus (originally from primates?)
HTLV	Often asymptomatic; adult T-cell leukaemia, neurological diseases	Worldwide with endemic foci	Human virus (originally non-human primate virus?)
Family: Poxviridae (DNA)			
Monkeypox	Smallpox-like	Africa (rainforest)	Rodent (squirrel)

* Transmitted by arthropod vector.
AIDS, acquired immunodeficiency syndrome; HF, Haemorrhagic fever; HIV, human immunodeficiency virus; HTLV, human T-cell leukaemia/lymphoma virus (human T-lymphotropic virus) types I and II.

tissue beneath it become part of the normal microbial flora; those that succeed in entering the underlying tissues become parasites. The first line of the body's defence against parasites must therefore be set up on its surface and must be aimed at preventing penetration at all costs.

There are two kinds of body surface, outer and inner (Fig. 21.3). The latter, although technically inside the body, is exposed to the external environment in the form of food, drink and air. It represents the surface of the gastrointestinal, respiratory and urogenital tracts. The two kinds are protected by different types of tissue: the outer surface by the skin and the inner by the mucosa. Immune mechanisms involved in skin and mucosal immunity are described in Chapter 18.

Skin

The skin is a highly inhospitable surface for microorganisms to colonize. Microorganisms grow best in a warm (37 °C), moist, neutral (pH 7) and nutrient-rich environment, and this the skin definitely does not provide. Its temperature is less than 37 °C, often much less; its surface is, with the exception of certain areas (scalp, armpits, groin), very dry; its pH is low (between 3 and 5); and its keratinized dead cells are no horn of plenty. Microorganisms that do prevail in taking hold of the cells immediately face the danger of being discarded when the cells are shed. Pores and folds of the skin are somewhat more hospitable in this regard, but they are protected by other means. Hair follicle-

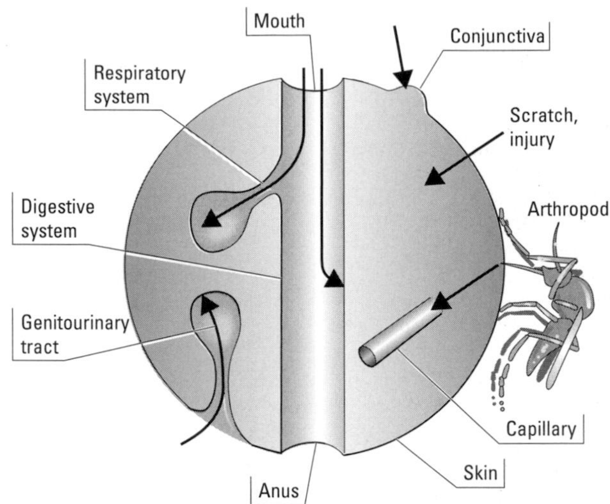

Figure 21.3 Outer and inner body surfaces. Sites of antigen entry are indicated by arrows. (Redrawn from Mims, C. A. (1977) *The Pathogenesis of Infectious Disease*. Academic Press, London.)

associated sebaceous glands secrete *sebum*, which contains lactic and fatty acids. Both substances acidify the environment and poison microorganisms. Furthermore, the environment contains *lysozyme*, which cleaves peptidoglycans in the cell wall of Gram-positive bacteria. These areas are also colonized preferentially by microorganisms of the *normal flora*, which have adapted to the harsh conditions of existence at body surfaces and with which a new invader must compete for nutrients and attachment sites. In this competition, the adapted residents invariably win.

All these features make the skin an extremely effective barrier that, as long as it remains intact, cannot be penetrated. However, it can be breached through wounds, breaks, abrasions, burns and insect bites. Parasites that have gained access to the underlying tissue then encounter the second line of defence, set up by the *skin-associated lymphoid tissue* (*SALT*; see Chapter 18).

In contrast to the skin with its desert-like conditions on the surface, the mucosa is much more congenial for any would-be colonizer. It provides plenty of moisture, a constant temperature of 37 °C and bountiful nutrients. None the less, microorganisms do not find it any easier to use the mucosa rather than the skin as a port of entry into the underlying tissues. For one thing, the epithelial cells of the mucosa are latched together by *tight junctions* (Fig. 21.4), which render the layer not only waterproof, but of course also bacteria-proof. For another, the epithelial cell layer renews itself continuously without disruption of its integrity, so that any microorganism attached to a cell gets a free ride off the body before it can make itself comfortable. The renewal is particularly rapid in the intestine, in which stem cells of the crypts continuously divide to produce epithelial cells that then move towards the tip of the villus, where they are shed into the lumen.

A third important protective mechanism is the secretion of *mucus* (*mucin*) by goblet cells strewn over the mucosal surface (see Chapter 3). Mucus is a thick, sticky substance that flows from the goblet cells in streaks over the surface like syrup from a jar. It is composed of polysaccharides and proteins that have two main functions: they lubricate the surface to prevent abrasions by particulate matter in the food and they entrap foreign particles, including microorganisms. Entrapment is enhanced by two factors, carbohydrates and secretory IgA. Some mucous carbohydrates are of the same type as those that bacteria exploit as their receptors for attachment to epithelial cells. Thus, instead of making contact with the mucosa, bacteria find themselves stuck in the mucin syrup. Secretory IgA binds with its Fab to antigenic molecules on the surface of the microbe and with its Fc to components of the mucus, thus achieving the same effect as the carbohydrates.

Blobs of mucus with ensnared microorganisms are expelled from the body by peristaltic movements of the intestine (see below) or by the action of *ciliated cells*. The latter are covered by hairs, or *cilia*, that wave rhythmically, like ears of wheat in the wind, and thus propel microscopic particles towards the body's openings.

Mucus also contains substances that kill microorganisms or inhibit their growth. They include *lysozyme* which, as mentioned earlier, degrades peptidoglycans of bacterial cell walls and thus makes bacteria more vulnerable to attack by other substances; *lactoferrin*, which scoops free iron before bacteria can get to it; and *lactoperoxidase*, which produces superoxide radicals toxic for most microorganisms (see Chapter 15).

Invaders that somehow have managed to avoid all these traps and obstacles and have reached the subepithelial layers become, analogously to the situation in the skin, the target of attack by the *mucosa-associated lymphoid tissue* or *MALT* (in the intestine the *gastrointestinal-associated lymphoid tissue* or *GALT*), parts of which are organized into Peyer's patches (see Chapter 18). A description of the various mucosal surfaces and their characteristics follows.

Eyes

About one-sixth of the eye's surface is exposed to the outer world: the transparent cornea covered by a mucous membrane, the *conjunctiva*. The membrane is kept moist by the continuous flow of secretions from lacrimal (tear-producing) and other glands; every few seconds, the lids

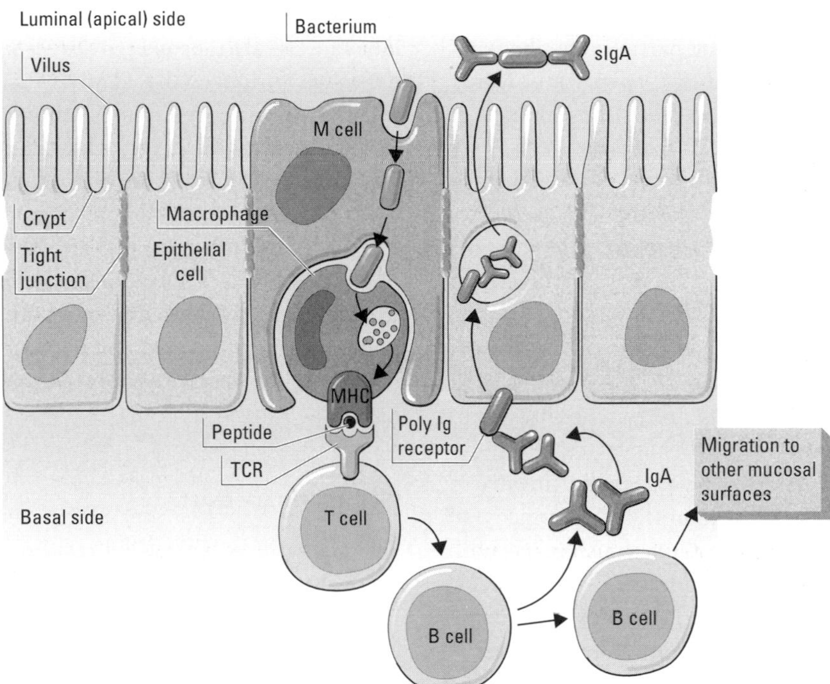

Figure 21.4 Handling of invaders (here a bacterium) by the mucosa-associated lymphoid tissue (MALT). The main components of MALT are M cells, macrophages, lymphocytes and mucosa-specific mast cells. M cells ingest microorganisms by phagocytosis and pass them on to the underlying macrophages. Macrophages digest the invaders and present, probably in the Peyer's patch (omitted for simplicity), the MHC-bound peptides to T lymphocytes. Activated T lymphocytes produce cytokines and activate B lymphocytes to produce IgA antibodies. IgA molecules are transcytosed and released as secretory IgA into mucus on the luminal surface. For details, see Chapters 8 and 18. (Based on Salyers, A. A. & Whitt, D. D. (1994) *Bacterial Pathogenesis. A Molecular Approach*. American Society of Microbiology Press, Washington, DC.)

pass over the conjunctiva (*blinking*) and, like a car's windshield wiper, wash away particles that might have soiled the conjunctival surface. This mechanical cleansing is supplemented by the antimicrobial action of lysozyme, lactoferrin and sIgA in secretions. The combined mechanical and chemical actions of the secretions normally keep the conjunctival surface clean; complications arise only when the conjunctiva is damaged or when defects occur in the secretory mechanisms. Infection of the conjunctiva is referred to as *conjunctivitis*, and one of its most severe forms is *trachoma* (Greek *trachoma*, rough, harsh) caused by *Chlamydia trachomatis*, a Gram-negative microorganism resembling rickettsiae and responsible for the formation of minute greyish or yellowish translucent granules beneath the eyelids. Trachoma, which can damage the cornea and cause partial or complete blindness, is as ordinary as the common cold in some parts of the world.

Respiratory tract

Air entering the respiratory system contains suspended particles of all kinds: smoke, soot, dust, pollen and microorganisms. More than 1000 million tons of particles are present in the earth's atmosphere and an average human being inhales some 10 000 microorganisms daily. Owing to several efficient cleansing mechanisms, however, the lungs normally remain sterile despite this bombardment of particles. In the *nose*, hairs entrap particulate material, including microorganisms, and the sneezing reflex expels it out of the airways. In the *mouth* and *throat*, the constant flow of saliva, which contains lysozyme, lactoferrin and sIgA, washes away the invaders. The nose, mouth and throat are also protected by resident microflora. In the *lungs*, the mucosa contains ciliated and mucus-secreting (goblet) cells in the epithelium and mucus-secreting glands in the subepithelial layers. Secreted mucus entraps particles not retained by the hairs in the nose, and the cilia then move the particles upward from the lungs to the back of the throat. In the upper tract, a similar mucociliary lining moves entrapped particles downwards to the throat, where they are then swallowed. Particles not removed by this *mucociliary escalator* may reach the alveoli, which have no cilia or mucus but are lined by macrophages. Most of the *alveolar macrophages* ingest and degrade the particles by phagocytosis *in situ*, but others move with the particles upwards into the throat using the mucociliary escalator. If macrophages alone cannot handle the invasion, the body quickly mobilizes the *granulocytic system*, so that within hours of infection a large number of neutrophils and other granulocytes enter the lungs and begin to eliminate the offending microorganism. sIgA becomes involved in defence when some of the macrophages process the antigen and present it in an appropriate form to T and B cells of the bronchial-associated lymphoid tissue.

When the cleansing mechanisms are functioning properly, most microorganisms have no chance to initiate an infection unless they are endowed with special means to avoid these mechanisms. For example, the surfaces of influenza viruses possess haemagglutinin, which reacts with sialic acid groups on the glycoproteins of epithelial cells, and by firm attachment to these cells the viruses avoid being swept away by the mucociliary escalators. When the cleansing mechanisms are damaged by destructive lesions of the respiratory system, caused for example by viral infections, heavy smoking or very dry air, the chance of infection increases.

Gastrointestinal tract

Microorganisms entering the gastrointestinal tract during eating and drinking are attacked by various enzymes (e.g. lysozyme in the saliva of the mouth, pepsin in the stomach juice and trypsin in the small intestine), acids (e.g. hydrochloric acid in the stomach) and bile (in the duodenum). Even if they escape chemical attack, microorganisms have little opportunity to settle down because everything is always in motion in the digestive system. In the small intestine, where motion is most intense, at least three kinds of movement can be recognized: *segmentation* (rhythmic contractions involving localized regions of the intestine), *peristalsis* (contractions travelling short distances along the length of the intestine), and *mucous membrane movement* (increase or decrease in mucosal folding and motility of the villi). The combined action of these three movements results in a constant mixing of particles in the intestinal lumen and a continual passage of intestinal contents towards the anus. In the large intestine (colon), movement slows down and it is here that many microorganisms manage to settle and establish the resident microflora. In humans, there are some 10^{11} bacteria per gram of colon or rectum content and in the rectum bacteria constitute about one-quarter of the faecal mass. The mucus covering the mucosa provides a mechanical, as well as immunological, barrier to the passage of bacteria through the intestinal wall. The small intestine is also protected by lysozyme, *cryptdins* and *defensins* produced by *Paneth cells* (defensins are also secreted by phagocytic cells). Paneth cells lie directly under the stem cells of the crypt, which they are believed to guard from infection. Cryptdins and defensins are peptides toxic for most bacteria (see Chapter 15).

Because of their openness and despite the high efficiency of their protective mechanisms, the respiratory and gastrointestinal tracts are the most vulnerable regions of the body in terms of invasion by pathogens. Indeed, most acute infectious illnesses are either respiratory or dysentery-like in nature.

Genitourinary tract

The *vagina* is colonized by resident microflora dominated by *Lactobacillus*, a Gram-positive bacterium that produces lactic acid. By reducing the pH, lactic acid prevents the growth of many other bacteria. *Lactobacillus*, with other members of the microflora, also protects the vaginal surface by forming a *biofilm*, a multilayer bacterial population embedded in a polysaccharide matrix attached to the mucosal surface. Biofilm prevents pathogens from gaining access to the mucosal surface. The *fallopian tubes* and the *uterus* are probably also normally completely sterile. Microorganisms are kept from entering the uterus through the cervix by a mucous plug in the cervical opening.

Microorganisms are prevented from entering the *bladder* by the sphincter action of the urethral opening. Any microorganisms entering the bladder are washed out during urination. The male urethra is longer and hence the bladder less accessible to bacteria compared with females.

Defences beneath body surfaces

When surface defence mechanisms fail to stop an infection and invaders reach the underlying tissues, another complex of defences is activated. These fall into two categories, non-adaptive and adaptive, which are described in this order. For the sake of clarity, both categories will be dissected further into individual mechanisms, although in reality many of these mechanisms operate in parallel with, and in interdependence on, one another. All the mechanisms are described in some detail in earlier chapters; here we bring them together in an attempt to provide an overall view of the immune system's functions during an infection. The description will apply primarily to infections by microorganisms, although some of it will also be applicable to macroparasites. The specific features of defence against macroparasites are dealt with later in this chapter.

Non-adaptive (inflammatory) responses

A parasite invading tissue underlying the body surface causes *tissue injury* either directly, for example by replicating in the cells and killing them, or indirectly by producing noxious substances (toxins) that damage or kill host cells. Substances released from dead or dying host cells (e.g. proteolytic enzymes) then attack other cells, thus augmenting the damage. The function of the non-adaptive defence system is to eliminate all the parasites, clear away the debris generated in consequence of their activities and repair the damage.

The tissue that the parasite has reached is likely to contain endothelial cells and platelets in its blood vessels (together with other blood cells), mast cells in the cuff around the blood vessels, as well as macrophages, fibroblasts and nerve fibres (Fig. 21.5). All these cells are involved in the earliest phases (within minutes of the invasion) of the response. They are joined rapidly (within the first 4 hours) by monocytes and slightly later by neutrophils emigrating from blood vessels. The tissue is bathed in a fluid derived largely from blood plasma as it seeps from the capillaries into the tissue, before returning back into the vessel. The fluid therefore contains most of the proteins normally present in the plasma, among them components of the four major activation systems: the coagulation (clotting), fibrinolytic, bradykinin and complement cascades. Each system consists of a set of proteins coordinated in their functions. Normally, these proteins are in an inactive form, but at a specific signal the first protein of the team is activated; it activates the second protein, which then activates the third member, and so on. The last members of the team then carry out a specific function: they form a clot that stops blood flow from a damaged blood vessel (*coagulation system*); they decompose (lyse) the clot when it is no longer needed (*fibrinolytic system*); they widen the lumen of blood vessels and increase capillary permeability (*bradykinin system*); or they participate in the destruction of the invading parasite (*complement system*). The systems interact with one another in a complex manner and thus form one supersystem. Some of the interactions are summarized in Fig. 21.6.

Coagulation system

Tissue damage caused by parasite invasion induces several responses almost immediately and simultaneously. The endothelial cells of the blood vessels, platelets and the plasma protein activation systems are among the first components to become involved. Endotoxin released from Gram-negative bacteria binds to receptors on the surface of *endothelial cells* and sets in motion a cascade of events that lead to the attachment of transcription factors to the AP-1 and κB sites in the enhancer region of a gene coding for *tissue factor* (TF) and expression of the factor on the cell surface (Fig. 21.7). TF is a membrane-anchored glycoprotein whose extracellular part consists of two immunoglobulin-like domains capable of binding factor VII, a serine protease of the coagulation cascade. The TF–factor VIIa complex (where factor VIIa is the activated form of factor VII) activates proteolytically factor X and thus initiates the *extrinsic pathway* of the cascade. Activated factor X activates *prothrombin* converting it to *thrombin*, an enzyme that converts *fibrinogen* to *fibrin*, which polymerizes into long, cross-linked fibres. Thrombin also binds to receptors on other endothelial cells, thereby stimulating them to express TF as well. Further expression of TF by endothelial cells (but also by other cells such as blood monocytes) is stimulated by cytokines such as tumour necrosis factor-α (TNF-α) and interleukin (IL)-1. Moreover, endothelial cells can also be activated by mechanical pressure and shear stress occurring during tissue injury. The activation of endothelial cells leads to the

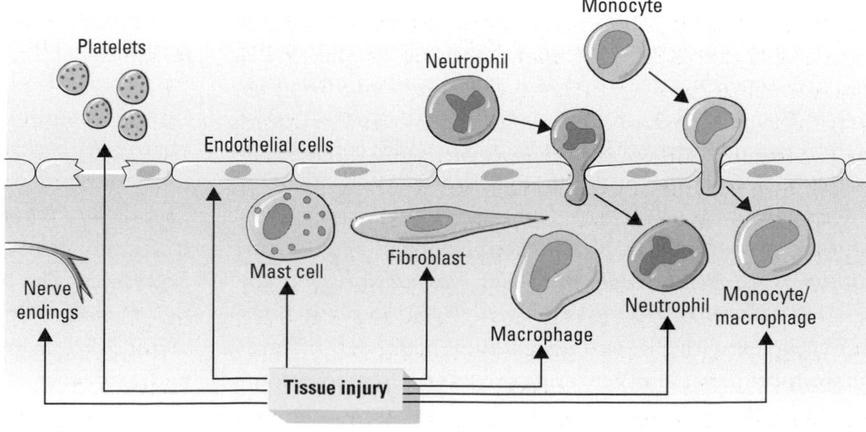

Figure 21.5 Cells involved in the early phase of non-adaptive response to tissue injury caused by a parasite.

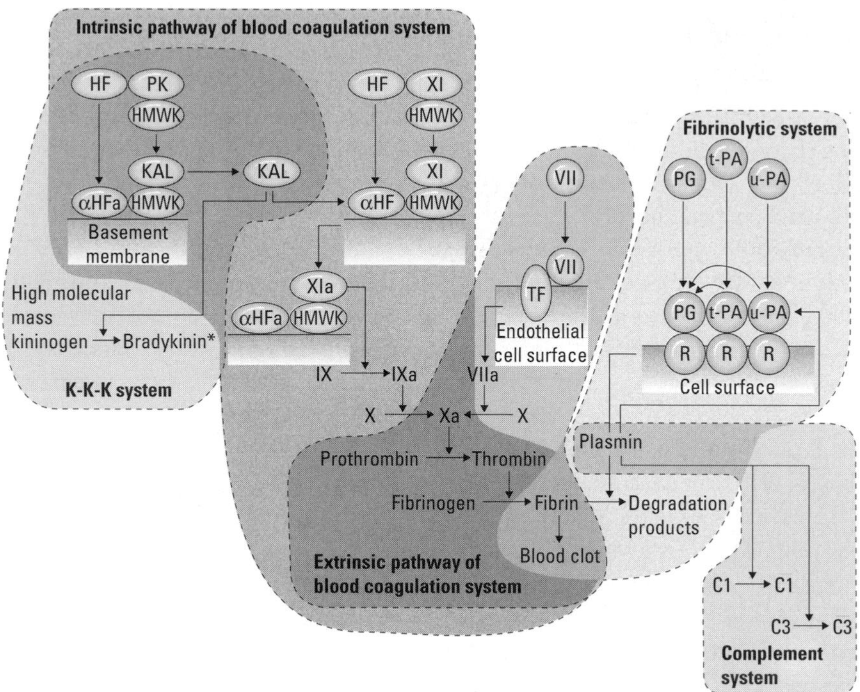

Figure 21.6 Relationships among the four activation systems based on blood plasma proteins. Symbols such as $\text{X} \xrightarrow{\text{XIa}} \text{Xa}$, indicate that inactive factor X is converted to active factor Xa by active factor XIa; *, in addition to bradykinin, two other fragments are produced which accelerate blood clotting. $\overline{\text{C1}}$ and $\overline{\text{C3}}$, activated C1 and C3 complement components; HF, Hageman factor; HMWK, high-molecular-mass (weight) kininogen; K-K-K, kallikrein–kininogen–kinin; KAL, kallikrein; PG, plasminogen; PK, prekallikrein; R, receptor; t-PA, tissue-type plasminogen activator; TF, tissue factor; u-PA, urokinase plasminogen activator.

expression of many other genes, whose products then become involved in various ways in the processes comprising the non-adaptive (and also adaptive) response (see Fig. 21.7 for a partial list).

Exposure of the basement membrane in the injured blood vessel supplies negatively charged surfaces necessary for the initiation of the *intrinsic coagulation pathway* ('intrinsic' because all its protein components are present in blood). The pathway also involves components of the *bradykinin* (*kallikrein–kininogen–kinin or K-K-K*) *system* and so the two are sometimes regarded as a single *contact activation system* (see Fig. 21.6). Initiation requires the participation of four main proteins: *Hageman factor* (HF, coagulation factor XII), a serine protease named after the patient in whose blood it was first identified; *prekallikrein* (PK), another serine protease, first isolated from pancreas (Greek *kallikreas*, pancreas); *high-molecular-mass (weight) kininogen* (HMWK), a protein that normally exists in plasma in a 1 : 1 complex with PK; and *coagulation factor XI*, the precursor form of yet another serine protease. These four components assemble on negatively charged surfaces such as collagen fibres and glycosaminoglycans of the basement membrane, heparin and bacterial lipopolysaccharides. HF binds to the surfaces first via positively charged amino acid residues of its heavy chain and is immediately joined by bimolecular complexes of HMWK and PK as well as HMWK and factor XI; the complexes attach to the surface via a histidine-rich, positively charged segment of the HMWK light chain. In the trimolecular HMWK–HF–PK complexes, HF activates PK, which in turn activates HF. Activated HF is cleaved either to αHFa (which remains surface bound) or to βHFa (which is released into the fluid phase); PK is cleaved into *kallikrein*, which is released into the fluid phase where it converts HMWK to a nine-residue peptide, *bradykinin*. Bradykinin effects smooth muscle contraction or relaxation and vasodilation; it is inactivated by peptidases. The freed kallikrein then activates factor XI in the trimolecular HF–HMWK–XI complexes. Activated factor XI activates factor X and the rest of this intrinsic pathway then proceeds as in the extrinsic pathway.

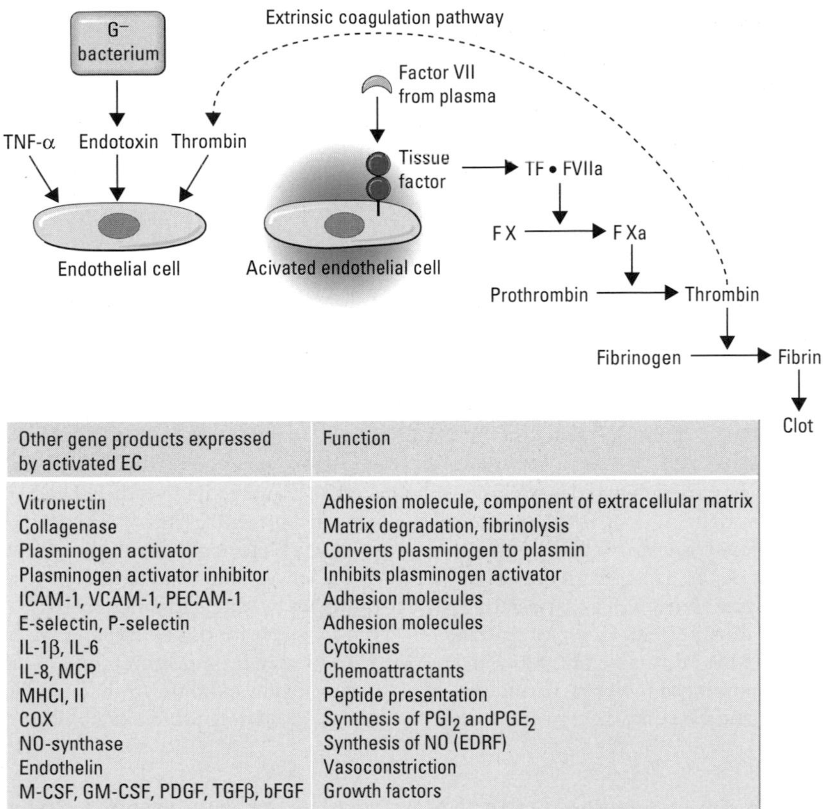

Other gene products expressed by activated EC	Function
Vitronectin	Adhesion molecule, component of extracellular matrix
Collagenase	Matrix degradation, fibrinolysis
Plasminogen activator	Converts plasminogen to plasmin
Plasminogen activator inhibitor	Inhibits plasminogen activator
ICAM-1, VCAM-1, PECAM-1	Adhesion molecules
E-selectin, P-selectin	Adhesion molecules
IL-1β, IL-6	Cytokines
IL-8, MCP	Chemoattractants
MHCI, II	Peptide presentation
COX	Synthesis of PGI_2 andPGE_2
NO-synthase	Synthesis of NO (EDRF)
Endothelin	Vasoconstriction
M-CSF, GM-CSF, PDGF, TGFβ, bFGF	Growth factors

Figure 21.7 Endothelial cell activation and initiation of the coagulation extrinsic pathway. bFGF, basic fibroblast growth factor; COX, cyclooxygenase; EC, endothelial cell; EDRF, endothelial-derived relaxing factor; F, factor (coagulation); GM-CSF, granulocyte–monocyte colony-stimulating factor; G^-, Gram-negative; ICAM, intercellular adhesion molecule; IL, interleukin; M-CSF, monocyte colony-stimulating factor; MCP, monocyte chemotactic protein; MHC, major histocompatibility complex; NO, nitric oxide; PDGF, platelet-derived growth factor; PECAM-1, platelet endothelial cell adhesion molecule; PG, prostaglandin; TF, tissue factor; TGF, transforming growth factor; TNF, tumour necrosis factor; VCAM, vascular cell adhesion molecule.

(Incidentally, factor XI and PK are related evolutionarily, encoded by genes presumably derived from the same ancestral gene.)

The extrinsic and intrinsic coagulation pathways are regulated by a set of inhibitors that include antithrombin, heparin cofactor II, tissue factor pathway inhibitor and protein C (Fig. 21.8). *Antithrombin* is a blood plasma glycoprotein that inhibits all active proteases of the coagulation system except factor VII, and it does so by forming tight equimolar complexes with the enzymes and blocking their catalytic sites. The inhibitory effect of antithrombin is greatly enhanced by *heparin*, which accelerates thrombin–antithrombin interaction by inducing a conformational change in the latter. *Heparin cofactor II* is, like antithrombin, a serpin, a serine protease inhibitor. It inactivates thrombin exclusively by posing as its substrate. Its action is enhanced by heparin and dermatan sulphate, the latter being, like heparin, a glycosaminoglycan. *Tissue factor pathway inhibitor* directly inhibits factor Xa and indirectly (with the participation of factor Xa) the TF–factor VIIa complex. Its activity, like that of the other two inhibitors, is augmented by heparin. *Protein C* is present in plasma in an inactive form and is activated by thrombin. But this activation proceeds slowly unless both factors are bound to their respective receptors on the luminal surface of vascular epithelium: thrombin to *thrombomodulin* and protein C to *endothelial-cell protein C receptor* (EPCR). The latter appears to be a member of the same protein family as the peptide-binding module of major histocompatibility complex (MHC) molecules. The thrombin–antithrombin complex activates receptor-bound protein C efficiently and activated protein C then binds another plasma component, *protein S*, while still attached to its receptor. The activated protein C–protein S complex then inactivates factors Va

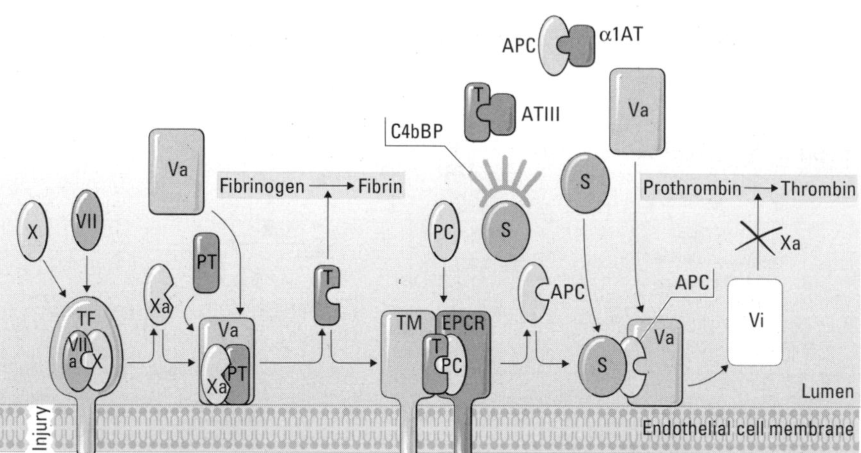

Figure 21.8 Regulatory mechanisms operating in the extrinsic coagulation pathway. From left to right: injury to the blood vessel leads to expression of the regulatory tissue factor (TF) on the endothelial cell surface. Tissue factor associates with the serine protease factor VIIa, which activates factor X. The serine protease factor Xa binds to another regulatory protein, factor Va, and the complex converts prothrombin (PT) to thrombin (T), which in turn catalyses the conversion of fibrinogen to fibrin. Thrombin binds to thrombomodulin (TM) and the complex converts protein C (PC), bound to its endothelial-cell protein C receptor (EPCR), to activated protein C (APC). Activated protein C in turn reacts with protein S (S) to accelerate the inactivation of factor Va. Inactivated factor Va (Vi) shuts down the conversion of prothrombin to thrombin by failing to function as a co-factor to factor Xa, which is responsible for this conversion. In the plasma, free thrombin is inactivated by antithrombin III (ATIII), activated protein C is inactivated by α_1-antitrypsin (α1AT) and protein S complexed with C4b-binding protein (C4bBP).

and VIIIa. *Factor Va* is involved as a co-factor in factor Xa-catalysed conversion of prothrombin to thrombin; hence its inactivation prevents the generation of factor Xa and thrombin. Thrombomodulin-bound thrombin itself is the target of another inhibitor, *antithrombin III*, which binds thrombin and the two then dissociate from thrombomodulin. Activated protein C is inhibited by complexation with either *protein C inhibitor* (PCI), *α_1-antitrypsin* (α_1-AT) or *α_2-macroglobulin*. Protein S circulates in complexes with *C4b-binding protein* (C4bBP), which bind in turn *serum amyloid P*, described later.

Each of the activation systems serves an important primary function, directly or indirectly concerned with defence against invaders and in more general terms with maintenance of the body's integrity. Each is, however, also involved in a number of secondary functions, at least some of which pertain to defence as well. The primary function of the coagulation system is to stop bleeding into the tissues. Each component of the system, however, also participates in a variety of other processes. Thrombin, for example, is not only a key enzyme in the formation of blood clots; it also activates platelets, triggers growth factor synthesis, promotes selected cell proliferation, causes synthesis and release of arachidonate metabolites, inhibits nerve cell growth and serves as a chemoattractant for neutrophils. Many different cell types express the seven-transmembrane-domain thrombin receptor and when activated by the ligand respond in a variety of ways, as we shall learn shortly. The same is apparently also true of several other coagulation system components: they too interact with their receptors to control cell proliferation and other functions. Thus, protein S binds to *Tyro 3*, a member of a family of tyrosine kinases expressed on the surface of endothelial cells, apparently to induce autophosphorylation of the receptor and to provide a mitogenic stimulus; factor Xa interacts with the *effector protease receptor-1* (EPR-1) to enhance prothrombin activation but also to promote lymphocyte proliferation; factor X interacts with Mac-1 (CD11b/CD18) on monocytes, not only to potentiate its own activation in the absence of TF, but also to facilitate the attachment and transmigration of monocytes across the endothelium; and so on. The business of the body's defence is emerging as an incredibly complex network of interactions involving dozens of different cell types and hundreds, perhaps thousands, of mediators and intercellular messengers.

Platelet activation

Thrombin produced in the coagulation cascade also becomes involved in the activation of *platelets*; some of the other stimuli that activate platelets are shown in Fig. 21.9. Platelets express a panoply of adhesion molecules: several integrins, P-selectin, platelet endothelial cell adhesion

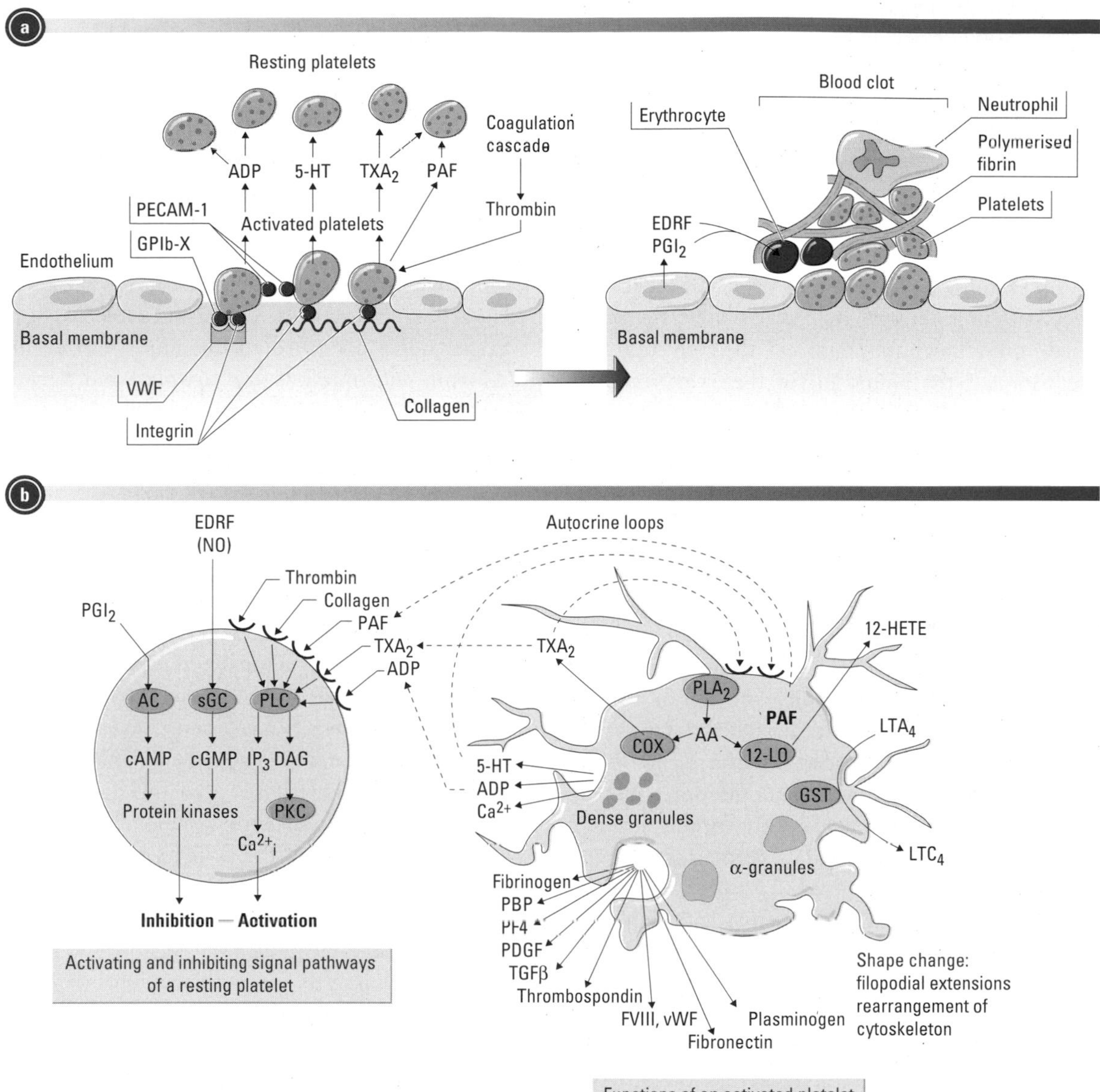

Figure 21.9 (a) Blood clotting and (b) platelet activation/inhibition. Explanation in the text. AA, arachidonic acid; AC, adenylate cyclase; ADP, adenosine diphosphate; cAMP, cyclic adenosine monophosphate; cGMP, cyclic guanosine monophosphate; COX, cyclooxygenase; DAG, 1,2-diacylglycerol; EDRF, endothelium-derived relaxing factor; FVIII, (coagulation) factor VIII; GP, glycoprotein; GST, glutathione-*S*-transferase; 12-HETE, 12-hydroxyeicosatetraenoic acid; 5-HT, 5-hydroxytryptamine (serotonin); IP_3, inositol 1,4,5-trisphosphate; 12-LO, 12-lipoxygenase; LTA_4, leukotriene A_4; LTC_4, leukotriene C_4; NO, nitric oxide; PAF, platelet-activating factor; PBP, platelet basic protein; PDGF, platelet-derived growth factor; PECAM-1, platelet endothelial cell adhesion molecule-1; PF4, platelet factor 4; PGI_2, prostaglandin I_2 (prostacyclin); PKC, protein kinase C; PLA_2, phospholipase A_2; PLC, phospholipase C; sGC, guanylyl cyclase; TGF-β, transforming growth factor-β; TXA_2, thromboxane A_2; vWF, von Willebrand factor. (b, modified from Ullrich, V., Hecker, G. & Schatz-Munding, M. (1991), in *Molecular Aspects of Inflammation* (Eds H. Sies, L. Flohe & G. Zimmer), p. 59. Springer-Verlag, Berlin.)

molecule-1 (PECAM-1, CD31, a member of the immunoglobulin superfamily) and glycoprotein Ib-IX (CD42, a member of a family characterized by a leucine-rich motif). These receptors normally do not bind their ligands, either because the interaction with them is of low affinity or because they do not have access to them. During tissue injury, however, thrombin (and other stimuli or *agonists*) activates platelets and thus converts the adhesion receptors from a low- to high-affinity state. Simultaneously, the rupture of blood vessels in the infected region exposes the basal membrane surrounding the endothelium of the vessel wall. The membrane is a layer of extracellular matrix composed mainly of tightly interwoven collagen and laminin fibres; it also contains *von Willebrand factor*, a large glycoprotein synthesized by endothelial cells. The factor is secreted into both the blood, in which it associates non-covalently with coagulation factor VIII and becomes one of the circulating plasma glycoproteins, and the matrix where it becomes immobilized. Activated platelets bind the immobilized von Willebrand factor via their glycoprotein Ib-IX receptors and the bound factor then also interacts with one of the high-affinity integrin receptors. This double contact causes the platelets to adhere strongly to the extracellular matrix. Moreover, the interaction of the receptors with their ligands leads to extensive cytoskeletal reorganization and thus spreading of the platelet over the matrix (Fig. 21.9). The adherent, activated platelets degranulate and release fibrinogen, fibronectin, vitronectin, osteopontin and additional von Willebrand factor (*release reaction*) into the matrix. (Another source of these components is blood plasma, in which they are normally present in soluble form.) All these components become attached to the matrix and serve as ligands of the various integrin receptors on platelets, both activated and resting. Some other platelet integrins also interact with matrix collagen and laminin. (PECAM-1 molecules of different platelets interact with each other or with glycosaminoglycans; P-selectin binds sialylated and fucosylated carbohydrates of specific leucocyte glycoproteins.) The net result of these interactions is the *spreading* of some platelets on the surface of the matrix and the *aggregation* of others (the latter is mediated by homotypic interaction or by fibrinogen and other soluble-form ligands forming bridges between receptors on different cells).

Among the substances liberated from platelet granules during the release reaction is also a non-metabolic pool of *adenosine diphosphate* (ADP), which then binds to resting platelets, thereby activating them and thus augmenting the reaction. The platelet aggregate enmeshed in the strands of polymerized fibrin is the *haemostatic plug* (haemostasis being the arrest of bleeding), the seed of an intravascular *clot* or *thrombus*. Other substances discharged from the granules include: *serotonin* (5-HT), a neurotransmitter that causes smooth muscle contractions either directly or via nerves; *platelet basic protein* (PBP), a cytokine proteolytically processed to form active mediators; *connective tissue activating peptide-III* (CTAP-III), a mitogen also referred to as low-affinity platelet factor 4 (LA-PF4); *β-thromboglobulin* (βTG), a fibroblast chemoattractant; *neutrophil attracting peptide-2* (NAP-2); *platelet factor 4* (PF4 or oncostatin A), which acts as a monocyte and neutrophil attractant, as an anticoagulant when bound to heparin, and inhibitor of blood vessel development; *platelet-derived growth factor* (PDGF), a cytokine that stimulates growth of connective tissue cells during wound healing and serves as a chemoattractant for fibroblasts, smooth muscles, monocytes and neutrophils; transforming growth factor-β (TGF-β), a pleiotropic cytokine that inhibits cell growth during tissue remodelling and wound repair; and molecules involved in platelet adhesion (*thrombospondin*, *fibronectin*, *factor VIII–von Willebrand factor complex* and *fibrinogen*; see Fig. 21.9).

Ligand occupancy of several types of platelet receptors leads to the release of intracellular Ca^{2+} ions and activation of membrane phospholipases, which then hydrolyse membrane phosphatidylcholine and phosphatidylinositol. Hydrolysis of phosphatidylcholine by phospholipase A_2 (PLA_2) produces 1-O-alkyl-*sn*-glycero-3-phosphocholine (lyso-PAF) and arachidonic acid (see Chapter 11). Lyso-PAF is then converted enzymatically to *platelet-activating factor* (PAF), which diffuses out of the cell, binds to other, resting platelets via a specific receptor (a seven-transmembrane-domain protein) and activates them. The liberated *arachidonic acid* is oxygenated by one of two enzymes, cyclooxygenase or 12-lipoxygenase (see Fig. 11.5). *Cyclooxygenase* converts the acid to endoperoxides (PGG_2 and PGH_2) and these transient intermediates are subsequently processed to several other products, of which the most important is *thromboxane* A_2 (TXA_2). Thromboxane is released, passively or actively, into the surrounding medium, binds to receptors on other platelets and generates a signal that mobilizes Ca^{2+} ions from intracellular stores. The free Ca^{2+} inhibits adenylate cyclase and thus lowers the level of cAMP, causing contraction of tubules, discharge of granules and platelet aggregation.

The other enzyme, *12-lipoxygenase*, processes arachidonic acid via intermediates to *12-hydroxyeicosatetraenoic acid* (12-HETE), which is released into the medium (see Fig. 11.5). It probably functions as a chemoattractant for neutrophils and smooth muscle cells; it also enhances TF expression on endotoxin-induced monocytes. Platelets lack 5-lipoxygenase and hence cannot produce leukotrienes from endogenous arachidonic acid. However, they can convert exogenously provided leukotriene A_4 to LTC_4 because they possess glutathione-*S*-transferase, the enzyme necessary for the conversion. The released LTC_4 serves as a chemoattractant that draws neutrophils to the clot (see Fig. 21.9); it also increases permeability of blood vessels.

Haemostasis

Clot formation (haemostasis) is regulated by several mechanisms ensuring that the process does not spread beyond the immediate area around the injured tissue. One of the regulatory mechanisms relies on arachidonates of the endothelium. Stimulation of endothelial cells activates membrane-bound phospholipases and these liberate arachidonic acid that is converted by cyclooxygenase into endoperoxides, just as in platelets. In endothelial cells, however, the endoperoxides are converted to *prostacyclin* (PGI_2 and other eicosanoids; see Fig. 11.5), which platelets are unable to produce. PGI_2 is then released to act on other platelets via specific receptors. PGI_2 bound to its receptor stimulates adenylate kinase, causing an elevation in cAMP levels and thus sequestration of Ca^{2+} ions into intracellular stores. Shortage of Ca^{2+} then inhibits platelet aggregation and suppresses the release reaction (see Fig. 21.9). Endothelial cells also use endoperoxides (PGG_2, PGH_2) released from platelets to increase the synthesis of PGI_2 and thus augment the inhibitory effects on platelets.

Further restraints are placed on platelet activities by the vascular endothelium via another mechanism. Endothelial cells contain the enzyme *nitric oxide synthase* (NOS) capable of converting, via intermediates, L-arginine into L-citrulline (in a reaction accompanied by the release of gaseous radical *nitric oxide*, NO; see Chapter 15). The enzyme is expressed constitutively at a low level (in contrast to macrophage NOS, which is inducible and encoded in a separate but related gene), but expression is increased by stimuli such as the neurotransmitter acetylcholine, bradykinin or shear stress acting on the endothelium. These stimuli cause an influx of Ca^{2+} ions, their binding to calmodulin and activation of NOS. The released NO is identical to what was originally described as *endothelial-derived relaxing factor* (EDRF), identified by its effect on smooth muscle (relaxation of the muscle fibres surrounding blood vessels and hence vasodilation). The newly synthesized NO diffuses to adjacent muscle cells where it activates guanylyl cyclase, which influences cyclic GMP (cGMP) levels. A cGMP-dependent protein kinase then initiates phosphorylation of myosin light chains and thus causes relaxation of contracted muscles. A similar sequence of events is also set in motion by NO diffusing into platelets. However, here the ultimate target of the sequence is apparently elements of the cytoskeleton and the end result is suppression of the release reaction and inhibition of platelet aggregation (see Fig. 21.9b).

Regulatory interactions also occur between platelets and neutrophils, which are brought with the bloodstream to the clot. The interactions are both stimulatory and inhibitory and involve not only arachidonate metabolites but also other molecules released from the two types of cells (Fig. 21.10). Platelets contain sufficient Ca^{2+} in their intracellular stores to activate their PLA_2 and thus to produce the endoperoxides PGG_2 and PGH_2 from arachidonic acid. In neutrophils, on the other hand, the intracellular Ca^{2+} supply may be too small for PLA_2 activation. But since platelets produce more endoperoxides than they need for their own use, they donate the surplus to neutrophils, which use it to produce LTA_4 via the 5-lipoxygenase pathway (this enzyme is also Ca^{2+} dependent but less than PLA_2 and the Ca^{2+} from intracellular stores is sufficient for it to function).

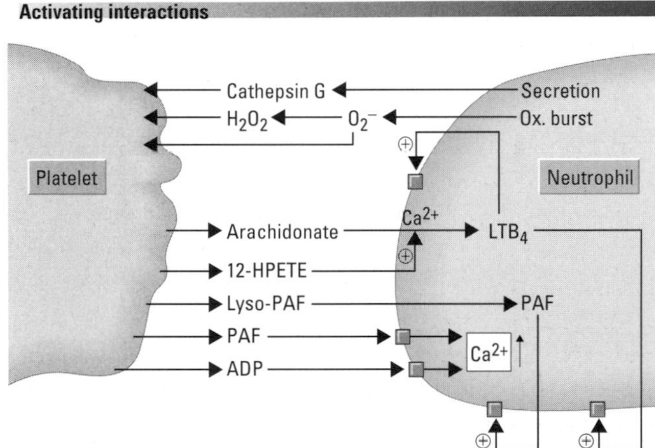

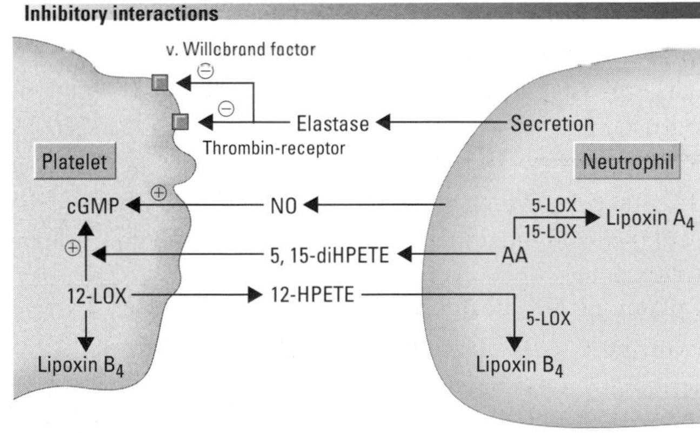

Figure 21.10 Molecular interactions between platelets and neutrophils. Explanation in the text. □, Receptor; (+), activation or upregulation; (–), inhibition or downregulation. ADP, adenosine diphosphate; cGMP, cyclic guanosine monophosphate; diHPETE, dihydroperoxyeicosatetraenoic acid; HPETE, hydroperoxyeicosatetraenoic acid; LOX, lipoxygenase; LTB, leukotriene B; NO, nitric oxide; Ox., oxidative; PAF, platelet-activating factor. (Modified from Ullrich, V., Hecker, G. & Schatz-Munding, M. (1991), in *Molecular Aspects of Inflammation* (Eds H. Sies, L. Flohe & G. Zimmer), p. 59. Springer-Verlag, Berlin.)

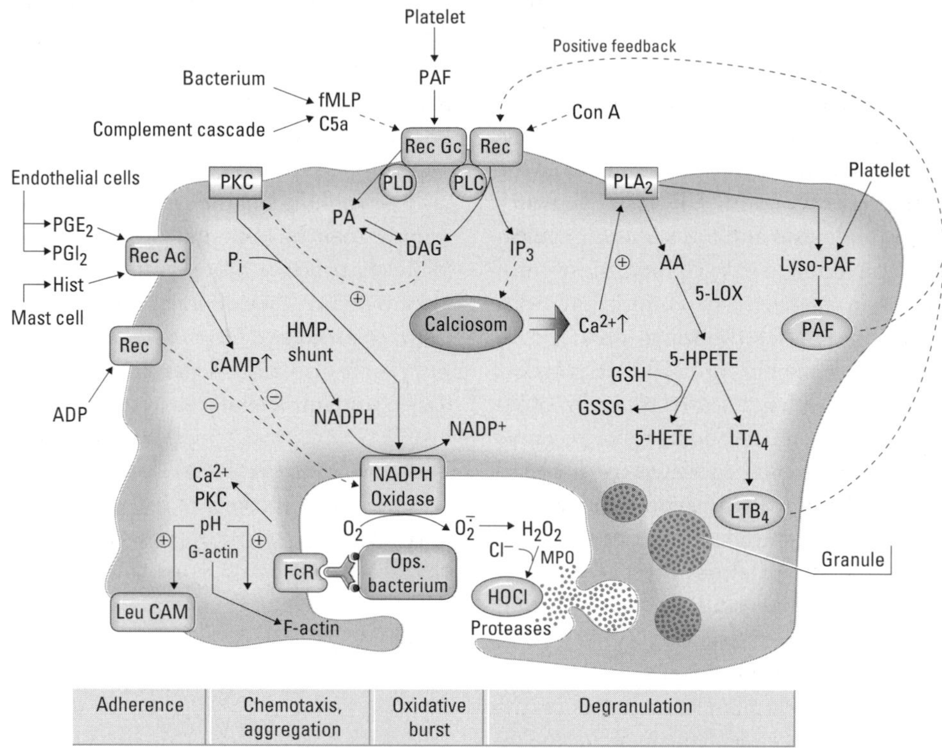

Figure 21.11 Stimulation and signal transduction in a neutrophil. AA, arachidonic acid; AC, adenylate cyclase; ADP, adenosine diphosphate; cAMP, cyclic adenosine monophosphate; Con A, concanavalin A; DAG, 1,2-diacylglycerol; FcR, Fc receptor; fMLP, N-formyl-methionyl-leucyl-phenylalanine; G, G-protein; GSH, glutathione; GSSG, glutathione disulphide; Hist, histamine; HMP, hexose monophosphate; HPETE, hydroperoxyeicosatetraenoic acid; IP_3, inositol trisphophate; LeuCAM, leucocyte cell adhesion molecule; 5-LOX, 5-lipoxygenase; LTA (B), leukotriene A (B); MPO, myeloperoxidase; NADPH and $NADP^+$, nicotinamide adenine dinucleotide phosphate, reduced and oxidized forms; Ops., opsonized; Pi, orthophosphate ion; PA, phosphatic acid; PAF, platelet-activating factor; PGE (I), prostaglandin E (I); PKC, protein kinase C; PLA_2, phospholipase A_2; PLC, phospholipase C; PLD, phospholipase D; Rec, receptor. (Modified from Ullrich, V., Hecker, G. & Schatz-Munding, M. (1991), in *Molecular Aspects of Inflammation* (Eds H. Sies, L. Flohe & G. Zimmer), p. 59. Springer-Verlag, Berlin.)

The released LTA_4 binds to specialized receptors on the same cell and the resulting activation signals lead to, among other things, opening of Ca^{2+} channels and influx of extracellular Ca^{2+} into the cell (Fig. 21.11). Platelets may also contribute to arachidonate metabolism in neutrophils in a different way. Using their 12-lipoxygenase they produce 12-hydroperoxyeicosatetraenoic acid (12-HPETE), some of which they export to neutrophils. In these cells, 12-HPETE potentiates the activity of 5-lipoxygenase, the enzyme that produces LTA_4 and LTB_4 (it ultimately also converts 12-HPETE to 5,12-dihydroxyeicosatetraenoic acid (5,12-diHETE)).

Platelets also produce lyso-PAF, only some of which is converted into PAF. The excess lyso-PAF diffuses into neutrophils where it is converted to PAF which, like LTA_4 and probably via the same receptors, stimulates the cell (Fig. 21.11). Once the neutrophil's PLA_2 is activated, the cell produces its own lyso-PAF and PAF, which then reinforce the autocrine stimulatory loop. However, neutrophils can be activated also by PAF provided by platelets.

LTB_4 and PAF are only two of several compounds that stimulate neutrophils; others include ADP provided by platelets, prostaglandin E_2 and PGI_2 contributed by endothelial cells, histamine supplied by mast cells, C5a derived from the complement cascade and fMLP[1] derived from microorganisms (see Fig. 21.11). Several activation

[1] Prokaryotes and the mitochondria of eukaryotic cells begin the synthesis of their polypeptides not with methionine, as in eukaryotes, but with the *N*-formyl derivative of methionine. Furthermore, eukaryotes usually remove the initial methionine residue once synthesis of the polypeptide is underway, whereas prokaryotes usually keep the formyl-methionine residue at the first position of their polypeptides. When microbial proteins are broken down into peptides, those derived from the N-terminus begin with the formyl-methionine residue; fMLP is therefore *N*-formyl-methionyl-leucyl-phenylalanine.

signals are also generated by the activities of the neutrophil associated with migration and phagocytosis; these are dealt with later in this chapter (see also Chapter 15; some of them are shown in Fig. 21.11). Cathepsin G, hydrogen peroxide (H_2O_2) and active oxygen radicals (O_2^-), in turn, can serve as platelet activation stimuli. In experimental set-ups, neutrophils are also activated by concanavalin A; *in vivo* the concanavalin A receptor presumably binds unidentified lectin-like molecules.

In addition to stimulatory signals, platelets and neutrophils also exchange *inhibitory signals*, which limit the activities of these two cells (see Fig. 21.10b). Two examples of the inhibitory signals involve NO and elastase. *NO* and *5,15-diHPETE* produced by the neutrophil influence the level of cGMP in the platelet, thereby initiating a signal cascade that inhibits the release reaction and limits platelet aggregation. *Elastase* secreted by neutrophils cleaves von Willebrand factor as well as the thrombin receptor at the platelet surface and so downregulates platelet aggregation.

The blood clot must not only be prevented from growing uncontrollably; ultimately it must also be removed so that blood circulation in the affected region can be restored. The basis of the elimination process is fibrinolysis, the degradation of fibrin strands by components of the *fibrinolytic system* (see Fig. 21.6). Degradation is accomplished by *plasmin*, a plasma serine protease derived by proteolytic cleavage from the enzymatically inactive *plasminogen*. The two enzymes that cleave plasminogen are *urokinase* and *tissue-type plasminogen activator* (t-PA). Plasminogen from the plasma binds to fibrin strands and to the surfaces of all cells that have been tested. Binding is of low affinity (K_d in the range of 100–200 nM) but the number of binding sites ('receptors') per cell is quite high (several million in the case of endothelial cells); it occurs between the lysine-binding site of plasminogen and terminal lysine residues of surface proteins. Surface-bound plasminogen is converted to plasmin by urokinase and t-PA, which are also surface bound to their respective receptors. Plasmin cleaves surface proteins and generates additional binding sites for plasminogen binding, thus amplifying the reaction. Plasmin also activates receptor-bound prourokinase to become a more efficient urokinase. Fibrinolysis is regulated by a number of proteins and glycoproteins, in particular by α_2-antiplasmin which inactivates plasmin (the free form much more rapidly than the cell-bound form).

At least one component of the fibrinolytic activation system is also involved in the *complement cascade*, thus tying these two systems together: plasmin can proteolytically activate both the C1 and C3 components (see Fig. 21.6). The complement cascade, however, is probably switched on very early in the response independently of the fibrinolytic system. Infection produces several stimuli that may activate either the alternative or the classical pathway (Chapter 12). Certain components of the parasite's cell surface, such as the polysaccharide moiety of the lipopolysaccharide (LPS) in Gram-negative bacteria, promote initiation of the alternative pathway.

The *classical pathway* can be activated by antibodies, and by C-reactive protein, mannose-binding protein, protein A and conglutinin, as well as by certain other lectins (see Chapter 12). Antibodies to specific antigens of the parasite appear, of course, much later in the response, but the host may possess *natural antibodies* that can bind to the invader's surface components. Natural antibodies are presumably either echoes of previous low-grade or inapparent infections or are the products of continuous exposure to microorganisms of the normal flora. They circulate with the blood and enter the tissues with other plasma proteins. Some may react or cross-react with antigens of the invading microorganisms and the Fc portion of the bound antibodies may bind the $C1qC1r_2C1s_2$ complex and thus turn on the classical pathway. *Mannose-binding protein* (MBP) is present in the plasma at low levels that increase dramatically later in the response. It binds to terminal *N*-acetylglucosamine, mannose, fucose or glucose residues of mannose-rich oligosaccharides in bacteria, viruses and yeasts. The bound MBP mimics C1q and thus activates the classical pathway without the participation of antibodies (see Chapter 12). The level of *C-reactive protein* in the plasma, like that of MBP, increases as the infection progresses. The protein binds with one site to phosphocholine residues on the surface of certain microorganisms and with another to C1q, which subsequently activates the $C1r_2C1s_2$ proenzyme and thus sets the classical pathway in motion. *Protein A* of some bacteria binds the Fc part of IgG molecules that happen to be circulating with the plasma, regardless of their antigenic specificity. The Fc region of the bound antibodies binds, in turn, the $C1qC1r_2C1s_2$ complex and activation of the classical pathway follows.

Conglutinin is another plasma protein with overall similarity to C1q, although not high enough for binding the $C1r_2C1s_2$ complex. Instead, conglutinin becomes involved in the complement cascade at the C3b stage (after the cascade has been activated by some other stimulus). It binds to carbohydrates exposed on iC3b and functions as opsonin. Both conglutinin and MBP, however, may bind to C1q collectin receptors, which are widely distributed among a variety of cell types. If they then recognize carbohydrates on the parasite's surface (conglutinin is, like MBP, a lectin), they may serve as opsonins without involving the complement cascade in the process.

Mast cell responses

Blood vessels constitute one focus of responses initiated by the invading parasite; the other is in the tissues and involves, in the early phase, mainly mast cells and macrophages. *Mast cells* of the connective tissue are often clustered along blood and lymph vessels, nerves and glandular ducts, especially in the gastrointestinal tract, respiratory tract and skin, areas the parasite is likely to enter during infection. Mast cells bear a number of receptors on their surfaces enabling them to respond to stimuli produced by the infection. Stimulation through different receptors may activate diverse intracellular signalling pathways and lead to distinct responses. Stimuli include neuropeptides, anaphylatoxins, ATP, formyl-methionine peptides, LPS, cytokines and, in the later stage of infection and especially in invasions by certain parasites, antibodies of the IgE (but also IgG) class (Fig. 21.12). The response may consist of the synthesis and release of lipid mediators, production of cytokines, receptor-mediated endocytosis and even phagocytosis, as well as the release of preformed mediators stored in intracellular granules (degranulation in Fig. 21.12).

Neuropeptides, exemplified by *substance P* (SP), are synthesized by neurons and used as neurotransmitters, substances released at a nerve terminal as a result of a nerve impulse and capable of transmitting the impulse across the synaptic gap by binding to receptors on another neuron, thereby exciting it. Parasite activities in the tissue lead to stimulation of local nerve endings and to the release of SP from nerve terminals. Some of the released SP binds to receptors on mast cells surrounding the terminals, thereby activating them. Activation leads to degranulation and cytokine production.

Of the three *anaphylatoxins* produced in the complement cascade, C5a stimulates mast cells most strongly, C3a less strongly and C4a weakly. The response to C5a stimulation includes the release of preformed mediators, whereas the response to C3a and C4a stimulation does not. C4a stimulation usually only enhances responses to IgE stimulation. The mast cell-stimulating *ATP* is provided by activated platelets and other cells, *formyl-methionine peptides* and *LPS* by microorganisms, and *cytokines* mainly by nerve cells, macrophages and lymphocytes. All three types of stimuli may lead to cytokine production by mast cells.

Lipid mediators synthesized by activated mast cells include PAF and arachidonic acid metabolites, mainly LTC_4 and PGD_2. Via these metabolites, mast cells communicate with smooth muscle cells, vascular endothelial cells, platelets, neutrophils, macrophages and other cells. The main effects of LTC_4 and PGD_2 are smooth muscle contraction and blood vessel dilation, respectively. The secretion of *cytokines* is a relatively recent discovery; mast cells were originally thought to bind cytokines, but not to produce them. In fact, activated mast cells secrete a plethora of cytokines, including IL-3, IL-4, IL-5, IL-8, granulocyte–monocyte colony-stimulating factor (GM-CSF), nerve growth factor (NGF), TNF-α, interferon-γ (IFN-γ) and leukaemia inhibitory factor (LIF). Different stimuli seem to lead to the production of diverse cytokines and the mast-cell surface is equipped with receptors for receiving cytokine-mediated signals from other cells. Mast cells are thus part of the cytokine network, enabling them to exchange messages with neurons, endothelial cells, macrophages, neutrophils, monocytes and lymphocytes. Because they also have receptors for the cytokines they secrete, they receive feedback information about their own activities. For example, mast cells secrete NGF and GM-CSF, which stimulate nerve growth but also have an autocrine effect on mast cells themselves. The main functions of mast cell-secreted cytokines include recruitment of neutrophils (via IL-8), induction of the acute-phase response proteins (more of which later) via

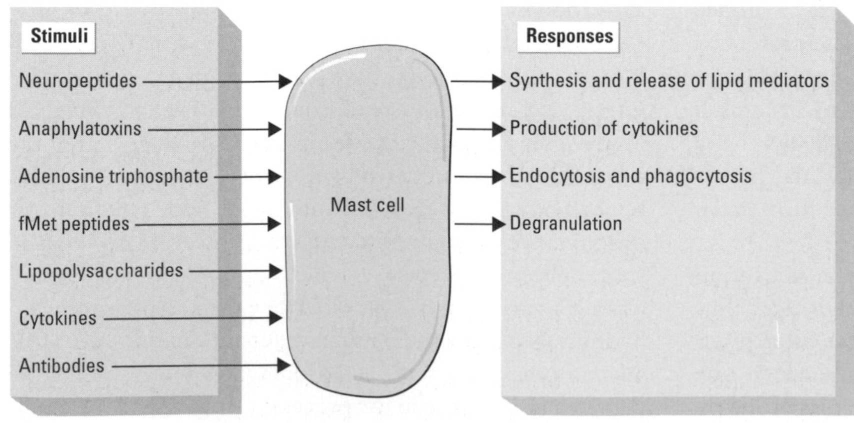

Figure 21.12 Mast-cell stimulators and mast-cell responses. fMet, formyl-methionine (peptide).

LIF, induction of E-selectin expression on vascular endothelial cells (via TNF-α) and induction of helper T (T_H)-cell differentiation (via IL-4), as well as integrin expression on Langerhans' cells.

Mast cells also possess *Fc receptors* not only for IgE but also for certain subclasses of IgG. The FcγRIII receptors can become involved in engulfment and phagocytosis of microorganisms. Engulfed bacteria can then be killed by some of the preformed mediators contained in mast-cell granules.

Most of the preformed mediators, however, are released by *degranulation* into the extracellular space, where they carry out a variety of functions. The three chief categories of preformed mediators are biogenic amines (histamine and serotonin; see Chapter 11), neutral proteases (chymase, tryptase and others) and proteoglycans (heparin). *Histamine* acts via its three receptors, H_1, H_2 and H_3, of which the first two are the most important. The receptors are expressed on monocytes, lymphocytes (T and B), neutrophils, endothelial cells, smooth muscle cells, glial and nerve cells, chondrocytes, hepatocytes and gastric parietal cells. All these cells may therefore, under certain circumstances, be stimulated by histamine and thus inducted into the response. Histamine-mediated effects include smooth muscle contraction, increase in vascular permeability, neurotransmission, regulation (positive or negative) of cytokine (IL-1, IL-2, IL-6, IL-8, TNF-α) production, regulation of natural killer (NK)-cell activity, regulation of acute-phase protein and complement component production, gastric acid secretion, hepatic glycogenolysis, gluconeogenesis and ureagenesis. *Serotonin* is present in the granules of only some species (e.g. rodents), usually bound to proteins. Its effects are described in Chapter 11. Released *chymase* inactivates bradykinin, attacks the basement membrane and activates the IL-1β precursor and angiotensin I (a peptide released by the action of the enzyme renin on a plasma protein: it stimulates smooth muscles of blood vessels). Released *tryptase* inactivates fibrinogen. *Heparin* forms the matrix of the secretory granule and provides the scaffolding to which many of the preformed mediators attach by ionic bonds. It also has anticoagulant and anti-complement effects.

Macrophage responses

No matter where a parasite has entered the body, it will invariably encounter *macrophages*. Parasites that have invaded the body via blood (by an insect bite for example) will be confronted by Kupffer cells lining liver sinuses and macrophages in the spleen. Parasites that have gained entrance through the lungs (with inhaled aerosol) will be accosted by macrophages lining the alveolar surfaces. If a parasite or its products have reached the nervous system, they will immediately run into microglial cells, and so on. In addition to macrophages, which reside in various tissues, the parasite will also encounter neutrophils. Much of the following description of macrophages also applies to neutrophils, the other *professional phagocytes*.

You will recall that macrophage precursors originate in the bone marrow, where they develop under the influence of GM-CSF and other cytokines into mature monocytes. After leaving the bone marrow, monocytes circulate in the blood for a brief period and then enter the tissues to become macrophages. In an unperturbed body, the recently immigrated cells downregulate a number of their genes and become settled. The pools of these *resident macrophages* are maintained both by local division and immigration from blood. In contrast to mast cells or platelets, for example, resident macrophages are by no means 'retired'. They are highly active metabolically, recycle their cell surfaces through endocytosis, synthesize and secrete proteins and other substances and, as they move about, continuously reorganize their cytoskeleton and microtubular networks. They also respond to numerous signals received via corresponding receptors. The signals include cytokines, lipid mediators, anaphylatoxins, chemokines, glucocorticosteroids, insulin, transferrin, lactoferrin, ligands on parasite surfaces, opsonins, antigens and others (Fig. 21.13). The responses mounted to these signals comprise secretion of cytokines, release of lipid mediators, secretion of complement components, secretion of coagulation factors, secretion of antiparasitic proteins, phagocytosis, production of reactive oxygen and nitrogen intermediates and antigen presentation (Fig. 21.13). Depending on the signal or combination of signals they receive, macrophages can exist in a number of functional states characterized by the expression of different sets of genes and different combinations of response. One particular state, that of highest alert, is often referred to as *activation* and the cells in that state as *activated macrophages*, although technically, of course, all other conditions are activations as well (see Chapter 19). Examples of different response combinations mounted to various signals are given below.

Macrophage involvement in the defence system is determined by its functional state. In essence, macrophages can participate in one or several of the following functions: chemotaxis, communication via cytokine and lipid mediator networks, regulation of coagulation and fibrinolysis, regulation of the complement cascade, regulation of extracellular enzymatic activities, regulation of acute-phase protein production, phagocytosis, killing of parasites and antigen presentation. A description of most of these

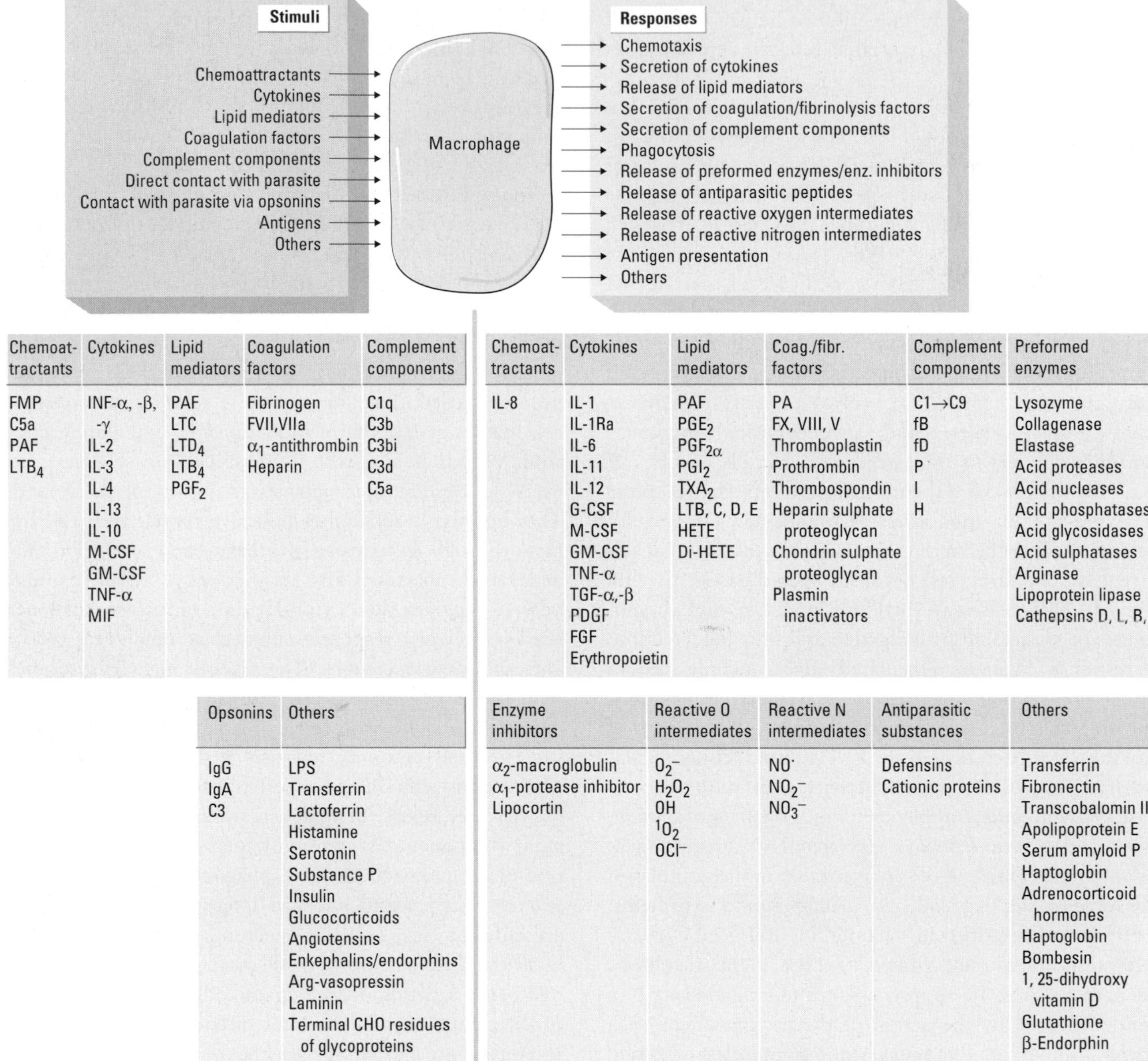

Chemoattractants	Cytokines	Lipid mediators	Coagulation factors	Complement components
FMP	INF-α, -β, -γ	PAF	Fibrinogen	C1q
C5a	IL-2	LTC	FVII,VIIa	C3b
PAF	IL-3	LTD_4	α_1-antithrombin	C3bi
LTB_4	IL-4	LTB_4	Heparin	C3d
	IL-13	PGF_2		C5a
	IL-10			
	M-CSF			
	GM-CSF			
	TNF-α			
	MIF			

Opsonins	Others
IgG	LPS
IgA	Transferrin
C3	Lactoferrin
	Histamine
	Serotonin
	Substance P
	Insulin
	Glucocorticoids
	Angiotensins
	Enkephalins/endorphins
	Arg-vasopressin
	Laminin
	Terminal CHO residues of glycoproteins

Chemoattractants	Cytokines	Lipid mediators	Coag./fibr. factors	Complement components	Preformed enzymes
IL-8	IL-1	PAF	PA	C1→C9	Lysozyme
	IL-1Ra	PGE_2	FX, VIII, V	fB	Collagenase
	IL-6	$PGF_{2\alpha}$	Thromboplastin	fD	Elastase
	IL-11	PGI_2	Prothrombin	P	Acid proteases
	IL-12	TXA_2	Thrombospondin	I	Acid nucleases
	G-CSF	LTB, C, D, E	Heparin sulphate proteoglycan	H	Acid phosphatases
	M-CSF	HETE	Chondrin sulphate proteoglycan		Acid glycosidases
	GM-CSF	Di-HETE	Plasmin inactivators		Acid sulphatases
	TNF-α				Arginase
	TGF-α,-β				Lipoprotein lipase
	PDGF				Cathepsins D, L, B,
	FGF				
	Erythropoietin				

Enzyme inhibitors	Reactive O intermediates	Reactive N intermediates	Antiparasitic substances	Others
α_2-macroglobulin	O_2^-	$NO^{\cdot}$	Defensins	Transferrin
α_1-protease inhibitor	H_2O_2	NO_2^-	Cationic proteins	Fibronectin
Lipocortin	OH	NO_3^-		Transcobalomin II
	$^1O_2$			Apolipoprotein E
	OCl^-			Serum amyloid P
				Haptoglobin
				Adrenocorticoid hormones
				Haptoglobin
				Bombesin
				1, 25-dihydroxy vitamin D
				Glutathione
				β-Endorphin

Figure 21.13 Macrophage stimulators and macrophage responses. Arg, arginine; CHO, carbohydrate; F(f), factor; FGF, fibroblast growth factor; FMP, formyl-methionine peptide; (di) HETE, (di) hydroxyeicosatetraenoic acid; INF, interferon; IL, interleukin; LPS, lipopolysaccharide; LT, leukotriene; M(G)-CSF, monocyte (granulocyte) colony-stimulating factor; MHC, major histocompatibility complex; MIF, migration inhibition factor; PA, plasminogen activator; PAF, platelet-activating factor; PDGF, platelet-derived growth factor; PG, prostaglandin; Ra, receptor antagonist; TGF, transforming growth factor; TNF, tumour necrosis factor; TX, thromboxane.

functions is given in the preceding chapters (see especially Chapter 15). Here, the picture is only broadened slightly.

A macrophage's place during an infection is at the centre of an invasion. Although some macrophages will probably be present at any site the parasite happens to invade, their numbers there will be bolstered by the deployment of cells from neighbouring areas. Macrophages are lured to the centre of infection by chemoattractants such as anaphylatoxins (mainly C5a) released from the complement cascade and by products released from disintegrating parasites, primarily formyl-methionine peptides.

Macrophages both receive and transmit signals in the form of *cytokines* (Fig. 21.14) and the secreted cytokines involve the macrophage in the cytokine network

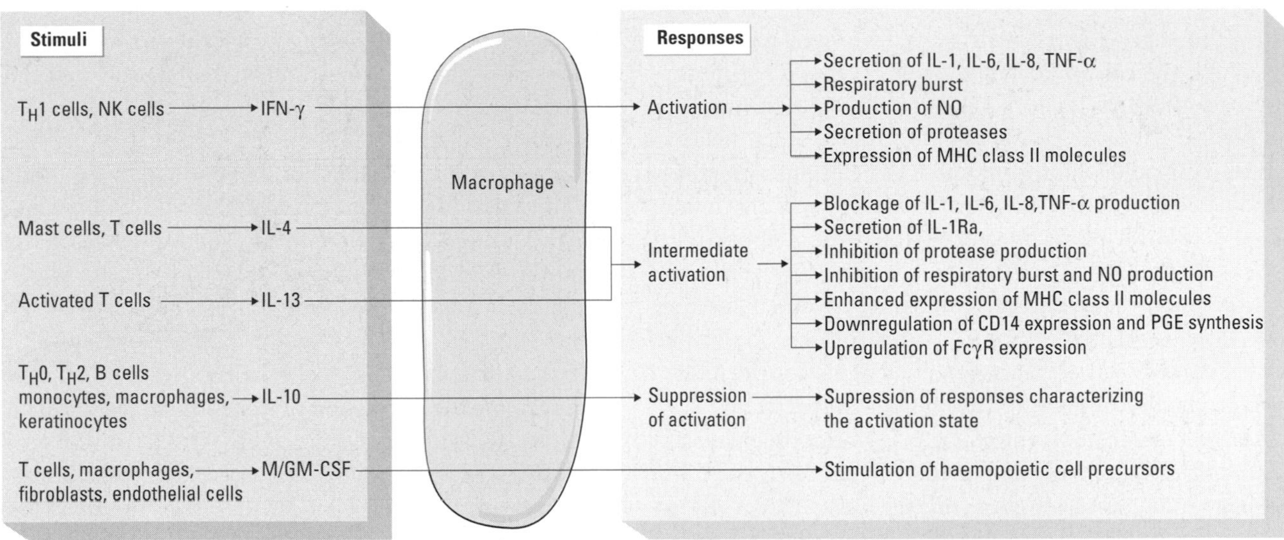

Figure 21.14 Responses induced by binding of cytokines to their receptors on macrophages (or their precursors). CD, cluster of differentiation; FcγR, Fcγ receptor; IFN, interferon; IL, interleukin; M/GM-CSF, monocyte/granulocyte–monocyte colony-stimulating factor; NK, natural killer; NO, nitric oxide; PG, prostaglandin; Ra, receptor antagonist; TNF, tumour necrosis factor.

(Fig. 21.15). They include IL-1 and IL-6, which become major stimuli for the production of acute-phase proteins (described later) and which also play an important part in lymphocyte activation and differentiation (IL-1 in T- and IL 6 in B lymphocyte activation); IL 8, a chemoattractant that lures neutrophils to the site of infection; IL-11, granulocyte colony-stimulating factor (G-CSF), monocyte colony-stimulating factor (M-CSF) and GM-CSF, which by stimulating haemopoietic precursor cells assure adequate replacements for the cells lost in combat; IL-12, which elicits IFN-γ production by NK cells and facilitates the development of T_H1-type lymphocytes in the later stages of defence; TNF-α, which can kill some of the infected cells and also activate cytokine production and promote MHC molecule expression; as well as TGF-β, which participates in wound healing and the formation of new blood vessels (angiogenesis).

As with cytokines, in the case of *lipid metabolites* macrophages are at both the receiving and producing end (see Fig. 21.13). They receive lipid-mediator signals from endothelial cells, mast cells, platelets and other cells and they synthesize lipid mediators *de novo* for their own use and to exert influence on other cells. The mediators comprise both PAF and arachidonic acid metabolites. Macrophage responses to PAF include chemotaxis, promotion of superoxide anion, IL-1, TNF-α, prostaglandin and

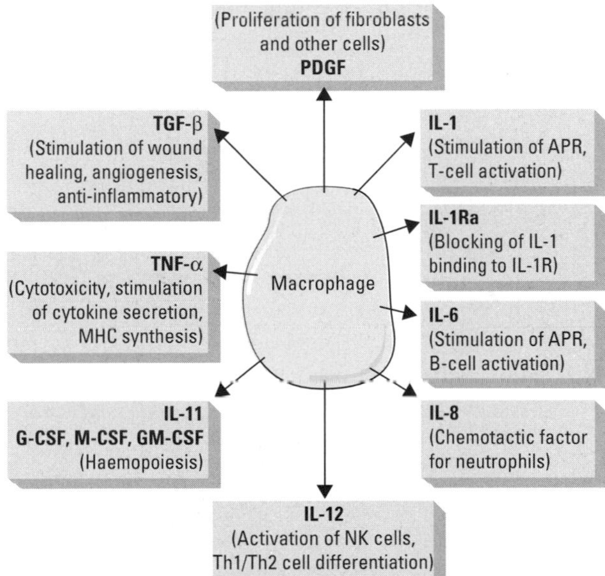

Figure 21.15 Cytokines produced by macrophages and their effects. APR, acute-phase response; GM-CSF, granulocyte–monocyte colony-stimulating factor; IL, interleukin; NK, natural killer (cell); PDGF, platelet-derived growth factor; R, receptor; ra, receptor antagonist; TGF, transforming growth factor; TNF, tumour necrosis factor.

leukotriene production, as well as enhancement of cytotoxic effects. The PAF produced by macrophages can act on platelets, neutrophils and monocytes/macrophages and induce a variety of responses in these cells (see Fig. 21.14). Macrophages can respond to LTC_4, LTD_4, LTB_4 and PGE_2 produced by other cells and they can release PGE_2, $PGF_{2\alpha}$, PGI_2, TXA_2, LTB_4, LTC_4, LTD_4, LTE_4, HETEs and diHETEs for use by other cells.

Macrophages *regulate the coagulation and fibrinolytic systems* by, again, receiving signals from and generating signals for the cascade. They possess receptors for fibrin, fibrinogen products, factors VII and VIIa, α_1-antithrombin and heparin. They secrete plasminogen activators, factors X, IX, VII and V, thromboplastin, thrombospondin, plasmin and fibrinolysis inhibitors. Macrophages also influence the cascades indirectly via cytokines and other factors. For example, TNF-α secreted by macrophages enhances the expression of TF and plasminogen activator inhibitor while downregulating expression of thrombomodulin on endothelial cells. These effects favour coagulation, facilitate fibrin production and are antifibrinolytic, respectively.

Macrophages have receptors for at least five fragments of the *complement cascade* components (C1q, C3b, iC3b, C3d and C5a) and synthesize and secrete the C1, C2, C3, C4, C5 components, factors B and D, properdin, C3b inactivator and C1-inhibitor. Complement components affect the migration, endocytosis, secretion and opsonizing functions of macrophages. Acid hydrolases secreted by macrophages affect the complement cascade by degrading certain complement components.

Macrophages produce numerous *enzymes*, some of which function at neutral pH (neutral proteases) and others at acidic pH (acidic proteases, see Fig. 21.13). Some enzymes act to degrade the structural components of blood vessel walls, basement membrane and connective tissue and are thus involved in the causation of tissue injury. Other enzymes hydrolyse components of the activation systems, while others still are involved in direct attack on the parasite (e.g. lysozyme and elastase). Enzyme activities are regulated by a set of *enzyme inhibitors* also produced by macrophages. The preformed enzymes are stored in cytoplasmic granules and released during phagocytosis into the phagolysosome and then into the extracellular space.

Some lipid mediators and cytokines (IL-1 and TNF-α in particular) released by macrophages are brought by blood to the liver and there they induce hepatocytes to synthesize a set of *acute-phase proteins*; these are described later.

Macrophages that have come face to face with parasites attempt to engulf these through *phagocytosis* and kill them by several mechanisms (see Chapter 15). Macrophage *antigen presentation* provides a link (one of several) between the non-adaptive and adaptive antiparasitic responses. It is described in the next section.

Neutrophil responses

Neutrophils present in the tissue at the time of parasitic invasion respond in a fashion similar to that of macrophages. Their numbers, however, are too small to cope with the infection effectively and so the call for reinforcement goes out from the infected site to the local blood vessels very quickly. Neutrophils that have reached the bloodstream from their place of origin, the bone marrow, normally circulate for about 6–12 hours. They then leave the bloodstream, presumably responding to continuous signals emanating at some basal level from the surrounding tissues. During an infection the effusion of signals from the invaded tissue intensifies considerably and the efflux of neutrophils towards this site increases tremendously. One set of signals (e.g. LPS, IL-1, TNF-α, thrombin, histamine, SP and others) activates the endothelial cells of local blood vessels to upregulate the expression of adhesion molecules such as Lewis^{a,x}, P-selectin, E-selectin, ICAM-1, -2, -3 and VCAM-1, all of which then interact with neutrophil adhesion molecules such as L-selectin, PSGL-1, β2 integrins, Mac-1, CD11c/CD18 and others to bring about tethering, rolling and finally tight adhesion between neutrophils and endothelial cells (see Chapter 9). Another set of signals consisting of the chemoattractants formyl-methionine peptides, C5a, LTB_4, PAF, MCP-1, IL-8, CTAP, Gro/MGSA, ENA-78 and others then establishes a concentration gradient that leads the transmigrating neutrophils into the tissue within the first 12 hours of the infection, producing the *polymorphonuclear infiltration*.

Once at the site, neutrophils behave similarly to macrophages but in a more restricted way in that they concentrate mainly on phagocytosis. Like macrophages, neutrophils initiate phagocytosis through direct or indirect contact with the parasite using the same or similar receptors and intermediaries. Engulfment is accompanied by the release of degradative enzymes and other active substances from cytoplasmic granules into the phagosome (Table 21.2) and by the production of nitrogen intermediates. Although the main function of the neutrophil is to kill the parasite, the cell also communicates with other cells via the cytokine internet both by responding to cytokines and by secreting a restricted range of cytokines (Fig. 21.16). Neutrophils that have fulfilled their task die and are drawn into the pus that forms at the site of an infection or in a wound.

The wave of polymorphonuclear infiltration is followed, 12–24 hours after the infection, by a wave of *mononuclear infiltration* dominated by *monocytes*, the blood-borne precursors of macrophages. Monocytes, like neutrophils, are removed from the circulation by signals intensifying the expression of adhesion molecules on endothelial cells (VCAM-1 interacting with VLA-4 on monocytes, in addition to those that interact with neutrophils) and by a stream of chemoattractants (MIP-1α, MIP-1β, MCP-1, RANTES and I-309, in addition to those that attract neutrophils; see Chapter 10). Following the chemoattractant gradient,

Table 21.2 Acute-phase proteins.

Major acute-phase proteins
Serum amyloid A
C-reactive protein
Serum amyloid P component
Complement proteins
C2, C3, C4, C5, C9
Factor B
C1-inhibitor
C4-binding protein
Coagulation proteins
Fibrinogen
von Willebrand factor
Proteinase inhibitors
α_1-Antitrypsin
α_1-Antichymotrypsin
α_2-Antiplasmin
Heparin co-factor II
Plasminogen activator inhibitor I
Metal-binding proteins
Haptoglobin
Haemopexin
Caeruloplasmin
Manganese superoxide dismutase
Other proteins
α_1-Acid glycoprotein
Haem oxygenase
Mannose-binding protein
Leucocyte protein 1
Lipoprotein (a)
Lipopolysaccharide-binding protein
Negative acute-phase proteins
Albumin
Prealbumin
Transferrin
Apolipoprotein A-I
Apolipoprotein A-II
α_1-human serum glycoprotein
Inter-α-trypsin inhibitor
Histidine-rich glycoprotein

monocytes enter the infected tissue and transform into macrophages: they shut down or downregulate the expression of some of their genes and activate others, depending on the signals they receive.

Inflammation

The molecular and cellular events taking place in the infected tissue are manifested outwardly by four or five characteristic changes that are especially apparent if the infection occurs near an observable body surface. Four of the five changes, redness (*rubor*), swelling (*tumor*), warmth (*calor*) and pain (*dolor*), were identified by the Roman physician Cornelius Celsus in AD 30 as the cardinal signs of *inflammation* (Latin *inflammare*, to set on fire). The fifth change, loss of function (*functio laesa*), was added by the second-century Roman physician Galen (Fig. 21.17). *Redness* of the inflamed site stems from changes in the *microcirculation*, the blood flow in the fine vessels (capillaries). Under normal conditions, only about 5–10% of all the capillaries in a resting tissue are open; the rest are closed by one of two mechanisms. First, each capillary has at its origin a thin layer of muscles, the *precapillary sphincter*, which, when constricted, prevents blood flow into the capillary. Second, fine arteries and arteriovenous capillaries are surrounded by a muscular cuff, the constriction of which closes them. The surface area of the capillary bed in humans is 630 m^2, but a large portion of the bed is closed; if all the capillaries were opened, the normal blood volume would increase considerably. At different times, different capillaries are open, and their opening and closing is probably controlled by the local concentration of oxygen, tissue metabolites and hydrogen ions. Following infection, microcirculation changes in the affected tissue. Substances liberated in the injured tissue paralyse the precapillary sphincter, so that most of the local capillaries open. The resulting flooding of the capillaries, *active hyperaemia* (in contrast to *passive hyperaemia* effected by an obstruction to blood

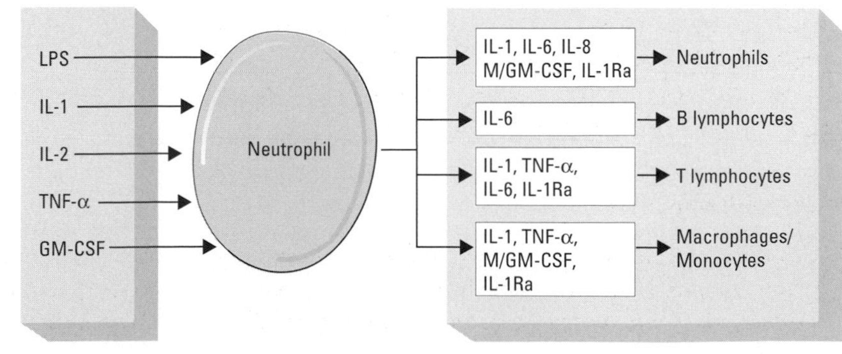

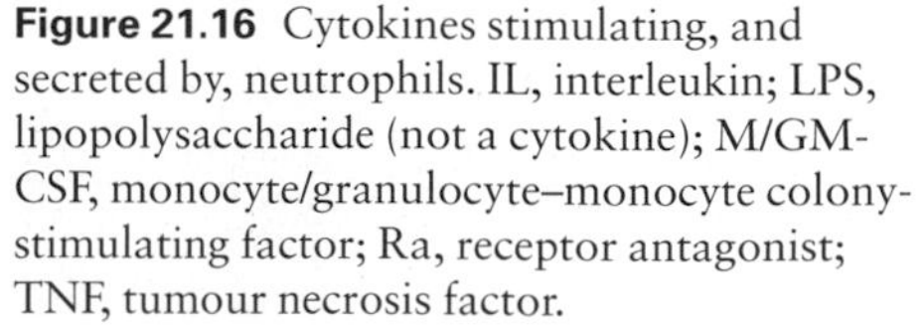
Figure 21.16 Cytokines stimulating, and secreted by, neutrophils. IL, interleukin; LPS, lipopolysaccharide (not a cytokine); M/GM-CSF, monocyte/granulocyte–monocyte colony-stimulating factor; Ra, receptor antagonist; TNF, tumour necrosis factor.

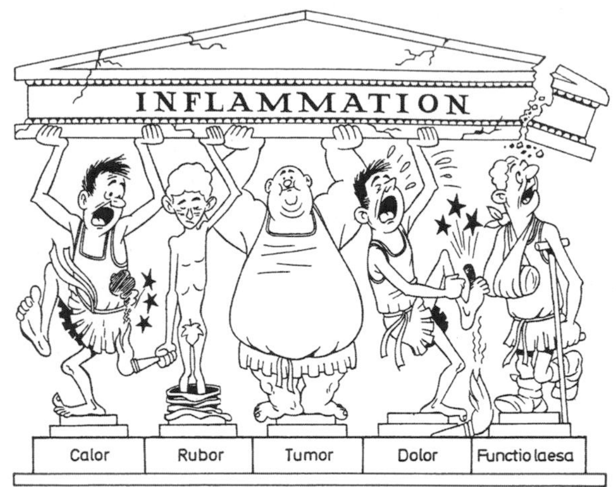

Figure 21.17 The five cardinal signs of inflammation. (According to Houck and Forscher, from Sandritter, W. (1986) *Allgemeine Pathologie*. Schattauer, Stuttgart.)

flow), causes the inflamed tissue to look red, a condition referred to as *erythema* (Greek, flush).

The changes in microcirculation lead to changes in *tissue temperature*. The normal temperature of tissues such as skin is between 30 and 32°C; that of resting limb muscle, for example, 34 or 35°C. The increased blood flow causes the temperature of the inflamed area to approach that of aortic blood: compared to surrounding normal tissue, the infected area seems warm.

Concurrent with these events, changes take place in the size of blood vessels in the infected tissue. The capillary wall is normally composed of flattened endothelial cells, with adjacent cells separated by a gap about 25 nm wide and filled with glycoproteins. During an infection, the injured tissue releases substances that stimulate, directly or indirectly, sympathetic nerve endings in the smooth muscle surrounding the arterioles, causing an active dilation of blood vessels (*vasodilation*); in addition, passive dilation also occurs because of increased blood flow in the arterioles. The main substances responsible for vasodilation are, in the early phase, histamine and serotonin released by tissue mast cells, and later prostaglandins, leukotrienes, PAF, bradykinin and complement components. The endothelial cells of dilated vessels separate from one another and the gaps between them enlarge to allow an outflow of fluid from the vessels into the tissue. The accumulation of protein-rich fluid, the *inflammatory exudate*, in the tissue causes tissue swelling, the *inflammatory oedema*. The pressure the oedema exerts on sensory nerve fibres in the tissue translates into signals that cause the feeling of *pain*. The main agents responsible for pain sensation are soluble mediators such as bradykinin and some of the arachidonic acid metabolites, which are capable of activating sensory pain fibres. The adaptive function of pain is believed to be to discourage use of the affected organ and hence prevent stress that would slow down the healing process.

The swelling immobilizes the tissue and is often responsible for the fifth cardinal sign of inflammation, *loss of function* of the affected organ. The leakage of fluid serves to dilute parasite-derived toxins and toxic metabolites produced by injured cells; it is also a means of dispersing substances that neutralize the toxins and aid in the destruction of the parasite.

The changes we have described thus far all occur locally, in the infected tissue and its vicinity. However, an infection may also affect regions of the body located at some distance from the invaded tissue. Distant sites are alerted to the infection by substances released from the injured tissue, primarily cytokines and prostaglandins. When introduced into the blood circulation, cytokines and other mediators can reach any site of the body within seconds to initiate a response in cells possessing the appropriate receptors. The local response is then augmented by a *systemic response*, i.e. one affecting the entire body system. Cytokines involved in the induction of the systemic response include IL-1, IL-3, IL-6, IL-11, TNF-α, LIF, MIP, GM-CSF, G-CSF, TGF-β, IFN-γ, oncostatin M (OSM) and ciliary neurotrophic factor (CNTF); the main participating prostaglandin is PGE_2. The cytokine and mediator targets are the immune system outside the infection site, bone marrow, central nervous system, pituitary gland and liver (Fig. 21.18).

The systemic effect on the *immune system* is mediated primarily by IL-1 and IL-6, which act mainly on T and B lymphocytes as part of the specific response to the infection (see next section and Chapters 16 & 17).

The main effect of cytokines on *bone marrow* is *leucocytosis*, an increase in both the total and relative numbers of circulating neutrophils. The increase is achieved by the action of the colony-stimulating factors GM-CSF and G-CSF, which promote the proliferation and differentiation of neutrophil precursors. Proliferation is sometimes so rapid that immature ('band form') cells may leave the bone marrow too early and circulate in the blood. Leukocytosis is a regulatory response to the massive emigration of neutrophils from the bloodstream at the site of infection. In certain parasitic infections, some cytokines may increase differentiation of other myeloid precursors in the bone marrow to produce eosinophilia or mastocytosis.

The main result of the effect on the *central nervous system* is the induction of *fever*. Substances that induce fever are known as *pyrogens*; those that induce it from inside the body are *endogenous pyrogens*. The most promi-

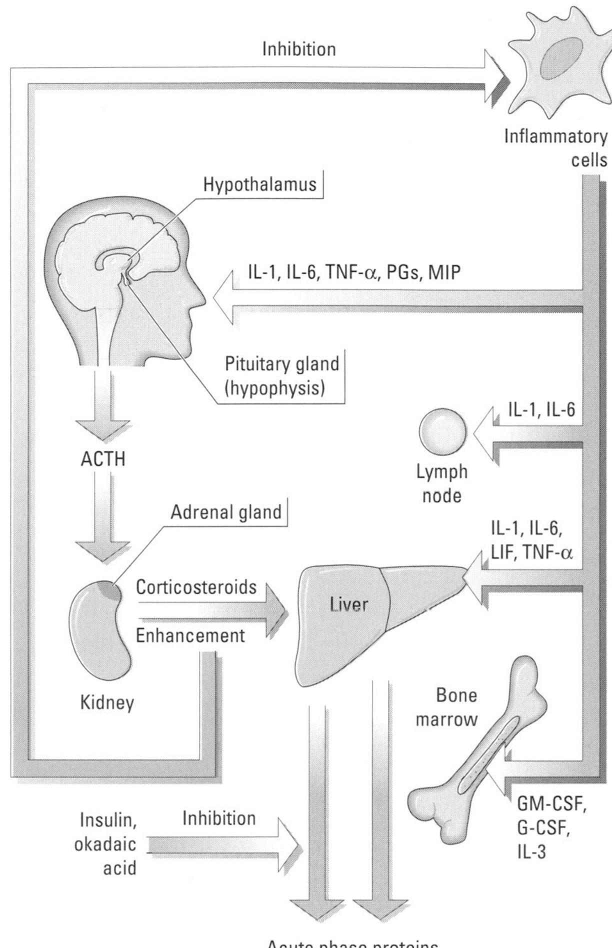

Figure 21.18 Systemic inflammatory response. ACTH, adrenocorticotropic hormone; GM/G-CSF, granulocyte–monocyte granulocyte colony-stimulating factor; IL, interleukin; LIF, leukaemia inhibitory factor; MIP, microphage inflammatory protein; PGs, prostaglandins; TNF, tumour necrosis factor.

nent pyrogen is IL-1; others include TNF-α, IFN-α and prostaglandins. IL-1 acts on the temperature-regulating centre in the hypothalamus, the deep-lying part of the brain that forms the floor and part of the lateral walls of the third ventricle. Stimulation of hypothalamic cells via IL-1 receptors leads to the local generation of arachidonic acid metabolites that then initiate nerve signals, leading to elevated heat production through increased metabolic rates. PGE_2 delivered from the infection sites acts directly on nerves. In principle, pyrogens elevate the body temperature by resetting the hypothalamic thermostat to a higher point. Fever is believed to be useful because at higher temperatures some parasites cannot reproduce, whereas certain immune responses (e.g. T-cell activation, T-cell cytotoxicity and antibody production by B lymphocytes) are enhanced.

The *pituitary gland* (*hypophysis*), which lies beneath the hypothalamus (see Fig. 21.18), responds to stimulation by IL-1 and TNF-α by the secretion of *adrenocorticotropic hormone* (ACTH), which in turn stimulates the cortex of the adrenal gland to secrete *corticosteroids* (glucocorticoids). A rapid rise in the level of corticosteroids is therefore often observed during the early phase of an infection. Corticosteroids downregulate IL-1 synthesis by macrophages and thus provide a negative feedback loop between the central nervous system and the immune system for the regulation of *de novo* cytokine synthesis. The primary effect of corticosteroids, however, is on protein synthesis by hepatocytes of the liver.

Acute phase response

In a healthy individual, the *liver* synthesizes a characteristic set of plasma proteins at a constant rate. During an inflammation the rate of synthesis changes, chiefly under the influence of IL-1 and TNF-α, in conjunction with corticosteroids produced by the adrenal gland. Some proteins are synthesized at a higher and others at a lower rate than normal; the increase is drastic for some proteins and modest for others. Most of the proteins are synthesized by hepatocytes, but some are also synthesized by monocytes, endothelial cells, fibroblasts and adipocytes (fat cells). The early set of reactions taking place during an inflammation is referred to as the *acute-phase response*; the plasma proteins whose profile changes during the response are termed *acute-phase reactants* (proteins) or *APRs*. The cytokine-driven synthesis of APRs is inhibited by the action of insulin and okadaic acid on liver cells (see Fig. 21.18). The net systemic effect of the acute-phase response is the general enhancement of body metabolism including increased protein catabolism, increased gluconeogenesis (the formation of glucose or glucose residues of glycogen from non-carbohydrate sources, especially protein-derived amino acids, chiefly in the liver under stimulation by corticosteroids) and negative nitrogen balance (the difference between the nitrogen intake and nitrogen output by the body).

APRs include components of the classical, alternative, lytic and regulatory *complement pathways*; at least two factors of the *coagulation system*, one (von Willebrand factor) involved in platelet–extracellular matrix interaction and another (fibrinogen) essential for clot formation and the healing process; several *proteinase inhibitors* necessary for the neutralization of lysosomal hydrolases released from activated macrophages and neutrophils; at least four *metal-binding proteins* required to prevent iron loss during infection, to minimize iron levels available to infecting microorganisms and to scavenge reactive oxygen intermediates; as well as an assortment of *other proteins* involved in a variety of infection-associated functions. The level of all these APRs rises moderately during the acute phase (from twofold to tenfold on average). The level of several proteins (albumin, prealbumin, transferrin and others) *decreases* during the acute phase (*negative APRs)*. Finally, the level of a few proteins escalates dramatically (up to 1000-fold) during the response (*major APRs*); in humans these include C-reactive protein, serum amyloid and serum amyloid A component.

C-reactive protein (CRP) was introduced in Chapter 12 in the context of its ability to bind C1q and thus activate the classical complement pathway without antibody involvement. It binds not only to C-polysaccharides of *Streptococcus pneumoniae* and to surface molecules of other parasites, but also to chromatin, histones and small nuclear ribonucleoprotein particles (snRNPs) and is therefore believed to function in the prevention of autoimmunity to nuclear antigens (see Chapter 25). Its other functions include opsonization for phagocytosis; enhancement of chemotaxis of neutrophils and macrophages; enhancement of NK-cell activity; modulation of platelet activation and enhancement of macrophage ability to kill tumour cells.

Serum amyloid P (SAP) is related to CRP in sequence (the two human proteins are identical in 51% of their amino acid residues); structure (both are *pentraxins*, proteins with a characteristic pentameric organization of identical subunits arranged into a single, in the case of CRP, or double, in the case of SAP, annular pentagonal discs); chromosome localization of their genes (the two genes are neighbours on human chromosome 1 and are, interestingly, flanked by genes coding for Fc receptors and for IFN-γ-inducible products); and functionally (both proteins are able to activate the classical complement pathway and to bind to chromatin and its components). In addition to circulating in plasma, SAP is also a normal component of basement membranes, where it binds fibronectin, heparan sulphate and dermatan sulphate and thus modulates blood coagulation.

Although similar in name, *serum amyloid A* (SAA) is unrelated to SAP. SAA is an apolipoprotein (protein component of a lipoprotein before it associates with a lipid) that binds the third fraction of high-density lipoprotein (HDL3). The association is believed to lead to displacement of apolipoprotein A1 from HDL3 and to act as a signal to redirect HDL3 from hepatocytes to macrophages, which then engulf cholesterol and lipid debris at the infected site. In this way macrophages are in a position to redistribute excess cholesterol for use in tissue repair or to excrete it. SAA may also have a feedback relationship with IL-1β and TNF-α (both of which induce SAA gene transcription), may inhibit thrombin-induced platelet activation and, by inhibiting the oxidative burst in neutrophils, may help prevent oxidative tissue damage. Human SAA is encoded in a cluster of at least three functional genes (*SAA1*, *SAA2* and *SAA4*) and one pseudogene (*SAA3*) on chromosome 11. The *SAA4* gene is expressed constitutively and is minimally influenced by the acute-phase reaction; the function of its product, C-SAA, is not known. Proteins encoded in the *SAA1* and *SAA2* genes (A-SAA) are nearly identical; they differ from C-SAA in 45% of their amino acid residues.

Both SAP and SAA tend to be deposited in tissues in large amounts. Because the deposits stain with the vital dye Congo red (sodium diphenyl-diazo-bis-γ-naphthylamine sulphonate) and when examined with a polarizing microscope retard light polarized in one plane differently from light polarized in another (they are birefringent, like starch), they are called *amyloids* (Greek *amylon*, starch; *eidos*, resemblance). In reality, however, they have nothing to do with starch, nor with each other. The only properties they share are hyaline (nearly transparent, glass-like) gross structure, fibrillar ultrastructure (parallel polypeptide chains arranged into β-pleated sheets), high refractivity (ability to refract light) and affinity for the Congo red dye. Several other proteins (e.g. myeloma proteins) are also known to form amylogenic deposits. Particularly susceptible to the formation of extracellular amyloid deposits are tissues in organs such as liver, kidney, spleen, heart and gastrointestinal tract. The disease characterized by the interstitial accumulation of amyloid fibres is referred to as *amyloidosis. Primary amyloidosis* occurs in the absence of a discernible preceding or concurrent disease (e.g. in Alzheimer's disease); *secondary* or *reactive amyloidosis* occurs secondarily to certain diseases, such as tuberculosis, leprosy, systemic lupus erythematosus or rheumatoid arthritis, diseases in which the inflammatory response becomes chronic (see below).

At the height of the inflammatory response, both local and systemic, the injured tissues begin to be *liquified*. The intracellular and extracellular digestion of dead or dying cells by neutrophils and macrophages produces a fluid that combines with the serous material exuded from the vessels. The resulting mixture, which includes dead neutrophils and other cells, is *pus*. A circumscribed collection of pus is referred to as an *abscess* (Latin *abscessus*, going away).

Healing phase

After the destruction of the invader, the inflammation begins to subside and the *healing phase* sets in. Hyperaemia gradually diminishes; leucocyte adhesion becomes less and less pronounced; individual blood vessels and the vascular pattern become normal once again; the inflammatory exudate diminishes, most of it being drained away by lymphatics into regional lymph nodes; and repair of the wound commences. The two main events in the repair process are the formation of new connective tissue by proliferating fibroblasts and the outgrowth of new capillaries (angiogenesis).

Even before the inflammation subsides, *fibroblasts* are seen to be moving into the injured area from the surrounding normal tissue where they exist in a dormant state. Guided by chemoattractants such as MCP-1, -2, -3, C5a, LTB_4 and others, they migrate by means of amoeboid movement along the strands of fibrin and distribute themselves throughout the healing area. At first they resemble tissue macrophages but then lose their oval shape and, after passing through a stellate stage, finally acquire their characteristic elongated appearance. During their morphological transformation they also change internally by developing an extensive rough endoplasmic reticulum and several Golgi complexes. Once fixed into position in the injured tissue, they begin to synthesize collagen and other components of the extracellular matrix (fibronectin, proteoglycans, tenascin). The synthesis of collagen requires ascorbic acid (vitamin C) for the conversion of proline and lysine into hydroxyproline and hydroxylysine, the two major constituents of collagen. This dependence on vitamin C explains why wounds do not heal in persons suffering from scurvy. The secreted collagen organizes itself into fibres, which are laid down somewhat haphazardly at first but later form bundles oriented with their longitudinal axes in the direction of greatest stress. As the collagen bundles become firmer, the fibroblasts gradually degenerate and attach closely to the bundles; the injured area transforms into *scar tissue*. At first the tissue is dense but later it loosens and acquires the normal appearance of connective tissue. The entire process, which requires the participation of many other cells in addition to fibroblasts, is coordinated by sets of cytokines and adhesion molecules. Most of the cytokines are secreted by macrophages and lymphocytes, but fibroblasts themselves secrete several cytokines by which they influence other cells (Fig. 21.19).

Nutrients for the growing scar tissue are supplied at first by the inflammatory exudate, but as the inflammation begins to subside the need for a direct blood supply arises and new vessels begin to grow into the site of injury. Stimulated by cytokines (IL-8, TNF-α, vascular endothelial growth factor (VEGF) and fibroblast growth factor (FGF), all produced by macrophages), the endothelial cells of the injured vessels begin to divide mitotically. The newly arising cells either force themselves between the existing ones, thus increasing the diameter or length of the vessel, or they bulge off and initiate formation of a new vessel. In the latter case, the dividing cells slip past one another, forming a bud that grows out of the existing vessel until it meets and fuses with a similar bud growing out of another vessel; thus a capillary loop is produced.

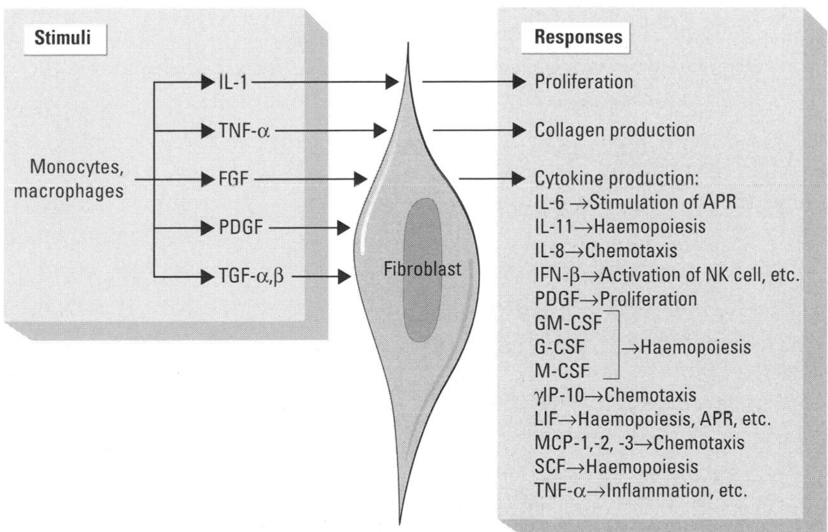

Figure 21.19 Fibroblast-stimulating cytokines and their effect. APR, acute-phase response; FGF, fibroblast growth factor; γIP-10, interferon-γ-regulated protein 10; GM-CSF, granulocyte–monocyte colony-stimulating factor; IL, interleukin; LIF, leukaemia inhibitory factor; MCP, monocyte chemoattractant protein; NK, natural killer; PDGF, platelet-derived growth factor; SCF, stem cell factor; TGF, transforming growth factor; TNF, tumour necrosis factor.

Chronic inflammation

Under normal circumstances, removal of the invader and the subsequent healing process are followed by a return to the preinfective state. The term *inflammation* is usually used for the entire episode, from initiation of the response to cessation of all extraordinary activities. To emphasize that the episode is of short duration, the qualifier 'acute' is often added to the designation, hence *acute inflammatory response* or *acute-phase response*. Highlights of the response are summarized in Fig. 21.20.

The response has two components, local and systemic. The former is characterized by polymorphonuclear and then mononuclear infiltration of the infected tissue. The latter is marked by the secretion of acute-phase proteins. An inflammation follows not only a parasitic infection but also, for example, mechanical or other tissue injury, even when it is not accompanied by microbial invasion. Whether of parasitic origin or not, inflammation runs a similar course, the specifics of which differ according to the type of injury and the type of affected tissue. Acute inflammation is over within a few days, or couple of weeks at most. However, if the agent responsible for the response persists, the inflammation may linger for months or even years. This *chronic inflammation* is caused by a low-grade but prolonged injury, the source of which can be any of the following.

- *Persistent parasitic infections*, exemplified by tuberculosis and leprosy (caused by mycobacteria), syphilis (caused by spirochaetes), histoplasmosis (caused by fungi) and schistosomiasis (caused by flukes).
- *Exogenous physical and chemical irritants*, such as inhaled particles of silica, asbestos, dust or fumes, for example beryllium compounds, as well as *endogenous irritants*, such as cholesterol crystals, unabsorbable sutures or splinters.
- *Hypersensitivity reactions* accompanying, for example, tuberculosis or autoimmune disease, such as thyroiditis and gastritis (see Chapter 25).
- *Unknown agents* involved, for example, in the case of *sarcoidosis* (Greek *sarx*, flesh), a disease characterized by the appearance of lesions in lymph nodes and various other organs, especially lungs, skin, spleen or eyes. The disease resembles tuberculosis but is not caused by the tubercle bacilli; its causative agent has not yet been identified.

In situations in which the body is unable to rid itself of the inflammatory agent, it settles for the next best thing, i.e. controlled surveillance of the agent's effects: no large amounts of chemical mediators are released, no massive influx of neutrophils into the area occurs and necrosis is maintained at a low level, being continually counterbalanced by an ongoing regeneration process. The most characteristic feature of chronic inflammation is the formation of *granulation tissue* or *granuloma*. In the early stages, the tissue is highly cellular, consisting of fibroblasts, monocytes, macrophages, lymphocytes, epithelioid cells (plump, polygonal cells with a central nucleus and eosinophilic cytoplasm, probably derived from macrophages) and giant cells (large, multinucleated cells originating from the fusion of several epithelioid cells). It is well vascularized and contains only a few fine collagen fibres. As the tissue ages, however, it matures into a tougher *fibrous tissue*, in which the cellularity and vascularity diminish greatly and the fibres thicken because of further collagen deposition. The term 'granuloma' derives from the observation that the tissue often forms a lump grossly resembling a tumour (the suffix *-oma* usually being reserved for tumours).

When chronic inflammation occurs in hollow organs (e.g. heart or small intestine), it may lead to the narrowing of orifices and tubes and to an obstruction, with all its consequences. In other situations it may result in shrinkage, scarring and distortion of an internal organ, caused by the loss of parenchymal cells and their replacement with fibrous tissue. For example, when acute viral hepatitis is followed by chronic hepatitis, it leads to cirrhosis (Greek *kirrhos*, tawny) or a fibroid induration of the liver, culminating in liver failure.

Adaptive response

The adaptive immune response takes place concurrently with the non-adaptive response; however, because it takes several days to develop, it affects the course of infection later than the non-adaptive response. Sometimes the non-adaptive response eliminates the infection well before the adaptive response can take part at all in the defence campaign. How often this happens is not known. The non-adaptive responses are at least as important for the protection of vertebrate bodies as the adaptive responses. Three observations support this conclusion. First, mutations that incapacitate or severely cripple the functions of the adaptive immune system occur with appreciable frequencies in both humans and animals. Virtually no mutations incapacitating the non-adaptive system are known. While this may be so in part because the non-adaptive response consists of many elements that can each take over the other's function, it may also be an indication that natural selection eliminates any such mutations immediately. Second, at least some of the animals with a non-functioning adaptive immune system survive for extended periods even in conditions that are not germ-free. By contrast, in the few instances in which one component of the non-adaptive system has been inactivated, individuals

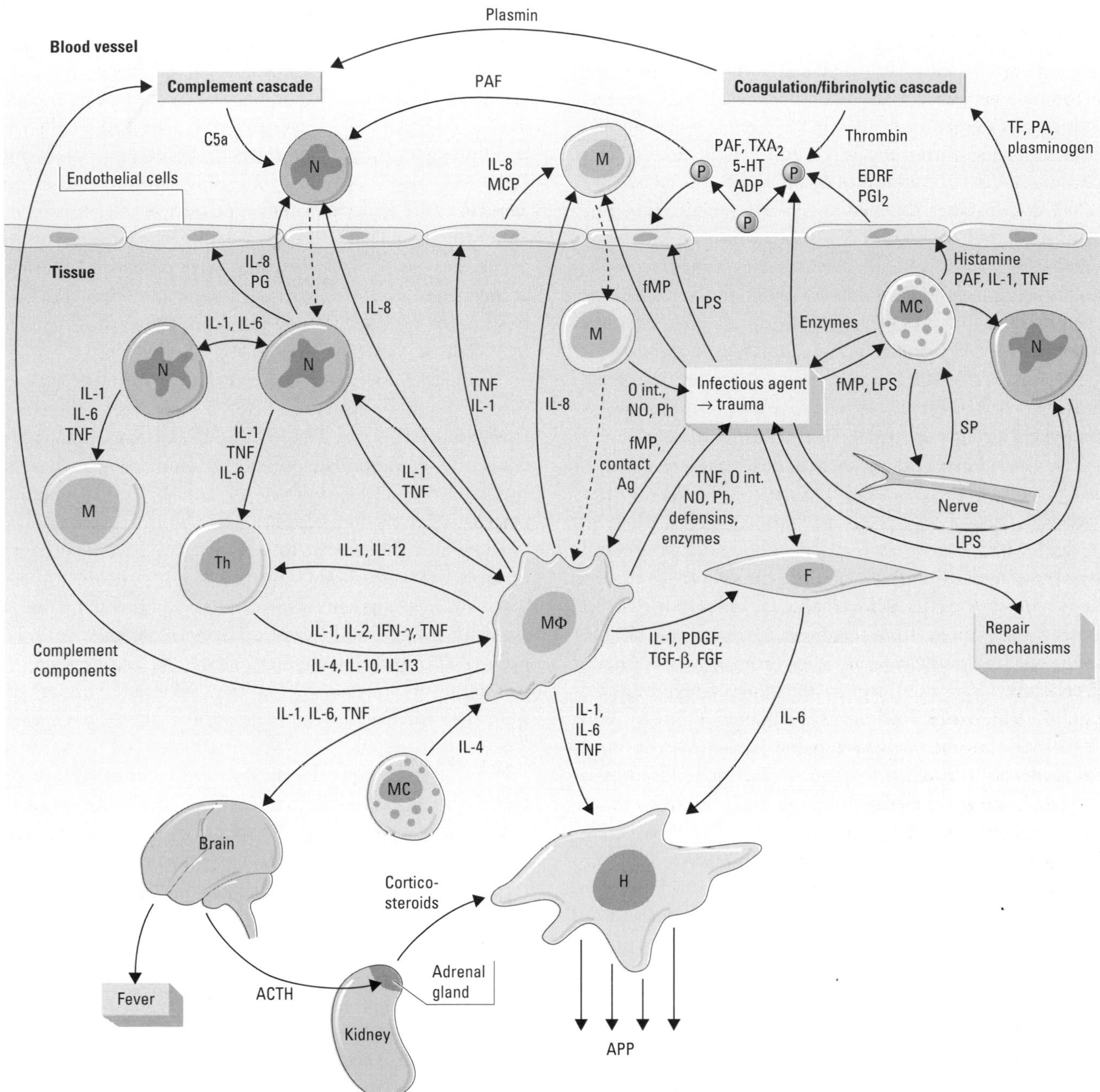

Figure 21.20 Some of the interactions and events taking place during the acute phase of the inflammatory response to an infection. Interactions characterizing the adaptive response have largely been omitted from this diagram. Solid arrows indicate interventions, broken arrows cell migrations. ACTH, adrenocorticotropic hormone; ADP, adenosine diphosphate; Ag, antigen; APP, acute-phase proteins; EDRF, endothelium-derived relaxing factor; F, fibroblast; FGF, fibroblast growth factor; fMP, formyl-methionine peptide; H, hepatocyte; 5-HT, serotonin; IFN, interferon; IL, interleukin; LPS, lipopolysaccharide; M, monocyte; MC, mast cell; MCP, monocyte chemoattractant protein; MΦ, macrophage; N, neutrophil; NO, nitric oxide; O, oxygen intermediate; P, platelet; PA, plasminogen activator; PAF, platelet-activating factor; PDGF, platelet-derived growth factor; PG, prostaglandin; Ph, phagocytosis; SP, substance P; TF, tissue factor; TGF, transforming growth factor; T_H, helper T lymphocyte; TNF, tumour necrosis factor; TX, thromboxane.

suffer from life-threatening parasitic attacks. For example, MBP is only one of a large number of acute-phase proteins and not even a major APR, yet when both copies of the gene encoding this protein are inactivated, affected children endure severe recurrent infections. (The fact that the mutation occurs with relatively high frequency, 17% in Caucasians, may be an indication that it has some selective value, for instance protection against extensive complement-mediated damage of host tissues during infections.) Third, most animals (all invertebrates) apparently rely exclusively on the non-adaptive system and yet have obviously no difficulty in coping with all the parasites they encounter. We have covered the adaptive response in depth in several preceding chapters; here therefore we simply provide a brief overview of the response in the context of the overall defence against a parasite infection

The central elements of the adaptive response are the *T and B lymphocytes*, the cells that express clonally antigen-specific receptors encoded in rearranging genes. There are subsets of both T and B lymphocytes, however, whose activities may actually be part of the non-adaptive response. These are the γ:δ T cells and the *B1* cells. Both express antigen-specific receptors from rearranged genes, but they are limited in the range of antigens they recognize. The *γ:δ T cells* are largely uniform in the type of receptors they express in a given epithelium (see Chapters 7 & 16). What these receptors recognize is not known, but according to one hypothesis the ligand is a self molecule shared by all the cells of a given epithelium (e.g. a heat-shock protein) and modified by the infection. The *B1* cells, which are present mainly in the peritoneal cavity, express immunoglobulin receptors that bind polysaccharides of bacterial capsules. The cells are activated independently of T cells but a second activation signal in the form of IL-5 (produced by mast cells, T cells or eosinophils) is necessary. The activated B cells secrete IgM antibodies, which then bind to the bacterial surface and initiate complement-mediated killing. It has been speculated that γ:δ T cells and *B1* cells are evolutionary relics of the transitional stage in the evolution from non-adaptive to adaptive form of response in early vertebrates.

The essence of the adaptive response is the specific recognition of structural motifs (antigens) present in the parasite but absent in the host. A parasite, especially a eukaryotic parasite, differs from the host in many thousands of such motifs, and if the host were to recognize all of them most of its lymphocytes would be activated. Such a massive response would clog the system, exhaust it and render the attack ineffective. (Incidentally, some parasites, as we learn later, use precisely this strategy to evade the host's immune response.) To prevent this, the immune system focuses on a limited range of antigenic determinants. Focusing is achieved by *antigen processing* in specialized antigen-presenting cells (APCs) and the presentation of selected antigen fragments to T lymphocytes by molecules encoded in the *MHC* genes. The interaction of activated T cells with B lymphocytes then concentrates the response of the B cells. Processing also solves the problem of access to the antigen. As long as the antigen is an integral part of the parasite, it is either totally inaccessible or accessible in a form not appropriate for lymphocyte activation. Since APCs are either professional or non-professional phagocytes, they are in a position to 'extract' the antigen from the parasite after its ingestion and destruction.

Although some antigen presentation may take place in the tissue parenchyma, the bulk of it occurs in the *lymph nodes* (Fig. 21.21; see Chapter 16). Parasites that manage to enter the bloodstream, either because they have overwhelmed the defence lines in the lymph nodes or because they have been introduced into the blood, e.g. by an insect bite, are brought into the *spleen* and there become the focus of an attack (Fig. 21.21). In the spleen, parasites or their fragments are ingested by macrophages in the white pulp as they exit the central arteriole. The antigens are then taken up by APCs of the white pulp, processed and presented to circulating T lymphocytes as they percolate through the pulp after entering it from the marginal sinus (see Chapters 3 & 16).

What happens next depends on a number of factors, primarily the nature of the parasite, the concentration of the antigen and the type of cytokines present in the local microenvironment. From the perspective of the adaptive response, there are two principal categories of parasites: extracellular and intracellular. *Extracellular parasites* normally multiply outside the host cell and, if small enough to be engulfed by phagocytes, remain in the phagosome until they are destroyed. *Intracellular parasites*, on the other hand, normally grow inside the host cell and some of them use phagocytosis as a means of reaching the cell's interior; they evade destruction in the phagosomes by escaping into the cytosol. Intracellular parasites include all viruses, some bacteria and certain protozoans; extracellular parasites make up the rest. The adaptive response to these two categories of parasites is dominated by two different types of CD4+ T lymphocytes: the T_H1 or T_H2 cells (Fig. 21.22). In both situations, the antigen is initially presented by class II MHC molecules to naive precursors of T_H cells (pT_H), circulating for a short time in the bloodstream after their generation in the thymus. The pT_H cells are capable of secreting IL-4, but possibly no other cytokine. They can differentiate into either T_H1 or T_H2 cells, depending on the stimuli they receive from other cells responding to the para-

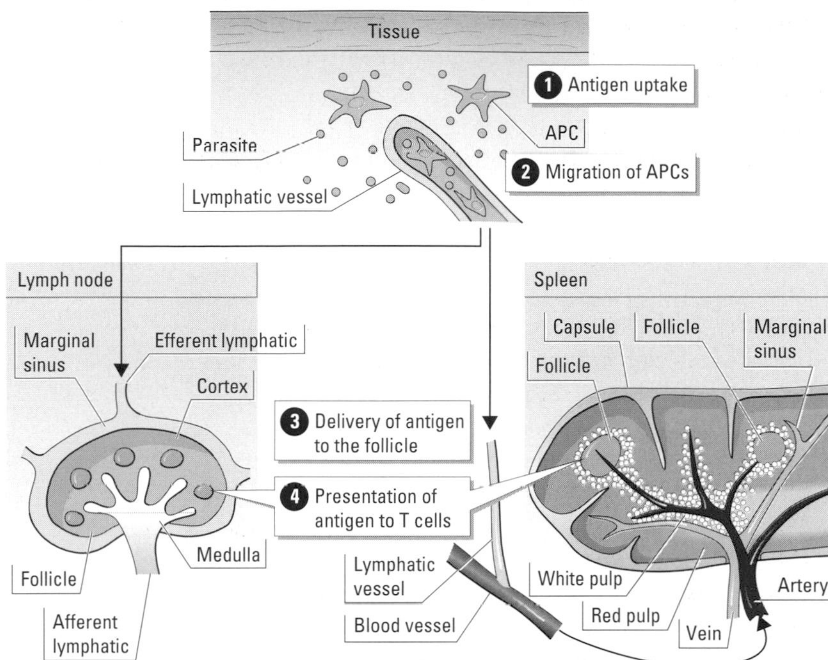

Figure 21.21 Initiation of adaptive immune response in the lymph node and spleen. APC, antigen-presenting cell. Consecutive stages are numbered.

site. During most infections, initially both T_H1 and T_H2 cells are generated but later one type prevails and actively suppresses differentiation of the other. Intracellular parasites activate macrophages to secrete several cytokines, among which IL-12 becomes essential for the further course of the response.

The initial response to extracellular parasites or their toxic products is implemented by IL-4 in the local microenvironment. The sources of IL-4 are activated mast cells (basophils) and activated $NK1^+$ T lymphocytes. Large extracellular parasites such as worms probably initiate the response by activating tissue mast cells and basophils in the manner described in the preceding section. Extracellular bacteria and other smaller parasites probably elicit the initial response by activating T cells. Exactly how they accomplish this is not clear, but very likely their activities induce an initial low-grade non-specific T-cell response that subsequently amplifies and switches to a specific response. IL-4 promotes differentiation of pT_H cells into T_H2 lymphocytes, which then secrete IL-4 (thus generating an amplification loop), IL-10, IL-5 and IL-13. These cytokines fulfil different functions. IL-10 and IL-13 block the differentiation of pT_H cells into T_H1 lymphocytes so that the response becomes dominated by T_H2 cells. IL-4 (and IL-13) promote involvement of B lymphocytes in the response, supporting their differentiation into antibody-secreting plasma cells and participating in the switch from one immunoglobulin class to another (Chapters 16 & 17). IL-5 draws eosinophils into the response, especially in infections by large parasites, and the activated degranulating eosinophils then spill their toxic cargoes onto the invaders. IL-4 also promotes the switch to production of IgE, which then binds by its Fc portions to the corresponding receptors on mast cells and basophils, involving them in the attack.

Because of this dichotomy in the response, intracellular parasites stimulate predominantly cell-mediated adaptive immunity (non-specific inflammatory response and lymphotoxicity), whereas extracellular parasites elicit a predominantly humoral response in which antibodies effect the elimination of parasites by activating the classical pathway of the complement cascade, by activating the release of toxic mediators from mast cells, basophils and eosinophils, or by some other means. The word 'predominant' needs to be emphasized here, because the division of labour is by no means absolute. Both cellular and humoral responses are initiated by most if not all parasites and both participate in the attack; it is only the degree of involvement of the two types of immunity that often differentiates the responses against intracellular and extracellular parasites. Another point needing emphasis is that the adaptive response runs in parallel to the non-adaptive response and that the two are intertwined so intimately (particularly through the cytokine network) that it is often not possible to classify a particular mechanism as being exclusively in one or the other category. Examples of the cytokine interconnections between adaptive and non-adaptive responses are given in Figs 21.23 and 21.24.

The elicitation of different types of response by intra-

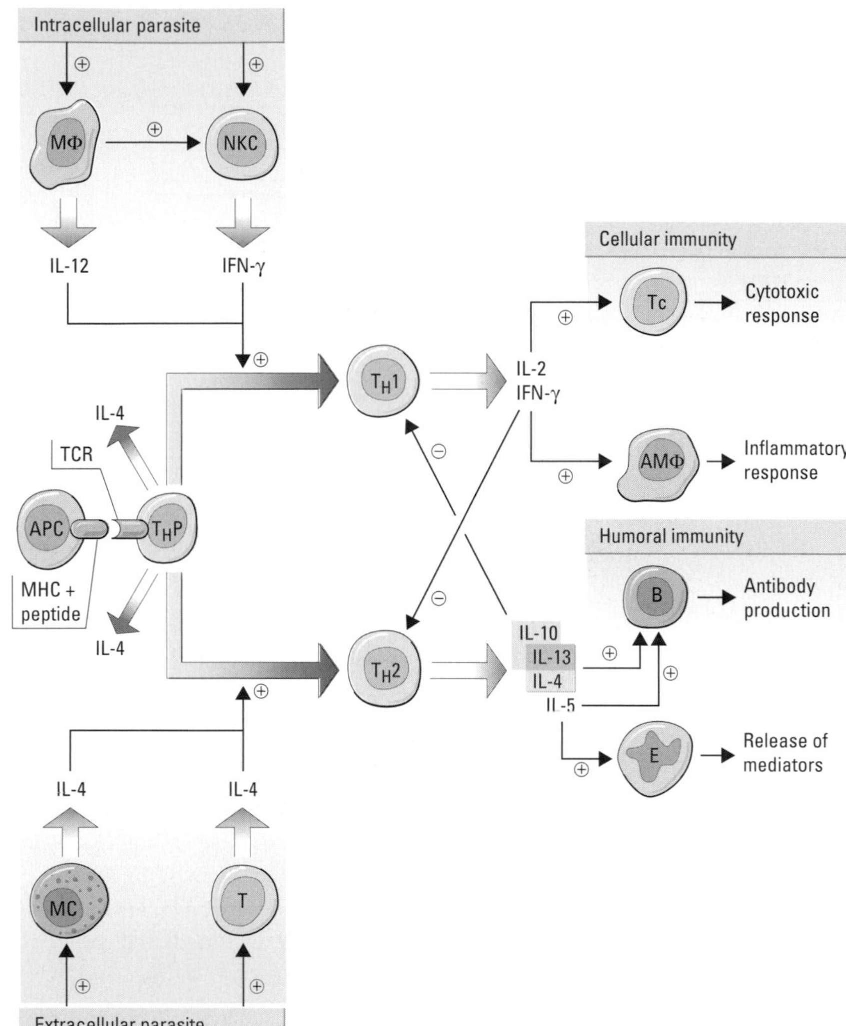

Figure 21.22 Principal dichotomy of the adaptive immune response initiated by intracellular and extracellular parasites. Thin arrows indicate the effect on cells, either stimulatory (+) or inhibitory (–); broad red arrows signify differentiation of cells; broad white/grey arrows signify production of cytokines. AMΦ, activated macrophage; APC, antigen-presenting cell; CK, cytokines; B, B lymphocyte; E, eosinophil; IFN, interferon; IL, interleukin; MC, mast cell; MHC, major histocompatibility complex; MΦ, macrophage; NKC, natural killer cell; T_H, helper T lymphocyte; T lulper cell precursor; T_C, cytotoxic T lymphocyte; TCR, T-cell receptor, T_HP, T helper cell precursor.

cellular and extracellular parasites constitutes evolutionary adaptations ensuring the most efficacious use of effector mechanisms: antibodies are effective against extracellular parasites and their toxic products but much less so against parasites hiding in the cell's interior. Activated macrophages and cytotoxic T (T_C) cells, on the other hand, are superb destroyers of infected cells but less effective against free parasites and their products. Another evolutionary adaptation to the two types of parasites is apparently the differential sensitivity of T_H1 and T_H2 lymphocytes to antigenic stimulation. It has been observed repeatedly that T_H2-cell responses are elicited even by class II MHC–peptide assemblages in which the two components associate with low affinity and by APCs with a low density of class II MHC–peptide assemblages on their surfaces. The initiation of T_H1-cell responses, on the other hand, requires high-affinity binding of peptides to class II MHC molecules and a high density of class II MHC–peptide assemblages on the surface of APCs. This difference makes sense when one considers the behaviour of extracellular and intracellular parasites. The former proliferate rapidly and cause damage almost immediately, and so response against them must be mounted as quickly as possible, even when the antigen concentration is still low. The latter, on the other hand, proliferate more slowly and cause damage only at a later stage of infection; the host has therefore time until a high threshold concentration of antigen is attained and high-affinity interactions can take place. This difference thus helps to channel the response against extracellular and intracellular parasites via the T_H2 and T_H1 arms of adaptive immunity, respectively.

The follicles in the cortex of the lymph node and in the white pulp of the spleen serve two purposes in the adaptive immune response: they promote the development of naive

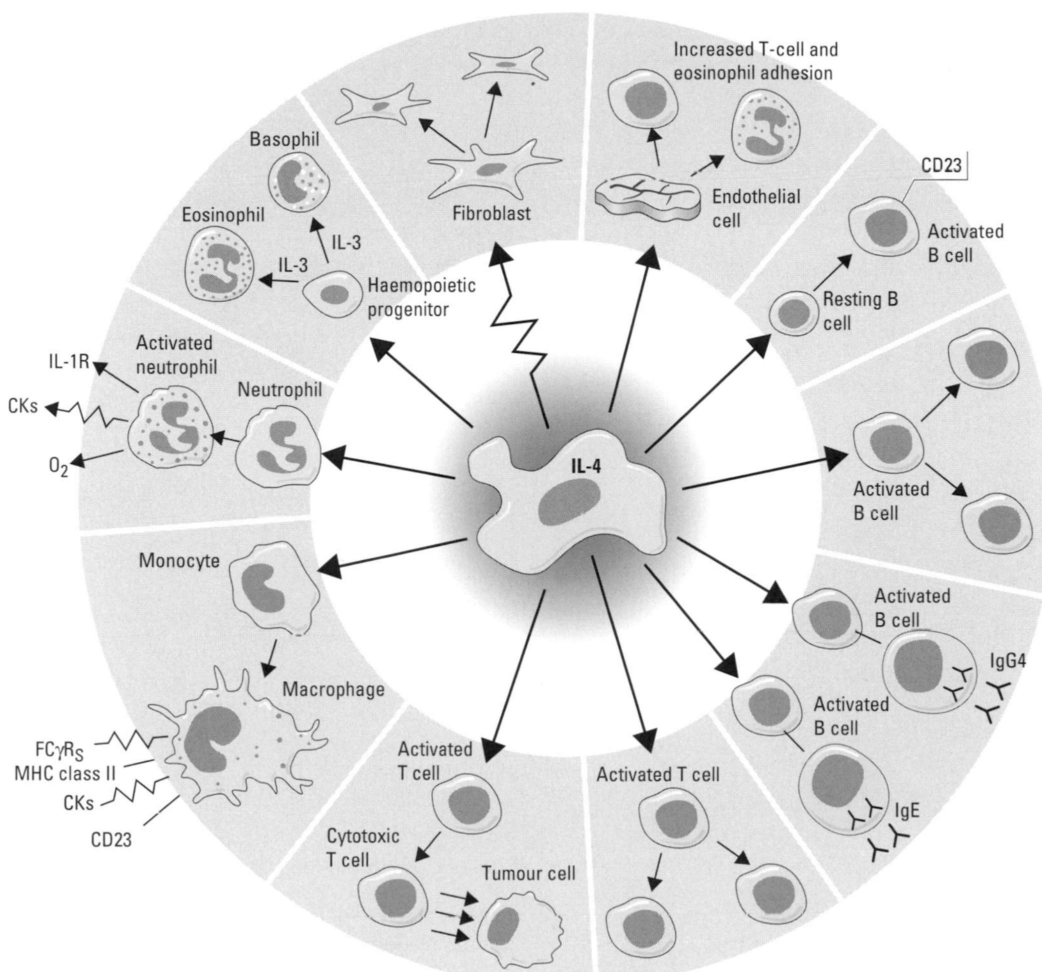

Figure 21.23 Pleiotropic effects of IL-4. Straight arrows indicate positive (stimulatory) effect, zigzag arrows negative (inhibitory) effect; straight lines denote upregulation, zigzag lines downregulation of expression. CD, cluster of differentiation; CKs, cytokines; IL, interleukin; MHC, major histocompatibility complex; O_2, oxygen intermediate; R, receptor. IL-4 increases the volume of *resting B cells* and induces hyperexpression of class II MHC and CD23 molecules, which are involved in antigen presentation to T cells; enhances growth and proliferation of *activated B cells* and induces isotype switch towards IgG4 and IgE antibody production; enhances the growth and proliferation of *activated T cells*, and promotes their differentiation into cytotoxic effector cells capable of killing tumour cells; upregulates the expression of MHC class II and CD23 molecules on *macrophages* and thus promotes antigen presentation, while downregulating the expression of Fcγ receptors and secretion of cytokines; inhibits the secretion of IL-8 and of other inflammatory cytokines and enhances the expression of both soluble and membrane-bound type II IL-1 receptor (anti-inflammatory effects) by neutrophils; promotes (together with IL-3) the differentiation of haemopoietic precursors into *eosinophils* and *basophils*; supports proliferation of *fibroblasts*; and downregulates the expression of ICAM-1 (intercellular adhesion molecule-1) and ELAM-1 (endothelial cell adhesion molecule-1) on *endothelial cells*, while upregulating the expression of VCAM-1 (vascular cell adhesion molecule-1) resulting in increased T-cell and eosinophil adhesion to blood vessel walls. (Redrawn from Banchereau, J. (1995) *Behring Institut Mitteilungen*, **96**, 58.)

pT_H cells into effector cells and provide the necessary microenvironment for interactions between T_H and B lymphocytes. The development of effector $CD4^+$ T_H1 cells (i.e. those that can activate macrophages) takes about 4–5 days to complete and involves both proliferation and differentiation of activated T-cell clones. The differentiation involves changes in the expression of genes, some being shut off and others, including those coding for cell-surface adhesion molecules, being activated. The differentiated effector cells then leave the lymph node or the spleen and enter the bloodstream. However, they circulate only until they happen to run into ligands on the endothelium to which their adhesion molecules can bind (Fig. 21.25). This occurs at a certain low level all over the body because endothelial cells express certain adhesion molecules (e.g. ICAM-2) constitutively and these bind their counterparts (e.g. LFA-1) on lympho-

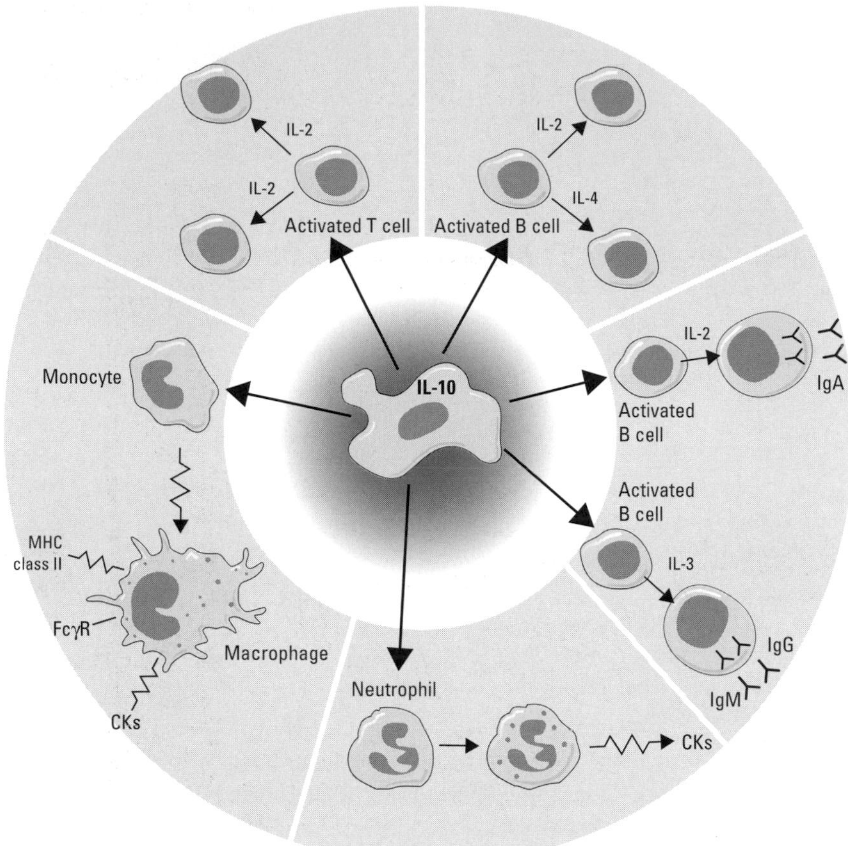

Figure 21.24 Pleiotropic effects of IL-10. Straight arrows indicate positive (stimulatory) effect, zigzag arrows negative (inhibitory) effect; straight lines denote upregulation, zigzag lines downregulation of expression of molecules. CKs, cytokines; FcγR, Fcγ receptor; IL, interleukin; MHC, major histocompatibility complex; IL-10 promotes (together with IL-2, IL-3 or IL-4) the proliferation, differentiation and class switch of *activated B cells*; inhibits the production of cytokines by *neutrophils*; upregulates the expression of class II and Fcγ receptors on *macrophages* while inhibiting the production of cytokines; and (together with IL-2) supports the proliferation and differentiation of *activated T cells*. (Redrawn from Banchereau, J. (1995) *Behring Institut Mitteilungen*, **96**, 58.)

cytes anywhere in the circulation. Emigration of lymphocytes initiated by contact with such molecules therefore takes place in various tissues independently of infection. However, if the tissue happens to be infected and the emigrating effector T lymphocytes encounter the antigen (on APCs) that stimulated their differentiation, they are activated to produce cytokines, including TNF-α, which then induce the endothelial cells of local blood vessels to express additional adhesion molecules (e.g. ICAM-1 and VCAM-1). This added expression of adhesion molecules increases the chances of an encounter with corresponding molecules (LFA-1 and VLA-4, respectively) on circulating T lymphocytes and thus enhances the emigration of lymphocytes into the tissues. Of course, in many instances the non-adaptive (inflammatory) response at the infected site generates TNF-α and activates endothelial cells before the first effector T lymphocytes arrive from the lymphoid organs. Because different tissues may induce the expression of different adhesion molecules on the endothelium of their blood vessels, migrant effector lymphocytes may home specifically to various parts of the body. However, lymphocytes cannot re-enter the lymph nodes because they lost, during their differentiation, L-selectin from their surfaces and therefore do not interact with the lining of high endothelial venules. Cells that have not encountered antigen undergo apoptotic death in the tissues.

The *interaction between activated B and activated T_H lymphocytes* (see Chapter 17) triggers a sequence of events that lead to the proliferation and differentiation (including immunoglobulin class switch) of the former (Fig. 21.26). Antibodies help to combat the infection by neutralizing the parasite and its toxic products; blocking the adherence of the parasite to host cells; opsonizing the parasite for phagocytosis; activating NK cells for the destruction of antibody-

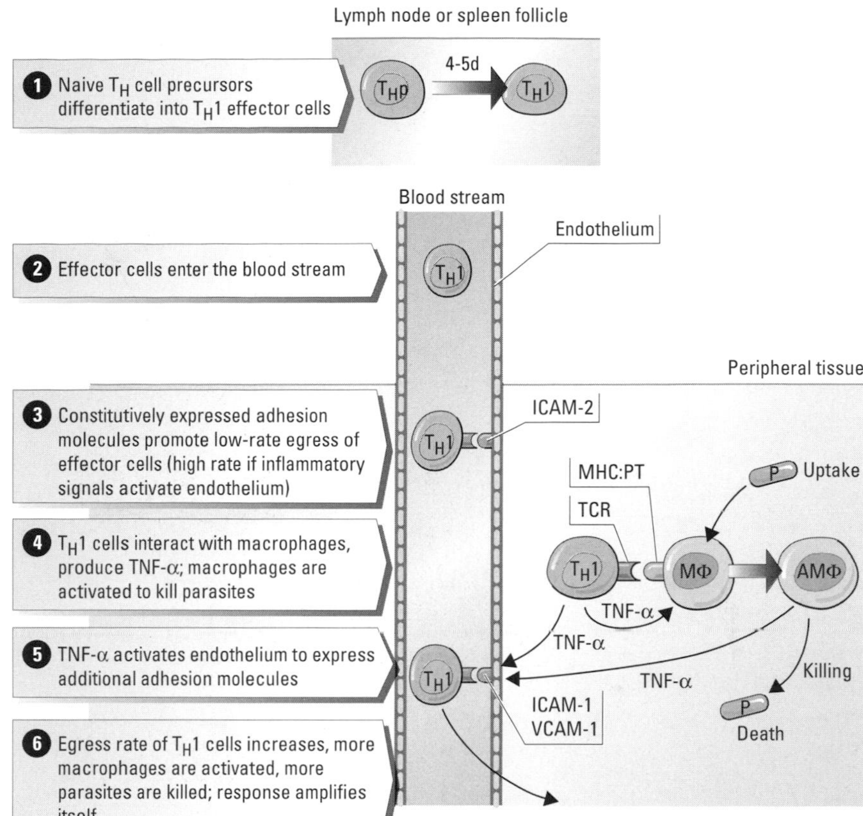

Figure 21.25 Development and action of effector helper T (T_H1) cells. Broad arrows indicate differentiation, thin arrows migration or secretion. AMΦ, activated macrophage; d, days; ICAM, intercellular adhesion molecule; MHC, major histocompatibility complex; MΦ, macrophage; P, parasite; PT, peptide; TCR, T-cell receptor; T_HP, helper T cell (precursor); TNF, tumour necrosis factor; VCAM, vascular cell adhesion molecule.

coated targets; activating mast cells (basophils and eosinophils) to release toxic mediators; and activating the classical pathway of the complement cascade.

Intracellular parasites such as viruses that multiply in the cytosol of the host cell also activate naive $CD8^+$ lymphocytes to differentiate into *effector T_C cells*. Model experiments *in vitro* have documented at least three modes of T_C-cell activation dependent primarily on the nature of APCs and their ability to provide co-stimulatory signals (Fig. 21.27). First, some APCs, such as dendritic cells with high co-stimulatory activity, interact with naive $CD8^+$ T_C cells without the participation of a third-party cell. In these interactions, class I MHC–peptide assemblages, as well as the CD80 and CD86 molecules of the APC bind the T-cell receptor (TCR)–CD8 complexes and the CD28 molecule of the T_C cell, respectively, and the activated T_C cell secretes IL-2 which then drives the differentiation into the effector cell. Second, the class II MHC–peptide assemblage of certain other APCs binds the TCR–CD4 complex of a T_H cell and induces the expression of CD80/CD86 on the APC. The class I MHC–peptide assemblage and the CD80 molecule of the same APC bind the TCR–CD8 complex and the CD28 molecule of a T_C cell and the activated T_C cells secrete IL-2 with an autocrine effect. Third, the class II MHC–peptide assemblage and the CD80/CD86 molecules of an APC bind the TCR–CD4 complex and the CD28 molecule of a T_H cell, respectively, and the activated T_H cell then secretes IL-2, which drives the differentiation of T_C cells activated by contact with the class I MHC–peptide assemblage of the same APC. Which of the three modes is used in the *in vivo* responses is not known.

At some point during the response, some of the activated T and B lymphocytes transform into *memory cells*, which then remain in the body after the infection has been abolished and all the effector cells have died. Memory cells deal quickly and efficiently with subsequent infections by the same parasite (see Chapters 16 & 17).

Six main groups of parasites exist: viruses, intracellular bacteria, extracellular bacteria, fungi, protozoan parasites and metazoan parasites. Although the host often uses all available means to defend itself against a parasite, the relative involvement of the individual defence components differs depending on the parasite. In the sections that follow we describe some of the idiosyncrasies of the response, particularly the adaptive response, against individual groups of parasites.

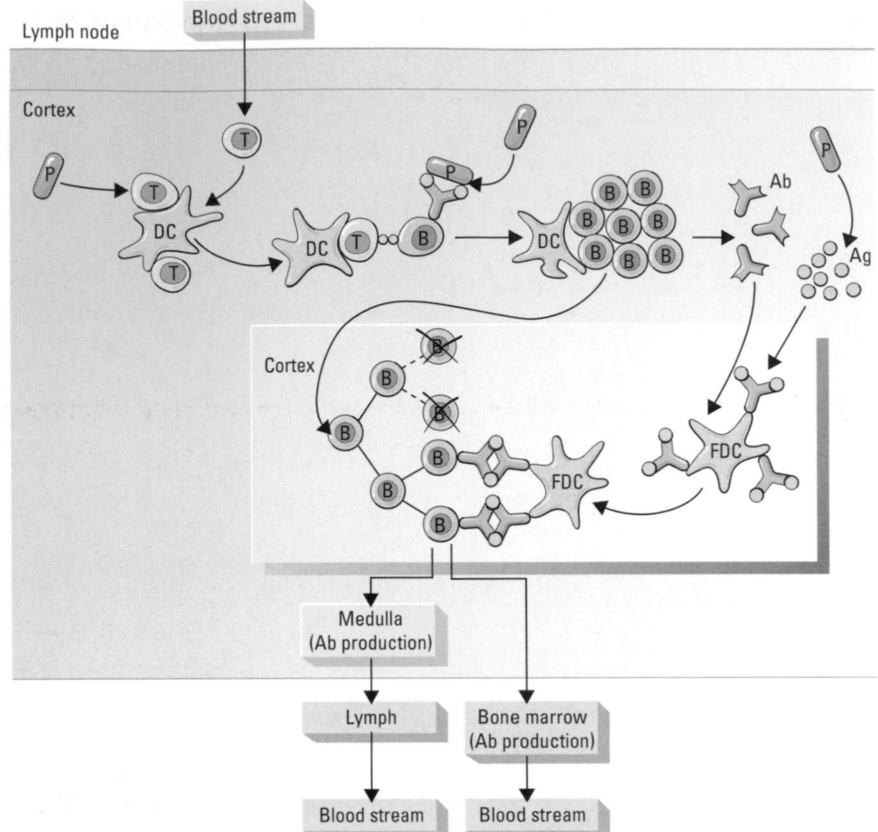

Figure 21.26 Activation of B lymphocytes and initiation of antibody response during an infection in a lymph node. Receptors on T cells and major histocompatibility complex molecules on dendritic cells are not shown. Immunoglobulin receptors are shown only on some B lymphocytes. Ab, antibody; Ag, antigen; B, B lymphocyte; DC, dendritic cell; FDC, follicular dendritic cell; P, parasite; T, T lymphocyte.

Defence against viruses

Characteristics of viral infections

Viruses are intracellular parasites that cannot grow or multiply outside a cell. They differ from all other parasites and, for that matter, from all other forms of life because they are not organized into cells. Although a far cry from the 'naked genes' they were once considered to be, they are more primitive than the most primitive cell and are able to replicate only by diverting the biosynthetic pathways of a cell to virus production. In contrast to all other life forms, among which, in each group, there are always some that can lead non-parasitic lives, all viruses are parasites.

Viruses range in size from 15 to 300 nm or more, and in shape from spherical through polyhedral to rod-shaped. A *virus particle*, or *virion*, consists of one or more molecules of nucleic acid (single-stranded RNA, double-stranded DNA or, rarely, single-stranded DNA) contained within a protein coat or *capsid* (the individual protein subunits of the capsid being the *capsomers*). The complex of nucleic acid and proteins, or *nucleocapsid*, can be either *naked* or enclosed by a lipoprotein *envelope*.

The life cycle of a virus can be divided into two phases, extracellular and intracellular. In the *extracellular phase*, the virus exists in the form of an inert, infectious virus particle. To be activated and so initiate the *intracellular phase*, the virus must reach its host, enter its body and then enter the body's cells. Some viruses enter the vertebrate body via skin, others via mucosal membranes and others still via blood during an arthropod or vertebrate bite. Some viruses multiply near the site of entry, spread from one cell to another by diffusion in intercellular spaces, cell contacts or secretions and excretions, and cause a *localized infection*, i.e. a single lesion or group of lesions in a particular organ. According to their target organs, localized infections are divided into *dermotropic* (affecting the skin), *neurotropic* (affecting the nervous system), *pneumotropic* (affecting the respiratory system) and so on. Other viruses also multiply at the site of entry, but then move to local lymph nodes and from there, via the lymph, reach the blood which disseminates them into various organs; they cause *generalized* (*systemic, disseminated*) *infection*. These viruses multiply and spread from one organ to the other. The presence of viruses in the blood is referred to as *viraemia*.

Before it can multiply, a virus must enter its target cell by

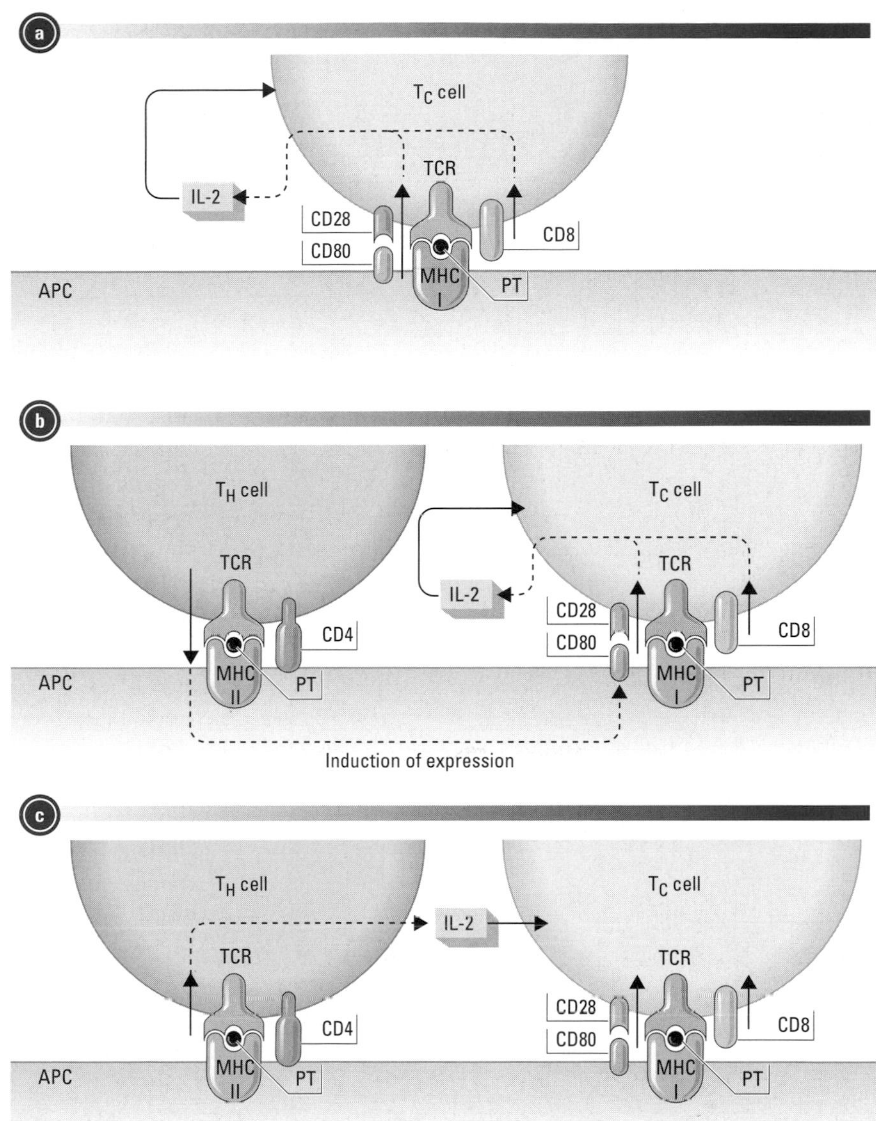

Figure 21.27 Three modes of cytotoxic T (T_C)-cell activation. Description in the text. APC, antigen-presenting cell; CD, cluster of differentiation (molecule); IL, interleukin; MHC I (II), major histocompatibility complex class I (II) molecule; PT, peptide; TCR, T-cell receptor; T_H, helper T cell.

interacting with specific receptors on the cell's surface (Fig. 21.28). Receptors include MHC class I (Semliki forest virus, simian virus 40) and class II (lactic dehydrogenase virus) molecules, CD4 and chemokine receptors (HIV), β_2-microglobulin (cytomegalovirus, herpes simplex virus), growth factor receptor (vaccinia virus), intercellular adhesion molecule-1 (rhinovirus), C3d receptor (Epstein–Barr virus) and many others. Using the receptor, the virus penetrates the cell by either fusing with the plasma membrane (in the case of enveloped viruses) or receptor-mediated endocytosis. Within the cell, lysosomal enzymes digest the capsid proteins (*uncoat* the virion) and expose the viral genome. What happens next depends on the particular type of virus. In DNA viruses the exposed viral DNA enters the nucleus and a part of it (the *early genes*) is transcribed, either by the host DNA-dependent RNA polymerase or, in the case of poxviruses, by viral transcriptase contained in the virion. The transcript is translated into enzymes needed for viral replication. These events are followed by transcription of *late viral genes* and translation of the transcript into viral structural proteins. These then assemble, together with the DNA, into virions, either in the nucleus or the cytoplasm depending on the type of virus. In the case of RNA viruses replication is more complicated. Also, the assemblage of virus particles is a complex process. Some viruses are released when the cell disintegrates; others bud out through the plasma membrane, thereby acquiring an outer membrane envelope that is composed primarily of host-cell

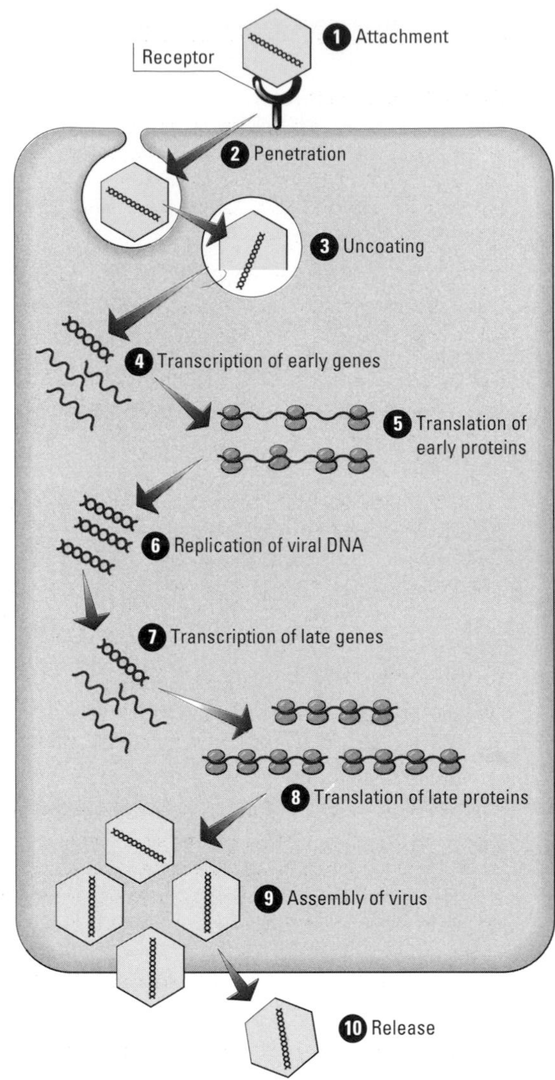

Figure 21.28 Multiplication cycle of a DNA virus.

membrane components. Some viruses (e.g. poxviruses) are confined to a single host species, while others (e.g. influenza virus) can be transmitted between species.

Viruses damage or kill host cells by shutting down cellular macromolecular synthesis, increasing the permeability of lysosomal membranes and thus effecting the release of lysosomal enzymes into the cytoplasm, inducing changes in the permeability of the plasma membrane, causing fusion of infected cells and the accumulation of virions that ultimately cause the cell to burst. Two types of infection can be distinguished, depending on the effect a virus exerts on the host cell: *cytopathic infections*, in which most of the infected cells are destroyed by viral multiplication; and *noncytopathic infection*, in which cells are lysed by the virus. (In some infections, however, the genetic material of the virus integrates into the genome of the host cell and behaves as if it were one of the cellular genes, causing no damage to the host.) A list of viruses responsible for major human diseases is given in Table 21.3.

Defence mechanisms

Mechanical protection

To initiate an infection, a virus must reach the right surface on or in the body and be able to stay there long enough to adsorb to the right cell. A respiratory virus must be inhaled with a droplet and land on the surface of the respiratory system; an enteric virus must be ingested with contaminated food or drink; an arbovirus must be injected into the blood by an insect sting; a dermotropic virus must be deposited on the skin by direct contact with an infected person or a contaminated object (fomite); and a neurotropic virus must enter the body, for example through an animal bite. Viruses that have landed in the right place may be prevented from infecting the host by one of several mechanisms: they can be removed by the mucociliary escalator; they can be prevented from attaching by the movement of the intestines; they can be wiped off the corneal surface; or they can be flushed from the urethra with urine. Those viruses that manage to stay put must be able to penetrate the mucosal layer, which contains a number of antiviral substances including antibodies (see below), and must find the receptors to which they will bind. If a virus that normally multiplies in epithelial cells gets this far, it has almost, but not quite, made it; all it has to do now is penetrate the epithelial cells. Viruses multiplying in other tissues must overcome several other obstacles before they reach their target organs. Because of the short duration of their journey, viruses infecting epithelial cells are highly successful parasites. Their success is further augmented by their effective use of a hit-and-run tactic: they enter epithelial cells, multiply rapidly in them, and exit by killing the cells. The whole attack is over within a few days, well before the body has had time to develop adaptive immunity. Furthermore, since the infection is limited to the epithelial layer and scarcely affects the underlying tissue, defence is limited primarily to non-immunological resistance mechanisms and to the action of interferons. Upon exiting from one focus of infection, the virus may be disseminated by the movement of the liquid or semi-liquid film on the mucosal surface, and fresh infectious foci may be established. Infections on wet surfaces, such as the mucosa of the respiratory system, are therefore usually more disseminated then infections on relatively dry surfaces, such as the skin.

Table 21.3 Major human diseases caused by viruses.

Principal transmission route	Virus	Properties of virus	Symptoms of disease
Respiratory	Influenza	ssRNA, myxovirus group, host-derived envelope	Inflammation of epithelial cells lining respiratory passages. Chills, fever, severe prostration, headache, muscle aches, dry cough. Sudden onset. Complications: secondary bacterial infections
	Common cold (rhinovirus)	ssRNA, picornavirus group	Mild upper respiratory inflammation. Nasal obstruction and discharge, sneezing, scratchy throat, cough, malaise. Complications: bronchitis
	Measles (rubella)	ssRNA, paramyxovirus group, host-derived envelope	First signs: acute respiratory inflammation, cough, fever and conjunctivitis. Later: oval eruption called Koplik's spot, measle rash, begins on the head and moves downward, eventually covering the entire body
	Mumps	ssRNA, paramyxovirus group	Acute inflammation of the salivary (parotid) gland and reproductive organs
Enteric	Poliomyelitis	ssRNA, picornavirus group	First signs: fever, headache, gastroenteric disturbances. Later: inflammation of the grey matter of the spinal cord, stiff neck and back, flaccid (soft, relaxed) paralysis of one or more muscle groups
	Hepatitis A (infectious hepatitis)	ssRNA, picornavirus group	Inflammation and necrosis of the liver, usually accompanied by jaundice. Short incubation period (15–40 days)
	Hepatitis B (serum hepatitis)	dsDNA, hepadna group	Transmitted by infected blood. Long incubation period (60–160 days); otherwise symptoms similar to those of hepatitis A; non-cytopathic; hepatocyte damage caused mainly by the immune response. Similar diseases caused also by several other viruses (non-A, non-B hepatitis)
Direct contact, fomites	Herpes simplex	dsDNA, herpesvirus group, host-derived envelope	Eruption of one or more groups of vesicles on the lips or on reproductive organs
	German measles (rubella)	ssRNA, togavirus group	Enlarged lymph nodes, fever, rash, usually mild
	Chicken-pox (varicella)	dsDNA, herpesvirus group, host-derived envelope	Sparse eruptions of papules, becoming vesicles and then pustules. Occurs usually in children only
	Smallpox (variola major)	dsDNA, poxvirus group	Ulceration of mucous membranes, skin lesions and eruptions, fever. The virus is now eradicated
Animal bites	Rabies	ssRNA, rhabdovirus group, host-derived envelope	Inflammation of the brain accompanied by paralysis delirium and convulsions
	Yellow fever	ssRNA, togavirus group	Headache, backache, fever, nausea and vomiting; liver damage accompanied by jaundice

ds, double-stranded; ss, single-stranded.

Phagocytosis

A virus that has crossed the epithelial layer of the body's surface on its way to remote target organs is like a soldier who has managed to get past the barbed wire: it now faces the real defenders in their trenches, the macrophages of the subepithelial tissues. Macrophages will try to ingest virus particles by phagocytosis and to destroy them inside their phagocytic vacuoles. But they do not always succeed; there are viruses that avoid being killed inside the phagocytic vacuoles. Viruses that have escaped the front-line macrophage assault are carried, with the lymph, into regional lymph nodes and filtered through a second macrophage entrenchment in the nodes' sinuses. Those viruses that slip through this second macrophage defence line as well are carried by the blood to various organs (such as the liver and spleen) that are rich in phagocytic cells. Here macrophages and histiocytes have one more chance to intercept the invader. The liver and spleen are also the main sites of capture for viruses entering the blood directly through insect stings or vertebrate bites. In addition to their function in phagocytosis, macrophages also contribute to the neutralization of the viral infection by cleaning up the destroyed cell debris and presenting viral antigens to T lymphocytes.

Antibody-mediated responses

Antibodies combat virus infection either immediately, at the site of virus entry, or later, when the infection spreads into the blood. At the port of entry, the defending antibodies are mostly of the IgA class, whereas in the blood other antibody classes take part in the defence. However, once a virus has gained access to the blood circulation, antibodies cannot prevent an infection; they merely help to contain it.

Antibodies act on viruses in two principal ways, directly or indirectly. In the direct way, they cause *virus neutralization*, i.e. abolition of viral infectivity. Antibodies can bind directly to virus particles and prevent their adsorption to cellular receptors; they may interfere with the penetration of a virus into a cell; or they may hinder proper uncoating of the virion. Antibodies can be assisted in their neutralizing role by *complement components* and, furthermore, the interaction of virus-bound antibodies with the full array of complement components, including the late-acting ones, may lead to lysis of virus particles. However, not all viruses are susceptible to antibody-mediated complement lysis.

In the indirect way, antibodies interact with viral antigens on the surface of the infected cell and mediate elimination of these cells, either through complement or through *antibody-dependent cell-mediated lysis*. Antibodies can also facilitate phagocytosis of virus particles or virus-infected cells (they have an *opsonizing effect*).

Exposure to some viruses (e.g. those causing smallpox, specific types of poliomyelitis, measles, mumps and yellow fever) induces lasting immunity; the antibodies protect the host against reinfection and individuals who have contracted diseases caused by these viruses rarely suffer a second attack. On the other hand, exposure to certain other viruses (e.g. influenza, common cold and other forms of poliomyelitis) does not protect individuals from subsequent bouts of the same illness. The reason for the absence of durable immunity is that the viruses exist in several different genetic variants; immunity to one variant does not prevent other variants from attacking the host.

T-cell-mediated responses

Once a virus infects a cell and disappears from intercellular spaces, it can no longer be recognized by the immune system. The only way of eliminating the virus is then to destroy the infected cell. This task is left to T lymphocytes and other cells. The mechanisms of T-cell activation in viral infections are still not well understood but it is assumed that the virus invariably infects some APCs such as lymphoid dendritic cells and B lymphocytes (Fig. 21.29). Some of the proteins synthesized by the virus in the cytosol of the infected cell are processed by the proteasomal machinery and some of the resulting peptides, bound to class I MHC molecules, are presented on the cell surface to naive $CD8^+$ lymphocytes. At the same time, some of the viral proteins are translocated into the endoplasmic reticulum and from there are delivered to the cell surface, only to be taken up

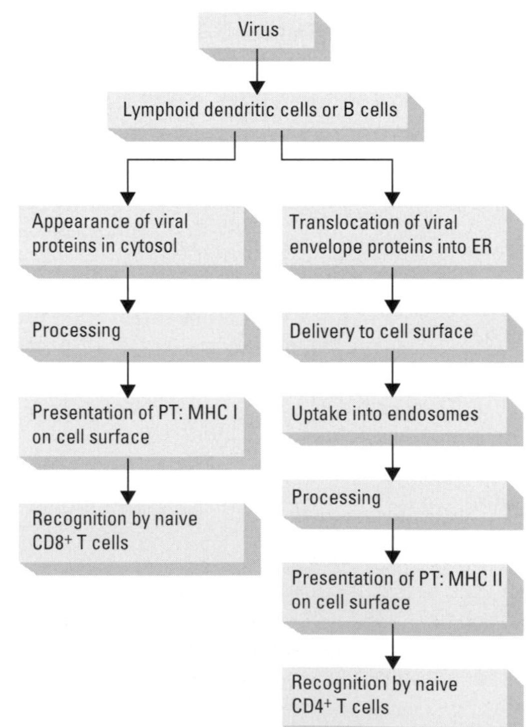

Figure 21.29 Activation of $CD4^+$ and $CD8^+$ naive T cells by virus-infected antigen-presenting cells (dendritic cells or B lymphocytes). ER, endoplasmic reticulum; MHC I (II), major histocompatibility complex class I (II) molecules; PT, peptide.

again into endosomes (see Chapter 6). They are then processed via the endosomal pathway, the resulting peptides bind to class II MHC molecules and the class II MHC–peptide assemblages are expressed on the surface of the infected APC. There they are recognized by naive pT_H cells which, in the presence of IL-12 and IFN-γ produced by stimulated macrophages and NK cells, differentiate into T_H1 effector cells. These produce IL-2, which then drives the differentiation of CD8+ T lymphocytes into T_C lymphocytes. The T_C cells recognize the class I MHC–peptide assemblages on the surface of the infected cells and kill the targets. Virus-specific T_C cells appear within 3–4 days and their activity peaks within 7–10 days of infection.

Activated T_H1 cells produce not only IL-2 but also IFN-γ, TNF-α and other cytokines. *IFN-γ* then induces an antiviral state in cells, while both IL-2 and TNF-α activate *NK cells*, which then produce large amounts of IFN-γ. NK cells also kill virus-infected target cells, which they may recognize by lowered expression of class I MHC molecules (the decrease being caused by the infecting virus) or by some other mechanism. *TNF-α* can also act directly on virus-infected cells and lyse them. Furthermore, *activated macrophages* have been shown to be able to destroy viruses that they have taken up by phagocytosis and to kill other virus-infected cells.

Defence against intracellular bacteria

Characteristics of bacterial infections

Bacteria are one-celled microscopic organisms that lack a well-defined nucleus and reproduce by division (fission) of parental cells. The bacterial cell can be surrounded by as many as three layers: plasma membrane, cell wall and capsule. According to their lifestyle, bacteria can be divided into *intracellular*, which spend most of their life inside host cells, and *extracellular*, which live outside host cells (and some have no hosts at all). Intracellular bacteria can be divided further into *facultative*, which do not depend absolutely on intracellular residency, and *obligate*, which are unable to survive outside host cells. Obligate intracellular bacteria have adapted to life within a cell to the degree that they lack many of the features characterizing other bacteria. They are therefore sometimes referred to as *atypical bacteria* and some were in fact taken earlier to be viruses.

Most intracellular bacteria (Table 21.4) enter the host's body through the mucosa in either the lungs (the airborne forms) or the intestine (the food-borne forms); only a few are introduced into the blood by the bites of ticks and mites. Once deposited at the mucosal membrane, they attach to epithelial cells and cross the epithelial cell layer either by

Table 21.4 Intracellular bacteria responsible for major infectious diseases.

Bacterium	Disease	Preferred port of entry	Preferred target cell	Intracellular location
FACULTATIVE INTRACELLULAR PATHOGENS				
Mycobacterium tuberculosis/M. bovis	Tuberculosis	Lung	Monocyte, alveolar macrophage	Phagosome, cytoplasm
Mycobacterium leprae	Leprosy	Nasopharyngeal mucosa	Unknown	?
Salmonella typhi/ S. paratyphi	Typhoid	Gut	Intestinal epithelial cell	Phagosome?
Brucella species	Human brucellosis, undulant fever, Malta fever	Mucosa	Macrophage	Phagosome?
Legionella pneumophila	Legionnaire's disease	Lung	Monocytes, macrophages	Coiled vesicle
Listeria monocytogenes	Listeriosis	Gut	Intestinal epithelial cell	Cytoplasm?
OBLIGATE INTRACELLULAR PATHOGENS				
Rickettsia prowazekii	Louse-borne typhus	Broken skin, mucosa	Endothelial cell	Cytoplasm
Rickettsia rickettsii	Rocky Mountain spotted fever	Blood vessels (tick bite)	Endothelial and smooth muscle cell	Cytoplasm
Rickettsia tsutsugamushi	Scrub typhus	Blood vessels	Endothelial cell	Cytoplasm
Coxiella burnetii	Q-fever	Lung	Mononuclear phagocytes and others	Phagolysosome
Chlamydia trachomatis	Urogenital infection	Urogenital mucosa	Columnar epithelial cell	Phagosome
Chlamydia trachomatis	Trachoma	Eye	Columnar epithelial cell	Phagosome
Chlamydia trachomatis	Lymphogranuloma venerum	Urogenital mucosa	Endothelial cell, lymphocytes	Phagosome

transcytosis (in the gut through M cells; endocytosis on one side of the cell and exocytosis on the other; see Fig. 21.4) or by being taken up by macrophages and ferried across the layer. They enter host cells by *phagocytosis* effected by either professional or non-professional phagocytes. *Professional phagocytes* (neutrophils and monocytes/macrophages) provide easy access for intracellular bacteria into cells, alas at a steep price. Phagocytosis by these cells is initiated by interaction between their mannose-type, galactose-type and fucose-type receptors and the corresponding sugar residues of the bacteria. Later, when the immune response is initiated, uptake is further facilitated by opsonins such as IgG, breakdown products of complement component 3 and fibronectin, which bind to their corresponding receptors on phagocytes. Once in the phagocyte, however, the bacteria become the target of attack by all the defence mechanisms these cells possess: acidification of the uptake vesicle, destruction by reactive oxygen and nitrogen intermediates, sequestration of intracellular iron, digestion by lysosomal enzymes and incapacitation by defensins and other similar molecules. Some bacteria have found ways of counteracting the offensive, however, and these have become disease-causing pathogens. The various mechanisms by which the intracellular parasite evades the attack are described later in this chapter. However, even bacteria that have learned to survive in the very hostile environment of a professional phagocyte cannot thrive in neutrophils, simply because the cells are short-lived: they normally die before the bacterium has time to reproduce. Most pathogenic bacteria that have chosen to live in professional phagocytes therefore parasitize monocytes and macrophages.

Other intracellular bacteria have turned to cells with a less hostile interior, the *non-professional phagocytes* such as epithelial cells, endothelial cells and lymphocytes. However, here the bacteria must find a way to get inside. Since these cells are normally non-phagocytic, they have to be compelled to ingest the bacteria. This is achieved by two types of molecules, adhesins and invasins, both of which were described earlier. *Adhesins* mediate the *attachment* of a bacterium (both intracellular and extracellular) to the host cell. There are two major types of bacterial adherence mechanism, one mediated by pili, the other by afimbrial adhesins. *Pili* are rod-like structures projecting from the surface of a bacterium and binding to sugar residues of the host cell's glycoproteins and glycolipids (Fig. 21.30a). *Afimbrial adhesins* are bacterial proteins not organized into rod-like structures and binding to the host cell's surface by an unknown mechanism. (Fig. 21.30b). *Invasins* also mediate attachment of a bacterium to a host cell, but they do more: they induce changes in the host cell's cytoskeleton, which lead to the formation of pseudopodia and thus to the engulfment of the bacterium (*invasion*). Some invasins bind to host-cell integrins, others to various receptors (e.g. epidermal growth factor receptor) and other cell-surface molecules. Even in the non-professional phagocyte, however, the intruders would normally be destroyed by some of the protective mechanisms that characterize professional phagocytes. Here, again, successful intracellular parasites have evolved evasive strategies. Some intracellular bacteria live, like viruses, in the cytosol; others take refuge in various intracellular vesicular compartments, including the most hostile—the phagolysosome (see Table 21.4).

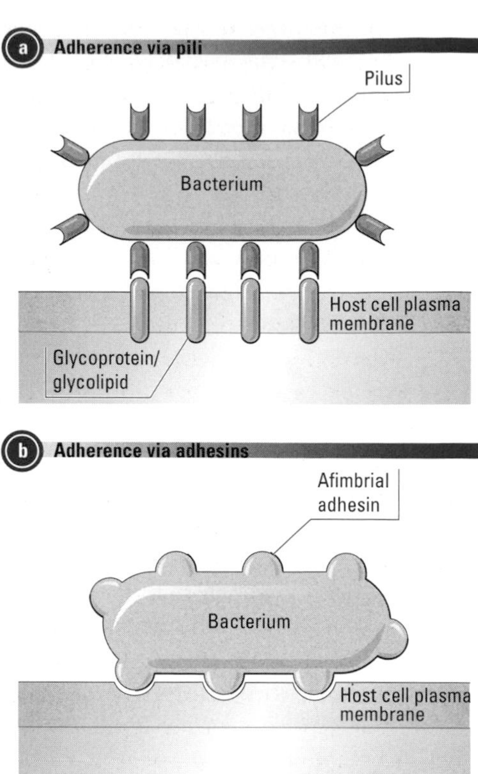

Figure 21.30 Two types of bacterial adherence mechanism.

Defence mechanisms

Intracellular bacteria face obstacles to successful infection similar to those confronting viruses. In the lungs most are removed by the mucociliary escalator; in the intestine their attachment is hindered by peristalsis. Once bacteria have reached the underside of the mucosal membrane, they are confronted by *monocytes* and *macrophages*, which engulf them, kill some and generate antigenic fragments from them. In the local lymph nodes the antigen is processed by APCs and presented to T_H2 *lymphocytes*, which then collaborate with *B lymphocytes* to produce antibodies. The early antibodies, most of them of the *IgA class*, function by interfering with the attachment of bacteria to the mucosa and with the invasion of epithelial cells by bacteria. In some infections (e.g. listeriosis or typhoid), monocytes also spread the antigen (bacteria) to distant organs such as spleen and liver and initiate systemic response.

The generated antigen also activates *intraepithelial T lymphocytes*, *α:β T cells* (presumably via MHC molecules on APCs) and *γ:δ T cells* (directly without the involvement of MHC molecules). Both types of lymphocyte are apparently involved in some non-standard forms of recognition of which their more conventional cousins are incapable and which may represent adaptations for dealing with certain bacterial forms, especially mycobacteria. Recognition can occur with or without the participation of MHC molecules; can involve class Ia, class Ib or class II molecules; and can be restricted to compounds characteristic of certain bacterial forms (*N*-formyl-methionine peptides occurring mostly in prokaryotes and rarely in eukaryotes; low-molecular-mass substances such as phosphorylated sugars or nucleotides, as well as other compounds peculiar to mycobacteria; Table 21.5; Fig. 21.31). Most of these cells are cytolytic for infected targets; some at least also produce cytokines involved in amplification of the response.

Cytokines produced by stimulated intraepithelial T cells, especially IFN-γ, in turn activate macrophages, induce the expression of class II MHC molecules on the surface of epithelial cells and help in the secretion and transport of IgA to mucosal surfaces. Monocytes and macrophages stimulated by the encounter with bacteria also produce cytokines and the entire cytokine network amplifies itself. Cytokines initiate infiltration of the infected site by inflammatory cells, activate macrophages and become involved in the formation of granulomatous lesions. A full-blown inflammatory response ensues.

The bulk of the attack on intracellular bacteria is carried out by cells: macrophages, NK cells and especially T lymphocytes. *Activated macrophages* kill bacteria they have ingested and some of the bacteria also before they are engulfed. However, some bacteria may escape digestion and establish themselves in macrophages or in other cells. These then become the focus of an attack by NK cells and T lymphocytes. As in the case of viral infection, both CD4+ and CD8+ *T lymphocytes* are activated during an infection by intracellular bacteria. Here, too, the pathways of antigen processing and presentation are not clarified yet, but the following mechanisms are believed to be involved. First, some of the bacteria are destroyed in the endosome and their proteins processed via the endosomal pathway; the resulting peptides appear on the cell surface bound to class II MHC molecules in order to stimulate CD4+ T lymphocytes. The conditions of the response are such that they favour the generation of T_H1 cells. Second, bacteria in the endosome secrete proteins that cross over into the cytosol, are processed there and the resulting peptides, bound to class I MHC molecules, are delivered to the cell surface to stimulate CD8+ T cells. Third, some bacteria may egress from the

Table 21.5 Variety of T lymphocytes involved in defence mechanisms against intracellular parasites.

T cell	Ligand	Function
TCR α:β CD4+	PT–MHC II	Help cytokine secretion
TCR α:β CD8+	PT–MHC Ia	Cytotoxicity
TCR α:β CD8+	fPT–MHC Ib	Cytotoxicity
TCR α:β CD8+	nPT–MHC Ib	
TCR α:β CD8+	nPT–CD1b	Cytotoxicity, IFN-γ production
TCR α:β CD4+NK1+	sPT–CD1b	IL-4 production, regulation of antimicrobial immunity
TCR α:β CD4−CD8−	nPT–CD1b	
TCR γ:δ	PT–MHC Ia	Cytokine secretion (T_H1-like pattern)
TCR γ:δ	PT–MHC II	Cytokine secretion (T_H1-like pattern)
TCR γ:δ	fPT–MHC Ib	Cytokine secretion (T_H1-like pattern)
TCR γ:δ	Protein (viral, self)	Cytokine secretion (T_H1-like pattern)
TCR γ:δ	IPPP	Cytokine secretion (T_H1-like pattern)

CD, cluster of differentiation; IFN-γ, interferon-γ; IL-4, interleukin-4; IPPP, isopentenyl pyrophosphate (also phosphorylated carbohydrates and nucleotidic pyrophosphodiesters from mycobacteria); PT, peptide; fPT, *N*-formyl-methionyl peptide; MHC, major histocompatibility complex (class Ia, class Ib or class II molecule); NK1, natural killer cell antigen-1; nPT, non-peptide (lipoarabinomannan from *Mycobacterium leprae*, mycolic acid from *Mycobacterium tuberculosis*); sPT, self peptide; TCR, T-cell receptor; T_H1, helper T cell type 1.

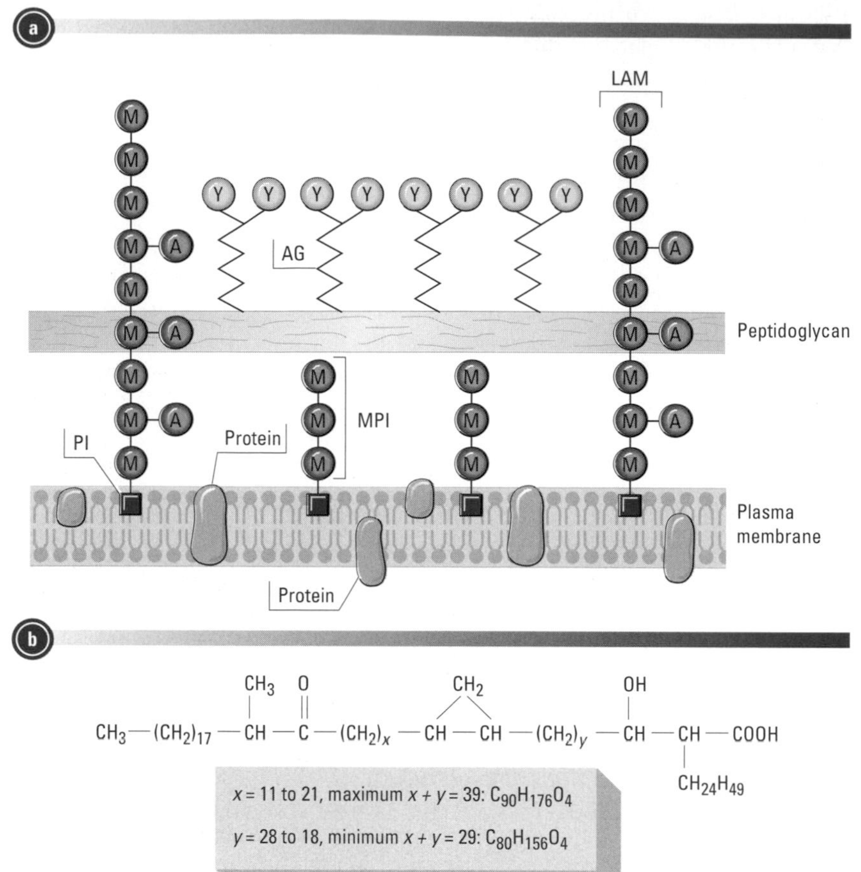

Figure 21.31 (a) Cell wall of a mycobacterium. (b) Structure of mycolic acid. A, arabinose; AG, arabinogalactan; LAM, lipoarabinomannan; M, mannose; MPI, mannophosphoinositide; PI, phosphoinositol; Y, mycolic acid.

vesicular compartment, enter the cytosol and secrete proteins that are then processed and the peptides presented in the context of class I MHC molecules to CD8+ T cells. Fourth, some non-secreted proteins of a destroyed bacterium may find their way into the cytosol and be processed by the class I pathway. How unconventional antigens (e.g. lipoarabinomannan and mycolic acid; see Fig. 21.31) find their way to (unconventional) MHC molecules is not known. Presumably they arise during degradation of bacteria in the endosome and then manage to reach the vesicles in which MHC molecules are being assembled. It appears that the complexation of ligands with the CD1b molecule takes place in the endosomal compartments (which normally serve the class II MHC pathway), even though CD1b is a class I-like molecule. T_H1 cells generated by these mechanisms help CD8+ T cells to differentiate into T_C cells, which then kill infected target cells. Although many different cytokines and various cell types participate in the response and their relative importance may vary depending on the bacterial species, in general IFN-γ and T_H1 lymphocytes are the key components of the adaptive immune response to intracellular bacteria.

An infection by intracellular bacteria can have one of three possible outcomes. First, the immune system succeeds in eliminating all invaders without substantial damage to host cells and so the infection causes no overt disease. Second, the immune system ultimately eliminates the parasite, but only after the latter has damaged host tissues; in this case clinical disease develops. Third, the immune response restrains the parasite but fails to eradicate it. Ultimately, a very labile balance between the activities of the bacterium and the host response is negotiated and the infection may persist. This *chronic infection* is usually accompanied by the formation of *granulomatous tissues* in which the host attempts to wall off the infected focus.

The course of an infection by *intracellular bacteria* is exemplified by the development of *tuberculosis* (TB), a disease caused by *Mycobacterium tuberculosis* (Fig. 21.32). The bacteria are spread from person to person by aerosols. When inhaled, the bacteria attach to the mucosa of the lungs, cross the epithelial cell layer and are engulfed by alveolar macrophages. The bacteria are killed only by activated and not unactivated macrophages, in which they can grow and multiply. In the infected but unactivated

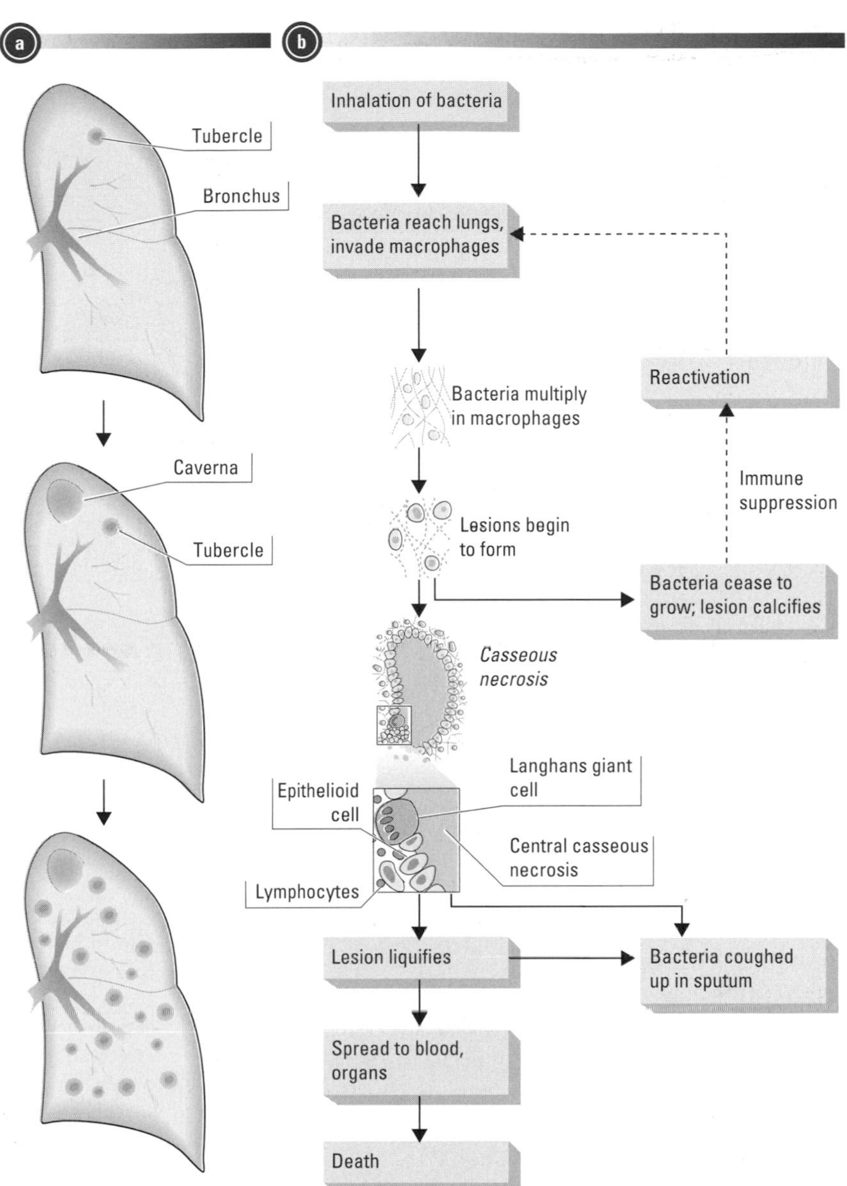

Figure 21.32 Infection by *Mycobacterium tuberculosis*. (a) Development of tubercles and a caverna in an infected lung. The ultimate stage (miliary tuberculosis) occurs in immunodeficient patients. (b) Steps in the pathogenesis of tuberculosis.

macrophage some of the proteins produced by the bacteria are processed via the endosomal pathway and bacterial peptides are presented on the cell surface by class II MHC molecules to naive CD4+ T cells. The precursor cells differentiate, in the presence of IFN-γ and IL-12 produced by other cells (macrophages and NK cells), into T_H1 cells that then secrete IFN-γ, IL-2, lymphotoxin and other cytokines. IFN-γ activates infected macrophages to destroy the engulfed bacteria. IL-2 promotes the differentiation of CD8+ T lymphocytes into T_C cells, which then also attack infected cells. Lymphotoxin kills infected macrophages that have been unable to rid themselves of the bacteria living in their vesicular compartments. The released bacteria are then ingested and killed by activated macrophages. IFN-γ also stimulates endothelial cells to bind circulating T lymphocytes and promote their migration towards the infected area. Other cytokines similarly prompt the convergence of blood monocytes on this area and their differentiation into macrophages. Lymphocytes and monocytes/macrophages thus accumulate at the site of infection.

In a healthy adult exposed to a relatively low number of bacteria, macrophages and T lymphocytes manage to stop the infection before it causes significant damage to the tissue. Memory T_H cells that remain in the body after the infection are responsible for the *positive TB skin test*: when a mixture of *M. tuberculosis* proteins (*purified protein derivative*, PPD) is inoculated into the skin, it stimulates T_H cells at the injection site to secrete cytokines that recruit neutrophils, monocytes and macrophages to this site. The leakage of fluid from the blood vessels together with the local inflammatory effects of cytokines cause redness and swelling (*erythema*) of the injection site; the deposition of fibrin causes its hardening (*induration*; see Chapter 23).

In infants and some adults unable to mount a rapid T-cell response, activated macrophages do not appear until much later. Unopposed by the macrophages, the bacteria thrive and their activities continue to attract new T lymphocytes, neutrophils, monocytes and macrophages to the infection site. The infected macrophage assumes a characteristic elongated shape called 'epithelioid' because it resembles the shape of an epithelial cell; the *epithelioid cells* arrange themselves concentrically forming a little nodule, the *tubercle* (see Fig. 21.32). Macroscopically the tubercle appears as a *granuloma*. As the tubercle grows, the cells in its centre fuse to form *giant cells* with dozens of nuclei at their periphery. The surface of the nodule becomes coated with a mantle of lymphocytes and proliferating fibroblasts. Isolated from the outside by this fibrous wall, cells in the core of the tubercle die, perhaps because of lack of oxygen. Initially, the central area in which the bacteria are growing has a thick, cheese-like consistency (*caseous necrosis*). As bacteria continue to grow, the necrotic area becomes more liquid, but ultimately the core may become calcified and give rise to the characteristic shadow visible on X-ray pictures of tubercular lungs. Some of the tubercles may rupture, discharging infectious bacilli to neighbouring areas and leaving a cavity in the lung parenchyma. As the disease progresses more of the parenchyma is destroyed, until a stage is reached at which the lung is no longer capable of supplying the body with sufficient oxygen. Expectorated sputum and droplets spread the bacilli to other individuals.

Defence against extracellular bacteria

Extracellular bacteria damage their hosts and cause disease by interfering with the body's physiological functions either directly or via exotoxins (Table 21.6). The host's defence must therefore be directed not only against the bacteria themselves but also against their exotoxins. The *non-adaptive response* follows largely the course described earlier in the general introduction to defence mechanisms. The *adaptive response* is dominated by humoral immunity based on antibody production.

The initiation phase of the adaptive response is still poorly understood (Fig. 21.33). Presumably some of the bacteria are engulfed and destroyed by macrophages and other phagocytes, the bacterial proteins processed via the endosomal pathway and the peptides presented on class II MHC molecules on the cell surface. Some bacterial debris is also excreted, taken up by other APCs, processed and again presented in the context of class II MHC molecules. The class II MHC–peptide assemblages are then recognized by TCRs of pT_H cells which, in the presence of IL-4, are activated to differentiate into *T_H2 cells*. The origin of IL-4 is obscure, but the cytokine is considered to have a variety of sources: mast cells and basophils stimulated by bacterial activities; α:β CD4+NK1+ T cells stimulated by self and other peptides complexed with CD1b molecules; various γ:δ T cells activated by *N*-formyl-methionine peptides in the context of class I MHC molecules; and T_H2 cells activated by other antigens. It is also possible that in the absence of T_H1-cell activity, pT_H cells differentiate into T_H2 cells without much need for IL-4. Finally, activated pT_H cells

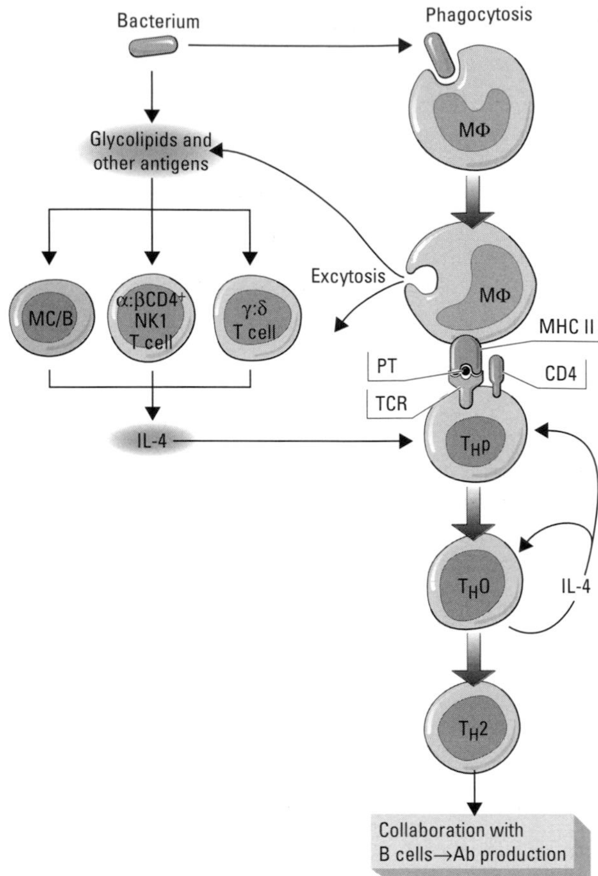

Figure 21.33 Stimulation of helper T (T_H2)-cell responses by extracellular bacteria. Thin arrows indicate production of molecules or their action on target cells; broad arrows indicate stages of cell differentiation. Ab, antibody; B, basophil; CD, cluster of differentiation; IL, interleukin; MC, mast cell; MHC II, major histocompatibility complex class II (molecules); MΦ, macrophage; PT, peptide; TCR, T-cell receptor T_HP, T helper cell precursor.

Table 21.6 Major human diseases caused by extracellular bacteria.

Bacterium	Disease	Symptoms
GRAM-POSITIVE COCCI		
Staphylococcus aureus	Boils	Focal, pus-containing lesions
	Osteomyelitis	Infection of the growing bone. Fever, chills, pain over the bone, muscle spasms around the area of involvement
	Food poisoning	Severe cramping, abdominal pain, nausea, vomiting and diarrhoea
Streptococcus pyogenes	Pharyngitis and scarlet fever	Inflammation of the mucous membrane of the pharynx. Sore throat, fever, chills, vomiting, headache, malaise. Red flush over various parts of the body
Streptococcus pneumoniae	Pneumococcal pneumonia	Inflammation of the respiratory tract, including lungs. Chills, pain in the chest, rust-coloured sputum, rapid breathing, abdominal pain, jaundice
GRAM-NEGATIVE COCCI		
Neisseria gonorrhoeae	Gonorrhoea	Infection of reproductive organs. Redness, swelling, penile or urethral discharge, frequent and burning urination
Neisseria meningitidis	Meningitis	Infection of the respiratory tract, nervous system and sometimes blood. Severe headaches, violent vomiting, high fever, delirium and rigid neck and back
GRAM-POSITIVE BACILLI		
Corynebacterium diphtheriae	Diphtheria	Infection of the respiratory tract. Sore throat, fever, vomiting, formation of ulcers and fibrous exudates (pseudomembranes) in the throat. Difficult breathing. Nerve and heart muscle degeneration
Bacillus anthracis	Anthrax	Pustules in skin. Infection of blood and lymph. Bleeding and serious effusions in the organs and cavities of the body
Clostridium tetani	Tetanus (lockjaw)	Toxins affecting the nervous system. Spasm of muscles and convulsions
Clostridium perfringens	Gas gangrene	Infection of wounds. Gassy swelling of the wounds, foul odour
Clostridium botulinum	Botulism	Toxins acting on the nervous system. Severe gastrointestinal upset, vomiting and diarrhoea, fatigue, disturbance of vision, paralysis
GRAM-NEGATIVE BACILLI		
Escherichia coli	Urinary tract infections, infantile gastroenteritis	Urinary pains. Diarrhoea and dehydration
Salmonella typhi, *S. paratyphi*	Typhoid and paratyphoid (enteric) fever	Infection of lymphoid tissues, ulceration, bleeding and perforations of intestinal walls. Fever, nausea, vomiting, severe abdominal pains, chills, diarrhoea
Shigella dysenteriae	Shigellosis (bacillary dysentery)	Infection of intestinal tract. Fever, nausea, vomiting, severe abdominal pain, blood in the stool, diarrhoea
Bordetella pertussis	Whooping cough (pertussis)	Infection of mucous membranes of respiratory tract and eyes. Cold-like symptoms, with characteristic cough followed by a whoop
Pasteurella pestis	Bubonic plague	Infection of blood, spleen, liver and lymph nodes. Enlarged inguinal lymph nodes (buboes). High fever, vomiting, hot dry skin, thirst, black spots on skin
Brucella abortus	Brucellosis (undulant fever)	General infection throughout the body. Periods of fever alternating with periods of normal temperature. Recurrent attacks, loss of weight, backache, weakness and insomnia
MISCELLANEOUS		
Vibrio cholerae	Cholera	Intestinal infection. Vomiting, diarrhoea, fluid loss, shock
Treponema pallidum	Syphilis (lues)	Infection of blood and nervous system. A hard, painless sore or chancre on the genitalia, variable types of skin eruption. Destruction of brain, heart, skin, bones and viscera

pass through a brief T_H0 stage in which they themselves produce IL-4 for their own use and for the stimulation of pT_H cells. Activated T_H2 cells then recognize bacterial peptides processed and presented to them by B lymphocytes in the context of class II MHC molecules. This launches B cells on the odyssey that ends with antibody-producing plasma cells as described earlier. IgM antibodies are the first to appear; IgG antibodies then follow. In a primary response, an appreciable level of IgG antibodies is not achieved until 5–7 days after infection.

B lymphocytes, however, respond not only to protein but also to carbohydrate and lipid antigens. Substances such as LPS of Gram-negative bacteria activate B lymphocytes directly without the involvement of T lymphocytes (Fig. 21.34). Carbohydrates consisting of repeated sugar residues can also stimulate antibody production by B lymphocytes independently of T lymphocytes or with the help of cytokines produced by non-specifically stimulated T cells. This is apparently the host's response to an attempt by some bacteria to protect themselves by cloaking their cells in a carbohydrate coat (the capsule; Fig. 21.34). The sugar coating masks the sites that professional phagocytes would otherwise be able to recognize by means of their receptors, and thus protects the bacteria from engulfment. However, antibodies to the carbohydrates opsonize the bacteria and thus render them palatable to professional phagocytes. Because in humans T-cell-independent B-lymphocyte responses do not develop until the age of 2 years, infants are

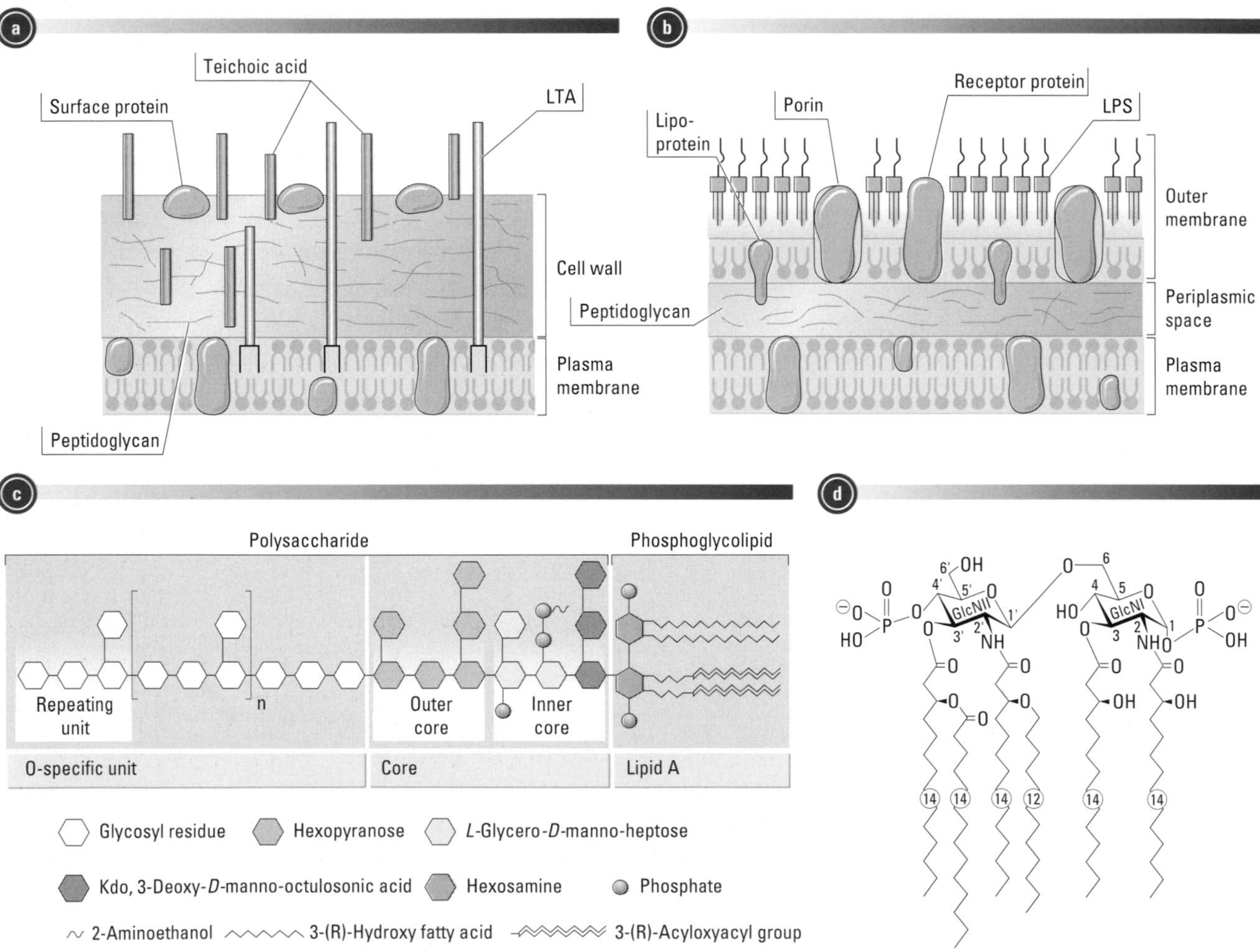

Figure 21.34 Sources of antigens in extracellular bacteria. (a) Structure of the cell surface of a Gram-positive bacterium. (b) Structure of the cell surface of a Gram-negative bacterium. (c) Structure of a lipopolysaccharide (LPS) from a Gram-negative bacterium; *n*, variable number of repeats. (d) Structure of the lipid A component of *E. coli* LPS. The numbers in circles indicate the number of carbon atoms in fatty acids. GlcN, glucosamine; LTA, lipoteichoic acid. (a and b, From Salyers, A. A. & Whitt, D. D. (1994) *Bacterial Pathogenesis. A Molecular Approach*. American Society of Microbiology Press, Washington, DC; c and d, from Rietschel, E. Th. *et al.* (1991), in *Molecular Aspects of Inflammation* (Eds H. Sies, L. Flohe & G. Zimmer), p. 207. Springer-Verlag, Berlin.)

particularly susceptible to infections by encapsulated bacteria.

Antibodies bound to the bacterial surface also activate the *complement cascade*; the assemblage of the membrane-attack complex on the bacterial membrane culminates in bacteriolysis. Some of the complement fragments liberated during activation act chemotactically, and so indicate the location of the bacteria to phagocytic cells. The complement cascade, particularly its alternative pathway, is also activated independently of antibodies, by bacterial products such as endotoxin. The union of antibodies with toxins neutralizes the latter, and toxin–antitoxin complexes are then removed by phagocytosis. However, if too many complexes form in a short time, they may cause an immune-complex disease and injure the host (see Chapter 23). In clinical situations, active immunization for protection against toxins is usually not carried out with native molecules but with toxins that have been treated (e.g. with formaldehyde) in order to destroy their toxic properties but to retain antigenicity. Such modified toxins are called *toxoids*.

Gram-negative intestinal bacteria primarily stimulate IgM production and these antibodies remain largely confined to the vascular system. They are particularly suited to agglutinating, lysing and opsonizing bacteria. However, most bacteria that produce acute infections mainly stimulate production of IgG antibodies, which are good precipitins and, in addition, diffuse readily to extravascular spaces. They are therefore best suited for toxin neutralization.

Defence against fungi

Fungi are plant-like organisms that lack the green pigment chlorophyll and grow on previously produced organic matter as *saprophytes*, i.e. they use dead organic matter as a source of food (Greek *sapros*, rotten; *phyton*, plant), or as *parasites* that obtain food from living bodies. A few are one-celled but most are many-celled, forming masses (*mycelia*) of tubular branching filaments called *hyphae* (Greek *hyphe*, a web). They reproduce asexually by generating one-celled spores, or sexually by the fusion of male and female gametes. There are some 40 000 fungal species, including yeasts, moulds, mildews, rusts, smuts and mushrooms; some 35–40 of these are capable of producing disease in humans (Table 21.7). The infection is spread by spores in the atmosphere or soil. When a spore is inhaled or picked up from the soil by bare feet, it begins to germinate on moist body surfaces and gives rise to a mycelium, which may either colonize the surface or spread through the body, causing a systemic infection. Examples of fungi that cause localized infections are *Microsporum*, *Trichophyton*, *Epidermophyton*, *Candida* and *Aspergillus*; representatives of systemically acting fungi are *Cryptococcus*, *Histoplasma*, *Coccidioides* and *Blastomyces*.

Resistance to fungal infections is mediated chiefly by T lymphocytes and the entire cellular arm of adaptive immunity. Most individuals with well-developed T-cell immunity systems readily contain the infection: the fungus grows rapidly at the port of entry for a week or two, causing an acute infection, but after this period T cells become sensitized to fungal antigens and attack the cells in which the parasite grows. Individuals with T-cell defects, on the other hand, are unable to cope with the infection, which then becomes chronic. The same thing happens in individuals genetically susceptible to fungal infections, newborns with incompletely developed immune systems or patients receiving immunosuppressive therapy. Antibodies often play only a secondary role in fungal infections.

Defence against protozoan parasites and macroparasites

Characteristics of protozoan parasites and macroparasites

Many researchers reserve the term *parasite* for protozoan parasites and macroparasites but refer to other parasites as *pathogens*. Protozoan parasites reproduce in the host's body (in the bloodstream, intestinal tract or internal tissues) and may spend at least a portion of their life cycle within host cells (erythrocytes, macrophages, fibroblasts, muscle cells). Macroparasites usually do not multiply in the vertebrate body but rather produce large numbers of eggs or larvae that develop in the external environment or in an intermediate host. Macroparasites comprise *endoparasites* (flatworms and round worms), which live inside the vertebrate body, and *ectoparasites* (ticks, mites, etc.), which live on the body's outer surface. They are a highly diverse group, each taxon having its own idiosyncrasies and distinct life cycle. Corresponding to this parasite diversity is the heterogeneity of defence reactions on the part of hosts. A description of responses against individual parasites is outside the scope of this book; instead, we simply point out the features common to many of them.

Parasites include some of humanity's greatest scourges (Table 21.8), which infect a large section of the human population and are responsible for life-threatening diseases such as malaria (some 300 million sufferers, annual mortality rate of 1–2 million), schistosomiasis (some 200 million sufferers, annual mortality rate of 800 000) and Chagas' disease (20 million infected persons, annual mortality rate

Table 21.7 Major human diseases caused by fungi.

Fungus	Disease	Manifestation of disease	Epidemiology
Candida albicans	Candidiasis	Member of normal flora of the mucous membranes in the respiratory, gastrointestinal and female genital tracts. Turns into a parasite in immunologically compromised individuals. Produces either systemic disease or localized lesions in the skin, mouth, lungs or vagina. Thrush, dermatitis	Present in most individuals
Cryptococcus neoformans	Meningitis	Infection via respiratory tract. Inflammation of brain and spinal cord membranes, sometimes accompanied by lesions of the skin and lungs	Bird faeces are the main source of infection
Blastomyces dermatitides	Blastomycosis	Infects lungs and disseminates into skin, bones, internal organs, brain and spinal cord membranes. Responsible for abscess formation and tubercle-like granulomas	Soil fungus in the Americas. Acquired by inhalation of dust
Histoplasma capsulatum	Histoplasmosis	Usually limited to lungs but may disseminate throughout the body. Lesions resemble tubercles	Soil fungus in the Americas. Abundant in bird and bat faeces
Coccidioides immitis	Coccidioidomycosis	Infection of the respiratory tract. Symptoms resemble pneumonia or tuberculosis. Sometimes also red nodules in the skin and other organs	Soil fungus; southwestern USA
Geotrichum candidum	Geotrichosis	Infection of the respiratory tract. Symptoms resembling chronic bronchitis; lesions in the mouth	Probably member of normal mouth flora
Epidermophyton sp.	Ringworm Tinea cruris Tinea pedis Tinea corporis	Skin infection of varying severity Jock itch Ringworm of foot (athlete's foot) Ringworm of smooth skin	Some species acquired from animals
Trichophyton sp.	Tinea capitis	Ringworm of the scalp	
Microsporum sp.	Tinea unguium	Ringworm of nails	
Aspergillus fumigatus	Aspergillosis	Skin, respiratory and general body infection	Birds

of 60 000). Parasites also infect substantial numbers of livestock and cause considerable economic loss. However, the highly virulent and dangerous species constitute only a small percentage; most parasitic infections either cause no disease at all or only mild symptoms.

Defence reactions

As in other responses, or perhaps even more so in the response to protozoan parasites and macroparasites, the host mobilizes a wide variety of defence mechanisms at its disposal. A brief description of some of these follows.

Incompatibility of conditions

If the chemical, physiological and nutritional conditions provided by the host are not appropriate, the parasite fails to survive or reproduce. An example of *chemical incompatibility* is the failure of *Plasmodium vivax* to infect erythrocytes lacking the Duffy blood group antigens. The Duffy antigen is a chemokine receptor via which the parasite enters the erythrocyte. *Physiological conditions*, such as pH, oxygen tension or concentration of various metabolites, allow plasmodia to invade only those cells that have reached a very specific stage of their development; cells in other stages are resistant to the infection. The effect of *nutritional conditions* can be seen when mice become relatively resistant to murine malaria by being kept on a milk diet, apparently because they are low in *p*-aminobenzoic acid, which the parasite requires as a growth factor.

Table 21.8 Major human diseases caused by protozoan parasites and macroparasites.

Organism	Disease	Symptoms	Transmission
PROTOZOA			
Entamoeba histolytica	Amoebic dysentery	Invasion of intestinal mucosa; ulceration of large intestine. May spread to liver, lungs and brain; causes abscesses	
Giardia lamblia	Giardiasis	Low-grade intestinal disease. Indigestion and dietary deficiencies	
Balantidium coli	Balantidiasis	Mild diarrhoea; severe ulcerations in mucosa of large intestine	Pig
Trichomonas vaginalis	Vaginitis (trichomoniasis)	Genitourinary infection in both sexes. Persistent vaginal or urethral discharge and inflammation	
Trypanosoma gambiense	Gambian trypanosomiasis	Blood (plasma) parasite	Tsetse fly (*Glossina* sp.)
Trypanosoma rhodesiense	Rhodesian trypanosomiasis	Intense headache, fever, insomnia; drowsiness, tremors, delusions, lethargy	Tsetse fly (*Glossina* sp.)
Trypansoma cruzi	South American trypanosomiasis	Blood (plasma) parasite. Swollen lymph nodes, fever, anaemia	Hemipteran bug *Triatoma* sp.
Leishmania donovani	Leishmaniasis (kala azar)	Blood parasite. Lesions on internal organs and skin	Sandfly *Phlebotomus* sp.
Plasmodium sp.	Malaria	Red blood cell parasite. Chills and fevers at regular intervals, followed by profuse sweating	Mosquito *Anopheles* sp.
Toxoplasma gondii	Toxoplasmosis	Blood parasite. Invasion of reticuloendothelial cells, leucocytes and epithelial cells. Fever and swelling of lymph nodes but may affect other organs as well. Transplacental infection	Widely distributed in animals and birds
METAZOA: FLATWORMS			
Schistosoma sp.(fluke)	Schistosomiasis (bilharziasis)	Enters through skin; develops in portal veins; multiplies in bladder or rectum. Inflammation of skin and bladder. Blood in urine	Several species of snail
Opisthorchis sinensis	Opisthorchiasis	Entry with contaminated food. Infection in bile passages. Irritation; secondary effects from toxic secretions	Snail, fish
Paragonimus sp.	Paragonimiasis	Entry with contaminated food. Lodging in duodenum and lungs. Tuberculosis-like symptoms. Coughing and blood-stained sputum	Crabs, crayfish, snail
Taenia sp. (tapeworm)	Taeniasis	Entry with contaminated food. Lodging in brain and liver. Gastrointestinal and nervous upsets. Anaemia and malaise	Cattle, pig
Dibothriocephalus latus (tapeworm)	Dibothriocephaliasis	Entry with contaminated food. Lodging in intestine. Gastrointestinal and nervous upsets. Anaemia, induced vitamin deficiencies. Diminished appetite, lowered vitality	Fish
METAZOA: ROUNDWORMS			
Ascaris lumbricoides	Ascariasis	Entry with food. Migration: intestine → blood → lungs → intestine. Inflammation of the lungs. Anaemia, fever, restlessness	
Ancylostoma duodenale	Hookworm disease (ancylostomiasis)	Enters through skin. Migrates from blood to lungs and then to intestine. Itching and localized eruption at site of entry Anaemia. Abscesses at site of intestinal attachment	

(*Continued on p. 584.*)

Table 21.8 (*Continued*).

Organism	Disease	Symptoms	Transmission
Trichinella spiralis	Trichinosis	Enters with food. Migration: intestine → blood → muscles. Abdominal pains, nausea, vomiting and diarrhoea, fever, oedema, muscular pains, pneumonia	Pig
Strongyloides stercoralis	Strongyloidiasis	Entry through skin. Migration: blood → lungs → intestine. Redness and intense itching, inflammation of lungs, abdominal pains, nausea, vomiting, diarrhoea and loss of weight	
Enterobius vermicularis (pinworm)	Enterobiasis	Entry with food, lodging in intestine and perianal region. Rectal irritation and anal itching	
Trichuris trichiura	Trichuriasis	Entry with food. Development in intestine. Nutritional and digestive disturbances. Anaemia and eosinophilia. Muscular aches and dizziness. Abdominal pains	
Wuchereria sp.	Filariasis	Entry through skin. Microfilariae in peripheral blood; adult forms in lymphatics and connective tissue	Mosquito *Culex* sp.
Onchocerca volvulus	Onchocerciasis (filariasis)	Entry through skin, lodging in skin. Nodules on face and neck, itching skin	Blackfly *Simulium* sp.
Loa loa	Loiasis (filariasis)	Entry through skin; lodging in subcutaneous connective tissue. Itching and swelling at infection site. Skin and eye irritations	Mango fly *Chrysops dimidiata*

Natural humoral immunity

Various protozoan parasites, including trypanosomes and leishmanias, are killed when incubated *in vitro* with fresh serum of many mammalian species. Presumably, normal serum of certain mammals contains factors that can lyse certain protozoan parasites *in vivo*. However, this does not mean that whenever a parasite is killed *in vitro* by serum of a given species, it cannot infect this species *in vivo*, for the parasite can escape the lytic action of the serum, for example by hiding inside the cell. *Humoral resistance factors* are probably natural antibodies, complement components, or both. For example, *Leishmania enrietti* is killed by normal guinea-pig serum because the serum contains natural antibodies directed against the β-D-galactosyl determinant of the parasite membrane, an antigenic configuration commonly found in nature.

Macrophages

Protozoan parasites and certain intermediate developmental stages of macroparasites fall into the size range of particles ingestible by phagocytic cells. Undoubtedly many protozoa are not pathogenic because they are phagocytosed and destroyed by macrophages when they manage to enter the vertebrate body. Destruction is effected by reactive oxygen intermediates and some of the other killing mechanisms operative in professional phagocytes. It does not require activation of the macrophage. Successful intracellular parasites such as *Toxoplasma*, *Leishmania* and *Trypanosoma*, however, have learned how to evade these mechanisms and they not only survive but multiply in macrophages. To kill these pathogenic parasites, the macrophage must be activated by exposure to IFN-γ and other cytokines and by the infection itself, which leads to production of TNF-α. Activated macrophages are presumably able to kill intracellular and extracellular parasites because of the heightened production of toxic oxygen and nitrogen intermediates. The reason macrophages often fail to eliminate all or even most of the parasites lies apparently in a failure of regulatory mechanisms. Either because of a defect on the part of the host or because of manipulative behaviour on the part of the parasite, the regulatory cellular and cytokine network may inhibit rather than stimulate macrophage activities.

Lymphocytes

For reasons not yet fully understood, individual parasites differ in the type of predominant T-cell response they elicit.

Some (e.g. protozoan parasites) stimulate predominantly T_H1-cell responses, whereas others (e.g. helminths such as schistosomes) activate mostly T_H2-cell responses. Some parasites (e.g. *Leishmania major*) induce either T_H1- or T_H2-cell responses, depending on the constitution of the host; the course of the infection then depends on whichever subset predominates. *T_H1 lymphocytes* help to activate macrophages and to differentiate $CD8^+$ precursors into T_C lymphocytes. T_C cells are believed to lyse target cells infected with protozoan parasites such as *Trypanosoma cruzi*, *Toxoplasma* and *Leishmania*. The first of these three parasites lives in the cytosol, where its antigens have direct access to the class I MHC processing pathway. *Toxoplasma*, by contrast, resides in specialized phagosomes and *Leishmania* within the phagolysosome. Antigens of these two parasites apparently reach the class I MHC processing pathway indirectly by one of the mechanisms described earlier for intracellular bacterial parasites. In malaria, $CD8^+$ T_C cells lyse *Plasmodium*-infected hepatocytes, which they reach with the help of specific homing adhesion molecules.

T_H2 lymphocytes produce cytokines that include IL-4, IL-5 and IL-3. IL-4 prompts activated *B lymphocytes* to switch to IgE antibody production, IL-5 promotes differentiation of bone marrow cell precursors into eosinophils and IL-3 (together with IL-4) stimulates mast cells and basophils. IgE antibodies bind via their Fc portions to the corresponding receptors on mast cells, basophils and eosinophils and via their Fab parts to antigens on the surface of parasites. *Mast* cells and *basophils* then degranulate and the released mediators increase infiltration of the infected site by monocytes/macrophages and eosinophils. The accumulation of eosinophils at the site is referred to as *eosinophilia*. *Eosinophils* bound to antibody-coated parasites also degranulate and release mediators that damage the parasite. The cells can be seen attaching to the worm's surface, flattening out, causing small lesions in the parasite's tegument (the layers covering the worm) and then migrating through the lesions into the worm's interstitial tissues. Ultimately, the eosinophils pry off the tegument and the worm dies. A particularly effective antiparasite mediator is the *major basic protein*, which resting eosinophils store in their crystalloid cores. Certain other mediators released from eosinophils act on mast cells and basophils to induce the release from these cells of the potent *eosinophil chemotactic factor-A* (ECF-A), which promotes eosinophilia. Stimulated mast cells and basophils also release IL-4 and IL-5, thus amplifying T_H2-cell responses. Eosinophils themselves produce a wide range of cytokines (e.g. IL-5, IL-1α) and express IL-2 receptors, CD4 molecules and HLA-DR molecules which enable them to function as APCs.

Antibodies

Degranulation of mast cells, basophils and eosinophils is only one mechanism by which antibodies participate in antiparasitic attacks; there are others as well. Antibodies can bind antigens on protozoal parasites, the antigen–antibody complexes can bind complement, and the lytic sequence of the complement cascade can kill the parasite. Antibodies can also bind to a protozoan parasite in the absence of complement and prevent it from infecting a host cell, a phenomenon akin to virus *neutralization*. Furthermore, antibodies can opsonize the parasite and facilitate its engulfment by macrophages. Finally, antibodies can mediate parasite killing by NK cells in the absence of complement (through *antibody-dependent cell-mediated cytotoxicity, ADCC*). All four functions have been demonstrated to operate against at least some parasites and in at least some experimental conditions. However, with the exception of a few protozoan parasites, such as *Plasmodium*, IgM, IgG and IgA antibodies do not play a *major* part in antiparasitic immunity.

Immunopathological consequences of parasitic infections

In situations in which the host fails to eliminate the parasite but the immune response against the parasite continues for long periods, the attack itself damages the body. We must thus distinguish two types of immune response: *immunoprotective*, which is aimed at the parasite; and *immunopathological*, which becomes misguidedly aimed at the host. Having described the former, we now turn to the latter. The nature of the damage to the body depends on the parasite, developmental stage of the disease and condition of the host. The principal effectors of the damage (*pathology*) are antibodies, immune complexes, eosinophils, T lymphocytes, cytokines, granuloma-associated phenomena and fibroblasts.

Antibodies

Chronic infections by the causative agents of diseases such as malaria, African trypanosomiasis, Chagas' disease and schistosomiasis are accompanied by polyclonal activation of B lymphocytes, T lymphocytes or both. Direct polyclonal activation of B lymphocytes leads to the production of a highly heterogeneous medley of antibodies, most of which have no specific affinity for the parasite. The plasma of the infected person then contains an elevated level of γ-globulins, i.e. it shows *hypergammaglobulinaemia*.

Polyclonal activation of T_H2 lymphocytes causes a similar effect indirectly via T cell–B cell interactions. Polyclonal activators can be parasites themselves, the substances they release (mitogens, superantigens) or host mechanisms triggered by the infections. Polyclonal responses interfere with the activities of the specific antibodies and jam and exhaust the immune system. They may also increase the expression of self epitopes to the level at which the immune system begins to notice them and mount *autoimmune reactions* (see Chapter 25).

Immune complexes

The massive destruction of certain parasites (e.g. trypanosomes in Chagas' disease) by antibodies and the shedding of antigens from living parasites into antibody-laden surroundings lead to the formation of large quantities of immune complexes. The physiological mechanisms that normally clear these complexes from the body are overwhelmed by this flood and the complexes begin to be deposited in blood vessels and organs such as the kidneys, where they interfere with the body's functions. The complexes also cause exaggerated complement activation and, directly or indirectly, the release of highly active inflammatory mediators (amines, peptides, lipids). The ensuing inflammatory response then greatly exacerbates tissue damage.

Eosinophils

Among polyclonally activated B lymphocytes are also cells that express IgE receptors on their surfaces and produce IgE antibodies. Only a small fraction of these antibodies is specific for the antigens of the parasite and hence protective; the others are potentially damaging to the host. Some of the antibodies may activate mast cells, basophils and eosinophils non-specifically, increase eosinophilia and cause degranulation of all those cells not on the surface of the parasite but in host tissues. The resulting tissue destruction becomes particularly dangerous when it affects tissues and organs such as the heart muscle fibres, skeletal muscles or the brain.

T lymphocytes

During an infection, T cells can contribute to host tissue injury either by providing help for antibody synthesis or through the production of cytokines (see below). T_C lymphocytes, too, may inflict considerable damage to host tissues in some infections (see Chapter 16).

Cytokines

T cell-produced cytokines stimulate monocytes and macrophages, which in turn secrete their own complement of cytokines. Macrophages can also be stimulated directly by parasites to produce cytokines without the involvement of T cells. When produced in excess, cytokines can be highly toxic to the host. For example, overproduction of TNF-α causes wasting (*cachexia*) in trypanosomiasis. Cytokines also contribute to the formation of granulomatous tissues.

Granuloma-associated phenomena

In some parasitic infestations, the body attempts to contain the infection by walling off the invader or its products (e.g. schistosome eggs). This process leads to the formation of granulomas, which can be harmful especially if formed in organs such as liver, intestine or bladder. In contrast to mycobacterial granulomas, which are initiated and whose growth is sustained chiefly by macrophage activities, granuloma formation stimulated by macroparasites is in the main a T-lymphocyte affair. Both T_H1 and T_H2 cells are apparently involved in the process, the relative role of the two depending on the particular parasite and the conditions of the infection. In a typical sequence of events, T lymphocytes recognize antigen presented by macrophages and produce IFN-γ, which in turn activates macrophages. The latter secrete IL-1, while T cells also produce IL-2 and both cytokines activate more T lymphocytes. Once activated, both T cells and macrophages become the source of additional cytokines including migration inhibitory factor (MIF), GM-CSF, IFN-γ, IL-4, IL-5, IL-10, TGF-β and TNF-α and also vasoactive peptides such as vasoactive intestinal peptide (VIP). The cytokines recruit various other cells (more macrophages, eosinophils, fibroblasts) to the initial cellular nest, which thus begins to grow. Subsequent giant-cell formation and matrix protein depositions lead to the development of granulomatous tissue.

Fibroblasts

Tissue injury stimulates wound-healing processes in which fibroblasts play the major part. These processes lead to the deposition of collagen and of other extracellular matrix components, i.e. *fibrosis*. The resulting scar tissue may obstruct blood and lymph vessels and reduce the functional effectiveness of affected organs. Fibrotic processes are regulated by a complex network of interactions between cells and their cytokines. Life-threatening forms of fibrosis occur in schistosomiasis, Chagas' disease and filariasis.

Evasion mechanisms used by parasites

We have hinted on several occasions in this chapter that parasites are able to evade the host's immune response by employing special mechanisms. We therefore conclude the chapter with a brief description of some of the tricks that parasites use. We cannot describe all of them because there are probably as many of them as there are parasites.

Anatomical seclusion

Many parasites play hide and seek with the host's immune system: they conceal themselves in cells and organs in which it is difficult for the immune system to spot them. In a way, intracellular parasitism itself can be viewed as an evasive manoeuvre because within a cell a parasite is inaccessible to an entire arm of the immune response, i.e. humoral immunity. However, some parasites go much further than this. A good example is *herpes simplex virus-1* (HSV-1), transmitted from person to person by oral contact, usually before 5 years of age. When the virus reaches the mucosa, it invades epithelial cells and multiplies rapidly in them, spreading from one cell to another. It kills the cells in this process, causing characteristic lesions of the gums, tongue and lips, which develop into painful ulcers. These activities of the virus mobilize the body's immune system, but before a full-scale attack can be mounted on infected cells and the virus, viral particles infect local sensory neurons and hide in them. Neural cells contain factors that shut down the synthesis of all viral proteins so that the virus becomes invisible to the immune system, because in the absence of its proteins no viral peptides can be displayed by class I MHC molecules (which are poorly expressed by neurons anyway). The virus can persist in this latent state for many years. However, when the immune system is temporarily impaired, for example by physical or emotional trauma, the virus is reactivated. It re-enters epithelial cells and multiplies quickly in them, but before the immune system can catch up with it, it goes back into hiding in the neurons. Several other herpesviruses are known to practise diverse variants of this game.

Antigenic shifts, drifts and variations

The most vulnerable part of a parasite is its surface because that is the target of any immune system. Adaptive immunity, especially its humoral arm, is highly efficient at storming parasite surfaces but it has an Achilles' heel: several days are needed to prepare and mount the offensive. Various parasites have been quick to exploit this weakness by altering their surfaces, so that by the time the host has developed the means of destroying them they are sporting a new disguise. There are several variants of this 'quick-change artist' strategy. The simplest is to integrate the surface switch into the parasite's overall developmental programme. The life cycle of most protozoan parasites and macroparasites consists of distinct stages, in each of which the parasites fit themselves out with a different coat. For example, *Plasmodium falciparum*, the causative agent of malaria, passes through several stages in the *Anopheles* mosquito and through at least three stages in the human body: cryptozoites in liver cells, merozoites and gametocytes in erythrocytes (Fig. 21.35). The antigenic properties of each of these forms are so different that antibodies produced against the surface antigens of one stage do not react with surface antigens of the next. Hence by the time the host is possibly able to destroy one form of the parasite, the invader has already reached the next stage.

Some parasites have evolved special genetic mechanisms that enable them to switch coats independently of their developmental programme. The mechanisms include high mutation rate, genomic reshuffling, gene transposition and genetic recombination. *High mutation rate* is a characteristic feature of many RNA viruses, including HIV and the influenza viruses. The multiplication cycle of these viruses requires that at a certain stage the single-stranded molecules constituting their genomes be transcribed into double-stranded DNA. This reverse transcription is catalysed by the enzyme *reverse transcriptase*. This enzyme, like any other copying apparatus, makes errors which, if uncorrected, become mutations, changes in the sequence of encoded proteins. In other systems, most of the errors are corrected by proof-reading enzymes and only the very few that have escaped the scrutiny of the proof-readers become mutations. In RNA viruses, however, proof-reading of DNA copies produced by the error-prone reverse transcriptase is often sloppy and the mutation rate of these genomes is therefore relatively high. In HIV, the mutation rate of the gene coding for the coat protein is so high that variants of the virus with distinct coats arise continuously even within a single infected person. The immune system, in this case, serves as an agent of selection favouring the emergence of new variants.

In the influenza virus, mutations are responsible for *antigenic drift*, the emergence of serologically novel strains to which the host population is not immune. Antigenic drifts occur when accumulating mutations modify one or more of the antigenic determinants of the haemagglutinin or neuraminidase molecules on the surface of a viral particle. As a result of the change, the new determinants may no longer

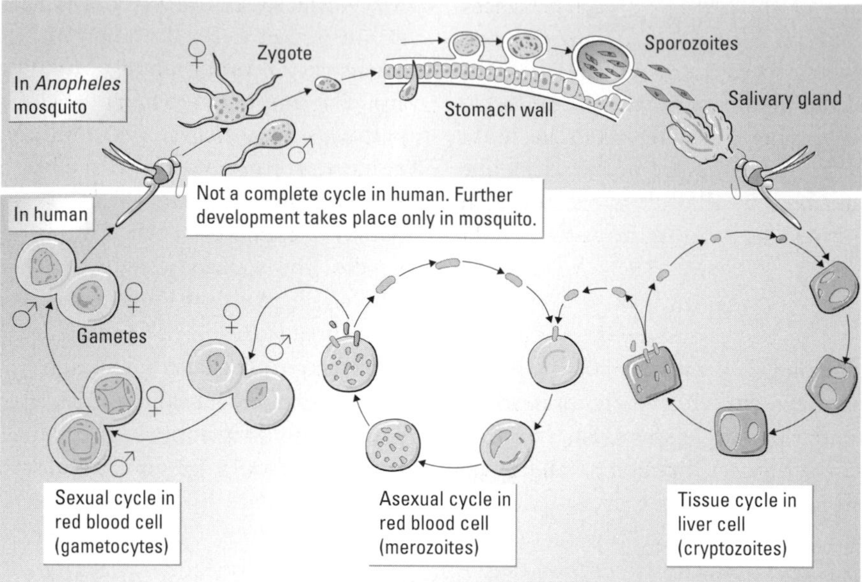

Figure 21.35 The life cycle of *Plasmodium*, the parasite responsible for malaria. *Plasmodium* parasites alternate between two hosts: a mammal (humans, monkeys) and an insect (mosquitoes of the genus *Anopheles*). Only the blood-sucking female mosquito transmits the protozoan; the male feeds on plant juices. When the mosquito bites a human, it injects an infectious form of the parasite, the *sporozoite*, with its saliva. The parasite enters the bloodstream, circulates in the blood for about 30 min, and then enters the liver and invades the parenchymal cells. Within the cell, the parasite enlarges and its nuclei divide without cell division. Then each nucleus surrounds itself with a portion of the cytoplasm, and the cell fragments into a number of *cryptozoites*. This form of non-sexual reproduction, in which the nucleus first divides into several parts and then the cell divides into as many parts as there are nuclei, is called *schizogony*. The infected liver cell then bursts and the cryptozoites leave and either infect another liver cell or enter the blood and infect red blood cells. Once in an erythrocyte, the parasite undergoes a process similar to that in the liver cell: it enlarges so that it almost completely takes up the volume of the erythrocyte, and divides by schizogony, producing *merozoites*, which are similar, if not identical, to cryptozoites (cryptozoites are sometimes also referred to as first-generation merozoites). The parasites then burst the erythrocyte and leave it to infect new erythrocytes and to produce new merozoites. By repeating the cycle, increasing numbers of parasites are produced, destroying more and more red blood cells. After several cycles, the invading merozoites do not undergo fission in some erythrocytes, but instead transform into either female or male *gametocytes*, which remain in the red blood cells until they are taken up by a mosquito. Once in the mosquito's stomach, the gametocytes leave the erythrocyte; male microgametocytes fuse with female macrogametocytes to form a zygote, which then enters the stomach wall and undergoes a meiotic division, accompanied by the reduction of chromosome number from diploid to haploid. The products of the division form rounded cysts in the stomach wall and the parasites multiply rapidly within the cyst, giving rise to as many as 10 000 sporozoites in about 3 weeks. Mature sporozoites break out of the cyst and wander about the body of the mosquito host, many coming to rest in the salivary glands, ready to be injected with the next mosquito bite and to start a new infection cycle. (Redrawn from Barnes, R. D. (1974) *Invertebrate Zoology*, 3rd edn. W. B. Saunders, Philadelphia.)

react with some of the antibodies directed against the original antigen and present in various individuals of a human population. The virus with the altered determinants will therefore possess a growth advantage and may cause a local outbreak of influenza until antibodies against the modified determinant are formed.

Genomic reassortment in the influenza virus leads to *antigenic shifts*. The virus, which is known to infect not only humans but also certain other mammals and birds, contains eight single-stranded RNA molecules. Although the RNA molecules of the individual species code for the same complement of proteins, the protein sequences, particularly those of haemagglutinin and neuraminidase, differ considerably. Normally the viruses are species specific, but occasionally a virus of one species infects another species, as is attested by the finding that farmers often have antibodies in their blood specific for pig, horse or duck influenza viruses. It is believed that in the rare instances in which a person is infected simultaneously by a human and an animal virus and the viruses happen to replicate in the same cell, genomic reassortment takes place during the assembly and packaging of viral ribonucleoproteins. Some of the particles budding from such a cell will then contain some RNA molecules of the human virus and others of the animal virus. If the reassorted particle retains genes necessary for the infection of human cells but acquires haemagglutinin- or neuraminidase-encoding genes of the animal virus, the new virus will find the human population totally unprepared because none of the antibodies present in the population will react against it. The antigenic determinants of the new virus will be entirely different from those of all other influenza viruses that may be present in the population: a major antigenic shift will occur. The virus will then cause a global outbreak of the disease or *pandemic*. Eventually, antibodies in resistant individuals will protect them from reinfection and the outbreak will be brought under control until another new virus with a reassorted genome enters the population. Influenza pandemics have a devastating effect on the human population. The 1918–19 pandemic is estimated to have killed 20–40 million people.

Gene transposition is responsible for *antigenic variation*, practised by African trypanosomes (*Trypanosoma brucei*, *T. rhodesiense*, Fig. 21.36). Antigenic variation occurs in the major constituent of the parasite's coat, the *variant-specific glycoprotein* (VSG; relative molecular mass 50 000), attached to the plasma membrane via a glycosylphosphatidylinositol (GPI) anchor. The protein part of VSG is encoded in a family of over 100 genes, which differ considerably in their coding sequence (except for the part specifying the last 50 amino acid residues of the protein). VSG is strongly immunogenic to the host and the immune system should therefore be able to control the infection easily; it should but it does not: the infecting parasite

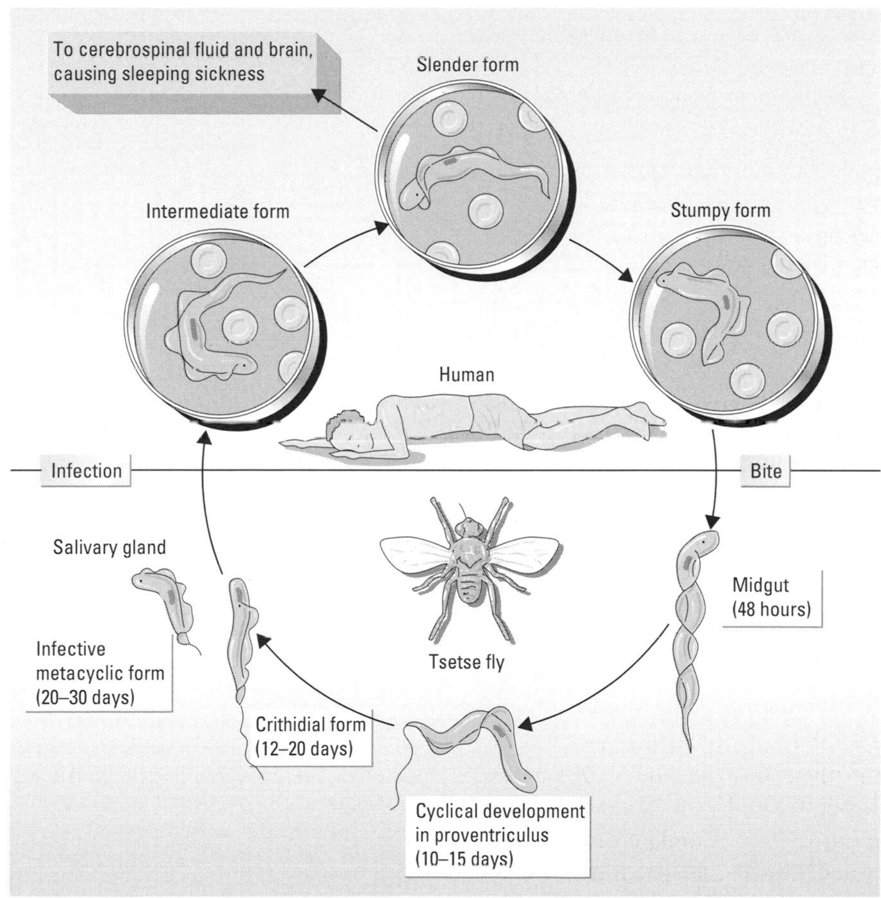

Figure 21.36 The life cycle of *Trypanosoma gambiense (rhodesiense)*, the parasite responsible for African sleeping sickness. The intermediate host of the parasite is the tsetse fly of the genus *Glossina*. During their 12–15 day sojourn in the fly, the trypanosomes multiply by binary fission in the midgut, then migrate to the salivary glands, transform into infective forms and are transmitted to humans in droplets of saliva as the fly sucks blood through the skin. After an incubation period of 6–7 days, trypanosomes begin to appear in large numbers in the blood. Later they invade lymph nodes, spleen and eventually the lymph fluid surrounding the nerves and brain, causing fever, severe headaches, sleepiness and paralysis. (From Klein, J. (1982) *Immunology: The Science of Self–Nonself Discrimination*. John Wiley & Sons, New York.)

catches the host unprepared, so the trypanosomes multiply unchecked for about a week. During this time, however, the host mobilizes its immune system and begins to produce antibodies against the antigen: antibodies lyse or agglutinate trypanosomes and the size of the parasite population rapidly declines. But then a few parasites emerge from the declining population, coated with molecules completely different from those of the preceding variant and therefore unassailable by the antibodies that the host has so laboriously produced. Unchecked by any defence mechanisms, the few multiply and flood the host, which must now start all over again with the production of a new antibody. When it manages to redirect production and antibodies begin to eliminate the second parasite variant, the trypanosomes change coats again, and so the process goes on. Since the new coat is always completely different from the preceding one, the previously produced antibodies are of no use. Behind each coat change is a transposition of one of more than 100 *VSG* genes to a position on the chromosome (near the telomere) at which it can be expressed (Fig. 21.37a). Before transposition, the gene is duplicated so that the size of the gene family stays the same. Because the individual genes differ greatly from one another, each transposition leads to the expression of an entirely different VSG on the surface of the trypanosome. The selection of a gene for transposition is apparently random.

Neisseria gonorrhoeae, the causative agent of gonorrhoea, achieves antigenic variation by a different mechanism still—*homologous recombination*. Variation occurs in the pilins, the protein subunits that comprise the shaft of the pilus. Pilins are encoded in several *pil* genes, some of which are expressed (*pilE*), while others are silent (*pilS*). Parts of the *pil* genes are highly conserved, whereas other segments, the *minicassettes mc1–mc6*, vary considerably in their sequence from one copy of the gene to another (Fig. 21.37b). It is believed that the two strands of the bacterial chromosome occasionally exchange segments of the *pilE* gene for corresponding segments of the *pilS* gene (Fig. 21.37c). This recombination replaces old minicassettes of the expressed gene with new ones and the bacterium thus comes into possession of pilins with entirely new antigenic properties. Because similar changes by the same or different mechanisms also occur in genes controlling other bacterial surface proteins, a collection of different variants arises. Some of the variants will be unaffected by the immune response the host has mounted against the old variants and will therefore be selected to grow and take over the population. This antigenic variation contributes to the lack of protective immunity in persons who have recovered from *Neisseria* infection; they can be reinfected by new variants of the bacterium.

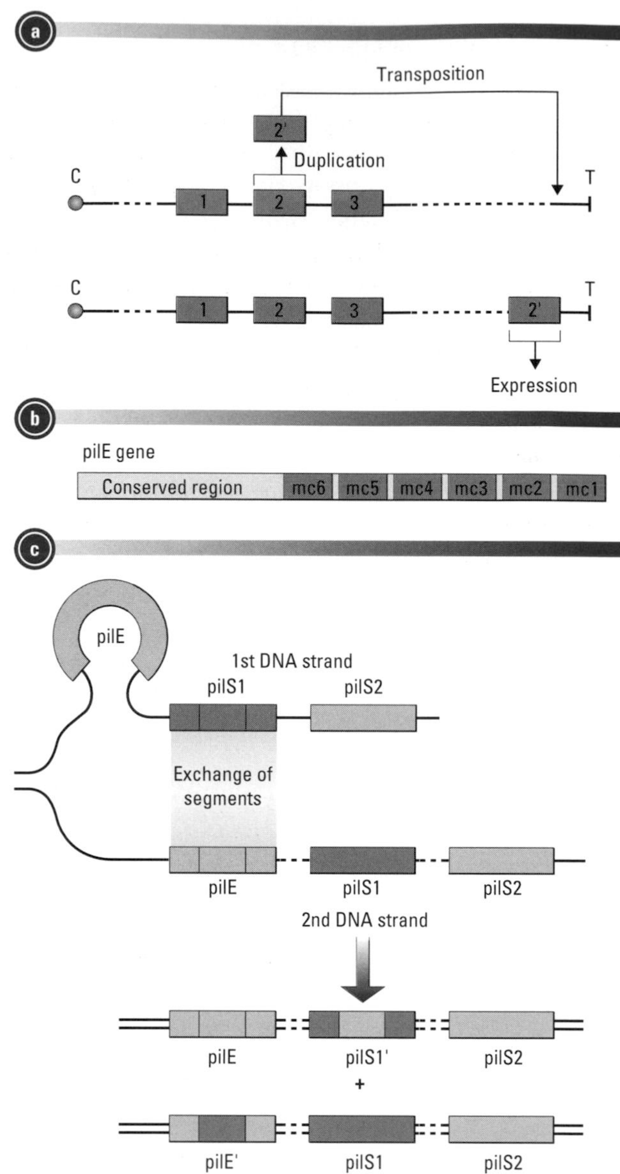

Figure 21.37 Examples of mechanisms responsible for antigenic variation in *Trypanosoma* (a) and *Neisseria* (b,c). In *Trypanosoma*, one of the telomere-distant genes (*1,2,3 . . .*) is duplicated and the copy is transposed to the vicinity of the telomere, where it is expressed. In *Neisseria*, the pilin-encoding gene (b) contains a conserved region and several variable segments (minicassettes, *ms1–ms6*). One DNA strand of a silent gene *(pilS)* undergoes an exchange of segments with the second strand of the expressed gene *(pilE)* of a replicating bacterial chromosome (c). After the completion of the replication, two double-stranded daughter chromosomes emerge, each of which appears to have undergone non-reciprocal recombination. Because assays for antigenic variation select for altered *pilE*, only one type of daughter chromosome is detected. C, centromere; T, telomere; (c) Is based on Salyers, A. A. & Whitt, D. D. (1994) *Bacterial Pathogenesis. A Molecular Approach*. Society of Microbiology Press, Washington, DC.

Antigenic disguise and mimicry

Yet another strategy used by parasites to escape detection by the immune system is to pretend that they are part of the host. This trick is used effectively by *schistosomes*, the flatworms that infect the small intestine and portal veins of vertebrates and cause *schistosomiasis*. The eggs released from the vertebrate host develop in fresh water into free-swimming larvae, *miracidia*, which then infect an intermediate host, a freshwater snail (Fig. 21.38). The larvae transform into *sporocysts* and these into *cercariae*, which then infect a vertebrate again. Following their attachment to human skin the cercariae discard the glycocalyx needed during their existence in fresh water and reveal the outer membrane, which carries parasite-specific antigens. The exposed antigens stimulate the host's immune response, but while the response is developing, the immature worm, the *schistosomulum*, makes its way to the blood vessels and there begins to cover itself with the host's molecules: red blood cell antigens (A, B, H) and molecules controlled by the MHC (both class I and class II). Blood plasma probably contains a low concentration of these molecules, which are continually shed from cells regenerating their surfaces. The schistosomulum picks up MHC molecules and completely coats its body with them, masking its own membrane antigens. By doing so, the parasite effectively causes the host immune system to regard it as a part of self. If such a host is re-exposed to new cercariae, the developing new schistosomules will encounter the immune response stimulated by the first infection and be killed, while the adult schistosomes already living in the body will remain untouched. This mechanism prevents superinfection by new parasites, while allowing old ones to persist for long periods in the body.

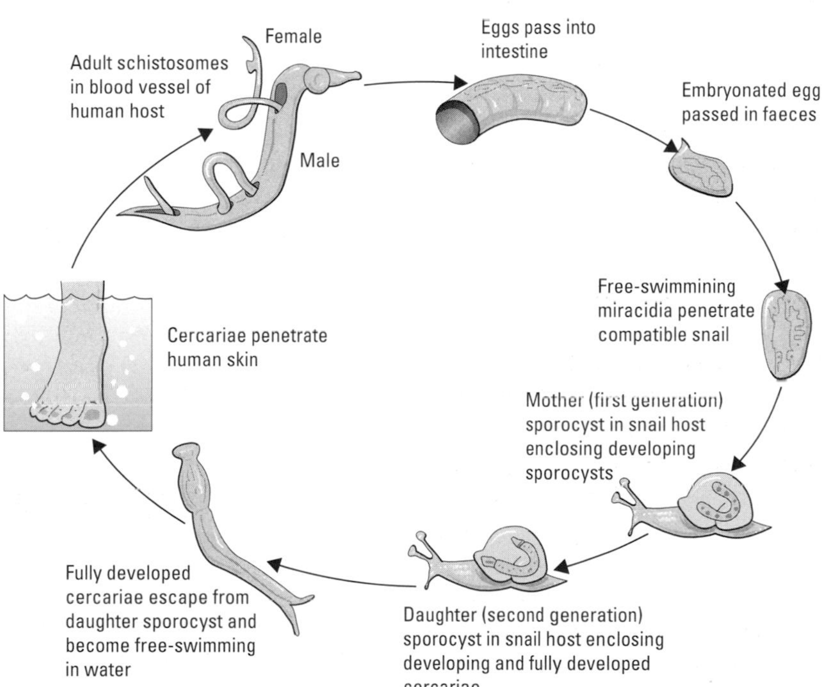

Figure 21.38 The life cycle of *Schistosoma mansoni*. The adult worms are of separate sexes, living in a most unusual arrangement: the male's body is split longitudinally (hence the name, from Greek *schistos*, split; *soma*, body) and in the groove thus formed resides the thread-like female. Eggs deposited by the female in the blood contain small, rapidly developing larvae which, by secreting digestive substances, aid the eggs in escaping from the blood vessels, through the tissues into the lumen of the intestine and out of the body with the faeces. However, some eggs enter the circulation and eventually become trapped in the lungs and liver, eliciting a granulomatous reaction from the host. If faeces are deposited in water, the fully embryonated eggs hatch and develop into ciliated, free-swimming larvae called *miracidia*. To develop further, the larvae must find an intermediate host, a freshwater snail. The miracidium bores into the snail and, upon reaching the snail's digestive tract, develops into a *mother sporocyst*, a simple sac-like structure in which germinal cells bud off internally and develop into a number of *daughter sporocysts*. Eventually the sporocysts transform into fork-tailed *cercariae*, which leave the snail and live in the water until they chance upon a human who happens to be bathing or working in the infested pond. On contact, the cercariae penetrate the human skin by a boring action that also involves enzymatic digestion, enter the bloodstream and let themselves be carried first to the lungs, then to the liver and finally to the intestinal veins. During this journey, the cercariae are gradually transformed into adult *schistosomulae*.

Frustration of the immune system

Parasite strategies described thus far are all aimed at either avoiding the attention of the immune system or keeping abreast of its effector activities. An entirely different strategy is to *interfere* with immune mechanisms and thus frustrate attempts to destroy the parasite. The targets of these interferences can be antibodies, complement components, cytokines and other immunologically important molecules, as well as cells—APCs, macrophages and lymphocytes.

Inactivation of antibody molecules

Parasites that have become coated with antibodies may attempt to neutralize the potentially lethal load by attacking it with their own enzymes. The attack is usually directed at the Fc region, the part of the antibody molecule most vulnerable proteolytically. If the antibody is bound to the parasite via its Fab regions, removal of the Fc regions prevents complement activation, with all its consequences; if it is bound by the Fc region, the cleaved fragments are released and may even interfere with other functions of the immune system. The former situation occurs, for example, in certain strains of *T. cruzi*; the latter with schistosome larvae.

Blockade of the complement cascade

Any one of the 30 or so complement components is a potential target for subversion by parasites and, since the components are functionally interdependent, by concentrating on one of them parasites may block the entire cascade. Subversion of several components has indeed been demonstrated. For example, vaccinia and herpes viruses produce proteins that bind C4b and thus inactivate the classical pathway. HSV produces proteins that bind C3b and thus block both the classical and alternative pathways. *Trypanosoma cruzi* and other parasites synthesize proteins that functionally mimic decay-accelerating factor (DAF), a natural inhibitor of the complement cascade. Certain forms of *Leishmania* escape complement-mediated lysis by inducing detachment of C5b–9 complexes from their surfaces before the membrane-attack complex can perforate any membranes. Finally, the worm *Taenia taeniaeformis* secretes substances that activate complement components in the fluid phase, where they cannot cause any damage, and thus depletes the cascade and prevents it from acting at sites where it *could* cause damage.

Meddling with the cytokine internet

Because the main purpose of the cytokine network is to regulate the immune response, any parasite that learns how to break into the network and to manipulate it to its own advantage will score a big win in the contest with the host. Not surprisingly, many parasites have evolved mechanisms that accomplish just that. A parasite can manipulate the network via either cytokine receptors or cytokines themselves. Both types of manipulation have been documented. A receptor, of course, functions when it is on the cell surface, connected to its signalling pathway. A receptor floating in the fluid phase is, with few exceptions, of no use; on the contrary, by binding cytokines and forming 'sterile' soluble complexes, it competes with the real receptor on the cell surface and thus prevents desirable responses from taking place. Several viruses use this strategy of incapacitating parts of the network by producing soluble receptor dummies. For example, some herpesviruses and poxviruses encode proteins that resemble receptors for IL-1β, TNF-α and IFN-γ except for the fact that they lack transmembrane and cytoplasmic regions. All three cytokines are, of course, important components of antiviral immunity, so by keeping them away from infected cells viruses increase their chances of completing their multiplication cycles undisturbed. Another example is provided by human cytomegalovirus, which produces a look-alike receptor for chemoattractants such as RANTES, MIP-1 and MCP-1. By preventing chemokines from reaching their real receptors on lymphocytes and monocytes, the virus prevents a large-scale influx of these cells to the site of infection.

Parasite interference with the cytokine itself can assume a variety of forms. The parasite can synthesize proteins that block the production of a mature cytokine (e.g. cowpox and vaccinia viruses synthesize serpins that prevent the pro-IL-1β converting enzyme from cleaving the intracellular IL-1β precursor into the mature secreted form); can alter arachidonic acid metabolism to prevent the production of certain chemoattractants (e.g. poxviruses synthesize proteins that block the production of LTB_4, a neutrophil chemoattractant); can bind the produced cytokine and thus prevent it from reaching the cytokine receptor (e.g. hepatitis B virus binds to cells that express IL-6 on their surfaces, preventing IL-6 release into the fluid phase); or can produce a cytokine look-alike that steers the immune response in a desired (from the parasite's perspective) direction (e.g. Epstein–Barr virus produces B-cell receptor factor 1, BCRF1, which resembles IL-10 and binds to IL-10 receptors to stimulate T_H2-cell responses and inhibits the appearance of T_H2 cells, thus avoiding the induction of inflammatory responses).

Influence on the expression of other immunologically important molecules

MHC molecules are frequent targets of a parasite's attempts to thwart antiparasitic immune responses. For example, several viruses downregulate the expression of class I MHC molecules and thus reduce presentation of viral peptides by infected cells. Certain adenoviruses synthesize glycoproteins that are retained in the endoplasmic reticulum where they bind class I heterodimers and so prevent their passage to the cell surface. One adenovirus inhibits the transcription enhancer of the class I genes. Mouse cytomegalovirus produces a protein that prevents the transport of peptide-loaded class I molecules into the medial Golgi compartment. Finally, human cytomegalovirus elaborates a class I-like protein (UL18) that competes with true class I polypeptides for β_2-microglobulin binding.

Human cytomegalovirus also produces a molecule that functions as an IgG-binding *Fc receptor*. The Fc regions of antibodies bound to these dummy receptors on infected cells or on virus particles are unavailable for binding complement or for binding to macrophages.

African swine fever virus (ASFV) encodes a homologue of the *adhesion molecule* CD2 and expresses it on the surface of ASFV-infected erythrocytes. The impostor is believed to interfere with T-lymphocyte and NK-cell functions mediated by the real CD2.

Invasion of cells of the immune system

Many parasites strike at the heart of vertebrate defence mechanisms by invading cells that would otherwise have posed the greatest threat to them: the lymphocytes and monocytes/macrophages. A notorious example of *lymphocyte* invasion is HIV, which targets CD4+ T cells and actually uses the CD4 molecule to enter the cells. Several other retroviruses are also lymphotropic. *Monocytes* and *macrophages* are invaded by a number of intracellular bacteria and protozoal parasites. All these parasites have evolved a set of protective mechanisms that allow them not only to evade hostilities once inside the cell but also to actually multiply there. Particularly striking examples of such adaptations are provided by mycobacteria.

To gain entry into macrophages, mycobacteria use either complement 1 and 3 receptors (CR1, CR3) or fibronectin and vitronectin receptors, none of which are connected to a signalling pathway that would activate oxidative burst reactions; mycobacteria avoid using Fc receptors, which *would* trigger these reactions. Once inside the macrophages, mycobacteria have a choice of several strategies allowing them to avoid antimicrobial activities that phagocytosis might otherwise initiate. They can inhibit fusion of the phagosome with lysosomes by an as yet not fully understood mechanism. However, some mycobacteria can survive and multiply even if fusion does occur and a phagolysosome is formed. They are then protected from the action of the released toxic substances by specialized mechanisms (see below). Mycobacteria can also escape from the phagolysosome into membrane-bound vesicles and use these as a kind of protective cocoon for replication. Finally, mycobacteria can disrupt the phagosome membrane and escape into the cytosol.

Most of the substances that protect mycobacteria from antimicrobial activities inside the host macrophage are concentrated in their cell walls. These contain special glycolipids and carbohydrate components, such as phenolic glycolipid-1 (PGL-1), mannosylated lipoarabinomannan (manLAM) and lipoarabinomannan terminated by arabinan residues (araLAM; see Fig. 21.31), which protect the bacteria at different stages of infection by modulating the release of macrophage-derived cytokines, blocking the activation of macrophages, inhibiting the production of reactive oxygen intermediates and scavenging these intermediates once they have been produced. In addition to resistance dependent on the cell wall, mycobacteria also produce several proteins that protect them against the hostile environment of the macrophage. These include the heat-shock proteins Hsp60 and Hsp70, as well as superoxide dismutase (SOD). The heat-shock proteins facilitate the refolding of mycobacterial proteins, while SOD limits the effects of reactive oxygen intermediates.

Mycobacteria also manipulate the host response by directly stimulating cytokine secretion from monocytes. The araLAM, manLAM and other components of the mycobacterial cell wall as well as several mycobacterial proteins are known to stimulate the secretion of TNF-α and IL-1β by macrophages. Virulent and non-virulent strains of mycobacteria often differ in the type of cytokines whose production they stimulate.

Further reading

Baumann, H. & Gauldie, J. (1994) The acute phase response. *Immunology Today*, **15**, 74–80.

Biron, C. A. & Gazzinelli, R. T. (1995) Effects of IL-12 on immune responses to microbial infections: a key mediator in regulating disease outcome. *Current Opinion in Immunology*, **7**, 485–496.

Bourin, M. C. & Lindahl, U. (1993) Glycosaminoglycans and the regulation of blood coagulation. *Biochemical Journal*, **289**, 313–330.

Britton, W. J., Roche, P. W. & Winter, N. (1994) Mechanisms of persistence of mycobacteria. *Trends in Microbiology*, **2**, 284–288.

Brook, D. R. & McLennan, D. A. (1993) *Parascript. Parasites and the Language of Evolution*. Smithsonian Institution Press, Washington, DC.

Cooper, A. M. & Flynn, J. L. (1995) The protective immune response to *Mycobacterium tuberculosis*. *Current Opinion in Immunology*, **7**, 512–516.

Erb, K. J., Holloway, J. W. & Le Gros, G. (1996) Mast cells in the front line. *Current Biology*, **6**, 941–942.

Esmon, C. T. (1995) Thrombomodulin as a model of molecular mechanisms that modulate protease specificity and function at the vessel surface. *FASEB Journal*, **9**, 946–955.

Ewald, P. W. (1994) *Evolution of Infectious Diseases*. Oxford University Press, Oxford.

Falus, A. & Merétey, K. (1992) Histamine: an early messenger in inflammatory and immune reactions. *Immunology Today*, **13**, 154–156.

Furie, B. & Furie, B. C. (1988) The molecular basis of blood coagulation. *Cell*, **53**, 505–518.

Gailit, J. & Clark, R. A. F. (1994) Wound repair in the context of extracellular matrix. *Current Opinion in Cell Biology*, **6**, 717–725.

Gallin, J. I., Goldstein, I. M. & Snyderman, R. (Eds) (1988) *Inflammation. Basic Principles and Clinical Correlates*. Raven Press, New York.

Geczy, C. L. (1994) Cellular mechanisms for the activation of blood coagulation. *International Review of Cytology*, **152**, 49–108.

Gerritsen, M. E. & Bloor, C. M. (1993) Endothelial cell gene expression in response to injury. *FASEB Journal*, **7**, 523–532.

Gordon, S., Clarke, S., Greaves, D. & Doyle, A. (1995) Molecular immunobiology of macrophages: recent progress. *Current Opinion in Immunology*, **7**, 24–33.

Halkier, T. (1991) *Mechanisms in Blood Coagulation, Fibrinolysis and the Complement System*. Cambridge University Press, Cambridge.

Hauschildt, S. & Kleine, B. (1995) Bacterial stimulators of macrophages. *International Review of Cytology*, **161**, 263–331.

Heinrich, P. C., Castell, J. V. & Andus, T. (1990) Interleukin-6 and the acute phase response. *Biochemical Journal*, **265**, 621–636.

Hormaeche, C. E., Penn, C. W. & Smyth, C. J. (Eds) (1992) *Molecular Biology of Bacterial Infection. Current Status and Future Perspectives*. Cambridge University Press, Cambridge.

Jones, B., Pascopella, L. & Falkow, S. (1995) Entry of microbes into the host: using M cells to break the mucosal barrier. *Current Opinion in Immunology*, **7**, 474–478.

Kaufmann, S. H. E. (1993) Immunity to intracellular bacteria. *Annual Review of Immunology*, **11**, 129–163.

Kovacs, E. J. (1991) Fibrogenic cytokines: the role of immune mediators in the development of scar tissue. *Immunology Today*, **12**, 17–23.

Lasky, L. A. (1992) Selectins: interpreters of cell-specific carbohydrate information during inflammation. *Science*, **258**, 964–969.

Lloyd, A. R. & Oppenheim, J. J. (1992) Poly's lament: the neglected role of the polymorphonuclear neutrophil in the afferent limb of the immune response. *Immunology Today*, **13**, 169–172.

Madigan, M. T., Martinko, J. M. & Parker, J. (1997) *Brock Biology of Microorganisms*, 8th edn. Prentice Hall International, London.

Marcus, A. J. & Safier, L. B. (1993) Thromboregulation: multicellular modulation of platelet reactivity in hemostasis and thrombosis. *FASEB Journal*, **7**, 516–522.

Marrack, P. & Kappler, J. (1994) Subversion of the immune system by pathogens. *Cell*, **76**, 323–332.

Marshall, J. S. & Bienenstock, J. (1994) The role of mast cells in inflammatory reactions of the airways, skin and intestine. *Current Opinion in Immunology*, **6**, 853–859.

Martin, D. M. A., Boys, C. W. G. & Ruf, W. (1995) Tissue factor: molecular recognition and cofactor function. *FASEB Journal*, **9**, 852–859.

Morse, S. S. (Ed.) (1993) *Emerging Viruses*. Oxford University Press, New York.

Pearce, E. J. & Reiner, S. L. (1995) Induction of T_H2 responses in infectious diseases. *Current Opinion in Immunology*, **7**, 497–504.

Powrie, F. & Coffman, R. L. (1993) Cytokine regulation of T-cell function: potential for therapeutic intervention. *Immunology Today*, **14**, 270–274.

Romani, L. & Howard, D. H. (1995) Mechanisms of resistance to fungal infections. *Current Opinion in Immunology*, **7**, 517–523.

Salyers, A. A. & Whitt, D. D. (1994) *Bacterial Pathogenesis. A Molecular Approach*. American Society of Microbiology Press, Washington, DC.

Schall, T. J. & Bacon, K. B. (1994) Chemokines, leukocyte trafficking, and inflammation. *Current Opinion in Immunology*, **6**, 865–873.

Schwartz, L. B. (1994) Mast cells: function and contents. *Current Opinion in Immunology*, **6**, 91–97.

Scully, M. F. (1992) The biochemistry of blood clotting: the digestion of a liquid to form a solid. *Essays in Biochemistry*, **27**, 17–36.

Shattil, S. J., Ginsberg, M. H. & Brugge, J. S. (1994) Adhesive signaling in platelets. *Current Opinion in Cell Biology*, **6**, 695–704.

Shukla, S. D. (1992) Platelet-activating factor receptor and signal transduction mechanisms. *FASEB Journal*, **6**, 2296–2301.

Smith, G. L. (1994) Virus strategies for evasion of the host response to infection. *Trends in Microbiology*, **2**, 81–88.

Stadnyk, A. W. & Gauldie, J. (1991) The acute phase protein response during parasitic infection. *Immunology Today*, **12**, A7–A12.

Steel, D. M. & Whitehead, A. S. (1994) The major acute phase reactants: C-reactive protein, serum amyloid P component and serum amyloid A protein. *Immunology Today*, **15**, 81–88.

Toft, C. A., Aeschlimann, A. & Bolis, L. (Eds) (1991) *Parasite–Host Associations. Coexistence or Conflict?* Oxford University Press, Oxford.

Valent, P. & Bettelheim, P. (1992) Cell surface structures on human basophils and mast cells: biochemical and functional characterization. *Advances in Immunology*, **52**, 333–423.

Warren, K. S. (Ed.) (1993) *Immunology and Molecular Biology of Parasitic Infections*, 3rd edn. Blackwell Scientific Publications, Boston, MA.

Zwilling, B. S. & Eisenstein, T. K. (Eds) (1994) *Macrophage–Pathogen Interactions*. Marcel Dekker, New York.

chapter 22 Defence against tumours

At the beginning of this century when immunology was beginning to flourish, researchers observed that tumours transplanted from one animal to another were usually destroyed after a short period of growth in the host. An immunological mechanism was postulated to be responsible. The tumours were thought to express unique tumour antigens that stimulated the host's immune system and initiated a response that eventually killed and eliminated the tumour cells. The reason the tumour was not rejected initially in the donor was thought to be an insufficiency of the immune response, possibly caused by the tumour itself.

Later studies demonstrated that the rejection of transplanted tumours was indeed immunologically mediated but was not stimulated by unique tumour antigens. The immune response was directed against antigens that were shared by tumours and normal tissues but which differentiated individuals of the same species. These findings seemed to herald the end of any rational prospects for tumour immunotherapy because, to an individual in which it arose, the tumour did not seem to present any new antigens that could stimulate the immune system.

The matter did not rest here, however. Later studies again raised hopes that true tumour antigens, expressed in neoplastic but not normal tissue, might exist after all and might even provide a means of destroying the tumour via an immune response. Riding mainly on these hopes, a whole subdiscipline of immunology developed—*tumour immunology*, the study of the immune response to tumours. The central question is: Does a spontaneously developing tumour induce immunological response? Or, put differently, does a spontaneously arising tumour express antigens that can stimulate an immune response in the individual in which the tumour develops?

Tumour antigens

Types

Immunologists distinguish between two types of tumour antigens: tumour-specific and tumour-associated. *Tumour-specific antigens* (TSAs) are true tumour antigens because they only occur on neoplastic cells and not on any normal cells at any stage of the individual's development. *Tumour-associated antigens* (TAAs) occur on neoplastic and normal cells but on the latter under conditions in which the individual does not become tolerant of them and can therefore (at least theoretically) respond to the tumour. A TAA may be expressed, for example, on early embryonic cells, at a stage when the immune system has not yet developed. The usual method of demonstrating tumour antigens is either by transplanting the tumour back to the same individual or by transplanting it to another individual with the same genetic constitution. If the tumour is rejected, it is thought to possess a unique antigen. Because of this method of detection, the antigens are often referred to as *tumour-specific transplantation antigens* (TSTAs) and *tumour-associated transplantation antigens* (TATAs).

Methods of demonstration

A tumour, if it expresses tumour antigens, could theoretically induce both humoral and cellular immunity, and one

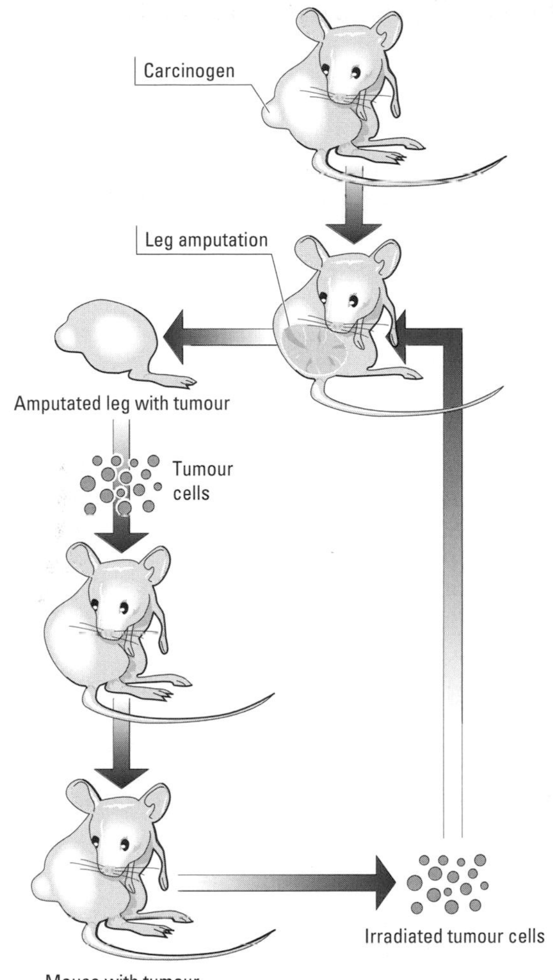

Figure 22.1 One of several methods used by immunologists in an attempt to demonstrate the existence of tumour-specific antigens. Explanation in the text. (Modified from Klein, J. (1982) *Immunology: The Science of Self–Nonself Discrimination*. John Wiley & Sons, New York.)

should therefore be able to demonstrate the antigens by both antibodies and sensitized T lymphocytes. However, the demonstration usually relies on rejection of the tumour, which is mediated mainly by T lymphocytes; successful demonstrations by antibodies are less frequent. In addition to the *in vivo* evidence of tumour rejection, the presence of tumour antigens can also be tested *in vitro* using cytotoxic T (T_C) lymphocytes to kill neoplastic target cells.

A growing tumour is rarely rejected spontaneously, however, and the *in vivo* demonstrations must therefore be carried out in oblique ways in which the tumour is removed, the individual sensitized to the neoplastic cells, and the tumour then transplanted back. The original method used to demonstrate the existence of TSAs was based on the gradual tightening of a thread around a tumour, thereby inducing necrosis and preventing the tumour from spreading further. When animals in which a tumour was 'strangled' were rechallenged with live cells (derived from the same tumour and stored for just this purpose), the grafts were frequently rejected, while the untreated individuals died of the tumour. Another method was to amputate the tumour-bearing leg of a mouse, irradiate the tumour cells to prevent their proliferation and inoculate them into the amputated mouse. Live-stored tumour cells were then inoculated into the same mouse (Fig. 22.1) and the immunized animal was shown to reject the tumour. A simpler method of demonstrating TSTAs is by transplanting tumours between genetically identical individuals of the same inbred strain.

Tumour-specific antigens

Three types of tumour have been used in attempts to demonstrate TSAs: chemically and virally induced tumours, and spontaneously occurring tumours. When *chemically induced tumours* were used, a striking observation was made: each tumour was antigenically unique so that immunity induced by one tumour did not protect the individual from the growth of another, although it did prevent the growth of the immunizing tumour. This observation applied to tumours derived from genetically identical individuals or even to multiple tumours originating in the same animal. Even when induced by the same chemical, different tumours expressed different antigens. Although the tumours may also express some cross-reacting or common antigens, these do not seem to be relevant to tumour rejection, unlike the unique antigens. At least some of the shared antigens might be virally encoded, since the tumours often become secondarily infected by oncogenic viruses.

The nature of *private TSAs* in chemically induced tumours is now finally becoming clear. It has been shown that even tumours with no sign of a TSTA can be induced to express the antigen by treating them with *N*-methyl-*N′*-nitro-*N*-nitrosoguanidine, a compound known to cause mutations. Variants can thus be derived from the original cells, which fail to produce tumours when inoculated into syngeneic mice and are therefore designated *tum⁻ variants* (in contrast to the original tum⁺ cells; Fig. 22.2). The failure of the tum⁻ variants to establish a tumour was shown to be caused by the rejection of the inoculated cells. By this criterion, the tum⁻ variant can be said to have acquired a TSTA by mutagen treatment. The genes coding for the TSTA have been cloned and shown to be present in normal cells as well. However, the tumour gene differs from the normal-cell gene by changes in the nucleotide sequence,

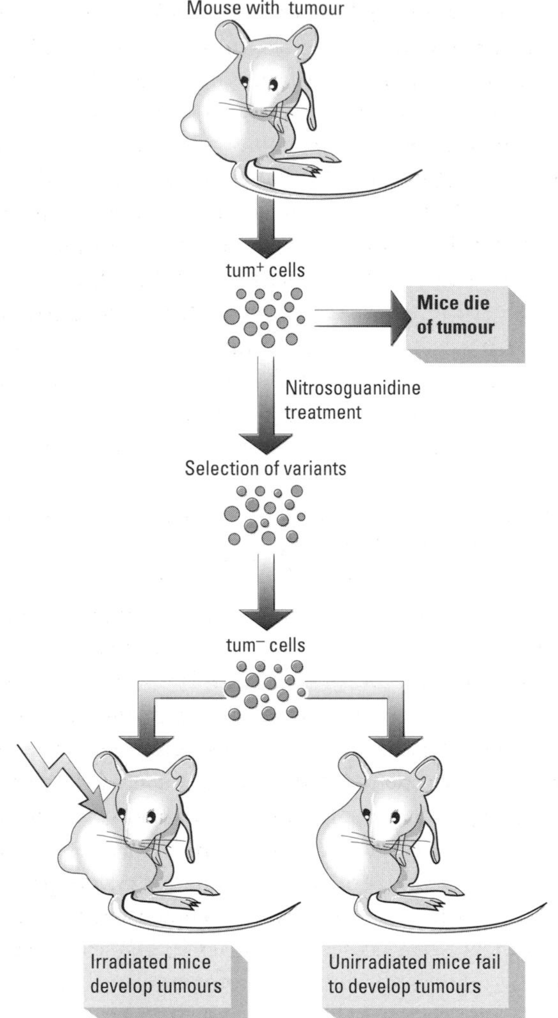

Figure 22.2 Procedure for the experimental induction of tumour-specific antigens. (Based on Boon, T. (1985) *Immunology Today*, 6, 307.)

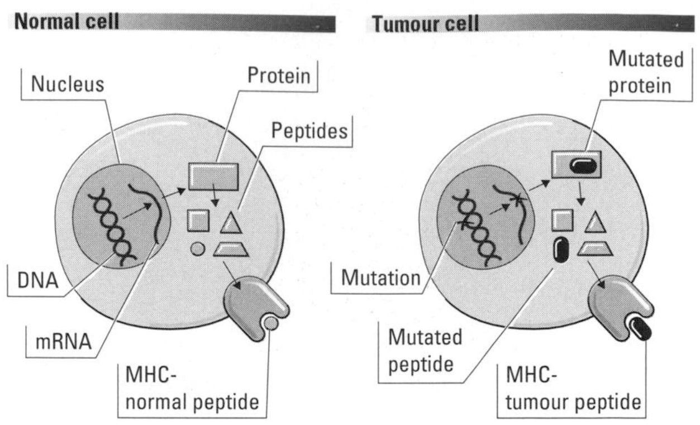

Figure 22.3 One of several mechanisms by which tumour-specific antigens may arise. A mutation in one of the tumour cells alters a cellular protein. A peptide derived from the altered protein is displayed on the cell's MHC molecule where it is recognized by T cells as foreign because it differs from the unaltered peptide to which the host is tolerant. Abnormal peptides may also be produced by the tumour cell as a result of differential processing of non-mutated proteins.

which translate into amino acid substitutions in the encoded protein. The TSTA of the tum− variant is therefore an epitope generated in the tumour cell by the mutations of a standard cellular gene. In the light of this observation, the TSTAs of chemically induced tumours can be explained as resulting from mutations in cellular genes. Chemical carcinogens are often mutagens as well, and carcinogenesis is therefore likely to be accompanied by the induction of mutations in a variety of cellular genes. Some of the mutations may lead to alterations in cellular proteins, and the altered peptides of the mutated cellular proteins can appear on the cell surface bound to major histocompatibility complex (MHC) class I glycoproteins and be recognized by T cells as foreign (Fig. 22.3). Since the probability is very low that the same mutation will occur in different tumours, each will have its private TSTA. The induced antigens resemble the minor histocompatibility antigens, which we discuss in Chapter 24. The fact that the TSTAs of chemically induced tumours (as well as the minor histocompatibility antigens) are peptides derived from intracellular proteins and exhibited at low density on the surface bound to MHC class I molecules explains why antibodies could not be produced against them.

In contrast to chemically induced tumours, *virally induced tumours* usually display TSAs shared by all tumours caused by the same virus. Unique tumour antigens may also appear on some virally induced tumours, but these are rare and difficult to demonstrate. The TSTAs of *RNA virus-induced tumours* can be detected both by antibodies and sensitized T lymphocytes. Detection by antibodies is complicated by the active production of virus particles, which bear the same antigens as the infected cells. RNA tumour viruses bud from patches of host-cell membrane into which they have inserted their spike proteins and glycoproteins, and the mature virions become enveloped in the spike-bearing portion of the membrane (Fig. 22.4). The usual targets of the antibodies are the shared epitopes on the gp70 components of the spikes. Since each virus has its own variant of the *env* gene that codes for the spike, cells infected by different viruses can be distinguished serologically. In addition, however, the *env* genes of some viruses may contain variable regions responsible for antigenic differences between individual viruses of the same species. Antibodies to several proteins encoded by the genomes of these viruses can be detected in the sera of infected subjects.

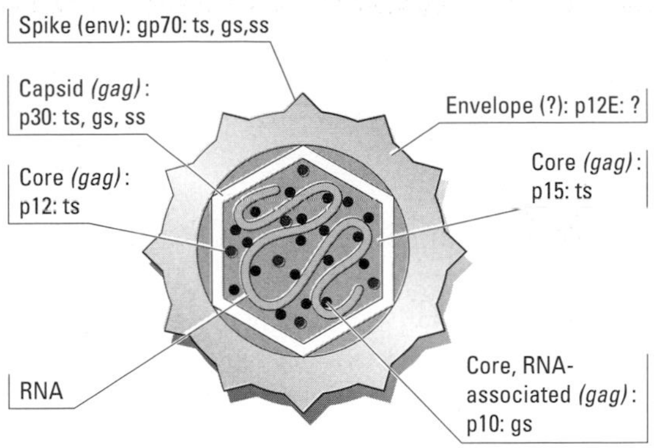

Figure 22.4 Antigens detectable in virally induced tumours and encoded in the genome of a mouse retrovirus. The antigens can be of three classes: type-specific (ts), group-specific (gs), and species-specific (ss); they can be borne by protein (p) or glycoprotein (gp) molecules of M_r 70 000, 30 000, 15 000, 12 000 or 10 000, and can be encoded in the *env* or *gag* genes of the viral RNA.

The TSAs expressed by *DNA virus-induced tumours* have been studied most extensively in two virus types: the papovaviruses, exemplified by polyoma virus and simian vacuolating virus 40 (SV40); and the herpesviruses such as Epstein–Barr virus (EBV), which has been implicated in the aetiology of two human malignancies, Burkitt's lymphoma and nasopharyngeal carcinoma.

While the study of chemically and virally induced tumours is important for understanding how tumours arise, the third category, *spontaneously occurring tumours*, is most relevant to the development of immunity against malignancies. Unfortunately, it has proved very difficult to demonstrate TSAs in spontaneous tumours. One possible reason for this difference between induced and spontaneous tumours is that the original neoplastic cell and its immediate progeny did at one time express a TSA, but later some of the progeny lost the antigen by random genetic variation. The TSA stimulated an immune response that led to rejection of those cells expressing the antigen. According to this explanation, the observed spontaneous tumours are the result of *immunoselection* favouring TSTA-negative neoplastic cells. An inverse relationship between tumour antigenicity and growth has indeed been observed. However, some investigators have challenged this explanation and provided evidence that tumour antigenicity is not influenced by immunoselection. Furthermore, the explanation does not account for the fact that induced tumours retain their TSAs despite immunoselection. An alternative possibility is that spontaneous tumours arise by a mechanism different from that operating in chemical and viral tumour induction and the former mechanism may lead to the appearance of TSAs at much lower levels or in less immunogenic forms. Nevertheless, several types of TSA have been demonstrated. One type constitutes *mutant forms of oncogenic proteins*. An *oncogene* is a virus-borne DNA segment capable of transforming a normal cell into a neoplastic cell, usually in combination with other factors. The segment is derived from the host cell and is incorporated into the viral genome accidentally during the viruses' sojourn in the host-cell genome. It represents an altered version of the cellular *protooncogene*, which controls some of the cell's functions, often those to do with proliferation. Different retroviruses carry various oncogenes, reflecting the sites in the host-cell genome the viral genome has visited: oncogenes are akin to stickers on a traveller's baggage. Individual oncogenes are designated by symbols, usually reflecting the virus rather than the cell from which they are derived.

One of the oncogenes, designated *Ras*, codes for a guanosine triphosphate (GTP)-binding protein (G-protein) critically involved in the signal transduction pathways of many receptors (see Chapters 10 & 16). Point mutations in the *Ras* gene may lead to expression of constitutive-active non-regulated forms of the Ras protein and thus to cell proliferation even in the absence of appropriate stimuli. Somatic mutations of *Ras* oncogenes occur in approximately 20% of all human cancers including 90% of pancreatic adenocarcinomas, 60% of follicular carcinomas of the thyroid, 50% of colon adenocarcinomas and 40% of myeloid leukaemias. The wild type of another oncogene product, p53, acts as a *tumour suppressor* by controlling the expression of a number of genes involved in cell proliferation. Some of the mutant forms of the protein are non-functional and thus unable to control cell proliferation; unregulated proliferation can then become the first step towards neoplasia. Mutations in p53 are present in about 50% of all human malignancies.

Fragments of mutant forms of the Ras and p53 proteins bind to MHC class I molecules and, if the bound peptide contains amino acid residues altered by the mutation, give rise to TSAs. T cells capable of recognizing such MHC–Ras or MHC–p53 assemblages have been demonstrated in cancer patients.

Another type of TSA is represented by the *idiotypic surface immunoglobulins of myelomas*, lymphoid tumours arising by malignant transformation of a single activated B-cell clone. These *myeloma-specific antigens* are expressed at high density on the tumour cell surface and are therefore potential targets of humoral responses.

Yet another example of a TSA is Bcr-Abl, an oncogenic protein found in 95% of patients with chronic myelogenous leukaemia (CML) and in 10–20% of patients with acute lymphocytic leukaemia (ALL). A hallmark of CML is the translocation of the c-*Abl* (named after Abelson murine leukaemia virus) protooncogene from chromosome 9 to the specific *breakpoint cluster region* (*Bcr*) on chromosome 22. This translocation gives rise to new fusion genes, one of which encodes a novel intracellular chimeric protein of relative molecular mass (M_r) 210 000. The Bcr-Abl protein is a constitutively active tyrosine kinase that stimulates the growth of haemopoietic progenitor cells and is essential for the pathogenesis of CML. The joining region of this fusion protein is therefore present only in the leukaemia cells, and MHC-bound peptides derived from this region serve as TSAs.

Tumour cells often express cell-surface glycoproteins that differ from their counterparts on corresponding normal cells in the structure of their oligosaccharide chains. The differences frequently involve sialic acid, which constitutes the terminal carbohydrate unit of the oligosaccharide chains. The differential glycosylation of tumour cell-surface glycoproteins may result from the altered activities of glycosyltransferases, the enzymes that catalyse the final phases of glycosylation reactions in the Golgi apparatus. Alternatively, it could result from an increase in synthesis of some of the surface proteins in the tumour cells. The proteins may overwhelm the glycosylation apparatus and as a result may be only incompletely glycosylated. Such altered forms of tumour cell-surface glycoproteins may also function as TSAs. An example of this category of TSA is the *epithelial mucin MUC-1*. The extracellular parts of members of this family of closely related glycoproteins are composed of between 20 and 125 tandem repeats of a 20 amino acid sequence rich in proline, serine and threonine residues. Most of the serines and threonines carry O-linked oligosaccharide chains. The mucin molecules on normal epithelial cells protrude far from the cell surface (over 100 nm) and serve as components of a thick coat protecting the epithelial surface from the harsh environment of the duct. In tumour cells of epithelial adenocarcinomas (i.e. tumours of breast, pancreatic and ovarian epithelia), some segments of the MUC-1 polypeptide are not O-glycosylated and these 'bare' parts are recognized by the immune system.

Tumour-associated antigens

TAAs can be regarded as abnormally expressed antigens of normal tissues. The two main categories of TAA are oncofetal and differentiation antigens. *Oncofetal antigens* are expressed during certain stages of embryogenesis but are either absent from normal adult cells or present at a very low concentration. They reappear in tumour cells or in connection with tumour growth, perhaps as a result of the derepression of certain host genes. These antigens are numerous but here we mention only two: α-fetoprotein and carcinoembryonic antigen.

α-Fetoprotein (α-FP) is an α-globulin secreted into the serum by normal embryonic liver cells. In human first-trimester embryos, it comprises 90% of the total serum globulin but its level declines rapidly after birth. The antigen reappears in patients with embryonal, pancreatic and hepatic carcinomas; in most other tumours, the levels of α-FP remain low. However, increased production of α-FP has been recorded in certain non-neoplastic diseases, such as acute viral hepatitis.

Carcinoembryonic antigen (CEA) was originally identified by a rabbit antiserum against a perchloric acid extract from a pool of human carcinomas. Following absorption with normal colon tissue, the antiserum formed a single precipitin line with extracts from other colon carcinomas. Subsequent studies revealed that the antigen detected by the antiserum was shared by human colon cancer cells and by cells of fetal gut, pancreas and liver up to the sixth month of gestation. The antigen is a glycoprotein with an M_r of 200 000–300 000; the molecule contains 50–70% carbohydrate, and is apparently part of the cell's mucous coating. Originally, clinicians hoped to use CEA to diagnose colon cancer, since the antigen was also detected in the serum of cancer patients. Unfortunately, it later emerged that a large percentage of normal individuals and patients with non-neoplastic diseases often had higher levels of serum CEA than colon cancer patients. However, CEA remains an important parameter in the surveillance of colon cancer patients in the postoperative phase. Lung and breast tumours may also contain tissue-specific CEAs.

Differentiation antigens are expressed in some tissues and absent in others; they reappear inappropriately in certain tumours. The expression of some of these antigens may attest to the cellular origin of the tumour. There are many examples of differentiation antigens in the various types of leukaemia. The best known of these is CD10 (CALLA; common acute lymphoblastoid leukaemia antigen), which is present on one of the most frequent types of leukaemia, originating from bone marrow preB cells. Similarly, most myeloid leukaemia cells carry the surface adhesive glycoprotein CD34, as do the early myeloid progenitors from which the malignant cells originate. CD10, CD34 and several other surface molecules are useful diagnostic markers.

Several TAAs have been characterized in *melanoma cells*. They include proteins such as the enzyme tyrosinase, glycoproteins gp75 and gp100 and Melan-A/MART-1 (melanoma antigen recognized by T cells) found in normal melanocytes and melanoma cells. Another group of melanoma-associated antigens is exemplified by a molecule called MAGE-1 (for melanoma antigen), a member of a family of related intracellular proteins of unknown function. It is expressed in testicular and placental tissues, most melanoma cells and also in a significant percentage of several other tumour types (bladder, mammary and prostatic carcinomas and sarcomas). Some of the peptides produced by processing of the 309-residue MAGE-1 protein bind to certain MHC class I molecules and the resulting assemblies then act as TAAs recognizable by the immune system. Several other melanoma-associated antigens of this kind have been discovered (groups called BAGE and CAGE; inspired by the MAGE designation).

Another TAA is a growth factor receptor called *HER-2/neu* (the name HER refers to its similarity to human epidermal growth factor receptor; neu derives from rat neuroblastoma oncogene). This transmembrane protein is weakly expressed on epithelial cells of many normal tissues. In a number of human cancers the gene encoding this receptor is amplified and the receptor itself is overexpressed about 50-fold as compared with normal cells. HER-2/neu overexpression correlates with the clinical outcome of breast cancer: patients expressing a high level of HER-2/neu run a greater risk of dying than patients who express low levels of the antigen. The difference in expression of this protein in normal and tumour cells makes it a potential target for immunotherapy.

Defence against cancer

Immune surveillance hypothesis

Once a tumour appears, the body seems to be helpless against it: cases of spontaneous remission are rare. Is it possible, however, that the diagnosis of cancer signifies a battle already lost, and that we are only very rarely aware of the body's victories? In other words, is cancer much more frequent than our statistics indicate, with the cancer cells being eliminated before they have a chance to multiply and get out of hand? Some cell biologists find it surprising that, given such ample opportunity in so many cell divisions, more aberrant cells than those actually detected do not arise. If the body really can battle with its own cells over which it has lost control, what kinds of defence mechanisms does it employ?

Several immunologists have suggested that the immune system does indeed prevent most tumours from arising. According to the once-popular *immune surveillance hypothesis*, T lymphocytes are continually patrolling body tissues, searching for aberrant cells that express antigens not found on normal cells. Any new neoplastic cell spotted by these T cells is attacked and eliminated. The tumours that do arise have somehow escaped immune surveillance, but if it were not for this surveillance tumour incidence would be much higher.

It is an attractive hypothesis, thought at first by immunologists to be supported by the known facts. The main prediction of the immune surveillance hypothesis is that abrogation of immune competence by neonatal thymectomy, irradiation, anti-lymphocyte serum treatment, or treatment with immunosuppressive drugs should increase the incidence of cancer in treated individuals. Also, an increased incidence of tumours should be observed in individuals with inherited immunodeficiencies. To a limited extent, this prediction has been borne out by experimental and clinical observations: in general, immunodeficient individuals do contract cancer more frequently than intact individuals. The difficulty is, however, that most of the neoplasias arising in such individuals are tumours of the lymphoid system. If the immune surveillance hypothesis were correct, one should observe a general increase in all kinds of tumours, not just lymphoid. The predominance of lymphoid tumours suggests that the increased incidence does not result from an immune surveillance failure, but from the treatment that immunodeficient individuals undergo. A further argument is that congenitally athymic mice, which have one arm of the immune system incapacitated, have the same tumour incidence as normal mice. However, there are counter-arguments to both these contentions: immunodeficient individuals do not survive long enough to show greater-than-normal incidence of cancer; and athymic mice are not completely devoid of T lymphocytes. Furthermore, these mice have a fully developed complement of natural killer (NK) cells which may play a dominant part in immune surveillance. The controversy continues but in the mean time enthusiasm for the immune surveillance hypothesis has waned.

Immune mechanism controlling tumour growth and metastasis

Failure to detect TSAs on spontaneous tumours has not deterred immunologists from exploring possible immune mechanisms by which neoplastic growth could be restricted, if not stopped altogether. The rationale for such studies is the belief that expression of TSAs may not be the only way of eliciting an immune response to tumours, a belief supported by the finding that some solid human tumours are found to be infiltrated by monocytes, lymphocytes and other cells at the time when the tumours are removed surgically. The developing mass is so out of place in the body that it must be recognized as foreign even without the involvement of antigen-specific T-cell receptors

(TCRs) and B-cell receptors (BCRs). The recognition can be expected to stimulate the components of non-adaptive immunity at least. In experimental situations, the participation of T lymphocytes, macrophages, NK cells, antibodies and immune complexes in antitumour immunity has indeed been demonstrated.

Strong evidence for the participation of *T lymphocytes* has been obtained for virally induced tumours. Most of these tumours, as has been mentioned, express viral antigens capable of eliciting T_C-cell responses, which lead to the rejection of the tumour *in vivo* and the lysis of target tumour cells *in vitro*. Moreover, there is a strong correlation between *in vivo* protection and *in vitro* cell-mediated destruction of *virally induced lymphomas*. The evidence for T-cell-mediated protection against *chemically induced tumours* is controversial. The outcome of protection experiments seems to depend on the assay system, the age and strain of the animals, the carcinogen and the transformed target cells. Generally speaking, T lymphocytes seem to be ineffective in preventing tumour development when the chemically induced tumours are transplanted from their primary host to syngeneic animals. As for *spontaneous tumours*, there is no convincing evidence that they can induce a T-cell response in primary or secondary hosts in the manner demonstrated for chemically or virally induced tumours.

Macrophages infiltrate the tumour site in large numbers, and when isolated from tumour-bearing animals they inhibit neoplastic cell growth *in vitro*. Agents known to inhibit macrophages, such as silica or anti-macrophage sera, accelerate tumour growth, whereas agents that stimulate macrophage activity, such as bacillus Calmette–Guérin (BCG) or *Corynebacterium parvum*, inhibit tumour growth when injected systemically or directly into the tumour.

Activated macrophages can restrict tumour growth by killing tumour cells through cytostatic or cytotoxic effects. In *cytostasis*, tumour cells stop their proliferation (which can be measured *in vitro* by the uptake of a DNA-seeking isotope); in *cytotoxicity*, tumour cells are lysed (as measured by isotope release). *In vitro*, the cytostatic effect can be detected as early as 4 hours after mixing tumour cells with activated macrophages and it peaks 12–24 hours after mixing. The cytotoxic effect, on the other hand, can only be detected 24 hours after cell mixing and is completed by 48–72 hours; it may be mediated by lysosomal enzymes released from activated macrophages. What determines the macrophage's course of action is not known; perhaps both effects are initiated at the same time but cytotoxicity takes longer to develop than cytostasis. Both effects are non-specific in the sense that macrophages do not discriminate among syngeneic, allogeneic and xenogeneic tumour cells. At the same time, however, they are also specific because activated macrophages discriminate between neoplastic and normal cells and act only on the former, perhaps because they recognize rapidly dividing cells. Macrophages also display a higher degree of specificity if appropriately *armed* by soluble factors. For example, antibodies are able to bind via their Fc regions to macrophages and via their combining sites to antigens on tumour cells, thus bringing the macrophage and its target together.

Tumour cells can also exert *suppressive effects* on macrophage-mediated antitumour immunity. They may release factors that decrease the chemotactic activity of macrophages and impair their ability to reach the site of inflammation. Macrophages in turn suppress the activity of the host lymphocytes. The outcome seems to depend on the balance between the stimulatory and inhibitory effects but unfortunately, more often than not, the latter appear to gain the upper hand.

NK cells are known to favour tumour cells as their targets *in vitro,* and several lines of evidence suggest that they also act on tumour cells *in vivo*. For example, athymic mice, which show high NK activity, are relatively resistant to the induction of primary tumours and to metastatic spread of NK cell-sensitive tumours. Mouse strains with high NK-cell activity are relatively resistant, while mouse strains with low NK-cell activity are relatively susceptible, to a small inoculum of NK cell-sensitive tumour cells. NK cell-deficient *beige* mice are unable to reject small inocula of NK cell-sensitive tumour cells and the clearance of tumours in certain hosts can be inhibited by antibodies specific for NK cells. All these observations suggest that NK cells participate in the clearance of certain tumour types. Unfortunately, in both cancer patients and tumour-bearing mice, NK cell activity is low and it is not clear whether this is the cause or the consequence of tumour growth.

NK-cell activity is greatly influenced by a variety of factors, in particular *interferons*. The release of interferons by activated lymphocytes or macrophages leads to the activation of NK-cell precursors and to the full manifestation of the cytolytic potential of these cells. This observation may, in part, explain the noted preference of NK cells for virally induced lymphoid tumours. Whether there are other cells which, like NK cells and macrophages, do not require prior immunization to be effective against tumours remains an open question.

Antibodies and other humoral components of the immune system can contribute to both the inhibition and promotion of tumour growth. Here, we consider only the former effect; the latter is discussed in the section that follows. Antibodies can inhibit tumour growth by binding complement, which then lyses neoplastic cells, or by binding to NK cells and macrophages, which then kill neoplastic targets. *Complement-mediated lysis* of tumour cells has been demonstrated *in vitro*; the degree to which it contributes to tumour rejection is not clear. Infusion of very high doses of antibodies into tumour-bearing animals may lead to the regression of certain tumours, but it is not known whether the effect is mediated by complement or by NK cells and macrophages. Sera of normal mice often contain *natural cytotoxic antibodies*, which can mediate complement-dependent lysis of tumour cells *in vitro*. The antibodies are largely of the IgM class, occur at increased levels in the sera of athymic mice and are believed to be produced in response to endogenous stimuli, perhaps viruses. A certain correlation exists between serum levels of these antibodies and host resistance to small tumour inocula.

Antibody-dependent cell-mediated cytotoxicity (ADCC) targeted at tumour cells can be effected by either NK cells or macrophages: the former lyse their targets, the latter cause target-cell death by a cytostatic effect. The relevance of ADCC to host protection against tumours *in vivo* is indicated by the presence of antibodies and macrophages in tumours and by the direct correlation between tumour regression and macrophage-mediated ADCC. It should be emphasized, however, that all the mechanisms of antitumour immunity discussed in this section have been mainly demonstrated in highly artificial experimental situations, often involving allogeneic tumours. The relevance of these findings to immunity against spontaneous tumours, which should be the actual subject of tumour immunology, is uncertain.

How tumours evade immunity

If immunity does develop against an arising neoplasm, the tumour can escape it by one of several mechanisms: immunoselection, antigenic modulation, the so-called 'sneaking through' mechanism, enhancement, production of blocking factors and immunosuppression. *Immunoselection* has already been alluded to. Although each tumour probably begins from a single cell and so represents a clone, the cells in this clone do not remain the same for long. As the tumour grows, additional changes occur, so that at any one time the tumour cell population is a heterogeneous mixture of different subclones. If some of the changes result in a decreased antigenicity, variants expressing low levels of surface antigens gain an advantage because of host immunity selection pressure. These variants can therefore take over and so increase the general immunoresistance of the tumour. The selective advantage of these tumour cells could result from not only a complete absence of antigens but also a decrease in their density on the plasma membrane. If the density drops below a certain threshold level, the tumour becomes 'invisible' to the immune system. A similar effect can be achieved by downregulation of MHC class I expression, whereby the density of the epitopes formed by peptides bound to MHC molecules falls below the threshold necessary for recognition by T_C cells. In such a situation, however, NK cells may substitute for T_C cells, as one of their functions is to eliminate cells with abnormally low MHC class I molecule expression (see Chapter 16).

Antigenic modulation was first demonstrated in the *Tla (thymus-leukaemia antigen) system* of class Ib MHC molecules. Mice immunized against Tla antigens and having high titres of cytotoxic Tla-specific antibodies might be expected to resist syngeneic Tla-positive leukaemias. Paradoxically, not only do these mice actually succumb to the tumours, but those malignancies recovered before the host's demise also lose their sensitivity to Tla-specific antibodies *in vitro*. The loss is only temporary because a single passage of the tumour in untreated syngeneic hosts leads to a complete reappearance of the antigens. This temporary loss of antigens after exposure to specific antibodies (antigenic modulation) is thought to occur either via shedding or via patching, capping and endocytosis of caps[1].

T lymphocytes of tumour-bearing individuals often display general systemic defects that make these cells much more difficult to stimulate than those of healthy subjects. Such T lymphocytes are poorly stimulated to blastogenesis by lectins, antigen-specific T_C cells are difficult to elicit *in vitro* and helper T (T_H) cells support antibody synthesis poorly. Similar defects are also observed in some cases of chronic inflammatory diseases and in subjects exposed to various forms of intense physical stress. It is thought that either tumour cells themselves or *suppressor macrophages* activated by the interaction with tumour cells secrete soluble mediators, such as prostaglandins, that act on T cells and render them hyporeactive. It may be that hyporeactivity is caused by conformational changes in the TCR complex and in the associated protein tyrosine kinases (see Chapters 7 & 16) that lead to aberrant signalling. Some of the defects seem to be due to abnormalities in the regulation of intracellular redox potential.

Researchers have noted that animals challenged with a

[1] Cross-linking of some cell surface antigens by antibodies may change their originally homogeneous distribution into accumulation within several areas (*patches*) or even a single spot called a *cap*. This *patching* and *capping* is dependent on the integrity of the actin cytoskeleton and is usually followed by internalization of the patches and caps. *Shedding* is a process in which cell-surface proteins are removed by proteolytic cleavage of their extracellular domains induced by various stimuli including cross-linking by antibodies.

low dose of neoplastic cells develop tumours more frequently than those inoculated with larger doses. This observation led to the formulation of the *'sneaking through' hypothesis*, according to which a few isolated tumour cells contain amounts of antigen that are too low to sensitize the host, but by the time significant immunity does develop the tumour is so large that it is already beyond the defence capabilities of the immune system. This simple hypothesis is difficult to prove or disprove experimentally.

In experimental situations, treatment intended to increase the host immune response sometimes has the opposite effect, i.e. it promotes tumour growth. This *immunological enhancement* usually occurs when animals are challenged with inactivated tumour cells before being inoculated with live cells. The increased tumour growth is mediated by serum antibodies. Enhancement is frequently encountered with allogeneically transplanted tumours; whether it also affects the growth of syngeneic tumours is less certain. The ability to enhance tumour growth can be transferred with the serum of the pretreated individual. Enhancement by transferred serum is referred to as *passive enhancement*, in contrast to *active enhancement* induced by pretreatment of the host with tissue. How enhancing antibodies act in preventing tumour rejection is not known. Some immunologists believe that they alter the tumour in some way, enabling it to escape the host's immune response (*efferent inhibition hypothesis*); others contend that the antibodies combine with antigenic material released from the tumour and thus prevent the material from sensitizing the host (*afferent inhibition hypothesis*); others still think that the antibodies or antigen–antibody complexes act on the lymphoid system, preventing it from mounting a cellular response against the tumour (*central inhibition hypothesis*). The actual mechanisms may involve a combination of any two or even all three of these postulated events. Another two possibilities are that tumours alter the homing pattern of antigen-reactive cells, and that antigen-reactive cells are opsonized by antigen–antibody complexes bound to them and phagocytosed by liver macrophages.

An important escape mechanism for most tumours is based on the inability of tumour cells to function as professional antigen-presenting cells (APCs). Even if tumour cells express sufficient numbers of MHC class I molecules, they lack the necessary adhesion and signalling molecules to provide co-stimulatory signals. Thus, the contact of precursor T_C or T_H cells with tumour cells leads to anergy rather than stimulation. Indeed, it is possible to enhance dramatically the immunogenicity of some tumour cells by making them express CD80, CD86 or other co-stimulatory molecules (Fig. 22.5).

Lymphocytes from tumour-bearing mice often kill tumour cells *in vitro*, but when serum from these mice is

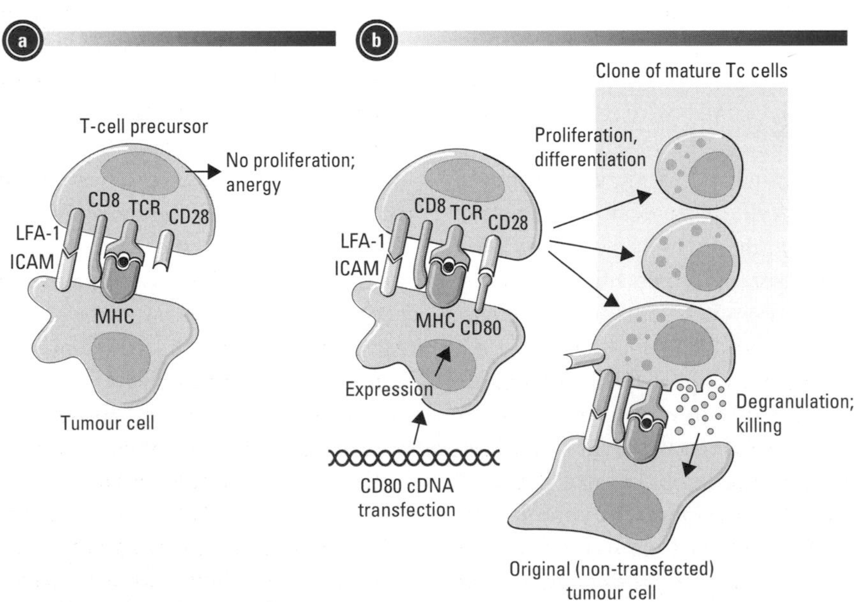

Figure 22.5 A strategy to enhance tumour immunogenicity. Most tumour cells do not express co-stimulatory molecules such as CD80 on their surface. Hence even if a tumour-specific antigen is recognized on their surface by T cells, the recognition results in inactivation rather than stimulation of the T cell (a). Tumour cells can be transfected with DNA coding for the co-stimulatory molecule and thus turned into an efficient antigen-presenting cell that can stimulate proliferation and maturation of specific cytotoxic (T_C)-cell clones capable of killing non-transfected tumour cells (b).

added to the test system cell destruction is terminated. This inhibition is attributed to *blocking factors* produced by the tumour-bearing mice, which are believed to be complexes of antigens and antibodies. The antigen of the blocking factors is presumably derived from the tumour cells by shedding. The function of blocking factors *in vivo* is poorly defined.

Some tumours may invade lymphoid tissues and so interfere with the normal immune response. Others may secrete soluble substances such as transforming growth factor β (TGF-β), which act as immunosuppressive factors by inhibiting lymphocyte proliferation. The result of both these actions is depression of the individual's ability to mount an immune response.

Prospects for cancer immunotherapy

Although considerable controversy remains regarding immune response to tumour cells, it is now generally accepted that immune cells are commonly present in tumours; that they are often directed against antigens displayed on tumour cells; and that some of these cells or their products can, under certain circumstances, damage or even kill tumour cells. These findings are sufficient to fuel hopes that immune mechanisms could some day be used to destroy cancer cells as soon as they appear. Numerous approaches have been suggested for manipulating the immune system to increase its effectiveness. We conclude this chapter with a brief description of some of these approaches.

One obvious possibility is to eliminate cancer cells by means of monoclonal antibodies that recognize TSAs. After binding to tumour cells, the antibodies eliminate them either by activation of the complement system or by opsonization followed by phagocytosis or NK-cell killing. To avoid antibody-induced antigen modulation, the use of monoclonal antibodies to which toxins or radioisotopes have been attached might be preferential (see Chapter 8). Such immunotoxins can kill cells quickly, even if the cell internalizes the surface antigen. However, the potential of tumour-specific monoclonal antibodies or immunotoxins *in vivo* appears to be limited, mainly because very few antigens sufficiently specific for tumours have thus far been found. One exception could be the *epithelial cell adhesion molecule (EPCAM)*, a surface antigen of tumours of epithelial origin. The antigen is broadly expressed on normal epithelial cells, but appears to be much more accessible on the surface of 'naked' tumour cells scattered as micrometastases in bone marrow. Patients treated with EPCAM-specific monoclonal antibody after surgical tumour removal had a significantly lower incidence of disease relapse compared with the untreated group. This approach appears to work best in cases of 'minimal residual disease', in which only small numbers of tumour cells remain after surgical removal of the large malignant mass.

Another potential target for treatment with monoclonal antibodies could be B-cell lymphomas that express idiotypic BCRs. Indeed, it has been reported that treatment with a monoclonal antibody recognizing the lymphoma's idiotype cured a patient. In most cases, however, this approach has only been partially successful at best, since after the initial remission of the tumour, variant cells that lost or changed their idiotype took over. Other possible targets include HER-2/neu, underglycosylated MUC-1 and possibly some tumour-specific glycolipids, which are expressed on tumour cells as intact surface molecules rather than as MHC-associated peptides. A potential problem with the therapeutic use of monoclonal antibodies of mouse or rat origin is the patient's immune response against xenogeneic immunoglobulins. This problem can be at least partially eliminated by *humanization of antibodies* (see Chapter 8).

A potential tool for targeting large numbers of T_C or NK cells at tumour cells could be the *bispecific antibodies* produced by *quadromas* or *tetradomas* (cells produced by the fusion of two hybridoma cells secreting monoclonal antibodies of different specificities; see Chapter 8). A bispecific antibody with one binding site specific for a tumour cell antigen and the other site for an antigen present on T cells (e.g. CD3) or NK cells (CD16) or both (CD2) should be able to bring together tumour cell and T_C cells or NK cells for non-specific killing. This approach works well in model systems, but here again a major obstacle is the lack of suitable TSAs. A potentially suitable target on tumour cells is the HER-2/neu protein.

The therapeutic use of tumour cell-specific antibodies and immunotoxins *in vivo* has thus far met with limited success. However, it is used extensively in the treatment of some types of leukaemia by *autologous bone marrow transplantation*. In this procedure, a sample of bone marrow is taken from a patient in the remission phase of the disease, in which only a few leukaemic cells remain in the body. The sample is then purged of leukaemic cells by means of monoclonal antibodies or immunotoxins directed at a leukaemia cell-surface molecule, which can be shared with some normal blood cells but not with haemopoietic stem cells. The patient is meanwhile given a high dose of γ-irradiation, which destroys not only leukaemic cells but also normal white blood cells, including stem cells. The purged bone marrow is then reintroduced into the patient to reconstitute the haemopoietic and immune systems free of leukaemia.

Some tumours are infiltrated by lymphocytes and other leucocytes. Although these cells in most cases seem to do little harm to the tumour (perhaps because they are anergized rather than stimulated), it is often possible to culture them and obtain clones of T_C cells from them that specifically recognize and kill tumour cells. In principle, therefore, it should be possible to boost cellular immune response against such a tumour in two ways: either by injecting interleukin (IL)-2 into the tumour, or by isolating lymphocytes from the patient's blood or tumour (*tumour infiltrating lymphocytes, TIL*), cultivating them *in vitro* with the tumour cells and IL-2 and then injecting them back into the patient. These treatments, too, have thus far met with limited success. This is also true for treatments that include injections of *Corynebacterium parvum* or *Candida* vaccines into a tumour; the injections elicit a local inflammatory response sometimes accompanied by tumour regression. When it occurs, the regression is probably due to TIL (and macrophage) stimulation by cytokines produced during the inflammatory response. On the other hand, bacillus Calmette-Guérin (BCG) has been used successfully in the treatment of bladder carcinoma: lavages (washes) of the bladder with BCG suspension following surgery have cured some 80% of patients. The treatment seems to lead to the activation of multiple mechanisms including T_H1 cell-mediated inflammation and killing by a special type of NK cell.

Recent advances in genetic engineering have opened up possibilities for innovative approaches to cancer immunotherapy. Thus, transfection with genes coding for co-stimulatory molecules such as CD80 and CD86 could provide means of turning tumour cells into efficient APCs (see Fig. 22.5). A similar effect could be achieved by transfecting tumour cells with genes encoding IL-2 or another cytokine, thus forcing them to produce large amounts of a T-cell stimulatory cytokine. Other cytokines produced locally by genetically manipulated cells might attract and activate cells of the non-adaptive immune system, such as eosinophils (stimulated by IL-4) or dendritic cells and macrophages (stimulated by granulocyte-monocyte colony stimulating factor (GM-CSF)). Yet another promising approach is to fuse tumour cells with efficient APCs and use the hybrids to stimulate tumour-specific T cells. All these methods have been tested experimentally and the results have been encouraging. The activity of tumour-specific T cells could be boosted, theoretically at least, by blocking their negative-regulatory receptors, such as CTLA-4.

It might also be possible to boost antigen presentation by tumour cells via heat-shock proteins of the gp96, Hsp70 and Hsp90 families. It has been shown that Hsp molecules isolated from tumour cells elicit antitumour response probably because they, like MHC molecules, bind peptides from cellular proteins, presumably including those derived from TSAs. Although Hsp molecules cannot present peptides to T cells, they can transfer them to the MHC glycoproteins of APCs.

Another technique is based on identification of peptides associated with the MHC proteins on the surface of tumour cells and recognized by T cells. In the most direct approach, MHC molecules are isolated from tumour cells and the peptides are eluted from them. The complex mixture is separated by high-performance chromatographic methods into individual fractions and these are then tested for their ability to sensitize cells to become targets of T_C-cell clones produced *in vitro* against the original tumour. The active peptides are then purified to homogeneity and their sequence determined. Once the peptides are identified, they can be synthesized in large amounts and used as *tumour peptide vaccines* for *in vitro* stimulation of T_C cells.

This method has been used in the case of several melanoma and carcinoma tumour antigens and many of the peptides have been identified. Most of them originated from cellular proteins also present in the normal counterparts of the tumour cells but some were derived from the MAGE-1, MAGE-3 and BAGE proteins. Other potential candidates for tumour peptide vaccines are mutants of Ras, p53, Bcr-Abl or MUC-1. T-cell clones (T_H1, T_H2 and T_C) recognizing assemblages of MHC proteins and peptides derived from tumour antigens are often obtained *in vitro* from tumour lymphocyte infiltrates. We face the challenge, therefore, of ways of activating these antitumour T cells and fully utilizing their potential. A possible danger is that these essentially autoreactive cells might also damage normal cells expressing small amounts of the target antigens. MUC-1-reactive T cells appear to violate the basic dogma of T-cell specificity by recognizing the unglycosylated segments of the MUC-1 polypeptide rather than MUC-1 peptides complexed with MHC molecules. Most of the MUC-1-specific clones are α:β TCR^+ and yet they have a B cell-like, MHC-independent pattern of recognition. These unconventional T cells appear to be stimulated by multiple contacts of their TCRs with the densely expressed, highly repetitive ligand. The existence of such unusual T cell makes sense from an evolutionary point of view since the mucin molecules protrude so far from the tumour cell surface that they effectively prevent any close contact between the tumour cell and T-cell surface, which would otherwise be necessary for conventional TCR–MHC molecule interaction.

Thus, the first step towards effective immunotherapy—the identification of some of the antigens recognized by T cells on tumour cells—has been achieved. The next few years should reveal whether the development of actual immunotherapeutic treatments will follow.

Further reading

Boon, T., Cerottini, J.-C., Van den Eynde, B., van der Bruggen, P. & Van Pel, A. (1994) Tumor antigens recognized by T-lymphocytes. *Annual Review of Immunology*, **12**, 337–365.

Chapman, P. B. & Houghton, A. N. (1993) Non-antibody immunotherapy of cancer. *Current Opinion in Immunology*, **5**, 726–731.

Cheever, M. A., Disis, M. L., Bernhard, H. *et al.*(1995) Immunity to oncogenic proteins. *Immunological Reviews*, **145**, 34–59.

Disis, M. L. & Cheever, M. A. (1996) Oncogenic proteins as tumor antigens. *Current Opinion in Immunology*, **8**, 637–642.

Dranoff, G. & Mullingan, R. C. (1995) Gene transfer as cancer therapy. *Advances in Immunology*, **58**, 417–454.

Finn, O. J., Jerome, K. R., Henderson, R. A. *et al.* (1995) MUC-1 epithelial tumour mucin based immunity and cancer vaccines. *Immunological Reviews*, **145**, 61–89.

Ghetie, M.-A. & Vitetta, E. S. (1994) Recent developments in immunotoxin therapy. *Current Opinion in Immunology*, **6**, 707–714.

Grabbe, S., Beissert, S., Schwarz, T. & Granstein, R. D. (1995) Dendritic cells as initiators of tumour immune responses: a possible strategy for tumour immunotherapy. *Immunology Today*, **16**, 117–121.

Hakamori, S. (1984) Tumor-associated carbohydrate antigens. *Annual Review of Immunology*, **2**, 103–126.

Hesketh, R. (Ed.) (1994) *The Oncogene Handbook*. Academic Press, New York.

Jackson, A. M. & James, K. (1994) Understanding the most successful immunotherapy for cancer. *Immunologist*, **2**, 208–215.

Jurcic, J. G. & Scheinberg, D. A. (1994) Recent developments in the radioimmunotherapy of cancer. *Current Opinion in Immunology*, **6**, 715–721.

Klein, E. & Mantovani, A. (1993) Action of natural killer cells and macrophages in cancer. *Current Opinion in Immunology*, **5**, 714–718.

Masucci, M. G. (1993) Viral immunopathology of human tumors. *Current Opinion in Immunology*, **5**, 693–700.

Melief, C. J. M., Offringa, R., Toes, R. E. M. & Kast, W. M. (1996) Peptide-based cancer vaccines. *Current Opinion in Immunology*, **8**, 651–657.

Nanda, N. K. & Sercarz, E. E. (1995) Induction of anti-self-immunity to cure cancer. *Cell*, **82**, 13–17.

Pardoll, D. M. (1993) New strategies for enhancing the immunogenicity of tumors. *Current Opinion in Immunology*, **5**, 719–725.

Ostrand-Rosenberg, S. (1994) Tumor immunotherapy: the tumor cell as an antigen-presenting cell. *Current Opinion in Immunology*, **6**, 722–727.

Riethmüller, G., Schneider-Gädicke, E. & Johnson, J. P. (1993) Monoclonal antibodies in cancer therapy. *Current Opinion in Immunology*, **5**, 732–739.

Robbins, P. F. & Kawakami, Y. (1996) Human tumor antigens recognized by T cells. *Current Opinion in Immunology*, **8**, 628–636.

Roth, C., Rochlitz, C. & Kourilsky, P. (1994) Immune responses against tumors. *Advances in Immunology*, **57**, 281–351.

Srivastava, P. K. & Udono, H. (1994) Heat shock protein–peptide complexes in cancer immunotherapy. *Current Opinion in Immunology*, **6**, 728–732.

Stevenson, F. K. & Hawkins, R. E. (1994) Molecular vaccines against cancer. *Immunologist*, **2**, 16–19.

Urban, J. L. & Schreiber, H. (1992) Tumor antigens. *Annual Review of Immunology*, **10**, 617–644.

Vallera, D. A. (1994) Immunotoxins: will their clinical promise be fulfilled? *Blood*, **83**, 309–317.

Van den Eynde, B. & Brichard, V. G. (1995) New tumor antigens recognized by T cells. *Current Opinion in Immunology*, **7**, 674–681.

Zier, K., Gansbacher, B. & Salvadori, S. (1996) Preventing abnormalities in signal transduction of T cells in cancer: the promise of cytokine gene therapy. *Immunology Today*, **17**, 39–45.

chapter 23

Allergies and other hypersensitivities

The vertebrate immune system has evolved to defend the individual against internal and external affronts and involves effector mechanisms designed to attack and destroy foreign bodies. Although the mechanisms possess built-in safeguards that normally direct the attack against non-self only, these are not completely foolproof and their failure or malfunction can lead to an attack on the individual's own tissues. Immunologically caused tissue injury is the subject of *immunopathology* and of the next three chapters.

Four principal situations exist in which the body can be attacked by its own immune system. These differ in the origin of the antigens that trigger the attack and in the mechanism as well as manifestation of the attack. The response can be set off by environmental antigens innocuous in a normal setting; by an infectious agent; by antigens on tissues derived from another individual; and by the individual's own antigens. The injurious reactions initiated by these four types of antigen are referred to as allergic, delayed-type hypersensitivity (contact sensitivity), allograft and autoimmune reactions, respectively. Allergic reactions are the subject of this chapter. To understand the term 'allergic', we describe briefly the historical context in which it arose.

Historical perspective

At the turn of this century, two French investigators, Paul J. Portier and Charles R. Richet, were commissioned by the Prince of Monaco to find a way of protecting swimmers in the Mediterranean Sea from the painful stings of the Portuguese man-of-war. Portier and Richet assumed correctly that the painful blisters were caused by a toxin injected through the animal's tentacles into the bather's skin and, since vaccination at that time was becoming a household word, decided to produce an antitoxin vaccine. They extracted the toxin from the sea creatures and inoculated it into dogs, expecting them to produce antibodies that would protect the recipients against a second challenge with the same toxin. To their great surprise, however, the opposite happened: not only were the dogs not protected, they became oversensitive. The second toxin injection elicited a state of shock from which most of the dogs failed to recover. Portier and Richet concluded that instead of inducing protection or *prophylaxis*, the treatment actually produced the opposite or *anaphylaxis* (Greek *ana*, away from; *phylaxis*, protection).

Soon after this, other investigators described further situations in which an inoculated substance induced increased sensitivity (*hypersensitivity)* instead of protection. Some of the substances were toxins, like that of the Portuguese man-of-war, but others were innocuous proteins such as ovalbumin. It seemed that an inoculated substance could induce two states in a recipient: protection (prophylaxis) and hypersensitivity (anaphylaxis). Both were *altered* states, because the recipient showed neither prophylactic nor anaphylactic response to the first encounter with the substance; it was only after the second exposure to the same substance that either a prophylactic or an anaphylactic response occurred. The German scientist, Clemens P. von Pirquet, thought that the two altered states should have a common name and in 1906 he suggested calling them *allergy* (Greek *allos*, other; *ergon*, work).

Gradually, however, scientists realized that there were also other hypersensitivity states that did not fit this classification. Three human diseases in particular, asthma, hay fever and eczema, seemed to fall out of line with anaphylaxis, which they otherwise resembled in some respects. *Asthma* is a condition characterized by shortness of breath caused by a constriction of the airways; *hay fever* is an inflammation of the lining of the nose leading to nasal obstruction and discharge; and *eczema* is an inflammation of the skin characterized by eruptions and reddening of the tissue. Asthma, hay fever and eczema resemble anaphylaxis in that they are forms of exaggerated sensitivity to certain substances but they also differ from anaphylaxis in one important aspect: while anaphylaxis can be induced in virtually all individuals manipulated in a certain way, asthma, hay fever and eczema only seem to afflict a certain low percentage of the human population and to occur in some families more frequently than in others. To distinguish the conditions involving hereditary predisposition from other hypersensitivities in which no hereditary component could be discerned, R.A. Cooke and Arthur F. Coca proposed calling the former *atopies* (Greek *atopos*, out of place) or *atopic diseases*. Other conditions also characterized by increased sensitivity and by hereditary predisposition are sometimes referred to as *intolerances*. *Food intolerance*, for example, is characterized by an adverse reaction to certain forms of food; only some food intolerances, however, have an immunological basis and these are often referred to as *food allergies*.

Some of these terms, originally introduced to denote certain hypersensitivity conditions, have in the meantime acquired a different meaning. This is particularly true of 'allergy', a term no longer used to refer to all prophylactic and anaphylactic responses. Instead, the word now denotes certain forms of hypersensitivity, although there is no longer agreement as to *which* forms the term should cover. 'Allergy' is sometimes used synonymously with 'atopy', but at other times is given a broader meaning. Virtually all possible meanings of the various terms can be found in the immunological literature. Anaphylaxis is sometimes equated with allergy, allergy with atopy, atopy is sometimes used to include food intolerance and at other times to exclude it, and so forth.

In an attempt to sort out the terminological muddle, P.G.H. Gell and R.R.A. Coombs proposed differentiating four types of hypersensitivity, which they referred to by the roman numerals I–IV. This classification takes into account the mechanisms by which the hypersensitivities exert their effects. Type I–III hypersensitivities are mediated by antibodies, whereas type IV is mediated by T lymphocytes; type I is mediated by IgE antibodies, whereas types II and III are mediated by IgM and IgG antibodies; and type II is mediated primarily by antibodies, whereas type III is mediated by antigen–antibody complexes. *Type I hypersensitivity*, also referred to as *immediate hypersensitivity* because its effects are recognizable within hours on rechallenge with antigen, is dependent on the binding of IgE antibodies to their receptors on mast cells and basophils. Cross-linking of the bound antibodies by antigen leads to the degranulation of these cells and to the synthesis of biologically active substances which, together with mediators released from the granules, effect an injurious form of inflammatory response. *Type II hypersensitivities* are antibody-dependent cytotoxic hypersensitivities. Antibodies of the IgM or IgG type, produced against antigens on the individual's own cells, in particular erythrocytes, leucocytes or platelets, bind to these antigens and the target cells are then phagocytosed, killed by natural killer (NK) cells in an antibody-dependent cell-mediated cytotoxic fashion or are lysed by complement that the bound antibodies activate. In *type III hypersensitivities*, immune complexes are formed in such large quantities that they cannot be cleared adequately by the reticuloendothelial system. The excessive complexes are deposited in the tissues, where they bind and activate complement and attract neutrophils, which then cause local tissue damage. Finally, in *type IV hypersensitivities*, particles such as tubercle bacilli sensitize T lymphocytes to produce cytokines upon secondary contact with the antigen. The cytokines initiate an inflammatory response that causes local tissue damage. Because the effects of the secondary encounter with the antigen are not seen until after a day or two, this form of response has been classified as *delayed-type hypersensitivity* (DTH).

Type I (immediate) hypersensitivity (mediated by IgE antibodies)	Anaphylaxis (no hereditary components)	
	Atopy	Hereditary component present
	Asthma	
	Hay fever	
	Eczema	
	Intolerance	
	Food allergy	
	Drug allergy	
Type II (cytotoxic) hypersensitivity (mediated by IgM and IgG antibodies)	Haemolytic disease of the newborn	
	Autoimmune haemolytic anaemia and certain other autoimmune diseases	
	Transfusion reactions	
	Hyperacute graft rejection	
Type III (immune complex) hypersensitivity (mediated by immune complexes)	Arthus reaction	
	Serum sickness	
Type IV (delayed-type) hypersensitivity (mediated by T lymphocytes)	Delayed-type hypersensitivity	
	Contact sensitivity	

Table 23.1 Relationships among various types of hypersensitivity.

Considerable overlap exists among the four types of hypersensitivity; in fact, the classification has done little more than put new labels on mechanisms that already had their own names. The various mechanisms may produce different effects but several also conspire to generate the same effect. In this sense, the classification is highly artificial: the only common feature of the four types of hypersensitivity is that they are all the result of exaggerated or inappropriate forms of beneficial immune response. A summary of the relationships among the various types of hypersensitivity appears in Table 23.1.

Type I hypersensitivities

Mechanisms of allergic (type I) reaction

The different types of allergy differ in their manifestation but all share the same underlying mechanisms (Fig. 23.1). All types are dependent on three key elements: mast cells, IgE and high-affinity IgE receptors (FcεRI). This dependence is most directly demonstrated by mouse mutants lacking some of these components. Mouse strains such as *white-spotting* (*W*) or *Steel* (*Sl*), deficient in mast cells (due to lack of the mast cell growth factor receptor c-kit or its ligand, respectively), are unable to mount anaphylactic responses. Similarly, mice with a disrupted gene coding for the FcεRI α subunit are resistant to local and systemic anaphylaxis. The situation is ambiguous with respect to the importance of IgE: mice with a disrupted *IgE* gene retain the capacity to mount systemic anaphylaxis indicating that under certain conditions, IgE can be replaced by other antibodies, probably IgG. In spite of this result, however, IgE appears to be the main immunoglobulin isotype involved in anaphylactic responses under normal conditions.

In the initial phase of an allergic reaction, antigen (here referred to as *allergen*) enters the body, is picked up by antigen-presenting cells (APCs), displayed by them in the context of class II major histocompatibility complex (MHC) molecules and recognized by helper T (T_H)- cell precursors. These are stimulated to proliferate and differentiate mainly into T_H2 cells, which help B lymphocytes differentiate into antibody-producing plasma cells (see Chapter 17). As in any other antibody-mediated response, the B cells that receive specific help from T_H cells are those that recognize the allergen via their surface receptors. Some of the cytokines produced by T_H2 cells, especially interleukin (IL)-4 and IL-13, stimulate the B cells to effect an immunoglobulin isotype switch and to produce IgE antibodies. The antibodies bind to high-affinity Fc receptors on the surface of mast cells in the connective tissue and mucosa, as well as to those on the surface of basophils in the circulation and mucosa. The receptors are also expressed on Langerhans' cells, eosinophils and monocytes (at a high level in atopic patients). The initial binding has no apparent effect on the cells; only when the allergen enters the body again in a certain way do problems arise. The multivalent allergen binds by one of its epitopes to one IgE molecule and by other epitopes to other IgE molecules on the same cell, thus forming a bridge between the IgE molecules (see Fig. 23.1). Since the antibodies are attached to Fc receptors, their bridging clusters the receptors. The allergen must have at least two epitopes (i.e. it must be bivalent) to be able to cross-link IgE molecules; the more epitopes it has, the better it clusters the receptors. Clustering of the receptors can also

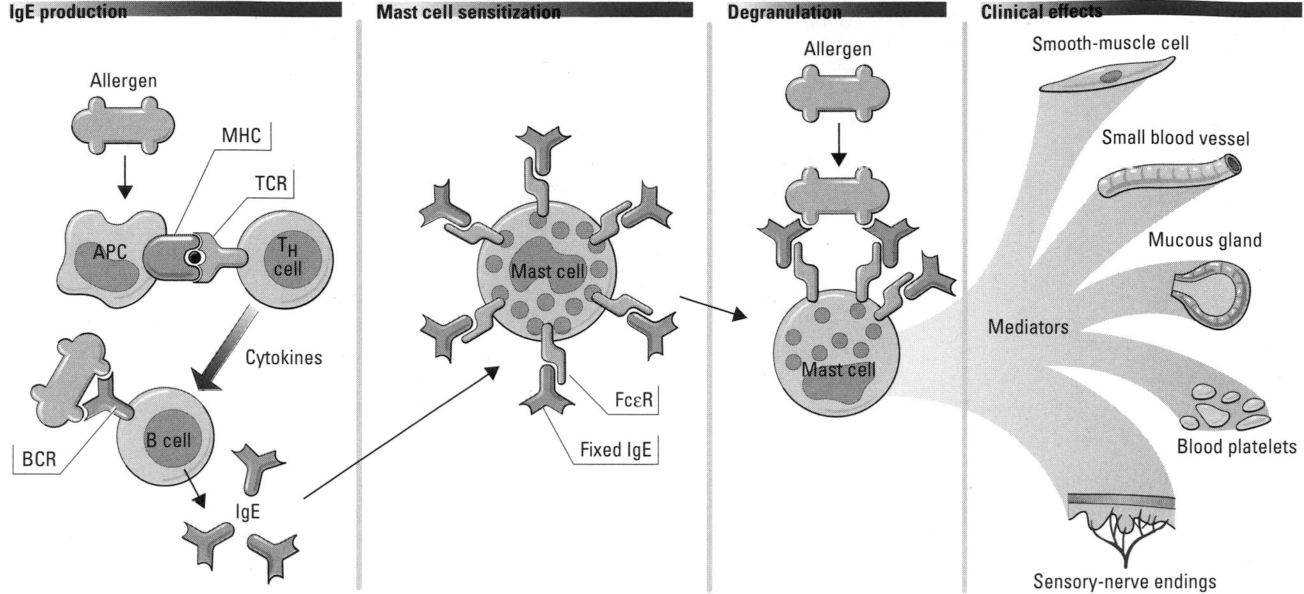

Figure 23.1 General mechanism underlying allergic reaction. First exposure to an allergen activates T and B lymphocytes and prompts the B lymphocytes to secrete allergen-specific IgE antibodies. The latter bind via their Fc regions to high-affinity Fcε receptors on mast cells and basophils, thereby sensitizing them. Upon a second encounter with the allergen, the cell-bound antibodies are cross-linked, Fcε receptors are clustered and mast cells and basophils are activated. The cells degranulate and the released mediators initiate reactions responsible for the clinical effects. APC, antigen-presenting cell; BCR, B-cell receptor, FcεR, Fc receptor for IgE; MHC major histocompatibility complex; TCR, T-cell receptor.

be achieved by means other than antigen: by antibodies specific for the bound IgE molecules; by antibodies specific for the Fc receptor itself; and by lectins which bind to carbohydrates on either the IgE or the Fc receptor molecules. However, allergic responses are initiated only when an allergen cross-links the IgE–FcεR complexes. As a result of FcεR cross-linking, aggregates form in the plasma membrane and cluster into patches containing thousands of receptor molecules. The aggregation immobilizes the receptor and probably also induces changes in the underlying cytoskeleton, to which the receptor molecules may be attached. Some of the antigen–IgE–FcεR complexes may be internalized. Aggregation of the receptors generates a signal that is eventually translated via intracellular events into degranulation of the cell.

The initial phase of the signal-transduction process is remarkably similar to signalling mechanisms used by antigen-specific receptors of T and B lymphocytes and by other Fc receptors. The β and γ subunits of the high-affinity IgE receptor contain, in their intracellular domains, the *immunoreceptor tyrosine-based activation motif* (ITAM), which is also present in the signal-transducing components of the T-cell receptor (the chains of the CD3 complex; see Chapter 7) and the B-cell receptor (the components of the CD79 complex; see Chapter 8). In the case of FcεRI, the Src-family kinase Lyn is associated with the ITAM sequence of the β chain. After allergen-induced aggregation of the receptors, several Lyn molecules are brought together so that they can phosphorylate each other. This autophosphorylation increases the catalytic activity of Lyn, which can then phosphorylate the intracellular parts of the β and γ chains and possibly also other proteins. The phosphorylated ITAM of the γ chain then binds another protein tyrosine kinase, Syk, which in turn phosphorylates other molecules such as the enzyme phospholipase C (Fig. 23.2). The following signalling pathways are in principle identical to those shown generally in Fig. 10.27. Another event occurring immediately after IgE receptor cross-linking is the attachment of the peptide ubiquitin to the cytoplasmic domains of the IgE receptor complex. This chemical modification probably markedly affects further non-covalent interactions of the receptor with intracellular components that may regulate the outcome of signalling. In addition to rapid protein phosphorylation, hydrolysis of phosphatidylinositol bisphosphate and rise of cytoplasmic Ca^{2+}, at least two other rapid biochemical changes are initiated as a result of FcεRI aggregation: methylation of membrane phospholipids and transient rise of intracellular cyclic adenosine monophosphate (cAMP). Methylation of phosphatidylethanolamine produces phosphatidylcholine and thus

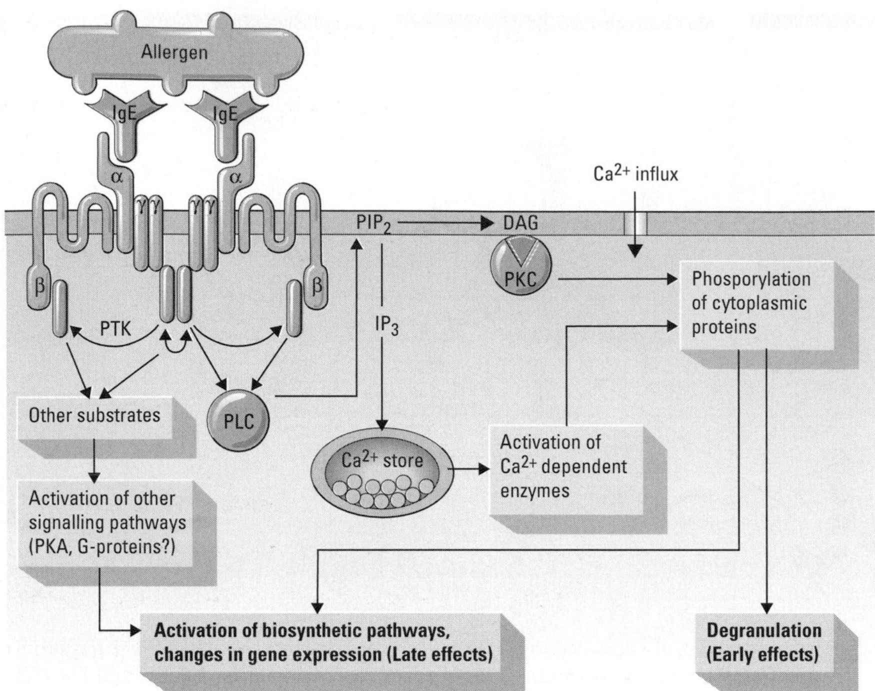

Figure 23.2 Mechanisms of mast cell activation and degranulation. FcεRI complexes bind IgE molecules and are cross-linked by the allergen. The associated cytoplasmic protein tyrosine kinases (PTKs), brought close together by the cross-linking, phosphorylate and thus activate each other. The activated PTKs phosphorylate other substrates and initiate several cascades of reactions principally similar to those triggered by other PTK-linked receptors (see Chapter 10). PLC, phospholipase C; PIP_2, phosphatidylinositol bisphosphate; IP_3, inositol trisphosphate; DAG, diacylglycerol; PKA, protein kinase A.

increases fluidity of the membrane and enhances permeability of Ca^{2+} channels. Inhibitors of methyltransferase, the enzyme responsible for phospholipid methylation, suppress the cytoplasmic Ca^{2+} influx and thereby inhibit mast cell degranulation. cAMP is produced by adenylate cyclase, another membrane-bound enzyme activated as a result of FcεRI aggregation. It activates protein kinase A, which phosphorylates cytoskeletal and cytoplasmic proteins needed for transport of granules and their fusion with the plasma membrane.

These, and possibly other, as yet unidentified mechanisms initiated by FcεRI aggregation, lead to *degranulation* of mast cells. The cytoplasmic granules fuse with the plasma membrane and release the *primary mediators* contained in them, a phenomenon similar to degranulation of phagocytes described in Chapter 15. Furthermore, signalling via FcεRI leads to activation of phospholipase A_2, an enzyme that initiates the synthesis of arachidonic acid-derived *secondary mediators* such as prostaglandin D_2 (PGD_2) and leukotriene A_4 (LTA_4) (see Chapter 11). Secretion of the secondary mediators is delayed after the rapid release of the primary mediators, but the effects of the secondary mediators last longer and are more pronounced.

The released biologically active substances are then responsible for the clinical manifestations of allergic reactions. The main mediators released or synthesized by *mast cells* are histamine, heparin, PGD_2 and the enzymes tryptase and acid hydrolases (β-hexosaminidase, β-glucuronidase, arylsulphatase, myeloperoxidase and superoxide dismutase). *Histamine* stimulates smooth muscle cells, vascular endothelial cells and nerve endings (Fig. 23.3). Its stimulatory action is opposed by the inhibitory effect of PGD_2 on most of these cells. *Heparin* exerts an inhibitory effect on platelets, which is opposed by the stimulatory effect of PGD_2. The released *enzymes* may generate additional mediators from precursor plasma proteins that have traversed the vessel walls, after these have been made permeable by the action of histamine. *Tryptase*, for example, generates anaphylatoxin (C3a) from the C3 complement component, and at the same time destroys high-molecular-mass kininogen, thereby pre-empting the generation of kinins and the activation of the intrinsic coagulation pathway (see Chapter 21). These events reinforce the antithrombocytic action of heparin and PGD_2. *Leukotrienes*, the secondary mediators secreted after a delay by mast cells, are much more potent bronchoconstrictors than

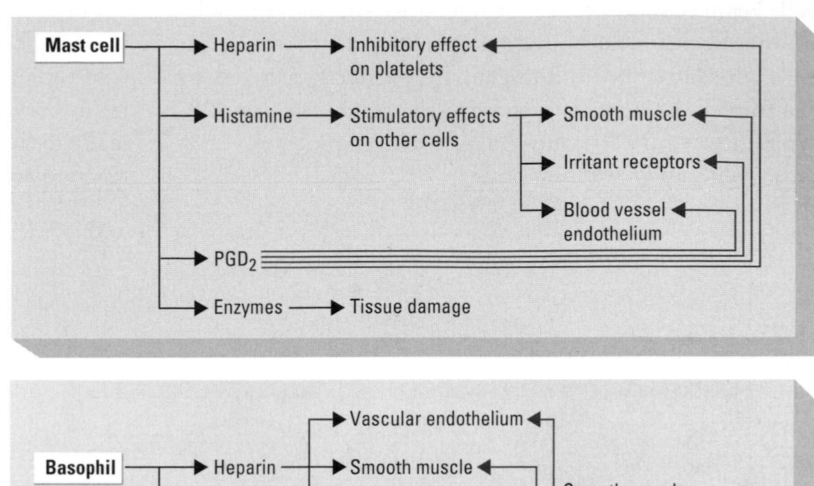

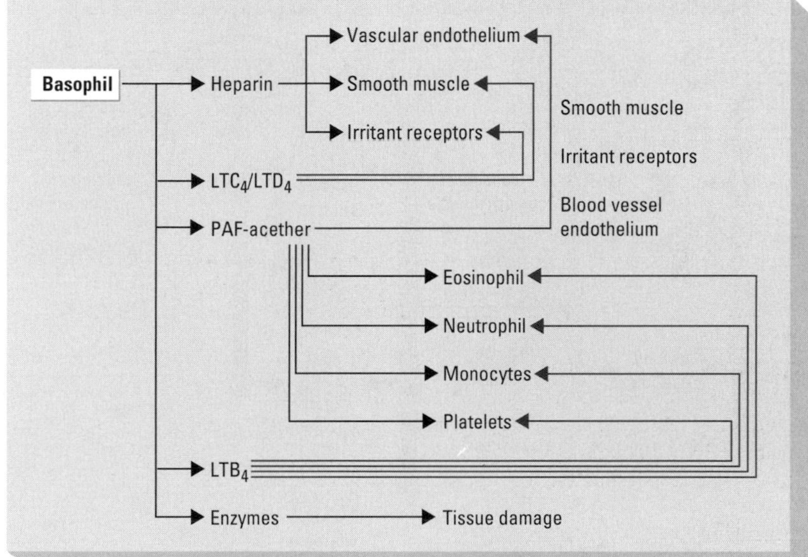

Figure 23.3 Activities of mediators released from mast cells during an allergic reaction. Red arrows indicate inhibitory action. LT, leukotriene; PAF, platelet-activating factor; PG, prostaglandin.

histamine; they also strongly stimulate mucous secretion in asthmatics.

Mediators released or synthesized by *basophils* include histamine, leukotrienes LTC_4, LTD_4 and LTB_4, platelet-activating factor (PAF-acether) and enzymes such as kallikrein, prekallikrein activator, Hageman factor activator, β-hexosaminidase and arylsulphatase (Fig. 23.4). The stimulatory action of histamine on smooth muscles and nerve endings is opposed by the inhibitory action of LTC_4/LTD_4, and that on vascular smooth muscles and vascular endothelium by PAF-acether. PAF-acether exerts a stimulatory effect on eosinophils, neutrophils, monocytes and platelets. This effect is opposed by the action of LTB_4. The activities of the released enzymes generate the anticoagulant plasmin, the vasodilator and spasmogen kinin, the procoagulant fibrin and the potent inflammatory agent bradykinin. Bradykinin can contribute to allergic reactions either directly or by the release of, and synergism with, other mediators.

The effects caused by these various mediators vary depending on the tissue exposed to the allergen. They include smooth muscle contraction, vascular leakage, hypotension, mucous secretion, weal and flare, itching, flushing and pain. These symptoms set in within minutes of secondary exposure to the allergen and abate within another 30–60 min; they constitute the *classical allergic reactions* (immediate hypersensitivity). In the past these manifestations were believed to be all there was to allergic responses. Now we know, however, that in reality they are followed by a more protracted response, the *late-phase reaction*, which sets in within 2–8 hours after stimulation and persists for 1 or 2 days and sometimes even longer.

The late-phase reaction is simply a particular form of inflammatory response (see Chapter 21) initiated by the release of synthesized mediators, in particular those that remain associated with the granular matrix (e.g. heparin, chymotrypsin/trypsin and inflammatory factors of anaphylaxis). Among the mediators are several with chemotactic activity for eosinophils, neutrophils, monocytes/macrophages and lymphocytes. Attracted by the mediators, these cells begin to infiltrate the inflammatory site, first the polymorphonuclear cells and somewhat later the mononuclear cells, the latter being attracted by products secreted by the former. A typical late-phase lesion contains some 30% lymphocytes, 30% neutrophils, 10% monocytes, 30% eosinophils and a few basophils.

Eosinophils may respond to the allergen either directly via cell-bound IgG and IgE antibodies or indirectly via C3d receptors. Upon degranulation, activated eosinophils release several enzymes as well as other substances normally toxic for invading parasites, but which in an allergic reaction attack the epithelial cells of the body (Fig. 23.5).

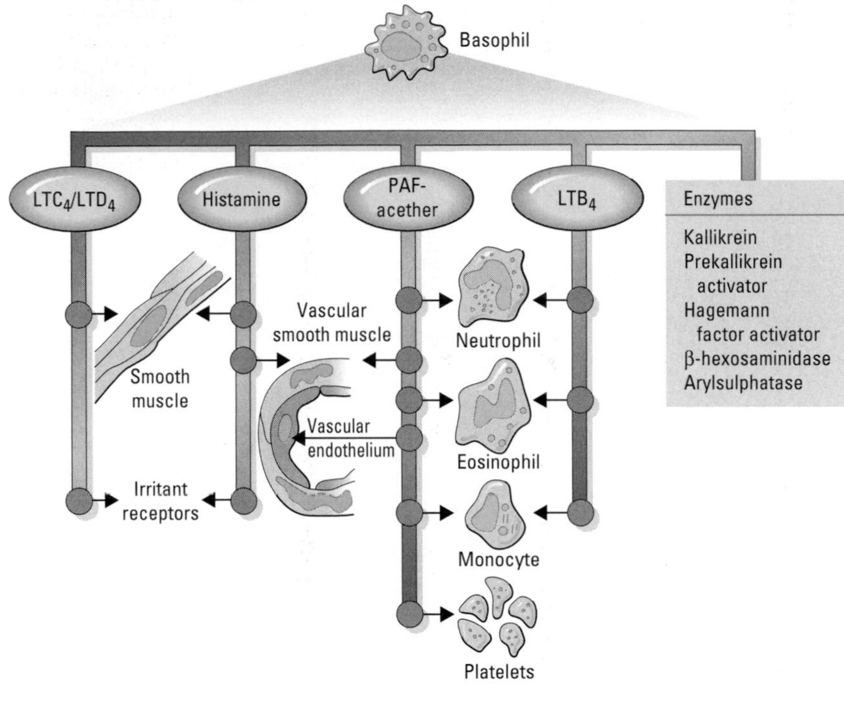

Figure 23.4 Activities of mediators released from activated basophils in allergic reactions. LT, leukotriene; PAF, platelet-activating factor. (Modified from Morley, J. *et al.* (1984), in *Allergy: Immunological and Clinical Aspects* (Ed. M. H. Less), p. 45. John Wiley & Sons, Chichester.)

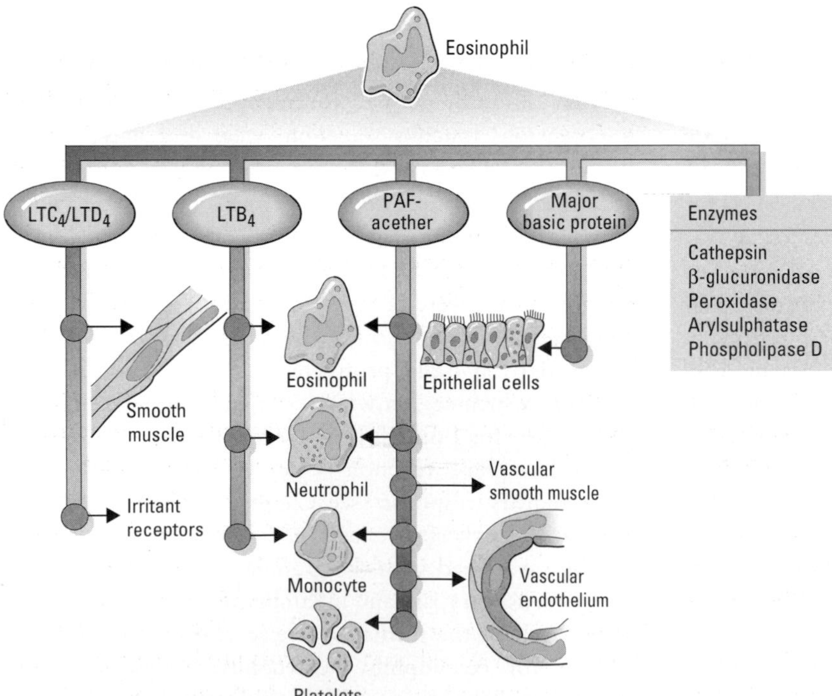

Figure 23.5 Activities of eosinophils in the late phase of the allergic reaction. LT, leukotriene; PAF, platelet-activating factor. (Modified from Morley, J. *et al.* (1984), in *Allergy: Immunological and Clinical Aspects* (Ed. M. H. Less), p. 45. John Wiley & Sons, Chichester.)

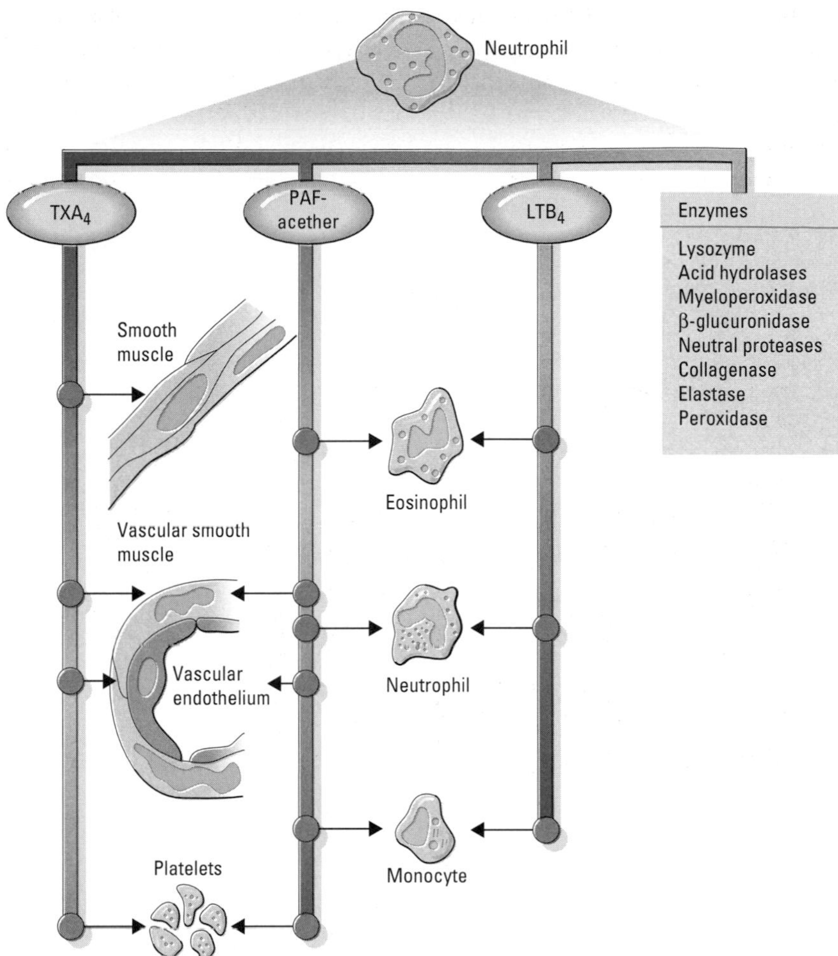

Figure 23.6 Activities of neutrophils in the late phase of the allergic reaction. LT, leukotriene; PAF, platelet-activating factor; TX, thromboxane. (Modified from Morley, J. *et al.* (1984), in *Allergy: Immunological and Clinical Aspects* (Ed. M. H. Less), p. 45. John Wiley & Sons, Chichester.)

Neutrophils may be activated by a number of immunological agents, including IgG antibodies, lymphokines, chemotactic peptides, thromboxane A_2, LTB_4 and PAF-acether (Fig. 23.6). Activated neutrophils secrete enzymes such as lysozyme, acid hydrolases, myeloperoxidase and elastase, which attack the tissue at the site of inflammation.

Monocytes and *macrophages* possess the high-affinity IgE receptor (FcεRI), the expression of which increases in atopic patients. Cross-linking of FcεRI can lead to direct monocyte activation accompanied by the release of cytokines and mediators. Monocytes and macrophages also possess low-affinity IgE receptors (CD23) but their function is not known. Activated macrophages produce an abundance of mediators: prostaglandins, thromboxanes, leukotrienes, PAF-acether, IL-1 and other cytokines and a variety of enzymes, some of which are directly toxic for the tissues (Fig. 23.7).

Lymphocytes are essential in the development of an allergic response (Fig. 23.8): B lymphocytes produce IgE and T_H2 cells are in a sense the major initiators of the response, since they produce IL-4 and IL-13 necessary for B-cell maturation and isotype switching to IgE. Furthermore, the interactions of low-affinity IgE receptors (CD23) on the surface of activated lymphocytes (B and T) with IgE or IgE-containing immune complexes seem to have regulatory functions, as described later in this chapter. IL-9 induces the expression of high-affinity FcεRI on mouse T_H cells and thus generates signals that regulate the response via feedback effects.

Finally, *platelets* become involved at different stages of the allergic reaction when they aggregate and are activated (Fig. 23.9). They can be activated directly or indirectly, in the latter case by adenosine diphosphate released from vascular *endothelial cells* upon their activation (Fig. 23.10). Among the mediators released from activated platelets are thromboxanes, serotonin, PAF-acether and a variety of tissue-damaging enzymes (Fig. 23.9). The complex interactions of all these cells and mediators produce the characteristic symptoms of the late-phase reaction, which include a

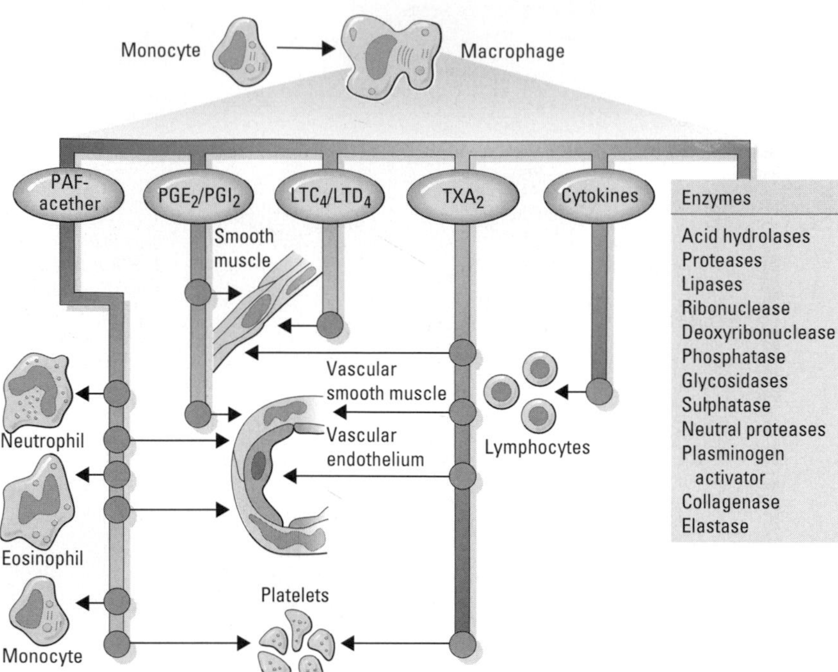

Figure 23.7 Activities of monocytes and macrophages in the late phase of the allergic reaction. LT, leukotriene; PAF, platelet-activating factor; PG, prostaglandin; TX, thromboxane. (Modified from Morley, J. *et al.* (1984), in *Allergy: Immunological and Clinical Aspects* (Ed. M. H. Less), p. 45. John Wiley & Sons, Chichester.)

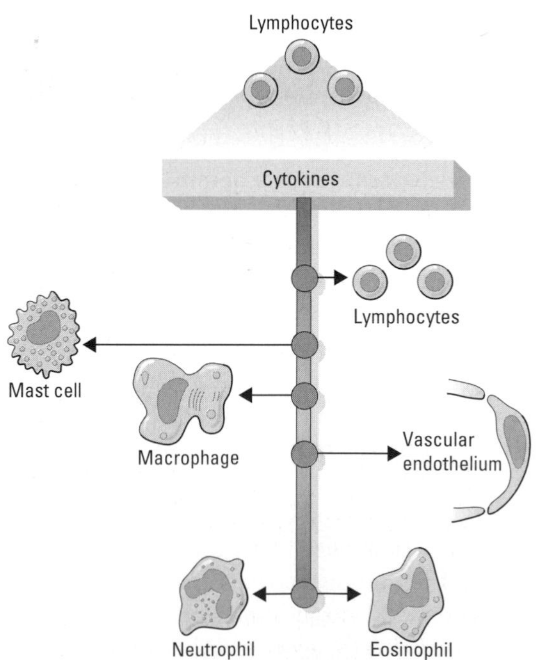

Figure 23.8 Activities of lymphocytes in the late phase of the allergic reaction. (Modified from Morley, J. *et al.* (1984), in *Allergy: Immunological and Clinical Aspects* (Ed. M. H. Less), p. 45. John Wiley & Sons, Chichester.)

burning tenderness, dysaesthesia (impairment of the touch sense), erythema and induration.

Allergic response is influenced by the *nervous system*, in both the acute and late phase. Many allergies are known to be affected by the physiological condition of the patient. In guinea-pigs, removal of the anterior hypothalamus (known to control the parasympathetic system) reduces the symptoms of experimentally induced IgE-mediated tissue injury, whereas removal of the posterior hypothalamus (known to control the sympathetic system) enhances these symptoms. The basic element of neurogenic control is the *reflex*, which consists of afferent input neurons, interneurons and efferent output neurons (Fig. 23.11). Afferent neurons end in sensory fibres in the peripheral tissue; interneurons form short fibres in the central nervous system (spinal cord); and efferent neurons end in the effector tissue or organ (smooth muscles, blood vessels, glands). Stimulated by heat, pressure or chemicals, sensory endings of afferent neurons generate impulses that are transmitted via interneurons to efferent neurons and lead to the release of neurotransmitters on the effector cells. Among the neurotransmitters are neuropeptides (substance P, vasoactive intestinal polypeptide) and acetylcholine (parasympathetic system), as well as noradrenaline (sympathetic system; Fig. 23.12).

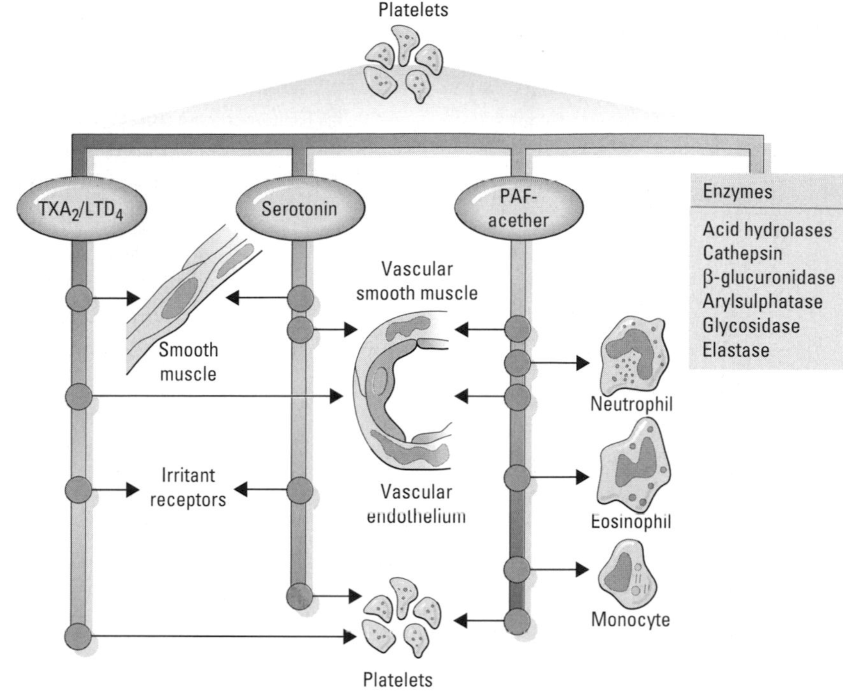

Figure 23.9 Activities of mediators released from platelets in the late phase of the allergic reaction. PAF, platelet-activating factor; TX, thromboxane. (Modified from Morley, J. *et al.* (1984), in *Allergy: Immunological and Clinical Aspects* (Ed. M. H. Less), p. 45. John Wiley & Sons, Chichester.)

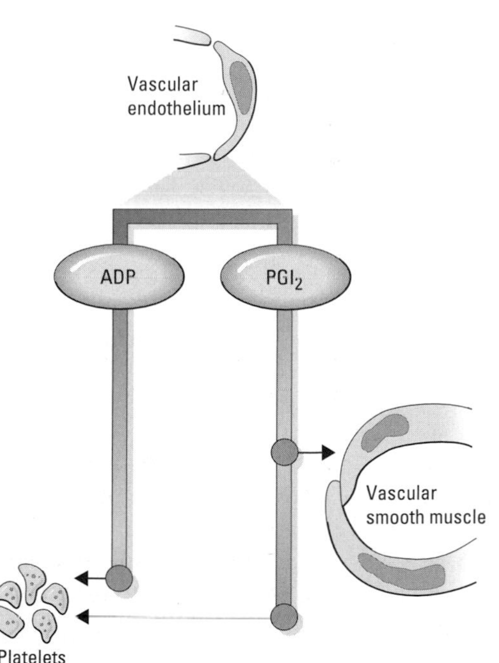

Figure 23.10 Activities of vascular endothelial cells in the late phase of the allergic reaction. ADP, adenosine diphosphate; PG, prostaglandin. (Modified from Morley, J. *et al.* (1984), in *Allergy: Immunological and Clinical Aspects* (Ed. M. H. Less), p. 45. John Wiley & Sons, Chichester.)

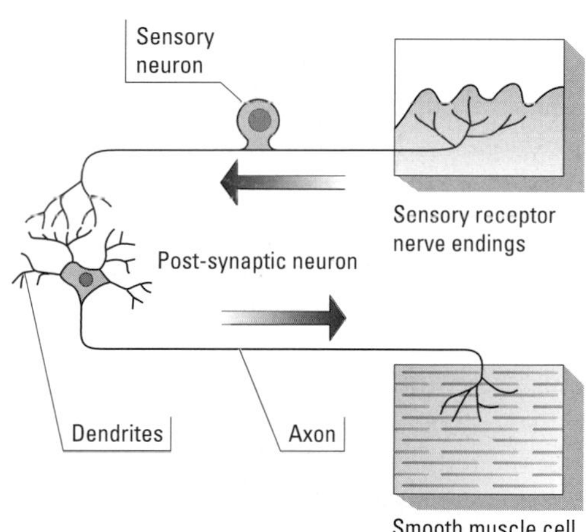

Figure 23.11 Simple reflex arc. (Modified from Morley, J. *et al.* (1984), in *Allergy: Immunological and Clinical Aspects* (Ed. M. H. Less), p. 45. John Wiley & Sons, Chichester.)

Neurotransmitters interact with their corresponding receptors on the effector cells and activate these via either cAMP (adrenergic receptors) or cyclic guanosine monophosphate (cGMP) (cholinergic receptors). The target cells of the neurotransmitters are mast cells, smooth muscle cells, epithelial and secretory cells, and the smooth muscle as well as

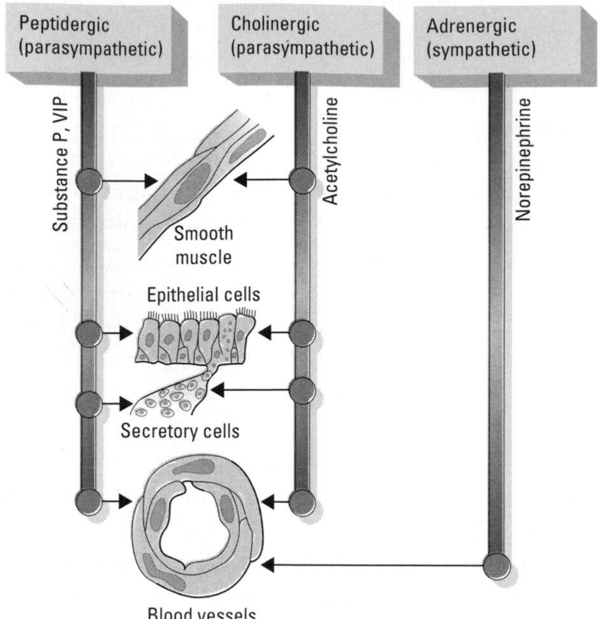

Figure 23.12 Participation of the nervous system in allergic reactions. VIP, vasoactive intestinal polypeptide. (Modified from Morley, J. *et al.* (1984), in *Allergy: Immunological and Clinical Aspects* (Ed. M. H. Less), p. 45. John Wiley & Sons, Chichester.)

endothelial cells of the blood vessels. Mast cells have both adrenergic and cholinergic receptors in their plasma membranes; smooth muscles, epithelial cells and secretory cells have peptidergic or cholinergic receptors and are therefore influenced by parasympathetic nerves, which may cause contraction (via acetylcholine and substance P) or relaxation (via acetylcholine or vasoactive intestinal polypeptide) depending on the site at which the transmitters are released.

In some situations, nerve signals do not need to pass through the central nervous system. Instead, an impulse induced at the terminal of one branch of nerve fibres may travel to the point of bifurcation of the nerve, bend back (reflect) there, and travel down the other branch to the effector organ (the impulse thus travels antidromically part of the way, i.e. in a direction opposite to that which is physiologically normal for the particular fibre). Such a response is referred to as an *axon reflex* (Fig. 23.13) but here reflex refers to the bending back of the signal; the response is not a true reflex in the sense in which neurobiologists normally use the word.

When IgE receptors on mast cells and basophils are aggregated under certain conditions, such as the absence of extracellular Ca^{2+}, the cells not only fail to release mediators but they also become *desensitized*: when Ca^{2+} is then added to such cells and permissive conditions are restored, degranulation still does not occur. If the initial conditions are such that only a few receptors are aggregated in the absence of Ca^{2+}, only these will be incapable of triggering the release reaction, whereas the remaining receptors aggregated subsequently in the presence of Ca^{2+} will induce degranulation from the same cells. Like activation, desensitization is initiated by aggregation of IgE receptors and appears to involve similar steps, all the way to the rise of intracellular Ca^{2+}. If a desensitized cell is exposed to an ionophore that directly raises intracellular Ca^{2+}, the desensitization state is abolished. Activation and inactivation processes apparently occur simultaneously in a cell: the balance between the two determines whether the cell will degranulate or become desensitized.

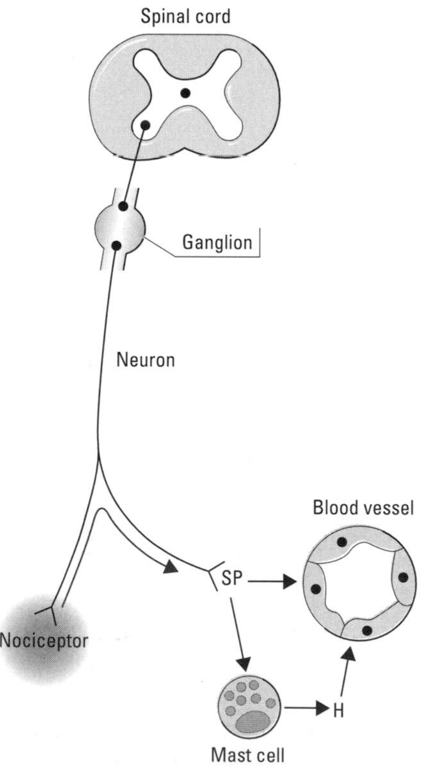

Figure 23.13 Axon-reflex model of neurogenic inflammation. Stimulation of polymodal nociceptors by heat, pressure or chemicals generates an impulse that is transmitted towards the spinal cord, but at the neuron's bifurcation point the impulse enters the other branch of the neuron and travels antidromically (in the direction opposite that which is physiologically normal) towards the effector organ. (*Nociceptors* are sense organs responsive to noxious stimuli that threaten to cause tissue damage.) In the organ, the impulse leads to the release of substance P (SP) or of other neuropeptides, which then act either directly on blood vessels or indirectly via mast cells and mast-cell mediators such as histamine (H).

Factors influencing allergic reactions

Nature of the allergen

It is not clear why some antigens have a tendency to elicit IgE responses and thus act as allergens. Genes encoding some of the allergens (e.g. various pollen substances, cat dander, house-dust mite, various food allergens) have been cloned and sequenced but no apparent common feature that could explain allergenicity has been found. Many allergens occur in multiple, closely related variant forms and it has been suggested that perhaps this microheterogeneity is related to allergenicity, but it is difficult to imagine how. One possible reason for allergenicity has been suggested based on the study of the major house-dust mite allergen *Der p*I. This protein of relative molecular mass (M_r) 30 000 is a cysteine protease produced in the midgut of the mite *Dermatophagoides pteronyssinus*, where it probably serves to digest food. It is incorporated in mite faecal pellets, which are common components of house dust. The protease cleaves a major membrane regulatory protein of IgE synthesis, the low-affinity IgE receptor (FcεRII; CD23) with considerable efficiency and specificity. As explained below, any processes leading to reduction in the amounts of surface CD23 and production of its soluble forms shift the IgE regulatory circuits towards increased IgE synthesis. Perhaps other allergens also interfere, at different levels, with homeostatic mechanisms regulating IgE synthesis.

Genetic factors

A genetic predisposition to allergic disease, especially to the triad asthma, hay fever and atopic dermatitis, has been recognized since the original studies of Cooke and Coca in 1923. The actual manner in which a genetic influence is exerted on the development of the diseases has, however, proved difficult to establish. Some of the difficulties lie in the definition of allergic disease, which varies according to the investigator; in obtaining accurate, relevant measurements; in the selection of subjects and methods of statistical analysis; in the purity of the allergen tested; and above all in the fact that the diseases are strongly influenced by environmental factors.

Three lines of study have been pursued: on populations, twins and families. Population studies have served to establish the prevalence, incidence and associations of the diseases. Studies on twins have been used to determine the relative influence of genetic and environmental factors on the development of the trait. Finally, family studies have provided information about the genes involved. The increased risk is manifested in four separately inherited characteristics: a predisposition to allergy in general; a predisposition to a particular disease (e.g. asthma); a predisposition to synthesize excess amounts of IgE; and a predisposition to an exaggerated IgE response to particular allergens.

General predisposition to allergy was first demonstrated by Cooke and Van der Veer in 1916, when they observed that 48% of their allergic patients had a family history of allergy, compared with only 14% of control subjects, and that children with two allergic parents developed allergies more frequently (68%; the range is now known to be 20–75%) than children with one allergic parent (51%; range 10–50%). The generality of the predisposition was indicated by the fact that children with asthma commonly had coincidental hay fever and often experienced atopic eczema in their infancy. The three diseases appeared, and continue to appear even now, to be closely associated.

At least two human genes are known to predispose to allergy. One is *IL4* or a gene in its vicinity. Polymorphism of the *IL4* gene correlates with increased IgE levels, which makes sense, since IL-4 is the cytokine that induces the IgE isotype switch. The *IL4* gene cluster on chromosome 5 also contains genes encoding IL-13 and IL-5 (a basophil differentiation factor). The second of the two predisposing genes codes for the FcεRI subunit β, and the gene is located on chromosome 11. A point mutation that replaces isoleucine for leucine at position 181 correlates with predisposition to allergy. This subtle change may alter the nature of the signal sent via FcεRI.

Predisposition to a particular disease has been studied most extensively with respect to asthma. Several reports indicate an exclusive predisposition to asthma, perhaps the best known of which is that carried out on the inhabitants of Tristan da Cunha, a small isolated island in the southern Atlantic Ocean. Most of the islanders are descendants of 15 original settlers, two or three of whom had asthma. When the population was examined in 1946, half of the residents had asthma but were free of other allergic diseases. In this partially inbred population, the predisposition to asthma was apparently inherited separately from the other forms of allergy.

Predisposition to produce excess IgE is often strong in some families. Raised IgE levels need not correlate with the actual occurrence of allergy, although they are known to be the second major allergy risk factor. The manner of inheritance is complex, heterogeneous and not well understood.

Predisposition to respond to a particular allergen has been associated with the human *MHC*, the human leucocyte antigen (*HLA*) complex. When humans are challenged with purified allergens and the response is measured by either the skin reaction or elevated production of IgE, individual differences often correlate with the person's *HLA* alleles. For example, individuals carrying *DRB*02* have been reported to respond to the ragweed allergen Amb a V more often than individuals who lack this allele, whereas individuals carrying *HLA-B*08* and *DRB1*03* alleles appear to be frequent responders to the ryegrass allergen *Lol p*I. Most of these data are controversial, however, since some investigators have failed to confirm associations reported by others.

Environmental influences

Of the many environmental effects on the development of allergic diseases, only a few are mentioned here: geographic region, season of the year, diet, infection and climate. The *effect of geographical conditions* is suggested by many anecdotal observations. For example, when a hurricane devastated Tokelan Island in the South Pacific in 1966, half of the population was resettled in New Zealand. Later, a comparison of the two populations revealed that asthma occurred with a frequency of 11% among the Tokelan Island children, but with a frequency of 25% among the New Zealand-born children. Evidence also suggests that children in urban areas have a higher frequency of asthma than those in rural regions. Generally, it does make a difference if someone susceptible to allergic diseases is either born in a high-risk allergy environment or moves to such an environment later in life.

Seasonal variation in the concentration of environmental allergens not only influences the frequency of occurrence but also predisposes to allergic diseases. In Finland, for example, children born in the period February–April run the highest risk of developing birch-pollen sensitivity, and those born in April–May are most likely to become sensitized to mugwort pollen. The minimal-risk months for all pollen allergies are July and August. It appears from these and similar studies that exposure to an allergy-favouring environment within the first 3–6 months of life increases the risk of developing an allergic disease later.

The degree to which a particular *diet* predisposes to the development of allergic sensitivity is controversial. Several studies have concluded that, for example, breast-fed children have a lower risk of developing allergic diseases than bottle-fed infants and that children fed a diet free of cows' milk and eggs develop allergic diseases less frequently than children on diets that include these two components. However, reports have also been published in which no difference in the frequency of allergic diseases has been found between the two groups of children.

The influence of *infection* is indicated by the observation that many patients first develop asthma or hay fever immediately after a viral respiratory illness. Since strong evidence for increased bronchial reactivity in asthma exists, it is believed that some respiratory virus infections cause temporary bronchial hyperreactivity and so predispose the patient to allergy. There is a striking increase in allergies in most developed nations, which is inversely correlated with the decrease in serious childhood diseases and which parallels greatly increased hygiene standards. Allergy is therefore one of the most typical 'civilization diseases'. It has been speculated that lack of exposure to some formerly common parasites (worms) during a critical period in childhood may be linked to allergy to innocuous environmental antigens. Parasitic infections are known to be accompanied by IgE responses and there seems to be an inverse correlation between total serum IgE levels and atopic disease in parasitized and control populations. Thus, too much hygiene in childhood may, paradoxically, be one of the factors contributing to the development of allergy.

The effect of *climate* and *microclimate* on the development of allergic diseases has been documented by numerous investigators. Changes in various climatic factors, such as temperature, humidity and barometric pressure, have been reported to activate allergic diseases, and damp houses have long been known to be detrimental for patients with asthma and hay fever. Various atmospheric pollutants, particularly sulphur dioxide, also clearly exacerbate asthma and hay fever. All these factors, however, are difficult to separate from other effects (this is true for *all* environmental effects) and so their role in *initiating* allergic disease remains unclear.

Nature of the defect

The fact that not everyone exposed to allergens becomes allergic and that certain individuals are genetically predisposed to developing the disease indicates that a certain defect or defects must underlie this condition. The nature of this defect, however, remains obscure. Since so many factors influence the development of the condition and so many components conspire in activating the disease, it is extremely difficult to distinguish cause from effect and to identify the one or a few root causes at the very beginning of the many complex chains and networks of interacting factors.

Since the diseases have a strong immunological component, immunologists like to think that a defect in the immune system is the primary cause of the allergic condition. A variety of immunological abnormalities are indeed associated with the condition. Neonatal and postnatal levels of serum immunoglobulin, particularly IgA, tend to be low in allergic individuals. Some 27% of allergic individuals, as opposed to 5% of healthy subjects, have a defect in yeast opsonization via the alternative complement pathway. Some 22% of allergic individuals, compared with 1% of healthy individuals, have low levels of the C2 component and of haptoglobin (the latter inhibits prostaglandin synthesis). Compared with healthy persons, allergic individuals often have a reduced number of T lymphocytes, in particular CD8+ T cells, a decreased responsiveness to mitogens and antigens *in vitro*, decreased autologous mixed lymphocyte reactivity (see Chapter 24) and decreased cytotoxic T-lymphocyte activity. Many allergic subjects have increased levels of IgE at birth and their basophils show a greater ability to release histamine. The latter property is revealed experimentally after treatment of basophils with heavy water (deuterium oxide, D_2O) *in vitro*. In healthy subjects, D_2O enhances histamine release caused by antigen and IgE; in allergic individuals it alone releases histamine from basophils. Several investigators have also reported that allergic individuals have a defect in the suppressor T-cell compartment. Levels of IgE have been claimed to increase when suppressor-cell number decreases and histamine has been reported to increase suppressor-cell activity. These findings, however, are controversial, as are suppressor cells in general. Two specific regulatory cytokines, *glycosylation enhancing* and *glycosylation inhibitory factors (GEF, GIF)* produced by regulatory T cells, have been described. They influence glycosylation of IgE and may be involved in IgE-regulatory circuits.

Among the best characterized of immunoregulatory mechanisms is that which operates via the *low-affinity IgE receptor* (FcεRII; CD23; see Chapter 8). Several types of cells, including B and T lymphocytes, monocytes and eosinophils, express constitutively low levels of CD23 in healthy individuals. Activation of these cells by inflammation and infection induces high levels of CD23 expression. In asthma patients, eosinophils, macrophages and epithelial cells of respiratory mucosa also express large amounts of CD23. Two slightly different isotypes of CD23, CD23A and CD23B, are produced by alternative transcription of a single gene and are differentially regulated. The lectin domains of the CD23 trimers act as Fc receptors by binding the $C_\varepsilon3$ domains of IgE; although this binding occurs via the lectin domain, it does not involve the carbohydrate moiety of IgE. CD23 expressed on the surface of IgE-producing B cells binds IgE and IgE-containing immune complexes. This binding provides a negative regulatory signal instructing these cells to shut down IgE synthesis. CD23 thus acts as a component of negative feedback regulation.

However, this is only one function of this remarkable molecule. It also acts as an adhesion molecule capable of binding to one of the complement receptors, CR2 (CD21), and to leucocyte integrins CD11b/CD18 and CD11c/CD18. In its interaction with CD21, the lectin head of CD23 binds the carbohydrate side-chains of CD21. CD23 is strongly expressed on the surface of follicular dendritic cells and its interaction with CD21 on the surface of B cells undergoing the germinal centre reaction (see Chapter 17) seems to play a part in B-cell stimulation and rescue from apoptosis.

Other functions of CD23 are carried out by soluble forms (M_r 37 000, 33 000, 29 000, 25 000 and 16 000) produced by proteolytic cleavage of the stalks of membrane molecules. These sCD23 molecules retain the IgE-binding lectin heads and act as pleiotropic cytokines. The largest of the sCD23 forms enhance IgE synthesis by B cells, in which T cell-dependent isotype switching to IgE has already taken place, probably by binding to membrane IgE and CD21.

The loss of CD23 from the cell surface and/or an increase in sCD23 concentration contribute to increased IgE synthesis. Since their increase can be induced by proteolytic activities of infectious agents and activated inflammatory cells, it is conceivable that these activities contribute to the development and perpetuation of allergy. In agreement with this proposed regulatory function of CD23, mouse mutants lacking this receptor exhibit increased levels of IgE in response to T cell-dependent antigens.

One powerful argument against the idea that an immunological defect is the *primary* cause of the allergic condition is that the same condition is often induced without the involvement of allergens, IgE, mast cells and basophils. Asthma, for example, can be induced by strenuous exercise. Because of this, some investigators argue that the primary cause of allergy is physiological rather than immunological. Perhaps the nerve endings in the smooth muscles, secretory glands and blood vessels of the target organs are genetically hyperactive in allergic patients and can be made hyperreactive by exaggerated stimuli in healthy individuals as well. Alternatively, the receptors on which these nerve endings act might be those that become hyperreactive. Thus the issue of the possible causes of the allergic condition remains wide open.

Anaphylaxis

We shall use the term 'anaphylaxis' to indicate hypersensitivity inducible in any individual of a given species by the appropriate antigenic challenge, and expressed by characteristic changes upon a second challenge with the same antigen. The changes, which include contraction of smooth muscles and dilation of capillaries, are caused by the release of pharmacologically active substances from mast cells and basophils after the combination of cell-bound antibodies with the antigen. The antigenic challenge inciting increased sensitivity is called *sensitization* (equivalent to 'immunization' in responses mediated by antibodies other than IgE), and the sensitizing substance is termed variously *sensitizing antigen*, *sensitizer*, *inducer*, *allergen*, or *anaphylactogen*; the substance actually evoking anaphylactic symptoms is called the *elicitor* and the immunized animal is referred to as *sensitive*, *hypersensitive* or *allergic*.

Sensitization can be accomplished in almost any manner, but for the actual response induction the antigen must be administered such that it comes into sudden contact with the sensitized tissue. Best results are achieved when the inducing dose is given intravenously or directly into the heart. To be effective, the antigen must be in soluble form. Cellular antigens, such as sheep red blood cells or bacteria, cause weak anaphylaxis. The amount of antigen required for sensitization varies widely, but for a particular situation it must fall within certain limits: too small a dose produces no response and too large a dose may result in protection instead of sensitization (see below). For the induction of anaphylactic symptoms, the *shock-inducing dose* must be considerably larger than the minimal dose needed for sensitization. It is important to allow enough time to elapse between the sensitizing dose and the inducing dose. However, the length of this interval varies greatly, depending on all the other conditions.

An animal that has survived administration of the shock-inducing dose is often temporarily refractory, in that further administration of the antigen does not produce anaphylaxis. This *desensitized state* can also be induced by administering repeated and closely spaced small-dose injections instead of a single, large shock-inducing dose. Each dose is too small to produce anaphylactic symptoms, but the repeated exposure gradually exhausts the supply of reactive antibodies. In some situations, desensitization may be caused by the preferential induction of blocking IgG instead of IgE antibodies. The desensitizing state is only temporary and, in most instances, lasts about 2 weeks, after which the state of increased sensitivity returns.

The ability to become anaphylactic has been demonstrated in birds, amphibians and fish, in addition to various mammals, and probably exists in all vertebrates; the specific form of anaphylaxis, however, varies from species to species. The main factors responsible for interspecies variation are different tissue distribution of mast cells and different contents of granules. The species in which anaphylaxis can be induced most easily and which has therefore been used in the bulk of experimental work is the guinea-pig.

The particular manifestation of the hypersensitivity state varies greatly, depending on the manner in which sensitization has been achieved and tested. The various forms can be classified according to whether sensitization occurs *in vivo* or *in vitro*, actively or passively.

Active systemic (generalized) anaphylaxis

This ensues when one injects an antigen intravenously, intraperitoneally or intradermally into an animal, and later challenges the recipient with an intravenous shock-inducing dose of the same antigen. The first injection induces IgE antibodies which then bind to tissue mast cells and basophils; the second injection provides antigen for the bridging of cell-bound IgE molecules, activation of mast cells and mediator release, leading to smooth muscle contraction and vasodilatation. The consequences of mediator release are strongest in tissues containing the largest quantities of mast cells. These differ according to species, so that each has a particular *shock organ* or organs in which the pathological changes are most pronounced. The manifestation of systemic anaphylaxis is also dependent on mast-cell distribution and composition. In guinea-pigs, administration of the shock-inducing dose leads to restlessness, ruffling of the skin, sneezing, coughing, itching, uncontrolled discharge of urine and faeces, breathing difficulty and violent convulsions, i.e. *anaphylactic shock*. The main pathological findings in such animals are constriction of bronchioles and hyperinflation of the lungs.

In humans, systemic life-threatening anaphylaxis occurs relatively rarely in genetically predisposed individuals; it can occur, for example, in response to insect venoms or to drugs such as penicillin. Penicillin contains a reactive lactam ring that forms covalent complexes with various blood plasma proteins that then elicit antibody responses. If IgE responses prevail, the patient becomes sensitized after first exposure to penicillin and anaphylaxis can occur during subsequent treatment with this drug. Anaphylactic reactions to insect venoms or drugs usually affect several organs simultaneously: skin (flushing, redness, rash, swelling), lungs (spasmodic narrowing of bronchi and laryngeal swelling), gastrointestinal tract (abdominal pains, nausea, vomiting, diarrhoea) and the circulatory system (fall in blood pressure and shock as a result of increased vascular permeability). Severe cases of anaphylaxis may result in death.

Passive systemic anaphylaxis

To induce *passive systemic anaphylaxis*, an animal is sensitized intraperitoneally against a given antigen and its serum is injected intravenously into a second animal, which is then challenged intravenously with the sensitizing antigen. The manifestations of passive systemic anaphylaxis are similar to those of active anaphylaxis. In *reversed passive anaphylaxis*, an antigen is injected intraperitoneally into an animal and the recipient is challenged intravenously 30–60 min later with serum containing IgE antibodies. Manifestations of this reaction are often shock and death.

Passive cutaneous anaphylaxis

Passive cutaneous anaphylaxis is a frequently used form of local anaphylaxis. Here, an animal is sensitized to an antigen and bled after the latent period. The antiserum is then injected intradermally into a second animal, and 4–6 hours later antigen and dye, such as Evans blue, are injected intravenously; 10 min later, blue spots appear in the skin at the injection site. In this instance, the passively administered IgE binds to mast cells in the skin and the antigen delivered by the bloodstream binds to the tissue-bound immunoglobulins. The subsequent mast-cell degranulation and mediator release cause an increase in capillary permeability and leakage of serum albumin together with the attached dye, and the area of reaction stains blue.

Active in vitro anaphylaxis (Schultz–Dale reaction)

In active *in vitro* anaphylaxis an antigen is injected into an animal that is then killed after 14 days. An organ containing a great deal of smooth muscle (e.g. small intestine, lung, tracheal ring or uterus) is removed and placed in a bath with buffered saline solution. One end of the organ is attached to the bottom of the bath and the other end is connected to a lever (Fig. 23.14). An antigen solution is then added to the bath and muscle contraction is recorded on a kymograph or polygraph.

Passive in vitro anaphylaxis

In passive *in vitro* anaphylaxis, sensitization is achieved by placing the intestine, lung or uterus of a non-sensitized animal into a bath containing serum of a sensitized animal and then incubating the bath for a period that allows binding of antibodies to the tissue. Exposure of the washed muscle to antigen solution then induces contraction of the stretched organ.

Treatment of allergic diseases

The best treatment for allergic diseases is prophylaxis, i.e. avoidance by the sensitized person of re-exposure to the sensitizing allergen. Before it can be avoided, however, the allergen must be identified by a skin test. Avoiding an allergen is relatively simple in drug and food allergies but more

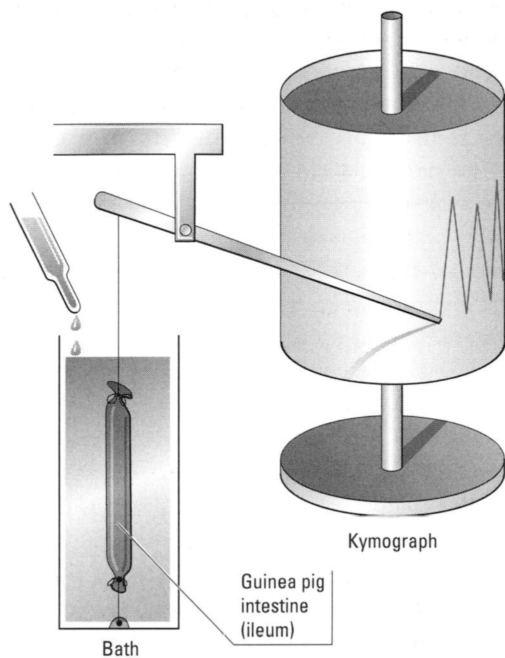

Figure 23.14 Method for measuring anaphylaxis *in vitro*. Addition of an antigen to the bath causes contraction of smooth muscles in the guinea-pig ileum, which is recorded on the kymograph drum. (Modified from Klein, J. (1982) *Immunology: The Science of Self–Nonself Discrimination*. John Wiley & Sons, New York.)

problematic in hypersensitivities to inhaled antigens. Necessary measures can include getting rid of a household pet, keeping a house relatively dust-free, installing air-conditioning or even moving to a new area. If these measures fail, it is necessary to resort to the use of medication. A large number of antiallergic drugs are now available, the different compounds which interfere with the various stages of the allergic reaction. *Antihistamines* block histamine receptors on the target cells. *Theophylline* inhibits the enzyme phosphodiesterase (which cleaves cAMP) and therefore maintains high cAMP concentration in mast cells, which inhibits degranulation. *Corticosteroids* inhibit histamine synthesis from histidine and stimulate synthesis of cAMP. *Sodium cromoglycate* increases membrane viscosity and thereby inhibits Ca^{2+} influx into mast cells.

Allergic diseases can also be treated by *immunotherapy*, the essence of which is the induction of unresponsiveness to specific allergens. Unresponsiveness can theoretically be achieved by elimination or anergization of allergen-specific T_H2 cells, by shifting the T_H1 vs. T_H2 cell balance in favour of the former by means of cytokine or cytokine antagonist treatments, by elimination of allergen-specific B cells or by inactivation of allergen-specific IgE. This last method involves the treatment of patients with antibodies specific for the Fc part of IgE antibodies; the treatment blocks IgE binding to the IgE receptor. It is thus far the only non-empirical method that has produced promising results. The empirical methods of immunotherapy involve desensitization (or rather hyposensitization) with a mixture of allergens. The patient is exposed repeatedly to this mixture, starting with low doses that do not induce a systemic allergic reaction, and increasing the dose gradually until even large doses, comparable with those to which the patient may be exposed naturally, no longer lead to allergy. Two such immunization protocols are used: perennial and preseasonal. In the *perennial method*, the patient, once made unresponsive, is kept in that state all year round by maintenance injections administered every 2–6 weeks. In the *preseasonal method*, frequent injections of increasing doses are given 3–6 months before the anticipated time of natural exposure to the allergen, such as pollen, and treatment is discontinued just before the pollen season begins. This is repeated every year. Attempts have been made to reduce the number of injections by incorporating the allergen into an adjuvant or by making it more immunogenic through chemical modification, but no encouraging results have been forthcoming.

Immunotherapy is used relatively successfully as a treatment for hay fever, allergic asthma and hymenopteran insect-sting anaphylaxis. One consequence of immunotherapy is the emergence of *blocking antibodies*, IgG antibodies specific for the allergens. They bind the allergen and thus make it unavailable to IgE antibodies, and since IgG–antigen complexes do not trigger degranulation of mast cells and basophils (or do so less efficiently) the allergic response is diminished. However, blocking by IgG antibodies is not the only positive result of immunotherapeutic treatment; it has been observed that after an initial increase, the immunizations gradually lead to a decrease in the level of IgE antibodies. Some form of partial immunological tolerance therefore seems to be induced by the treatment quite apart from the appearance of blocking antibodies. *Desensitization* of the patient is never absolute; it merely reduces the symptoms of the allergic reaction, and full symptoms eventually return after the treatment is discontinued. The empirical procedures presumably work because the allergen is presented under conditions other than those that normally result in T_H2-cell response and allergy.

Type II hypersensitivities (induced by alloimmunization and mediated by antibodies)

Type II hypersensitivities involve antibody-mediated destruction of cells, which occurs when antibodies that coat the cells either activate the classical pathway of complement or bind to Fc receptors on phagocytes and NK cells. The antibodies can arise either as a result of an autoimmune reaction or by allogeneic immunization. Antibody-mediated autoimmune diseases are dealt with in Chapter 25. A description of transfusion reactions and of one example of antibody-mediated damage resulting from feto-maternal immunization follows. The response to an allogeneic transplant is described in Chapter 24.

Transfusion reactions

It has been known since the turn of this century that humans can be classified into four *blood groups*, depending on whether their erythrocytes carry the A antigen, the B antigen, both or neither. The antigens are sugar residues at the termini of oligosaccharide chains attached to a variety of lipids, proteins and complex carbohydrates. They occur not only on erythrocytes but also on mucus secreted by several glands. Attachment of the terminal residues to the oligosaccharides is catalysed by two glycosyltransferases, products of allelic genes. The precursor structure (a trisaccharide called *substance H*, composed of *N*-acetylglucosamine, galactose and fucose) to which the terminal residues of *N*-acetylgalactosamine (the A antigen) or galactose (the B antigen) are added is controlled by a gene at another locus. The A, B and H antigens occur also in many animals, plants and microorganisms, so that throughout their lives humans are continually exposed to antigens that they do not carry. As a result, individuals of blood group A have B-specific antibodies in their blood, B-group individuals have A-specific antibodies and A-negative, B-negative individuals (blood group O) possess both A- and B-specific antibodies. Individuals of the fourth blood group, AB, being tolerant of both antigens, lack both antibodies. The antibodies are mostly of the IgM class and hence are efficient activators of the classical complement pathway. Transfusion of blood between ABO-incompatible individuals would lead to coating of the donor erythrocytes by antibodies, complement activation and haemolysis. These effects are avoided by ABO-matching of the donor with the recipient. Human erythrocytes, however, carry more than 600 other antigens and matching for all of these is neither possible nor necessary, since the corresponding human blood does not contain the corresponding *natural antibodies* to most of these. Nevertheless, antibodies specific to some of these other blood group antigens can form on repeated exposure (transfusion) of the recipient to the same antigen. Most of these antibodies are of the IgG class and so bind via their Fc parts to the Fc receptors on macrophages and via their combining sites to the antigens on erythrocytes. The macrophages then proceed to destroy the transfused erythrocytes and to elicit a *transfusion reaction* characterized by fever, anaemia and increased bilirubin level.

Haemolytic disease of the newborn

The second major system of human blood group antigens was discovered with antisera produced by the immunization of rabbits and guinea-pigs with rhesus monkey erythrocytes. The antisera were shown to agglutinate erythrocytes of some human individuals only and the antigens responsible for the reaction were designated Rh. Forty-nine of these *Rh antigens* are now known, all encoded in alleles at two closely linked loci (*RHD* and *RHCE* on chromosome 1) and all borne by protein molecules specified by the *RH* loci. The individual Rh antigens are designated by letters in one terminology and by numbers in another.

The 85% of humans who possess the RhD antigen are usually referred to as Rh^+, because D is the most prevalent of all the 49 antigens. The remaining 15% of humans are Rh^- because they lack the D antigen. In situations in which a Rh^- mother carries a Rh^+ child in her uterus, a small number of fetal red blood cells may pass into the mother's circulation, particularly during delivery when the placenta separates from the uterine wall (Fig. 23.15), and induce the formation of RhD-specific antibodies in the mother. If a significant level of Rh antibodies builds up, those of the IgG class can pass through the placenta during subsequent pregnancies, enter the fetal circulation, attack Rh^+ fetal erythrocytes and cause *haemolytic disease of the newborn*, which is characterized by severe anaemia. In an attempt to compensate for the loss of mature erythrocytes, the fetal haemopoietic system begins to release immature erythroblasts into the blood, a condition known as *erythoblastosis fetalis*. Another consequence of the attack is the accumulation of excessive amounts of fluid in fetal tissues, organs and

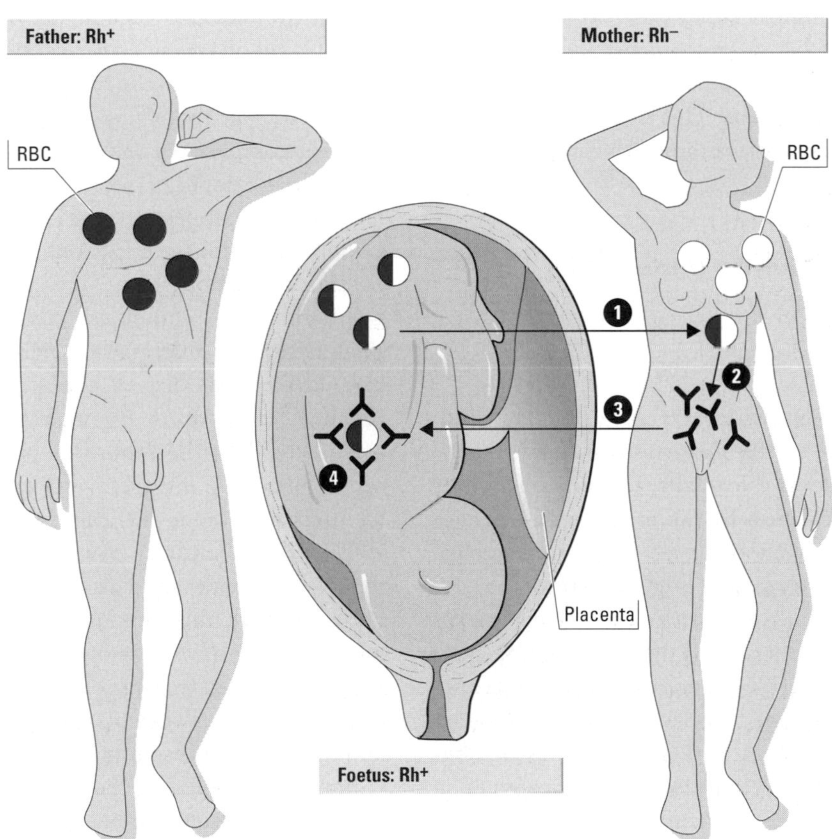

Figure 23.15 Haemolytic disease of the newborn (erythroblastosis fetalis). (1) A foetus has inherited the RhD antigen of its red blood cells (RBC) from the father; both are therefore Rh-positive (Rh^+). During the first pregnancy (delivery) some fetal RBCs enter the mother's circulation via the placenta. (2) The immune system of the mother, who is Rh-negative (Rh^-), produces antibodies (Ab) against the RhD antigen. (3) During the second pregnancy, the RhD-specific antibodies cross the placenta and attack the erythrocytes of the fetus. (Based on Ahlheim, K.-H. (Ed.) (1984) *Wie funktioniert das? Der Mensch und seine Krankheiten*. Bibliographisches Institut Mannheim, Meyers Lexikon Verlag.)

cavities, a condition referred to as *hydrops fetalis*. Futher symptoms are enlarged liver and spleen and generalized swelling. Some of the affected fetuses may be aborted, others delivered stillborn and yet others born alive but with severe defects, particularly in the central nervous system, where considerable damage is caused by the deposition of bilirubin in ganglia. Haemolytic disease of the newborn does not always develop in every Rh^- mother carrying a Rh^+ fetus. Usually the first pregnancy is not affected, but in later pregnancies, as the titre of Rh antibodies increases, the chances of haemolytic disease of the newborn also increase. A mild form of haemolytic disease of the newborn may occur in cases of RhD compatibility and ABO incompatibility between the mother and fetus.

The disease can be prevented by giving the mother anti-RhD IgG fraction intramuscularly at the time of delivery (within 60 hours). These passively administered antibodies prevent sensitization of the mother's lymphoid system and thus the production of RhD antibodies. The mechanisms of desensitization appear to be based on the negative regulatory interactions of immune complexes with both B-cell receptors and Fc receptors on antigen-specific B cells (see Chapter 17). The passively administered antibodies are then eliminated by natural decay. This treatment reduces by 95% the risk of an anamnestic response during subsequent pregnancies.

Type III hypersensitivities (induced by immune complexes)

Principle

The interaction of antigens with their corresponding circulating antibodies leads to the formation of *antigen–antibody (immune) complexes*. Normally, immune complexes are removed from circulation by the mononuclear phagocyte system, particularly in the liver (by Kupffer cells), spleen and lungs, but if formed in large quantities they are deposited in various tissues. Deposited immune complexes bind and activate complement, and the C3a and C5a fragments so generated bind to basophils in the blood and cause their degranulation. Immune complexes may also interact directly with basophils and platelets (via the immunoglobulin Fc regions) and cause their degranulation. Some of the released mediators, in particular histamine and 5-hydroxytryptamine, cause retraction of endothelial cells and so increase blood vessel permeability and lead consequently to the deposition of more immune complexes. The activated platelets aggregate and initiate the formation of small clots on the collagen of the exposed basement membrane beneath the endothelial cell. Other mediators attract neutrophils, which then attempt to phagocytose the deposited complexes. The tissue-bound complexes cannot be easily engulfed, however, and the macrophages spill their lysosomal contents over the tissue. Normally, the released lysosomal enzymes would be inactivated quickly by substances in the serum, but since the serum is to a great extent excluded from the contact zone between the phagocytes and the tissue cells, the enzymes have enough time to attack the tissue. The resulting tissue damage leads to a form of hypersensitivity that involves IgG rather than IgE antibodies. The hypersensitivity manifests itself in a characteristic tissue response described shortly.

Immune complexes are deposited preferentially in certain sites throughout the body: the kidney glomerulus, the joints, the lungs and the skin. Reasons for this preference may vary from organ to organ. The kidney accumulates immune complexes because the blood pressure in the glomerular capillaries is four times higher than in other capillaries and because the glomerulus retains immune complexes by a simple filtering effect. Similarly, immune complexes may also accumulate on other body filters: the ciliary body of the eye, where aqueous humour forms, and the choroid plexus in the brain, where cerebrospinal fluid is produced. The characteristics of the diseases that lead to immune-complex deposits may also determine the deposit site. Systemic lupus erythematosus, for example, is characterized by the appearance of DNA-specific antibodies (see Chapter 25), and since DNA has affinity for collagen in the basement membrane of the glomerulus most of the DNA–anti-DNA complexes accumulate in this organ. In rheumatoid arthritis, plasma cells produce immunoglobulin-specific antibodies in the synovium of the joint and immune complexes then initiate an inflammatory response at this site. Why the deposition of immune complexes only occurs in certain diseases is not known. Possible contributory factors include the affinity of the antibodies and the valency of the antigen (low-affinity antibodies combining with low-valency antigens may form complexes that the body has difficulty clearing); the participation of complement (binding of C3b and C3d to immune complexes solubilizes deposited complexes and the lack of appropriate complement involvement may have the opposite effect); and the nature of the antigen, as pointed out earlier.

Immune complexes form frequently in autoimmune diseases such as systemic lupus erythematosus and rheumatoid arthritis; in low-grade persistent infections such as those characterizing leprosy, malaria, African trypanosomiasis and viral hepatitis; and on repeated exposure of body surfaces, such as the lungs, to antigenic material such as pigeon antigens (leading to *pigeon fancier's disease*) or fungi from mouldy hay (leading to *farmer's lung disease*). The experimental models of these situations are the Arthus reaction and serum sickness.

Arthus reaction

In 1903, N. Maurice Arthus and Maurice Breton described an experiment in which at intervals of several days they repeatedly injected normal horse serum subcutaneously into rabbits, and after the fifth or sixth injection observed a skin reaction characterized by firm induration, swelling, abscess formation and necrosis. It was not necessary that the site of the last injection coincided with that of previous injections; the reaction could be observed at any site where the last injection was made. The phenomenon, now referred to as the *Arthus reaction*, is not peculiar to rabbits; similar reactions were also observed in guinea-pigs, rats, dogs and humans. The traditional explanation (Fig. 23.16) has been that repeated injections induce the formation of precipitating antibodies specific for horse proteins. As the antigen diffuses from the injection site through the tissue and into the regional blood vessels, it combines with the antibodies and insoluble antigen–antibody complexes form locally in the venules. These immune complexes are deposited between and beneath the endothelial cells, where they activate complement. Chemotactic factors liberated from the complement cascade attract neutrophils and platelets to the reaction site. Neutrophils adhere to the tissue-bound immune complexes via their C3 receptors (CR1) and attempt to phagocytose them. However, since the complexes are attached to a non-phagocytosable substrate (the basement membrane), phagocytosis is incomplete and the phagosome remains open to the exterior, releasing lysosomal enzymes into the surrounding medium. The enzymes attack the basement membrane and the tissue surrounding it, with collagenases disrupting collagen fibres, neutral proteases destroying the ground substance and elastases degrading elastic fibres. The proteases also generate additional C5a from C5, which initiates degranulation of neutrophils. Mediators released from the granules promote further neutrophil accumulation and degranulation. Some of the mediators act on mast cells and basophils causing their degranulation, thus further exacerbating the inflammatory reaction. Some of the complement components activated by the deposited immune complexes act on platelets, causing them to clump and to release clotting factors, and these, too, then amplify the inflammation. The extensive tissue damage manifests itself externally in local reddening, swelling and necrosis, characteristic signs of the Arthus reaction. A *reversed Arthus reaction* can be induced by administering the antibody intradermally and introducing the antigen intravenously. A *passive Arthus reaction* is induced by administering the antibody intravenously into a

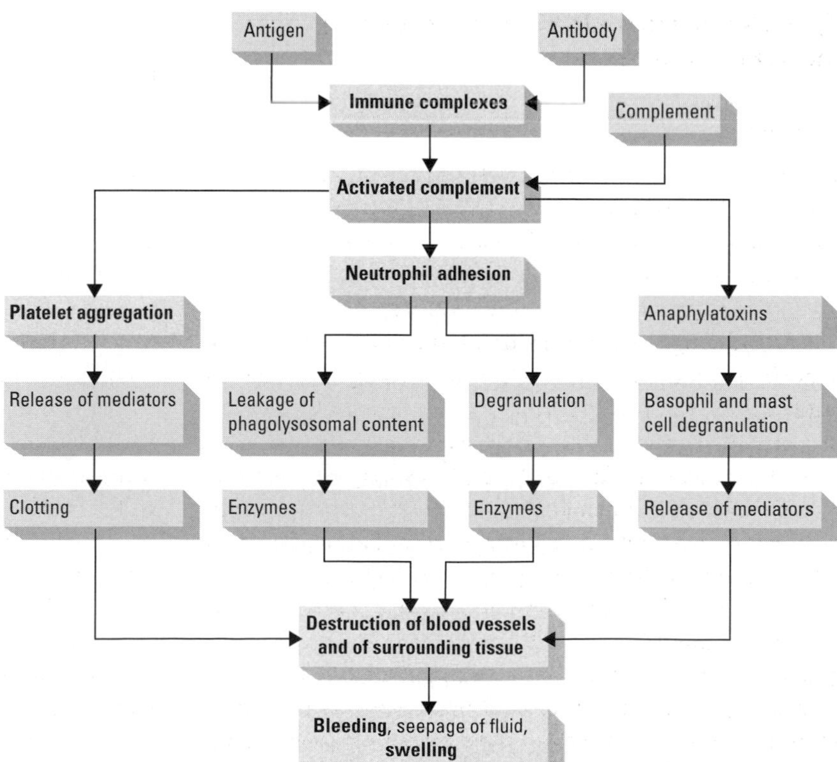

Figure 23.16 Major mechanisms leading to the Arthus reaction: traditional view. More recent results indicate that binding of immune complexes to Fc receptors on neutrophils is the primary cause of neutrophil degranulation.

non-immunized recipient and challenging this recipient by an intradermal injection of antigen.

The traditional explanation of Arthus reaction, based mostly on complement activation by immune complexes, has been challenged by recent experiments with mice in which the Fc-receptor subunit γ (a necessary component of most known Fc receptors) was eliminated by targeted gene disruption. These mice had a normally functioning complement system and responded normally to other inflammatory stimuli but they did not manifest the Arthus reaction. Hence initiation of the Arthus reaction and probably also of other forms of type III hypersensitivity is critically dependent on the activation of FcγR-bearing cells (most likely mast cells) by immune complexes, and the release of mediators attracting and activating neutrophils. Complement activation may be only a supplementary mechanism leading to a similar outcome.

Serum sickness

At the end of the nineteenth century it was realized that infectious diseases such as diphtheria could be cured by the injection of an antiserum produced in another species (e.g. horse) and specific for the bacterial toxins. The injection of xenogeneic sera into human beings therefore became a relatively common practice. It was soon noticed, however, that some of the serum recipients developed undesirable reactions, particularly when large quantities of sera were introduced (in excess of 10 ml). This *serum sickness* was characterized by the occurrence of rashes of the urticarial type commencing at the injection site, accompanied by fever, swelling of lymph nodes near the injection site and pain in the joints. In the most severe cases, particularly when serum injections were continued following the appearance of serum sickness, recipients fell into a state of shock and some died. The mechanism of serum sickness is probably similar to that of the Arthus reaction, only more generalized. The immune complexes formed by the interaction of antibodies with the serum protein antigens are deposited in blood vessels not only near the injection site but also in the kidneys, heart and joints; as a result, these organs also become involved in the reaction.

Studies on experimental animals, particularly the rabbit, led to the recognition of two forms of serum sickness, acute and chronic. *Acute serum sickness*, also referred to as *acute immune complex disease* (AICD), results from a single, intravenous injection of a large dose of xenogeneic protein antigen, such as bovine serum albumin (BSA; 250 mg/kg). As antibodies begin to form some 7 days after the injection, they combine with the antigen still circulating in the blood, thereby generating immune complexes with M_r between 300 000 and 500 000 (mostly of the Ag_2Ab type, though Ag_2Ab_2 or Ag_3Ab_2 complexes also occur; Fig. 23.17). Concurrent with the appearance of immune complexes in the circulation, characteristic lesions develop in the kidneys, blood vessels and skin, reaching a maximum at about 10 days after injection, when free antigen becomes practically undetectable in the serum. The type of lesions in the *kidney* depends on the size of immune complexes (Figs 23.18 & 23.19). If the serum contains a large antigen excess, the complexes are small and therefore pass readily not only through the endothelial layer lining the capillaries in the kidney glomerulus but also across the underlying basement membrane. The complexes thus end up outside the blood vessels under the epithelial cells that surround them. The

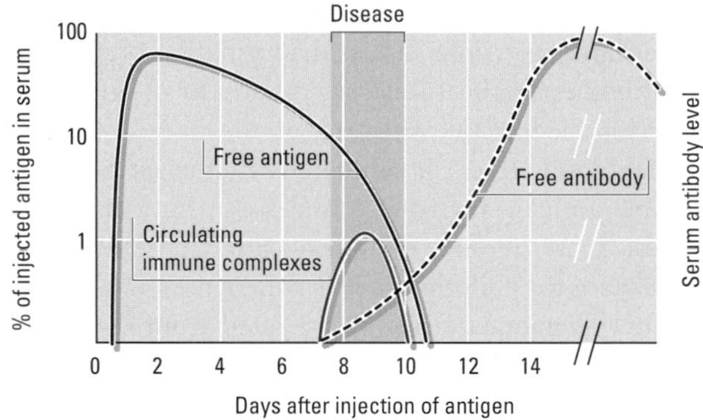

Figure 23.17 Relationship between antigen, antibodies, immune complexes and serum sickness.

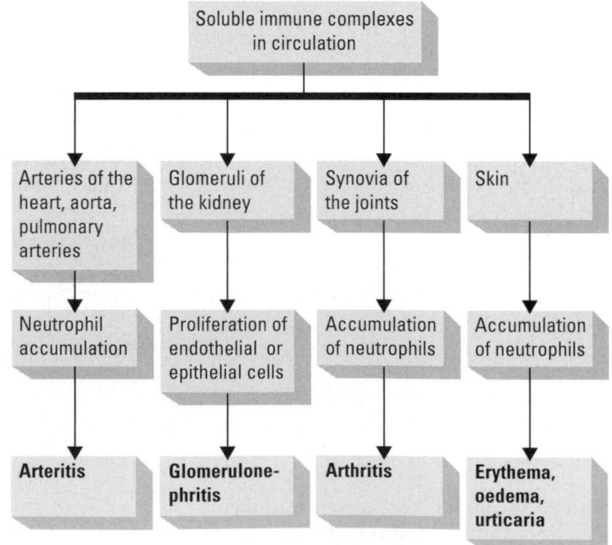

Figure 23.18 Consequences of immune-complex deposition in serum sickness.

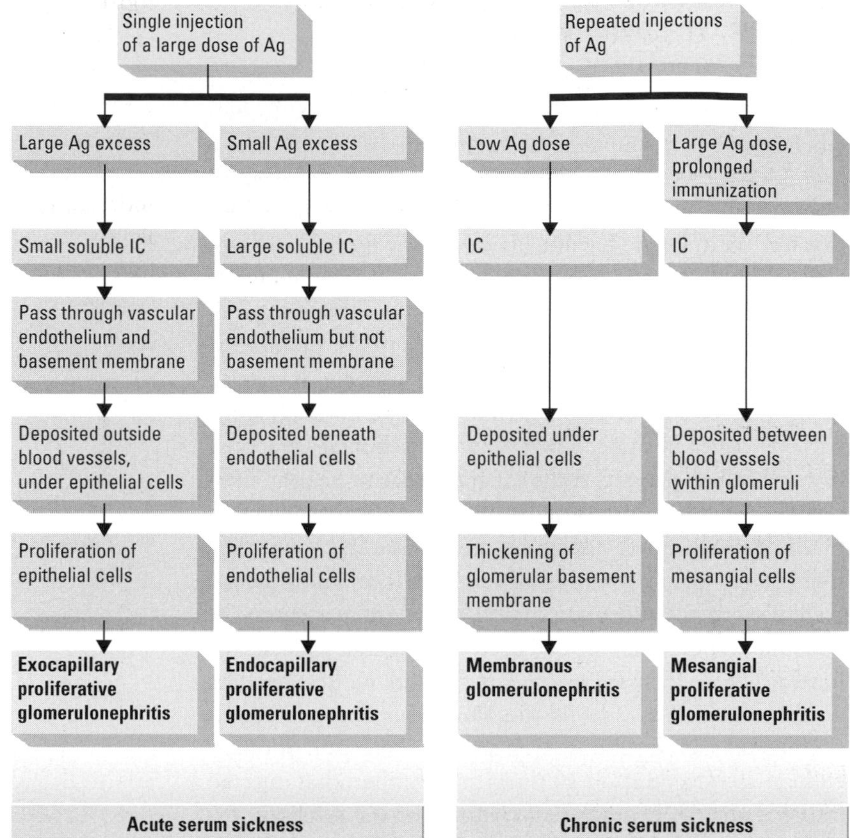

Figure 23.19 Various forms of serum sickness induced by immune-complex (IC) deposits in the kidney, depending on the antigen (Ag) dose and the immunization schedule.

immune-complex deposits stimulate the epithelial cells to swell and proliferate. On the other hand, if the serum contains a small antigen excess, the large soluble immune complexes penetrate the endothelial layer but not the basement membrane and are therefore deposited inside the blood vessels under the endothelial cells. Here again the deposits stimulate the endothelial cells to swell and proliferate. Simultaneously, the tissue-bound complexes outside and inside the blood vessel activate the complement cascade and through it initiate an inflammatory response that leads to kidney damage, i.e. to *glomerulonephritis* (Greek *nephros*, kidney). There are many kinds of glomerulonephritis associated with different diseases; the one characterized by cell proliferation is referred to as *proliferative glomerulonephritis*, and it is either *exocapillary* (characterized by proliferation of epithelial cells outside the blood vessels) or *endocapillary* (characterized by proliferation of endothelial cells inside the blood vessels). Inflammation of the kidney glomeruli disturbs their normal filtering function and leads to the appearance of proteins in the urine (proteinuria) between 8 and 11 days after the injection.

Deposition of immune complexes in the *joints*, *arteries* and *skin* may cause an Arthus-type response characterized by neutrophil accumulation and infiltration in the afflicted tissue and consequent tissue destruction. The resulting lesions in the joints lead to *arthritis* and those in the arteries to *arteritis*. Tissue destruction in the skin leads to reddening, swelling and rash.

Chronic serum sickness results from repeated injections of antigen. The main immune-complex deposit site is the kidney; joints, arteries and skin are rarely involved. The outcome (the form of glomerulonephritis) depends on the antigen level in the circulation. At low antigen doses, immune complexes are deposited mainly on the basement membrane of the blood vessels, thus leading to their thickening, characteristic of *membranous glomerulonephritis*. At high antigen doses, immune complexes penetrate the basement membrane and enter the mesangium (the tissue filling the space between the individual capillary loops) of the glomerulus, where they stimulate the proliferation of mesangial cells, characteristic of *mesangial proliferative glomerulonephritis*. Deposits of immune complexes in either acute or chronic serum sickness can be demonstrated by immunofluorescence.

Delayed-type hypersensitivity and contact sensitivity

Delayed-type hypersensitivity was discovered by Robert Koch, one of the founders of modern microbiology. While searching for a vaccine against tuberculosis, Koch extracted a number of substances from the causative agent of this disease, the tubercle bacillus *Mycobacterium tuberculosis*. One of the extracts, *tuberculin*, which was subsequently identified as a lipoprotein residing in the outer membrane of the bacillus, seemed at first a good candidate for the vaccine and Koch promoted it as such. Unfortunately, it proved later, to Koch's great embarrassment, to be nothing of the sort. However, he noticed that tuberculin elicited a response in tuberculous patients different from that in healthy individuals and suggested using the extract for early diagnosis of the disease. Koch tested his preparations by injecting them subcutaneously and observed both local and systemic responses to the inoculation in tuberculous patients. The systemic response manifested itself in fever and malaise; the local reaction consisted of a red, indurated, painful swelling at the inoculation site in the skin. Healthy individuals showed no such reactions, even after the injection of tuberculin at a concentration 10 times greater than that injected into patients. A characteristic feature of the swelling, the *tuberculin reaction*, was that it developed some 24 hours after inoculation (Fig. 23.20). Later, investigators demonstrated that the swelling was accompanied by local tissue destruction, and they classified it as one of the hypersensitivities that arise when the immune system over-reacts, causing harm to the body. It was then that the term *delayed-type hypersensitivity (DTH)* was introduced to designate this phenomenon. In the classification of hypersensitivities suggested by Coombs and Gell in 1963, DTH was designated as *hypersensitivity type IV*. Both designations are misleading, however, because DTH has very little in common with other hypersensitivities.

Following Koch's pioneering work, immunologists demonstrated a similar reaction to culture fluids from bacteria other than *M. tuberculosis* (e.g. *Salmonella typhi*, *Brucella abortus* and *Pfefferella mallei*) and to proteins of non-bacterial origin (e.g. egg-white or serum albumin). The course of the reaction was principally the same (Fig. 23.21).

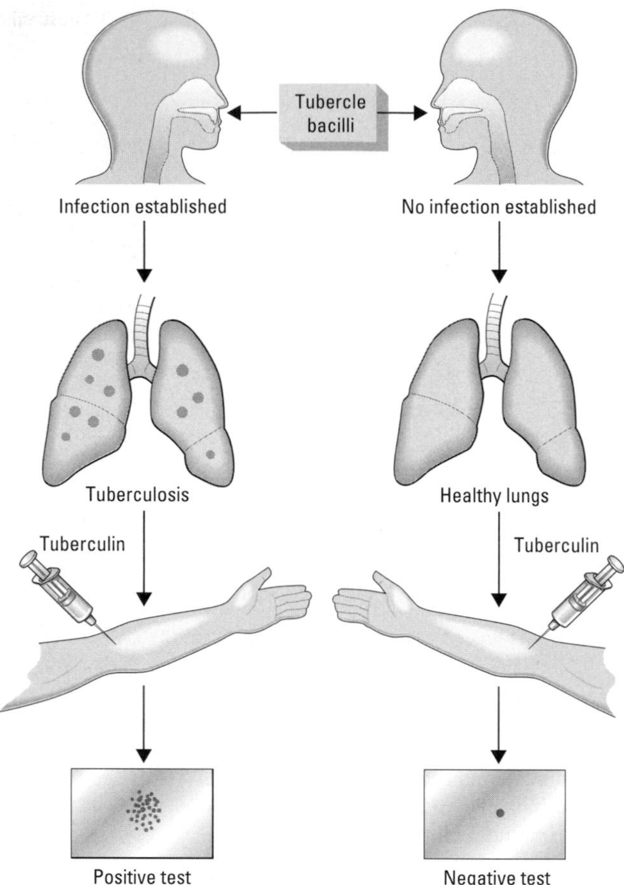

Figure 23.20 Tuberculin skin test for the delayed-type hypersensitivity reaction in individuals infected with tubercle bacilli.

Methods of detection

DTH reactions occur in individuals previously exposed (sensitized) to a given antigen. In humans, this sensitizing antigen is derived from the microorganisms responsible for the disease (e.g. tuberculin from *M. tuberculosis*, typhoidin from *S. typhi* and abortin from *B. abortus*), and sensitization occurs as a result of a chronic infection. In animals, sensitization is achieved by injection of an antigen emulsified in complete Freund's adjuvant into the skin. In both humans and animals, hypersensitivity is tested by the injection of the antigen dissolved in physiological salt solution into the skin (either intradermally or subcutaneously). In the guinea-pig, the experimental animal favoured in DTH research, immunologists test the reaction in the following way. They shave the skin and inject the antigen intradermally into the sensitized animal. They then measure the thickness of the skin fold at the injection site periodically with calipers and compare it with that of another site into which they had injected physiological salt solution without antigen. Thickening of the site of antigen injection in comparison with the control site is taken as evidence of DTH reaction.

Although sensitization for DTH always occurs *in vivo*, actual testing of the reaction can be carried out *in vitro*. One *in vitro* test is based on the observation that DTH effector

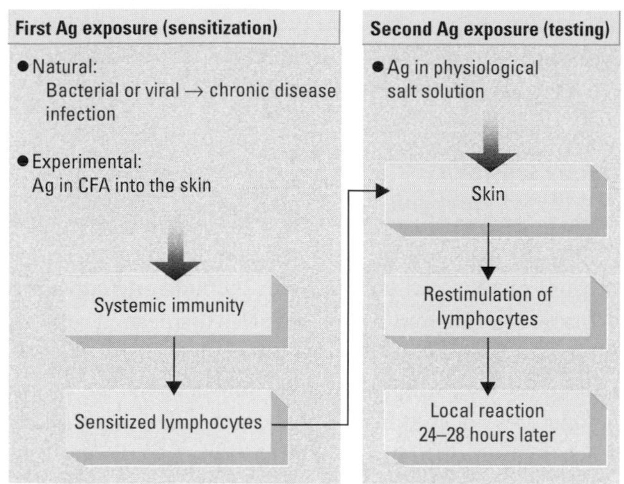

Figure 23.21 Principle of the delayed-type hypersensitivity reaction. Ag, antigen; CFA, complete Freund's adjuvant.

cells produce factors, such as lymphotoxin, that kill innocent bystander cells (i.e. cells that happen to be within the factor's action range). In this test, lymphocytes removed from mice 1 week after sensitization are added, together with antigen, to a culture of target fibroblasts. After 72 hours of incubation, the time needed for release of the factor by the lymphocytes and killing of the fibroblasts, target-cell survival is compared with that of a control culture.

Conditions for induction and detection of DTH

DTH can be induced by a wide variety of natural and synthetic proteins; decisive evidence for induction of DTH by other substances is not available. Claims that DTH can be elicited by polysaccharide injection have been made, but in none of these experiments has the presence of contaminating proteins been excluded rigorously, and whenever a pure polysaccharide was used no DTH could be obtained. Synthetic polypeptides containing L-amino acids do induce DTH, whereas those composed of D-amino acids (optical isomers absent in natural proteins) do not.

To induce DTH, a protein must be presented to the organism in a particular way. In a natural situation, some infectious diseases are accompanied by DTH and others are not, but the reason for this difference is not known. Diseases accompanied by DTH are chronic and frequently associated with the formation of granulomatous tissues. It seems that the microorganism or parasite must be able to lodge itself into a particular tissue in such a way that it provides the host with a particular type of antigenic stimulus. In an experimental situation, DTH sensitization occurs only when the sensitizing injection is given in adjuvant, preferably of the complete type.

Manifestation

DTH can manifest itself either locally or systemically. The characteristic feature of the *local reaction* is the development, within about 48 hours in humans or 24 hours in guinea-pigs, of a swelling at the site of subcutaneous or intradermal injection of the antigen. In contrast to the soft, fluid-filled swelling that accompanies some of the immediate-type hypersensitivities, swelling in the DTH skin reaction is firm because it is caused by the dense accumulation of cells at the site of injection. On subsequent days, skin in the swollen area becomes necrotic and eventually sloughs off, leaving a shallow ulcer that heals quickly. Histological examination of the swollen area reveals an accumulation of mononuclear cells, especially around small blood vessels. About 80–90% of the mononuclear cells are monocytes (the rest being lymphocytes) and this massive monocyte infiltration of the skin lesion is one of the most characteristic features of DTH. Although granulocytes can also be found in the swollen area, they are usually only a minor component of the classic DTH reaction. Mononuclear cells are brought into the skin by the bloodstream. Histological sections of lesions at later reaction stages reveal extensive tissue damage. Another local manifestation of DTH is the appearance of a milky-white opacity in the cornea of the eye. In guinea-pigs, this *corneal reaction* appears about 24 hours after the injection of antigen into the sensitized animal and it correlates well with development of the skin reaction.

The *whole-body (systemic) reaction* occurs in cases in which large quantities of the antigen enter the bloodstream. Its symptoms are fever, malaise, backache, joint pain and reduction in the number of circulating lymphocytes (lymphopenia). Severe cases of systemic reaction may result in shock, and even death, several hours after the antigen injection (as opposed to immediate hypersensitivity, in which shock occurs within minutes of antigen administration). The events leading to shock may be initiated by the combined action of immune cells and antibodies. Unsensitized individuals tolerate antigen doses many thousands of times higher than those tolerated by sensitized individuals.

Mechanism

Important information about the mechanism of DTH can be gained by the *transfer of the reaction* from sensitized to normal individuals. To this end, immunologists remove lymph node, spleen or thoracic duct cells from the sensitized animal about 1 week after sensitization and inject them intravenously into an unsensitized animal, preferably of the same strain as the cell donor. They then challenge the second recipient by intradermal injection of the antigen about 24 hours after the transfer.

These experiments have demonstrated conclusively that DTH is essentially dependent on a subset of T lymphocytes, originally called T_{DTH}. In modern terminology, they are identical to T_H1 cells. As discussed in Chapters 15 and 16, the major function of this T_H subset is to collaborate with monocytes and macrophages, so that activated macrophages are produced which effectively kill intracellular bacteria and attack larger parasites. The local manifestation of DTH after injection of the antigen is thus nothing more than the secondary (anamnestic) T_H1 cell response of the immunized individual: the antigen is picked up by skin APCs (Langerhans' cells, macrophages), its fragments are displayed on their surface bound to MHC class II molecules and are recognized by a small number of mature, fully differentiated T_H1 cells present in the body because of previous immunization. The T_H1 cells are stimulated by contact with the antigen to secrete cytokines, which act directly on the tissues *in situ* but mostly cause local inflammation characterized by the accumulation of monocytes. The accumulation is largely a response to the action of interferon-γ, which activates monocytes, stimulates their emigration from local veins to the tissue and induces them to turn into activated macrophages. The latter release lysosomal hydrolases, reactive oxygen intermediates and cytokines (IL-1, tumour necrosis factor (TNF-α)) that damage the surrounding tissue. Experimental DTH thus mimics a physiological defence reaction against an infectious agent, eliciting a response based on T_H1 cells and activated macrophages. The tissue damage characteristic of DTH contributes to the pathogenesis of diseases such as tuberculosis. The characteristic delay between the injection and the reaction occurs because it takes a relatively long time until the antigen is processed and recognized by T_H1 cells and until the monocytes accumulate in the tissue and damage it. These are all slow processes compared with the rapid mast cell degranulation following the interaction of IgE antibodies with allergen. DTH is an experimental system often used in studies of T_H1 cell-based immune mechanisms and of immune regulatory mechanisms in general. Its advantage is that DTH can be measured relatively easily and semi-quantitatively *in vivo*.

Since 1955 it has been repeatedly reported that DTH specific to various antigens can be transferred passively from a sensitized recipient by dialysable leucocyte extracts, the *transfer factor*. This was said to be of low molecular mass (a few thousand) but still exhibiting specific affinity for the antigen. Despite numerous studies and attempts (reportedly successful) to use it therapeutically, the factor's nature and even its existence remains in doubt.

Contact sensitivity

Contact sensitivity is a form of DTH in which the target organ is the skin and the response is induced by prolonged exposure or repeated contact with the inducing substance. In contrast to tuberculin-type sensitivity, a dermal reaction, contact sensitivity is predominantly epidermal.

All contact sensitivity-inducing substances have at least two features in common: a low molecular mass, which allows them to diffuse through the skin, and the ability to combine with amino acid side-chains and thus form protein conjugates. The substances are usually not immunogenic, but when bound to proteins are capable of stimulating lymphocytes. They include drugs, excretions of certain plants and industrial products, such as chromate, nickel, turpentine, varnish, various resins, cosmetics and hair dyes. One of the best-known examples of contact sensitivity-inducing plant products is urushiol from the leaves of poison ivy, *Rhus toxicodendron* (Fig. 23.22). Urushiol (from Japanese *urushi*, lacquer; a similar oil is also secreted by the Asiatic lacquer tree, *R. vernicifera*) is a mixture of non-volatile catechol derivatives. Other urushiol-secreting plants are the primrose *Primula obconica* and poison oak *Toxicodendron radicans* (Fig. 23.22). When one touches poison ivy or primrose leaves, some of the oil sticks to and then diffuses into the skin, initiating the reaction.

For experimental induction of contact sensitivity, immunologists usually use various nitro- or chloro-substituted benzenes that combine easily with proteins, e.g. trinitrophenol (TNP), dinitrochlorobenzene (DNCB) or dinitrofluorobenzene (DNFB) (Fig. 23.23). The skin of experimental animals is repeatedly 'painted' for several days with solutions of these substances. After a few weeks the reaction is tested by rubbing a small amount of the solution into the skin and then measuring the diameter of the swelling after an additional 24 hours. However, sensitization can also be accomplished by intradermal, subcutaneous, intravenous, intraperitoneal or oral administration of the sensitizing chemical. The non-cutaneous routes usually produce a good sensitizing reaction only when the chemical is applied in complete Freund's adjuvant.

A mild form of contact sensitivity is characterized by reddening (erythema) and swelling (oedema) of the skin; more severe sensitivity by the formation of blisters (vesiculation), which may break and leave raw, weeping areas. In humans, the blisters may cover the whole body except for the palms and soles, which are spared because the thickness of the

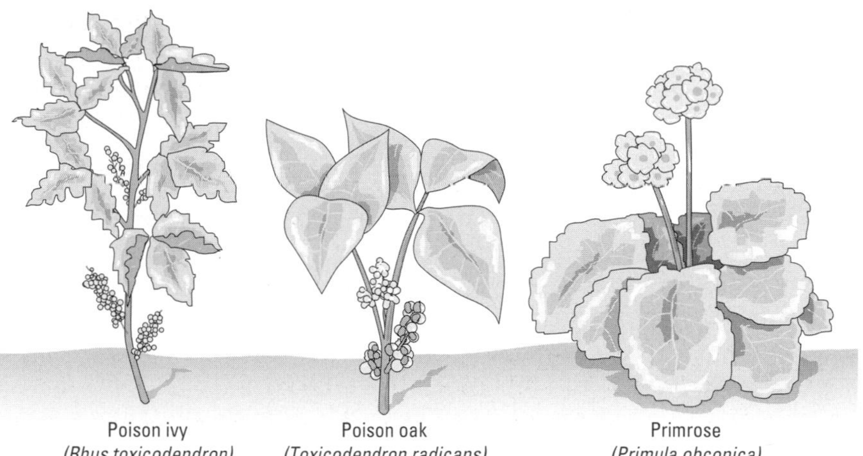

Figure 23.22 Plants whose secretions cause contact sensitivity in humans. (From Klein, J. (1982) *Immunology: The Science of Self–Nonself Discrimination*. John Wiley & Sons, New York.)

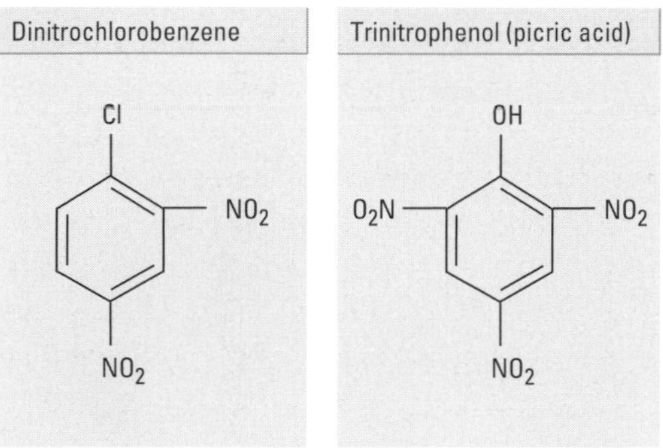

Figure 23.23 Two examples of chemicals (haptens) that can cause contact sensitivity.

cornified epithelium interferes with the penetration of sensitizing chemicals. In contrast, eyelids and genital regions, with their relatively thin skin, are usually the most susceptible areas. The lesions reach their maximum at 24–48 hours and subside over a period of several days. Severe forms of contact sensitivity are sometimes referred to as *allergic contact dermatitis* or *allergic eczematous contact dermatitis*. Prolonged exposure to the sensitizing substance may lead to a chronic condition characterized by thickening of the skin, scaling and lichenification (leathery induration).

The mechanism of contact sensitivity is essentially the same as that of classical DTH. The difference is that in the former the antigen is generated by covalent binding of the sensitizing substance to the recipient's proteins, whereas in the latter the entire antigen is of exogenous origin. The modified self proteins are processed by APCs and the peptides carrying the covalently attached hapten are recognized by T_H1 precursors. From this point on, the contact sensitivity reaction is identical to classical DTH.

As with DTH, partial or complete desensitization of sensitive individuals can be accomplished by a systemic or parenteral application of the sensitizing chemicals. However, like DTH, the desensitization is only of short duration.

Further reading

Beaven, M. A. & Baumgartner, R. A. (1996) Downstream signals initiated in mast cells by FcεRI and other receptors. *Current Opinion in Immunology*, **8**, 766–772.

Casolaro, V., Georas, S. N., Song, Z. & Ono, S. J. (1996) Biology and genetics of atopic disease. *Current Opinion in Immunology*, **8**, 796–803.

Daser, A., Meissner, N., Herz, V. & Renz, H. (1995) Role and modulation of T-cell cytokines in allergy. *Current Opinion in Immunology*, **7**, 762–770.

Huang, S.-K. & Marsh, D. G. (1993) Genetics of allergy. *Annals of Allergy*, **70**, 347–358.

Jardieu, P. (1995) Anti-IgE therapy. *Current Opinion in Immunology*, **7**, 779–782.

Marshall, J. S. & Bienenstock, J. (1994) The role of mast cells in inflammatory reactions of the airways, skin and intestine. *Current Opinion in Immunology*, **6**, 853–859.

Norman, P. S. (1993) Modern concepts of immunotherapy. *Current Opinion in Immunology*, **5**, 968–973.

Paul, W. E., Seder, R. A. & Plaut, M. (1993) Lymphokine and cytokine production by FcεRI+ cells. *Advances in Immunology*, **53**, 1–29.

Ravetch, J. V. (1994) Fc receptors: rubor redux. *Cell*, **78**, 553–560.

Romagnani, S. (1994) Regulation of the development of type 2 T-helper cells in allergy. *Current Opinion in Immunology*, **6**, 838–846.

Shirakawa, T., Li, A., Dubowitz, M. *et al.* (1994) Association between atopy and variants of the β subunit of the high-affinity immunoglobulin E receptor. *Nature Genetics*, 7, 125–129.

Sutton, B. J. & Gould, H. J. (1993) The human IgE network. *Nature*, **366**, 421–428.

Valenta, R. & Kraft, D. (1995) Recombinant allergens for diagnosis and therapy of allergic diseases. *Current Opinion in Immunology*, 7, 751–756.

Zweiman, B. (1993) The late-phase reaction: role of IgE, its receptor and cytokines. *Current Opinion in Immunology*, 5, 950–955.

chapter 24 Allograft reaction

Transplantation

Concepts

When a gardener cuts a sprout or a shoot and fixes it to a rootstock, we call this *grafting*[1] or *transplantation* (Latin *trans*, across, over; *planta*, a sprout). Surgeons have always striven to function like gardeners, and not only remove tissues and organs but replace them with tissues from other parts of the body, or better still from another individual. Over the last several decades techniques have been perfected to the degree that surgeons can now transplant virtually any tissue or organ in a manner that should in theory result in success. If the operation nonetheless often fails, it is not for want of surgical skill but because of the body's immunological attack against the transplant. Since individuals of the same species differ in their genetic constitution and therefore also in the proteins and other constituents of their bodies, a graft presents a set of foreign proteins to the recipient, which the immune system recognizes as *allogeneic antigens* and so mounts a response, an *allograft reaction*, against them. To the frustration of surgeons, this reaction often destroys the graft, no matter how perfect the grafting was. Allograft reaction is therefore an instance in which the immune system has a harmful rather than beneficial effect on the body.

Transplantation, or grafting, is the transfer of living cells, tissues or organs from one part of the body to another or from one individual to another. The transferred cells, tissues or organ is the *graft* or *transplant*. The individual who donates the graft is the *donor* and the one who receives it is the *recipient* (*host*). Grafts placed in the same anatomical position normally occupied by the tissue are *orthotopic* (Greek *orthos*, straight; *topos*, a place), whereas those placed in an unnatural position are *heterotopic* (Greek *heteros*, different). An example of a heterotopic graft is a piece of skin taken from the buttock and placed on the face. Grafts taken from and placed back on the same individual are *autogeneic* (*autografts*); grafts transplanted between genetically identical individuals (for instance, between mice of the same inbred strain) are *syngeneic* (*syngrafts* or *isografts*); grafts transplanted between genetically different individuals of the same species (for example, between two different inbred strains) are *allogeneic* (*allografts or homografts*); and finally, grafts transplanted between individuals of two different species are *xenogeneic* (*xenografts* or *heterografts*).

The fate of a graft is determined by the genetic relationship between donor and host. Each species has a set of *histocompatibility* (*transplantation*) *genes* coding for

[1] The word 'graft' is probably derived from Latin *graphium*, a stylus, and refers to the fact that the shoot is often sharpened into the form of a stylus before it is attached to the rootstock.

histocompatibility (*transplantation*) *antigens* that determine compatibility or incompatibility of tissue transplants. In general, grafts exchanged between animals that do not differ in their histocompatibility genes are *accepted* (i.e. they heal in place and survive indefinitely), whereas those transplanted between individuals differing in their histocompatibility (*H*) genes are *rejected* (destroyed). Rejection is brought about by the *allograft reaction*, the immune response against histocompatibility antigens. The complex of immunological phenomena leading to the rejection of grafts in unsensitized recipients is the *first-set reaction*; immunological response to a graft by a sensitized recipient is the *second-set reaction*. Depending mainly on the speed, but also on other characteristics, immunologists distinguish three types of graft rejection. *Hyperacute rejection* is the destruction of the graft within hours or even minutes of transplantation. *Acute rejection* is the destruction of the graft within the first few days after grafting. Finally, *chronic rejection* is a slow, gradual destruction of the graft extending over weeks or even months after transplantation.

In most situations, the allograft reaction is a one-way process: the host reacts against the graft, but the graft cannot react against the host (*host-vs-graft reaction* or HVGR). In some situations, however, grafts containing significant numbers of immunocompetent lymphoid cells mount a *graft-vs-host reaction* (GVHR), which may occur simultaneously with HVGR.

An important quantitative measure of the allograft reaction is the *survival time*. Even when transplanted under exactly the same conditions, across the same H-antigen difference and to genetically homogeneous recipients, all grafts are not rejected at the same time. Rejection is influenced by many environmental factors, which cause some grafts to be rejected sooner than others. The range of individual survival times can vary from a few days in the case of strong H antigens to several months in the case of weak H antigens. It has therefore become customary to express the length of graft duration in terms of the *median survival time (MST)*, i.e. the time between transplantation and rejection of 50% of the grafts.

Genetics of graft rejection

The primary genetic rule of transplantation is that *a graft is rejected whenever it possesses H antigens absent in the recipient*. This rule can be expanded into five *laws of transplantation*.

- Grafts within an inbred strain (syngeneic grafts) succeed.
- Grafts between different inbred strains (allografts) fail.
- Grafts from either inbred parent strain to the F_1 hybrid succeed, but grafts in the reverse direction fail.
- Grafts from F_2 or subsequent F generations to the F_1 hybrid succeed.
- Grafts from either inbred parent strain succeed in some members of an F_2 generation, but fail in others. Also, grafts from one inbred parent strain succeed in some members of a back-cross generation produced by crossing the F_1 hybrid to the opposite parent strain, and fail in others.

The laws are based on the assumption that *H* genes are co-dominant so that an F_1 hybrid expresses both alleles at each *H* locus. This assumption is supported by a large body of experimental data.

There are several exceptions to the rules, the most important being that they do not apply to transplantation between individuals of different sexes. Since both the Y and X chromosomes code for H antigens, the presence of sex-linked histocompatibility genes must be taken into account in a grafting experiment. To allow for sex difference, the transplantation laws must be modified as follows.

- Within an inbred strain, grafts from females to males succeed, whereas grafts from males to females may be rejected.
- Grafts from the female parent to a male or female F_1 recipient succeed, whereas grafts from the male parent to a male or female F_1 recipient may be rejected.

Histocompatibility antigens

Allograft reaction is stimulated by antigens expressed on the cell surfaces of the graft, the *histocompatibility antigens*. Both donor and recipient carry the same *H* loci but may differ by carrying different alleles at these loci, which translate into different protein variants. Mutational differences between corresponding alleles can determine that the donor has an epitope on a given protein different from that of the recipient and the epitope is then recognized by the recipient's immune system in the HVGR (the opposite situation occurs in the GVHR).

Histocompatibility antigens fall into two categories, major and minor. The *major histocompatibility loci* are nearly all found in a single chromosomal region, the *major histocompatibility complex* (*MHC*); the *minor histocompatibility* (*MIH*) *loci* are scattered all over the genome. Both major and minor H antigens can cause graft rejection but they do so at different speeds. A difference between the donor and the recipient at the *MHC* usually leads to rapid rejection of the exchanged grafts, whereas a difference at a single minor *H* locus usually leads to slow rejection, although the combined effect of several minor *H* loci may lead to a rejection as rapid as that elicited by an *MHC* disparity. The vigorousness of allograft reaction, however, is a highly unnatural criterion for classifying antigens and brings together elements that in reality are totally unrelated.

Elucidation of the biological function of the MHC (see Chapter 6) has led to an understanding of the difference between MHC and MIH antigen function in graft rejection. If the graft and recipient differ in allelic forms of their MHC proteins, the cells of the graft will display a large number of peptide–MHC molecule assemblages that differ from those expressed on the recipient's cells. The many complexes will be recognized by numerous T-cell clones (called *alloreactive T lymphocytes*; see later in this chapter) and the recipient's immune response will appear to be strong. A single minor H antigen, on the other hand, usually represents a single amino acid difference from the recipient's corresponding protein. It will therefore generate only one or very few peptide–MHC molecule assemblages and stimulate very few T-cell clones so that the response will appear to be weak. However, if donor and recipient differ in several MIH antigens, a number of peptides bound to MHC molecules will be generated, many T-cell clones will be stimulated and the graft will be rejected rapidly.

Over 50 *MIH* genes have been identified, scattered over the entire mouse genome. Very few have so far been cloned and identified. One of these well-characterized MIH antigens is the *H-Y antigen* (histocompatibility antigen controlled by the Y chromosome), which is responsible for the rejection of male grafts by female recipients of the same inbred strain. The H Y antigen is identical to the product of the *Smcy* gene (selected mouse cDNA on the Y chromosome), coding for a ubiquitously expressed intracellular, evolutionarily conserved protein of relative molecular mass (M_r) 170 000 whose function is not known. The SMCY protein is 85% identical to the product of another ubiquitously expressed gene (expressed both in male and female tissues), *Smcx*. At least one undecapeptide derived from the SMCY protein, which differs from the homologous SMCX protein fragment, binds to some MHC proteins (e.g. human HLA-B7) and can be recognized by alloreactive T lymphocytes. In some mouse inbred strains male grafts succeed in female recipients probably because some MHC proteins do not bind any peptides originating from the SMCY protein.

Another human MIH antigen called HA-2 has been identified as a complex of the MHC protein HLA-A2.1, with a nonapeptide derived from a polymorphic region of one species of myosin.

Mechanisms of allograft reaction

The recipient's immune system perceives the graft as though it were an infected part of its own body. Consequently, all immune mechanisms involved in antiparasite immunity may also participate in graft rejection. The major difference is that most grafts, in contrast to parasites, also contain antigen-presenting cells (APCs) and other cells that may contribute to the reaction.

Sensitization

Principally, there are two ways in which host lymphocytes become exposed to and sensitized by graft antigens. These are exemplified by two kinds of transplant, skin and kidney, the former a popular experimental system and the latter a common clinical model. In the *skin-grafting* procedure, a patch of recipient skin is replaced by a similarly shaped patch of donor skin. At the beginning, the graft does not contain any functioning blood vessels but is in close contact with the lymphatic capillaries of the host's underlying tissue, and the extended wound area itself stimulates lymphatic flow. Unprimed lymphocytes are brought with the blood to the wound area and encounter H antigens on APCs (dendritic cells, macrophages, vascular endothelial cells) present in the graft. Activated lymphocytes leave the graft with the lymph and enter the nearest (regional, draining) lymph node, where they begin to proliferate and differentiate. Some APCs also migrate to the draining lymph nodes and there activate cytotoxic T (T_C) and helper T (T_H) cells. Maturing effector cells leave the node with lymph, enter the thoracic duct and the bloodstream, and are brought with blood back to the graft. Once the blood supply has been re-established to the graft, lymphocytes invade the transplant. Some lymphocytes leave the blood vessels, enter the parenchyma and begin to proliferate directly in the graft. This pathway of sensitization is called *peripheral* because it mainly involves the graft and regional lymph nodes.

The APCs of the recipient also contribute to the development of the allograft reaction: cell debris generated in the graft is phagocytosed by the recipient's macrophages or dendritic cells, the graft-derived proteins are processed and the resulting peptides displayed on the recipient's MHC molecules where they are recognized by the recipient's T lymphocytes. Some graft-derived proteins are also recognized by antigen-specific receptors of the recipient's B lymphocytes which, upon receiving the necessary signals from activated T_H cells, differentiate into plasma cells and produce antibodies.

In contrast to a skin graft, in which vascularization is delayed and established only by the ingrowth of the recipient's blood vessels, in *kidney grafts* the major blood vessels are sutured together with those of the recipient so that the transplanted organ presents a large surface area of donor epithelium to the blood cells of the host (Fig. 24.1).

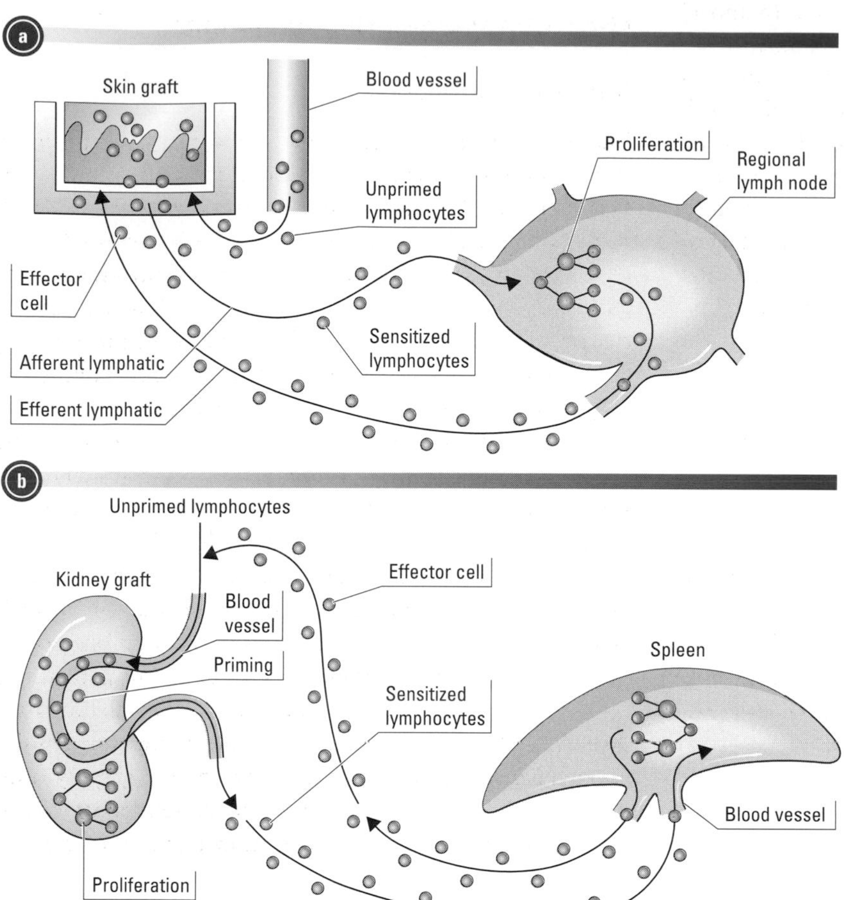

Figure 24.1 Two pathways of sensitization in the allograft reaction. (a) Peripheral pathway. (b) Central pathway. (Modified from Klein, J. (1986) *Natural History of the Major Histocompatibility Complex*. John Wiley & Sons, New York.)

Unprimed lymphocytes are brought into the kidney graft in blood vessels and encounter antigen on the lining endothelial cells. Most of the lymphocytes are transported with the blood to the spleen, but some leave the blood vessels and enter the kidney parenchyma. These migrating cells then either re-enter capillaries and, like the bulk of lymphocytes, are brought into the spleen, or they remain in the parenchymal interstices because their normal return route through lymphatics draining the organ is blocked. If they encounter the antigen on efficient APCs, which provide the necessary co-stimulatory signals, they may then proliferate in the kidney and develop into effector cells directly in the organ. Most sensitized lymphocytes, however, end up in the spleen where they undergo further development. The lymphocytes enter the marginal zone, which is a region rich in fixed macrophages required (as APCs) for functional maturation of the sensitized cells. The lymphocytes then enter the periarteriolar lymphoid sheath where they proliferate. Potential effector cells leave the spleen via sinuses and enter the bloodstream, which eventually brings them back into the kidney graft. This pathway of sensitization is called *central*.

Graft destruction

The allograft reaction has two components, non-specific and specific. The *non-specific component* is the recipient's response to the surgical trauma of the grafting procedure. It is the same kind of response as that induced by a splinter lodged in a finger or by an abrasive wound on the knee. The series of changes that occur in the tissue following an injury represent *inflammation,* characterized by an invasion of *inflammatory cells* from the bloodstream into the wound. These cells are of two kinds, polymorphonuclear and mononuclear leucocytes. The cellular response is accompanied by the liberation of a number of mediators such as serotonin, Hageman factor, plasmin, kinin, and many others. All these substances contribute to wound healing (see Chapter 21).

The non-specific component is common to all graft responses; it also occurs after the transplantation of autologous or syngeneic tissues. The *specific component*, on the other hand, is characteristic of the reaction against allogeneic and xenogeneic grafts. Executors of the attack are cells (cellular immunity) and soluble factors (humoral immunity). The *specific cellular response* is initiated by T lymphocytes activated by graft antigens but it also involves natural killer (NK) cells, neutrophils and other cells. Both T_C and T_H1 cells participate in the response: T_C cells use their perforin- and Fas-based cytotoxic mechanisms to attack and destroy graft cells; T_H1 cells initiate the inflammatory reaction of delayed-type hypersensitivity, leading to the recruitment of monocytes and macrophages into the graft. NK cells, presumably alerted by the absence in the graft of MHC molecules present in the recipient, may also attack the graft in the early phase of the response. Neutrophils are mainly responsible for clearing the wound or removing damaged cells and cellular debris in the late phase of the allograft reaction.

The *humoral immune response* against the graft is initiated by antibodies, which contribute in several ways to graft destruction. They bind to graft cells and their Fc parts interact with the Fc receptors of macrophages, neutrophils and NK cells. Activated macrophages and neutrophils phagocytose some of the graft cells and spill toxic substances over others. NK cells kill graft cells attached to them via the antibody–Fc receptor bridge. Antibodies also activate the complement cascade and the products of this activation opsonize target cells for phagocytosis, induce the release of histamine from mast cells and hydrolytic enzymes from neutrophils, attract granulocytes and monocytes into the graft, and activate Hageman factor of the blood clotting pathway (the factor can be activated directly, however, by endothelial cell damage; see Chapter 21).

Immune complexes formed by antibodies and soluble antigens or membrane fragments also contribute to blood clotting. Massive clots in the capillaries cause an immediate infarction of the organ, leading to hyperacute rejection of the graft. (Hyperacute rejection occurs when the recipient has pre-existing serum antibodies against graft antigens, such as those against the ABO blood group or MHC antigens.) Hageman factor induces the generation of kinin, which further increases vascular permeability and promotes the accumulation of fluid in the tissues and thus the formation of oedemas.

The activated complement cascade may also terminate in the assemblage of the membrane attack complex, leading to osmotic lysis of the cell. This type of damage is probably only of minor importance, however, because nucleated cells possess several mechanisms that protect them from complement lysis. Together, these complex changes ultimately lead to resolution of the grafted tissue—rejection of the transplant.

Organ transplantation in humans

Kidney transplantation

The main causes of kidney failure are glomerulonephritis (inflammation of the glomeruli), pyelonephritis (inflammation of the renal pelvis, the funnel-shaped structure in which urine is collected from the tubuli before it is carried on to the ureter and into the bladder) and polycystitis (the formation of multiple cysts of varying size). Any of these three diseases may lead to irreversible damage of the kidney tissue, the parenchyma, and if that happens to both kidneys the only two ways of keeping the patient alive are regular haemodialysis or kidney transplantation. *Haemodialysis* consists of passing the patient's blood through a *haemodialyser (artificial kidney)*, an apparatus used to remove toxic wastes accumulating in the blood. Although a patient can live for a long time totally dependent on the artificial kidney, his or her life can hardly be considered normal. Under these circumstances, kidney transplantation is often a welcome alternative because, if successful, the patient can return to a more-or-less normal life. The two methods are complementary, however, because most patients require initial haemodialysis before they are fit for surgery and, furthermore, if rejection occurs the patient must return to haemodialysis until a new transplantation can be performed.

The two sources of kidney grafts are cadavers and living donors. In the former, the kidney must be removed immediately after the donor has been pronounced clinically dead and must be submerged promptly in a physiological salt solution cooled to 4 °C. The kidney is then perfused with a preservation fluid, which is pumped into the renal artery until the venous effluent is clear and the kidney cortex pale. The perfused kidney is placed into a sterile bag containing a physiological salt solution and packed in ice in a thermally insulated container. Machines are now available that carry out these perfusion–preservation steps automatically. The kidney from a living donor is infused to promote discharge of urine, cooled and transplanted immediately.

During the operation, both of the recipient's kidneys are removed to preclude the danger of the disease spreading from the affected kidney to the transplant. One of the kidneys is then replaced by the graft: the main blood vessels of the graft and the recipient are connected and the ureter of the graft is implanted into the recipient's bladder.

Kidneys can be transplanted between family members (a living donor provides one of his or her kidneys to the patient) or between unrelated individuals (cadaveric donors). The influence of *HLA* matching is different in these two situations. If we designate the paternal *HLA* haplotypes a and b and the maternal haplotypes c and d, then the donor and the recipient within a single family can be matched for two haplotypes (e.g. $a/d \rightarrow a/d$), one haplotype (e.g. $a/d \rightarrow a/c$) or no haplotype (e.g. $b/d \rightarrow a/c$). In this situation, matched haplotypes mean identical alleles at all loci rather than similar alleles at some loci. The survival rate of grafts correlates with the degree of *HLA* identity: the longest-surviving grafts are those matched for two haplotypes, followed by those matched for only one haplotype, and the shortest surviving are those mismatched for both haplotypes (Fig. 24.2). However, even among completely mismatched grafts, 80–90% are still functioning 1 year after transplantation. These results indicate that the *HLA* complex is the most important, but not the only, genetic factor determining the survival rate of a kidney transplanted between related individuals. Other factors are presumably the non-*HLA* histocompatibility loci for which complete matching is a practical impossibility. However, the effect of these minor H antigens can be controlled by immunosuppressive therapy, as discussed at the end of this chapter.

HLA matching between unrelated individuals influences the outcome of kidney transplantation less markedly. Some surgeons are so unimpressed by the effect that they prefer to match recipients for sex, age and health status, rather than for *HLA*. The main reason for the difference is that *HLA* haplotypes matched between related individuals are truly identical, whereas those matched between unrelated individuals are usually merely similar. So great is the *HLA* allelic and haplotypic polymorphism that to find identical haplotypes among unrelated individuals is extremely difficult. Nevertheless, even in kidney transplantation from unrelated donors, grafts matched as closely as possible in their *HLA* haplotype with the recipient have a clearly better chance of long-term survival (Fig. 24.2). While 75% of grafts with no mismatches in HLA-A, -B and -DR from the recipient survive for at least 3 years, only 65% survive for this period if they are fully mismatched. The benefits of HLA matching are even less in case of organs such as the heart.

Transplantation of other organs

In addition to the kidney, many other organs have been transplanted in humans: liver, lung, spleen, pancreas, intestine, tendon, bone, cartilage, blood vessels, larynx, cornea, skin, heart and bone marrow (Fig. 24.3). The success rate has been variable but generally lower than in the case of kidney (with the exception of cornea). Over 20 000 kidney, about 5000 liver and some 3000 heart transplantations are performed each year worldwide, the 5-year success rate being 70–80%, 40–50% and 60–70%, respectively.

Bone marrow transplantation is the treatment of choice for some inborn or acquired deficiencies of haemopoiesis, immunodeficiencies and leukaemia. Its aim is to replace the malfunctioning haemopoietic system of the recipient by functional stem cells capable of restoring normal haemopoiesis. Though technically simple, bone marrow transplantation presents a formidable immunological problem: not only is the graft highly vulnerable to attack by the host's immune system, but some of the bone marrow cells, mainly T lymphocytes, can also attack the host. This graft-vs-host response is discussed later in this chapter. The HVGR can in most cases be eliminated by heavy irradiation, which completely destroys all the patient's immunocompetent and stem cells. Severe GVHR is best prevented

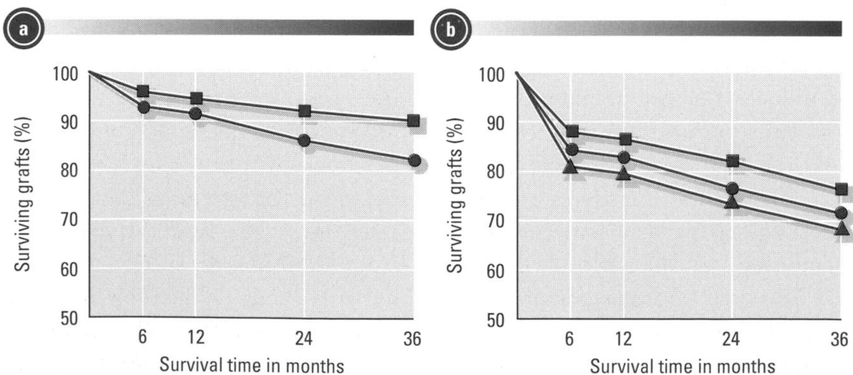

Figure 24.2 Survival of human kidney graft. (a) Related donors: upper curve, match in both haplotypes; lower curve, match in one haplotype (three HLA molecules). Data on cases where both haplotypes are mismatched are difficult to obtain, as very few such transplantations are performed. (b) Unrelated donors: upper curve, no or one mismatch; middle curve, three mismatches; lower curve, six mismatches. (Based on Suthanthiran, M. & Strom, T. B. (1994) *New England Journal of Medicine*, **331**, 365.)

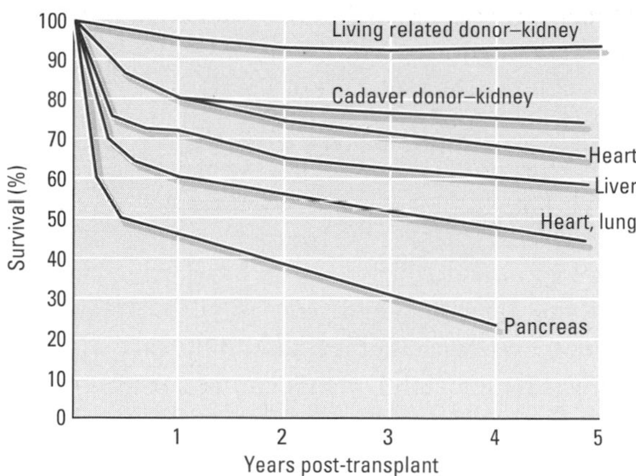

Figure 24.3 Survival of organ grafts. (Modified from Shell, A. G. R. (1987) *Transplantation Proceedings*, **19**, 2782.)

by *HLA* matching and effective immunosuppression. Another possibility is to purge the graft of immunocompetent cells with the help of monoclonal antibodies that bind to mature lymphocytes and their precursors but not to stem cells. Antibody-coated cells can be removed, for example by complement lysis or the paramagnetic bead method (see Chapter 5). Of course, an ideal solution would be to have a method for isolation of stem cells free of more differentiated T cells, or even to have a method for *in vitro* expansion of these stem cells before transplantation. The difficulty with these methods is that the number of pluripotent stem cells is very small and their biology is poorly understood.

Xenotransplantation

The major obstacle in human organ transplantation is the lack of suitable donors. An obvious way of overcoming this difficulty is to use animal instead of human donors. The donor species can be evolutionarily either relatively close (*concordant*, e.g. great apes or baboons) or distant (*discordant*, e.g. pigs). The problem with this approach, however, is that such *xenogeneic transplantation (xenotransplantation)*, especially in the case of discordant donor species, often leads to hyperacute rejection caused by natural antibodies reactive mainly with carbohydrate antigens of xenogeneic cells. The main targets of these antibodies, the endothelial cells of the graft blood vessels, are rapidly destroyed by complement-mediated attack. If it were possible to eliminate hyperacute rejection, there is a good chance that the rest of the rejection reaction could be controlled by immunosuppressive drugs. Moreover, host T cells might have certain problems in attacking xenogeneic cells, since some of the T-cell adhesion and signalling molecules needed for T-cell stimulation and effector functions appear to be species specific in that they do not bind well to xenogeneic receptors. One possibility of solving the hyperacute rejection problem is to produce transgenic pigs lacking the targeted carbohydrate antigens on their endothelial cells, or pigs expressing large numbers of molecules capable of blocking complement activation. Yet another possibility is to find effective inhibitors of natural antibodies or to block their synthesis. The potential danger of xenotransplantation is that grafts might introduce into the human population new viruses with potentially devastating effects.

Privileged sites

Certain sites in the body offer special privileges to a graft by protecting it from the allograft reaction. Grafts placed in these *privileged sites* survive longer than those at other sites, sometimes permanently. The sites include the anterior chamber of the eye, cheek pouch of the Syrian hamster, brain, cornea, retina of the eye, cartilage, testicle, ovary, prostate, mammary and subcutaneous fat pads, matrix of hair follicles, pregnant female uterus and placenta. It was once thought that these sites owed their privileged status to their isolation from the immune system. Some of these sites possess blood–tissue barriers, which are difficult to penetrate by cells of the immune system, and lack lymphatic drainage. It is now known, however, that this explanation is an oversimplification and that privileged sites are protected not only by barriers but also by active mechanisms. Antigenic materials introduced into privileged sites, such as the anterior chamber of the eye, elicit a systemic state of immunity characterized by the absence of elements responsible for inflammatory responses (T_H1 cells and complement-fixing antibodies) and by the stimulation of T_H2-cell responses. This phenomenon has been termed *anterior chamber-associated immune deviation (ACAID)*. It has been proposed that after injection of antigen into the eye, intraocular dendritic cells pick up the antigen and deliver it via blood to the splenic white pulp where MHC class I-restricted, $CD8^+$, antigen-specific regulatory and effector T cells are activated. The cytokine products of these regulatory cells (interleukin (IL)-4, IL-10, transforming growth factor-β (TGF-β)) then inhibit activation of T_H1 cells. The reason this type of T cell is stimulated and not the T_H1 cells apparently has to do with the cytokine microenvironment of the white pulp, possibly created by dendritic cells arriving from the eye.

Privileged sites should be distinguished from *privileged tissues*. The former are body regions in which grafts of foreign tissue survive longer than in non-privileged sites. Privileged tissues resist immune rejection even when grafted into conventional (non-privileged) sites. For example, testis cells grafted from C57BL/6 mice into the renal capsule, a non-privileged site, of genetically disparate BALB/c mice survive indefinitely.

Mechanisms that enable privileged tissues to escape destruction by allograft reaction include concealment of their surface under a layer of proteoglycans, strongly reduced expression of classical MHC glycoproteins and secretion of immunosuppressive cytokines and corticosteroids. Liver, which in a sense is also an immunoprivileged organ, produces soluble MHC class I molecules that may bind to antigen-specific T cells and anergize them.

Another mechanism that protects both privileged sites and privileged tissues is based on cunning use of the Fas ligand. Activated T lymphocytes express on their surfaces the 'death receptor' Fas. However, the cells of privileged tissues, such as Sertoli cells of the testes or cells of the anterior eye chamber, express the Fas ligand (FasL) which, when bound to the Fas receptor, causes the T lymphocyte to self-destruct. Thus, when T cells attempt to kill cells of the privileged tissue, they receive instead a signal to undergo apoptosis. The effect of FasL has been demonstrated conclusively in experiments with mice bearing the *gld* mutation, which do not express FasL. Testis cells of these mice are rapidly rejected when transplanted into genetically disparate mice and the privileged status of the anterior eye chamber of *gld* mice is compromised.

The existence of mechanisms that prevent inflammatory responses in immunologically privileged sites and tissues makes sense from the evolutionary point of view because such responses would have fatal consequences in organs such as the gonads, the central nervous system or the eye. These sites have instead evolved to use protection mechanisms based largely on non-inflammatory humoral and non-adaptive responses. For example, in the brain a dense network of macrophage-like *microglial cells* appears to be the major system eliminating damaged cells and protecting the organ from infections.

Surgeons have been quick to take advantage of privileged sites and to use them to achieve long-term survival of transplants. Thus corneal grafts are among the most successful transplants that, without immunosuppression, survive even in genetically incompatible donor–recipient combinations. The privileged status of the brain is currently being explored in attempts to correct conditions such as Parkinson's disease, in which there is a defect in the production of brain neurotransmitters. Small (fetal) allogeneic brain fragments implanted in the brain not only survive but continue secreting neurotransmitters. The effectiveness of this procedure for treatment of Parkinson's disease is, however, highly controversial.

In vitro correlates of the allograft reaction

Mixed lymphocyte reaction

Immunologists and cell biologists have long known that lymphocytes are difficult to grow *in vitro*. At some point they noticed, however, that it made a difference whether the culture was set up from lymphocytes of a single individual or whether it was a mixture of lymphocytes from two different individuals. In the former instance, the lymphocytes all died within a few days; in the latter, they not only stayed alive but some even eventually divided. Before dividing, however, cells in this *mixed lymphocyte (leucocyte) culture* (MLC) underwent changes characteristic of mitogen- or antigen-stimulated lymphocytes, such as an increase in the synthesis of proteins, RNA and DNA and enlargement into blasts (*blast transformation*). It became obvious that the cells were undergoing *mixed lymphocyte (leucocyte) reaction* (MLR), the response of lymphocytes from one individual to antigens on the lymphocytes of the other individual. The three hallmarks of the response are synthesis of macromolecules, blast transformation and proliferation. Later, it could also be demonstrated that the cells need not come from different individuals: under certain circumstances, lymphocytes can respond to other cells from the same individual. Depending on the genetic relationship of the cells in the mixture, we can therefore distinguish allogeneic, xenogeneic, syngeneic and autogeneic (autologous) MLR. The first of these four has been studied most extensively because immunologists expected it to provide a rapid test predicting donor–recipient compatibility for organ transplantation. This expectation has been borne out only to a certain degree.

In *allogeneic MLR*, T lymphocytes of individual A recognize, via their antigen-specific receptors, MHC molecules on the cells of individual B, and are thereby stimulated. In an A + B mixture of untreated cells, A cells respond to B antigens and B cells respond to A antigens, producing a *two-way MLR*. To turn this complex response into a simpler *one-way reaction* in which only A cells respond to B antigens, lymphocytes derived from individual B must be prevented from responding. The three principal ways of achieving a one-way MLR are, first, by using a mixture of parental and F_1 cells (the F_1 cells cannot respond to the parental cells but the parental cells can respond to antigens of the F_1 cells inherited from the other parent); second, by mixing tolerant B cells with non-tolerant A cells; and third, by inactivating B cells in such a way that they stay alive but are unable to divide. The two commonly used methods of cell inactivation are X-ray irradiation and mitomycin C treatment. *X-rays* break DNA strands and thus interfere with normal mitotic divisions. *Mitomycin C*, an antibiotic derived from *Streptomyces caespitosus*, cross-links DNA strands and thus prevents their separation during replication. Both X-irradiated and mitomycin-treated cells are activated but progress in their cycle only as far as the S phase and then stop. They stay alive long enough to stimulate the untreated cells. In a one-way MLR, untreated cells are the *responders* and inactivated cells the *stimulators*.

In *primary MLR* (Fig. 24.4), achieved by the single exposure of responding cells to stimulators, increased protein synthesis can be detected within 24 hours of mixing. DNA synthesis and cell proliferation begin to mount within 2 or 3 days, peak at 4–6 days, and then decline rapidly. After 1 week in culture, the activated lymphocytes begin to revert to small, resting cells and then die, unless they are restimulated with the same antigen. The kinetics of the response may vary, however, depending on conditions and details of the system used. When fresh stimulating cells are added to a culture that has just undergone a primary response, a new burst of activity occurs, more rapid than that following the first stimulation: the number of blasts in this *secondary MLR* peaks at about 3 days after restimulation, and some 90% of the cells remaining after the primary MLC transform into blasts, in contrast to a mere 5% of cells transformed in the primary culture. Only the stimulated cells from the primary culture seem to survive and multiply, whereas the unstimulated cells die. Restimulation can then be repeated often and a series of consecutive peaks of blast transformation can be obtained. When restimulation is discontinued, the cultured lymphocytes die after about 3 weeks.

Cells responding in MLC are mostly CD4+ lymphocytes. Although CD8+ lymphocytes are also activated, they proliferate to a much lesser extent than CD4+ lymphocytes, so the bulk of the response can be attributed to the latter cells. Since CD4+ lymphocytes preferentially recognize class II MHC molecules, allogeneic class II antigens are the main stimulators of MLR. Under standard conditions, only the proliferative response to class II alloantigens is detected in MLR, but by adjusting the conditions properly a response to class I alloantigens can also be demonstrated. Response to alloantigens other than those controlled by the *MHC* is, with one exception, difficult to detect, and some investigators doubt whether it exists at all. Alloantigens controlled by the *Mls* (mixed lymphocyte stimulation) locus in the mouse (see Chapter 13) constitute the one exception.

Stimulators of MLR need not be lymphocytes; any other cells that express MHC class II, adhesion and co-

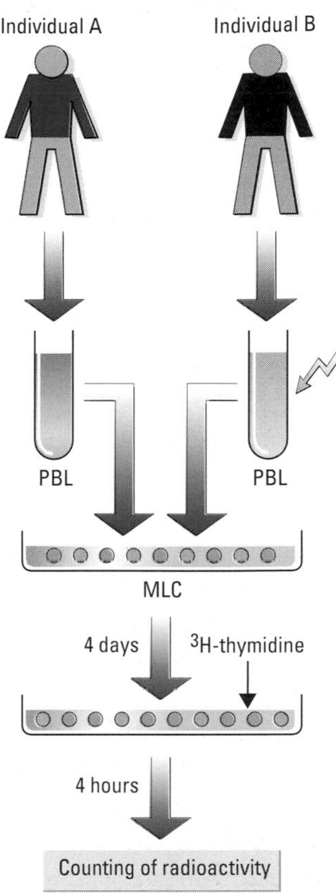

Figure 24.4 Assay for measuring mixed lymphocyte reaction (MLR). MLC, mixed lymphocyte culture; PBL, peripheral blood lymphocytes; ⚡ γ-rays.

stimulatory molecules can carry out this function as well. Among the best MLR stimulators are therefore dendritic cells, macrophages and activated B and T lymphocytes.

The T-cell receptors (TCRs) involved in the recognition of alloantigens appear to be the same as those normally used for the recognition of other foreign antigens. T-lymphocyte clones recognizing foreign antigens in the context of self MHC molecules often cross-react with allogeneic MHC molecules. Cross-reactivity is frequent and is probably the reason why so many lymphocytes (some 5%) respond to MHC alloantigens in the primary MLC: the *alloreactivity* draws on a pool of lymphocytes that normally recognize peptides derived from foreign antigens and bound to self MHC molecules but that also happen to recognize allogeneic MHC molecules loaded with self peptides originating mainly from membrane proteins.

T lymphocytes can be stimulated in several ways under the conditions of MLC *in vitro* (and presumably also *in vivo*). If we designate the stimulator and responder cell MHC molecules as S and R respectively, then in a one-way MLR alloreactive responder T cells can be stimulated by the recognition of allogeneic MHC molecules (S) loaded with self peptides on stimulator APCs. Second, stimulator APCs may take up fragments of responder cells, process them and expose MHC molecules (S) on their surface loaded with peptides derived from the responder's antigens. Third, responder APCs can take up fragments of stimulator cells, process them and express responder MHC molecules (R) on their surface loaded with peptides derived from the stimulator cell antigens. This manner of alloantigen perception is sometimes called *indirect recognition*. Activated responder T lymphocytes may therefore include cells recognizing alloantigens in the first, second or third manner, and their ratio both *in vitro* and *in vivo* may depend on a number of factors, such as the nature of the allogeneic MHC molecules, the degree of dissimilarity between the R and S MHC molecules, the presence of non-MHC polymorphic molecules, and the presence and activity of APCs in the stimulator cells (or in the graft *in vivo*).

In the standard MLR assay, one compares thymidine incorporation in an allogeneic mixture with that in a syngeneic or autologous mixture. Since syngeneic cells are obtained from genetically identical individuals, theoretically they should not be stimulated to incorporate thymidine. In practice, they always show some degree of stimulation, attributed to non-specific factors such as the slight mitogenic effect of the serum in which they grow. This non-specific stimulation is considered to be the 'background', which must be subtracted from the incorporation value in allogeneic mixtures so that the value of the specific stimulation can be obtained.

However, not all proliferation in control experiments is the result of non-specific stimulation. At least four situations have been described in which mixtures of genetically identical cells give a proliferative response comparable with that observed in allogeneic mixtures. These situations occur when (i) adult thymocytes are mixed with autologous spleen cells; (ii) adult lymph node cells are used as stimulators; (iii) human peripheral blood lymphocytes are mixed with neoplastic cells from *MHC*-identical siblings, B-lymphoblastoid cell lines or mitogen-stimulated autologous lymphocytes; and (iv) a T-cell-rich fraction isolated from human peripheral blood lymphocytes is mixed with a B-cell-rich fraction. Of these four conditions, the second and the fourth have been studied most extensively. The former is referred to as the *syngeneic MLR* (SMLR) and the latter as *autologous MLR* (AMLR). The nature of SMLR and AMLR is controversial. All investigators agree that class II molecules are involved, but they disagree on the manner of involvement. Some researchers believe that class II molecules alone stimulate the autoreactive clones, whereas others speculate that class II molecules bind peptides derived from xenogeneic antigens. The latter could be derived from two sources: the culture medium (particularly fetal calf serum, FCS, added to the culture) and the ingredients used to fractionate cell populations prior to the MLR, particularly sheep red blood cells (SRBC) used to rosette human peripheral blood lymphocytes and bovine serum albumin (BSA) used in density gradient centrifugation. Components of the serum, BSA or SRBC fragments presumably are taken up by the stimulating cells, which then act as APCs, displaying the foreign peptide bound by self class II molecules.

Cell-mediated lymphocytotoxicity

A standard MLC activates not only rapidly proliferating $CD4^+$ lymphocytes but also modestly proliferating $CD8^+$ cells, which include the precursors of T_C cells. Activation of T_C lymphocytes can be demonstrated by the lysis (or rather apoptotic disintegration) of appropriate target cells. There are thus two read-out systems for the MLC. In one, the proliferation of cells is measured by the incorporation of isotopes into replicating DNA (standard MLR assay); in the other, the *cell-mediated lymphocytotoxicity* (CML) assay, killing of target cells is determined by isotope release. In the standard CML assay (Fig. 24.5), lymphocytes from two different individuals are incubated for 5 days in a one-way MLC and the surviving cells are then mixed with target cells and incubated for another 4 hours. The targets are either tumour or normal lymphocyte blasts induced by concanavalin A, bacterial lipopolysaccharide or some other mitogen. The targets are labelled with $Na_2{}^{51}CrO_4$, which is taken up by the cells and reduced to Cr^{3+}; the latter remains trapped inside the cells but is released upon their killing. The release of radioactive chromium from the destroyed cells is then a measure of the CML reaction.

Since $CD8^+$ lymphocytes mainly recognize class I MHC molecules, most CML is directed against class I alloantigens. However, a modified CML procedure also reveals T_C lymphocytes specific for class II alloantigens. As far as is known, MHC alloantigens are the sole targets of the T_C-cell response. All other antigens (e.g. minor histocompatibility antigens) can serve as T_C-cell targets only when presented as peptides bound to class I MHC molecules. Full activation of at least some of the T_C-lymphocyte clones depends on cytokines provided by stimulated T_H lymphocytes. For this reason, T_C lymphocytes can be more easily generated when helper T lymphocytes are activated simultaneously. A difference between the responder and the stimulator at both class I and class II loci is therefore required under certain culture conditions to obtain a satisfactory CML response: $CD4^+$ cells in the culture respond to class II alloantigens and

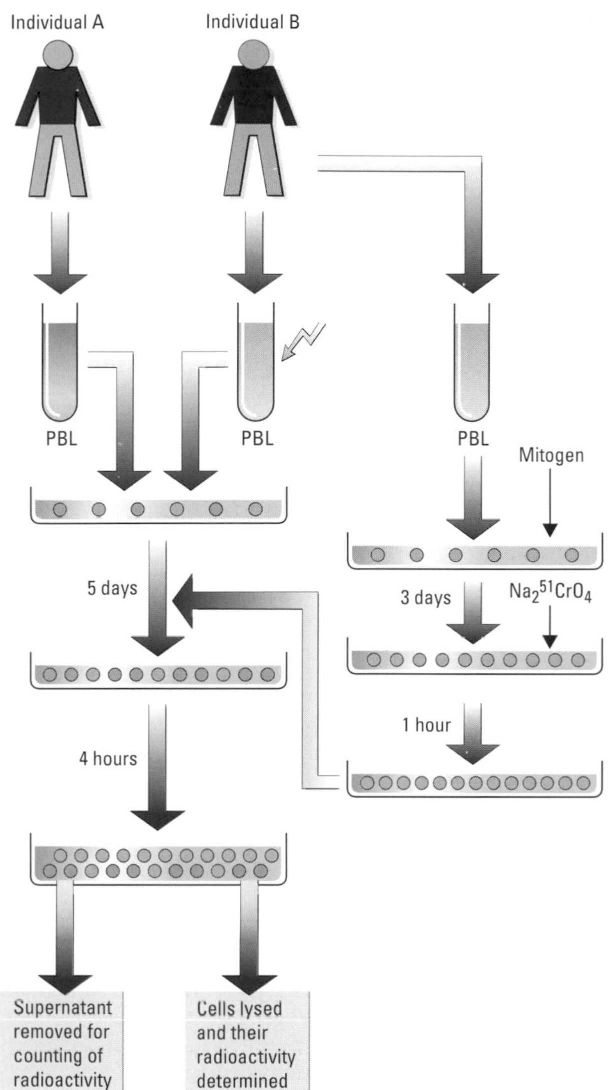

Figure 24.5 Assay for measuring cell-mediated lymphocytotoxicity (CML). PBL, peripheral blood lymphocytes; irradiation by X-rays.

produce cytokines that $CD8^+$ cells, responding to class I alloantigens, use for the full development of their cytotoxic potential. Collaboration between class II-specific T_H cells and class I-specific T_C cells thus takes place in some cultures. In other cultures, class I-specific T_C lymphocytes are generated apparently without help from class II-specific T_H lymphocytes.

A specific form of alloreactivity may be caused also by NK cells. As described in Chapters 7 and 16, these cells use a unique receptor system to detect abnormal cells deficient in expression of MHC class I molecules. Different subsets of NK cells carry different combinations of inhibitory receptors recognizing various sets of MHC class I molecules (isotypes, allelic forms) present in the individual. When NK cells of such an individual come in contact with allogeneic cells, at least some NK cells may attack them because their inhibitory receptors are unable to bind with sufficient affinity to some of the allogeneic MHC class I molecules. Different NK cell subsets may substantially differ in their alloreactivity, depending on the spectrum of inhibitory receptors expressed on their surface. NK-cell alloreactivity is responsible also for the phenomenon of *hybrid resistance* to parental bone marrow transplantation. According to the classical laws of transplantation, F_1 hybrids of two parental inbred strains, A and B (differing in *MHC* haplotype), should accept tissue grafts from the A and B strains. This is generally true, but in some strain combinations bone marrow grafts from the parental strains are rejected by the $(A \times B)$ F_1 hybrid, rejection being mediated by the recipient's NK cells. The latter may perceive the A or B strain cells as abnormal because A-strain cells do not express B molecules and vice versa. The intensity of the rejection depends on the degree of dissimilarity between the A and B haplotype, as perceived by NK-cell inhibitory receptors. The reason why only grafts of lymphoid cells and not of other tissues are rejected by this mechanism is probably the high level of MHC class I molecule expression on lymphocytes and their bone marrow precursors. Changes in the level of expression can therefore be profound and hence more easily detected by NK cells on these than on other tissues.

Graft-vs-host reaction

Terms and definitions

GVHR ensues when allogeneic or semi-allogeneic lymphocytes (graft) are inoculated into a recipient (host). Of course, if the host's immune system is working properly, it beats the graft in mounting an immunological attack and destroys the inoculum. To observe GVHR, one must therefore use hosts that cannot respond immunologically to the graft. These can be embryos or neonates with incompletely developed immune systems; adults with immune systems destroyed by irradiation or by some other means; F_1 hybrids genetically incapable of reacting against the inoculum of parental lymphoid cells; two adult animals whose blood circulation systems have been joined surgically and who are therefore exposed to masses of foreign lymphocytes; and individuals who have been made tolerant of prospective grafts (Fig. 24.6). In all these situations, alloreactive T lymphocytes of the graft recognize alloantigens (MHC molecules loaded with self peptides) on the surface

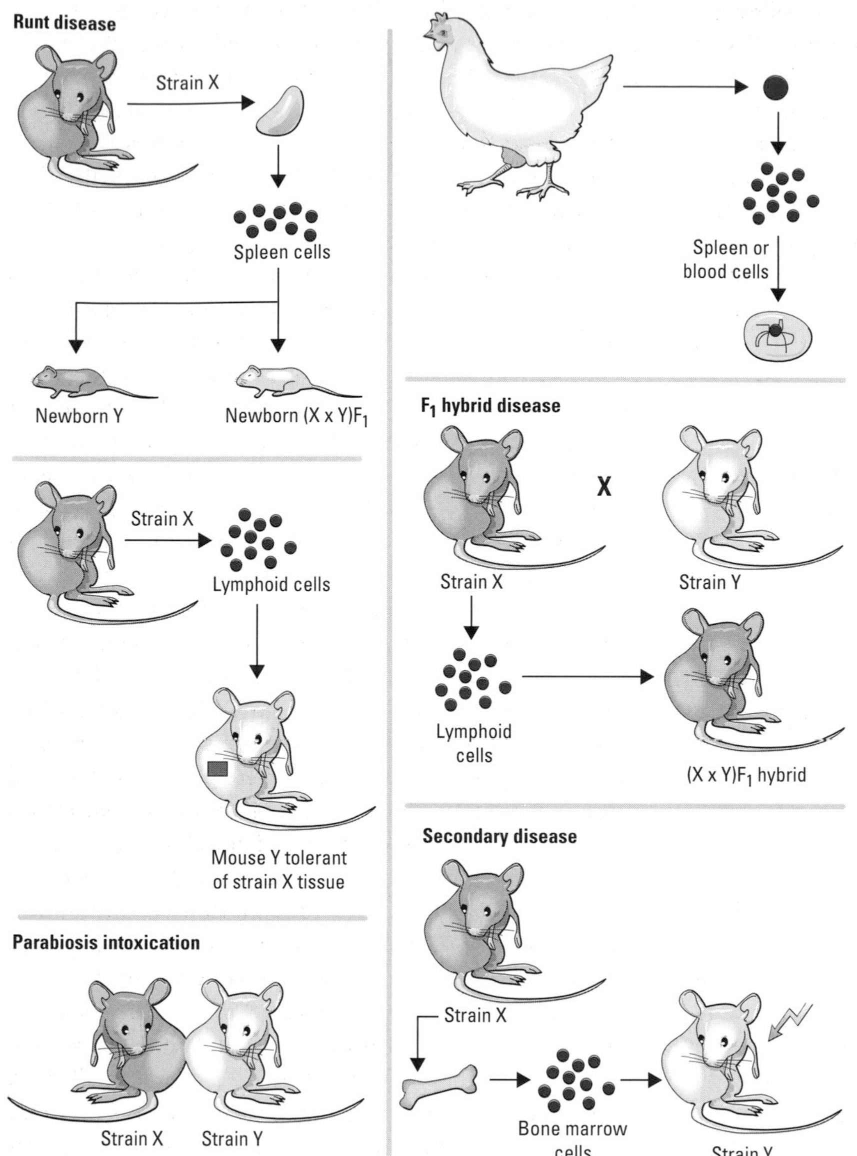

Figure 24.6 Experimental situations leading to the induction of graft-vs-host reaction. (Modified from Klein, J. (1982) *Immunology: The Science of Self–Nonself Discrimination.* John Wiley & Sons, New York.)

of the host's APCs, become activated and then attack various host tissues via T_H1- and T_C-cell-based mechanisms. Details of the GVHR differ depending on the experimental or clinical situation. When GVHR manifests itself outwardly by the deteriorating health and even death of the affected individual, one speaks not of a reaction but of *graft-vs-host disease* (GVHD). Some of the specific forms of GVHD also have their own names (Fig. 24.6): *runt disease* (the reaction ensuing when allogeneic lymphocytes are inoculated into newborn animals); *F_1 hybrid disease* (provoked by the inoculation of parental lymphocytes into adult F_1 hybrids); *secondary disease* (triggered by the inoculation of parental lymphocytes into lethally irradiated individuals); and *parabiosis intoxication* (the reaction resulting from cross-circulation of peripheral blood between two immunologically competent allogeneic individuals joined surgically).

Pathology of human GVHD

The cardinal signs of GVHR in animals are weight loss and general runting, diarrhoea, enlargement of the liver and of various lymphoid organs and severe anaemia. These vary depending on the strength of the antigenic stimulus, the number of inoculated cells, the age of the host at the time of grafting and the animal species. In humans, GVHD often follows the transplantation of bone marrow, primarily in patients treated for severe combined immunodeficiency, aplastic leukaemia or anaemia. It may also occur following blood transfusion into immunodeficient recipients. GVHD occurs in two forms, acute and chronic. *Acute GVHD* is found in 35–50% of patients who received *HLA*-identical bone marrow transplants. It has a sudden onset, usually within the first 2–10 weeks after transplantation, a rapid, severe course and is of relatively short duration. It is manifested by a body rash that sometimes develops rapidly into a form similar to toxic epidermal necrolysis. Other symptoms are diarrhoea, enlargement of liver and spleen, jaundice, arrhythmias, increased excitability of the central nervous system and infiltration of cells into the lungs. Approximately one-half of patients suffering from moderate or severe GVHD die, usually not because of the disease itself but because of uncontrollable bacterial, fungal or viral infections accompanying it. Treatment of acute GVHD consists of placing the patient in protective isolation and suppressing the initial natural immune responses with methotrexate, corticosteroids, antithymocyte globulin, cyclosporin or monoclonal antibodies. Fully developed GVHD is very difficult to control by any known treatment. Therefore, every effort must be made to prevent it by using genetically well-matched grafts or by the elimination of T lymphocytes from transfused bone marrow.

Chronic GVHD develops between 3 and 18 months after bone marrow transplantation and occurs in about 45% of long-term survivors. Its incidence is higher in older patients and in those who had previously experienced an episode of acute GVHD. It is lethal in a small proportion of patients and the main cause of death is again bacterial and fungal infection. Its main targets are the same organs as in acute GVHD but it affects, in addition, tear and salivary glands. Common symptoms include chronic diarrhoea and wasting. Because of similar aetiology, the clinical state induced by chronic GVHD resembles that of certain autoimmune diseases. Most cases of chronic GVHD can be partially controlled by immunosuppressive treatment.

Prevention of allograft reaction

Allograft reaction is a great source of frustration for a transplant surgeon: no matter how skilful his or her work, the reaction manages eventually to spoil its fruits. To minimize the effect of this undesired form of the body's defence, the surgeon enlists the help of *immunosuppressive agents*, which are capable of lowering the immune response. An ideal immunosuppressive agent would reduce the vigorousness of the allograft reaction but not affect other forms of the immune response. Such a specific immunosuppressive agent has, however, not yet been discovered. What is more, immunologists have had a hard time even devising an agent that non-specifically affects cells of the immune system alone. Most agents now in use not only lower the body's general resistance to infection but also have other undesirable side-effects. At high doses, these agents are toxic for immune as well as many other cells; at low doses, they do not have the desired biological effect on immune cells. Thus the surgeon is always walking the thin line between administering too much or too little of a given agent.

Immunosuppressants can influence defence reactions either specifically or non-specifically. Among the many non-specific immunosuppressants used to control the rejection of organ grafts the most powerful at present is the antibiotic *cyclosporin A* (CsA), which is produced by the fungus *Trichoderma polysporum*. CsA is a cyclic peptide composed of 11 amino acid residues, most of which do not occur in proteins (Fig. 24.7). The drug acts specifically on T lymphocytes: it binds to the M_r 17 000 protein *cyclophilin*, an enzyme involved in correct polypeptide chain folding. The cyclophilin–CsA complex binds to the heterodimeric enzyme *calcineurin* (phosphatase 2B), which regulates the activity of transcription factors involved in *IL2* gene expression in activated T cells (Fig. 24.8). Because of its toxicity it is necessary to monitor CsA level in patients' blood during treatment. A completely unrelated fungal metabolite called *FK506* (see Fig. 24.7b) has similar effects and even a mechanism of action similar to CsA. A structural analogue of FK506, *rapamycin* (see Fig. 24.7c), was initially found to have antibacterial, antifungal and antitumour activities and was later also identified as a potent immunosuppressant. Although rapamycin binds to a protein related to cyclophilin, its mechanism of action is different from that of CsA or FK506; it inhibits cell-cycle progression in activated T cells at the late G_1 stage, while CsA and FK506 inhibit an earlier stage, the G_0 to G_1 transition. These immunosuppressive drugs must be taken by patients lifelong to prevent eventual graft rejection.

Other drugs, such as azathioprine (Imuran), cyclophosphamide and methotrexate, block proliferation of activated T cells. *Azathioprine* is an inhibitor of synthesis of a key nucleotide metabolite, inosinic acid. *Cyclophosphamide* is an alkylating agent covalently cross-linking the DNA double helix and thereby preventing its replication. *Methotrexate* blocks biosynthesis of purine nucleotides. All these drugs have strong side-effects because they affect all dividing cells in the body.

Corticosteroids (prednisone, prednisolone, methylprednisolone) are powerful immunosuppressants, but they too have significant side-effects. They are steroid hormone derivatives that, because of their hydrophobic nature, pass through the plasma membrane and in the cytoplasm bind to receptor molecules that transport them to the nucleus.

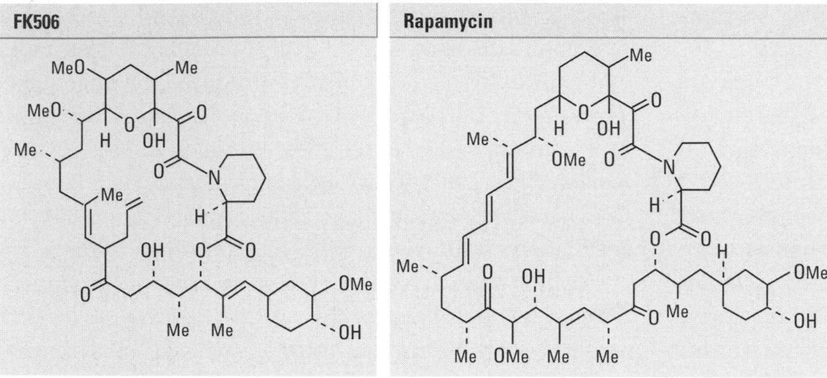

Figure 24.7 Structure of commonly used immunosuppressants. CsA, cyclosporin A. (Modified from Bierer, B. E. *et al.* (1993) *Current Opinion in Immunology*, 5, 763.)

There the complexes bind to regulatory sequences of specific genes and influence their transcription. One of the proteins translated from the transcripts is IκBα, which binds in the cytoplasm to the transcription factor NF-κB and thereby blocks its activity. Inhibition of NF-κB activity blocks activation of the *IL2* gene and therefore activation of T cells. The corticoid–receptor complexes also prevent another general transcription factor, AP-1, from binding to its target genes. One of the genes inhibited by blocking of the AP-1 factor codes for the secreted protease collagenase, a major contributor to tissue damage in inflammation. The overall effect of corticosteroid treatment is powerful suppression of inflammation, inhibition of T-cell activation and induction of apoptosis in immature thymocytes.

Other non-specific immunosuppressive agents include ionizing radiation and antilymphocyte serum. The former (no longer used) took advantage of the sensitivity of lymphocytes to γ-rays. The patient received repeated doses of irradiation that destroyed lymphocytes in lymphoid organs but did not affect significantly the function of the bone marrow. Once immunosuppressed, the patient received the graft which was then tolerated to some degree by the recovering immune system.

Antilymphocytic serum (ALS) or its γ-globulin fraction (antilymphocytic globulin, ALG) is produced by the inoculation of human lymphocytes into a rabbit or some other animal. When injected into the patient it seems to remove preferentially mature T lymphocytes from circulation. Although ALS treatment often significantly prolongs transplant survival, it also renders the patient highly susceptible to infection. A more modern version of ALS uses monoclonal antibodies, usually of mouse origin and specific for T-cell surface molecules such as the CD3 complex of the TCR. The antibodies, which upon inoculation rapidly deplete T lymphocytes, are often used during rejection crisis, when an organ graft begins to be rejected despite immunosuppression by CsA or other drugs. When the crisis is past, treatment is discontinued to prevent patients from producing antibodies against the mouse immunoglobulin. In the future it may be possible to replace mouse antibodies by humanized or otherwise engineered antibodies (see Chapter 8).

Attempts are also being made to use monoclonal antibodies targeted at activated T lymphocytes and unreactive with all other cells of the immune system. Indeed, it has been reported that monoclonal antibodies specific for CD25, a component of the high-affinity IL-2 receptor expressed on activated but not resting T cells, are in some cases effective immunosuppressants preventing graft rejection, GVHD and some autoimmune diseases. Immunosuppressive effects have also been described for monoclonal antibodies against adhesion molecules such as LFA-1, ICAM-1 and CD2.

Ultimately one would like to obtain *specific immunosuppression* by agents that would prevent a response against

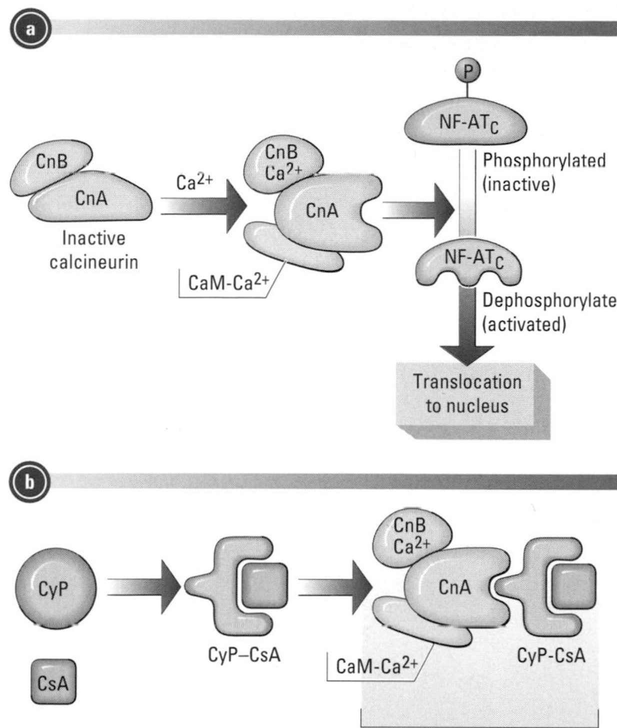

Figure 24.8 Immunosuppressive action of cyclosporin A. (a) An important part of the T-cell receptor (TCR) signalling pathway in T cells is the phosphatase calcineurin (Cn), which in its inactive state is composed of two subunits, CnA and CnB. As a result of TCR-triggered activation, cytoplasmic concentration of Ca^{2+} is increased; Ca^{2+} binds to the protein calmodulin (CaM) and to CnB. CaM–Ca^{2+} forms a complex with calcineurin, which becomes enzymatically active. One of its substrates is the phosphorylated inactive protein NF-AT_c, which upon dephosphorylation translocates to the nucleus where it binds to the transcription factor complex NF-AT_n. The binding initiates transcription of several genes including those encoding IL-2 and IL-2R. Transcription of these genes is a critical step towards cell proliferation. (b) Cyclosporin A binds to the cytoplasmic protein cyclophilin (CyP), thereby changing its conformation in such a way that the CyP–CsA complex tightly binds to the active calcineurin and inhibits its enzymatic activity. As a result, NF-AT_c is not activated and *IL2* and *IL2R* gene transcription is blocked. The other immunosuppressant, FK506 (and also rapamycin), binds to the FK506-binding protein (FKBP), which is similar to CyP, and the complex also inhibits calcineurin activity. CyP and FKBP belong to a family of immunophilins that are involved in proper folding of nascent polypeptide chains and protection of cells from heat shock.

the graft while permitting all other responses to proceed normally. Some possibilities being considered or tested include the use of antagonistic peptides, antibodies or other ligands binding to the CD4 and CD8 co-receptor molecules and interfering with CD28-mediated co-stimulatory signals (see the discussion on tolerance induction in Chapter 20). Given the complexity of allograft reaction, the development of such specific treatments is extremely difficult.

Further reading

Azuma, H. & Tilney, N. L. (1994) Chronic graft rejection. *Current Opinion in Immunology*, **6**, 770–776.

Bierer, B. E., Holländer, G., Fruman, D. & Burakoff, S. J. (1993) Cyclosporin A and FK506: molecular mechanisms of immunosuppression and probes for transplantation biology. *Current Opinion in Immunology*, **5**, 765–769.

Chao, N. J. (1992) Graft versus host disease following allogeneic bone marrow transplantation. *Current Opinion in Immunology*, **4**, 571–576.

Dorling, A. & Lechler, R. I. (1994) Prospects for xenografting. *Current Opinion in Immunology*, **6**, 770–776.

Galili, U. (1993) Interaction of the natural anti-Gal antibody with α-galactosyl epitopes: a major obstacle for xenotransplantation in humans. *Immunology Today*, **14**, 480–482.

Goulmy, E. (1996) Human minor histocompatibility antigens. *Current Opinion in Immunology*, **8**, 75–81.

Kahan, B. D. (1992) Immunosuppressive therapy. *Current Opinion in Immunology*, **4**, 553–560.

Kaufman, C. L., Gaines, B. A. & Ildstad, S. T. (1995) Xenotransplantation. *Annual Review of Immunology*, **13**, 339–368.

Krensky, A. M. & Clayberger, C. (1994) The induction of tolerance to alloantigens using HLA-based synthetic peptides. *Current Opinion in Immunology*, **6**, 791–796.

Lanier, L. L. (1995) The role of natural killer cells in transplantation. *Current Opinion in Immunology*, **7**, 626–631.

Möller, G. (Ed.) (1994) Xenotransplantation. *Immunological Reviews*, **141**, entire volume.

Rosenberg, A. S. & Singer, A. (1992) Cellular basis of skin allograft rejection: an *in vivo* model of immune-mediated tissue destruction. *Annual Review of Immunology*, **10**, 333–358.

Rowe, P. M. (1995) Xenotransplantation: from animal facility to the clinic? *Molecular Medicine Today*, **2**, 10–15.

Sherman, L. A. & Chattopadhyay, S. (1993) The molecular basis of allorecognition. *Annual Review of Immunology*, **11**, 385–402.

Sigal, N. H. & Dumont, F. J. (1992) Cyclosporin A, FK-506 and rapamycin: pharmacologic probes of lymphocyte signal transduction. *Annual Review of Immunology*, **10**, 519–560.

Streilein, J. W. (1995) Unraveling immune privilege. *Science*, **270**, 1158–1159.

Sykes, M. (1993) Novel approaches to the control of graft versus host disease. *Current Opinion in Immunology*, **5**, 774–781.

von Boehmer, H. (1995) Female anti-male attack. *Nature*, **376**, 642.

Waldmann, H. & Cobbold, S. (1993) Monoclonal antibodies for the induction of transplantation tolerance. *Current Opinion in Immunology*, **5**, 753–758.

Waldmann, H., Cobbold, S. & Hale, G. (1994) What can be done to prevent graft versus host disease? *Current Opinion in Immunology*, **6**, 777–783.

Wecker, H. & Auchincloss Jr, H. (1992) Cellular mechanisms of rejection. *Current Opinion in Immunology*, **4**, 561–566.

chapter 25

Autoimmunity and autoimmune diseases

Concepts

Any body protein and many carbohydrates and lipids, as well as nucleic acids, are potential antigens. The body is capable of constructing T-cell receptors (TCRs) or B-cell receptors (BCRs) that can recognize these antigens and initiate an immune response against them. Many of the body's components are therefore potential *autoantigens* (self antigens, autologous antigens) capable of inducing *autoimmunity* (Greek *auto*, 'self'), humoral or cellular. Hence, autoimmunity is an immune response against components of self. It may or may not have adverse effects on the body, and if it does the pathological changes it induces constitute an *autoimmune disease*. Clinical immunologists designate as autoimmune all those diseases in which they can demonstrate the presence of either antibodies or T lymphocytes reactive with autoantigens. Self-reactive antibodies are referred to as *autoantibodies* and the self-reactive cells as *autoreactive T lymphocytes*.

We know from Chapter 20 that the body has devised ways, collectively called tolerance, of avoiding immune response against self components. Autoimmunity is therefore a failure of tolerance.

Mechanisms and causes of autoimmunity

There is nothing special about autoimmune mechanisms; they are the same ones that play beneficial roles in normal, protective immunity, i.e. humoral (antibody)-based mechanisms and cytotoxic T (T_C) and helper T (T_H1) (inflammatory) cell-mediated mechanisms. There appear to be no autoimmune diseases caused by IgE-activated atopic mechanisms. We noted in previous chapters that immune response against foreign antigens often leads to tissue damage, which may in some cases be more serious than the damage caused by the pathogen itself. In these instances, however, the primary target of response is the pathogen and the tissue damage is essentially an undesired by-product of the protective attack on foreign antigens. By contrast, in autoimmune reactions the targets of attack are self components of the body, although foreign antigens may play a triggering role. Hence in autoimmune disorders, certain cells or tissues are perceived by the system as infected and all efforts are made to eliminate the non-existing infection.

The occurrence of autoimmune diseases indicates the presence in the body of autoreactive lymphocyte clones which can, under certain circumstances, become activated. As discussed in Chapter 20, a major mechanism of self tolerance is deletion or functional silencing (anergization) of the clones recognizing autoantigens. T-cell clones recognizing any antigens that occur in the thymus are physically eliminated by the process of negative selection. Similarly, many B-cell clones recognizing soluble or cell-surface-bound self molecules die by apoptosis if they meet the autoantigen during early stages of their development. Negative selection, however, does not operate in instances in which the level of the potential autoantigen in the thymus (for T cells) or bone marrow (for B cells) is too low to trigger apoptotic signalling. Many tissue-specific molecules do not occur at all in the thymus and the bone marrow. T-lymphocyte clones recognizing such molecules survive the early process of negative selection, but when they encounter the autoantigens in the periphery they usually become anergized or are even induced to die, because the confrontation nearly always involves cells that cannot provide the co-stimulatory signals necessary for positive stimulation. Similarly, B cells recognizing self structures in peripheral tissues are anergized rather than activated because they do not receive co-stimulatory signals from T_H cells. Theoretically therefore there should be no autoreactive lymphocytes in the mature immune system. However, this is not the case, for at least five reasons.

1 Some self molecules are expressed at levels below the sensitivity threshold of lymphocytes. These autoantigens are ignored by the immune system and the potentially autoreactive clones are not eliminated.

2 Some molecules, such as those expressed at immunologically privileged sites (see Chapter 20), are protected by a barrier from contact with lymphocytes.

3 Some epitopes are normally hidden from the immune system (*cryptic epitopes*) and tolerance towards them is not established. Under normal circumstances, self proteins are cleaved either in the cytosolic or vesicular processing pathways into a certain set of peptides, some of which bind to major histocompatibility complex (MHC) molecules; clones of T cells expressing receptors for these peptide–MHC molecule assemblages are either anergized or eliminated by negative selection. Under altered circumstances (e.g. infection, inflammation, recruitment of novel types of antigen-presenting cells such as activated endothelial cells, etc.), different sets of MHC-bound peptides may be generated because of quantitative or qualitative changes in protein expression, in the activities of processing proteases and in the accessibility of MHC molecules. The new sets can then be recognized by T-cell clones that were not eliminated by negative selection.

4 Autoreactive clones made tolerant by anergization can be reactivated under some circumstances.

5 Some autoreactive clones may be kept in check by regulatory mechanisms involving, for example, the elusive suppressor T cells, and when these mechanisms fail the clones may become active.

The immune system therefore contains at all times a large number of lymphocyte clones that in certain situations can react with self antigens.

What, then, activates potentially autoreactive but normally silent lymphocyte clones? Unfortunately, there is still no definitive answer. Agents have been identified that induce autoimmune diseases in animal models and there are a few examples of human autoimmune diseases in which the effector has tentatively been identified. For most autoimmune diseases, however, the causes remain unknown. A description of the factors that have been identified and that may contribute to the development of autoimmunity follows.

Molecular mimicry

The main assumption of the *molecular mimicry hypothesis* is that some epitopes on foreign antigens are sufficiently similar to certain self epitopes to become the target of immune response elicited by the former. Thus, an epitope generated by the binding of a virus peptide to MHC class I molecules may be recognized by a T-cell clone, which is thereby stimulated and becomes involved in elimination of the viral infection. The TCR of that T-cell clone, however, may cross-react with an epitope formed by a self peptide and an MHC molecule. This self epitope is expressed at a subthreshold level and so its presence is normally ignored by the immune system — the corresponding T-cell clone is not anergized. After stimulation by the foreign epitope, however, mature effector T cells are able to attack not only the virus-infected cells but also cells expressing the cross-reactive autoantigen (Fig. 25.1). One might expect this type of autoimmunity to wane after the infection is abolished. However, once the autoimmune reaction is triggered, it may perpetuate itself: the local inflammation induced by it can enhance expression of the autoantigen on antigen-presenting cells and so mimic a real, persistent infection. Numerous similarities between amino acid sequences of various self proteins and antigens of pathogens have been noted (Table 25.1) but in no instance, with the exception of rheumatic fever triggered by streptococcal antigens, has a causal relationship between molecular mimicries and autoimmune diseases been proven. Among the microbial antigens most frequently implicated in autoimmunity induced by molecular mimicry are heat-shock proteins. These are so similar between evolutionarily very distant organisms that cross-reactivity between microbial and human peptides is likely to occur.

Uncovering of sequestered antigens or cryptic epitopes

An injury or infection may temporarily release molecules normally inaccessible to the immune system, which can then stimulate autoimmune attack on the cells carrying

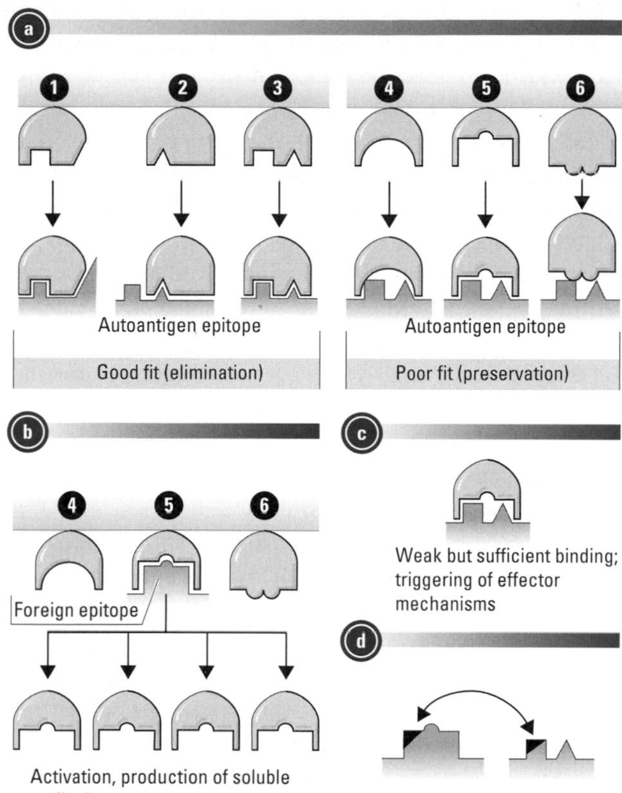

Figure 25.1 Molecular mimicry as a trigger of autoimmunity. (a) The original repertoire of antibody-combining sites (B-cell receptors, BCRs) contains sites (1, 2, 3) that bind an autoantigen epitope so strongly that immature B cells carrying these autoreactive BCRs will be eliminated or anergized. BCRs of other B cells (4, 5, 6) bind weakly or not at all to this (and any other) autoantigen; these cells are therefore spared. BCR no. 5 binds partially to the autoantigen but the interaction is too weak to trigger anergization of this clone. The absence of appropriate helper T cells also prevents positive stimulation of this clone at the stage of mature B cell. (b) During an infection, some BCRs (here no. 5) recognize certain epitopes of the pathogen and the recognition leads to the production of large quantities of antibodies. (c) The antibodies bind weakly to the autoantigen. Binding triggers effector mechanisms leading to tissue damage and local inflammation that may further stimulate autoimmunity against previously cryptic autoantigens. (d) One part of the foreign epitope is similar to (mimics) a part of the autoepitope (black regions).

them. Similarly, local trauma or inflammation may change the pattern of self-protein processing and lead to the presentation of novel epitopes that also become targets of an attack. Most injuries are probably accompanied by a temporary immune reaction to some of the sequestered proteins or cryptic epitopes, but such reactions usually disappear after the wound heals, the original conditions are re-established and the potential autoantigens become sequestered again. Under certain circumstances (genetic predisposition, unknown environmental factors), however, the normal homeostatic mechanisms fail and the autoimmune reaction may perpetuate itself. It has been observed repeatedly that in the early phase of an autoimmune disease lymphocyte clones generally react with only very few autoantigen epitopes. Later, clones reactive with more and more auto-epitopes are recruited so that in the fully developed disease a number of tissue components become the target of the response. This *determinant spreading* phenomenon can be explained by assuming that as the autoimmune reaction progresses, new previously cryptic epitopes are uncovered: these enhance the reaction and thus lead to the unmasking of more cryptic epitopes, and so on, generating a vicious circle that amplifies the response. Determinant spreading makes it difficult to identify the primary autoantigen or epitope that triggered the process; by the time the disease is diagnosed, the originally activated clones may be completely overwhelmed by those that have arisen later in the process. A similar phenomenon is also observed in allergic diseases. Here the patient often becomes progressively hypersensitive to more epitopes or even new allergens as the disease progresses.

Table 25.1 Sequence similarities between microbial proteins and human host proteins. Immunological cross-reactivity between proteins in each pair has been demonstrated. Amino acid sequences are given in the single-letter code (see Appendix 1). (Modified from Oldstone, M. B. A. (1987) *Cell*, 50, 819.)

Protein	Residue	Sequence
Human cytomegalovirus IE2	79	PDPLGRPDED
HLA-DR molecule	60	VTELGRPDAE
Poliovirus VP2	70	STTKESRGTT
Acetylcholine receptor	176	TVIKESRGTK
Papilloma virus E2	76	SLHLESLKDS
Insulin receptor	66	VYGLESLKDL
Rabies virus glycoprotein	147	TKESLVIIS
Insulin receptor	764	NKESLVISE
Klebsiella pneumoniae nitrogenase	186	SRQTDREDE
HLA-B27 molecule	70	KAQTDREDL
Adenovirus 12 E1B	384	LRRGMFRPSQCN
α-Gliadin	206	LGQGSFRPSQQN
Human immunodeficiency virus p24	160	GVETTTPS
Human IgG constant region	466	GVETTTPS
Measles virus P3	13	LECIRALK
Corticotropin	18	LECIRACK
Measles virus P3	31	EISDNLGQE
Myelin basic protein	61	EISFKLGQE

Experimental autoimmunity can be triggered reproducibly by immunization of animals with autoantigens normally hidden from the immune system. For example, autoimmune encephalitis can be initiated by immunization with myelin basic protein or even crude brain extract under conditions favouring local inflammatory reaction (administration in complete Freund's adjuvant). Similarly, experimental rheumatoid arthritis can be provoked by immunization with collagen. Autoimmune diseases are also induced following injury of immunologically privileged sites. For example, symphathetic ophthalmia (severe inflammation of the middle, vascular part of the eyeball) develops following eye injury, and orchitis (inflammation of the testis) following vasectomy.

Activation of potentially autoreactive T-cell clones by superantigens

Autoimmune reactions may also be triggered by superantigens (see Chapter 13) produced by some microorganisms. Superantigens are polyclonal activators that can, among other things, stimulate clones previously anergized by the encounter with an autoantigen or clones that ignored the potential autoantigens because of their low expression or sequestration. Superantigens have been shown to be responsible for autoimmune reactions following streptococcal and mycoplasma infections. On the other hand, however, exposure to common infections may also protect against some autoimmune diseases: mice genetically predisposed to insulin-dependent diabetes mellitus (IDDM) develop the disease more frequently when kept under germ-free conditions compared with those exposed to viral infections. Similarly, transgenic mice manipulated genetically to become predisposed to autoimmune encephalitis develop the disease spontaneously only when kept under sterile conditions. The reasons for the protective effects of infections are unknown.

Genetic factors

Familial associations and the susceptibility of inbred mouse strains to certain autoimmune diseases indicate that the development of autoimmunity depends on genetic factors. The association of many autoimmune diseases with certain *MHC* genotypes is discussed in Chapter 6. Two inbred mouse strains in particular, NOD and NZW, have proved to be useful models in the study of autoimmune diseases. The non-obese diabetic (NOD) strain is highly susceptible to the spontaneous development of IDDM. The major susceptibility gene *Idd-1* has been mapped within the *MHC*, but its identity has not been established. It does not seem to be one of the class I or class II genes; candidate genes include *Tnfa* and *Tnfb* in the class III region. The same region also controls allergic orchitis and contains the gene encoding myelin oligodendrocyte glycoprotein, which may be a critical antigen in multiple sclerosis. Other genes contributing to IDDM susceptibility in NOD mice appear to be those encoding interleukin (IL)-2 and the high-affinity Fc receptor for IgG (FcγRI)[1]. New Zealand black (NZB) strain mice are prone to spontaneous development of systemic lupus erythematosus (SLE) but the genes involved have not been identified. Other strains known to have defective genes for Fas or Fas ligand (the molecules participating in the induction of apoptosis), or to overexpress the antiapoptotic molecule Bcl-2, also develop systemic autoimmunity. Hence genes controlling the elimination of autoreactive clones by apoptosis may also be important in the aetiology of some human autoimmune disorders.

Genetic factors alone, however, are not sufficient to effect an autoimmune disease. This conclusion is supported by the observation that identical twins do not develop an autoimmune disease such as IDDM concordantly: when one of the twins is affected, the other develops the disease in only about 30% of cases. Similarly, only a fraction, albeit relatively large, of mice of a susceptible inbred strain develops the disease. There must therefore be other factors, probably environmental, which in conjunction with genetic predisposition precipitate the disease. Among such factors may be infection, as already mentioned, and the subject's hormonal status. Many autoimmune diseases occur predominantly in females (multiple sclerosis, SLE) and others in males (ankylosing spondylitis). Moreover, disease intensity correlates in some instances with oestrogen and progesterone levels.

Failures of immune regulation

It has been hypothesized that some autoimmune diseases are caused by an impairment of negative regulatory T cells (suppressor T cells) that normally inhibit potentially autoreactive clones, but little experimental evidence exists at present in support of such a mechanism. Mice that lack $CD8^+$ T cells (which should include the enigmatic suppressor T cells) as a result of either gene-knockout or anti-CD8 antibody treatment have an incidence of autoimmune experimental encephalitis similar to that of mice with normal $CD8^+$ T-cell levels. On the other hand, there is no doubt that cytokine-based regulatory interactions do play a part in autoimmunity. The balance between T_H1 and T_H2 subsets is certainly a factor in the development and maintenance of the disease, just as it is in normal protective immunity. For example, it is possible to inhibit the development

[1] Susceptibility to human IDDM appears to be directly linked to MHC class II (*DQ*) genes, as discussed in Chapter 6.

of diabetes in rats by the transfer of a T_H2-like subset of CD4+ T cells. The mechanism seems to involve IL-4 and IL-10 production that inhibits interferon-γ secretion and the development of T_C and T_H1 autoreactive clones. IL-4 treatment also prevents diabetes in NOD mice. The T_H1-type response to a supposedly major human IDDM autoantigen, glutamic acid decarboxylase, is characteristic for subjects at risk, in contrast to the prevailing T_H2-type response in controls. All these observations point to the importance of T_H1 vs. T_H2 regulatory mechanisms in autoimmune disorders.

An experimental multi-organ autoimmune disease, caused most probably by the failure of normal regulatory interactions, develops in mice thymectomized neonatally (between days 2 and 5 after birth). T cells produced by the immature prenatal thymus appear to be incompletely self tolerant, while T cells leaving the thymus later are able to suppress this autoreactivity. When these more mature T cells are missing, the autoreactive clones attack self tissues.

Causes of tissue damage

Autoimmunity develops into a disease when components of the immune system begin to damage the body. This need not happen in all cases of autoimmune reactions. Autoantibodies to many self molecules are commonly found in sera of healthy individuals and some immunologists consider them to be important regulatory components of homeostatic networks. The mechanisms of tissue damage vary according to the types of autoimmune disease. In some diseases the damage is caused by autoantibodies via complement activation or deposition of large amounts of immune complexes. Alternatively, autoantibodies may either block the normal function of physiologically important receptors or inappropriately stimulate the receptors by binding to them and mimicking the action of a natural ligand. In other diseases, tissue damage is caused by autoreactive T_C or T_H1 cells effecting cytotoxic or delayed-type hypersensitivity (DTH) damage, respectively. In the section that follows we give examples of some autoimmune diseases, their manifestations and possible causes.

Examples of autoimmune diseases

Diseases caused mainly by autoantibodies

In *systemic lupus erythematosus*[2] autoantibodies are produced against DNA and other nuclear components (histones, ribonucleoproteins). These antibodies form large quantities of immune complexes with the abundant antigens; the complexes are deposited in joints and in the walls of blood vessels in the renal glomeruli, where they activate phagocytes and initiate complement activation. This process induces local inflammation and tissue damage that releases more antigen from the damaged cells and worsens the condition. The disease can manifest itself in nearly any organ. The patients (four times more frequently women than men) often suffer from chronic fever, wasting and fatigue, joint pains, a rash on body parts exposed to sunlight, nephritis (inflammation of the kidney), mental disturbances and anaemia. Chronic glomerulonephritis may eventually cause kidney failure that ultimately kills the patient. Some mouse strains such as NZB develop spontaneously an SLE-like disease. The primary autoantigens driving the pathogenic autoimmune response in humans and mice are probably nucleosomes (complexes of DNA with histones), which commonly occur in serum after apoptotic cell destruction. Insufficient apoptosis of autoimmune B cells may be one of the factors contributing to the development of the disease.

Immune complex deposition on blood vessel walls, complement activation and the ensuing chronic inflammation is also responsible for tissue damage in polyarteritis nodosa (in which the triggering antigen is hepatitis B virus surface antigen (HBsAg)) and poststreptococcal acute glomerulonephritis incited by streptococcal antigens. *Polyarteritis nodosa* is an inflammation of the medium-sized and small arteries in kidney, muscles, gastrointestinal tract and heart; it is accompanied by chronic fever, cough, pain in the legs and the formation of painful subcutaneous nodules. *Poststreptococcal acute glomerulonephritis* is a severe inflammation of kidney glomeruli occurring in children 5–28 days after infection with a nephritogenic strain of group A haemolytic streptococci.

Patients suffering from *Graves' disease* produce autoantibodies to the thyroid-stimulating hormone (TSH) receptor that mimic the action of the natural ligand (TSH) and stimulate excessive production of thyroid hormones. The elevated levels of thyroid hormones are responsible for increased basal metabolic rate, increased heart rate, nervousness, heat intolerance and excessive sweating, which are some of the symptoms of Graves' disease (named after the Irish physician Robert James Graves (1796–1863)). The disease is relatively frequent, affecting between 0.1 and 0.5% of the population.

In *myasthenia gravis*, autoantibodies to the acetylcholine receptor at the neuromuscular junction block signal trans-

[2] Opinions on the origin of the designation 'lupus erythematosus' (literally 'red wolf') differ. According to one, the name was introduced because the pattern produced by the facial reddening that accompanies the disease resembles a wolf's head; according to another it stems from the likeness of the facial ulceration to a wolf bite. The adjective 'systemic' is used to point out that the disease can involve almost any part of the body.

mission from nerve endings to muscle. This leads to muscular weakness (Greek *mys*, muscle; *asthenia*, weakness) and eventual death due to the loss of proper respiratory muscle function (clinicians use the adjective *gravis*, Latin for 'dangerous', to indicate serious conditions). Similarly, blocking autoantibodies to insulin receptors may cause some cases of *insulin-resistant diabetes*. Autoantibodies to thyroid antigens such as thyroglobulin (a thyroid hormone) and thyroid peroxidase are the cause of *Hashimoto's thyroiditis*, named after the Japanese surgeon Hakaru Hashimoto (1881–1934). The antibodies bind to these proteins and thereby interfere with iodine uptake in the thyroid and thyroid hormone production. The thyroid becomes the target of an inflammatory response (hence 'thyroiditis'), which destroys the gland's normal architecture. The thyroid attempts to regenerate and this process, together with the inflammatory infiltration, leads to an enlargement of the gland, called *struma* (Latin *struo*, to pile up) or *goitre* (Latin *guttur*, throat). The goitre disappears in the ultimate stages of the disease when the gland is completely destroyed. Hashimoto's thyroiditis can be treated successfully by the administration of thyroid hormones. In *autoimmune haemolytic anaemia*, patients have autoantibodies to some of their erythrocyte surface antigens (Rh, I and H antigens). The autoantibody-coated erythrocytes are then lysed by complement. *Pernicious anaemia* is caused by autoantibodies to *intrinsic factor*, a membrane protein of intestinal epithelial cells, which is involved in transport of vitamin B_{12}. A shortage of this vitamin, which is necessary for erythropoiesis, leads to anaemia.

Autoantibodies to the basement membrane collagen of renal glomeruli and alveoli of the lung are the cause of *Goodpasture's syndrome* (named after US pathologist Ernest William Goodpasture (1886–1960)). Complement activation at these sites leads to rapid kidney damage and pulmonary haemorrhage. Autoantibodies to the epidermal adhesion molecule cadherin cause *pemphigus vulgaris* in which patients suffer from large painful skin blisters (Greek *pemphigos*, a thing filled with air, blister; Latin *vulgaris*, common, not rare). Autoantibodies to the major platelet adhesion molecule gpIIb/IIIa (β3 integrin) cause thrombocyte depletion and abnormal bleeding in *autoimmune thrombocytopenia purpura*. In *acute rheumatic fever*, autoantibodies reactive with cardiac muscle surface antigens are produced after previous streptococcal infection, presumably because of cross-reactivity between bacterial antigens and autoantigens.

Diseases caused by autoreactive T cells

In other autoimmune diseases, T-cell-mediated tissue damage is the main pathogenic factor. Of these, IDDM, rheumatoid arthritis (RA) and multiple sclerosis (MS) are the best known.

In *IDDM*, insulin-producing β cells of the pancreatic islets of Langerhans are destroyed by CD8+ T_C cells, probably with some contribution from inflammatory T_H1 cells. This relatively common, juvenile form of diabetes has its usual onset in children between 10 and 14 years of age and affects around 0.25% of the population. Patients suffer from poor tolerance of glucose, a condition that can be successfully treated by replacement therapy (administration of insulin). The primary autoantigen in IDDM is not known, but likely candidates are the enzyme glutamic acid decarboxylase (expressed at high levels in the β cells and in the brain) and heat-shock protein Hsp 60. The critical factor triggering IDDM is unknown but it is hypothesized that it may be local inflammation in the pancreas, caused perhaps by a viral infection. This leads to inappropriate MHC class II expression and autoantigen fragment presentation to CD4+ T_H-cell clones that escaped tolerance induction, perhaps due to sequestration and crypticity of the autoantigen under normal conditions. Activated T_H cells support the development of autoantigen-specific T_C cells that gradually destroy the β cells. By the time IDDM is diagnosed nearly all β cells have been destroyed, which leaves little room for therapeutic intervention. In patients who received pancreatic transplants from their identical twins, β cells in the transplant were rapidly destroyed by an invasion of β-cell-specific CD8+ T_C cells.

The involvement of HLA-DQβ chains in IDDM is discussed in Chapter 6. Although it seems that the presence of amino acid residues other than aspartic acid at position 57 confers susceptibility to the disease, the critical peptide (possibly originating from glutamic acid decarboxylase or Hsp 60) presumably bound to the DQ molecule has not been identified.

Experimental autoimmune encephalitis (EAE), believed to be an animal model of human multiple sclerosis, is produced by immunization of mice or rats either by brain extract or by purified protein components (peptides) of myelin (the insulating sheath of nerve axons), i.e. myelin basic protein (MBP), proteolipid protein (PLP), myelin-associated glycoprotein (MAG) and myelin oligodendrocyte glycoprotein (MOG). The immunization stimulates inflammatory T_H1-cell clones that attack nervous tissue. They recognize autoantigenic peptides bound to MHC class II glycoproteins on microglial cells or activated endothelial cells and create inflammatory DTH-like conditions that lead to the destruction of myelin (demyelination). Even if elicited by means of a single peptide, the disease is ultimately characterized by the presence of a spectrum of T-cell clones specific for various components of myelin (*determinant spreading*). Although T-cell clones specific for MBP have been demonstrated in patients with multiple sclerosis, it is not known whether these clones cause the disease. The symptoms of *multiple sclerosis* are highly variable, depending on the affected parts of the central nervous system. Patients often suffer from motor, visual or hearing defects, spasms and mental disturbances. The disease can be reliably diagnosed by visualization of characteristic plaques in the central nervous system using nuclear magnetic resonance.

Rheumatoid arthritis, the most prevalent human autoimmune disease, is characterized by fever, malaise, fatigue, pain, stiffness and later deformation of joints, granulomas in subcutaneous and other tissues, vasculitis and ocular damage. The disease is probably caused by T_H1 $CD4^+$ cells reacting with fragments of joint antigens such as a collagen or a heat-shock protein bound to MHC class II molecules. The T_H1 cells initiate inflammation in the joint, causing DTH-like damage. The disease and related inflammatory arthritides (reactive arthritis, ankylosing spondylitis) are probably triggered by microbial infections, such as *Chlamydia*, *Yersinia* or mycobacteria. The diseases can sometimes be positively influenced by antibiotic treatment, indicating that a persistent infection is involved. Rheumatoid arthritis is also characterized by the occurrence of autoantibodies reactive with immunoglobulins called *rheumatoid factor*. Some of the tissue damage is caused by the deposition of immune complexes and complement activation. Symptoms resembling rheumatoid arthritis can be induced in mice by immunization with collagen.

Psoriasis (skin disease) is caused by the infiltration of epidermis by activated T cells and monocytes. The cells release proinflammatory cytokines that induce hyperproliferation of epidermal cells. The primary trigger of this relatively frequent disorder, characterized by scaling skin lesions, is unknown.

Treatment of autoimmune diseases

As in the case of allergy or transplantation, the aim of autoimmune disease treatment is to suppress the undesired immune response. Immunosuppressants that interfere with graft rejection (cyclosporin A, corticosteroids, antibodies to T-cell antigens) are also effective in some autoimmune diseases. Such a non-specific approach, however, compromises the patient's defence against infections. Efforts are therefore being made to replace them by more specific methods. Antibodies against activated T-cell-surface molecules, such as CD25 (a subunit of the IL-2 receptor) or gp39 (ligand of the CD40 receptor), or antibody conjugates with potent toxins (immunotoxins) have been reported to have therapeutic effects without grossly immunocompromising the treated subject. Other potential, partially selective, immunosuppressants are cytokines conjugated to toxins and cytokine antagonists (antibodies to cytokines, soluble forms of cytokine receptors or substances binding to the cytokine receptors but unable to trigger signalling). An even more specific approach is *T-cell vaccination*. When T cells infiltrating the tissues affected by T_H1-mediated autoimmune diseases (e.g. EAE) were isolated, expanded *in vitro*, fixed with glutaraldehyde and injected into animals, the disease was either markedly ameliorated or permanent remission was achieved. Similar beneficial effects were observed when peptides from variable regions of autoreactive TCRs were used instead of the fixed T cells. Presumably this vaccination leads to stimulation of T cells recognizing and destroying the autoreactive cells (anti-idiotypic T cells).

Development of rational specific therapies requires identification of the key autoantigens. This is difficult especially in the case of diseases caused by autoreactive T cells, in which the antigen is a peptide associated with an MHC molecule. The recently developed methods of direct analysis of the peptides bound to MHC molecules should, at least in theory, be a straightforward solution to this problem. However, relatively simple immunotherapies might be developed even without detailed knowledge of the autoantigen. It is possible, for example, to significantly improve the condition of some patients with rheumatoid arthritis by feeding them chicken collagen. Similarly, EAE could be inhibited by inhalation of the encephalitogenic peptide of MBP. The onset of diabetes in NOD mice can be delayed or prevented by parenteral administration of pancreatic autoantigens (insulin, glutamic acid decarboxylase). These treatments presumably induce mucosal tolerance (see Chapter 20), not only of the administered substance but of antigens (including the elicitor of the disease) expressed in the particular organ or tissue.

Further reading

Charlton, B. & Lafferty, K. J. (1995) The T_H1/T_H2 balance in autoimmunity. *Current Opinion in Immunology*, 7, 793–798.

Elson, C. J., Barker, R. N., Thompson, S. J. & Williams, N. A. (1995) Immunologically ignorant autoreactive T cells, epitope spreading and repertoire limitation. *Immunology Today*, **16**, 71–76.

Kikutani, H. & Makino, S. (1992) The murine autoimmune diabetes model: NOD and related strains. *Advances in Immunology*, **51**, 285–322.

Kuchroo, V. K., Das, M. P., Brown, J. A. *et al.* (1995) B7-1 and B7-2 costimulatory molecules activate differentially the

T_H1/T_H2 developmental pathways: application to autoimmune disease therapy. *Cell*, **80**, 707–718.

Martin, R., McFarland, H. F. & McFarlin, D. E. (1992) Immunological aspects of demyelinating diseases. *Annual Review of Immunology*, **10**, 153–187.

Merriman, T. R. & Todd, J. A. (1995) Genetics of autoimmune disease. *Current Opinion in Immunology*, 7, 786–792.

Naparstek, Y. & Plotz, P. H. (1993) The role of autoantibodies in autoimmune disease. *Annual Review of Immunology*, **11**, 79–104.

Nepom, G. T. (1995) Glutamic acid decarboxylase and other autoantigens in IDDM. *Current Opinion in Immunology*, 7, 825–830.

Nousari, H. C. & Anhalt, G. J. (1995) Bullous skin diseases. *Current Opinion in Immunology*, 7, 844–852.

Rõcken, M., Racke, M. & Shevach, E. M. (1996) IL-4-induced immune deviation as antigen-specific therapy for inflammatory autoimmune disease. *Immunology Today*, **17**, 225–231.

Song, Y.-H., Li, X. & Maclaren, N. K. (1996) The nature of autoantigens targeted in autoimmune endocrine diseases. *Immunology Today*, **17**, 232–238.

Stanley, J. R. (1993) Cell adhesion molecules as targets of autoantibodies in pemphigus and pemphigoid, bullous diseases due to defective epidermal cell adhesion. *Advances in Immunology*, **53**, 291–326.

Thorsby, E. (1995) HLA-associated disease susceptibility: which genes are primarily involved? *Immunologist*, **3**, 51–58.

Wucherpfennig, K. W. & Strominger, J. L. (1995) Molecular mimicry in T cell-mediated autoimmunity: viral peptides activate human T cell clones specific for myelin basic protein. *Cell*, 80, 695–705.

chapter 26 Immunodeficiency diseases

In this chapter we examine what happens when components of the adaptive part of the immune system fail (for defects in the non-adaptive components of the immune system see Chapters 12 & 15; rare immunodeficiencies caused by defects of major histocompatibility complex (MHC) glycoprotein expression are described in Chapter 6). This knowledge has been gleaned from studies on patients who suffer various inherited disturbances in the development of their immune system or whose immune system has been disturbed by environmental factors (infections, irradiation), i.e. patients suffering from immunodeficiency diseases. Immunodeficiency diseases usually manifest themselves by a marked susceptibility to certain types of infections that often threaten the life of the patient. Some immunodeficiency diseases predispose to the development of certain forms of autoimmunity. Corresponding to the two principal causes, immunodeficiency diseases can be divided into *inherited* and *acquired*.

Inherited immunodeficiencies

Several immunodeficiency diseases are caused by defects in genes residing on the X chromosome and are manifested mostly in males. Since males have only one X chromosome, if they inherit the defective chromosome from the mother they will suffer from the disease. Females, who have two X chromosomes only one of which carries the defective gene, are usually only partly immunodeficient. The reason behind the partial immunodeficiency of heterozygous females is the phenomenon of X-chromosome inactivation. In each cell one X chromosome is randomly inactivated; when this happens to the normal chromosome, the cell has no functional gene coding for the particular immunological trait. Half of the immune cells in the heterozygous female are therefore defective.

Immunodeficiencies caused by B-cell and immunoglobulin synthesis defects

Patients affected by *X-linked agammaglobulinaemia (XLA)* have virtually no B cells and therefore hardly any immunoglobulins either; as a result, they are highly susceptible to many types of infection. The disease begins to manifest itself in affected males at the age of 5 or 6 months, presumably because up until this stage, boys are protected by antibodies passively transferred from their mothers. First described by O. C. Bruton in 1952, this disease was later shown to be caused by a defective gene on the X chromosome and the gene coding for Bruton's tyrosine kinase (Btk). The absence of this enzyme blocks the development of B lymphocytes at the preB-cell stage, probably because of defective signalling via the preB-cell receptor (see Chapter 8) necessary for immunoglobulin gene rearrangement. However, Btk is also involved in signalling via the B-cell receptor and via some cytokine and Fc receptors. A structurally similar kinase, Itk, appears to be involved in signalling via the CD28 receptor on T cells (see Chapter 16). A defect in the *Btk* gene is also present in the immunodeficient *Xid* mouse strain.

A defect in antibody production is responsible for the X-

linked hyper-IgM syndrome, which is characterized by normal B- and T-cell development and high levels of serum IgM but absence of immunoglobulins of other isotypes. Patients suffering from the syndrome are unable to respond to T-dependent antigens and apparently have no B-cell memory. This makes them susceptible to bacterial infection and infestation by eukaryotic parasites. The defect is, however, in helper T (T_H) rather than in B cells. The former fail to express CD40L, the ligand of the B-cell co-stimulatory receptor CD40 (see Chapter 17). Because of defective T_H cells, B cells do not receive proper help, there is no development of germinal centres, no isotype switching and therefore no differentiation into memory B cells or plasma cells producing high-affinity antibodies.

The most common defect in the humoral branch of the immune system is *selective IgA deficiency*, which occurs in approximately 1 in 800 persons. The affected individuals have almost no serum IgA but, somewhat surprisingly, most are healthy, while only some are predisposed to respiratory infections. A few are also prone to inhalation allergies and can be in danger of developing serious anaphylactic reactions after blood transfusions, since they produce antibodies to IgA which is a foreign protein to their immune system. The genetic basis of this disorder has not been precisely determined, it almost certainly involves several genes including *HLA-DQB*, an unknown gene in the *MHC* class III region and additional genes within the *IGHC* region.

Common variable immunodeficiency (adult acquired agammaglobulinaemia) is characterized by decreased concentrations of IgG and IgA (and in some cases also of IgM) and is probably related to selective IgA deficiency, as it seems to have a similar, poorly defined genetic cause. In most cases patients have normal B-cell and immunoglobulin levels in their youth but these decrease later in life, leading to infections of the respiratory and digestive tract.

Immunodeficiencies caused by T-cell defects

Patients with *DiGeorge syndrome* have multiple developmental defects including abnormal facial characteristics (Fig. 26.1), anatomical heart abnormalities and an underdeveloped parathyroid gland and thymus. The one thing these defects have in common is that before the twelfth week of gestation, the anlages (embryonic foundations) of the affected organs (aortic arch near the heart, parathyroid gland and thymus, all derived from the third and fourth pharyngeal pouches) all happen to be located in the same region of the embryo. In addition to other serious manifestations (e.g. low parathormone level causing dysregulation of calcium homeostasis), the patients have an abnormally low number of T cells, and hence a deficient cellular arm of immunity. The defect is caused by the deletion of a gene in the chromosome 22q11 region, which apparently directs cell migration in the pharyngeal pouches of the embryo. Hemizygosity at this locus (the presence of a locus on only one of the homologous chromosomes, the other being deleted) causes the *velocardiofacial syndrome*, which overlaps clinically with DiGeorge syndrome but does not include defective development of the thymus. An analogous syndrome has been created in mice by targeted disruption of the *HOX* (homeobox) *1.5* gene.

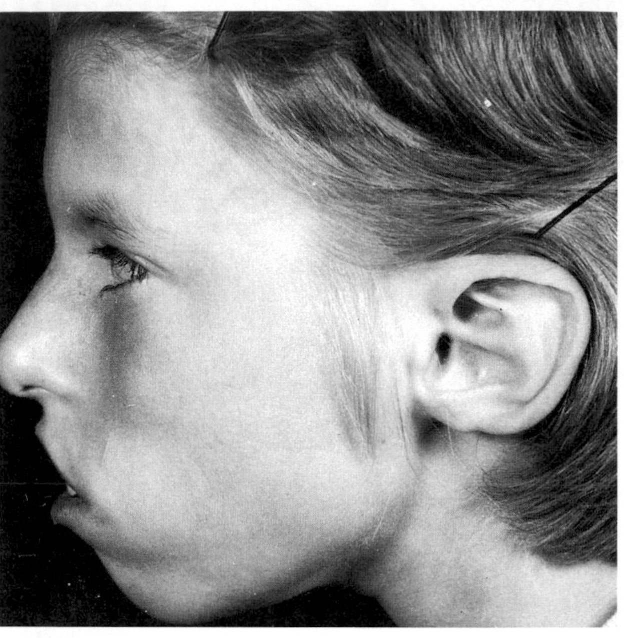

Figure 26.1 DiGeorge syndrome. Note the shortened philtrum (the groove in the midline of the upper lip) resulting in a fish-shaped mouth, low-set, notched ear pinnae, and shortened jaw. Not clearly visible are the eyes, set wide apart. (Photograph courtesy of Dr Fred S. Rosen.)

Another genetically determined developmental defect characterized by the lack of thymus occurs in *nu/nu* mice. It is controlled by a recessive *nude* gene on chromosome 11. The homozygotes are hairless ('nude') and have no thymus, apparently because the differentiation pathway transforming pharyngeal pouches into the epithelial thymus anlage is genetically blocked. In the absence of thymic epithelium, T-lymphocyte precursors fail to mature and the mice have a greatly reduced ability to develop cellular immune reactions. (One consequence of deficient cellular immunity is that these mice can accept and grow almost any kind of graft, be it fowl skin with feathers or a human tumour.) Treatment of *nu/nu* mice with interleukin (IL)-7 restores normal development of their T cells, indicating that under suitable conditions extrathymic sites may provide the envi-

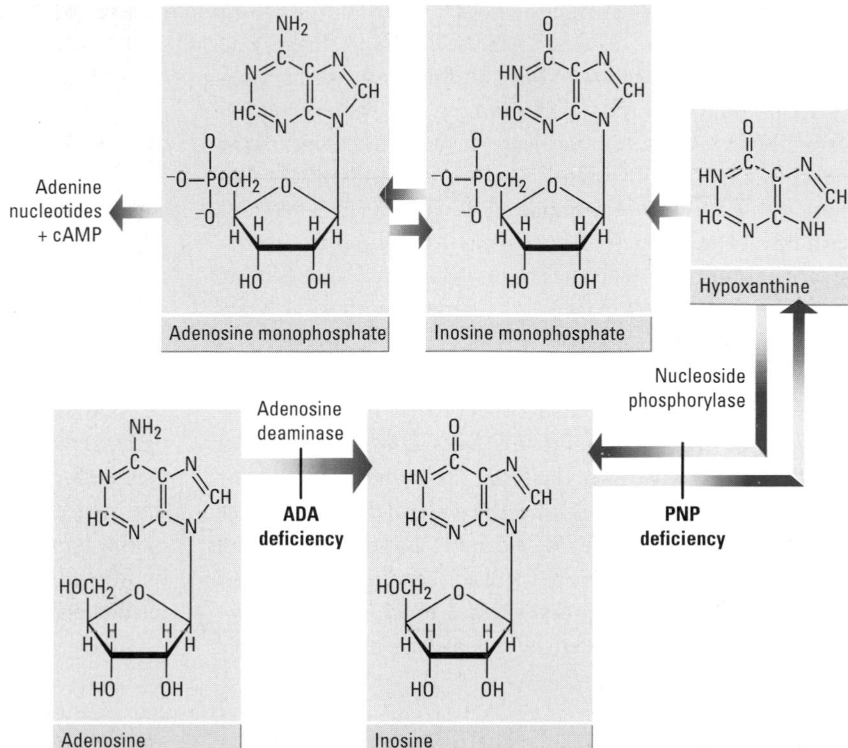

Figure 26.2 The pathway of adenosine metabolism and the sites blocked in adenosine deaminase (ADA) and purine nucleoside phosphorylase (PNP) deficiencies.

ronment necessary to induce T-cell maturation. The *nude* gene encodes a transcription factor of the winged-helix family expressed specifically in the skin and thymus. The nude mouse is an important model for investigating many topics in immunology, virology and oncology.

Adenine deaminase (ADA) deficiency has a variable phenotype, depending on the nature of the mutation affecting this enzyme of nucleotide metabolism. Nucleotide metabolites that are substrates of this enzyme (Fig. 26.2) appear to be toxic for developing T cells, so that ADA deficiency causes a blockage in the development of thymocytes at an early stage and therefore the absence of T cells in the immune system. ADA is non-covalently associated with CD26, a surface protein of activated T cells, that is enzymatically (proteolytically) active itself. A phenotype similar to that of ADA deficiency is also observed in individuals deficient in another enzyme of nucleotide metabolism, purine nucleotide phosphorylase (PNP). PNP deficiency affects cytotoxic T (T_C) cells in particular.

X-linked severe combined immunodeficiency (SCID) is characterized by defective T-cell differentiation, while B-cell maturation is unaffected. The disorder is caused by mutations in the gene encoding the γ chain of a group of cytokine receptors (for IL-2, IL-4, IL-7, IL-9 and IL-15; see Chapter 10), leading to the blockade of multiple cytokine signalling pathways. The critical cytokine is probably IL-7, which is necessary for early thymocyte development. The severe phenotype in X-linked SCID contrasts with the mild phenotype accompanying defects in the *IL-2* gene, which occur in humans or which can be created by targeted gene disruption in mice. A similar severe phenotype (lack of T cells but not B cells) is observed in rare cases of autosomal SCID caused by defects in the gene encoding the Jak-3 kinase, the enzyme used as a signalling device by the γ-receptor subunit. Another form of autosomal SCID is caused by nonfunctional ZAP-70 kinase, which is involved in T-cell receptor (TCR) signalling. It is characterized by the absence of $CD8^+$ but not $CD4^+$ T cells. The encoding gene is on chromosome 16.

Some rare T-cell immunodeficiencies may also be caused by mutations in genes encoding components of the TCR/CD3 complex, specifically the CD3γ and CD3ε chains. Patients with the CD3γ defect have reduced numbers of $CD8^+$ T cells, an observation that suggests the existence of possible interactions between CD8 and CD3γ.

A number of immunodeficient mouse strains have been created in which specific genes have been disrupted ('knocked out'). Some results of this type of experiment have been surprising, while others have confirmed the functions ascribed to specific molecules in the immune system. For example, IL-2-deficient mice undergo normal T- and B-lymphocyte development, indicating that IL-2 is, at least to some extent, dispensable. Knocking out the gene for interferon-γ causes marked defects in macrophage and natural killer (NK)-cell functions, and increases susceptibility to pathogens normally cleared by T_H1-based mechanisms. Mice lacking tumour necrosis factor-α receptor type 1 are, as expected, resistant to endotoxin (lipopolysaccharide) but have severely impaired resistance to infections with intracellular bacteria such as *Listeria monocytogenes*. Severe immunodeficiency has been observed in mice lacking the protein tyrosine kinase Lck associated with CD4, CD8 and TCR. This defect blocks thymocyte development and the few mature T cells that do develop are non-functional. Immunodeficiencies are also observed in mice with disrupted genes for CD4, CD8, CD28, CD40 or IgD molecules. Surprisingly, mice lacking the adhesion receptor CD2, as well as those lacking the T- and B1-cell-surface molecule CD5, appear to be normal. Another surprising result is that mice defective in the IL-2 receptor γ chain (used by several cytokine receptors) show a much milder phenotype than humans affected by a similar defect (X-linked SCID).

Other genetically determined immunodeficiencies

Ataxia telangiectasia is an autosomal recessive disorder characterized by loss of the ability to coordinate muscles controlled by the cerebellum (cerebellar ataxia), dilation of capillaries in facial skin and eyeballs (oculocutaneous telangiectasia; Greek *telos*, end; *angeion*, vessel; *ektasis*, a stretching out), hypersensitivity to ionizing (but not ultraviolet) radiation, lung infections, reduced number of T cells, defective T_H-cell activity, increased incidence of certain tumours and reduced serum levels of certain immunoglobulin classes (IgA, IgE and IgG2). Some of the immunological defects can be explained by the underdevelopment of the thymus, which remains embryonic in appearance or is missing altogether. The neurological disorders are caused by progressive neuronal degeneration, which begins at an early age when the child starts to walk. The dilation of venous capillaries begins around the conjunctivae of the eyes, then spreads to the eyelids, ears and neck. Other common features of the disease are premature greying of the hair, atrophy of the skin, endocrine abnormalities involving a number of organs, increased levels of serum α-fetoprotein and glucose intolerance. Hallmarks of this disorder are DNA fragility and chromosomal translocations mainly involving *TCR* and *IG* loci in lymphocytes. The defective *ATM* gene is localized on chromosome 11q22–23. The coding portion of the gene is very large (about 12 kb) and its function can be affected by at least 40 different mutations. One section of the ATM protein is similar to phosphatidylinositol 3-kinases, enzymes involved in mitogenic signal transduction, meiotic recombination and cell-cycle control. Another part of the protein resembles another group of proteins whose function is to block the cell cycle in cells whose DNA has been damaged by ultraviolet radiation or X-rays. Epidemiological studies indicate that a single copy of the defective gene (ataxia patients have two defective copies) increases the risk of breast cancer. It is estimated that one woman in five who develops breast cancer is a carrier of the defective gene.

Wiskott–Aldrich syndrome is a severe X chromosome-linked immunodeficiency disorder affecting both the cellular and humoral branches of the immune system, but patients also suffer from eczema, autoimmunity, increased incidence of tumours and thrombocytopenia, which causes severe bleeding. A typical feature of this disease is 'baldness' of the lymphocytes, a lack of microvilli formed by actin bundless. The primary defect is in a gene encoding a 502-residue protein that probably acts as a transcription factor.

Autosomal recessive SCID is characterized by the absence of T and B lymphocytes and the presence of NK cells. It is phenotypically similar to mouse SCID and also to mouse immunodeficiencies caused by disruption of the *RAG1* or *RAG2* genes, which encode components of the machinery responsible for the rearrangement of *TCR* and *IG* genes. Autosomal recessive SCID is caused by a gene on chromosome 8, which codes for a DNA-dependent protein kinase ($DNA\text{-}PK_{CS}$). This enzyme forms a complex with an abundant nuclear heterodimeric protein Ku, which binds to broken ends of DNA. The latter can arise as a result of radiation damage or after excision of intervening sequences during *IG* and *TCR* gene rearrangement. $DNA\text{-}PK_{CS}$ phosphorylates a number of substrates including the tumour suppressor p53 and the products of *RAG* genes, but its exact function in DNA repair and gene rearrangement is unclear.

Acquired (secondary) immunodeficiencies

Temporary or permanent immunodeficiencies often accompany various infectious diseases, malignancies, malnutrition and stresses of various kinds, including post-injury trauma and surgery. Ionizing radiation and many drugs may also adversely affect leucopoiesis in bone marrow or have toxic effects on mature leucocytes, especially in the case of immunosuppressive drugs used to prevent organ graft rejection or to treat autoimmune diseases.

The *acquired immune deficiency syndrome (AIDS)* is at present by far the most serious immunodeficiency disease. About 1.5 million people worldwide suffer from this inevitably fatal illness. The number of people infected by the

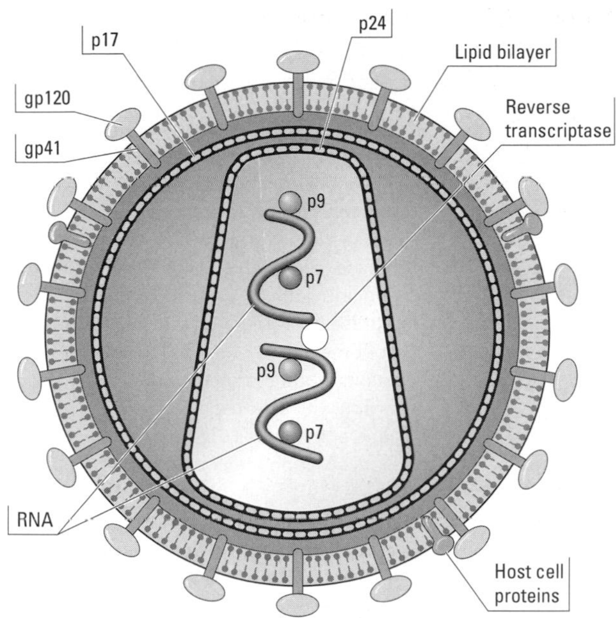

Figure 26.3 Human immunodeficiency virus (HIV) virion. The envelope is a phospholipid bilayer derived from the host-cell plasma membrane. The major surface protein is a complex of transmembrane gp41 and gp120, which interact with the CD4 receptor of the host cell and subsequently with the CKR co-receptors. Each gp41/gp120 knob is composed of three pairs of these molecules. The viral core (nucleocapsid) consists of two layers, the outer formed by protein p17 and the inner by protein p24. The core contains two identical RNA molecules that carry the virus's genetic information. Associated with the viral RNA are nucleoid proteins p7 and p9 as well as one molecule of reverse transcriptase and certain other proteins such as the enzymes protease and integrase (not shown here; see Fig. 26.5). The virion also contains small amounts of captured host-cell proteins, such as membrane components (e.g. MHC glycoproteins) in the envelope as well as some proteins of cytoplasmic origin in the nucleocapsid (not shown).

virus causing AIDS is probably higher than 25 million and increases daily by about 5000. The disease is characterized by a greatly reduced number of CD4+ T cells, functionally defective antigen-presenting cells (dendritic cells) but normal or increased number of B cells and elevated serum immunoglobulin levels. Patients suffer from infections that healthy individuals can normally ward off without any problems. The infections include those caused by bacteria (*Mycobacterium tuberculosis*, *Mycobacterium avis*, *Haemophilus influenzae*, *Salmonella*), fungi (*Candida*, *Cryptococcus neoformans*), protozoan parasites (*Toxoplasma*, *Microsporidium*, *Leishmania*, *Pneumocystis*) and viruses (herpes simplex, varicella zoster, cytomegalovirus) that are normally combated by T_H1-type responses. Patients with AIDS also suffer from otherwise rare tumours such as Kaposi's sarcoma or non-Hodgkin's lymphoma, as well as neurological disorders and cachexia (wasting).

The causative agent of AIDS is *human immunodeficiency virus-1 (HIV-1)* or the closely related HIV-2 (Fig. 26.3). These are *retroviruses* (see Chapters 13 & 22) belonging to the group of non oncogenic *lentiviruses* (Latin *lentus*, slow), which can persist over a long period in the infected cells and eventually kill them. HIV is transmissible by sexual contact or by contaminated blood. HIV infection has three major phases (Fig. 26.4). The first is a typical acute phase lasting a few weeks immediately after exposure to the virus. During this phase, large numbers of CD4+ T lymphocytes and macrophages are infected, large numbers of virus particles can be found in body fluids and the patients often display symptoms similar to mild influenza. The body of the infected individual mounts vigorous humoral and cell-mediated responses against HIV, leading to the production of a high level of antibodies and a plethora of virus-specific

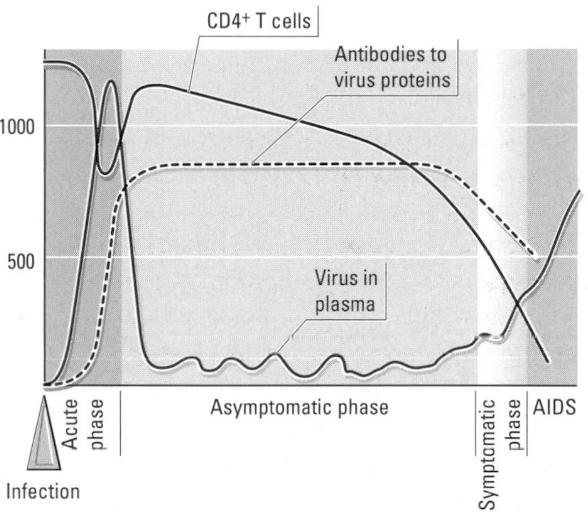

Figure 26.4 Progression of a typical human immunodeficiency virus (HIV) infection. A few weeks after infection the patient suffers a mild influenza-like disease accompanied by a transient drop in CD4+ T-cell numbers and the development of an immune response (acute phase). The response (cytotoxic T (T_C) cells and antibodies) causes a marked decrease in viraemia but fails to eradicate the infection. During the following relatively long asymptomatic phase (1–10 years), antibody and T_C-cell levels remain high and virus concentration in the blood fluctuates around a relatively low mean; the fluctuation reflects expansion of virus variants and their suppression by immune reactions. During this phase the CD4+ T-cell count slowly but steadily decreases. After it drops below 500/μl, opportunistic infections begin to occur and viraemia increases. This symptomatic phase usually lasts 2–3 years. The last phase, that of fully developed AIDS, is usually shorter than 1 year and is characterized by CD4+ T-cell counts below 200/μl and by a decrease in antibody and T_C-cell levels.

T_C- and T_H-cell clones. This response, however, rarely succeeds: only very few individuals manage to rid their bodies of the virus. In most cases the infection becomes latent. In this second phase, which may last many years, the patient remains healthy and the number of infectious virus particles in blood plasma drops to a very low level. However, even during this period a slow but steady decline in the number of CD4+ T cells continues, the titre of antibodies to HIV proteins in serum remains high and HIV-specific T_C cells are readily demonstrable. When the number of CD4+ T cells drops to under 500/μl (normal values are around 1200/μl), immunodeficiency and other symptoms become manifest. When the CD4+ T-cell count decreases to below 200/μl, the patient is said to have AIDS. The length of the asymptomatic phase varies from less than 1 year to more than 10 years. The factors that affect this variation and contribute to the second phase and thus to the appearance of AIDS are largely unknown, but simultaneous infections by bacteria or other viruses may be involved. In the terminal phase of the disease, CD4+ T cells disappear almost completely, severe pathological changes in the structure of secondary lymphoid organs occur, the number of infectious virus particles increases and the patient usually succumbs to a secondary infection.

The HIV particle consists of a core and an envelope. The core contains the viral RNA genome surrounded by several proteins encoded by the *gag* gene and one molecule of the enzyme reverse transcriptase (see Fig. 26.3). The virus envelope consists of a phospholipid bilayer studded with two non-covalently linked glycoproteins, gp120 and gp41. The glycoproteins are produced by the cleavage of the primary product (gp160) of the viral *env* gene. In addition to these two genes (*gag* and *env*), the HIV genome contains seven other genes coding for enzymes (reverse transcriptase, protease and integrase) and several regulatory proteins (Fig. 26.5, Table 26.1). The HIV RNA genome is flanked at both ends by *long terminal repeats* (LTR) involved in integration into the host genome. The transcript of the *gag* and *pol* genes is translated into a large polyprotein precursor, which is then cleaved into the mature proteins by the viral protease (the latter being part of the polyprotein).

The envelope glycoprotein gp120 binds specifically to the CD4 surface molecule expressed on a subset of T lymphocytes and also present in lower amounts on monocytes and macrophages. Recall that the major function of CD4 is to serve as the co-receptor of MHC class II glycoproteins during contact between a T cell and an antigen-presenting cell (APC) (see Chapters 7 and 16); CD4 is also the receptor of IL-16 (see Table 10.2). CD4 thus serves as the primary receptor for HIV. However, binding of HIV to CD4 alone is not sufficient to enable fusion of the viral envelope with the cell membrane. To achieve this step, that is crucial for infection of the cell, the envelope gp120 must subsequently bind to a co-receptor on the cell surface. Several chemokine receptors (CKR) have been identified as HIV co-receptors.[1] Since the viral envelope contains a number of host cell-membrane proteins such as MHC glycoproteins and several adhesion molecules, it is possible that these, too, participate in attachment of the virion to host cells. The complex of gp120 with CD4 formed during the initial contact of HIV with the cell surface subsequently attaches to the CKR co-receptor. Formation of this ternary complex (gp120-CD4-CKR) brings the lipids of the viral envelope and cell plasma membrane into its proximity and thus enables fusion of the membranes, which is followed immediately by the contents of the viral particle being discharged into the cytoplasm. Two major CKR co-receptors of HIV have been identified: CC-CKR-5 (a receptor specific for the CC-chemokines RANTES, MIP-1α and MIP-1β) expressed mainly on macrophages, and CXC-CKR-4. CXC-CKR-4 is also called CXCR-4, fusin or LESTR (for leucocyte-expressed seven-transmembrane-domain receptor) and is expressed mainly

Table 26.1 HIV proteins and their functions.

Gene	Products	Functions
gag	p17	Forms outer layer of nucleocapsid (viral core)
	p24	Forms inner layer of nucleocapsid
	p7	Component of viral core
	p9	Component of viral core
pol	p64, p51	Reverse transcriptase and RNase (p64)
	p10	Protease (cleaves the primary polyproteins gag and pol)
	p32	Integrase (integration of viral cDNA into host genome)
env	gp41	Transmembrane protein; participates in virus fusion with the host cell
	gp120	Ligand of host cell's CD4
vif	p23	Enhances virion infectivity
vpr	p15	Unknown
tat	p14	Strong transcription activator
rev	p19	Participates in the production and transport of unspliced viral RNA
nef	p27	Regulates viral replication
vpu	p16	Participates in virus budding and release

[1] Chemokines are a group of cytokines exhibiting, among other activities, strong chemotactic effects on phagocytes and other leucocytes. Included among the 30 or so identified chemokines are IL-8, RANTES, MIP-1α, MIP-1β and others (see Chapter 10). Chemokines can be divided into two major groups called CC- and CXC-chemokines based on characteristic features of their primary structure. Receptors for chemokines all belong to the seven transmembrane-spanning receptor superfamily (STSR-SF) and send signals via associated cytoplasmic trimeric G-proteins (Chapter 10).

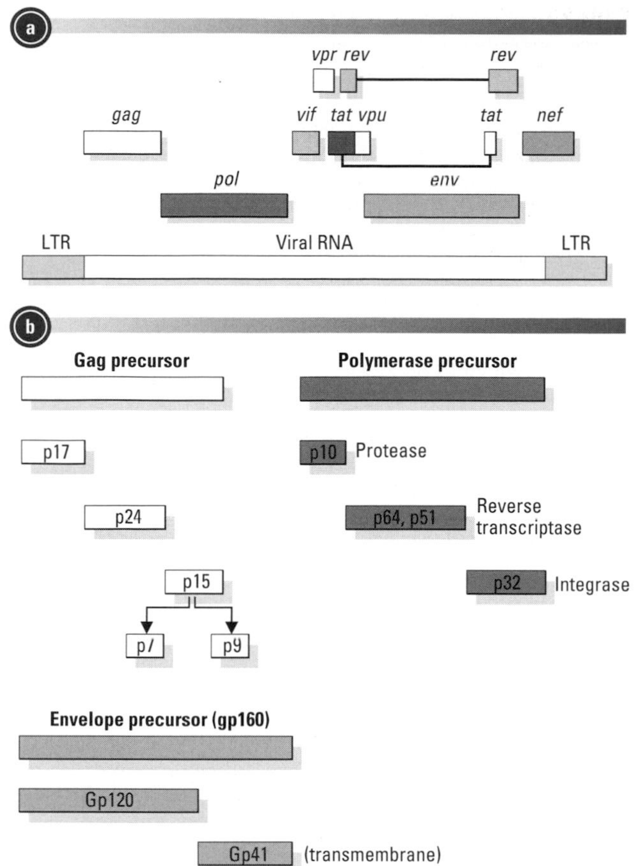

Figure 26.5 Human immunodeficiency virus-1 (HIV-1) genome (a) and its protein products (b). The entire genome (9749 nucleotides) is organized into nine partially overlapping genes (some of the RNA segments can be read in two or three different frames so that the coding capacity of the small genome is increased). The genes are flanked by *long terminal repeats* (LTR), which do not encode any proteins but function in viral integration into the host-cell genome and in regulation of viral genome expression. The gene products and their functions are listed in Table 26.1. Note that two of the genes (*rev* and *tat*) are split into two separate exons brought together by the splicing of RNA transcripts. Primary translation products of three of the largest genes (*gag*, *pol*, *env*) are polyproteins that are subsequently cleaved into final products by the viral protease (*gag*, *pol*) or by a host-cell protease (*env*).

on T cells. It binds the CXC-chemokine that is termed stromal cell-derived factor-1 (SDF-1). The essential role of CKR co-receptors in HIV infection is illustrated by the fact that individuals deficient in expression of the CC-CKR-5 are highly resistant to the infection. The respective chemokines (RANTES, MIP-1α and MIP-1β) effectively block HIV infectivity presumably because upon binding to the CKR they interfere with its gp120 co-receptor function.

After penetration into the cytoplasm, reverse transcriptase copies viral RNA into double-stranded DNA, which enters the cell nucleus and integrates into the host-cell DNA as a *provirus*. When the host cell is activated, the cell's transcription factors (mainly NF-κB) initiate transcription of the integrated viral genome. Transcription, which is greatly enhanced by two viral proteins (tat and rev), leads to the production of all components of new virions, which assemble at and bud from the cell surface.

The proportion of infected CD4+ T cells in the blood is around 10%; large numbers of infected CD4+ T cells are also present in lymphoid tissues even in the latent, asymptomatic phase of the disease. Infected T cells die rapidly (average lifespan 2.2 days) either because of cytopathic effects of the virus or because they are destroyed by the immune system. The dying cells, however, are immediately replaced by newly formed cells so that most of the healthy T cells observed in blood are actually newcomers that have not yet been infected. This observation explains the progressive loss of memory T cells known to be associated with the infection. Although the immune system is, in the first phase of HIV infection, able to replace the lost infected CD4+ T cells, the increasing difference between clearance and renewal of these cells gradually results in net decrease of their number. This process gives a superficial impression of latency, but actually it is a highly dynamic race. Many HIV-infected and some neighbouring uninfected T cells fuse *in vitro* upon interaction of viral gp120 and cellular CD4 molecules and the giant multinucleated *syncytia* die. No evidence exists, however, for syncytia formation *in vivo*.

Why is the immune system eventually unable to deal with the infection? The first reason is that the virus infects cells that are of crucial importance to the regulation of the immune system. The second reason is that HIV uses multiple ways of avoiding immune response, the main one being that it mutates frequently in a host and constantly produces new variants. Some of the variants are abortive because of defects in vitally important proteins, but others may be functionally neutral. The peptides derived from the variant proteins may either fail to bind to MHC molecules or the complexes may not be recognized by T-cell clones expanded in response to the earlier variants. Some HIV variant peptides may even act as TCR antagonists that efficiently switch off certain T-cell clones (see Chapter 16). HIV variants also change their gp120 and gp41 epitopes so that they are no longer recognized by antibodies formed against earlier variants. Although the CD4-binding site remains apparently unchanged in all variants, antibodies against this site do not form for some reason. HIV variability is such that each patient carries a large collection of different viruses and no two separate isolates from the same patient are identical.

Table 26.2 Possible mechanisms contributing to HIV pathogenicity and escape from immune control.

Phenomenon	Comments
Induction of syncytia	Many HIV-infected cells fuse together *in vitro* to form large, multinucleated, non-viable syncytia. The phenomenon is probably not important *in vivo*
Direct cytopathic effect	Activation of latently infected CD4+ T cells leads to massive production of new virions accompanied by destruction of the host cell. The destroyed cells are replaced by an increased rate of thymocyte maturation. Some HIV proteins (tat, gp120) stimulate apoptosis
Cytotoxic killing of infected cells	HIV-infected cells are recognized by T_C cells and killed (a desirable but dangerous defence mechanism to stop infection)
Destruction of uninfected bystander cells	Free gp120 binds to CD4 on uninfected activated T cells and after internalization and processing some gp120 peptides bound to MHC proteins may be recognized by T_C cells
Antibody-mediated destruction of infected and bystander cells	Infected cells expressing gp120 on their surface bind antibodies and may be destroyed by complement, ADCC or phagocytosis. The same can happen to uninfected T cells that bind gp120 to their surface
Inactivation of CD4+ T cells by gp120	gp120 (either as part of a virion or released in a soluble form) binds to CD4. The resulting altered signal via the TCR inactivates the T cell
Destruction or incapacitation of APCs	APCs infected by HIV are either destroyed by some of the above mechanisms or are functionally changed so that they are less efficient
Destruction of thymus stromal cells	Thymus epithelial and dendritic cells are destroyed by an unknown mechanism; thymocyte development is impaired
Shift of T_H1 vs. T_H2 balance	Infection of APCs may change their properties in such a way that T_H2-cell development is preferred to T_H1-cell development; this contributes to an inadequate response to opportunistic infections
Loss of T-cell memory	Activated CD4+ T cells are continuously removed by some of the above mechanisms, so that memory cells cannot be established. The immune system is dominated by freshly formed naive T cells
Damage by autoantibodies produced by polyclonal B-cell activation	gp120 acts as a polyclonal activator of V_H3-positive B cells, and leads to the production of potentially autoreactive antibodies
Escape by antigenic variation (including antagonist peptide variants)	Error-prone mechanisms of HIV replication produce large numbers of mutants that continually escape humoral and cytotoxic immune mechanisms. Other variants are responsible for the development of drug resistance. Some escape variants either produce no peptides binding to host-cell MHC molecules or produce antagonist peptides that inactivate T-cell clones specific for other HIV variants

ADCC, antibody-dependent cell-mediated cytotoxicity; APCs, antigen-presenting cells; HIV, human immunodeficiency virus; MHC, major histocompatibility complex; T_C, cytotoxic T cell; TCR, T-cell receptor; T_H, helper T cell.

The mechanisms responsible for HIV pathogenicity have not been firmly established; some possibilities are listed in Table 26.2. The only non-human species that can be infected with HIV is the chimpanzee. Curiously, the infected animals, for unknown reasons, do not develop AIDS. A virus closely resembling HIV, simian immunodeficiency virus (SIV), infects African green monkeys and causes an immunodeficiency similar to human AIDS. In addition, several other retroviruses cause immunodeficiencies similar to AIDS, but these are usually accompanied by lymphoproliferative disorders. They include mouse leukaemia virus, which causes mouse AIDS (MAIDS), and feline leukaemia virus.

Possible immunodeficiency therapies

Some inherited or acquired immunodeficiencies, especially those characterized by antibody deficiencies, can be treated relatively successfully by a substitution therapy involving infusions of immunoglobulin preparations in combination with antibiotics. Since these preparations usually contain antibodies to various pathogens, they provide at least partial protection from infections.

A more radical therapy is bone marrow transplantation. It provides the only chance for survival for individuals with severe immunodeficiencies caused by defects in the normal development of certain types of leucocytes.

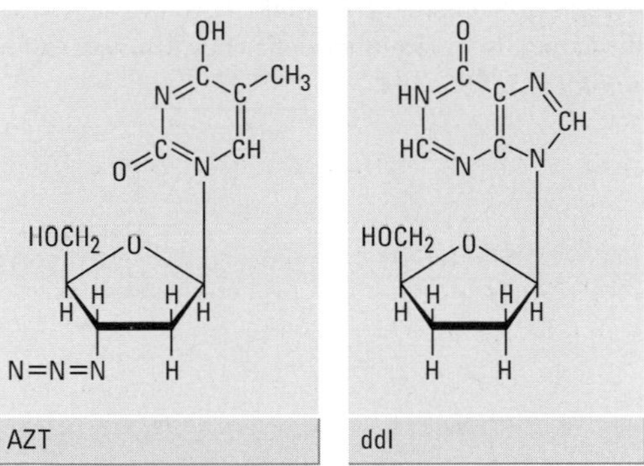

Figure 26.6 Nucleotide analogues used to treat human immunodeficiency virus (HIV) infection. AZT (3′-azido-deoxythymidine; zidovudine) and ddI (2′,3′-dideoxyinosine; didanosine) are synthetic analogues of natural DNA building blocks, deoxynucleotides. They lack a hydroxyl group in the 3′ position of the deoxyribose part of the molecule. When the analogues are incorporated by reverse transcriptase into the growing cDNA chain, the chain cannot grow further because there is no acceptor OH group in the 3′ position for the next nucleotide. HIV reverse transcriptase, in contrast to host-cell DNA polymerase, actually prefers AZT to normal thymidine. The drug thus efficiently inhibits viral replication and considerably less host-cell DNA synthesis. However, reverse transcriptase variants arise that do not accept AZT and thus lead to drug resistance.

Until very recently no really effective treatment for AIDS was available. Efforts were made to inhibit the entry of HIV into cells, to block some essential step of its life cycle or to manipulate the immune system so that it eliminates the infection before the devastating disease can develop. Attempts to use soluble CD4 to block the virus–CD4 interaction have failed, presumably because of insufficient affinity of soluble CD4 for gp120. During recent years the only drugs that had a certain positive effect were those interfering with the reverse transcription of HIV RNA. These are nucleotide analogues such as 3′-azido-2′,3′-dideoxythymidine (AZT; zidovudine) and 2′,3′-dideoxyinosine (ddI; didanosine) (Fig. 26.6), which after incorporation into the growing DNA chain interrupt its further extension because they lack the required hydroxyl group at the 3′ position of the carbohydrate ring. Unfortunately, during treatment variants of HIV arise, whose reverse transcriptases have become resistant to the drugs. The use of mixtures of two or more therapeutics of this type appears to be superior because it keeps the virus concentration in the body at a substantially decreased level for much longer periods than a single nucleotide analogue. Several inhibitors of the HIV protease (whose commercial names are ritonavir, indinavir and saquinavir, for example) appear to be even more effective. Perhaps the most efficient HIV chemotherapy at present is the use of a mixture of two reverse transcriptase inhibitors and one or two protease inhibitors. Such treatment decreases the patient's viral load to undetectably low levels. However, several years will be needed before the therapeutic potential of this promising new generation of virostatics is fully evaluated. New possibilities for the development of another type of HIV therapeutics arose after the discovery of the CKR co-receptors: the cytokines naturally binding to these CKRs or their analogues might effectively block the spread of infection.

Immunotherapeutic approaches to the prevention or treatment of HIV infection are not practical at present because knowledge of how the virus interacts with the immune system is highly inadequate. All attempts to develop an HIV vaccine have thus far been unsuccessful.

Further reading

Bloom, B. R. (1996) A perspective on AIDS vaccines. *Science*, **272**, 1888–1890.

Cournoyer, D. & Caskey, C. T. (1993) Gene therapy of the immune system *Annual Review of Immunology*, **11**, 297–329.

Fischer, A. & Arnaiz-Villena, A. (1995) Immunodeficiencies of genetic origin. *Immunology Today*, **11**, 510–514.

Haynes, B. F., Pantaleo, G. & Fauci, A. S. (1996) Toward an understanding of the correlates of protective immunity to HIV infection. *Science*, **271**, 324–328.

Kindt, T. J. & Hirsch, V. (1995) The ideal animal model for AIDS: a continuing search. *Immunologist*, **3**, 26–31.

Kindt, T. J., Hirsch, V. M., Johnson, P. R. & Sawasdikosol, S. (1992) Animal models for acquired immunodeficiency syndrome. *Advances in Immunology*, **52**, 425–474.

Knight, S. C. (1995) A problem of antigen presentation? *Current Biology*, **4**, 1131–1134.

Levy, J. A., Mackewicz, C. E. & Barker, E. (1996) Controlling HIV pathogenesis: the role of noncytotoxic anti-HIV response of CD8+ T cells. *Immunology Today*, **17**, 217–224.

Möller, G. (Ed.) (1994) Genetic basis of primary immunodeficiencies. *Immunological Reviews*, **138**, entire volume.

Möller, G. (Ed.) (1994) HIV and its receptors. *Immunological Reviews*, **140**, entire volume.

Mosmann, T. R. (1994) Cytokine patterns during the progression to AIDS. *Science*, **265**, 193–194.

Poignard, P., Klasse, P. J. & Sattentau, Q. J. (1996) Antibody neutralization of HIV-1. *Immunology Today*, **17**, 239–246.

Richman, D. D. (1996) HIV therapeutics. *Science*, **272**, 1886–1888.

Weiss, R. A. (1996) HIV receptors and the pathogenesis of AIDS. *Science*, **272**, 1885–1886.

Wells, T. N. C., Proudfoot, A. E., Power, C. A. & Marsh, M. (1996) Chemokine receptors—the new frontier for AIDS research. *Chemistry and Biology*, **3**, 603–609.

Wilkinson, D. (1996) Cofactors provide the entry keys. *Current Biology*, **6**, 1051–1053.

Yeung, R. S. M., Penninger, J. & Mak, T. W. (1993) Genetically modified animals and immunodeficiency. *Current Opinion in Immunology*, **5**, 585–594.

chapter 27 Immunoprophylaxis

Immunology evolved from attempts to develop ways of protecting people and animals from infectious diseases. From such efforts researchers eventually learned about the existence of the immune system and realized that immunity was the best method of defence. Immunoprophylaxis (protection by immunological means) continues to be one of the propelling forces in immunological research, even though immunology has become a basic science discipline which, in addition to its utilitarian mission, also deals with fundamental biological problems.

The effort to protect human populations from communicable diseases has been highly successful. The widespread use of immunoprophylaxis has led to global eradication of one disease (smallpox), the near elimination of several other diseases in developed countries (poliomyelitis, rubella, tetanus, diphtheria and measles) and a dramatic reduction in the incidence rates of other illnesses still.

To induce immunity against a specific infectious agent, an individual is *immunized* against it, either actively or passively. In *active immunization*, the individual is exposed to the causative agent or parts thereof; in *passive immunization*, the individual receives protective molecules (antibodies) or cells (lymphocytes) produced in another individual. The preparation of parasites or of their fragments used to induce active immunity against a communicable disease is a *vaccine*. An alternative to a vaccine is *toxoid*, a bacterial toxin that has been rendered harmless without losing its ability to induce immunity, usually in the form of *antitoxins* (antibodies to toxins). To some clinicians, however, antitoxin is a preparation of antibodies from the serum of animals immunized with a specific antigen and used to achieve passive immunity.

The parasites contained in a vaccine cannot be used in their natural form because they might induce a disease instead of preventing it. They must therefore either be killed or used in an attenuated form. *Attenuated* forms are designated parasites that multiply in their hosts without causing disease. They are genetic variants of pathogenic forms that, by mutation or some other change, have lost a particular property normally required for pathogenicity. Following administration of a vaccine, the attenuated microorganisms multiply in the recipient until the immunity, which they have induced in the meantime, eliminates them. *Subunit vaccines* are purified components of a parasite, such as envelope proteins of a virus.

Vaccination works because of *immunological memory*. Response to the vaccine stimulates T and B lymphocytes, some of which become memory cells capable of responding swiftly and efficiently should they later encounter the parasite in its *virulent* (non-attenuated) form. In some cases, vaccination establishes an antibody level in the plasma sufficient to eliminate the parasite even before it becomes the target of the secondary response initiated by memory cytotoxic T (T_C) and B cells. This type of protection is essential, for example, in poliomyelitis, because infection of and damage to neurons must be prevented at all costs.

Most vaccines are *prophylactic*, i.e. they are used before the real infection occurs; the state of immunity they induce effectively prevents contraction of the disease. However, in some cases *therapeutic* vaccination is used to elicit or accelerate immune response to a dangerous pathogen that has already invaded the body.

Certain *risks* are associated with vaccination, but they are outweighed by its benefits. In some rare cases, the live attenuated vaccine may cause disease in highly susceptible, immunodeficient individuals. In other cases, adverse anaphylactic reactions can occur, mainly because of the presence of contaminants originating, for example, from the cells in which the parasite used for vaccination was propagated. A major risk has been that some live vaccines have lost their efficiency after inappropriate storage and thus have failed to provide the expected protection. A critical vaccine component may sometimes induce tolerance instead of immunity in some individuals, as apparently happened with the measles vaccine introduced in the 1960s.

Passive immunization

Therapeutic or prophylactic passive immunization can be provided by the application of serum or immunoglobulins obtained from human or animal donors who recover from the disease or who are intentionally immunized. Passive immunization is used in either immunodeficient patients unable to make their own antibodies or individuals who become acutely exposed to a noxious agent (a venom or an infectious microorganism). Horse or rabbit antisera or immune globulins raised against bacterial, snake or other animal toxins are commonly used to treat affected individuals. The treatment, however, is associated with a risk of anaphylactic reactions and can be used only in individuals who have not received serum of that particular species before. Another form of passive immunization involves the use of pooled human immunoglobulins from many normal or immunized donors. This preparation can be administered either intramuscularly or, after careful removal of any aggregates, intravenously. Immunoglobulin preparations are used to provide general protection for immunodeficient patients or for individuals exposed (or at high risk of being exposed) to diseases such as hepatitis A or B, rabies or tetanus.

Active immunization

Successful active immunizations against major infectious diseases have been based mostly on attenuated viruses or bacteria, and in some cases also on killed microorganisms. Generally, live attenuated vaccines provide better and longer-lasting immunity but they may pose certain dangers, as mentioned earlier. Live vaccines are usually also more sensitive to storage conditions. Attenuation has traditionally been achieved by growing the microorganism for several generations in unnatural host cells *in vitro*. Adaptation to these conditions leads to selection of mutants that have lost the pathogenicity of the original wild type but still have a limited ability to replicate in the human host and to elicit an immune response. A more rational alternative is manipulation of microorganisms using methods of recombinant DNA.

The optimal vaccination scheme must be empirically established in each particular case. Important factors are dose, site of application, number of doses and intervals between them. Age is also an important factor. Infants up to the age of 1 year, for example, contain maternal antibodies that may interfere with the vaccine's efficiency. A brief description of some live attenuated vaccines follows.

Vaccinia virus was long used as protection against smallpox, but now that the disease has been eradicated (the last case was recorded in 1970 in Somalia) this type of vaccination has been abandoned. The last few samples of the smallpox virus are being kept in a few laboratories and it is heatedly argued that these too should be destroyed. The structure of the smallpox virus genome has been determined and so any of its genes could be reconstructed if needed.

Measles virus attenuated by growth in chicken embryos or dog kidney cells is given as a single subcutaneous dose at the age of 15 months and provides lifelong protection. The same is also true for *mumps* and *rubella* viruses. Attenuated *poliomyelitis vaccine* (a mixture of viral strains I, II and III grown in monkey kidney cells) is given usually in three peroral doses and provides lifelong protection. Vaccines made of inactivated poliomyelitis virus are also in use. Poliomyelitis is considered to be the next target for complete eradication.

A single subcutaneous dose of attenuated *yellow fever* virus provides protection for about 10 years.

An attenuated strain of *Mycobacterium bovis* (bacillus Calmette–Guérin, BCG) is used in a single subcutaneous dose given to individuals who belong to groups at risk for tuberculosis. The latter includes persons who do not have antibodies against mycobacterial antigens produced in response to a natural infection. BCG has been the most widely used live vaccine: over 2.5 billion people have been immunized and only relatively few serious complications have been observed.

In a number of other cases killed subunit vaccines have been used successfully. To increase immunogenicity, such vaccines are usually administered with an adjuvant (aluminium hydroxide). *Diphtheria toxoid* adsorbed on alum is given to children in four or five intramuscular doses and provides protection for about 10 years. *Hepatitis B vaccine* is presently made from recombinant viral surface antigen (HBsAg) obtained in engineered yeasts. Three doses provide protection for about 5 years. Killed *pertussis bacteria* are given as part of a triple vaccine (diphtheria, tetanus, pertussis) in three intramuscular doses and protect for about 5 years. Killed bacteria are also used in the case of vaccination against *cholera*, *plague* and *typhoid* (in all cases only partial and short-term protection is generated) and inactivated viruses are used in the case of *influenza* and *rabies*. Therapeutic vaccination (usually simultaneously with passive immunization with antibodies) is used when rabies infection is suspected. In this case, the development of natural infection is so slow (up to 2–3 months) that it is possible to produce sufficient amounts of antibodies by a suitable immunization scheme to halt the disease before it can manifest itself. In several other cases vaccines are based on purified pathogen antigens, such as the polysaccharide antigens of *Haemophilus influenzae*, *Neisseria meningitidis* or *Streptococcus pneumoniae*.

Development of new types of vaccines

Despite the success rate of vaccination in the suppression of numerous infectious diseases, a number of problems remain. First, many serious diseases exist for which there are no suitable vaccines. These include malaria, schistosomiasis, trypanosomiasis, viral diseases such as AIDS, the respiratory disease caused by respiratory syncytial virus (RSV) and severe diarrhoea caused by rotaviruses and by *Shigella*. In most of these cases even exposure to natural infection does not provide protection against a subsequent infection; in some cases the primary infection is not resolved by the immune system, the patients remain chronically infected and suffer from repeated outbursts of the disease. Conventional vaccination procedures essentially mimicking natural infection apparently fail for the same reasons: the parasites have learned how to avoid immunity (see Chapter 21). The challenge is to make use of our understanding of the immune system and parasite biology to devise more sophisticated vaccination procedures. In a number of other infections, existing vaccines are imperfect in that they either do not provide protection for a sufficiently long time or are not able to elicit protective immunity in a high proportion of vaccinated individuals. Tuberculosis is a good example of this category.

Second, adverse effects occur after some vaccinations in a minority of recipients. The ideal situation would be to have completely safe, inexpensive, stable and highly efficient vaccines, several of which could be combined so that a minimal number of vaccinations would suffice to induce long-lasting immunity to many different pathogens. For obvious reasons, perorally active vaccines would be preferable to those needing to be injected.

Recent progress in molecular biology and in the understanding of the basic principles of immunity raise hopes that these problems could be solved by placing some of the largely empirical procedures on more rational grounds. We conclude this book with a brief discussion of some avenues of research into the development of a new generation of vaccines that are currently being explored.

Recombinant vaccine vectors

Common experience has taught us that the best vaccines are based on live attenuated pathogens. To avoid some of the problems associated with the development of such vaccines, attempts are being made to insert one or several genes of a pathogen into a non-pathogenic virus or bacterium that could then be safely used as a live vaccine (Fig. 27.1). It should even be possible to develop a recombinant vector microorganism expressing genes of several pathogens simultaneously. A number of recombinant live vaccines are now in various stages of development. One of the most promising is based on vaccinia virus, which was used successfully against smallpox. This virus tolerates insertions of large pieces of foreign DNA and replicates in the host-cell cytoplasm. Major disadvantages of this vector are: (i) the possibility of disseminated disease in immunodeficient patients; (ii) the limited possibility of using vaccinia-based vaccines repeatedly because the strong immune response elicited against the initial vaccinia virus antigens will rapidly inactivate any subsequent inoculum; and (iii) the weak immunogenicity of the antigens expressed by the vaccinia virus. Some of these disadvantages can be largely avoided by using drastically attenuated vaccinia variants such as the NYVAC strain recently developed by genetic engineering. Possible alternatives to vaccinia virus are several closely related avian viruses (avipoxviruses). These produce an abortive infection in humans (i.e. they infect cells but do not spread further) and are not strongly immunogenic, so they can be used repeatedly. The question is whether the virus could be made to express the inserted foreign genes strongly. Experimental vaccines against rabies and measles based on modified canarypox virus are presently being tested.

Another potential viral vaccine vector could be provided by adenoviruses. Here again, foreign genes can be inserted into the relatively small viral genome and the recombinant vaccine could be given perorally. Adenovirus-based vaccines are thought to be particularly promising for generating mucosal immune responses. There are, though, some concerns about the safety of adenovirus-based vectors with respect to their possible cell transformation potential (i.e. their ability to induce tumours under some conditions). However, it may be possible to remove the tumour-inducing

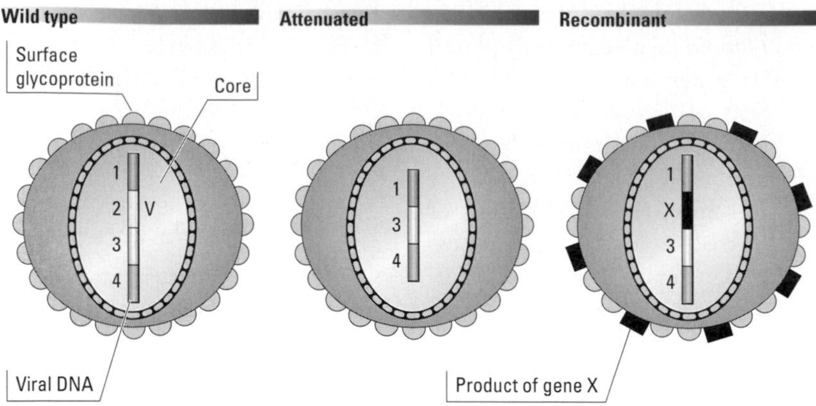

Figure 27.1 The use of engineered virus vectors for vaccination. Wild-type virus possessing four genes in its genome is made harmless but still capable of cell infection by the elimination of the virulence gene (here gene no. 2, V). A gene from another virus or bacterium (here X) can be introduced into the genome of such a vector and be expressed either on the surface or inside the recombinant virus particle.

part by genetic engineering of the virus. Other currently explored viral vector systems include poliovirus and herpesviruses (herpes simplex virus, cytomegalovirus and varicella virus).

Several bacteria are also being tested as potential vaccine vectors. Among these, a variety of different *Salmonella* species, such as the mouse pathogen *Salmonella typhimurium* and the human *Salmonella typhi* strain Ty21a (currently used as an oral vaccine against typhoid), have been studied most extensively. These strains survive for a relatively long time in the gut, interact with gut-associated lymphoid tissues and elicit strong IgA production as well as cellular immune responses. *Salmonella*-based vectors are therefore most promising for the development of vaccines against diseases requiring a strong mucosal immune response for protection. *Salmonella* (and other bacteria) can carry the foreign gene either integrated in their genome or in the form of an epigenetic element (plasmid). Integration within the genome ensures stable expression for long periods, whereas integration into the plasmid may yield very high expression for a short time only. The level of expression vs. its duration may be important parameters contributing to the final outcome of the immune response. Recombinant *Salmonella* strains expressing antigens of *Bordetella pertussis*, surface antigen of hepatitis B virus (HBsAg), *Escherichia coli* toxin subunits, *Plasmodium* antigenic repeat sequences, *Vibrio cholerae* lipopolysaccharide antigens and *Shigella* antigens have been tested in animals and some also in human clinical trials, with encouraging results.

Another bacterial vector currently being explored is BCG (attenuated *M. bovis*). Strong and lasting antibody responses were elicited to the OspA antigen of *Borrelia burgdorferi* (causative agent of Lyme disease) when it was expressed in the membrane of recombinant BCG. Other antigens expressed in BCG and yielding encouraging results in animal vaccination include the surface protein PspA of *Streptococcus pneumoniae*, a glycoprotein antigen of the protozoal parasite *Leishmania* and an antigen of simian immunodeficiency virus. In the last two cases protective cellular (helper T (T_H1) or T_C cell-mediated) responses could be elicited.

Other attenuated bacteria (*Shigella*, *Vibrio*, *Listeria*) and even protozoal parasites (*Leishmania*) are being developed as potential recombinant vaccine vectors. Finally, attempts are also being made to use genetically engineered plants for the production of antigens suitable for vaccination. For example, tobacco plants have been produced that express HBsAg in an immunogenic, easily purifiable form. It may even be possible in the future to produce edible plants expressing microbial antigens suitable for peroral vaccination.

Nucleic acid vaccines

Inoculation of antigen-encoding plasmid DNA intramuscularly can result in prolonged antigen expression and the generation of humoral and cellular immune responses. The foreign DNA is apparently not incorporated into the host genome and a similar result can also be achieved when mRNA encapsulated in liposomes is injected instead of DNA. In another variant of this *genetic vaccination*, DNA-coated microscopic gold particles have been used to elicit protective immunity against influenza in mice. These micro-bullets are loaded in an apparatus, appropriately called a gene-gun, that shoots them at high velocity so that they penetrate the thin layers of tissue and deposit their DNA in the cells of mucosal, muscle or other tissues. Genetic vaccination would eliminate all inconveniences of antigen purification, pathogen attenuation and the risks associated with the use of live vectors in immunocompromised individuals.

Development of new carriers and adjuvants

Theoretically, it would be best to use only small parts of a microbial antigen (epitope) for immunization and thus minimize the risk that potentially autoreactive lymphocyte clones would be activated. Antigenic fragments are poorly immunogenic, however, and must therefore be coupled to suitable carriers and used with adjuvants to elicit strong responses. The carrier molecule serves as a source of T_H-cell epitopes expressed on the surface of antigen-presenting cells (APCs). The epitopes induce carrier-specific T-cell help necessary for efficient B-cell priming. The traditionally used carrier molecules for experimental immunizations include tetanus toxoid, bovine serum albumin, ovalbumin or keyhole limpet haemocyanin (KLH), to which peptides or other poorly immunogenic antigens (haptens) can be linked by glutaraldehyde or other cross-linkers. An ideal carrier molecule should not elicit a significant antibody response to itself, while providing a strong helper effect for the antibody response to the attached hapten. The carrier must also work well in all individuals of a population expressing different major histocompatibility complex (MHC) class II allelic forms. In other words, it must, when processed by the APC, produce peptides capable of binding to products of various MHC class II alleles. *Universal (promiscuous) peptides* capable of binding to products of almost any *MHC* class II alleles have indeed been described. It should therefore be possible to synthesize a molecule consisting of repeats of such peptides, which would serve as an optimal carrier. One candidate for the ideal primer is the group of mycobacterial heat-shock proteins (Hsp70). Another candidate is the *multiple antigen peptide system*, consisting of multiple clusters of the antigenic epitopes attached to a small oligolysine core. Such a system can contain multiple copies of a single epitope (peptide) or different epitopes attached to the same macromolecule.

Hapten–carrier conjugates must be mixed with *adjuvants* to achieve sufficient immunogenicity. An ideal adjuvant should help to deliver the antigen to APCs in a form that provides efficient, protracted stimulation; it should also non-specifically stimulate APCs or lymphocytes. It must not, however, cause undesirable polyclonal activation or inflammation. The classical adjuvants have largely been developed by an empirical process with some rationalizations based on the understanding of how the immune system works. They include precipitated aluminium hydroxide, mineral oil emulsions and suspensions of killed mycobacteria. Newly developed adjuvants with superior immunostimulatory properties and minimal noxious side-effects include: *liposomes* encapsulating the antigen; *microcapsules*, consisting of an inner reservoir of antigen surrounded by an outer biodegradable polymer wall through which the antigen is slowly released in the lymphoid tissue; *immunostimulatory complexes (ISCOMs)*, generated by mixing the antigen with a biocompatible detergent saponin (Quil A, from the bark of the South American tree *Quillaja saponaria*), cholesterol, phosphatidylcholine and oil-based emulsions containing biodegradable materials such as squalene oil, non-ionic block polymers, surfactants and derivatives of muramyl dipeptide or lipid A. Immunopotentiation can also be achieved by attaching a peptide to a lipidic tail, which apparently enhances uptake by APCs, or to the non-toxic subunit of cholera toxin.

The outcome of vaccination can also be potentiated by the administration of cytokines that can either be included into the antigen–adjuvant mixture or produced by a recombinant attenuated microorganism, as discussed above. Immunopotentiating effects have been demonstrated for interleukin (IL)-1, IL-2 and IL-12 co-administered with the vaccine. Certain low-molecular-mass substances, such as vitamin E or a short peptide derived from IL-1, have also been reported to have immunopotentiating effects.

Further reading

Arnon, R. & Horwitz, R. J. (1992) Synthetic peptides as vaccines. *Current Opinion in Immunology*, **4**, 449–453.

Bergquist, N. R., Hall, B. F. & James, S. (1994) Schistosomiasis vaccine development. Translating basic research into practical results. *Immunologist*, **2**, 131–134.

Connell, N., Stover, C. K. & Jacobs Jr, W. R. (1992) Old microbes with new faces: molecular biology and the design of new vaccines. *Current Opinion in Immunology*, **4**, 442–448.

Del Giudice, G. (1992) New carriers and adjuvants in the development of vaccines. *Current Opinion in Immunology*, **4**, 454–459.

Donnelly, J. J., Ulmer, J. B. & Liu, M. A. (1994) Immunization with polynucleotides. A novel approach to vaccination. *Immunologist*, **2**, 20–26.

Haq, T. A., Mason, H. S., Clements, J. D. & Arntzen, C. J. (1995) Oral immunization with a recombinant bacterial antigen produced in transgenic plants. *Science*, **268**, 714–716.

Lanzavecchia, A. (1993) Identifying strategies for immune intervention. *Science*, **260**, 937–944.

Mekalanos, J. J. & Sadoff, J. C. (1994) Cholera vaccines: fighting an ancient scourge. *Science*, **265**, 1387–1389.

Möller, G. (Ed.) (1992) Antibodies in disease therapy. *Immunological Reviews*, **129**, entire volume.

Möller, G. (Ed.) (1994) Immunoglobulin treatment: mechanisms of action. *Immunological Reviews*, **139**, entire volume.

Nussenzweig, R. S. & Long, C. A. (1994) Malaria vaccines: multiple targets. *Science*, **265**, 1381–1382.

Pardoll, D. M. & Beckerleg, A. M. (1995) Exposing the immunology of naked DNA vaccines. *Immunity*, **3**, 165–169.

Plotkin, S. A. (1994) Vaccines for varicella-zoster virus and cytomegalovirus: recent progress. *Science*, **265**, 1383–1385.

Rabinovich, N. R., McInnes, P., Klein, D. L. & Hall, B. F. (1994) Vaccine technologies: view to the future. *Science*, **265**, 1401–1404.

Siber, G. R. (1994) Pneumococcal disease: prospects for a new generation of vaccines. *Science*, **265**, 1385–1387.

Staats, H. F., Jackson, R. J., Marinaro, M., Takahashi, I., Kiyono, H. & McGhee, J. R. (1994) Mucosal immunity to infection with implications for vaccine development. *Current Opinion in Immunology*, **6**, 572–583.

Stover, C. K. (1994) Recombinant vaccine delivery systems and encoded vaccines. *Current Opinion in Immunology*, **6**, 568–571.

Ulmer, J. B., Sadoff, J. C. & Liu, M. A. (1996) DNA vaccines. *Current Opinion in Immunology*, **8**, 531–536.

Appendix 1: Amino acids and their symbols

Amino acid	Three-letter symbol	One-letter symbol
Hydrophobic (non-polar)		
Alanine	Ala	A
Valine	Val	V
Leucine	Leu	L
Isoleucine	Ile	I
Proline	Pro	P
Phenylalanine	Phe	F
Tryptophan	Trp	W
Methionine	Met	M
Uncharged polar		
Glycine	Gly	G
Serine	Ser	S
Threonine	Thr	T
Cysteine	Cys	C
Tyrosine	Tyr	Y
Asparagine	Asn	N
Glutamine	Gln	Q
Acidic		
Aspartic acid	Asp	D
Glutamic acid	Glu	E
Basic		
Lysine	Lys	K
Arginine	Arg	R
Histidine	His	H

Further three-letter symbols: Asx, Glx = either acid or amide.
Further one-letter symbols: B = Asx, Z = Glx, X = undetermined or non-standard amino acid residue.

Appendix 2: CD molecules

CD molecule	Synonyms	M_r (×10^{-3})	Expression	Structural features	Ligands	Functions
CD1a	T6	49 + 12 (b2m)	Thymocytes, Langerhans cells	IG SF	TCR	MHC class Ib antigen-presenting molecule
CD1b		45 + 12	Thymocytes, dendritic cells	IG SF	TCR	MHC class Ib antigen-(lipid) presenting molecule
CD1c		43 + 12	Thymocytes, Langerhans cells, dendritic cells, B-cell subset	IG SF	Probably TCR	MHC class Ib antigen-presenting molecule
CD1d		37	Intestinal epithelial cells	IG SF	Probably TCR	MHC class Ib antigen-presenting molecule
CD2	T11, LFA-2, E-rosette receptor	45–55	Thymocytes, T and NK cells	IG SF	CD58, CD48, CD59(?)	Adhesion and signalling receptor
CD2R	T11.3	45–55	Activated T cells	IG SF	See CD2	See CD2 (activation-dependent form)
CD3	T3	27 (γ chain) 20 (δ chain) 20 (ε chain) 16 (ζ chain) 22 (η chain)	Thymocytes, T cells Thymocytes, T cells Thymocytes, T cells Thymocytes, T cells Thymocytes, T cells	IG SF IG SF IG SF		Components of the TCR complex, necessary for signal transduction
CD4	T4	55	Thymocytes, T-cell subset, monocytes (weak)	IG SF	MHC class II, IL-16, HIV	Coreceptor for MHC class II; signalling (association with cytoplasmic PTK Lck)
CD5	T1	67	Thymocytes, T and B1 cells	Scavenger R type A family	CD72	Adhesion, signalling (negative?) receptor
CD6	T12	110	Thymocytes, T and B cell subset	Scavenger R type A family	ALCAM	Adhesion receptor
CD7	gp40	40	Thymocytes, T cells	IF SG	Unknown	Unknown
CD8	T8	32(α), 32(β) Cystine-linked heterodimer α : β or homodimer α : α	Thymocytes, T cell subset	IG SF	MHC class I	Coreceptor for MHC class I; signalling (association with cytoplasmic PTK Lck)
CD9	p24	24	Pre-B cells, thrombocytes	Tetraspan SF	Unknown	Unknown
CD10	CALLA, enkephalinase, neutral endopeptidase	100	Lymphoid progenitors, granulocytes			Ectoenzyme (endopeptidase)
CD11a	LFA-1 (αL chain)	180 (+ assoc. CD18)	Leucocytes	Integrin SF	CD50, CD54, CD102	Adhesion receptor
CD11b	Mac-1, CR3 (αM chain)	170 (+ assoc. CD18)	Myeloid cells, NK cells	Integrin SF	CD54, iC3b, fibrinogen, factor X, LPS, β-glucans, CD23	Adhesion, complement receptor
CD11c	gp150, CR4 (αX chain)	150 (+ assoc. CD18)	Myeloid cells	Integrin SF	CD54, iC3b, fibrinogen	Adhesion, complement receptor

(*Continued.*)

CD molecule	Synonyms	M_r (×10^{-3})	Expression	Structural features	Ligands	Functions
CDw12		90–120	Myeloid cells, thrombocytes	Unknown	Unknown	Unknown
CD13	Aminopeptidase N	150	Myeloid cells	Type II membrane protein	Coronaviruses	Ectoenzyme (aminopeptidase); probably plays a role in surface antigen processing
CD14	LPSR	55	Myeloid cells	Leucine rich glycoprotein family; GPI anchor	LPS, other bacterial complex carbohydrates	Activation receptor for LPS
CD15	Lewis-x (Le^x) (3-fucosyl *N*-acetyl lactosamine)	Epitope present on various glycolipids and glycoproteins	Granulocytes	Oligosaccharide	Selectins	Adhesion ligand
CD15s	Sialyl-Lewis-x	see CD15	Many different cells	Oligosaccharide	Selectins	Adhesion ligand
CD16a	FcγRIII	50–70	NK cells, monocytes	IG SF	Immune complexes	Phagocytic and ADCC Fc receptor
CD16b	FcγRIII (GPI-anchored)	50–70	Granulocytes	IG SF	Immune complexes	Phagocytic Fc receptor
CDw17	Lactosylceramide		Myeloid cells, thrombocytes	Glycolipid	Unknown	Unknown
CD18	β2 integrin subunit	95 (+ CD11a, b or c)	Leucocytes	Integrin SF	See CD11a, b, c	Common subunit of leukocyte (β2) integrins (adhesion molecules)
CD19	B4	95	B cells	IG SF	CD77?	Component of a B-cell coreceptor (CR2 complex)
CD20	B1	33–37	B cells	FcR β chain family; probably 4 TM domains		Probably a component of membrane Ca^{2+} channel
CD21	CR2	140	B cells, follicular dendritic cells	CCP SF	C3d, C3dg, EBV, CD23, IFN-α	Component of a B-cell coreceptor (CR2 complex); adhesion molecule
CD22	BL-CAM	130 (α-form) 140 (β-form)	B cells	IG SF	Sialoglycoproteins	Adhesion receptor
CD23	FcεRII Blast-2	45	B-cell subset, activated macrophages, follicular dendritic cells	C-type lectin SF; type II membrane protein	IgE, CD21, CD11b, c	Low-affinity IgE receptor (regulator or IgE production); adhesion ligand; soluble forms have cytokine-like activities
CD24	BA-1, HSA (mouse)	35–45	B cells, granulocytes	Extremely glycosylated peptide (31 amino acids); GPI-anchored	Selectins?	Unknown
CD25	Tac, IL-2Rα	55	Activated T cells, B cells and monocytes	CCP SF	IL-2	α-subunit of high-affinity IL-2R
CD26	Dipeptidyl peptidase IV (DPP IV)	110	Activated and memory lymphocytes, macrophages	Type II membrane protein	Collagen	Ectoenzyme (protease); adhesion molecule; associated with adenosine deaminase
CD27		$(50–55)_2$	T cell subset	TNFR SF	CD70	Activation cytokine receptor
CD28	Tp44	$(44)_2$	T cells, plasma cells	IG SF	CD80, CD86	Major costimulatory receptor of T cells
CD29	β1 integrin subunit	130 (+ CD49 α subunits)	Many different cells	Integrin SF	See CD49	Common subunit of β1 integrins (VLA antigens); adhesion receptor

CD molecule	Synonyms	M_r (×10−3)	Expression	Structural features	Ligands	Functions
CD30	Ki-1	105	Activated lymphocytes	TNFR SF	CD30L	Cytokine receptor
CD31	PECAM-1, gpIIa	130	Lymphocyte subsets, myeloid cells, thrombocytes, endothelia	IG SF	Glycosaminoglycans, αVβ3 integrin, CD31 (homotypic binding)	Adhesion receptor
CD32	FcγRII	40 (six forms known)	Myeloid cells, B cells, thrombocytes	IG SF	Immune complexes	Negative regulation of B cells; phagocytic Fc-receptor
CD33	gp67	67	Myeloid progenitors, monocytes	IG SF	Sialoglycoproteins	Adhesion receptor
CD34		105–120	Progenitor cells, endothelial cells	Sialomucin family	Selectins	Adhesion ligand
CD35	CR1	160–250 (four different forms)	Most leucocytes, erythrocytes, follicular dendritic cells	CCP SF	C3b, iC3b, C4b	Complement receptor type 1; involved in phagocytosis and endocytosis of immune complexes
CD36	gpIV, gpIIIb, OKM5	88	Monocytes, thrombocytes	Scavenger R group B family	Oxidized LDL, thrombospondin, collagen I and IV, phospholipids	Adhesion receptor; involvement in phagocytosis of apoptotic cells
CD37		35–50	B cells, weakly T cells, monocytes	Tetraspan SF	Unknown	Unknown
CD38	T10	45	Thymocytes, pre-B cells, activated lymphocytes	Type II membrane protein	Moon-1 (M_r 120 000)	Ectoenzyme (NAD^+ glycohydrolase, ADP ribosylcyclase, ADP ribose hydrolase)
CD39		80	B cell subset, activated T cell subset, activated NK cells, macrophages, dendritic cells	2 TM segments; similarity to yeast guanosine diphosphatase	Unknown	Probably ectoenzyme
CD40		50	B cells, monocytes, dendritic cells	TNFR SF	CD40L	Costimulatory receptor of B cells; induction of affinity maturation and memory
CD41	gpIIb, αIIb integrin chain	120 + 22 (+ β chain CD61)	Thrombocytes	Integrin SF	Fibrinogen, fibronectin, von Willebrand factor, thrombospondin	Complex of CD41/CD61 (gpIIb/IIIa) is the major thrombocyte adhesion receptor
CD42a	gpIX	23	Thrombocytes		von Willebrand factor	Adhesion receptor (complex with CD42b, c)
CD42b	gpIb-α	135	Thrombocytes		See CD42a	See 42a
CD42c	gpIb-β	22	Thrombocytes		See CD42a	See CD42a
CD43	Leukosialin, sialophorin	95–135 (cell type-dependent glycosylation forms)	Leucocytes	Sialomucin family	CD54, selectins(?)	Adhesion and activation receptor (may act as antiadhesion molecule)
CD44	Pgp-1, H-CAM	80–95	Leucocytes, erythrocytes	Cartilage link family	Hyaluronic acid, collagen	Adhesion receptor
CD45	Leucocyte common antigen (LCA), T-200	170–220 (splice variants)	Leucocytes	Protein tyrosine phosphatase	Possibly CD22	Regulation of activation (intracellular tyrosine phosphatase domain)
CD45RA, B, C, O	Splice variant forms of CD45 (see Fig. 16.5)					
CD46	MCP	55, 63 (splice variants)	Many different cells	CCP SF	Measles virus	Complement regulatory protein (membrane cofactor of Factor I)

(*Continued.*)

CD molecule	Synonyms	M_r (×10−3)	Expression	Structural features	Ligands	Functions
CD47	IAP	47–52	Many different cells	IG SF, 5 TM domains	Thrombospondin	Component of β1 and β3 integrin complexes (adhesion receptors)
CD48	Blast-1, Hu Lym-3	45–50	Leucocytes	IG SF; GPI-anchored	CD2	Adhesion ligand
CD49a	VLA-1, α1 integrin chain	210 (+β1 chain, CD29)	Activated T cells, monocytes	Integrin SF	Collagen, laminin	Component of the VLA-1 (α1β1) adhesion integrin
CD49b	VLA-2, α2 integrin chain, gpla	170 (+β1 chain, CD29)	B cells, monocytes, thrombocytes	Integrin SF	Collagen, laminin, echovirus 1	Component of the VLA-2 (α2β1) adhesion integrin
CD49c	VLA-3, α3 integrin chain	125 + 30 (+β1 chain, CD29)	B cells	Integrin SF	Fibrinogen, laminin, collagens	Component of the VLA-3 (α3β1) adhesion integrin
CD49d	VLA-4, α4 integrin chain	150 (+β1 chain, CD29 or +β7 chain)	Leucocytes	Integrin SF	Fibronectin, CD106 (ligands of the α4β1 complex); MAdCAM, fibronectin (ligands of the α4β7 complex)	Component of the VLA-4 (α4β1) and α4β7 adhesion integrins
CD49e	VLA-5, α5 integrin chain	135 + 25 (+β1 chain, CD29)	Memory T cells, thrombocytes, monocytes	Integrin SF	Fibronectin	Component of the VLA-5 (α5β1) α5 adhesion integrin
CD49f	VLA-6, α6 integrin chain	120 + 30 (+β1 chain, CD29; or +β4 chain)	Thrombocytes, memory T cells	Integrin SF	Laminin	Component of the VLA-6 (α6β1) and α6β4 adhesion integrins
CD50	ICAM-3	130	Many different cells	IG SF	LFA-1	Adhesion and activation receptor
CD51	VNR α-chain, αV integrin chain	125 + 25 (+β3 chain, CD61; or +β1, β5, β6, β8 chains)	Thrombocytes, endothelial cells, fibroblasts	Integrin SF	Vitronectin, fibronectin, fibrinogen, thrombospondin, von Willebrand factor	Component of several integrin adhesion molecules
CD52	Campath-1	20–30	Leucocytes	Extremely glycosylated peptide (12 amino acids); GPI-anchored	Unknown	Unknown
CD53	OX-44 (rat)	32–40	Leucocytes	Tetraspan SF	Unknown	Unknown
CD54	ICAM-1	90	Many different cells	IG SF	LFA-1, CR3, CD43, rhinoviruses	Adhesion ligand
CD55	DAF	70	Many different cells	CCP SF; GPI-anchored	CD97, echoviruses	Complement regulatory protein (accelerates decay of C3 convertase)
CD56	NKH-1, isoform of N-CAM	175–185	NK cells	IG SF	CD56 (homotypic interaction)	Adhesion receptor
CD57	HNK-1, Leu-7		NK cells, T-, B-cell subsets, neurons	Sulphated carbohydrate epitope attached to various glycoproteins and lipids	Unknown	Unknown
CD58	LFA-3	40–65	Many different cells	IG SF; TM and GPI-anchored forms exist	CD2	Adhesion ligand
CD59	Protectin	18–20	Many different cells	Ly-6 SF	C8; possibly CD2	Complement regulatory protein (inhibits C9 polymerization on MAC)
CDw60	Acetylated ganglioside GD3		T-cell subset, thrombocytes, monocytes	Glycolipid	Unknown	Unknown

CD molecule	Synonyms	M_r (×10⁻³)	Expression	Structural features	Ligands	Functions
CD61	gpIIIa, β3 integrin chain	110 (+ αIIb chain or + αV chain)	Thrombocytes, macrophages	Integrin SF	See CD41, CD51	See CD41, CD51
CD62E	E-selectin, ELAM-1	115	Activated endothelial cells	C-type lectin SF, CCP SF	Carbohydrate epitopes on GlyCAM-1, CD34 and other glycoproteins	Adhesion receptor
CD62L	L-selectin, LAM-1, LECAM-1	75	Leucocytes	C-type lectin SF, CCP SF	Carbohydrate epitopes on GLyCAM-1, CD34 and other glycoproteins	Adhesion receptor
CD62P	P-selectin, PADGEM	150	Activated thrombocytes, activated endothelial cells	C-type lectin SF, CCP SF	Carbohydrate epitopes on PSGL-1 and other glycoproteins	Adhesion receptor
CD63	ME491	30–60	Many different cells intracellularly (lysozome membrane); surface of activated cells	Tetraspan SF	Unknown	Unknown
CD64	FcγRI	72	Monocytes, macrophages	IG SF	IgG, immune complexes	High affinity IgG phagocytic and activation receptor
CD65	Ceramide dodecasaccharide		Myeloid cells	Glycolipid	Unknown	Unknown
CD65s	Sialylated form of CD65					
CD66a	BGP, NCA	160–180 (alternatively spliced forms)	Neutrophils	IG SF (CEA family)	Unknown	Probably adhesion receptor
CD66b	Previously CD67	95–100	Granulocytes	IG SF (CEA family); GPI-anchored	Unknown	Unknown
CD66c	NCA50, NCA90	90	Granulocytes	IG SF (CEA family); GPI-anchored	Unknown	Unknown
CD66d	CGM1	30	Neutrophils	IG SF (CEA family)	Unknown	Unknown
CD66e	CEA	180–200	Colon epithelium	IG SF (CEA family)	Unknown	Probably adhesion receptor
CD66f	PSG			IG SF (CEA family); secreted protein	Unknown	Unknown
CD67	renamed to CD66b					
CD68	Macrosialin	110	Monocytes, macrophages	Sialomucin family	Oxidized LDL, phospholipids	Possibly a scavenger receptor
CD69	AIM, EA1	28 + 34 (dimer of differentially glycosylated subunits)	Activated lymphocytes, macrophages	C-type lectin SF; type II membrane protein	Carbohydrate epitopes	Unknown
CD70		29 (and oligomers)	Activated lymphocytes, macrophages	TNF SF; type II membrane protein	CD27	Membrane-bound cytokine
CD71	Transferrin receptor; T9	$(95)_2$	Activated and dividing cells	Type II membrane protein	Transferrin	Uptake of Fe^{2+} via transferrin
CD72		$(42)_2$	B cells	C-type lectin SF; type II membrane protein	CD5	Ligand of regulatory receptor CD5

(Continued.)

CD molecule	Synonyms	M_r (×10^{-3})	Expression	Structural features	Ligands	Functions
CD73	ecto-5′-nucleotidase; L-VAP-2	69	Subsets of T and B cells, endothelial cells	GPI-anchored		Ectoenzyme (5′-nucleotidase); adhesion molecule
CD74	Ii	33, 35, 41, 45 (splice forms)	Monocytes, B cells	Type II membrane protein		Surface form of the MHC class II invariant chain (Ii)
CDw75			B cells	Sialylated carbohydrate epitopes	Possibly CD22	Unknown
CDw76			B cells, T-cell subset, endothelial cells	Sialylated glycolipid	Possibly CD22	Unknown
CD77	Globotriaosylceramide Gb3; P^k blood group antigen		Germinal centre B cells undergoing apoptosis	Glycolipid	CD19(?), verotoxin	Unknown
CDw78	Ba; an MHC class II epitope		B cells, monocytes	IG SF	Probably TCR	A conformationally determined MHC class II subpopulation of unknown function
CD79a	mb-1, Igα	32 (+ CD79b)	B cells	IG SF	Unknown	Component of the BCR complex involved in signalling
CD79b	B29, Igβ	37 (+ CD79a)	B cells	IG SF	Unknown	See CD79a
CD80	B7-1, BB1	60	Activated B cells, monocytes, dendritic cells, activated T cells	IG SF	CD28, CTLA-4	Costimulatory ligand for CD28; inhibitory ligand for CTLA-4
CD81	TAPA-1	26	Many different cells	Tetraspan SF	Unknown	Component of the CR2 complex
CD82	R2, C33, IA4, 4F9	40–60	Many different cells	Tetraspan SF	Unknown	Possible suppressor of metastasis
CD83	HB15	45	Dendritic cells, activated lymphocytes	IG SF	Unknown	Unknown
CD84		74	B cells, monocytes, thrombocytes	Unknown	Unknown	Unknown
CD85		120	B cells, monocytes	Unknown	Unknown	Unknown
CD86	B7-2, B70	80	Activated B cells, monocytes, dendritic cells	IG SF	CD28, CTLA-4	See CD80
CD87	uPA-R	45–55	Myeloid cells, endothelial cells	Ly-6 SF; GPI-anchored	Urokinase plasminogen activator (uPA)	Surface protease receptor involved in cell migration
CD88	C5aR	40	Myeloid cells, smooth muscle cells	STSR SF	C5a	Chemotactic and activation receptor
CD89	FcαR	55–70	Myeloid cells, subsets of T and B cells	IG SF	IgA, immune complexes	IgA receptor involved in phagocytosis
CDw90	Thy-1	25–35	Progenitor subsets, neurons; T cells (in rodents)	IG SF; GPI-anchored	Sulphated glycoproteins	Probable adhesion receptor
CD91	α2-macroglobulin receptor	515 (α-chain) + 85 (β-chain)	Monocytes	β-chain transmembrane, α-chain extracellular	α_2-macroglobulin	Receptor of multiple ligands including α2-macroglobulin-proteinase complex, plasminogen activators, chylomicrons, lipoprotein lipase
CDw92		70	Myeloid cells, thrombocytes, endothelial cells	Unknown	Unknown	Unknown

CD molecule	Synonyms	M_r ($\times10^{-3}$)	Expression	Structural features	Ligands	Functions
CD93		120	Myeloid and endothelial cells	Unknown	Unknown	Unknown
CD94	KP43	40 (+assoc. NKG2 subunits)	NK cell, T-cell subset	C-type lectin SF	Some allelic forms of HLA-B	NK-cell receptor
CD95	Fas, APO-1	43	Many cell types	TNFR SF	FasL	Induction of apoptosis
CD96	Tactile	160	T cells, NK cells	IG SF	Unknown	Unknown
CD97		74, 80, 89	Myeloid cells, activated lymphocytes	STSR SF; EGF-like domains; RGD-motif	CD55	Unknown
CD98	4F2	40 + 80	Lymphocytes subpopulations, thrombocytes	Type II membrane protein (β-chain)	Unknown	Unknown
CD99	E2, MIC2	32	Many cell types	Collagen-like repeats	Unknown	Possibly adhesion molecule
CD99R	Restricted CD99	32	T-cell subset	See CD99	See CD99	See CD99 (a form of CD99)
CD100	p150	$(150)_2$	Many cell types	IG SF, semaphorin family	Unknown	Unknown
CDw101	V7, p126	$(120)_2$	Myeloid cells, T-cell subset	IG SF	Unknown	Unknown
CD102	ICAM-2	55–65	Many cell types	IG SF	LFA-1; CR3	Adhesion ligand
CD103	HML-1, αE integrin chain	150 + 25 (+ assoc. β7 chain)	Intestinal epithelial lymphocytes	Integrin SF	E-cadherin	Adhesion receptor
CD104	β4 integrin subunit	220 (+ assoc. α6 chain)	Epithelial, endothelial cells; trophoblast; Schwann cells	Integrin SF	Laminin, epiligrin	Adhesion receptor
CD105	Endoglin	$(95)_2$	Endothelial cells, activated macrophages, subset of bone marrow cells	Type II membrane protein	TGF-β	Low affinity TGF-β receptor; possibly adhesion molecule
CD106	VCAM-1	95, 100	Endothelial cells	IG SF	VLA-4 (α4β1) and α4β7 integrin	Adhesion ligand
CD107a	LAMP-1	110	Activated thrombocytes	Mucin	Unknown	Unknown; lysosomal membrane protein translocated to activated cell surface
CD107b	LAMP-2	120	Activated thrombocytes	Mucin	Unknown	See CD107a
CDw108		80	Some T-cell lines, erythrocytes (weakly), activated lymphocytes	GPI-anchored	Unknown	Unknown; carries the JMH blood group
CDw109		120–165	Endothelial and activated T cells, thrombocytes	GPI-anchored	Unknown	Unknown
CD110–CD113	So far unassigned					
CD114	G-CSFR	130	Granulocytes, monocytes	CKR SF	G-CSF	A component of activation and differentiation cytokine receptor
CD115	M-CSFR c-Fms	150	Monocytes, macrophages	IG SF, PTKR SF	M-CSF	Activation and differentiation cytokine receptor
CD116	GM-CSFR α-chain	75–85 (+ β-chain KH97)	Myeloid cells	CKR SF	GM-CSF	Activation and differentiation cytokine receptor

(*Continued.*)

CD molecule	Synonyms	M_r (×10−3)	Expression	Structural features	Ligands	Functions
CD117	SCFR, c-Kit	145	Haemopoietic progenitors, mast cells	IG SF, PTKR SF	SCF	Differentiation and proliferation cytokine receptor
CD118	So far unassigned; reserved for IFN-α/βR					
CDw119	IFN-γR α-chain	90–100	Myeloid cells, B cells	IFNR SF	IFN-γ	Activation cytokine receptor
CD120a	TNFR I	50–60	Many cell types	TNFR SF	TNF-α, LT	Receptor of apoptotic signal; cytokine receptor
CD120b	TNFR II	77–85	Myeloid cells	TNFR SF	TFN-α, LT	Activation cytokine receptor
CD121a	IL-1R type I	80	Thymocytes, T cells	IG SF	IL-1α, IL-1β, IL-1Ra	Activation cytokine receptor
CDw122	IL-2R β-chain	75	NK cells, activated T and B cells	CKR SF	IL-2, IL-15	A component of high-affinity IL-2R and IL-15R activation receptors
CDw123	IL-3R	70	Stem cells, monocytes, B cells	CKR SF	IL-3	A component of high-affinity activation cytokine receptor
CD124	IL-4R α-chain	140	T and B cells, haemopoietic precursors	CKR SF	IL-4, IL-13	Activation and differentiation cytokine receptor
CDw125	IL-5R α-chain	60	Eosinophils, basophils	CKR SF	IL-5	A component of high-affinity activation and differentiation cytokine receptor
CD126	IL-6R α-chain	80 (+ CDw130)	Many cell types	CKR SF	IL-6	Activation and differentiation cytokine receptor
CD127	IL-7R α-chain	75 (+ IL-2R γ-chain)	Lymphoid precursors, T cells, monocytes	CKR SF	IL-7	Differentiation and activation cytokine receptor
CDw128	IL-8R	58–67	Neutrophils, basophils, T-cell subset	STSR SF	IL-8	Chemotactic and activation receptor
CD129	So far unassigned					
CD130	gp130	130	Many cell types	CKR SF		Common β-chain of IL-6R, IL-11R and several other cytokine receptors
CDw131	Common β-chain	120	Various cell types	CKR SF		Common β-chain of high affinity activation receptors of IL-3, IL-5 and GM-CSF
CD132	Common γ-chain	64	Various leucocytes	CKR SF		Common γ-chain of high affinity activation receptors of IL-2, IL-4, IL-7, IL-9 and IL-15
CD133	So far unassigned					
CD134	OX40	50	Activated T cells	TNRF SF	OX40L	Activation receptor of the membrane-bound cytokine OX40L
CD135	FLT3, flk-2	130–150	Progenitor cells	IG SF, PTKR SF	FLT3 ligand	Activation receptor of the membrane bound cytokine FLT3 ligand
CDw136	MSPR	150 + 40	Epithelial cells, some hematopoietic cell lines	PTKR SF	MSP, HGF-1	Activating cytokine receptor

CD molecule	Synonyms	M_r ($\times 10^{-3}$)	Expression	Structural features	Ligands	Functions
CDw137	4-1BB	30	Activated T cells	TNFR SF	4-1BBL	Receptor of the membrane-bound cytokine 4-1BBL
CD138	Syndecan-1	150–250	Plasma cells	Proteoglycan; glycosamino-glycan side-chains	Unknown	Unknown
CD139		220 + 250	B cells	Unknown	Unknown	Unknown
CD140a	PDGFR (α-chain)	180	Many cell types	IG SF, PTKR SF	PDGF	A component of activating cytokine receptor
CD140b	PDGFR (β-chain)	180	Endothelial cell, stromal cell lines	IG SF, PTKR SF	PDGF	A component of activating cytokine receptor
CD141	Thrombomodulin, fetomodulin	100	Myeloid, endothelial cells	C-type lectin SF	Thrombin	Receptor for thrombin; regulates coagulation
CD142	Tissue factor	45	Monocytes, endothelial cells	CKR SF, FNIII type domains	Factor VII	Receptor for factor VII of the coagulation cascade; an inducer of extrinsic pathway of the coagulation
CD143	ACE, peptidyl dipeptidase A	170	Endothelial, epithelial cells	Peptidyl peptidase family	Angiotensin	An ectoenzyme (peptidyl dipetidase) cleaving angiotensin
CD144	VE-cadherin, cadherin 5	135	Endothelial cells	Cadherin family	CD144	Homophilic adhesion molecule
CDw145		25	Endothelial cells	Unknown	Unknown	Unknown
CD146	MUC 18, S-endo, MCAM	118	Endothelial cells, activated T, smooth muscle cells	IG SF	Unknown	Probably adhesion molecule
CD147	Neurothelin, basigin, M6	50–60	Many cell types	IG SF	Unknown	Unknown
CD148	p260, HPTP-eta, DEP-1	260	Many cell types	Type III receptor protein tyrosine phosphatase	Unknown	Protein tyrosine phosphatase
CDw149	MEM-133	120	Leucocytes	Unknown	Unknown	Unknown
CDw150	SLAM, IPO-3	75–90	Thymocytes, subsets of lymphocytes	IG SF	Unknown	Regulation of T-cell response
CD151	PETA-3, SFA-1	27	Leucocytes (immature), endothelial cell, platelets	Tetraspan SF	Unknown	Unknown
CD152	CTLA-4	$(44)_2$	Activated T cells	IG SF	CD80, CD86	Negative regulator of T-cell activation
CD153	CD30L	40	Activated T cells	TNF SF	CD30	Membrane bound cytokine
CD154	gp39, CD40L	39	Activated T cells, mast cells	TNF SF	CD40	Membrane bound cytokine
CD155	Poliovirus R	80–90	Monocytes, progenitor cells	IG SF	Poliovirus	Unknown
CD156	ADAM-8	69	Monocytes, neutrophils	Distintegrin-, metallo-proteinase-, cysteine-rich- and EGF domains	Unknown	Probably involved in extravasation of leucocytes

(*Continued.*)

CD molecule	Synonyms	M_r ($\times 10^{-3}$)	Expression	Structural features	Ligands	Functions
CD157	BSF-1, Mo5	42–45	Monocytes, granulocytes, bone marrow stromal cells	ADP-ribosyl cyclase family; GPI-anchor	Unknown	Ectoenzyme (ADP-ribosyl cyclase, cADPR hydrolase)
CD158a	p58.1/p50.1	58, 50	NK cells	IG SF	MHC class I	NK cell inhibitory receptor of MHC class I
CD158b	p58.2/p50.2	58, 50	NK cells	IG SF	MHC class I	NK cell inhibitory receptor of MHC class I
CD159 and CD 160	So far unassigned					
CD161	NKR-P1A	$(40)_2$	NK, T-cell subset	C-type lectin SF	Unknown	Probably NK cell activating receptor
CD162	PSGL-1, CD62 ligand	$(110)_2$	Leucocytes	Mucin	CD62L, CD62P	Ligand of endothelial cell selectins
CD163	KiM8	130	Monocytes	Scavenger R family	Unknown	Unknown
CD164	MGC-24	$(80)_2$	Leucocytes, epithelial cells	Sialomucin family	Unknown	Adhesion molecule
CD165	AD2, gp37	37	NK and T-cell subset, platelets, thymocytes	Unknown	Unknown	Unknown
CD166	ALCAM	100	Many cell types	IG SF	CD6	Adhesion ligand

ACE, angiotensin converting enzyme; ADAM, a disintegrin and metalloprotease; ADCC, antibody-dependent cellular cytotoxicity; ADP, adenosine diphosphate; AIM, activation-inducing molecule; ALCAM, activated leucocyte cell adhesion molecule; BCR, B-cell receptor; BGP, billiary glycoprotein; b2m, β_2-microglobulin; CALLA, common acute lymphoblastoid leukaemia antigen; CAM, cell adhesion molecule; CCP, complement control protein; CD, cluster of differentiation; CEA, carcinoembryonic antigen; CKR, cytokine receptor; CR, complement receptor; CTLA, cytotoxic T-lymphocyte antigen; DAF, decay accelerating factor; DEP, high cell density-enhanced phosphatase; EBV, Epstein–Barr virus; EGF, epidermal growth factor; ELAM, endothelial–leucocyte adhesion molecule; GM–CSF, granulocyte–monocyte colony stimulating factor; gp, glycoprotein; GPI, glycosylphosphatidyl inositol; HGF, hepatocyte growth factor-like; HPTP, hematopoietic protein tyrosine phosphatase; HSA, heat stable antigen; IAP, integrin-associated protein; ICAM, intercellular cell adhesion molecule; IFN, interferon; IG, immunoglobin; IL, interleukin; L, ligand (e.g. CD40L); LAMP, lysozyme-associated membrane protein; LDL, low density lipoprotein; LECAM–1, lymphocyte–endothelial cell adhesion molecule; LFA, leucocyte function antigen; LPS, lipopolysaccharide; LT, lymphotoxin; L–VAP, leucocyte–vascular adhesion protein; MAC, membrane attack complex; MAdCAM, mucosal addresin cell adhesion molecule; MCAM, melanoma cell adhesion molecule; MCP, membrane cofactor protein; M-CSF, monocyte colony stimulatory factor; MHC, major histocompatibility complex; MSP, macrophage stimulating protein; NAD, nicotinamide dinucleotide; NCA, nonspecific cross-reactive protein; N-CAM, neural cell adhesion molecule; PADGEM, platelet alpha granule membrane glycoprotein; PDGF, platelet-derived growth factor; PECAM, platelet and endothelial cell adhesion molecule; PSGL, P-selectin glycoprotein ligand; PTK, protein tyrosine kinase; R, receptor; SCF, stem cell factor; SF, superfamily; SLAM, surface lymphocyte activation molecule; STSR, seven transmembrane superfamily receptor; TAPA, target of antiproliferative antibody; TCR, T- cell receptor; TGF, transforming growth factor; TM, transmembrane; TNFR, tumour necrosis factor receptor; VCAM, vascular cell adhesion molecule; VLA, very late activation antigen; VNR, vitronectin receptor.

Index

Page references in *italics* refer to Figures and those in **bold** refer to Tables.